Chinese Pulse Diagnosis:
A Contemporary Approach

Chinese Pulse Diagnosis
A CONTEMPORARY APPROACH

Leon I. Hammer, M.D.

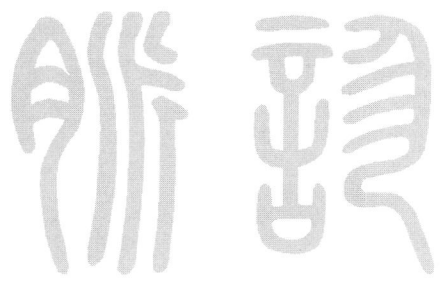

EASTLAND PRESS ❖ SEATTLE

©2001 by Eastland Press, Incorporated
Illustrations copyright ©2001 by Robert Heffron and
Bruce Wang

Published by Eastland Press, Incorporated
P.O. Box 99749, Seattle, WA 98199 USA

No part of this book may be reproduced or transmitted
in any form or by any means without the prior written
permission of the publisher.

Library of Congress Control Number: 2001131458
International Standard Book Number: 0-939616-25-4
Printed in the United States of America

2 4 6 8 10 9 7 5 3 1

Book design by Gary Niemeier
Illustrations by Marie Dauenheimer and Bruce Wang

The spirit of this book is dedicated to the memory of my son Kirin.

The inspiration for and substance of this book is dedicated to the memory of my teacher, a modern master of Chinese pulse diagnosis, Dr. John H.F. Shen.

Human life depends on the pulse. The ten pulse types parallel the types of song. Therefore, healing requires knowing the pulses, and then knowing what song to use as a remedy.

Laying on of hand confers wisdom. Thus, Moses laid his hand on Joshua to give him wisdom. The Torah says, 'Joshua, son of Nun, was full of the spirit of wisdom because Moses had laid his hands upon . . . him.' Joshua thus became a man 'who has wind-spirit in him.' This meant that he knew how to determine each person's wind-spirit, which is manifested in that person's pulse.

—*The Stories of Rabbi Nachman of Breslov*

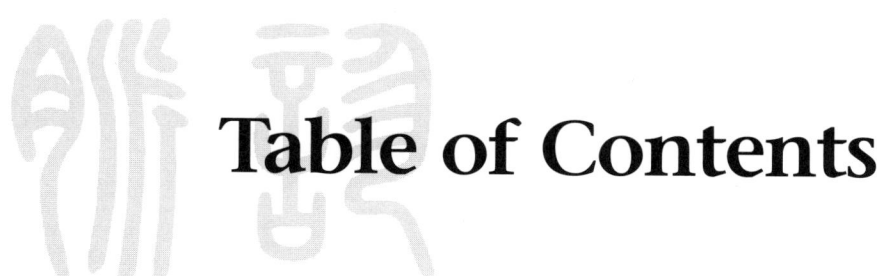

Table of Contents

FIGURES AND TABLES ····· *viii*
FOREWORD ····· *xi*
AUTHOR'S NOTE ····· *xiii*
ACKNOWLEDGEMENTS ····· *xiv*
PREFACE ····· *xvi*
INTRODUCTION ····· *xix*

Chapter 1   Preliminary Reflections, 1
Chapter 2   Pulse Positions Through History, 17
Chapter 3   Basic Axioms and Other Considerations, 31
Chapter 4   Taking the Pulse: Methodology, 53
Chapter 5   Classification and Nomenclature of Pulse Qualities, 87
Chapter 6   Rhythm and Stability, 109
Chapter 7   Rate, 147
Chapter 8   Volume, 175
Chapter 9   Depth, 229
Chapter 10   Size: Width and Length, 287
Chapter 11   Shape, 307
Chapter 12   Individual Positions, 383
Chapter 13   The Three Depths and Common Qualities Found Uniformly over the Entire Pulse, 453
Chapter 14   Uniform Qualities on Other Large Segments of the Pulse, 495
Chapter 15   Qualities as Signs of Psychological Disharmony, 539
Chapter 16   Prognosis and Prevention, 595
Chapter 17   Interpretation, 621
              Appendix: Case Illustrations, 647

EPILOGUE ····· *683*
ENDNOTES ····· *687*
APPENDIX 1: PULSE QUALITIES: SENSATION AND INTERPRETATION ····· *731*
APPENDIX 2: GLOSSARY ····· *747*
APPENDIX 3: BIBLIOGRAPHY ····· *757*
PULSE INDEX ····· *761*
GENERAL INDEX ····· *765*

Figures and Tables

FIGURES

Fig. 2-1: Pulse positions according to Hammer, 24
Fig. 2-2: Pulse positions according to Shen, 25
Fig. 2-3: Special Lung position, 26
Fig. 2-4: The three depths, 29
Fig. 3-1: Normal pulse wave, 38
Fig. 4-1: Pulse record, 58
Fig. 4-2: Wave comparisons, 68
Fig. 4-3: The eight depths, 69
Fig. 4-4: Both hands, 71
Fig. 4-5: Left Special Lung position, 71
Fig. 4-6: Left Neuro-psychological position, 72
Fig. 4-7: Left distal position, 73
Fig. 4-8: Large Vessel position, 73
Fig. 4-9: Mitral Valve position, 74
Fig. 4-10: Heart Enlarged position, 74
Fig. 4-11: Distal Liver Engorgement position, 74
Fig. 4-12: Left middle position, 75
Fig. 4-13: Liver Ulnar position, 75
Fig. 4-14: Liver Radial Engorgement position, 76
Fig. 4-15: Gallbladder position, 76
Fig. 4-16: Left proximal position, 77
Fig. 4-17: Large Intestine position, 77
Fig. 4-18: Left Pelvis/Lower Body position, 78
Fig. 4-19: Right Special Lung position, 78
Fig. 4-20: Right Neuro-psychological position, 79
Fig. 4-21: Right distal position, 79
Fig. 4-22: Pleura position, 80
Fig. 4-23: Esophagus position, 80
Fig. 4-24: Right middle position, 81
Fig. 4-25: Spleen position, 82

Fig. 4-26: Stomach-Pylorus Extension position, 82
Fig. 4-27: Right proximal position, 83
Fig. 4-28: Small Intestine position, 83
Fig. 4-29: Right Pelvis/Lower Body position, 84
Fig. 5-1: Normal pulse wave, 91
Fig. 6-1: Hesitant Wave quality, 126
Fig. 6-2: Change in Qualities, 134
Fig. 6-3: Change in Intensity, 136
Fig. 6-4: Change in Amplitude, 139
Fig. 6-5a: Rhythm flowchart, 143
Fig. 6-5b: Rhythm flowchart (detail), 144
Fig. 6-6: Stability flowchart, 145
Fig. 7-1: Rapid flowchart, 172
Fig. 7-1b: Rapid flowchart (detail), 173
Fig. 7-2: Slow flowchart, 174
Fig. 8-1: Hollow Full-Overflowing quality, 180
Fig. 8-2: Flooding Excess quality, 191
Fig. 8-3: Inflated quality, 193
Fig. 8-4: Suppressed quality, 201
Fig. 8-5: Yielding at qi depth quality, 203
Fig. 8-6: Diminished at qi depth quality, 204
Fig. 8-7: Absent at qi depth quality, 205
Fig. 8-8: Spreading quality, 206
Fig. 8-9: Yielding partially Hollow quality, 206
Fig. 8-10: Diminished at blood depth quality, 207
Fig. 8-11: Flooding Deficient Wave quality, 207
Fig. 8-12: Diffuse quality, 209
Fig. 8-13: Reduced Substance quality, 210
Fig. 8-14: Flat quality, 211
Fig. 8-15a: Feeble (early stage) quality, 216
Fig. 8-15b: Feeble (later stage) quality, 217
Fig. 8-16: Absent quality, 217
Fig. 8-17: Muffled quality, 226
Fig. 8-18: Volume flowchart, 228
Fig. 9-1: Cotton quality, 236
Fig. 9-2: Floating quality, 240
Fig. 9-3a: Empty quality (early stage), 248
Fig. 9-3b: Empty quality (middle stage), 248
Fig. 9-3c: Empty quality (later stage), 249
Fig. 9-4a: Yielding Empty Thread-like quality (early stage), 254
Fig. 9-4a: Yielding Empty Thread-like quality (later stage), 254
Fig. 9-5a: Leather quality (early stage), 255
Fig. 9-5b: Leather quality (later stage), 255
Fig. 9-6: Scattered quality, 257
Fig. 9-7: Minute quality, 258
Fig. 9-8: Leather-like Hollow quality, 263
Fig. 9-9: Deep quality, 269

Fig. 9-10: Firm quality, 282
Fig. 9-11a: Hidden Excess quality, 283
Fig. 9-11b: Hidden Deficient quality, 283
Fig. 9-12: Depth flowchart, 286
Fig. 10-1: Thin quality, 295
Fig. 10-2: Long quality, 301
Fig. 10-3: Short quality, 303
Fig. 10-4: Width flowchart, 304
Fig. 10-5: Length flowchart, 305
Fig. 11-1: Slippery quality, 314
Fig. 11-2: Violin (nonfluid qualities: Taut, Tense, Tight, Wiry), 328
Fig. 11-3: Ropy quality, 360
Fig. 11-4: Choppy quality, 361
Fig. 11-5: Smooth and Rough Vibration qualities, 366
Fig. 11-6: Shape flowchart, 381
Fig. 11-7: Qualifying terms and anomalous qualities flowchart, 382
Fig. 13-1: The three depths, 458
Fig. 13-2: The eight depths, 459
Fig. 13-3: Progression of heat and toxicity in the blood, 478
Fig. 13-4: Blood Unclear quality, 480
Fig. 13-5: Blood Heat quality, 481
Fig. 13-6: Blood Thick quality, 482
Fig. 13-7: Tense Hollow Full-Overflowing quality, 483

TABLES

Table 1-1: Comparison of pulse terminology in English, 8-9
Table 2-1: Historical correlations among pulse positions and organs, 20
Table 5-1: Characteristics of the Normal pulse, 92
Table 5-2: Qualities classified according to sensation (Hammer), 99
Table 5-3: Qualities classified according to Chinese condition (Hammer), 99
Table 5-4: Nine principal categories of qualities, 99
Table 6-1: Classification of arrhythmias, 114
Table 14-1: Similar qualities bilaterally at same position, 535
Table 15-1: Pulse qualities and associated psychological states, 592
Table 17-1: Methodology for interpretation, 643
Appendix 1: Pulse Qualities: Sensation and Interpretation, 731

Foreword

What is more natural than to stroke the forehead of a sick child to discover a fever, or palpate the rise and fall of the chest of someone who has lost consciousness to assess whether the breath remains lively? Is it any less natural to lay one's fingers on a vessel to feel the slight thump that signifies life, and, while lingering there, note rhythms and tides, the melodious and discordant strains of the body's chorus?

Leon Hammer has constructed a monumental diagnostic praxis for our times. Through the medium of apprenticeship with the venerable John H. Shen, after two decades of clinical experimentation, Dr. Hammer makes transparent, teachable, and achievable what has remained, until now, a formidably esoteric, mystifying methodology mired in confusing ambiguities and perpetuated dogmas. Even without direct linguistic access to the Chinese source literature, he has peeled away the murky debris of stereotyped rituals and abstruse doctrines to reveal the core of traditional insight, providing us with a contemporary technology for acquiring *skillful means*. By systematizing Dr. Shen's idiosyncratic approach, he enables access to many more hands and minds. Perhaps his most stunning achievement has been to re-establish—as the ancient physicians must have originally done—a concrete link between the conceptual language of pulse diagnosis and somatic reality: actual felt sensations becoming once again the basis for the vocabulary of qualities, and, more importantly, readable, real-time artifacts of organismic process.

This treatise is a comprehensive commentary on the history of *pulsology* as well as a philosophically and pragmatically coherent manual. Like the universally revered classics, it is destined to become a dog-eared, perennial repository of didactic knowledge, clinical insight, and practical guidance—a touchstone in developing a deeper appreciation of the utility and validity of traditional Chinese diagnostic methods, and thus, of the value of Chinese medicine as a whole.

With time, with reflection, and with use, this source becomes a bridge that forms a living link between mind and substance, inner and outer, sensing and comprehending, past and future, art and science. As much as this work represents two decades of unrelenting intellectual effort in first compiling, and then cogently organizing a colossal stockpile of information into learnable skills, it springs from the heart of a dedicated physician bent on assisting those who suffer and would be healed, and those who would be healers.

Having persevered for nearly a decade under the tutelage of Dr. Hammer, I still struggle to alloy a complex system of terms, techniques, and heuristic principles with my day-to-day work with patients. Though mastery appears to me as a mirage, the persistent practice of this method deepens my understanding of the people who come to me, enhancing my effectiveness. Out of this pursuit, the original excitement, idealism, and conviction that drew me into the practice of this medicine have been renewed: the more I dig, the more I reap, the further I realize I need to seek.

However one may prefer to represent it, life is of the body, and so is medicine. What more intimate and profound entry is there into any person's life than to touch them? To feel the pulse is to learn the cadence of that life. Leon Hammer offers us a path to mastery, not only for *the masters,* but for any of us with the passion and determination to study, to see, to feel, and, perhaps, even to know.

—Efrem Korngold, L.Ac., O.M.D.

The Pulse: An Aqueous Geology

Wading into the river of the
soul, ordinary clamor
evaporates. Poised on the wrist
with wing-tipped touch,
fingers navigate currents
grasping secrets buried beneath
waters of memory or words.
The body encodes the mind,
within tissue,
through fluid soil—
each tributary deposits
silt on its bottom,
amassing layers of
sedimentary history,
a palpable geology.
Chanting
on the shore,
oceans echo
gurgling estuary
fed from mountain mouth,
plunging toward a red sea,
percussive beats undulating
below bony landmarks.
The story spills:
there is no silence,
rather a flood
of whispers we teach
ourselves to hear.

—Harriet Beinfield, L.Ac.

Author's Note

The exterior of the body is a communication center of almost infinite capacity. Incalculable patterns of potentially decipherable messages are transmitted from the interior to the surface, a few of whose codes have been rendered intelligible over the millennia by a few aware beings through revelation, investigation, and experimentation, across the spectrum of civilizations, primitive, ancient, and recent.

It should therefore come as no surprise that so many different, even apparently contradictory, systems of reading the messages all appear to be correct. Each is describing a different aspect of reality which no human model could ever totally encompass. These systems were conceived by a cosmic intelligence to bring into consciousness in many different ways the important internal physiologic news of the moment. This remarkable, steady stream of constantly changing information conforms to no man-made theory, eight principle or five element. Nor is the system that I am presenting here constrained to fit into a theory. The locations, sensations, and interpretations are based on clinical experience.

The process of gaining new insight into these communication systems continues today and in our times and will never cease unless the creative spirit is silenced. Let us hope and pray and vigilantly watch over that spirit which wakens us to the infinite sources of wisdom. Chinese pulse diagnosis is one of the most enduring and profound of this multitude of insights to whose unceasing evolution this book is committed.

Acknowledgements

The pulse, and Chinese medicine in general, have traditionally been taught by following a master, just as I did with Dr. John H.F. Shen over a period of many years. This has been described in Tibetan theology as the way of the Sadhami. In recent times, both in China and in the West, Chinese medicine is taught in schools with relatively large classes, much as Western medicine is taught, with didactic and practical classroom experience and clinical work in the hospitals or clinics.

Since it is rarely feasible for one person to follow a master, and because I was sought out to instruct in the pulse by students of Chinese medicine, I have developed an alternative system of teaching in small groups, developing new methods and techniques along the way with the help of my students. This method of teaching seems to attract a certain number of students for whom (I assume) touch has become an important way of gathering information, and who have an unceasing thirst to be more complete in themselves and their work despite the obstacles.

This book began as a manual for my students when I started to experiment with teaching the pulse to small groups of acupuncture practitioners. I am deeply grateful to many of these gifted people who have enhanced my ability to transmit this art–science and transform it into a better diagnostic tool.

It began with Elaine Stern, almost two decades ago. Jason Elias, Lonny Jarrett, Mona Tempkin, Maribeth Bunn, Rory Kerr, Stuart Watts, Edith Davis, Cara Frank, Gary Kaplan, Jack Daniels, Lila Wah, Karen Kisslinger, Will and Bobbie Morris, Robert Heffron, Brian La Forgia, Joseph Thomas, Ann-Marie Hemken, Andrea Ford, Giulio Picozzi, Kathleen Leavy, Bill Chesser, Scott Maloney, Liz Pelzner, David Cook, and Kevin Ergil have followed in the frustrating effort to create these seminars. The limit of twelve practitioners to a seminar means that they are not financially profitable. It is therefore a labor of love for each of them in the service of pursuing and assimilating the finer essences of Chinese medicine wherever they can find it. Gratitude to my long-suffering wife Ewa is endless for, among many reasons, her dedication to the successful organization of these seminars.

I want to thank Kathleen Leavy and David Bole for introducing this pulse work as part of the curriculum at the Dragon Rises School of Oriental Medicine, and for their support of this work over the years.

I wish to express my special appreciation to my longest continuous student and associate, Robert Heffron, M.D., who, with Marie Dauenheimer, contributed the graphic representations of the principal pulse qualities in this book. I am also grateful for his valuable advice over the years. He is an outstanding teacher with a great grasp of the sensory and interpretive aspects of this system of pulse diagnosis.

I also wish to thank others who are certified to teach this system, or are on the path to certification. In particular, Brian La Forgia has pursued a mastery of this work for many years. He teaches it so well, and transmits to his students a balanced spirit of inquiry and humility ineluctable to the success of this work and the practice of Chinese medicine. I am grateful to Robbee Fian, another fine teacher, who has given me much needed spiritual support and wise counsel during the past few years, and to Susan Goldstone, who has embraced this work with great passion and intelligence. Phyllis Bloom has studied this method almost from the beginning and has provided me with many searching and valuable questions, always in the spirit of the further development of this work, for which I am endlessly grateful. Fortunately, many other fine hearts and minds are working to complete the difficult road to certification as teachers.

I wish especially to express my thanks to Eastland Press for publishing this book, and to the dedicated editing of Dan Bensky and John O'Connor, who have stimulated my thinking and contributed immeasurably to the accuracy and readability of this text. I also wish to thank Nissi Wang and Rory Kerr for their editorial contributions.

Preface

This book is, in part, intended to be used as a reference work. For this reason there is an inevitable amount of repetition where I felt it necessary to convey the material in a particular section most comprehensively. Special terms which are encountered by the reader prior to their exposition in the text—such as 'qi wild'—are defined in the glossary at the back of the book. And for those who would gainfully read this work as a textbook, from front to back, many of the references to the literature have been placed in endnotes so as not to disturb the flow or interrupt the presentation of the principal material in the text.

This book is organized into seventeen chapters and follows the format by which it is taught in our seminars, through an advancing hierarchy of complexity. Chapter 1 considers general issues of terminology, classification, tradition versus revision, and the sense of touch. Chapter 2 looks at the pulse from an historical perspective in terms of positions and depths. Chapter 3 discusses special considerations such as age and gender, acute versus chronic, and diagnosis and prevention, among other topics. Chapter 4 provides a step-by-step procedure for taking the pulse. Chapter 5 focuses on the Normal pulse and the special nomenclature governing the description of the pulse.

The middle chapters (6 through 11) are concerned with individual pulse qualities, which are there discussed in detail. Chapter 12 is concerned with these qualities at each position. Chapter 13 looks at the three depths, and uniform qualities that can be found over the entire pulse. Chapter 14 examines those qualities that are found uniformly over large segments of the pulse, such as the entire left or right side, or all of the three burners. Chapter 15 addresses the relationship of the pulse to psychology, and Chapter 16 the relationship between the pulse and prognosis. Chapter 17 is a summary of all that came before, demonstrating how to bring this material together to satisfy our fundamental objective: to make a rational diagnosis based on reliable information from the pulse, and to formulate a treatment strategy. This process is illustrated through sample case histories drawn from my seminars.

On my website, *www.dragonrises.org,* is an examination which covers many of the important aspects of this pulse system. I encourage all serious students to take this examination, which I call the Personal Contemporary Chinese Pulse Diagnosis Self-Assessment Document. The website will also provide a forum for communicating with other students and instructors in an ongoing dialogue, to find news of seminars, and articles of common interest.

With regard to this system of pulse diagnosis, some have suggested that the model is more relevant to a treatment modality based on herbs, since my teacher, Dr. John H.F. Shen, was himself an herbalist. However, I used it with considerable benefit for many years when acupuncture was virtually my only treatment modality. While it is of great value to herbal medicine because of its emphasis on the state of the internal organs and their interrelationships—rather than just the circulation of qi in the channels—I have found it to be of equal value in the practice of acupuncture.

Wang Shu-He observed in the preface to *The Pulse Classic* that "The mechanisms of the pulse are fine and subtle, and the pulse images are difficult to differentiate."[1] As I move around the country, with my fingers guiding others to discover pulse qualities, the most frequent comment I hear, echoing those of Wang Shu-He, is "That *is* subtle!" The message I wish to leave is how much *more* subtle Chinese medicine is than the student ever imagined. No lifetime is long enough for even the most talented to discover all that the pulse has to teach.

Anton Jayasuriya[2] noted that "To add to his other difficulties, the novice realizes that pulse diagnosis may only be learnt from experience at the bedside under the tutelage of an experienced traditional practitioner for many long years." To this he added:

> Pulse diagnosis is a time-consuming and extremely difficult art to master, but perhaps it is well worth the effort. Many obscure ailments are due to some kind of imbalance in the body energy which are difficult to detect by the usual methods of Oriental and Western diagnosis, and pulse diagnosis may be very helpful in the diagnosis of such obscure disorders.

The seminars that I conduct have demonstrated to me that the interpretations which are found in the literature (and in this book) are greatly limited in terms of what we have yet to learn about their meaning. Each class enlarges my awareness as I listen to the new correlations with qualities, previously never suspected, emerging from the practitioners and their patients. Although this information may be unique to a particular person, it may also apply to many others.

My own "experienced traditional practitioner" was Dr. Shen; my deepest regret is that this book was not written by him, and that the seminars which inspired it are mine instead of his. He was the undisputed master and architect of all the advancements made in the understanding and interpretation of the pulse that are embodied in this book. With his recent death, a body of knowledge has gone with him which I could scarcely absorb, given the depth of his understanding and the limitations of time, language, and cultural differences with which we were mutually burdened.

Since he chose not to make a more extensive written record of this unsurpassed and uncommon wisdom, it was left to others to make the effort. The content of this book is, therefore, an attempt to pass on some of the most extraordinarily creative augmentations of the Chinese medical tradition in generations, by one of the great Chinese physicians of the twentieth century. Dr. Shen's legacy can enrich this diagnostic medium far beyond what is known and described in our current literature, or taught today in the principal centers of education of Chinese medicine. Compared to what he has taught publicly or placed in print,[3] I can attest from personal experience that there is no aspect of Chinese medicine on which Dr. Shen could not expound for hours—even days—and still not exhaust the subject.

What is included here is a record of what Dr. Shen actually taught and demonstrated to me on a day to day basis, in the context of an extensive clinical practice over a period of eight intensive years. During this time, we would meet two to three days a week seeing thirty or more patients daily. This was followed by another fifteen years of less intensive interaction. Nevertheless, the reader should be aware that what I have recorded may vary somewhat from his published and publicly spoken statements on the subject of the pulse. In preparing this book I have spared no effort to reconcile these two sources of information.

My contribution has been to appreciate the excellence of Dr. Shen's work, and to dedicate myself to this learning. Around this core of information I have built and recorded my own body of experience and information, developed new ways of teaching in groups, and organized this knowledge for future generations.

As Dr. Shen often observed, the information discussed here consists of generalities, abstractions of the truth. The truth for any patient can only be found by placing these abstractions in the field of that person's constitution and life experiences. The essence of Chinese medicine is, after all, the expression and unfolding of this challenge: to diagnose the person and not the disease.

By itself, the pulse is a remarkable diagnostic instrument, the jewel in the crown of diagnosis. However—and this cannot be repeated too often—pulse diagnosis was always meant to be used in the context of looking, listening, asking, and all of the other diagnostic modalities involving touch. No experienced practitioner, especially Dr. Shen, would suggest otherwise. In this context it is important to appreciate that whenever there is a disparity between the pulse and other diagnostic parameters, one must weigh the possibility of a more serious illness.

It is important that every assertion stated in this book be tested by as many practitioners as possible so that the information becomes ever more refined and encompassing of the world in which we live and function. Even as you learn, learn first to trust your fingers and your senses, which this discipline will never cease to advance.

The critical link between the information in this book and the practical use of that information in the clinic is the ability to accurately identify qualities on the pulse. The object is to find a common language of felt sensation and terminology. This can be done only by hands-on instruction in a seminar setting, and it is my hope that during the remainder of my lifetime I will have the opportunity to teach this to many more practitioners and students.

---

1. Wang Shu-He, *The Pulse Classic,* trans. Yang Shou-Zhong (Boulder, CO: Blue Poppy Press, 1997) *xi.*
2. Anton Jayasuriya, *Textbook of Acupuncture Science* (Sri Lanka: Chandrakanthi Industrial Press, 1981) 517.
3. John Shen, *Chinese Medicine* (New York: Educational Solutions, 1980).

Introduction

It is the intention of this book to reawaken an awareness of the importance of pulse diagnosis within the practice of Chinese medicine. It has been my experience that diagnosis in general, and the art-science of the pulse in particular, has been neglected.

What is the potential value of pulse diagnosis at the dawn of the twenty-first century? In 1992 I participated in a conference in Japan, the purpose of which was to explore the healthcare system of the future. Apparently, the Japanese government had concluded that their current healthcare system was dysfunctional. The participants were representatives of a wide variety of 'traditional medicines' from many countries, even from the Sami Laplander culture. Following the presentations, the concluding statements emphasized that the direction of future healthcare in Japan must stress self-help and prevention.

Increasingly, people and governments are acknowledging the failure of modern medicine to provide affordable and efficient health care. The trend is toward finding medical systems which emphasize the cheapest and most effective medicine: wellness and prevention.

Prevention depends entirely on an exquisitely sensitive diagnostic scheme which is capable of accessing the process of disease close to its inception. In our time the only marginally available diagnostic instrument of which I am aware that embodies this sensitivity is the art and science of the Chinese pulse. The Ayurvedic and Tibetan models, similarly suited for this task, are simply too inaccessible outside of their countries of origin, and the excellent Korean system has limited exposure in the West.

Yet the tradition of Chinese pulse diagnosis is rapidly disappearing. In China as well as in the West, diagnosis is increasingly the purview of biomedicine, with acupuncture and herbs relegated to the role of a biomedical technique. Acupuncturists are flocking to the sides of medical doctors in hospitals, an environment in which there is no time for the lengthy 'asking, looking, listening, and touching' examinations required in traditional Chinese medicine.

The catalog of an American acupuncture school that I recently read offers 2,700 hours of instruction, of which only 60 hours involve diagnosis. Having abandoned those aspects of Chinese medicine that define them as physicians, acupuncturists have reduced themselves to mere technicians in a powerful medical system in which they are being swallowed whole. Their identity as physicians is disappearing. This book is an attempt to revitalize traditional diagnosis by renewing the concepts and practices of pulse diagnosis to make them vitally relevant for modern times and modern practice. The object is to reestablish those aspects of traditional Chinese medicine that distinguish the practitioner as a physician.

The Normal pulse is a sensitive and precisely measurable standard of health. It enables us to detect early deviations from health. It provides us with a preventive medicine. All of these capabilities are lacking in our modern healthcare system.

This growing recognition of the importance of the development of an effective preventive medical system to contemporary healthcare systems renders pulse diagnosis as potentially the most significant single body of current medical knowledge. However, it is only as useful as the proficiency with which it is practiced. What we must acknowledge is that, despite its enormous potential for good, without the skills which have largely been lost today, the value of Chinese pulse diagnosis becomes irrelevant.

The enormous body of knowledge which can be discerned by touch at the radial arteries would have been unknown to me had I not had the great good fortune to meet a master of this tradition in 1974. Dr. John H.F. Shen's capacity to use the pulse diagnostically left me little choice but to follow him after our first meeting. His lifelong study of the pulse, and his extraordinary ability to use it to plumb the depths of his patients, has left many observers in disbelief, certain that this wizardry is primarily intuitive. It is not.

Over the years of our association, Dr. Shen demonstrated to me, logically and reasonably, exactly how he arrives at his conclusions. He was quick to point out that the interpretation of the pulse is influenced by body type, history, and a perspective based on changes in the pulse over time. His interpretations are therefore an integration of what is at his fingertips together with many other elements of perception and interaction. The mystery is how one person's intelligence can combine such global awareness of what is seen, heard, and touched over a lifetime of study and practical experience to fathom the human enigma with an accurate and original perspective.

There is, therefore, a wealth of information available from the pulse that I have found unmentioned in the literature, and rarely hinted at in any of the current teaching institutions with which I am familiar. It is my intention to share this information, and the techniques required to access it, with all who wish to learn.

Beginning with my retirement from active practice in 1990, I started the task of organizing all that I had learned from Dr. Shen concerning the pulse, and integrating this knowledge with my own experience and that of other available sources in the English language. A review of the literature available in English has been as complete as possible.

While the source of this book is primarily the contribution of Dr. Shen, the organization of the material into an original classification system based on sensation and clinical experience is primarily my own. The interpretation does vary from that of Dr. Shen's. It represents an attempt to bring his work, my experience and perspective, and the work of others past and present into an accessible, meaningful, and richer blend of clinical significance.

This material is intended to be used in conjunction with small group seminars; it can never be a substitute for hands-on learning. The object of a seminar is to establish the parameters of the Chinese pulse on the radial artery, to identify qualities, to establish priorities in observation, to interpret qualities, to clinically relate qualities, depths, and positions, to integrate pulse diagnosis with other modalities, and to study patients, conditions, and pulse configurations in greater depth.

The final purpose of this book, and of the seminars with which it is associated, is to preserve the subtlety of this art-science so that it may serve to fulfill its potential as an instrument of early diagnosis and prevention. My hope is to enhance the tradition by increasing the refinement of diagnostic information with a system of classification that is more manageable for the practitioner of the twenty-first century. I hope this book will serve as a watershed in the modern application of the art and science of pulse diagnosis, to make it a more effective clinical tool for the modern practitioner.

CHAPTER 1

Preliminary Reflections

CONTENTS

Tradition and Revision, 3
Terminology, 6
Classification and Nomenclature, 6
    General comments, 6
    Specific issues in classification, 7
    Classification by sensation or by condition, 7
    ▪ Table 1-1: Comparison of pulse terminology in English, 8-9
    Differentiation of qualities, 10
Contemporary Chinese Pulse Diagnosis in the Context of Modern Practice, 10
    Time, 10
    Significance, 10
Potential for Pulse Diagnosis, 11
Limitations of Pulse Diagnosis, 12
The Pulse and Other Methods of Diagnosis, 13
The Practitioner, 14
The Senses, 14
    Touch, 14
Theory, 15
Reflection, 15

CHAPTER 1

Preliminary Reflections

The method of pulse diagnosis described in this book, which I call Contemporary Chinese Pulse Diagnosis, is, in my experience, superior for obtaining the greatest amount of physiological and psychological information about an individual. This is not to say, however, that it is the only valid system of pulse diagnosis, either within or outside of Chinese medicine. In fact, pulse diagnosis was highly developed in other traditional cultures including Ayurvedic, Egyptian, Persian, Arabic, Hebrew, and, to a lesser extent, Greek.[1] I have had the opportunity to study several approaches to Chinese pulse diagnosis, and have found that each is valid within a particular sphere of sometimes mutually exclusive information.

Early in my career I used the pulse intuitively with considerable success, accessing information that is less available to me now that I am formally indoctrinated. Education can be a deadly necessity requiring one to live with paradox somewhere on a thin line between wisdom and dogma. Yet thousands of years of experience is not to be discarded without some risk.[2]

Tradition and Revision

There are two broad traditions in Chinese medicine. One involves the abstract and highly theoretical court medicine which was recorded in books that have come down to us through the ages as the classics. The other is a more informal, often clan-based, medicine grounded more in practical experience. This tradition was rarely recorded for posterity since it lacked the approval of the official court physicians. Its jealously-guarded secrets were handed down from generation to generation as part of an oral tradition. Yet it is this more practical, experience-based medicine that has served the Chinese people through the millennia, to a large extent independent of the classical tradition.

To be sure, the system of pulse diagnosis set forth in this book draws from the classical tradition. But it is grounded as well in the oral tradition of Chinese medicine, with its emphasis on learning through actual experience. My teacher, Dr. John H.F. Shen, was himself a physician in the lineage of the Ding (Ting) clan.

What I have found too frequently in the literature are uncritical duplications of observations first recorded two thousand years ago in terminology that modern practitioners find difficult to decipher. I have also found that the classical Chinese pulse systems seem to be largely limited by theoretical models that tend to disregard observations that don't fit within those models. I approach Chinese medicine with the most profound respect and gratitude for tradition. Yet much of what has come down to us as scripture does not stand the test of clinical scrutiny. It is just as important, or more so, to respect the messages from our own fingers, with thorough confirmation by the patient, when those messages differ from dogma. As Dr. Shen frequently reminded me, the people who created tradition were themselves, after all, only people, just like us.

Let me illustrate this point with an example from *The Pulse Classic (Mai jing)*, written by Wang Shu-He in the second century. No one has had a greater influence on Chinese pulse diagnosis than Wang, who was chief physician to the royal family. Here is his description of the Choppy pulse quality:

> It is fine and slow, coming and going with difficulty and scattered or with an interruption, but has the ability to recover.[3]

Commentators on the pulse have repeated this description word for word for nearly two millennia.[4] Yet in certain important respects it is very misleading, because the words that Wang uses to describe the pulse—fine, slow, scattered, interrupted—are themselves distinct pulse qualities whose significance differs markedly from that of the Choppy quality. Just because these other qualities may, on occasion, coexist simultaneously with the Choppy quality on the pulse is not to say that they mean the same thing. They may represent a related, but distinct, condition, or signify one etiology, but not the condition itself.[5]

The failure to properly distinguish each of these qualities has led to much confusion.[6] For example, Wang correctly associates the Choppy quality with blood stasis or stagnation. It is well-known that many conditions will affect the flow of blood, and because there are many etiologies for blood stagnation, one might reasonably (and correctly) expect that there would be a different quality associated with each. Yet by lumping so many qualities together under the rubric of just one quality—Choppy—suggests that they all mean the same thing. They don't. To take just one example, the Slow quality often signifies qi deficiency, and qi deficiency and blood stagnation are often found together, since qi moves the blood. It would therefore be correct to say that qi deficiency is one cause or etiology of blood stagnation. But it does not follow that the Slow quality —a sign of qi deficiency—is therefore a sign of blood stagnation, any more than the Choppy quality—a sign of blood stagnation—is a sign of qi deficiency. Obviously, to treat a patient with qi deficiency for non-existent blood stagnation could be very harmful to his health.

As remarkable as his work is in many other respects, in this case Wang simply erred by failing to distinguish between qualities which are potentially associated with an etiology of blood stagnation, or a related condition, and the quality (Choppy) which signifies the condition of blood stagnation itself. This error underlines the need to study the classics with a critical eye, testing what they say against what we as practitioners find in the clinic.

Another type of mistake can be found in what are traditionally classified as the 'hard' pulse qualities—such as Tight and Wiry—which are associated with disorders that do not reflect modern clinical experience. No doubt the associations attributed to these pulses were correct at the time they were made. Yet the Tight pulse,[7] which in the classical literature is almost always associated with stagnation due to internal cold, is in our times more often found in connection with moderate heat from deficiency.

The term Tight in this context requires some explanation. I have found that there is a progression of diminishing flexibility and increasing hardness—a distinction that is absent from the traditional literature—from Normal to Taut to Tense to Tight and to Wiry, and that each of these qualities conveys different information (see Chapter 11). With moderate internal cold the pulse reflects the sensation which we call Tight, and with extreme pain, Wiry, which is very hard, like a metal wire.

Li Shi-Zhen, on the other hand, describes a Tight pulse as being "like a tightly stretched rope and feels twisted" and "vibrates to the left and right."[8] But in my experience, in the progression of loss of flexibility, a Tight pulse feels thinner and harder than a "stretched rope"—a quality which we call Tense—and does not feel "twisted." Only in extreme cases of life-threatening cold such as hypothermia have I found a pulse quality like that described by Li at the level of the bone, and which I call Hidden Excess.

Similarly, the Wiry quality is traditionally associated with malarial disorder, yet no mention is made of what is currently its most common pattern associations: severe deficiency of yin-essence and/or pain, early diabetes, and early hypertension at the left middle and proximal positions.

The severe, acute medical disorders mentioned by the ancients, which are characteristic of pre-industrial agricultural societies, such as malarial disorder and internal cold obstruction, are rarely seen today by most practitioners in the centrally-heated West. These accounts are translated from the distant past and are not necessarily based on current practice.[9] Instead, in the West we are today confronted with chronic disease largely based on stress, either emotional, physical, or chemical. And most acute medical symptoms here are treated with biomedical modalities. Thus, the interpretation of these pulse qualities has changed as we have moved from acute to chronic phases of disharmony.

This view is reflected in the following passage by the noted contemporary Chinese physician Deng Tietao:

> Modern physicians disagree about the location of the viscera and bowels of the inch, bar and cubit positions; some agree with traditional descriptions and others disagree. Those who disagree argue that perpetual knowledge is not reliable, while those who agree cannot produce objective evidence. We believe... that a further step should be taken in deeper research of the topic.[10]

To base treatment on interpretations of pulses that are inconsistent with contemporary living conditions is dangerous. Interpreting a Tight pulse to mean that there is cold stagnation, when in fact there is heat from deficiency, is obviously not in the patient's best interest. The classification and interpretation of these qualities in this book are, I believe, more in keeping with current clinical experience, allowing for a more logical and rational treatment program.

The study of pulses, like all of Chinese medicine, is dynamic and growing, as it has been from its inception two millennia ago. Chinese medicine is circular. The polarities that create the movement around and across this circle are relative and not absolute. The circle is a symbol and realization of unity, continuity, strength, dynamic fluidity, centeredness as a core of the absolute, yet with the unending capacity for expansion and contraction.

For this reason, Chinese medicine is mutable. It can change to meet the requirements of the new physical and psychological stresses that have accompanied the clock, the assembly line, the jet engine, and the communications revolution. It is limited in its development only by the far reaches of the expanding universe. This book is the record of the participation of one man and his student in the amplification of that circle of wisdom, in and of our times.

At the risk of being accused of heresy, I admonish current and future generations of practitioners to respect and to consider, yet also to question, every assertion made since antiquity, including those in this book. An ongoing integration of new and old, as with Dr. Shen and others, is the proper avenue to a vital and effective model of pulse diagnosis.

Terminology

Only the pulse qualities, the special complementary pulse positions, and the names of the organs in the traditional medical system are capitalized in this book. Terms unique to Dr. Shen, such as 'qi wild' and 'Heart nervous,' are enclosed by single quotation marks. Most of these terms are referenced to Chapter 14 of my book *Dragon Rises, Red Bird Flies*, and are also defined in the glossary to the present volume.

The term *principal position* refers primarily to the six major traditional individual positions—the distal, middle, and proximal positions of the radial pulse on the left and right wrists. I also use the term *complementary position* to refer to those parts of the anatomy and physiology that Dr. Shen or I have discovered to be represented on the pulse either proximal, distal, medial, or lateral to, or between the distal, middle, and proximal principal positions.

The term *level* refers to the three burners—upper, middle, and lower. The term *depth* refers to the vertical qi, blood, and organ layers of the pulse from (respectively) the top, which is just below the surface of the skin, to the bottom of the pulse, which is still well above the bone. The term *function* is used in this book to refer to the natural function of an organism or one part of the organism. *Yin organ* refers to a solid organ, and *yang organ* refers to a hollow organ.

Although I recognize the importance of initially distinguishing the terms *pattern* and *disharmony* from pathology, disease, and illness, I believe that the time has passed for practitioners of Chinese medicine, reading a work intended only for themselves, to continue to require these distinctions. I use these terms with the understanding that we are all speaking the same energetic language.

Classification and Nomenclature

GENERAL COMMENTS

There is a crisis in Chinese medical terminology, from the extreme of pedantic translation, such as 'vacuity' for deficiency and 'replete' for excess, to the Latinized forms of usage. For the student, especially the American student, this crisis creates confusion and discouragement.

The naming of pulse qualities is no less bewildering. One source, for instance, translates the Choppy quality as 'difficult,' a term that tells us nothing about the sensation or the meaning of this quality. Another example is the term 'soft' (or 'soggy'), which again tells us nothing about sensation or interpretation. I have renamed this quality as it feels, Yielding Empty Thread-like. Indeed, the literature abounds with terminology that is confusing, misleading, and contradictory.[11]

Table 1-1 provides a comparison of the most widely used English terms for the principal pulse qualities. It is presented to illustrate the current confusion in nomenclatures, which discourages students of Chinese medicine from the study of the pulse. One of my goals in this book is to present a uniform nomenclature based on sensations easily recognized by those who are familiar with the English language. Many of the qualities described in this book are not among those listed in the table below. In part, this is because I have identified many more qualities than appear on the list, and in part, because my sensory descriptions and interpretations are often different from those listed. For example, the sensory descriptions provided by some authors of qualities such as Tight and Wiry are unrelated to anything that a native English speaker would commonly associate with those words.

Perhaps the Wiry quality is the most challenging for the student of traditional Chinese medicine studying the system described in this book, since the term is used to describe a wide variety of sensations including one which actually feels like a very tense rope rather than a thin, hard, immalleable substance like a metal wire. The Chinese interchange wiry with 'string taut' and 'bow string,' which indicates that the confusion is possibly in the translation from Chinese to English. While I have considered such terms as steely, rigid, and flinty as substitutes for Wiry in order to reduce the confusion, I have not found a better term to describe what is actually felt. Nonetheless, the quest to reconcile our terminology with other systems which I find much less accurate will continue.

SPECIFIC ISSUES IN CLASSIFICATION

Apart from the difficulty of organizing a body of knowledge that far exceeds the work of any one person on this subject, a large problem has been to reconcile Dr. Shen's English terminology with that found elsewhere in the literature. For example, he uses the term Overflowing to mean what others refer to as 'full.' His widespread use of the term 'full' in our communications is not described elsewhere, so I have coined a new term, Inflated, to encompass the sensation and special meaning of this pulse quality. This conundrum is an ongoing challenge.

Archaic language which modern practitioners find difficult to decipher and relate to the sensations accessed from the pulses of their patients makes the ancient and traditional pulse diagnosis texts unapproachable and clinically impractical.[12] Students in my classes have expressed a clear preference for a simpler, less ambiguous nomenclature based on sensations easily transposed into an easily understood modern language.

For example, to most of my students the term 'sinking' implies a process of something moving from the surface to the depths. However, the sensation felt as the sinking quality is accessed only at the organ depth, which is the innermost functional part of the pulse. This pulse is resident at the organ depth, and therefore is not in the process of sinking. Furthermore, the clinical interpretation of the sinking quality implies a chronic condition that has already reached deeply and profoundly into the most crucial areas of the physiology. For this reason, the term Deep is substituted for sinking.

An important task has been to correlate the many different terms for the same quality and to create a new logical terminology for our times. While attempting to clarify, I have tried to incorporate the incredible nuances that make Chinese medicine so uniquely valuable. The subtleties may seem initially intimidating, but the rewards—even for the novice—quickly outweigh these concerns for those who persist.

CLASSIFICATION BY SENSATION OR BY CONDITION

Pulse classification should be organized on the basis of the most immediate and relevant message perceived by the clinician through the act of palpation. The nomenclature used here is therefore based on sensation rather than on clinical interpretation.

We access the pulse first through our senses before our mind makes associations with those sensations. We *perceive* Tight before we *think* heat from deficiency, although with experience the two become nearly synonymous. Furthermore, before we make the diagnostic leap and attach final meaning to what we feel, we usually consult other signs such as the tongue, eyes, and color, as well as the symptom picture.

One example is the quality elsewhere referred to as 'big' or 'large.' Descriptions of the physical sensation associated with this quality in the literature emphasize its width. For example, Wu Shui-Wan notes that it is "twice as wide as a normal pulse."[13] Neither big nor large clearly conveys that width is the principal identifying sensation. Therefore, instead of either word, I use the term Wide, which corresponds more accurately with the felt sensation. For the sake of coherence, I use Wide and Thin to describe the qualities that are subsumed under the aegis of width. These terms describe the two extremes of sensation in terms of width, and only coincidentally in terms of excess and deficiency of blood, conditions often associated with these qualities.

Table 1-1 Comparison of pulse terminology in English

Chinese	*The Pulse Classic* Wang Shu-He, trans. Yang Shou-Zhong	*The Web That Has No Weaver* Ted Kaptchuk	*Practical Diagnosis in Traditional Chinese Medicine*, Deng Tietao, trans. Marnae Ergil	*Pulse Diagnosis* Li Shi-Zhen, trans. Hoe Ku Huynh
Fú 浮	Floating	Floating	Floating	Floating
Chén 沉	Deep	Sinking	Deep	Deep
Chí 遲	Slow	Slow	Slow	Slow
Shuò 數	Rapid	Rapid	Rapid	Rapid
Xū 虛	Vacuous	Empty	Vacuous	Empty
Shí 實	Replete	Full	Replete	Full
Huá 滑	Slippery	Slippery	Slippery	Slippery
Sè 澀	Choppy	Choppy	Rough	Choppy
Cháng 長	---	Long	Long	Long
Duǎn 短	---	Short	Short	Short
Hóng 洪	Surging	Flooding	Surging	Flooding
Dà 大	---	Big	Large	Big
Wēi 微	Faint	Minute	Faint	Minute
Jǐn 緊	Tight	Tight	Tight	Tight
Huǎn 緩	Moderate	Moderate	Moderate	Leisurely
Xián 弦	Bowstring	Wiry	String-like	Wiry
Kōu 芤	Scallion-stalk	Hollow	Scallion stalk	Hollow
Gé 革	Drumskin	Leather	Drumskin	Leather
Láo 牢	---	Confined	Confined	Firm
Rú 濡	Soft (?)	Soggy	Soggy	Soft
Ruǎn 軟	---	---	---	---
Ruò 弱	Weak	Frail	Weak	Weak
Sàn 散	Dissipated	Scattered	Scattered	Scattered
Xì 細	Fine	Thin	Fine	Fine
Xiǎo 小	---	---	Small	---
Fú 伏	Hidden	Hidden	Hidden	Hidden
Dòng 動	Stirring	Moving (Spinning Bean)	Stirring	Moving
Cù 促	Skipping	Hurried	Skipping	Hasty
Jié 結	Bound	Knotted	Bound	Knotted
Dài 代	Interrupted	Intermittent	Regularly Intermittent	Intermittent
Jí 急	---	---	Racing	---

Chinese	*The Essentials of Chinese Diagnostics* Manfred Porkert	*The Chinese Pulse Diagnosis* Wu Shui-Wan	*Acupuncture: The Ancient Art of Chinese Healing* Felix Mann	C.S. Cheung & Jenny Belluomini
Fú 浮	Superficial	Floating	Floating	Floating
Chén 沉	Submerged	Deep	Sunken (Deep)	Sinking
Chí 遲	Slowed down	Slow	Slow	Slow
Shùo 數	Accelerated	Rapid	Rapid	Rapid
Xū 虛	Exhausted (Depleted)	Empty	Empty	Deficient
Shí 實	Replete	Full	Full	Excess
Huá 滑	Slippery	Slippery	Slippery	Slippery
Sè 澀	Grating	Choppy	Choppy (Rough)	Difficult
Cháng 長	Long	Long	Long	Long
Duǎn 短	Brief	Short	Short	Short
Hóng 洪	Flooding	Overflowing	Overflowing	Tidal
Dà 大	Large	Big	---	Large
Wēi 微	Evanescent	Minute	Minute	Diminutive
Jǐn 緊	Tense	Tight	Tight	Tight
Huǎn 緩	Languid	Slowed-down	Slowed-down	Leisurely (Relaxed)
Xián 弦	Stringy	Wiry	Bowstring	Bowstring
Kōu 芤	Onion stalk	Hollow	Hollow	Leek stalk
Gé 革	Tympanic	Leather	Leather	Leather
Láo 牢	Fixed	Firm	Firm (Hard)	Prison
Rú 濡	Frail	Weak-Floating	Weak-Floating	Soft
Ruǎn 軟	Soft	---	---	---
Ruò 弱	Infirm	Weak	Weak	Weak
Sàn 散	Dispersed	Scattered	Scattered	Scattered
Xì 細	Minute	Fine	Fine	Small
Xiǎo 小	Small	---	---	Small
Fú 伏	Recondite	---	Hidden (Buried)	Hidden
Dòng 動	Mobile	Moving	Moving	Agitated
Cù 促	Agitated	Hasty	Hasty	Accelerated
Jié 結	Adherent	Knotted	Knotted	Nodular
Dài 代	Intermittent	Intermittent	Intermittent	Replacement
Jí 急	Racing	---	Fast (Hurried)	Rushing (Swift)

DIFFERENTIATION OF QUALITIES

Most sources list between nineteen and twenty-eight pulse qualities. Table 5-2 (see Chapter 5) summarizes my own classification of the qualities, categorized according to sensation, and organized according to clinical experience. (As an exercise for my own comprehension of pulse diagnosis, I have also classified the qualities according to their associated conditions; see Table 5-3.)

Most students who attend my seminars come because what they are experiencing in their consulting rooms does not coincide with what they read in textbooks, which perpetuates rather than tests the information handed down through the ages. At first glance, the system subscribed to in this book seems more complicated than others. It is, however, simpler because it corresponds to what is at one's fingertips, especially in relationship to the presenting clinical condition. Over the years I have been able to demonstrate the value of these finer diagnostic differentiations to reach a more rational and successful treatment program. Furthermore, students have absorbed these distinctions with less difficulty than anticipated, and with a growing and lasting appreciation of their clinical application. Besides, it has been noted that in Ayurvedic and Unani medicine, as many as six hundred different pulse varieties have been identified.[14]

Contemporary Chinese Pulse Diagnosis in the Context of Modern Practice

TIME

How much time does one require to obtain an accurate reading of the pulse? This question arises almost purely from the time/cost considerations of a pressured practice, both at acupuncture school clinics and in the private practice of Chinese medicine.

I personally require approximately thirty to forty-five minutes for teaching purposes during seminars and the patient's initial visit, and about five to ten minutes during subsequent visits. Dr. Shen required less than five minutes. Students have reported using as little as ten minutes. The answer seems to lie within the general pace of the individual. Therefore, one should be encouraged to view this approach to pulse diagnosis as potentially cost effective once one has achieved a reasonable level of competence.

Furthermore, students from many different schools of acupuncture theory and practice, which vary considerably from my own, have found this method of pulse diagnosis to be both compatible with and helpful to their own practices, which vary considerably from my own.

SIGNIFICANCE

Each examination reveals layers of information about rhythm, rate, organs, substances, body systems and areas, and activities. Until we see these findings within the context of the process of disease from birth to death, the sum of this information will seem overwhelming. Pulse examination is a readout of the life process at the time, however early, of that investigation in the person's life. When done correctly, it is an extremely sensitive tool available for the creation of a preventive medicine.

Of importance to the beginner is that this system is organized such that the most straightforward and easily accessed information can be usefully applied by the neophyte, even without the deeper subtleties available to the more experienced practitioner. For example, even the beginner should be able to gain information about the basic substances (qi, blood, yin, essence, yang) and activity (heat and cold) of the body, which will be helpful in prescribing the proper treatment.

Each pulse finding is real and requires ultimate attention. Some findings are more relevant than others to the current complaint, which is to be determined by experience and by relating the pulse to other signs and symptoms.

Potential for Pulse Diagnosis

Neither palpation of the pulse nor, for that matter, any other single diagnostic technique represents the sole vehicle that will lead us to the truth about the state of an individual's health. Yet the pulse can deliver a tremendous amount of information. Let us examine the kinds of information an experienced practitioner of pulse diagnosis can expect to obtain using this methodology.

In terms of the past, one should be able to learn something about the person's constitution, the course of his or her life, previous illnesses, emotional state, and habits (e.g., work, exercise, nutrition, drugs—both recreational and medicinal—and sex).

In terms of the present, one should be able to ascertain information about the individual's lifestyle and habits; overall body condition, or true qi; the strength of one's constitution; balance in terms of the relationship of the various organ systems to each other, and between them and external factors; whether the condition is hot or cold, active or passive, internal or external, deficient or excessive, stagnant or weak; the extent to which the problems that confront the individual are due more to the amount, balance, rhythm, or circulation of fundamental substances such as qi, yin, blood, fluid, essence, or spirit; and the stage of disease. The pulse should tell us about the function of what Dr. Shen referred to as the 'nervous system,' 'circulatory system,' 'digestive system,' and 'organ systems.'[15]

The pulse should also tell us much about the mind and the spirit, in terms of mental status and behavioral style, methods of coping, stability, worry, guilt, fear, depression, mania, tension, and frustration, recent and past emotional (and physical) trauma, recent and past sadness, psychotic and/or epileptic tendencies, disappointments, and unexpressed anger.[16] Central nervous system and auto-immune diseases can also sometimes manifest on the pulse.

Because it immediately reveals so much on an emotional level, pulse diagnosis has been, for my patients, an objective reading of their emotional state, which bypasses the usual resistance to interpretation that one encounters in psychotherapeutic practice.

Furthermore, Dr. Shen demonstrated that the pulse offers a sensitive and reliable tool for assessing the course of treatment. From one session to the next, one can quickly access the most subtle responses (or lack thereof) to treatment, and thus make the treatment itself part of the ongoing reassessment of the diagnosis.

Most importantly, for the patient's future, one should be able to practice preventive medicine by reasonably extrapolating from what one has felt in the past and the present to predict future physical conditions and possible diseases, even many years hence. At the other end of the spectrum, the pulse is capable of indicating imminent death (see Chapter 16).

New diseases and new problems associated with a modern civilization, so very different from the agricultural society that spawned the original Chinese medicine, have begun to show consistencies in pulse diagnosis. The 'ceiling dripping' Scattered pulse of AIDS, and the various 'qi wild' pulses associated with immune deficiency disorders, are among the few recently identified syndromes that seem to have characteristic pulse pictures.

Hopefully, with the information provided in this book and the skills developed in pulse seminars, practitioners will be equipped to explore new worlds, expand the purview of Chinese medicine, and serve future generations.

Limitations of Pulse Diagnosis

Pulse diagnosis is an individually-developed art form, a blend of learning skills, intuition, a form of meditation, of being in touch simultaneously with the deepest parts of oneself and another. It requires both an ability to trust one's senses and years of practice, especially with a master. As Amber[17] observed:

> The pulse is the symphony of the body and the only way it can be played and understood [heard] is by practice and more practice. The best instructions, however elaborate, cannot teach the student much. The way to learn the pulse is to examine as many patients as possible and observe the peculiarities and characteristics of each one for himself. The help of a teacher who understands his subject is almost a necessity.

Pulse diagnosis is not subject to the Western scientific model. In some ways it is perhaps the most fickle of all the diagnostic modalities. It is temporarily more easily affected by ephemeral influences than is the tongue or other forms of diagnosis. It can be affected transiently by emotion, acute illnesses, activity, medications, diet, a full bladder, an imminent or concurrent menstrual flow, biorhythms, seasons of the year, and even the time of day. The quality of the practitioner's energy can also have a fleeting influence. However, I wish to emphasize the *transient* nature of these influences through which the experienced practitioner can, nevertheless, find the enduring, authentic qualities and message.

Furthermore, the quality that appears on the pulse depends on the condition of the body at the time of the event that caused the quality to appear, the intensity of the event, its location in the body, and the time that has passed since it occurred. For example, a trauma to the chest might create an Inflated quality in a strong person, and a Flat quality in a weaker person, in the upper burner positions. If, however, the trauma is overwhelming, even the strong person will show a Flat pulse, and with time and/or diminished body condition, both the Inflated and Flat pulse will ultimately become Feeble-Absent.

Another consideration is that the meaning of a quality may differ depending on where it is found on the pulse. Slipperiness at the organ depth of the left middle position can mean a Liver infection; at the blood depth it can be a sign of blood toxicity or excess viscosity (elevated cholesterol); over the entire pulse it could signal pregnancy or Heart qi deficiency. The interpretation may even vary in the same position, depending on the other qualities and conditions that accompany it. A Slippery quality, for example, at the left distal position (Heart and Pericardium, according to my tradition) will vary in its clinical significance depending on a number of factors. If the Slipperiness in the Heart pulse is rather general, and the pulse rate is Normal or a little Slow, most likely the condition is one of phlegm blocking the orifices of the Heart. In biomedical terms this may correspond to depression, epilepsy, or schizophrenia. If the pulse is Slippery and Rapid, the condition might be phlegm–fire, which is associated with mania. If the Slipperiness is acute, the pulse very rapid, and there is high fever, the person may have myocarditis. If, let us say, the Slipperiness is felt only in one small area on the lateral side of the pulse in the left distal position, rather than generally throughout this position, the condition is more likely to be a mitral valve defect.

Since it is affected by so many ephemeral influences, I myself must initially examine the pulse for at least a half hour. I repeat: pulse diagnosis is a meditative process. The more one empties one's mind and focuses with steady, serene concentration on the sensations at one's fingertips, the closer one comes to reality. One must take the pulses of many people and ask many questions. It is only with experience that one can quickly differentiate the authentic from the transient aspects of what one is feeling.

Some of the claims made about the pulse have been challenged by practitioners through the ages. One such physician was Xu Da-Chun, who excoriated doctors of his and other times for exaggerating the power of the pulse, to say, for example, on the basis of the pulse whether a person is good or bad, or when they will be promoted, or "in what year someone will acquire a fortune, and of what size."[18] I am also reminded of the characterization of Dr. Shen's skill in diagnosing the cause of a disease as being intuitive or wizard-like, which I continually hear as I travel about and meet people who are familiar with his work. For years I challenged every one of his assertions. But he demonstrated to me concrete findings from the pulse that led to his conclusions, most of which I have been able to replicate over the years in my own practice. It is perfectly understandable that to those without the skill, the use of the pulse in this manner would seem to be either impossible, or outright sorcery.

The Pulse and Other Methods of Diagnosis

No single modality was ever intended to be used alone, in isolation from other diagnostic methods. The practitioner integrates the pulse with other diagnostic guides: looking, listening, asking, and the other forms of touching. If, for example, the left middle position is Tight and the right middle position is Feeble-Absent, the problem could have begun at either position, even though the general rule is that the problem begins where the quality is most deficient or reduced. If the patient was tense before he or she developed digestive symptoms, then the condition is the familiar one in which the Liver is attacking the Spleen/Stomach. However, if the patient experienced digestive symptoms well before he or she was aware of the tension, then the Spleen/Stomach has affected the Liver, or (in Dr. Shen's terms) the 'digestive system' has affected the 'nervous system.'

Whenever there is a disparity between the pulse and other sources of diagnostic information, a more serious situation is usually at hand. If the symptoms and the pulse differ, the pulse is generally more accurate when interpreted by an experienced practitioner, unless the other diagnostic signs—such as the tongue, eyes, color and turbidity of urine, bowel movement patterns, types of sputum, preferences for hot and cold, color, and thirst patterns—are more in agreement with the symptoms. In that case, the diagnosis should lean in the direction indicated by the symptoms.

For example, the pulse may indicate an internal deficient cold disorder with a Slow rate and a Thin, Feeble, or Empty quality, but the symptoms suggest a hot disorder with fever, dryness, and irritability. In such a case, the symptoms may be favored as the true diagnosis if the tongue is red and dry, the urine scanty, dark, and burning, the eyes red and face flushed, and if the patient is constipated, with a preference for cold and an aversion to warmth. On the other hand, if the tongue is pale and wet, the urine is diluted and pale, the eyes show no heat signs, the face is pale, and the patient has diarrhea and expresses a preference for warmth and an aversion to cold, this would be compatible with a diagnosis that agrees with the pulse. Often cold and hot disorders coexist, and our management decision would rest with treating both, with emphasis on the one that shows the most severe signs and symptoms. More often, both conditions exist simultaneously; the pulse often reveals both, with the emphasis on the one which is most emergent.

In certain situations, false cold or false heat may be present. For example, if the pulse is Rapid and Tense, and the patient experiences chills and feels very cold, there may be, depending on the other symptoms, a condition of damp-heat in the Gallbladder, known biomedically as cholecystitis. Another example of false cold is a person whose hands and feet are cold, but whose pulse, especially at the Liver position, is Tense. Frequently, with Liver qi stagnation, the circulation to the extremities is diminished.

In a condition of circulatory shock, which is one of great weakness, the pulse is very Rapid but Feeble, yet the patient feels extremely hot on the outside and is sweating profusely. Here again is a situation in which the pulse and the symptoms differ, with the pulse being more meaningful.

Despite all of these conundrums, the pulse is ultimately the most important diagnostic tool available to a practitioner of Chinese medicine, but only if one is willing to focus, practice, search, and be patient.

The Practitioner

In Chinese medicine the practitioner is traditionally the only diagnostic instrument. His or her intelligence, intuition, experience, common sense, and sensory awareness are the tools with which he or she accesses the inner human world. In the West, those of us who have chosen to practice this profession are unique in this culture, inasmuch as we have undertaken a task that operates largely outside of the burgeoning mechanical and electronic technology in which our society has become more deeply immersed over the past three centuries.[19] In contrast to the physician of even my childhood, as well as my own training as a medical student, today's biomedically-trained physicians depend almost entirely on machines and negligibly upon the rich blend of attributes that I have mentioned above.

The objective of a Chinese diagnostician—to blend seemingly unrelated, disparate information into a unified picture of the whole person—is a talent that is not encouraged or developed by the scientific model. Biomedical physicians are not trained to seek the relationship between a hemorrhoid and angina as an expression of a single systemic process, perhaps blood stagnation. The emphasis is on the differential and not the integral mental process. By contrast, as Amber observes,

> The taking of the pulse may call for some mechanical skill, but the interpretation of its story is an art.... Scientific facts by themselves are useless unless they are integrated and properly interpreted. Most diseases are dynamic chain reactions which affect the whole organism, not just a part.[20]

Those who require unity[21] and a deep personal connection to their work through their senses as well as their intelligence, and for whom impersonal detachment is anathema, are people who will be drawn to and gratified by the practice of Chinese medicine and its premier diagnostic treasure, pulse diagnosis.

The Senses

The practitioner of Chinese medicine has eyes with which to look, ears to listen, nose to smell, tongue to taste and to ask, and hands to touch and feel. In my experience, one or more of these senses in each of us is more highly developed than the others. Touch is easily my strongest sensory apparatus. Of the four trunks of Chinese diagnosis—looking, listening, touching, and asking—I especially depend on the latter two, and upon listening in the particular fashion that was the core of my training as a psychoanalyst and psychiatrist.

Other practitioners should, in a similar manner, depend primarily on their own innate gifts. If touching is not one of these, it should not become a source of frustration or of feelings of inadequacy. Developing competency with the pulse can instead become an opportunity to expand one's capacities in this lifetime. That is what I attempt to do with looking and listening.

TOUCH

Touch is obviously the sensory modality with which we are involved in our study of the pulse. However, touch is important in Chinese medicine in many other ways. Palpation of the skin tells the Chinese doctor a great many things about the patient. For example, dry and/or rough skin can be a sign of blood deficiency, yin deficiency, or fluid stagnation. If the skin tends to be swollen without leaving an indentation on pressure, the problem is one of yang deficiency of the Spleen; an indentation would implicate the Kidneys and/or the Heart. If the skin tends to be moist, there is probably a deficiency of protective qi. If the skin is thin, there is usually deficiency, often a clue to a deficient constitution; and if it is thick, the condition is probably one of excess, such as fluid stagnation. If the skin is cold, it usually suggests deficiency, although in specific areas it may be associated with cold from excess; and if it is hot, this is another indication of excess. By feeling the texture of the hair or of the nails we can ascertain the state of the blood and the yin, as well as the Kidneys and Liver.

In addition, the surface of the body can be palpated diagnostically for tenderness superficially and deeply along the channels of energy; at the alarm points on the ventral surface of the body; the back associated points on the dorsal surface; and tender non-channel points—*ashi* ("oh yes!"), trigger points—all of which tell us something about the states of excess and deficiency in the organ and channel systems.

Over the millennia many systems of abdominal diagnosis have been developed—Chinese, Japanese, Korean, and Vietnamese. With regard to the choice of herbal preparations, the Japanese Kanpo herbalists have a separate and elaborate system of abdominal diagnosis.[22]

When feeling the pulse, although I am using my fingers, I often express myself in terms of sound, as if I were listening rather than feeling. Amber concurs:

> The Chinese use sounds to describe their pulse findings, e.g., music of the lute, the rustles of the reeds, etc. But time does not permit of an extensive treatment of this glorious symphony of the body to which some people are tragically tone-deaf.[23]

He adds, "The Unani physician was required to study music so that he could distinguish the different sounds and tones of the pulse." Of course, the sound associations of a person in the twenty-first century will likely be different from those of a Chinese physician writing in the second century B.C.

Theory

Theories abound concerning the rationalization of the pulse as an image of the organism. None that I have heard over the years is convincing enough to bear repeating here. But I will make one exception out of respect for Amber, who writes:

> The Chinese intimated but never directly concluded that the pulse is controlled by the brain. It is the author's opinion, based on his own observations supported by many years of clinical practice, that what affects the nervous system affects the pulse. [Furthermore,] the polarity of the body—its plus and minus factors—is also revealed by the pulse, again through the brain, which is the electrical power house, and through the liver, which is the chemical factory of the body. Here are two different energy systems working independently of each other and yet paradoxically closely interrelated.[24]

If I have missed a more cogent explanation, I welcome being informed.

Reflection

The diversity of diagnostic modalities in Chinese medicine is great. However, it would be fair to say that, over the long period of time during which Chinese medicine has been practiced, the pulse has been considered, on the one hand, to be the most revealing mode for assessing the general and specific condition of a patient,[25] and on the other, perhaps the most difficult to master and communicate to others. Nevertheless, if studied and applied in gradual increments, it will provide ever-increasing joy and the most profound satisfaction to the practitioner of Chinese medicine.

CHAPTER 2

Pulse Positions through History

CONTENTS

Historical Considerations, 19
    Wang Shu-He, 19
        ■ Table 2-1: Historical correlations among pulse positions and organs, 20
    Nei Jing, Li Shi-Zhen, and Dr. John H.F. Shen, 21
    Classic of Difficulties (Nan Jing), 22
Principal and Complementary Individual Positions, 22
    Principal positions, 23
    Complementary positions, 23
        ■ Fig. 2-1: Pulse positions according to Hammer, 24
        ■ Fig. 2-2: Pulse positions according to Shen, 25
        ■ Fig. 2-3: Special Lung position, 26
Rolling the Fingers on the Pulse, 26
    Middle position (burner) qualities, 26
    Literature, 26
    Contemporary Chinese pulse diagnosis, 27
    Musculoskeletal positions, 28
The Three Depths, 28
■ Fig. 2-4: The three depths, 29

CHAPTER 2

Pulse Positions through History

Historical Considerations

Opinions regarding the significance of the six positions of the pulse have varied from the *Inner Classic (Nei jing)* over two thousand years ago right up to the present time. Table 2-1 shows some of these differences, the principal ones being whether there were two or three depths, and their interpretation; and the precise locations of different organ systems and areas of the body at the six positions on the wrists.

There is nothing sacrosanct about the associations between the organs and the six positions. While the radial artery is close to the surface and offers an extraordinary opportunity to receive information, it can be, and has been, accessed in many different ways, at different times and in different cultures, each yielding a somewhat different set of information. These traditions (Chinese, Ayurvedic, Tibetan) become set over time and with repeated use, but they are not exclusive and represent only one partial, albeit useful, segment of what the organism is trying to communicate. Naturally, the message systems and the messages overlap.

I believe that the pulse is only one aspect of a larger abstraction in which living organisms are understood in their totality as broadcast systems which can be accessed as if on an infinite number of bands of the electromagnetic spectrum, and that messages coming from one band can be linked to others in endless ways to produce diagnostic systems of endless variety. There are systems of the pulse that leave out the part of the pulse we use entirely and begin further up the arm. Who knows how many models have come and gone and what accidents of history have retained some and lost others? As already mentioned, there is strong evidence that the ancient Hebrews had a very sophisticated pulse system based on sounds, as did the Arab-Iranians (Unani). They probably exchanged information when the Jews were exiled in Babylon.

WANG SHU-HE

The Pulse Classic (Mai jing),[1] written in the second century by Wang Shu-He, has had a profound influence on the practice of pulse diagnosis. In Wang's system, the deeper

Table 2-1 Historical correlations among pulse positions and organs

	Nei Jing c. 100 BC	Nan Jing c. 200 AD	The Pulse Classic Wang Shu-He Late 2nd century	Pulse Diagnosis Li Shi-Zhen 1564	Collected Treatises Zhang Jie-Bin 1624	John H.F. Shen* Late 20th century
LEFT WRIST POSITION						
Distal,						
Superficial:	Sternum	Arm tai yang	Small Intestine	—	Pericardium	**
Deep:	Heart	Arm shao yin	Heart	Heart	Heart	Heart/Pericardium
Middle,						
Superficial:	Diaphragm	Leg shao yang	Gallbladder	—	Gallbladder	**
Deep:	Liver	Leg jue yin	Liver	Liver	Liver	Liver/Gallbladder
Proximal,						
Superficial:	Abdomen	Leg tai yang	Bladder	—	Bladder/Lg. Int.	**
Deep:	Kidney	Leg shao yin	Kidney	Kidney (Life Gate)	Kidney	Kidney/Lge Intestine
RIGHT WRIST POSITION						
Distal,						
Superficial:	Chest	Arm yang ming	Large Intestine	—	Sternum	**
Deep:	Lungs	Arm tai yin	Lungs	Lungs	Lungs	Lungs
Middle,						
Superficial:	Spleen	Leg yang ming	Stomach	—	Stomach	**
Deep:	Stomach	Leg tai yin	Spleen	Spleen	Spleen	Stomach/Spleen
Proximal,						
Superficial:	Abdomen	(Text unclear)	Triple Burner	—	T. Burner/Sm. Int.	**
Deep:	Kidney	(Text unclear)	Kidney (Life Gate)	Kidney (Life Gate)	Kidney	Bladder/Sm. Intestine

* This selection does not include the complementary pulse positions in the Shen system.

** In the Shen system the superficial depth is associated with qi, the middle depth with blood, and the deep depth with the parenchyma of the yin organs.

pulse at any position reflects the yin organ associated with that phase or element, and the superficial pulse represents the yang organ. To some extent—with respect to the left and right middle pulses, and the left distal pulse—this principle was followed by Zhang Jie-Bin in his seventeenth-century work *Collected Treatises of [Zhang] Jing-Yue (Jing yue quan shu).*[2]

Having used Wang Shu-He's reference field for four years prior to encountering Dr. Shen, I have some basis for comparing the two methods. Those who have been exposed to both methods agree that in terms of the patient's physical, mental, and emotional states, Dr. Shen's interpretation of the pulse is clinically more complete and far richer in content than what can be learned through the Wang Shu-He method.

With regard to what we have historically ascribed to a single position on the pulse, we have had a choice. Either the entire position represents aspects of the qi, blood, and yin (parenchyma) of a solid organ, as with Li Shi-Zhen and Dr. Shen, and to a certain extent the *Inner Classic,* or it represents the solid (deep) and hollow (superficial) organ pairs (e.g., Lung/Large Intestine) of an element (metal). Wang, in my opinion, mistakenly chose the element pairing to fit a theoretical model—the five elements (phases)—rather than the clinical model which emphasizes the qi, blood, and yin aspects of the solid organ itself (in this example, the Lung). Joseph Needham agrees that the triumph of abstract phase energetics over clinical practice was lamentable for Chinese medicine.[3]

Having spent time over several years with students of the five element school, it is my impression that they subscribe to the Wang Shu-He interpretation of the pulse. However, many of them seem to be feeling the yang organ superficial to what would be called the qi depth by Dr. Shen and by contemporary practitioners in China. The yin organ seems to be accessed somewhere between the qi and blood depths, generally while the patient is lying down. According to some of them, their interpretations are more of the ethereal and astral bodies than of the material body. It is my feeling that the two methods cannot be compared and that each is valid in its own area of concern. The five-element school interpretation is more ethereal and spiritual than Dr. Shen's, whose purview is more mental, emotional, and material.

In this regard, Jiang Jing[4] makes an interesting observation:

> If the pulse wave moves above the superficial level, it indicates a higher expression, at which point the situation is totally emotional. If it goes lower than the deep level, it shows deeper hiding and means that the situation has totally adopted organic characteristics.... If a person has a chronic emotional blockage you can usually pick it up on the superficial level of the pulse. Once it progresses to the organic level it will be stored as a deeper stress.

The acerbic Liao Ping, writing in his commentary to the *Classic of Difficulties (Nan jing)*, noted that

> The lofty and inappropriate [application] of the Five Phases originated from this book [*Nan jing*]. [It resulted from] a mistaken reading of the *Nei jing* which was combined with the [doctrine of the] Five Phases. Consequently, the medical community of subsequent times believed that anybody who could utter empty talk was a competent person.... How can liver and gall generate the heart? The generation and destruction among the Five Phases [refers to] influences not to form.[5]

Kato Bankei, in his commentary to the same passage of the *Classic of Difficulties (Nan jing)*, adds further criticism to Wang Shu-He:

> Statements such as 'the heart [corresponds to] the inch [section] of the left [hand] and the lung [corresponds to] the inch [section] of the right hand' were first released like a whirling dart by Wang Shu–ho from the Western Chin. All the authors of the T'ang, Sung, Yuan, and Ming [eras] followed his signal flag. Increasingly, they acted contrary to all reason; increasingly [their ideas] became more numerous and confused.... Finally, in the middle of the Ming [era], Chao Chi-tsung and Li Shih-chen crushed what had become too numerous and disorderly, with the intention to devise a concise [system of diagnosis].[6]

While I believe that the above criticisms are important and demonstrate the lack of unanimity regarding the credibility of the five element (phase) system, even in the *Classic of Difficulties (Nan jing)*, the system is of great value when applied with common sense rather than as dogma, which is still often the case today.

NEI JING, LI SHI-ZHEN, AND DR. JOHN H.F. SHEN

At the dawn of the twenty-first century we find two prevailing schools of pulse diagnosis. One, in Europe and parts of America, favors the Wang Shu-He interpretation, and the other, in China, reflects the perspective of the renowned Li Shi-Zhen, author of the sixteenth-century work *The Pulse Studies of Bin Hu (Bin hu mai xue)*. As interpreted by Dr. Shen[7] and illustrated in Fig. 2-1, the pulse positions which I subscribe to lean more toward the work of Li Shi-Zhen, with some concepts reflecting the interpretations of Zhang Jie-Bin, and others drawn from the *Nei jing*.

The interpretations of the *Nei jing*[8] and those of Li Shi-Zhen[9] place the emphasis almost entirely upon the yin organs as the significant energetic factors to be considered in diagnosis. Here, the importance of the yang organs is relegated to a relatively minor place in the spectrum of energy with regard to health and disease. This is in keeping with my own view of the yang organs as conduits to and from the yin organs on a material, mental, and spiritual level. However, in the pulse model taught in this book, each yang (hollow) organ is represented on the pulse by a complementary position accessed by rolling the finger.

Dr. Shen, Li Shi-Zhen, and others also challenge the position of the Triple Burner in the Wang Shu-He system. The position's connection with water metabolism suggests an association with the Bladder/Kidney, but since there are *three* burners, there is no single position for it in any other system except that of Wang Shu-He and Zhang Jie-Bin. Furthermore, all of the functions of the Triple Burner involve the entire organism simultaneously. This includes controlling the separation of the pure from the impure by all of the involved organs (Lungs, Kidneys, Spleen, Small Intestine, Large Intestine) and by the internal duct of the Triple Burner; the Triple Burner's role in the distribution of the *yuan* (source) qi to the source points at birth; and its capacity as social harmonizer on a mental-emotional level. I assess the function of the Triple Burner based on the appearance of the same unusual quality bilaterally at the same burner, and on whether or not there is a coherence of qualities among the burners.

The pulse position between the upper and middle burners, for which Dr. Shen uses the term 'diaphragm,' is implied by the *Nei jing* system, wherein the left distal superficial position refers to the sternum and the left middle to the 'diaphragm.' (Zhang Jie-Bin correlates the sternum with the superficial pulse in the right distal position.) These pulses and their interpretation by Dr. Shen have proven to be clinically reliable in my practice.[10]

CLASSIC OF DIFFICULTIES (NAN JING)

In essential agreement with Wang Shu-He, although expressed somewhat differently in terms of the six channels or stages, is the form attributed to the *Classic of Difficulties (Nan jing)*. In a discussion about positions, Paul Unschuld has a wonderful note concerning the "Tenth Difficulty" in the section entitled "Movements": "Although this difficult issue appears to impart straightforward data, it has, nevertheless, caused considerable confusion among commentators."[11]

Consistent with Unschuld's remark, the ensuing, very serious discussion leads one down the unavoidably humorous, intricate pathways of a human mind faced with the task of fitting one paradigm (the five phases) to a diagnostic tool—the pulse—whose development had a separate, pragmatic, and clinically-based history. The result is akin to a Robert Benchley essay, a Rube Goldberg cartoon fantasy, or the medieval preoccupation with how many angels could sit on the tip of a needle.

Principal and Complementary Individual Positions

Dr. Shen cites two general types of individual positions that I have labeled the principal individual positions and the complementary individual positions (Figs. 2-1 and 2-2). My version of these positions and terminology (Fig. 2-1), which is based on my own experience and the requirements of teaching in a communicable nomenclature, varies somewhat from Dr. Shen's.

PRINCIPAL POSITIONS

The principal positions are the six traditional ones, with three at each wrist, and with some variations discussed in Chapter 4. For Dr. Shen, each represents a major yin organ except for the right middle and proximal positions, which represent the Stomach and Bladder respectively. However, even here I find that only when there is a specific disharmony of excess in these yang organs—such as excessive heat, damp-heat, and pain—do these positions truly reflect their condition. I have found that the right middle position primarily reflects the Spleen in conditions of deficiency, and primarily the Stomach in conditions of excess.

Likewise, for the right proximal position, I find that the position reflects Kidney yang unless there is some active pathology in the Bladder, whose signs then override the Kidney yang signs. The other exception is severe Kidney yin deficiency, which can sometimes express itself with a Tight or Wiry quality at the right as well as the left proximal position.

When the left proximal position reveals hard qualities, such as Tight or Wiry, it is communicating yin-essence deficiency. When this position is Feeble or Absent it is more a sign of Kidney yang deficiency. Both proximal positions can therefore depict deficiency of Kidney yang and Kidney yin energies. When both conditions exist simultaneously, the left proximal position will more likely reflect the yin deficiency and be Tight, while the right proximal position is more likely to reflect the yang deficiency and be Feeble. However, in either position the qualities can change from Tight to Feeble when both conditions exist simultaneously.

The right distal position can be used to locate the different lobes of the material lung, and simultaneously, the site of disharmony in the energetic Lung. In my experience this is accomplished more readily and accurately by using the Special Lung position, as illustrated in Figs. 2-1 and 2-2. However, if an Inflated quality is greater when rolling the fingers proximally from the right distal position, and less when rolling distally from the right middle position, it is a sign of pathology in the pleura. Another sign of injury to the pleura is a Rough quality as the finger is rolled distally from the right distal to the Diaphragm position.

COMPLEMENTARY POSITIONS

I have found the twenty-two complementary positions to be very accurate and useful in the clinic. The positions described in this book are my own versions of those to which I was introduced by Dr. Shen. They include the Neuro-psychological, Pericardium, Mitral Valve, Large Vessels, Heart Enlarged, Diaphragm, Special Lung, Pleural, Liver Enlargements (distal, radial, and ulnar), Large Intestine, Esophagus, Gallbladder, Spleen, Stomach-Pylorus Extension, Small Intestine, and the Pelvis/Lower Body (my term for the pelvis, low back, lower extremities, ovaries, fallopian tubes, uterus, and prostate). Complementary positions seem to be recognized in Korean pulse diagnosis as well.[12]

It is interesting to note that, like Dr. Shen, Zhang Jie-Bin's notation places the Large Intestine in relationship to the left proximal position, and the Small Intestine in relationship to the right proximal position, although at a more superficial level. It is also of interest that Dr. Shen's positioning of the Pericardium is somewhat in agreement with Zhang Jie-Bin.

The bilateral Special Lung position (Fig. 2-3) has been an exceptionally rich source of information concerning the past and present condition of the Lungs, unobtainable from the regular Lung pulse in the right distal position. This area, unmentioned as far as I know in any reference other than Dr. Shen's, will be expanded upon in the section

Fig. 2-1 Pulse positions according to Hammer, based on the Shen model. Arrows indicate the direction in which the finger should be rolled to assess the given pulse.

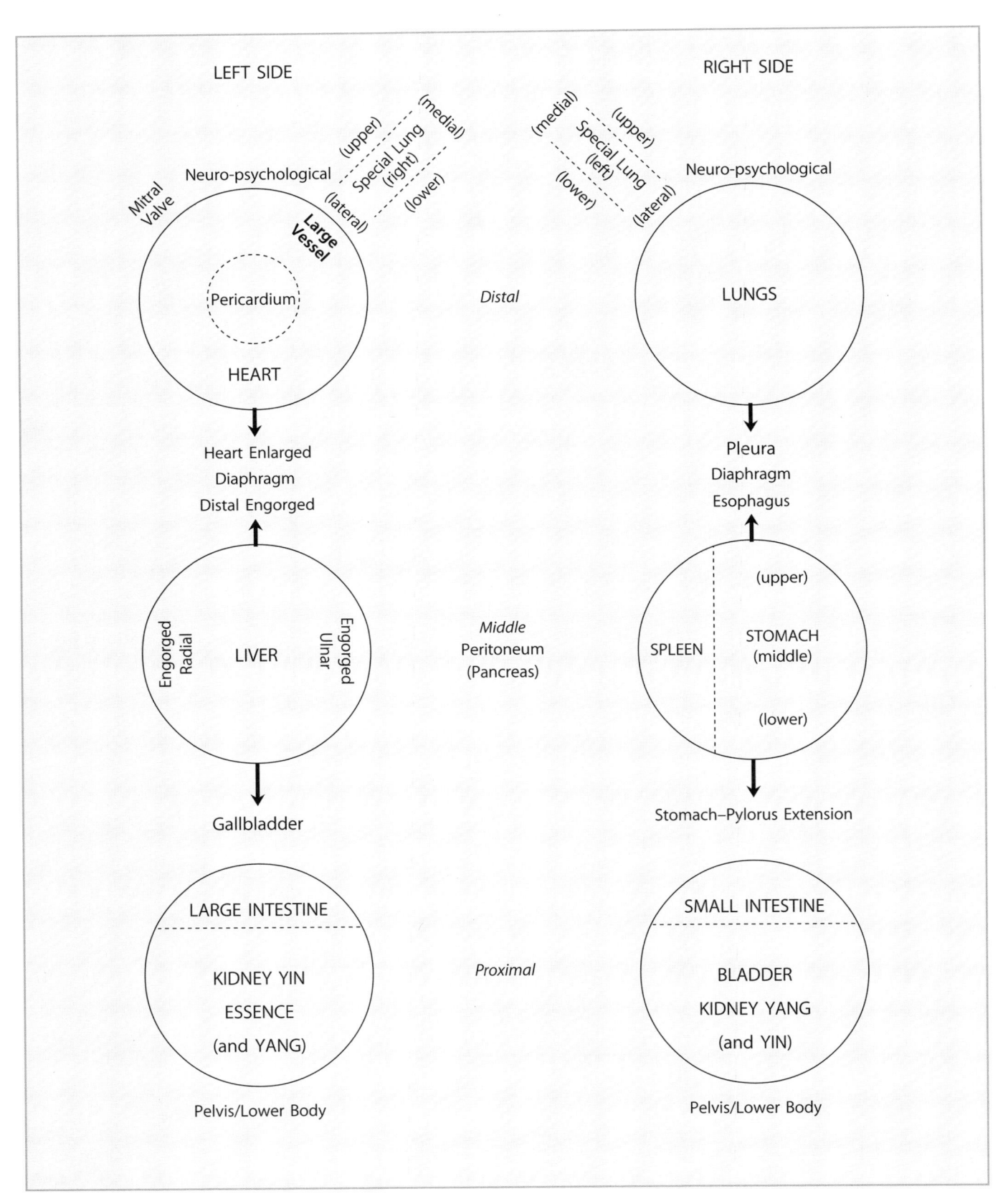

LEFT SIDE

Distal:
- Mitral Valve / Neuro-psychological / Special Lung (right) (upper/medial/lower) / Large Vessel / Pericardium / **HEART**
- ↓ Heart Enlarged, Diaphragm, Distal Engorged

Middle:
- Engorged Radial / **LIVER** / Engorged Ulnar
- ↓ Gallbladder

Proximal:
- LARGE INTESTINE
- **KIDNEY YIN ESSENCE (and YANG)**
- Pelvis/Lower Body

Middle: Peritoneum (Pancreas)

RIGHT SIDE

Distal:
- Neuro-psychological / Special Lung (left) (upper/medial/lower) / **LUNGS**
- ↓ Pleura, Diaphragm, Esophagus

Middle:
- SPLEEN | **STOMACH** (upper/middle/lower)
- ↓ Stomach–Pylorus Extension

Proximal:
- SMALL INTESTINE
- **BLADDER KIDNEY YANG (and YIN)**
- Pelvis/Lower Body

Fig. 2-2 Pulse positions according to Shen. Asterisks denote pulse positions differentiated by quality.

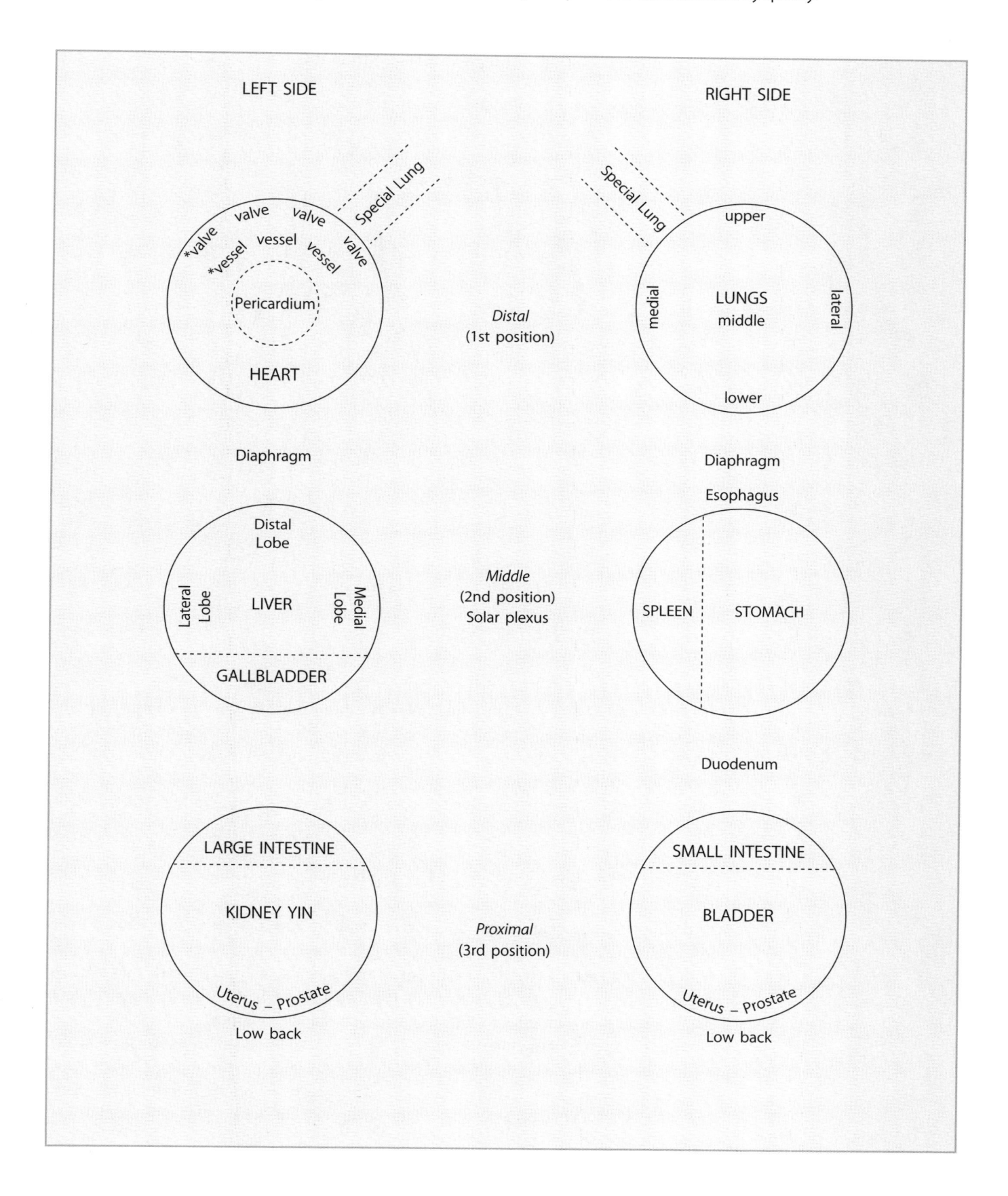

LEFT SIDE — RIGHT SIDE

Distal (1st position)

Left: Special Lung; valve, valve, valve, *valve; vessel, vessel, vessel, *vessel; Pericardium; HEART

Right: Special Lung; LUNGS — upper, middle, lower; medial, lateral

Diaphragm — Diaphragm
Esophagus

Middle (2nd position) Solar plexus

Left: Distal Lobe, Lateral Lobe, LIVER, Medial Lobe, GALLBLADDER

Right: SPLEEN | STOMACH

Duodenum

Proximal (3rd position)

Left: LARGE INTESTINE; KIDNEY YIN; Uterus – Prostate; Low back

Right: SMALL INTESTINE; BLADDER; Uterus – Prostate; Low back

related to the right distal position in Chapter 12. The Special Lung position runs distally at an angle from approximately the position of L-9 *(tai yuan)* toward a point on the transverse crease of the wrist, just distal and radial to PC-7 *(da ling)*. The position of this vessel that carries this pulse is highly variable within this area.

Fig. 2-3 Special Lung position (right hand)

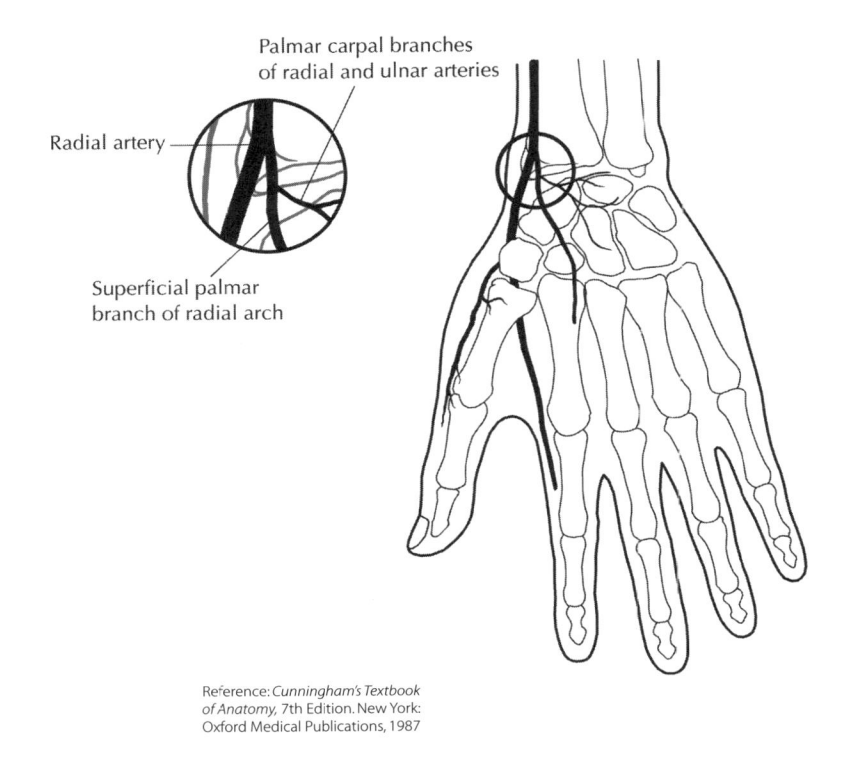

Palmar carpal branches of radial and ulnar arteries
Radial artery
Superficial palmar branch of radial arch

Reference: *Cunningham's Textbook of Anatomy,* 7th Edition. New York: Oxford Medical Publications, 1987

The distinction of qi, blood, and organ depths is not informative in the complementary positions, as it is in the principal positions. However, they do have superficial and deep aspects. The qualities also frequently have different interpretations in these positions than in the principal positions. For example, a Tight quality at the Large Intestine position usually indicates an overactive, irritable, or inflamed intestine rather than yin deficiency. (See discussion of complementary positions in Chapters 4 and 12.)

Rolling the Fingers on the Pulse

Instruction in pulse diagnosis in the current literature and in acupuncture schools does not include teaching the necessity of moving the fingers within, around, and between positions for a more complete assessment of the diagnostic signs. Instead, students are taught to access the pulse positions in a rigid manner with the finger(s) fixed in one place. The only movement is a vertical one in order to access depth.

From Dr. Shen I learned that moving or "rolling" the fingers is an essential aspect of pulse diagnosis, without which one misses detailed diagnostic information. I have since discovered, as cited later in this chapter, that this facet of Dr. Shen's technique has been a prominent aspect of Chinese pulse diagnosis through the ages, and is found in Korean medical practice as well.

MIDDLE POSITION (BURNER) QUALITIES

The pulse qualities of the middle burner (middle position) tend to expand into the other positions, especially into the distal position. This is partly due to anatomical considerations. The abdominal area represented by the middle position is much less confined than the chest (distal position), and somewhat less confined than the pelvis (proximal position). The qi in the middle burner is therefore anatomically freer to expand. This overflow from the middle to the distal and proximal positions is also partly due to the fact that the Liver stores the blood, which is so often at some stage of heat, and therefore expansive. For these reasons it is necessary to roll the fingers distally in order to properly access the qualities in the upper burner. (For additional discussion, see Chapter 4.)

LITERATURE

Figure 2-2 shows Dr. Shen's system of pulse location, in which the fingers are rolled within the position up and down and sideways.[13] Except for Dr. Shen's book, this technique was not mentioned in any source with which I was familiar[14] until I came upon excerpts from the work of George Soulié de Morant (passed on to me by J.D. Van Buren thirty years ago[15]) and the more recent publication of the translation of Soulié de Morant's book. These references indicate that this technique was known and practiced in China up to the first third of the twentieth century, but has since been neglected. Its practice is also implied in the *Classic of Difficulties (Nan jing)*.[16] It is even referred to by Wang Shu-He[17] and recently by Deng Tietao,[18] who refers to Zhen Jia-Shu's "lifting, seeking, pressing and pushing."

The Soulié de Morant reference[19] on this subject is particularly interesting since European pulse diagnosis, derived from Soulié de Morant's translations, is built around Wang Shu-He's system, which nowhere indicates the positions into which Soulié de Morant suggests rolling the fingers. Somewhere between Soulié de Morant and Ferreyrolles, and their student Lavier, this material was lost. And Lavier is the most immediate teacher of the generation of acupuncturists who have created the current acupuncture communities in Europe.

Giovanni Maciocia[20] also confirms that the method of rolling the fingers is not unique to Dr. Shen:

> Nearly all ancient Chinese texts on pulse diagnosis say that the pulse is felt not by keeping the fingers absolutely still on the artery, but by moving the fingers in five different ways: (1) lifting tells you whether the pulse is Floating; (2) pressing (down) tells you whether the pulse is Deep; (3) searching (not moving the finger) is used to count the rate; (4) pushing (from side to side) tells you about the shape of the pulse (Slippery, Hollow, Leathery, Wiry); and (5) rolling (distally and proximally) tells you whether the pulse is Long or Short. Actually, in the past, *wai* and *nei* did not refer to superficial and deep, but to lateral (strangely corresponding to the *zang* organs) and medial (strangely corresponding to the *fu* organs). This also somewhat coincides with Dr. Shen's technique of distinguishing lateral and medial aspects of the pulse by moving the finger from side to side.

Contemporary Chinese Pulse Diagnosis

When first studying our method of pulse diagnosis, much time should be devoted to learning to identify the complementary positions through the technique of rolling the fingers. These special positions are either medial and lateral to, between, or at the distal and proximal aspects of the six principal positions.

Originally, Dr. Shen said that certain positions would show no qualities if they were normal. I have found this to be true for some but not for others, and about one I am uncertain. With regard to the Large Vessel position, it is clearly best if there are no qualities. This is also true for the Mitral Valve, Diaphragm, Liver Engorged, and Spleen positions. The position about which I am unsure is the Neuro-psychological. I am certain that an Absent quality at the Special Lung position is a sign of grave danger.

With the other complementary positions, Dr. Shen stated that to be considered normal, they should have the same quality as the principal position. I have found this to be true for the Stomach-Pylorus Extension. With the Intestine positions I have found that the commonly encountered Tight quality at the proximal positions is frequently found at the Intestine positions, but that there is a subtle difference that can be discerned with experience. I feel that the Gallbladder, Pelvis/Lower Body, and Intestine positions must be judged independently of the principal positions with which they are associated. An Absent quality at the proximal position is a sign of pathology, and at the Pelvis/Lower Body position on the same side it is also a sign of pathology; it is not normal simply because it is the same as its associated proximal position.

The question has been raised as to why the yang organs, such as the Large Intestine and Small Intestine, are sections of a yin organ position, and do not have a position of their own, except for the Stomach, which occupies the right middle position. This question is asked in light of the two-depth system found in the *Classic of Difficulties (Nan jing)* and Wang Shu-He, in which the yang organs are assigned their own superficial positions contiguous to the deeper yin organs. With respect to the right middle position and the Stomach, the answer quite simply is experience. My own view, for example, varies slightly from Dr. Shen's in that the interpretation of the position is more a function of the qualities than of fixed positions of Stomach and Spleen. For example, I find that qualities in the right middle position which suggest stagnation and heat are more closely related to the Stomach, and those representing deficiency are signs of Spleen qi deficiency. I also correlate the left proximal position generally with both Kidney yin and/or yang, depending on whether the quality is harder or more yielding, and the right proximal position with Kidney yang, unless there are signs of a more acute process, in which case I would consider disharmony in the Bladder, Large and Small Intestine, or genital organs (including the prostate).

The interpretation of the pulse positions to which I subscribe (Fig. 2-1) is based on the work of Dr. Shen. As noted in Table 2-1, and mentioned above, Li Shi-Zhen, and to some extent Zhang Jie-Bin and the *Inner Classic (Nei jing)*, are the known antecedents of this orientation. The positions recorded in Fig. 2-1 are based on my own experience and other sources, and vary somewhat from those of Dr. Shen (Fig. 2-2), which depict pulse positions based on his book.[21] While he does not include the 'lobes of the Liver' in his configuration, he has nonetheless written that "the outward position is related to the exterior part of the Liver."[22] The inevitable language difficulties encountered over the years are undoubtedly responsible in part for this and other differences.

From my own clinical experience I now consider the presence of these complementary positions to indicate engorgement of the Liver, and designate them by location as distal, lateral, and medial.

MUSCULOSKELETAL POSITIONS

Our system of pulse diagnosis emphasizes the organs. However, by rolling the fingers to the radial side of the area between the burners, one can detect musculoskeletal disorders. I have tended to ignore these positions while teaching since patients readily volunteer the existence of musculoskeletal pain or discomfort. I am inclined to save my talent as a pulse diagnostician for less obvious disorders.

The pulse is generally very Tight when there is musculoskeletal pathology. The Tight quality at these positions is also a sign of pain. Above and radial to the distal positions we access the neck. Radial to the area between the distal and middle positions is the shoulder girdle. Radial to the area between the middle and proximal positions we access the hip, and radial to the area between the proximal and Pelvis/Lower Body positions is the knees.

The Three Depths

Another critical disparity between pulse diagnosis in Europe and America on the one hand and that of Dr. Shen and current East Asian practice on the other, involves the existence in the latter system of three depths (Fig. 2-4), and in the former of two depths. (The reference to 'three depths' is somewhat misleading. In the system proposed in this book there are actually eight depths, and in the Korean pulse system, nine.) This will be thoroughly examined in Chapter 13.

Fig. 2-4   The three depths

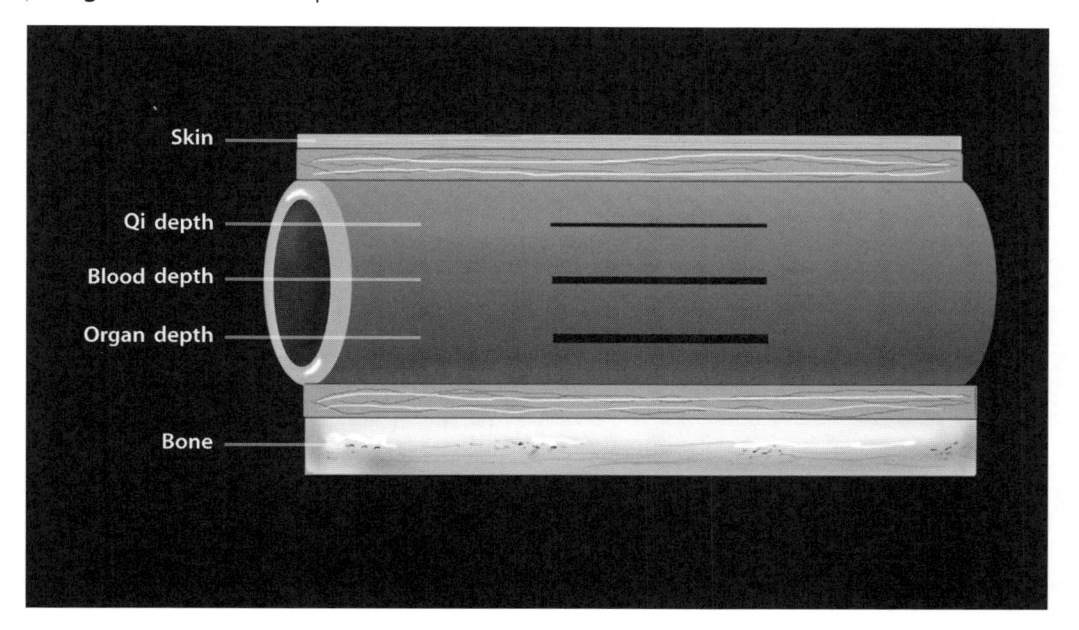

CHAPTER 3

Basic Axioms and Other Considerations

CONTENTS

The Pulse and Chinese Physiology, 33
    Combinations of pulse qualities that seem paradoxical, 33
    Paradox as a sign of illness, 33
    Pulse qualities are predictors of pathology, 34
    Positive and negative signs, 34
    Pulse as life record, 35,
    The hard and yielding pulses in acute and chronic conditions, 35
    Relationship between hard and pliable qualities, 35
The Pulse and Western Physiology, 35
Large Segment and Small Segment Pulse Signs, 36
    Large segments, 36
        Rhythm, 36
        Rate, 36
        Stability, 37
            Separation of yin and yang, 37
            Changes in Qualities, 37
            Changes in Intensity, 37
            Changes in Amplitude, 38
        Wave Form, 38
        ■ Fig. 3-1: Normal pulse wave, 38
    Small segment, 39
Quantity vs. Quality, 39
Conditions and Circumstances that Affect Pulse Qualities and Interpretation, 40
    Environment and etiology, 40
    Age at onset of qi deficiency, 40
    Age and the interpretation of qualities, 40
    Gender, 41
    Body condition, 41

            Vulnerability, 41
            Foundation, 42
                    Abuse of the foundation, 42
                    Proximal pulses and the foundation, 43
                    Emotions and the foundation, 43
        History, 43
        Organ systems and body areas, 44
        Position, Sensation, and Similarity, 44
        Position and interpretation, 44
        Immediate obscuring factors, 45
        Recreational substances (drugs), 45
Origin of Disharmony, 45
        Chronic, 45
        Acute, 45
Focus of Interpretation, 46
Overlapping Pathologies and Qualities, 46
        Acute, 46
        Chronic, 47
Feng Shui and Social Factors, 47
The Seriousness of Disharmony, 48
        Consistency, 48
        Response to treatment and rest, 48
Stagnation, 48
Restoration of Equilibrium and Qualities Associated with Stages of Disharmony, 49
Balance, 50
The Preeminence of the Cardiovascular System in the Disease Process, 50

CHAPTER 3

Basic Axioms and Other Considerations

In this chapter we will summarize a number of basic axioms and considerations underlying pulse diagnosis. These are encountered repeatedly in the discussion of individual pulse qualities, which make up the preponderance of this book.

The Pulse and Chinese Physiology

COMBINATIONS OF PULSE QUALITIES THAT SEEM PARADOXICAL

The pulse is a precise instrument for transmitting signals about the organism of which it is a part. Frequently, the method of transmission does not meet our definition of logic and for this reason is at first difficult to accept. For example, during a pulse examination, as finger pressure is increased from the qi through the blood depths to the organ depth, a Hollow quality at the blood depth is evident. Depending on other factors, this can signify the presence of blood deficiency or of hemorrhaging. However, during the same examination, as pressure is released from the organ to the qi depth, the blood depth could fill out and become Wide if a quality of Blood Heat or Blood Unclear is also present. Therefore, we have two entirely different sensations at the same blood depth, depending on whether we are applying pressure or releasing it. While this may seem to be illogical, it is nonetheless true. In order to learn from the pulse we must be flexible about our deeply-held concepts and free ourselves to see things as they are, not as they should be.

PARADOX AS A SIGN OF ILLNESS

This subject is covered more thoroughly in Chapter 17, and in summary form in Chapter 16. Two simple examples of what we mean are, first, a very high temperature and a very low pulse rate, or a very low temperature and very high pulse rate. These are signs of physiological chaos ('qi wild') of the most serious kind, frequently found in the terminal yin stage of illness. Secondly, in an acute disease the pulse should be Robust and Pounding, and in a chronic disease the pulse should be Reduced. If the pulse and the disease correspond, the prognosis is better than when they are incompatible or paradoxical.[1]

PULSE QUALITIES AS PREDICTORS OF PATHOLOGY

The representation of the physiology of qi, blood, yin, and essence in the pulse is not an exact replica of the actual physiological state of the organism (see Chapter 6). In chronic conditions there is a time lag between the two, which is often significant. The pulse presents a pathological picture that always appears somewhat worse than the pathological reality. This is because the pulse is accessing a physiology and pathology at a level subtler than the threshold for symptoms or the diagnostic tools of biomedicine. This lag between the two remains until the pulses associated with impending death appear, when the pulse signs and the underlying reality are finally unified.

Correlations have been recognized between what is palpated and what concretely occurs in physiology. Since the Chinese pulse signs are several steps ahead of the physiology of the organism in terms of the outward manifestations of disease, the pulse is thereby an instrument for prediction and prevention. The diagnostic challenge is to correctly match the sign with the fact.

For example, with a Feeble-Absent or Empty pulse, the patient, though possibly unwell, is still functioning and therefore has a considerable reservoir of true qi. An Absent quality is a relative measure of yin organ deficiency, and does not imply that there is no qi in the yin organ. The yin organs are still performing their tasks well enough to sustain life. However, it is important to note that the implication of the Absent quality is that the person will be ill within a year or two, and of the Empty quality that the person will be ill within six months to a year. The development of most chronic diseases is a process, and usually a slow one.

Turning to another example, if the left proximal position related to Kidney function is Tight, the relationship of this sign to the physiology of the Kidney is that, while Kidney yin is significantly diminished, the Kidney organ system is still performing and has not completely shut down in terms of controlling, storing, and supplying yin. But while the Tight quality does not mean that the yin organ is non-operational, it does alert us to examine and correct a harmful process before the organ function is permanently altered. Therefore, the pulse becomes, perhaps most importantly, a prognosticator and the foundation of a preventive medicine.

POSITIVE AND NEGATIVE SIGNS

The pulse record is a statement of a person's condition somewhere along the continuum from birth to death. Since we must all die at some time the picture is not usually pretty, since the record is telling us how we are dying and how far along we are in the process.

However, it also tells us of our *strengths*. Intact proximal positions (lower burner) tell us that we have root, ground on which to stand and heal. Intact middle positions (middle burner) tell us that we can restore and cleanse ourselves. Intact distal positions (upper burner) tell us that we can reach out to the world with awareness of our creative being, with the strength to communicate and protect our being, and to maintain mental and emotional stability despite the "slings and arrows of outrageous fortune" with which we are constantly bombarded.

Even with signs of Heart disharmony, a Normal rhythm tells us that there is strength to recover. Normal complementary positions inform us that the pathology found in the associated principal positions is not as serious as it must first seem and that the chances of restoration are good.

PULSE AS LIFE RECORD

Above all, remember this: An accurate pulse record is a precise and faithful catalog of a person's physiology and pathology at a given moment in life. It is the royal road to early diagnosis and prevention. This is the true reality of who we are along the passage from birth to death, and upon which management is more fruitfully guided than by any other diagnostic parameter or by the therapeutic pursuit of symptoms.

THE HARD AND YIELDING PULSES IN ACUTE AND CHRONIC CONDITIONS

At any position the quality of an acute condition can supersede the quality of a chronic condition. For example, with Kidney yang deficiency the quality of the pulse at the right and left proximal positions can be Deep, Feeble, or even Absent. If, however, an acute Bladder damp-heat condition (infection) develops, the right proximal position can appear Tight, and a Normal or Slow rate might accelerate and become Rapid. Likewise, on the left proximal position, an acute fulminating colitis or prostatitis can change the Reduced quality there to a Tight, Flooding Excess, Robust Pounding, Slippery, and Rapid pulse.

RELATIONSHIP BETWEEN HARD AND PLIABLE QUALITIES

In general, the yin gives the body substance and suppleness and the yang gives the body expansiveness and force. When yin becomes deficient, the pulse becomes Hard. When yang (qi) is deficient, the pulse becomes Yielding.

When two conditions exist simultaneously and affect the same position, the harder qualities can override the more yielding and pliable (softer) qualities. For example, if there is an initial deficiency of Kidney yang, both right and left proximal positions can be Feeble-Absent. If a Kidney yin condition develops along the way, the quality can change to Tight, masking the Kidney yang condition. However, under these circumstances, especially at the left proximal position, the pulse will often change from Tight to Feeble-Absent as the finger is held on that position. Ultimately, in the most advanced chronic qi-deficient state, the Feeble-Absent quality will again be the dominant one in that position.

It is important to remember that the condition whose pulse quality is displaced still exists. When a pulse sign associated with stagnation and heat from excess (Tense) changes to a sign of yin deficiency and heat from deficiency (Tight), the pattern of stagnation and heat from excess continues to exist, although it now may not be the dominant clinical consideration, which, for the organism's survival, has shifted to relieving the yin deficiency.

The Pulse and Western Physiology

The past three decades during which I have been involved with Chinese medicine have witnessed the promulgation of many biophysiological theories of Chinese medicine and the pulse. None has stood the test of time. Amber has given considerable thought to these issues, and discusses pulse diagnosis in terms of wave mechanics and hydraulics of the "amplitude or volume of the individual wave" and of the cardiovascular system.[2]

I have no objection to such efforts made to bridge the gap between the two physiological models. However, it is my impression that trying to explain one in terms of the other misses the essential point that they are in fact complementary, and that each can help fill the gaps in the other.

Like Einstein's analogy of reality as a watch that can be observed but never opened, a model of reality must not be confused with the truth. Its only value is its usefulness, not its appeal. Chinese medicine has an integrated theory of health and of relationships that biomedicine desperately requires in order to accommodate its ever-burgeoning accumulation of unrelated information.[3]

Large Segment and Small Segment Pulse Signs

LARGE SEGMENTS

The large segments of the pulse include rhythm, stability, and rate, as well as uniform qualities that are found over the entire pulse, at one or another of the three burners, or on one side of the wrist. The large segments also include the qi, blood, and organ depths of the entire pulse.

The tendency to focus only on individual positions and qualities, rather than also on the larger divisions, is a fundamental error in the teaching and practice of pulse diagnosis. In and of themselves, the qualities of the smaller segments are unreliable indicators. While it is important to study the individual positions and qualities, it is the larger aspects of the pulse that are the key to successful diagnosis. It is here that a condition is first manifested, and where its effect on the entire organism can best be assessed.

In the following passage, Deng Tietao[4] refers to the larger picture of qualities over the entire pulse and its reference to the smaller segments of the individual positions:

> After determining the location of the three fingers, a single finger adding pressure and palpating the pulse image, or three fingers divided and feeling the pulse from first to last, is called 'single pressing.' Three fingers applying pressure, palpating and pressing simultaneously, is called 'combined pressing.' Single pressing breaks the wrist pulse down into three parts and determines which channel or organ is distressed. Combined pressing examines the condition of the five viscera, six bowels and entire body. First use combined pressing and then single pressing.

Rhythm, stability, and rate are aspects that take precedence over other qualities or combinations of qualities in terms of diagnosis and treatment. Deviations from the norm among these parameters are generally the most critical in determining the seriousness of disharmony and the sequence of treatment. Frequently, when the rhythm, instability, and rate of the pulse are brought into order and balance, the other qualities and signs will themselves change.

Rhythm

Rhythm is the most significant measure of Heart and circulatory function. Instability in the emperor (Heart) is tantamount to chaos in the empire and anarchy among ministers and subjects. Unless rhythm is attended to first, all other efforts may be in vain. As described in Chapter 6, irregularity of rhythm is considered in terms of whether it occurs at rest or during movement, whether or not the rate can be perceived, whether the changes in rate are small or large, and whether its irregularity is constant or occasional.

Rate

Classically, the rate of the pulse has been correlated with conditions of heat or cold. Thus, a uniformly Rapid pulse is interpreted to mean a condition of heat or hyperactivity, while a uniformly Slow pulse is usually indicative of a condition of cold and hypoactivity. The rate increases with acute external pathogenic heat, but less so with generalized yin deficiency; it decreases with acute external pathogenic cold and with conditions of chronic qi and yang deficiency.

In my experience, however, *alteration from the Normal rate is more often a sign of significant and far-reaching processes than just heat and cold; it is most frequently associated with the heart and with circulation.* Hence, changes in rate from the norm are more often the result of either a shock to the heart *in utero*, at birth, and emotional shock during life, and/or some alteration in the circulation of blood and qi due to factors outside of, but ultimately affecting, the heart. When there is severe deficiency, it is important to remember that the pulse can sometimes be temporarily very Rapid—especially upon exertion—due to the instability of the qi, particularly the qi of the heart.

Stability

By stability we mean the capacity of an organism to return easily to equilibrium after stress, and its capacity to maintain operational parameters within optimally functional limits over time. Apart from the regularity of the pulse, stability is associated with the steadiness of the amplitude, intensity, qualities, and rate of the pulse, as well as the balance of yin and yang, and among the pulse positions.

SEPARATION OF YIN AND YANG

Differences between pulse qualities in which yin and yang are in contact, and those in which they are not in contact, must be considered. One way of understanding deficiency is to distinguish between that which occurs with yin and yang in contact, and the more serious variety, in which yin and yang are not in contact. The qualities associated with each can occur over the entire pulse, or just in one position.

An example of a quality in which yin and yang are still in contact is the Feeble quality. This is a sign of significant deficiency wherever it is found, whether just in one position or over the entire pulse. A quality in which yin and yang are out of contact is the Empty quality. When it is found in just one position, it is a sign of extreme dysfunction in the organ associated with that position. But when it is found over the entire pulse, yin and yang are out of contact in the organism as a whole. This condition is referred to as 'qi wild,' wherein the person is at great risk for serious debilitating illnesses such as cancer, severe auto-immune disease, a degenerative illness of the central nervous system, or psychosis. While the 'qi wild' state is one which affects the entire organism, when yin and yang are separated in one organ, this can eventually destabilize the entire system and thereby lead to a 'qi wild' state throughout the organism.

CHANGES IN QUALITIES

A Change in Qualities is a sign that yin and yang are separating. When the qualities are changing in one position, it is a sign of extreme dysfunction in the Organ which that position represents. When they are changing in many positions, it is a sign of a serious imbalance in which the patient is at great risk of life-threatening disease or severe mental illness. I have also observed the latter situation in seriously mentally ill patients who are on heavy medication.

CHANGES IN INTENSITY

Intensity is the buoyancy, elasticity, and resilience of the pulse wave. It is an expression of the condition of the qi, blood, and yin-essence of the organism. Strong intensity is a sign of healthy qi, blood, essence, and yin. Diminished intensity indicates deficiency in one or all of these fundamental energic resources.

Consistent, ongoing Changes in Intensity can involve the entire pulse, as well as specific areas. Over the entire pulse, this sign is indicative of either circulatory or Heart problems, the etiology and implications of which depend on factors discussed in Chapter 6. A Change in Intensity in one position is most often a sign of the separation of yin and yang of the organ associated with that position, or less often, a transition in the energy of that organ or area, from better to worse or vice versa.

The significance of a Change in Intensity over the entire pulse will be considered under the discussion of individual qualities. For now, we can say that they may be divided into two general categories, one in which the instability in intensity is always present (blood circulation), and the other when the instability in intensity is not consistently present (qi circulation).

CHANGES IN AMPLITUDE

Amplitude is the height to which the pulse is generated from organ to qi depth or beyond, and is a measure of the yang force, which is roughly equivalent to the basal metabolic functional heat of the organism. High amplitude reflects a strong yang force, while low amplitude is a mark of diminished yang force and basal metabolic heat. Only recently have I been able to consistently differentiate between Changes in Intensity and those in Amplitude. While they are related, I feel that they are physiologically distinct.

Wave form

The wave associated with a Normal pulse is a sine wave or bell curve, as illustrated in Fig. 3-1. Deviations from this norm are indications of pathology discussed more fully in Chapters 4, 8, and 13. The Hollow Full-Overflowing wave is similar to the sine wave except that it rises above the qi depth and theoretically begins at the blood depth. The first part of the Flooding pulse wave rises gradually from the organ depth like the sine curve and then falls off precipitously once it reaches the top. The Hesitant quality feels like a single narrow line without the rise and fall of the sine wave, as if there is a split second hesitation between beats. While the Hesitant quality is classified with the abnormal wave forms, its abnormality is its lack of a wave.

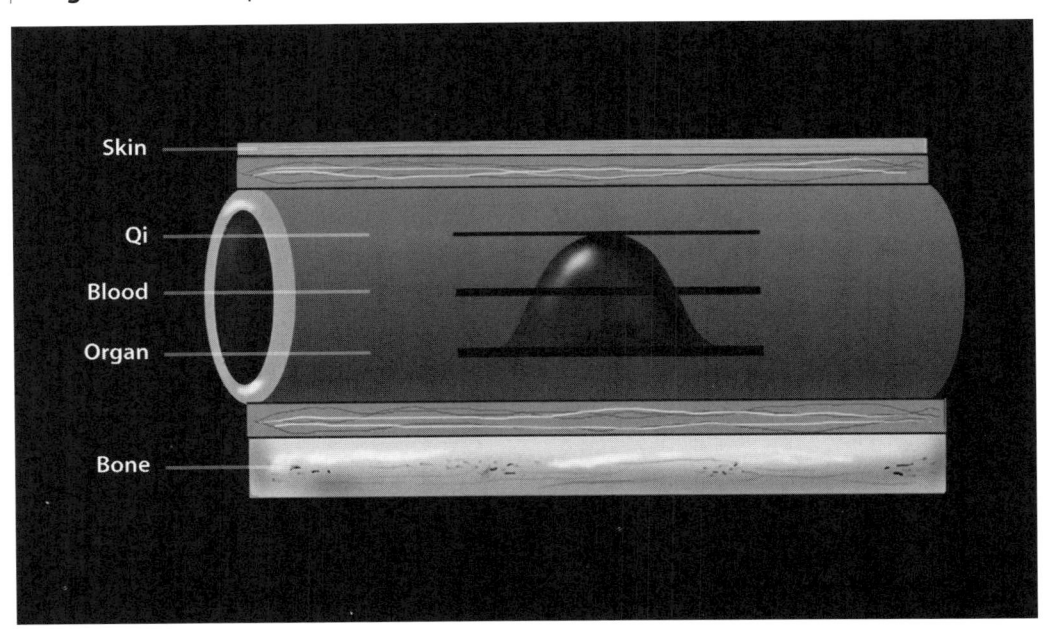

Fig. 3-1 Normal pulse wave

SMALL SEGMENT

Here the critical and dominant factor is the yin organ. The entire position at each depth is a reflection of the integrity of that organ. While the organ depth is the repository of information about the qi, blood, and yin of the yin organ, the qi depth tells us about its contribution to the total true qi, and the blood depth about the organ's contribution to the total blood of the organism. When the qi and blood depths are inaccessible at a particular individual position, the yin organ is no longer making a full contribution to the total function. It is retaining the qi and blood for its own survival, a manifestation that we palpate at the organ depth.

Quantity vs. Quality

Many systems of pulse diagnosis notate only a *quantity* of impulse at each position, such as "two plus" for a moderately strong pulsation, or "two minus" for moderately weak pulsation. In these systems, little regard is given to the *qualities*, such as Tense or Feeble. The quantitative measure of the pulse conveys none of the subtlety that has made the pulse the foundation of Chinese medical diagnosis since antiquity. Only a study and recording of the shades of quality will serve this purpose.

In the context of the pulse scheme expounded in this book, the other systems that assess and record quantity are also often misleading. For example, a pulse that has what some would call a yang (Excessive) or Pounding quality is easily misinterpreted as a sign of strength. In fact, a Reduced Pounding quality can be a sign that the organism is overworking to compensate for severe deficiency.

One of the most common errors that practitioners who emphasize quantity make is misinterpreting the hard qualities as signs of excess or strength. In fact, the hard Tight and Wiry qualities are signs of deficiency, more specifically of yin-essence deficiency. It is a fallacy to assume that all deficiency is either a weak (Feeble-Absent), Deep, or Slow pulse. Treatments based on these false assumptions will create more problems than they solve.

Jiang Jing[5] seems to support this view:

> Students of pulse diagnosis often make rudimentary mistakes by considering a strong pulse as an indication of a strong organ.... More often than not, a strong pulse should be looked at more closely to discover what big changes are taking place in the organ.

Elsewhere,[6] in discussing the "string" pulse, he observed:

> The energy becomes tense and agitated, but in reality it is also a deficient, passive and negative pulse since it does not contain a normal level of energy; sometimes creating friction and tension which lead to heat... it is just being very urgent and very desperate in its action to continue its activities or function. That is its present condition, so there is not much left, but it tries to continue. If this activity is very clear, the organ is being worked excessively in relation to the capacity it has left.

The nature of the quality inherently depicts and encompasses the quantity. Flooding-Excess or Full-Overflowing qualities are by definition expressions of overabundant quantity, and Absent or Empty qualities are likewise statements of deficient quantity. For many qualities, such as Robust Pounding or Changing Intensity, we can indicate the degree with a numbering system, from one to five, with one being the least and five the most.

Conditions and Circumstances that Affect Pulse Qualities and Interpretation

ENVIRONMENT AND ETIOLOGY

Environmental and cultural considerations have played a considerable role in the form and substance of Chinese medicine. For example, qualities which I classify as Reduced, such as Diffuse, Reduced Substance, Deep, and Feeble-Absent, as examples of qi deficiency due to chronic disease, can have underlying conditions of excess. In ancient times this was more common when interior cold was a common condition due to earthen floors, the lack of central heating and insulation, and the widespread unavailability of warm clothing and footwear. Today, however, conditions of excess causing blockage of circulation of qi and blood and false deficiency are rare. While I have chosen to emphasize the chronic deficiencies rather than the infrequent excesses as etiology, excess must be considered if there are signs supporting its presence, such as a very Rapid rate, high temperature, acute pain, and a Robust Pounding and Flooding Excess wave.

AGE AT ONSET OF QI DEFICIENCY

The causes of qi deficiency are usually a combination of factors including an impoverished environment (inadequate nutrition, shelter, clothing), overwork, exercise beyond a person's energy, drug abuse, premature or excessive sex, or constitutional deficiency. When one or more of these factors—such as impoverishment or even abuse—begin between birth and five years of age, the associated quality as later palpated in the adult is the Interrupted Yielding-Hollow or Intermittent Yielding-Hollow. When they begin between five and ten years of age, the expected quality in the adult would be Interrupted or Intermittent; between ten and fifteen, Yielding-Hollow Full-Overflowing (entire pulse); and between fifteen to twenty years, the Empty pulse. After the age of twenty, the Feeble-Absent pulse quality is more likely to be encountered.

AGE AND THE INTERPRETATION OF QUALITIES

In the course of the disease process, time is a factor in the progression of qualities. For example, it generally takes more than half a lifetime to develop the pulse qualities associated with deficiency. Should these qualities—such as Feeble-Absent (qi deficiency) or Tight (yin deficiency)—occur in a young person, one must seek explanations other than those associated with the normal wear and tear of the aging process. An adolescent with a Feeble-Absent pulse quality, in the absence of extreme deprivation, probably has a constitutional deficit. A young person with a generalized very Tight pulse is more likely to be in general pain than suffering from yin deficiency.

Furthermore, after reviewing my records, I am now forced to consider children's pulses differently from those of adults, where the same degree of chaos may reflect their immaturity and state of constant change, rather than a serious disease. However, each case must be considered on an individual basis, since I have seen other cases in which this chaos was pathognomonic of serious disease.

Dr. Shen classifies the pulses of people who overwork or over exercise on the following rough time line, based on the age during which the overwork occurred.

To 5 years:	Interrupted or Intermittent Yielding Hollow
5 to 10 years:	Interrupted or Intermittent

10 to 15 years:	Yielding Hollow Full-Overflowing and Slow (entire pulse)
15 to 20 years:	Empty
20 to 40 years:	Feeble-Absent
40 to 65 years:	Deep and Feeble-Absent
65 and older:	Deep and Absent

GENDER

A very Thin pulse in a man and a very Wide pulse in a woman are inappropriate signs, since men tend more toward heat from excess and women more toward blood deficiency. A Thin pulse quality in a man represents a greater degree of deficiency than when found in a woman, and a Wide pulse in a woman represents more heat from excess than would the same pulse in a man.

BODY CONDITION

The diagnostic significance of a pulse quality can be affected by other factors. Two important ones are body condition, discussed here, and history, which follows.

Vulnerability

Given similar antecedent life events, the pulse positions at which a problem will appear in any given patient depend to some extent upon the vulnerability of that person's organ systems. The disharmony will occur in the most deficient organ. If, for example, a person does heavy physical work after eating, the Inflated quality will appear in either the Stomach or the Intestines position, depending upon which organ is weakest. Likewise, if a person is angry and the Lungs are weaker than the Liver, even though it is the Liver which is commonly associated with anger, it is the Lungs that will be affected first.

This vulnerability of organ systems depends on three variables. The first is 'constitution,' which Dr. Shen defines as having three aspects: heredity, pregnancy, and delivery. 'Body condition,' in his terminology, is more specifically determined by experiences between birth and approximately the age at which a person is fully grown, years when the individual is largely dependent upon the behavior of others—parents, and parent surrogates. After this age, which Dr. Shen specifies as eighteen for women and twenty for men, the term 'life' is used to mean those adult habits and lifestyles that affect a person's well-being such as work, sex, drugs, exercise, and nutrition. At this point, the term 'body condition' means the sum total of all the above.

Dr. Shen specifically requested that, were I to write a book reflecting his views, the following should be emphasized. The body, he says, is like a car. If the body condition is good, it is like owning a fine car. Theoretically, one can drive a fine car more often and for longer distances than a cheap car and it will still function well. The cheaper car will break down sooner under the same circumstances. However, the condition of the car, like the body, also depends on who uses it and how it is used. If an expensive car is misused, it may not last as long as a cheap car that is carefully driven and well cared for.

From my own perspective, the issue is whether the level of activity is within or beyond one's energy. If one performs within one's capabilities and listens to the messages that presage overuse, one can stay free of disease. If one ignores this inner intelligence and forewarning, one invites illness. Therefore, the point is not whether one should or should not participate in sports or sex, for example, but rather that one should tailor the activity to stay within one's capabilities.

Foundation[7]

The foundation for all human function is Kidney qi, yin, yang, and essence. Kidney energy is as complex as the human central nervous system: there are almost an infinite variety of Kidney functions, each reflecting its own aspect of the nervous system, as well as the endocrine system. Summing it up as Kidney yin, yang, essence, and qi is a massive oversimplification. That is why one small aspect of the central nervous system can malfunction and the rest remain intact.

No one would disagree that Kidney energies are closely bound with the archaic substrate of all existence, the genetic code which organizes it into form and substance, and the force which brings it into life.

What I had learned earlier from European sources concerning the origins of Kidney energies is that the universal cosmic energies of pure yang or spirit combine with the pure yin or essence to form the source or *yuan* qi. The source qi is stored in the Kidneys of both male and female and is mobilized at conception. Managed by Triple Burner energies, the source qi provides the template and force of ontology, the development of the fetus, and brings qi to the source points of the channels to be distributed to the rest of the organism. It is then stored again in the Kidneys where it manifests during life as essence.

Information about Kidney energies is hard to come by. While I was in China in 1981 I made a special effort to obtain more information from the traditional doctors with whom I was in contact at the Guan An Men Hospital in Beijing. They seemed curiously resistant to my inquiries and delegated the task of studying the archives to a young student.

In China I learned of the concept that the Kidney yin and yang are derived from essence. The combined function of Kidney yin and yang is Kidney qi. Kidney yin-essence controls the pituitary gland and Kidney yang-essence controls the thyroid and parathyroid. The adrenal medulla is Kidney yang-essence and the adrenal cortex is Kidney yin-essence. Kidney yang-essence supports Spleen qi and is therefore indirectly in control of the enzyme function of the pancreas. The endocrine function of the pancreas—insulin production—is not specifically cited, though evidence from the pulse points to Kidney yin-essence. The combined Kidney yin and yang is Kidney qi-essence, which controls the general growth and development of the organism. Supported by stored Kidney essence, Kidney qi represents the foundation upon which rest the function of all organ systems throughout life.

Kidney essence is more often associated with Kidney yin. However, its functions cross over between yin and yang since it is the origin of both. It controls the development of the central nervous system (marrow).[8] Kidney yin and yang-essence nourishes the central nervous system throughout life, and Liver yang nourishes the peripheral nerves. Kidney essence also has a yang aspect in terms of sexual function involving both the testes and ovaries. Kidney essence and yin control the development of bone and bone marrow, and thereby an important aspect of hemopoetic function. All yin and yang deficiency involves some deficiency of essence in the form of yin-jing and yang-jing, since developmentally, essence precedes both.

ABUSE OF THE FOUNDATION

The Kidneys are profoundly affected by constitutional and congenital factors. Since Kidney qi, yin, yang, and essence are the functional foundation for all the other organ systems, they are quickly exhausted in a life marked by abuse.

The Deep pulse quality is a sign of the depletion of qi, which, for the reason just suggested, would explain the usually deeper position of the proximal positions. This certainly explains why the proximal positions are deeper in older people. However, during my thirty years of Chinese medical practice, it is clear that the pulses in these positions are becoming deeper and more feeble in younger and younger people.[9]

PROXIMAL PULSES AND THE FOUNDATION

It is my clinical impression that deficiencies of Kidney essence, yin, and yang can be found at both the left proximal position, with Kidney yin accompanied by a Tight quality, Kidney yang by a Feeble-Absent quality, and Kidney essence by a Wiry pulse quality. While both proximal positions can indicate both yin and qi-yang deficiency, the yin deficiency will tend to show up first at the left proximal position, and the qi-yang deficiency at the right proximal position. When both occur simultaneously, the left might be Tight and the right Feeble, or they may both reflect Change in Qualities, from Tight to Feeble.

This position, therefore, tells us a great deal about the origin of a disorder, since the Feeble-Absent quality in all but the aged is usually associated with a constitutional etiology; the Tight quality with an etiology which has occurred later in life, usually overworking of the 'nervous system'; and the Wiry quality with the extreme of yin-essence deficiency, as a sign of pancreatic and/or circulatory dysfunction, or pain the lower burner. This is important both for treatment as well as the advice we give to patients regarding changes in lifestyle.

If the proximal positions are Feeble-Absent in a person of a relatively young age, the etiology is frequently constitutional; it is important that this patient understand that he or she does not have the innate strength, without becoming ill, to do certain things that others can do easily. I have found this to be one of the most liberating pieces of information for people who have lived a lifetime burdened by a sense of inferiority because they were not performing as expected by parents and peers. They are relieved to be released from the guilt and to be free of the burden of performing disabling activities which enervate them and lead to symptoms.

If the etiology is not constitutional and begins at a later stage of development, the pulse is more often Tight from overworking of the mind and nervous system, or Wiry in the extreme instances of abuse, and one can delineate the habits which create the excesses and the symptoms about which the patient complains. Changes in addictive and ego-based lifestyle patterns are then the focus of treatment. Here there is usually more resistance to change.

EMOTIONS AND THE FOUNDATION

The propensity toward depression is rooted in Kidney energy deficiencies. Depressions which begin early in life and are independent of circumstance have been referred to as endogenous depressions; in my opinion, these are rooted in constitution, intrauterine exigencies, and very early-life misfortune, all closely associated with Kidney essence deficiency. This and other aspects of emotional life and Kidney energies are discussed in Chapter 15.

HISTORY

By history we are referring to specific events throughout life, including *in utero* and at birth. For example, a Flat pulse in the distal position may result from a birth delivery complicated by the umbilical cord being wound around the neck after the head is outside of the mother's body. Usually both distal positions are involved, and less often only the left distal position. In such cases, the proximal Kidney positions would probably be Feeble-Absent. Thus, a search for history of birth trauma is often fruitful when these pulses are encountered.

A Flat pulse in the distal positions could also mean that the person had a trauma to the chest when they were in poor physical condition. Pain or a horizontal red line under the eyelid or a purple blister on the edge of the tongue would, for example, be a supporting sign of physical trauma to the chest.

A Flat pulse at the left distal position could also mean that the Heart has closed due to a severe emotional trauma about which the person is in a state of denial. Or the emotional trauma may have occurred at a stage of growth when the body was still immature and unable to cope. The loss of a parent or other significant person at an early age is an example.

The real etiologic event can be determined by history and through other diagnostic signs and symptoms in conjunction with the pulse, and is significant in terms of intervention. Identifying the true cause is also important for instituting a treatment plan. For example, treating a prior emotional shock, which usually affects the Heart, is significantly different from treating a prior physical shock to the overall circulation, or an event that occurred during delivery, which almost always involves treating Kidney energies as well other relevant interventions.

ORGAN SYSTEMS AND BODY AREAS

As a rule, pathologies in areas of the body such as the chest or pelvis, as opposed to disharmony in a yin or yang organ alone, are distinguishable when the same quality appears bilaterally at the same position, or bilaterally between the distal and middle positions (diaphragm), or laterally between all positions (musculoskeletal disorders). This is discussed in Chapter 14.

POSITION, SENSATION, AND SIMILARITY

The sensations of the pulse qualities are generally consistent, but some qualities will *feel* somewhat differently at different positions. For example, a Tight pulse at the Pericardium on the left distal position feels more like a sharp point sticking the finger when compared to the longer, more string-like Tight sensation on the left middle and proximal positions.

Qualities with a similar sensation (Rough) are sometimes difficult to distinguish. Relying on experience and percentages, they are therefore sometimes ascribed interpretations based on where they are found. For example, a Rough Vibration pulse in the Special Lung position is a sign of loss of lung aveolar function. However, a seemingly similar but actually different sensation is called Choppy in the Pelvis/Lower Body position, where it is a sign of blood stagnation.

The qualities Slippery, Spreading, and 'separating' are frequently confused. The Slippery quality slides rapidly under the finger(s) in one direction, and is not associated with finger pressure. Spreading describes a quality where there is no qi depth, and the blood depth separates on finger pressure. This quality is a sign of moderate qi and some blood deficiency. The organ depth is present. The term 'separating' is a sensation in which, on pressure, the pulse moves in two directions—distally and proximally—at the same time, away from the center of the finger. It is a modifying term and not a quality per se; it can be one aspect of the Empty, Hollow, or Spreading qualities.

POSITION AND INTERPRETATION

Interpretation of the qualities is generally consistent, but the same quality sometimes has a different *meaning* from position to position. A Slippery quality at the organ depth of the left middle position can mean infection; in the Mitral Valve complementary position it can indicate blood flowing backwards (prolapse) in the mitral valve and qi deficiency of the Heart; in the left distal position it represents phlegm 'misting' the Heart; in the right middle position, Spleen dampness or stagnant food; over the entire pulse at all depths, pregnancy, Heart qi deficiency, or elevated lipids; and at the middle blood depth, it can reflect turbulence in the blood vessels. A Muffled quality in the left distal position is associated with depression. The same quality over the entire pulse or at other positions might indicate a malignant tumor.

Choppy also has slightly different meanings at different positions. At the Gallbladder position it is a sign of necrosis of the gallbladder wall. At the Stomach-Pylorus Extension position it is associated with severe gastritis and ulcer, and at the Intestine positions, with fragility of the inflamed mucosa and micro-bleeding. However, in most of the principal positions and at the Pelvis/Lower Body position it is a clear sign of blood stagnation in the tissues.

IMMEDIATE OBSCURING FACTORS

The Robust Pounding, very Rapid, Interrupted, and Intermittent qualities, as well as medications and both stimulating and excessively calming substances, aerobic exercise, physical and emotional trauma, and heavy lifting can obscure the real pulse. Overeating will also temporarily obscure the real pulse, but much less significantly than the other factors.

RECREATIONAL SUBSTANCES (DRUGS)

The cooling substances such as marijuana, heroin, and LSD drain yang, especially the yang of the Liver, and lead to an Empty quality at the left middle position. LSD has been associated with a Muffled quality at the Neuro-psychological position. Cocaine at first gives rise to heat from excess in the Liver, causing Tense, Robust Pounding, and even Flooding Excess qualities at the left middle position. The fire reaches the Heart where it causes the same qualities at the left distal position with a very Tight quality at the Pericardium position. Later in the process, as the fire burns itself out in the Liver and the Heart, both the left middle and distal positions become Wiry, a sign of extreme yin-essence deficiency. The amphetamines act in a similar manner.

Origin of Disharmony

CHRONIC

A useful and very general guide to the etiology of a chronic disharmony is that the organ that has a Feeble-Absent quality, or the pulse position that reflects the greatest chaos ('qi wild'), is where the problem began; while the organ that has a hard (Taut, Tense, Tight, or Wiry) pulse quality is where the problem presently resides. The former has affected and created the disharmony in the latter. For example, with Liver-Spleen disharmony, the pulse at the left middle position might have Changing Qualities or Intensity, while the right middle position could be Tight, Inflated, or even Hollow or Slippery. The inability of the Liver to move the qi in the digestive system is due to deficiency, which is generally not acknowledged, manifested in a slowing of function and the accumulation of qi (distention, as reflected in the Inflated quality), and cold gastritis or ulcer (the Hollow and Slippery qualities). In five-phase terms, the Spleen is violating the Liver, since wood is not strong enough within the mutual controlling cycle to control the Spleen, thus causing the energy to stagnate or move in the reverse direction.

ACUTE

Acute patterns show a different pulse picture. The origin of the acute problem might present itself on the pulse with a more Tense, Rapid Tight, Robust Pounding or Flooding Excess quality, whereas the organ affected might also have a non-fluid quality of slightly less hardness. Returning to the example of the Liver and the Spleen, if acute hepatitis causes stagnation and severe excess heat in the Liver, this stagnant qi and excess heat will be directed away from the Liver to the most vulnerable organ. If that organ system is the Spleen/Stomach (Liver attacking the Spleen), the pulse quality in that position will also be more Tense or Tight than usual, with hyperactivity and heat symptoms such as gastritis.

Although these are rules of general application, the other parameters of diagnosis must also be attended to in order to make a conclusive evaluation.

Focus of Interpretation

In searching for the organ system suffering the greatest functional distress, the focus is on the positions that show the greatest Change in Intensity, Amplitude, and Qualities, or that show Empty qualities.

Overlapping pathologies and qualities

The sequences in the process of a chronic disease from qi stagnation to the various stages of qi and blood deficiency (see Chapter 13), and from qi stagnation to progressive yin deficiency (see Chapter 11), often occur concurrently. Changes in all principal pulse qualities that track these progressions take place simultaneously. Therefore, those qualities moving in the direction of qi and blood deficiency, such as Diminished, Thin, or Feeble, may appear at the same time as those reflecting yin deficiency, such as Tight and Wiry. Often the harder sensations, Tight and Wiry, will override the more pliable qualities, such as Feeble. For example, if we have a condition of Kidney qi deficiency—usually signaled by a Deep, Feeble, or Absent quality in the proximal positions—at the same time that we also have Kidney yin deficiency—signaled by a Tight quality—the proximal position is more likely to reflect the harder Tight quality than the softer Feeble quality until the qi deficiency becomes overwhelming. When, through therapy, we relieve the Kidney yin deficiency and the Tight quality disappears, we may be surprised to find a Feeble quality at the proximal positions, requiring that we then treat the deficient Kidney qi. More often the qualities change back and forth from Feeble-Absent to Tight, informing us of the simultaneous presence of both conditions.

ACUTE

In terms of treatment, acute conditions usually take precedence over chronic ones unless the latter present an immediate threat to life. When an acute sign appears, ongoing treatment for chronic conditions should be reduced or interrupted temporarily until the acute condition is resolved. Acute disorders are usually accompanied by sudden changes in pulse qualities. For example, if a less serious pulse quality such as Floating suddenly predominates or combines with other signs and symptoms that suggest a pattern of wind-cold or wind-heat, clinically speaking the newly-appearing quality temporarily overrides the treatment of more serious pulse signs, such as Empty. Treatment of a patient with a pulse signifying an ongoing severe deficiency, such as the Feeble quality, would also become secondary to the treatment of other pulse qualities of acute heat, such as Rapid Flooding Excess qualities in the proximal positions, reflecting fulminating colitis or prostatitis. However, the sudden worsening of the deficiency would take precedence over the acute heat disorder. Again, together with symptoms of abdominal discomfort, the sudden appearance of a bilateral very Tight-Wiry quality in the middle position could represent an acute digestive disorder. Treatment of this disorder would take precedence over a pulse with, for example, consistent Change in Intensity over the entire pulse, indicating a serious chronic condition involving the Heart and circulation. However, should the pulse become suddenly Interrupted, the Heart condition would take precedence.

Within the category of acute signs there is a hierarchy as well. A Leathery-like Hollow quality, especially if it is Rapid, represents imminent bleeding and is an immediate threat to life. When it appears it will take precedence over all other qualities. Other pulse qualities that signify acute states—apart from Floating, Flooding-Excess, Leather-like Hollow, and Tight (pain)—are Bean (Spinning), Smooth Vibration (sudden worry), very Slow (hypothermia), very Rapid (febrile states or Heart shock), suddenly very Rapid with very low fever, suddenly very Slow with very high fever, and suddenly Interrupted-Hollow (acute serious heart failure).

In acute diseases, the organs associated with positions with the most robust or hard qualities are probably the source ('root'), and the less robust or hard qualities are secondary ('branch'). For example, a very Tense-Tight quality at the left middle (Liver) position can cause a mildly Tense Inflated quality (stagnation) at the right middle (Spleen-Stomach) position in the syndrome known as Liver attacking Spleen (the 'controlling cycle' of the five phases). In this case, the symptoms would again be in the organ-associated secondary aspect of the process with more acute indigestion, abdominal pain, and signs of Stomach heat such as penetrating frontal headaches, mouth ulcers, bad breath, nausea, and vomiting.

CHRONIC

With chronic illness the hierarchy of pulse qualities classified according to seriousness is based on the degree of deficiency or stagnation which each quality represents. Thus, an Empty quality representing chaos would be a more serious sign than a Deep or Feeble-Absent quality, which are signs of severe qi deficiency.

In treating chronic illness, several conditions are often dealt with at the same time. For example, although the Muffled quality at the left distal position is not as serious as the Interrupted quality, it may be necessary to overcome the qi stagnation which the former represents before completely regulating the rhythm, if the symptoms associated with the Muffled quality dominate the clinical picture. While the cause of an arrhythmia, such as Heart qi deficiency, should be treated to restore harmony to the Heart, the initial thrust should attempt to undo the qi stagnation if, for example, the person is very depressed.

A Muffled quality in the Pelvis/Lower Body position could also take precedence over an Empty quality over the entire pulse—generally a serious sign—if the Muffled quality gives reason to suspect malignancy in the pelvis

The organs showing the greatest chaos or deficiency are most likely to be reliably identified with the etiology—or root—of a chronic disease process. Often in chronic disease, but less reliably, those positions (and organs) associated with the harder qualities (very Tense-Tight-Wry) may reflect the secondary—or branch—issues. We often find the highest degree of current compelling symptomatology in those organs associated with these branch-related organs. One example is cardiac asthma in which the left distal and Heart related complementary positions can show signs of considerable deficiency (Feeble-Absent, etc.), while the right distal (Lung) and Special Lung positions are Tense-Tight, Slippery, Inflated and have Rough Vibration. The obvious symptoms are Lung related, though the root condition lies in the Heart.

Feng Shui and Social Factors

It is my impression that certain pulse qualities appear more frequently in some parts of the earth than others. I first noticed this on my initial visit to the earthquake-prone San Francisco Bay area, confirmed by subsequent visits over a nine year period, where I found 'qi wild' qualities to be ubiquitous. In North Carolina practitioners tell me that the Slippery qualities at the Neuro-psychological position, normally very rare, are quite common.

During a three day pulse seminar there were nine patients who showed enormous Changes in Intensity and Amplitude over their entire pulses. It became incumbent to go beyond the concepts of Heart qi deficiency to question if there might not be a common thread in the community which could account for this instability. In fact, the single unifying event in the lives of all these people was the breakdown of their social structure in the wake of the departure of many major companies, which had been the economic mainstay of the community for as long as a century. People were being forced to move, marriages were coming unraveled, and in one instance a longstanding intentional community was being disbanded, with its members unprepared for life in the outside world.

They all shared the experience of a 'broken heart.' The implications for future heart disease, especially among the vulnerable, is unpredictable. But the presence of Changes in Intensity and Amplitude certainly warranted closer scrutiny in this population for heart problems.

The Seriousness of Disharmony

CONSISTENCY

Broadly speaking, qualities that appear consistently are signs of a greater disharmony than those that appear occasionally. For example, a pulse that shows an *occasional* Change in Rate at Rest is sometimes a sign of Heart qi agitation. However, a *consistent* Change in Rate at Rest is an early sign of significantly deficient Heart qi and blood.

RESPONSE TO TREATMENT AND REST

A condition that responds to a moderate period (1-2 weeks) of absolute rest, or that changes after a short period of treatment, is a qi (functional) disease rather than an organic disease. By the latter, Dr. Shen means pathology in the biomedical sense such as infarction, cancer, or other gross and microscopic parenchymal changes. With regard to healing, Dr. Shen views it as an "up and down process" analogous "to the waves of the ocean." Within this cycle of rise and fall in the progress toward health, one expects the "up" waves to gradually predominate.

Stagnation

Based on Dr. Shen's ideas, I have developed a concept of qi stagnation in terms of pulse qualities which includes the Taut and Tense qualities, the Inflated quality, as well as the Flat, Cotton, Muffled, Dead, Short, Bean (Spinning), Firm, and Hidden Excess qualities. Stagnation can be due to excess or deficiency. All of the above distinctions are clinically relevant in terms of diagnosis, prognosis, and treatment and are discussed in detail in Chapters 8 through 11, and in Chapter 13.

Dr. Shen classifies the Stagnant pulse as one with a diminished wave form. I use the term Flat instead, because it describes the sensation, and because Dr. Shen has delineated several other types of stagnant qualities in addition to Flat.

The condition most commonly associated with the term stagnation is the one for which the Taut and Tense qualities are signs. With these qualities, there are two opposing and usually strong forces within an area or organ. Here, the irresistible force engages the immovable object. The classic example is Liver qi stagnation in which the qi wants to move and spread, but is opposed and restrained, usually by repressive emotional forces.

The Inflated quality is a sign of qi or heat trapped in an area or organ in which the qi was initially robust. The Flat stagnant condition is one in which qi is unable to enter an area or organ in which the qi is deficient. Thus, the Flat and Inflated qualities can have similar etiologies, but very different body conditions. The a priori condition of the Flat quality is deficient qi, and the a priori condition of the Inflated quality is robust qi. Trauma and shock are common etiologies.

The Cotton quality reflects a profound sense of resignation, or a major physical trauma, in which the free flow of qi at the surface of the body is smothered or suppressed throughout the entire body, especially at the protective and qi levels of circulation. Dr. Shen calls it the 'sad pulse.' The Muffled and Dead qualities are related to potential, imminent, or present tumor formation, or other life-threatening disease. The Firm, Hidden Excess, and Short Excess qualities are associated with severe internal cold. The Short Excess quality can also involve qi, blood, or food stagnation between yin organs. The Bean (Spinning) quality is found in cases of severe fright and intense pain.

Restoration of Equilibrium and Qualities Associated with Stages of Disharmony

Each pulse quality is a sign of the body's attempt to restore equilibrium, or of its failure to do so. For example, a Rapid or Reduced Pounding pulse can be a reflection of overwork whereby the organism tries to compensate for a body that has gone beyond its energy in one way or another. And an Empty pulse is a sign that the compensatory restorative measures are failing.

Flooding Excess and Floating qualities are associated with acute disharmonies. With Flooding Excess the body is attempting to eliminate heat that is accumulating in an organ, as with acute hepatitis, and the Floating quality is an attempt to eliminate heat or cold that is invading from the exterior. Both of these qualities reflect the body's effort to restore equilibrium.

The early stages of chronic disease are almost entirely due to interference with normal function, a process which we call stagnation, and which frequently goes unobserved in the clinic. The Taut and Tense qualities are most common at this stage, with the Inflated quality being somewhat less common. Attempts to resolve the stagnation lead to the accumulation of heat necessary to overcome the stagnation, which in turn is reflected in such qualities as Tense and a mild degree of Robust Pounding, representing the body's effort to eliminate the heat.

At the next stage the body tries further to eliminate the heat so as to restore equilibrium. If it is unable to do so through normal channels—the intestines, urine, skin, and lungs—some of the heat will enter the blood, which is reflected in the Blood Heat pulse. This can progress to the Blood Thick and Hollow Full-Overflowing qualities. The pulse may also become more Rapid.

If the body's efforts to eliminate the heat are unsuccessful, it must provide fluids (yin) to balance the heat. This will gradually deplete the yin, especially the Kidney yin, which is the principal source. The qualities change to Tight and Wiry, and may also be a little Rapid. At the blood depth the Slippery quality will appear as a sign of turbulence. Later, as the heat affects the walls of the vessels, a Rough Vibration quality will appear at the blood depth. When heat accumulates, blood begins to stagnate, a process that presents with the Choppy qualities, especially in dependent areas such as the pelvis.

Over time this attempt to overcome stagnation and eliminate heat depletes qi as well as yin. We move to a Diminished or Yielding quality at the qi depth, followed by Spreading, Flooding Deficient Wave, Diffuse, Reduced Substance, and then Deep and Feeble-Absent. The final step in the process of qi depletion is represented by the pulse qualities associated with the separation of yin and yang, such as the Empty qualities (e.g., Empty, Scattered) and Changes in Qualities, as well as those associated with damaged parenchyma, such as Rough Vibration, Unstable, and Nonhomogeneous. Blood deficiency usually accompanies qi deficiency, which is represented on the pulse by a Thin quality.

Balance

Balance in general refers to a condition in which all parts of a whole maintain a harmonious relationship with each other, such that the function of each augments rather than overshadows the others. Balance leads to symmetry and harmony.

Conceptually and operationally, balance overlaps with, and is closely related to, stability, as discussed above. The distinction here is that, with regard to balance and the pulse, we are referring to the relationships among the different positions, that is, the harmony among the various yin organs, rather than harmony within a yin organ. In my opinion, balance is a function of the Triple Burner. With stability, we are referring to a consistency in function such as rhythm, rate, amplitude, intensity, and quality, and in the relationship of yin and yang. Both stability and balance, of course, influence the function of the entire organism.

Whenever there is a great disparity between the pulse and other sources of diagnostic information, we are usually dealing with a more serious situation. Also, under ordinary circumstances, a Feeble-Absent quality over the entire pulse only indicates vulnerability, while a pulse that has a different quality at each position as well as at each depth points to chaos. Chaos is disease and is the most serious of all disorders. It is encountered with alterations of rhythm either over the entire pulse, or in one position, where it is experienced as the Unstable quality. Other manifestations of a 'qi wild' chaotic physiology are found in cases where there are frequent changes in amplitude, intensity, or qualities, with widely varying qualities from one position to another (balance), and where yin and yang are functionally separated, as with the Empty, Scattered, and Hollow qualities.[10]

The Preeminence of the Cardiovascular System in the Disease Process

It has been my experience over the past twenty-five years that the two systems which seem to bear the brunt of both constitutional deficits and self-abuse are the Heart and the Kidneys. Unexpectedly but irrefutably, the cardiovascular system is the one which shows signs of depletion of qi, yin, and blood at an earlier age, and far exceeding that of any other system, including the Kidneys. Because the Kidneys are associated with storing the essence, upon which all other systems draw when under stress, we have come to expect that they would be the first organ to show signs of depletion. However, this is not borne out by the pulse, which shows that the Heart—the emperor—is the critical system. I have also observed that, perhaps because of this lofty status recognized and endowed by the ancients, a large number of disorders—as diverse as gynecological, neurological, headaches, and arthritis, as well as chronic fatigue syndrome, but including any pathology—are due primarily to deficits in Heart (cardiovascular) function. This diagnostic discovery has assisted a great many patients to recover from conditions that were previously resistant to treatment. By adding small amounts of herbs for the Heart and circulation to other formulas, some students report great success in treating sinusitis, migraines, arthritis, neurologic and circulatory manifestations of diabetes, and depression.

I include this section on the cardiovascular system because the ubiquitous finding of early heart pathology with this pulse method seems incredible to most students. Considering that diseases of the heart and circulation are the single largest cause of death in this country, it must accordingly be regarded as the single most important pulse sign. I cannot tell you how many times patients and friends whose pulses have revealed the process of cardiovascular disease were told by their cardiologists that this was impossible, and who, not many years later, underwent bypass surgery, or the installation of pacemaker, stent, or balloon. Most are kind enough to remind me that I had warned them, yet few preferred my advice to that of the cardiologist at the time.

CHAPTER 4

Taking the Pulse: Methodology

CONTENTS

Time Required for Examination, 57
The Pulse Record, 57
Ideal Conditions for Pulse-Taking, 57
■ Fig. 4-1: Pulse record, 58
Subject's Position, 59
Practitioner's Position, 59
Taking the Pulse, 59
    Locating the principal impulse, 59
    Rolling the fingers on the pulse, 60
    Contemporary Chinese Pulse Diagnosis technique, 60
        Broad, closer, and closest focus, 60
        Congruency and paradox, 61
        Calibration, 611
    Amber and Shen techniques, 61
    Finger placement, 62
        Longitudinal location, 62
        Direction, 62
Depth And Level, 62
    Depth, 62
    Finger pressure and the three depths, 62
    Complementary positions and the three depths, 63
    Level, 63
        Middle position qualities, 63
Qualities, 64
Procedure, 64

Broad focus, 65
    Gender and age, 65
    Rhythm and rate, 65
        True arrhythmias, 65
        Pseudo-arrhythmias and amplitude, 66
    Uniform qualities over the entire pulse, 66
        Iatrogenic-related qualities, 66
        Stability or instability, 67
        Width and hardness, 67
Closer focus, 67
    Wave form, 67
    Uniform qualities on the two sides, 67
        Uniform left side, 67
            Fig. 4-2: Wave comparisons, 68
        Uniform right side, 68
        Intensity alternating between sides, 68
        Qualities alternating between sides, 68
    Depths, 68
        Fig. 4-3: The eight depths, 69
        Above the qi depth, 69
        Qi depth, 70
        Blood depth, 70
        Organ depth, 70
        Below the organ depth, 70
Closest focus, 71
    Principal individual and complementary individual positions, 71
    Fig. 4-4: Both hands, 71
        Left principal and complementary positions, 71
            Left Special Lung position, 71
            Fig. 4-5: Left Special Lung position, 71
            Left Neuro-psychological position, 72
            Fig. 4-6: Left Neuro-psychological position, 72
            Left distal, Pericardium, and Large Vessel positions, 72
            Fig. 4-7: Left distal position, 73
            Fig. 4-8: Large Vessel position, 73
            Mitral Valve position, 73
            Fig. 4-9: Mitral Valve position, 74
            Left Diaphragm, Heart Enlarged, and distal Liver Engorgement positions, 74
            Fig. 4-10: Heart Enlargement position, 74
            Fig. 4-11: Distal Engorgement position, 74
            Left middle position, 75
                Principal left middle position, 75
                Fig. 4-12: Left middle position, 75
                Lateral and medial engorgement of the Liver, 75
                Fig. 4-13: Liver Ulnar Engorgement position, 75
                Fig. 4-14: Liver Radial Engorgement position, 76
                Gallbladder position, 76
                Fig. 4-15: Gallbladder position, 76
            Left proximal position, 76
                Principal left proximal position, 76

- Fig. 4-16: Left proximal position, 77
- Large Intestine position, 77
  - Fig. 4-17: Large Intestine position, 77
- Left Pelvis/Lower Body position, 78
  - Fig. 4-18: Left Pelvis/Lower Body position, 78
- Right principal and complementary positions, 78
  - Right Special Lung position, 78
    - Fig. 4-19: Right Special Lung position, 78
  - Right Neuro-psychological position, 78
    - Fig. 4-20: Right Neuro-psychological position, 79
  - Right distal (regular Lung) position, 79
    - Fig. 4-21: Right distal position, 79
  - Right Diaphragm, Pleura, and Esophagus positions, 80
    - Fig. 4-22: Pleura position, 80
    - Fig. 4-23: Esophagus position, 80
  - Right middle position, 81
    - Principal right middle position, 81
      - Fig. 4-24: Right middle position, 81
    - Spleen position, 81
      - Fig. 4-25: Spleen position, 82
    - Stomach-Pylorus extension and Duodenum positions, 82
      - Fig. 4-26: Stomach-Pylorus Extension position, 82
    - Peritoneal position, 82
  - Right proximal position, 82
    - Principal right proximal position (Bladder position), 82
      - Fig. 4-27: Right proximal position, 83
    - Small Intestine position, 83
      - Fig. 4-28: Small Intestine position, 83
  - Right Pelvis/Lower Body position, 83
    - Fig. 4-29: Right Pelvis/Lower Body position, 84
- Similar qualities found bilaterally at same position (burner), 84
- Musculoskeletal positions, 84
- Rate on exertion, 84
- A reminder, 85

The learning process, 85

CHAPTER 4

Taking the Pulse: Methodology

Time Required for Examination

In preparing for the first pulse examination the patient should be alerted to the need for setting aside 30-45 minutes for this purpose. This will alleviate the problem of being pressed for time, which interferes with the practitioner's concentration. With any new procedure based on very fine and subtle measurements, time, practice, and patience are required for mastery. With a reasonable amount of training, the time required for the initial examination should approach 15-20 minutes, and follow-ups about five minutes.[1]

The Pulse Record

There are many possible ways of constructing a pulse record that differ from the one I prefer, which is presented in Fig. 4-1. Some people prefer to have the page organized according to the left and right hands, and others according to burner. The important thing is that the record include everything that the original form requires.

Ideal Conditions for Pulse-Taking

Patients should be advised to abstain, within the margins of safety, from all medications, and especially all stimulants, before pulse examination. Most medications suppress the pulse wave by causing it to become totally uniform, thus obscuring most of the nuances of pulse diagnosis. Stimulants such as coffee also eliminate the subtleties of the pulse by creating artificial Full-Overflowing, Tense, Robust Pounding, and Bounding qualities.

It is recommended[2] that the patient observe the following behavior prior to the examination. One is to be rested for one-half hour beforehand. In addition, pulse-taking should not be conducted following a large meal (especially one high in fat), or if the patient is excessively hungry, has a distended bladder or is constipated, or is fatigued or emotionally upset. Anatomical abnormalities on the radial artery, very severe atheroscle-

Fig. 4-1 Pulse record

P = Present   ---- = Absent   (1 → 5) = Difficulty of access by degree: 1=low, 5=high

Name:		Gender:	Age:	Date:	Refer:
Weight:	Height:	Occup:			

Rhythm

First Impressions of Uniform Qualities

Entire Pulse:

Sides, LEFT:

RIGHT:

Rate/Min.   Begin: End: W/Exer:

OTHER RATES DURING EXAM:

Three Depths

ABOVE QI DEPTH:

QI:

BLOOD:

ORGAN:

Wave:

Principal Positions

Distal Position

LEFT (Pericardium):

RIGHT:

Middle Position

LEFT:

RIGHT:

Proximal Position

LEFT:

RIGHT:

Three Burners

Same Qualities Bilaterally

UPPER:

MIDDLE:

LOWER:

Other:

Complementary Positions

Neuro-psychological

LEFT:

RIGHT:

Heart

MITRAL VALVE:

LARGE VESSELS:

ENLARGED:

Lung

Special Lung

LEFT:

RIGHT:

Pleura:

Diaphragm

LEFT:

RIGHT:

Liver

Engorged

RADIAL:

ULNAR:

DISTAL:

Gallbladder:

Spleen-Stomach

ESOPHAGUS:

SPLEEN:

STOMACH-PYLORUS EXTENSION:

PERITONEAL CAVITY (PANCREAS):

DUODENUM:

Intestines

SMALL:

LARGE:

Pelvis/Lower Body

LEFT:

RIGHT:

rosis, and meditation can also distort the pulse. Amber discusses other factors including exercise, foods and tastes, seasons and climates, color and sound, among others.[3] Jayasuria deplores our inattention, "especially in Western countries... to these pitfalls.... The result is improper diagnosis and poor results."[4] Indeed, most practitioners give little consideration to these factors in their daily clinical procedure.[5]

The patient's respiration should be even and not excited, and both the patient and examiner should be rested and calm. Pulse-taking at its best is a form of meditation for the practitioner, and is sometimes experienced this way by the patient.

As for when the pulse should be taken, in general, it should be performed before rather than after a meal. However, there are many other suggestions in the literature for the timing of the examination. Amber, for example, reports that the physician should "consider the auspicious moment for his undertaking and... decide which of the ten celestial stems started the first month of the year. Their constellations determine the day on which the examination [is] to take place."[6]

Nowadays the practitioner must be prepared to take the pulse at any time of the day or night, and under any circumstance. The pulse should be examined when the patient's and practitioner's mental and physical states are their calmest. At the same time, the practitioner should develop the ability to distinguish the transient qualities of the pulse from the enduring ones, and to use even unusual circumstances—such as changes in the pulse during activity and rest—in order to enhance the diagnosis.

Subject's Position

Traditionally, the pulse is taken with the patient in a seated position, and the wrist held at about the same level as the heart. Usually the patient's wrist rests on a thin pillow on a table about thirty inches high. In the standing or reclining position, the arm is adjusted so that the wrist and heart are in the same plane. The patient's comfort is the preeminent consideration.[7]

Practitioner's Position

I am particularly impressed by the fact that practitioners seem unaware of how uncomfortable they are when they take the pulse. Yet in order to access the subtleties that are possible with this model of pulse diagnosis, it is imperative that the practitioner be completely comfortable and relaxed. This is accomplished by resting the arm on the table such that it is totally supported, and having one's arm at approximately right angles to the patient's arm. The only exception is when accessing the distal positions, at which time the practitioner's entire arm must be lifted. Become aware of your arm and the level of fatigue and discomfort created by positions other than the recommended ones!

Taking the Pulse

LOCATING THE PRINCIPAL IMPULSE

The single most important exercise in taking the pulse is locating the principal impulse. The principal vessel must be palpated directly in the middle of its path in order to communicate messages which are reproducible by another practitioner and which can be meaningfully compared.

The principal impulse is located where one accesses the strongest impulse. If one palpates off to the side of the vessel the qualities will vary considerably from those at the vessel's center. This accounts for most of the differences in the findings between myself and my students when we compare findings on the same pulse. The two radial arteries may be entirely medial, central, or lateral, or one side may vary from the other, and even some positions may vary from others on the same side. Statistically, more vessels and positions tend to be accessed medially. The point is that one must take the time to find the strongest impulse in each position.

ROLLING THE FINGERS ON THE PULSE

As mentioned in Chapter 2, the ineluctable necessity of moving the fingers within, around, and between positions for a more complete assessment of the pulse is fundamental to the methodology espoused in this book. Rolling the fingers is essential because, as stated earlier, the qualities in the middle burner tend to expand and overflow into the other positions, especially into the distal position. Thus, in order to obtain an accurate reading of the upper burner, the index finger must be rolled distally toward the thenar eminence and scaphoid bone where the qualities are accessed with the medial (radial) side of the index finger, rather than the flat of the pad.

Rolling the fingers is also necessary to access the complementary positions. As previously noted, Dr. Shen originally said that certain positions would show no qualities if they were Normal. I have found this to be true for some but not for others, and about one I am uncertain. With regard to the Large Vessel position, it is clearly best if there are no qualities. This is also true for the Mitral Valve, Diaphragm, Liver Engorged, and Spleen positions. The position about which I am unsure is the Neuro-psychological. I am certain that an Absent quality at the Special Lung position is a sign of grave danger, an interpretation not shared by everyone.

With the other complementary positions, Dr. Shen stated that to be considered Normal, they should have the same quality as the principal position. I have found this to be true for the Stomach-Pylorus Extension. With the Intestine positions I have found that the commonly encountered Tight quality at the proximal positions is frequently found at the Intestine positions, but that there is a subtle difference that can be discerned with experience. I feel that the Gallbladder, Pelvis/Lower Body, and Intestine positions must be judged independently of the principal positions with which they are associated. An Absent quality at the proximal position is a sign of pathology, and at the Pelvis/Lower Body position on the same side it is also a sign of pathology; it is not Normal because it is the same as its associated proximal position.

CONTEMPORARY CHINESE PULSE DIAGNOSIS TECHNIQUE

Broad, closer, and closest focus

As will be shown in the discussion of interpretation (Chapter 17), our examination consists of three stages. They are the broad focus, the closer focus, and the closest focus. The broad focus includes the rhythm, rate, and qualities found uniformly over the entire pulse. The closer focus involves the qualities found uniformly at the different depths, sides, and burners. The closest focus are the individual principal and complementary positions.

Rather than beginning and ending with the closest focus, I recommend that, at the beginning of each session, the pulse of both wrists be taken at the same time. With the practitioner and subject facing each other across a narrow table, the practitioner's left hand palpates the subject's right wrist, and the right hand palpates the subject's left wrist.

The purpose of assessing both wrists simultaneously at the outset is to evaluate the broader and closer focus, which involve the overall state of the patient's substances, stability, heart-circulation, balance, and strength. From this assessment we have an almost immediate sense of the condition of the *qi* (intensity, amplitude, force and Flooding

Deficient wave, qi, and organ depths); *blood* (width, blood depth [thick or hollow], Full-Overflowing wave); *yin and essence* (hardness, fluidity [Slippery]); *Heart-circulation-shock* (rhythm, rate, Change in Intensity, Rough Vibration); *Stability* (Empty, Change in Qualities); *balance* (mental: Change in Rate at Rest; sides: husband-wife; wave: Hesitant); *signs of potentially serious illness* (Muffled, Ropy; Flooding Excess Wave); and *area* rather than organ pathology (uniformity of qualities at the burners).

The closest focus can now be approached as part of a larger picture of this person, rather than as isolated pieces of information of specific organs. We see the blood stagnation in the lower burner (Choppy quality) in the context of the information we already have in the first fifteen minutes or less of the examination. We already know the overall ability of the Heart-circulation and/or qi to move the blood, the heat in the blood, or the overall blood deficiency. This larger diagnostic perspective of the specific finding in the closest focus leads us to a more effective therapeutic strategy. (See case illustrations appended to Chapter 17.)

Congruency and paradox

The initial impression also prepares one to compare the overall pulse qualities in relation to the condition of the body. A very Wide pulse in a very thin person, and a very Thin pulse in a very heavy person, is usually an indication of greater disharmony than when the Thin pulse is found in a thin person and a Wide pulse in a heavy person. Also, by using both hands simultaneously, the practitioner can tune in more quickly to the incongruities that portend more serious disorders—a paradoxically Thin pulse in a man, and a Wide pulse in a woman—thereby facilitating other important adjustments in assessment.[8]

Calibration

There are important calibrations that one can make from the broader focus or first impression. A Wide pulse generally tends to be more elastic, and a Thin pulse less elastic. The less elastic qualities are associated with yin deficiency. Thus, a Thin pulse will feel less elastic, and suggest more yin deficiency, than would a pulse of normal width. With a Thin pulse, therefore, one adjusts one's thinking to take into account the possibility that this person is less yin deficient than if the pulse were of normal width, or even Wide. The practitioner would accordingly make this adjustment in interpreting all of the individual positions.

Another example of the importance of calibration made on the first impression (broader focus) is the assessment of the blood depth. A woman who attended one of our seminars presented with a Thin pulse. She also had a filling-out of the left middle position, rather than the normal diminishment, as finger pressure was released from the organ depth to the blood depth. However, the filling-out was very subtle. In fact, it was overlooked by even the experienced students. This slight increase in substance at the blood depth on release of the pressure would be interpreted as a 'blood unclear' condition (see glossary). However, one had to take into account the fact that, were her pulses of normal width, it would have filled out even more; and in fact her condition was probably 'blood heat,' which has a different etiology, pathology, and treatment than 'blood unclear.' This differentiation could be further developed using other parameters of diagnosis.

AMBER AND SHEN TECHNIQUES

According to Amber, the order of pulse-taking differs according to gender: "In the man, the left pulse is taken first; in the woman, the right. Here the procedure is the reverse of the Ayurvedic and Unani practice."[9] Dr. Shen had no set procedure, and palpated with either of his hands, whichever was closest to the wrist. I do not suggest this approach for anyone less experienced than he.

FINGER PLACEMENT

Longitudinal location

I advise against the method, recommended in the literature,[10] of placing the middle finger on the styloid process. The position of the muscle-ligament attachments (abductor pollicis brevis) between the styloid process and the scaphoid bone varies considerably and is therefore not a reliable guide for finger placement. Instead, I recommend using the scaphoid bone as the guide so that one becomes accustomed to the essential maneuver of rolling the index finger distally for an accurate reading of the upper burner. Again, this is necessary because the qualities of the middle position expand and overflow into the distal position. Thus, when beginning the pulse-taking procedure, the index finger should be placed contiguous to the scaphoid bone. In this manner, the index finger can easily be rolled under the bone to access the distal position with the lateral side of the index finger.

With respect to the other fingers, the middle finger goes in the middle or second position on or near the radial styloid process and contiguous to the distal index finger, and the ring finger falls into place adjacent to the middle finger. In addition, I have found that by placing the thumb in an opposing manner against the ventral aspect of the patient's hand at about LI-5 *(yang xi)* provides greater control, and enhances the capacity to access the subtleties of the pulse. Control is also augmented by using only the index finger, without touching the subject elsewhere with the hands, when searching for the Neuro-psychological, Mitral Valve, and radial Liver Engorgement positions.

If the subject is large, the practitioner's fingers should be spread out slightly more. If the practitioner's fingers are larger than the patient's, the fingers should be somewhat more compressed. It should be remembered that the most sensitive part of the finger is the center of the small area between the nail and the flat pad of the finger.

Direction

The radial artery, which we palpate in our model of pulse diagnosis, runs and is explored longitudinally, from distal to proximal. The middle and proximal positions are examined in this direction. The distal positions, however, are explored horizontally, from lateral (radial) to medial (ulnar), along the radial edge of the index finger.

Depth and Level

DEPTH

Depth refers to the vertical dimensions of the pulse on the radial artery, from the ventral to the dorsal aspect. While we commonly speak of three depths as the principal vertical areas of inspection, there are actually eight.

FINGER PRESSURE AND THE THREE DEPTHS

The most common mistake in pulse-taking, which is taught in the schools and even done by many experienced practitioners, is the tendency to press too deeply, thus obliterating the true pulse. When the bone or tendon has been reached, the physiological value of Chinese pulse diagnosis has been significantly lost. At the other end of the spectrum, many practitioners from the European schools press too lightly and never reach the organ depth, or even the blood depth, as defined in this system. The boundaries of the pulse in the Chinese model are exact and extremely subtle; the key to the depths of the pulse is in the fingers, wrist, and arm of the practitioner. It should be noted that the distance between the surface and the qi depth, and between the depths themselves, is perhaps less than one thirty-second of an inch. The greatest distance is between the skin and the qi depth, and between the organ depth and the bone. The only variation is weight dependent. With a heavy person the entire pulse (i.e., all three positions on both wrists) is normally slightly deeper; therefore, heavier pressure is applied to find the qi depth. With a thin person, the qi depth is accessed more superficially. The distances between the depths would, however, be constant under all circumstances.

It is a common error to assume that the qi depth is where one first feels the pulse, and to then access the other depths with that first encounter as a benchmark. The qi depth is not necessarily where the impulse is first found. In fact, the qi depth is at a predetermined pressure. If nothing is found there, the qi depth is Absent. If a pulse wave is felt before exerting that particular amount of pressure, then a Floating, Flooding Excess, or Hollow Full-Overflowing pulse is present, which is a sign of some disharmony. These degrees of pressure are a relatively impartial tool by which the patient's pulse is subject to an unbiased measurement, capable of objective comparison with every other person.

COMPLEMENTARY POSITIONS, QUALITIES, AND THE THREE DEPTHS

The three depths—qi, blood, and organ—do not apply to the twenty-two complementary or distal positions. In these positions one can discern deeper and more superficial sensations, but they do not correspond to qi, blood, and organ. The interpretation of qualities at the complementary positions (e.g., Tight = inflammation) also varies from that at the principal positions (Tight = yin deficiency).

The Special Lung position, Gallbladder, Stomach-Pylorus Extension, and Pelvis/Lower Body positions are best accessed by moving the finger up and down and distal to proximal, because the several different qualities one will find in these positions are found in different parts of the position, either superficial or deep and distal or proximal. Also, in the complementary positions, especially the Neuro-psychological and Mitral Valve positions, the qualities are sometimes ephemeral; one must therefore move around the position with a very light touch and/or wait.

LEVEL

Level refers to the horizontal dimensions of the radial artery, from the wrist toward the elbow. There are three levels: the upper burner, which is most distal, the lower burner, which is most proximal, and the middle burner, which is between the other two.

Middle position qualities

The pulse qualities of the middle burner (middle position) tend to dominate and overflow into the other positions, especially into the distal position. Partly this is due to anatomical considerations. The abdominal area represented by the middle position is much less confined than the chest (distal position), and somewhat less confined than the pelvis (proximal position). The qi in the middle burner is therefore anatomically freer to expand.

Partly this overflow from the middle position to the distal positions is due to the nature of the qi and blood in the organs of the middle burner. According to Dr. Shen, the qi in the middle right position and gas in the digestive lumen are equivalent. Gas, he says, is the qi in the Stomach. Because qi is yang energy, it is expansive by nature. This is translated by the communication system between organs and areas to the pulse by the movement of the sensation in the right middle position, especially toward the right distal position, and to a much lesser extent to the right proximal position.

This natural tendency is exaggerated when the the qi in the Stomach and Intestines is stagnant, or expands further when there is heat from excess in this system. (The Inflated pulse quality is identified with this process.)

The middle position on the left side is associated with the Liver and Gallbladder. There are two aspects of Liver function which contribute to the tendency of the qualities of the middle positions to overflow, especially to the distal positions. The first is the Liver's function of spreading the qi throughout the body, which contributes to expansiveness of qi from the natural anatomical configuration of the abdomen and middle burner. Perhaps the most celebrated disharmony in Chinese medicine involves the inhibition of this continuous spreading process by a variety of etiologies, especially repression of emotion, particularly anger. When qi thereupon stagnates and is unable to flow freely through the body it will accumulate in the Liver; this will be expressed in the invasion of the distal positions (especially) by whatever qualities are present at that time in the middle burner. For example, depending upon the stage of the stagnation (see Chapter 11), we might feel Taut, Tense, or Tight qualities in the distal positions, which, upon examination, we find are simultaneously the same qualities at the left middle position.

The second aspect of Liver function that contributes to the overflow of the middle position pulse is that of storing the blood. When heat from excess in the Liver develops as it attempts to overcome qi stagnation, the blood stored in the Liver will expand, and the pulse will accordingly overflow (Hollow Full-Overflowing). Heat in the blood of the Liver thereby contributes to the tendency of the middle pulse position to fill a greater space than that occupied by the other two positions.

For these reasons it is necessary to roll the fingers distally from the conventional upper burner position in order to properly access the qualities in the upper burner.

Qualities

The classification of qualities is made according to sensation:

- Hardness or pliability is a function of yin.
- Force (strength or weakness) is a function of qi or yang.
- Width (narrow or wide) is a function of blood.

The degree of presence of a quality is measured on a scale of one to five, with five being the greatest degree and one the least.

Procedure

Before introducing the actual pulse-taking procedure, it should be noted that there are certain uniform or overall pulse qualities that may obscure or conceal other qualities, or make them more difficult to discern. Among these are the Robust Pounding, Uniformly Tense, very Rapid, very Slow, Muffled, Heavy Cotton, very Thin, Ropy, very Deep, Interrupted, and Intermittent pulses. The same is true of certain medications, stimulants (e.g., caffeine), and excessively calming substances (e.g., marijuana), as well as aerobic exercise, physical and emotional trauma, and heavy lifting. Less significantly, the pulse picture may be temporarily affected by overeating, and in a severely deficient person, by sexual activity.

Below is an outline of the methodology of pulse examination followed in this book. (See also Chapter 17 for elaboration.)

- **Broad focus**

  Rhythm, rate at rest (after movement, tested only at the end of the examination), and the uniform qualities over the entire pulse (i.e., simultaneously at all three positions and depths on both sides)

- **Closer focus**

  The three depths, the two sides, and the wave form

- **Closest focus**

  The individual principal and complementary positions, and bilaterally at the three burners

Again, the pulse is accessed with the fingertips at the center of the small area between the nail and the flat pad of the finger. Exceptions to this rule are the Special Lung position, distal positions, the Neuro-psychological, Large Vessel, Mitral Valve, Diaphragm, medial and lateral Engorgement of the Liver, Gallbladder, Large and Small Intestine, Pelvis/Lower Body, and the Stomach-Pylorus Extension positions—all of which require rolling of the fingers. In addition:

- For the Special Lung position, use the flat part of the index finger.
- For the distal positions, use the radial side of the index finger, which is rolled under the scaphoid bone and then lightened up slightly to access the upper burner. Most important is to distinguish the impulse coming from the middle burner, which is felt on the ventral surface of the index finger, from the impulse coming from the upper burner, which is felt on the radial edge.
- For the Gallbladder and Stomach-Pylorus Extension positions, use the ulnar side of the middle finger.
- For the Pelvis/Lower Body position, use the ulnar side of the ring (fourth) finger.
- For the Neuro-psychological, Mitral Valve, Liver Radial Engorgement, and Special Lung positions, use one finger alone.

The description and interpretation of pulse characteristics in the sections below are highly abbreviated, and are intended only to provide an overview. A more comprehensive discussion of each aspect is presented in later chapters.

BROAD FOCUS

Gender and age

These are discussed in Chapter 3 and are the two single most important pieces of information, since qualities and conditions which are natural signs at certain ages are not at others. A Ropy quality at age eighty would not arouse the same concern as it would at age thirty. We have already alluded to the gender issue with regard to the width of the pulse. Weight and height are important because we would find it paradoxical for a large, heavy person to have a Thin and Superficial pulse, or a small, light person to have a very Wide and Deep pulse.

Rhythm and rate

TRUE ARRHYTHMIAS

The pulse-taking process is initiated by assessing the rate of the pulse on both wrists simultaneously in order to note irregularities in the rhythm or differences in the rate between the two sides. In terms of rhythm, these include Changes in Rate at Rest, and the Interrupted and Intermittent qualities. Changes in Rate at Rest are a useful indicator of emotional instability.

With rate, the usual qualities are Normal, Rapid, or Slow in varying degrees. Sometimes the rate is indiscernible because the rhythm is too irregular. In the modern era, a Rapid or Slow rate is mostly indicative of Heart and circulatory function, and of emotional states, and far less often of heat or cold from excess.

At the end of the examination, the resting rate should be taken again, and then a final reading immediately after exertion, to observe whether the rate increases, remains the same, or decreases. To measure the rate on exertion, have the subject rotate their arm at the shoulder vigorously ten to fifteen times, then measure the rate for ten seconds and multiply by six. Substantial change in the rate between rest and exertion is significant with regard to Heart function (see Chapter 6). This should be repeated at least once to ensure accuracy.

PSEUDO-ARRHYTHMIAS AND AMPLITUDE

The Hesitant Wave, Change in Intensity and Amplitude, and Unstable qualities mimic true arrhythmias (see Chapter 6).

Uniform qualities over the entire pulse

The next step is to obtain a quick impression of other qualities that are uniform over the entire pulse or just on one side. This initial overall impression is made while taking the pulse on both wrists simultaneously. The purpose here is to get a sense of the qualities that are uniform over the entire pulse (all three positions on both sides) and on other large segments of the pulse, such as the three burners, and over each wrist. These have special significance to the diagnosis which is different than when the same qualities are found in only one position (see Chapter 13). Among the questions we should ask when examining the entire pulse: Is it Deep, Normal, or Superficial? Is it Thin or Wide, Pounding with or without spirit and force (Robust or Reduced)? Is it resilient or easily compressible, continuous or fragmented (Long, Scattered, or Short)? Or is it Feeble-Absent, Empty or Hollow Full-Overflowing, or balanced or unbalanced between the three depths and six positions?

In asking these questions, we are partially assessing the person and their condition in terms of excess and deficiency. With deficiency the concern is whether it is of qi, blood, or yin, whether the person is still able to maintain a semblance of function, and which systems are more or less capable of contributing to this function. With excess the concern is its extent and whether we are dealing with heat, cold, dampness, or qi stagnation, either alone or in some combination.

In answering these questions, we are attempting the important task of differentiating the big picture (the entire pulse) from the small picture (the individual positions) in terms of diagnosis.

Qualities found uniformly over the pulse include the following: Floating, Tense, Tight, Pounding, Thin, Cotton, Deep, Smooth and Rough Vibration, Slippery, Reduced Substance, Ropy, Muffled, Spreading, Change in Intensity, Amplitude, or Qualities, Blood Heat, Blood Unclear, Blood Thick, Hollow Full-Overflowing, Suppressed, Flooding Excess, Flooding Deficient and Hesitant Wave.

Iatrogenic-related qualities

Pharmaceuticals can affect the pulse in a variety of ways. As an example, some commonly used diuretics cause a flattening of the very top of the Normal wave, as if the wave is about to fully hit the finger and just stops short of the totality of the surge. This is a Suppressed quality. Some cardiac and antihypertensive medications cause the Robust Pounding quality at the organ depth (due usually to heat from excess) to diminish quickly at the blood and qi depths. Steroids usually cause the pulse to become Slippery. Anti-depressants reduce or eliminate the Cotton quality, and I have heard of the Muffled quality associated with anti-psychotic drugs.

STABILITY OR INSTABILITY

A general impression is obtained of Changes in Qualities, Amplitude, and Intensity. Wherever there are large Changes in Qualities and Amplitude over the entire pulse, the integrity of qi is usually highly compromised by chaos ('qi wild' or circulation out of control) with often precarious emotional states. Consistent Changes in Intensity are related to the Heart and circulation. Inconsistent changes in Intensity are associated with Liver qi stagnation, which is easily affected by daily stresses.

WIDTH AND HARDNESS

While a pulse quality is naturally comparable from one person to another, the same quality can also vary slightly from one person to another. For example, as previously mentioned, the evaluation of the hardness or pliability of qualities must be made with an overall allowance for the general width (breadth) of the individual pulse. Pulse qualities are, in a sense, most productively evaluated within the context of an individual's own energetic gestalt. It should also be remembered that women's pulses are generally thinner than men's. Normally the organ depth has the greatest width and substance, decreasing steadily as one releases finger pressure to the blood and qi depths and above.

CLOSER FOCUS

Wave form

The Normal wave form resembles a sine or bell curve which stays between the organ and qi depths. Unusual wave forms include the Hollow Full-Overflowing, Flooding-Excess, and Flooding-Deficient qualities, the Suppressed quality, and the Hesitant quality. The Hollow Full-Overflowing quality has the correct shape but exceeds the qi depth. (See Fig. 4-2.)

Uniform qualities on the two sides

The large segments of the pulse are assessed to identify uniform qualities on each side separately. For example, is one side in all three positions Feeble, Tight, or Slippery? These findings are clinically significant and are detailed in Chapter 14.

UNIFORM LEFT SIDE

The most common uniform qualities to be found on the left side are Tense, Tight, Yielding, Spreading, Diffuse, Reduced Substance, Vibration, Deep, Feeble, Hollow, Hollow Full-Overflowing, Slippery, Change in Intensity, and Cotton. A slightly Feeble Deep quality with a Thin Tight quality at the pulse's most superficial aspect is found when the 'nervous system' affects the 'organ system.' When moderate, persistent worry is the etiology, superficial Smooth Vibration is found over the entire left side. Rough Vibration on the left side only is a sign of parenchymal damage to the vital yin organs.

Fig. 4-2 Wave comparisons

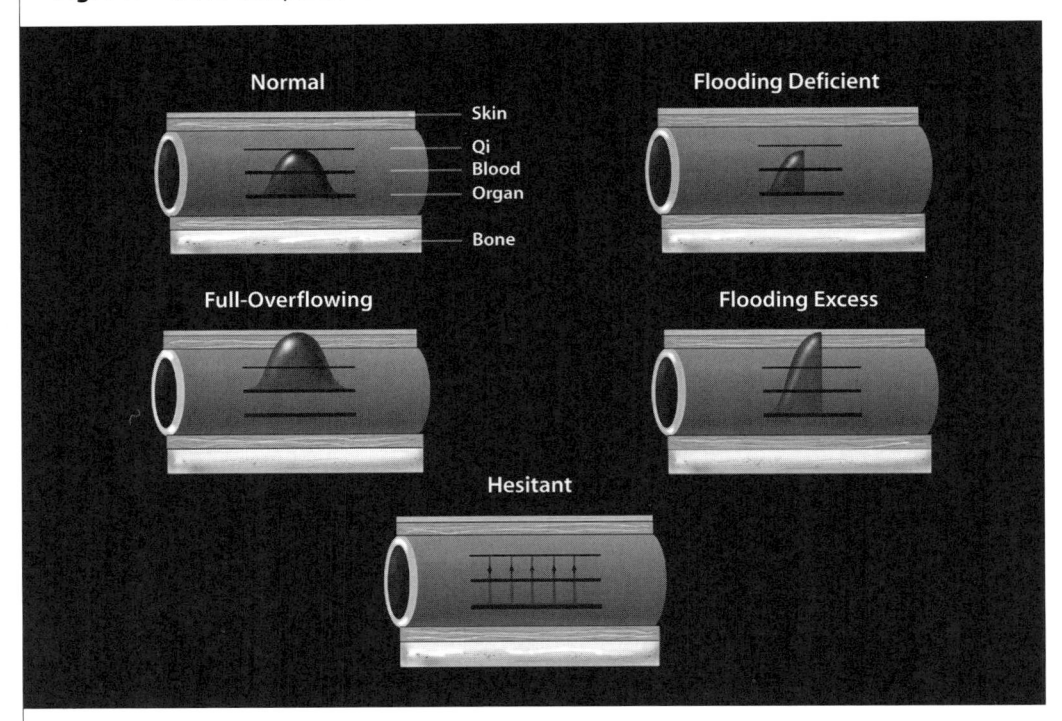

UNIFORM RIGHT SIDE

The common qualities found uniformly on the right side are Tense, Tight, Yielding, Reduced Substance, Deep, Feeble, and Cotton. A Slippery quality is also encountered uniformly, but much less often. A Thin Tight quality at the pulse's most superficial aspect is found when a person eats too quickly.

INTENSITY ALTERNATING BETWEEN SIDES

When palpating both left and right radial arteries simultaneously the intensity may seem at first to increase on one side and diminish on the other, and then reverse. This is associated most often with a current, significant interpersonal conflict, and less often with a situation in which the person has worked or exercised beyond their capacity for a period of weeks prior to the examination.

QUALITIES ALTERNATING BETWEEN SIDES

When the qualities on the left and right sides switch places throughout the examination, this is a sign of the separation of yin and yang and a serious 'qi wild' condition (see Chapter 6).

Depths

As previously mentioned, there are actually eight depths in our system (Fig. 4-3). There is an above-the-qi depth between the skin and the qi depth; the qi depth; and the organ depth, which can be subdivided into three: between the organ depth and the bone (Firm quality) and just above the bone (Hidden quality). Whereas the qi and blood depths involve the contribution of a particular yin organ to the total organism of qi and blood, the organ depth is again divided into qi, blood, and organ informing us respectively of the state of the qi, the blood, and the parenchyma of that organ. The full use of this division of the organ depth is being explored.

Fig. 4-3 The eight depths

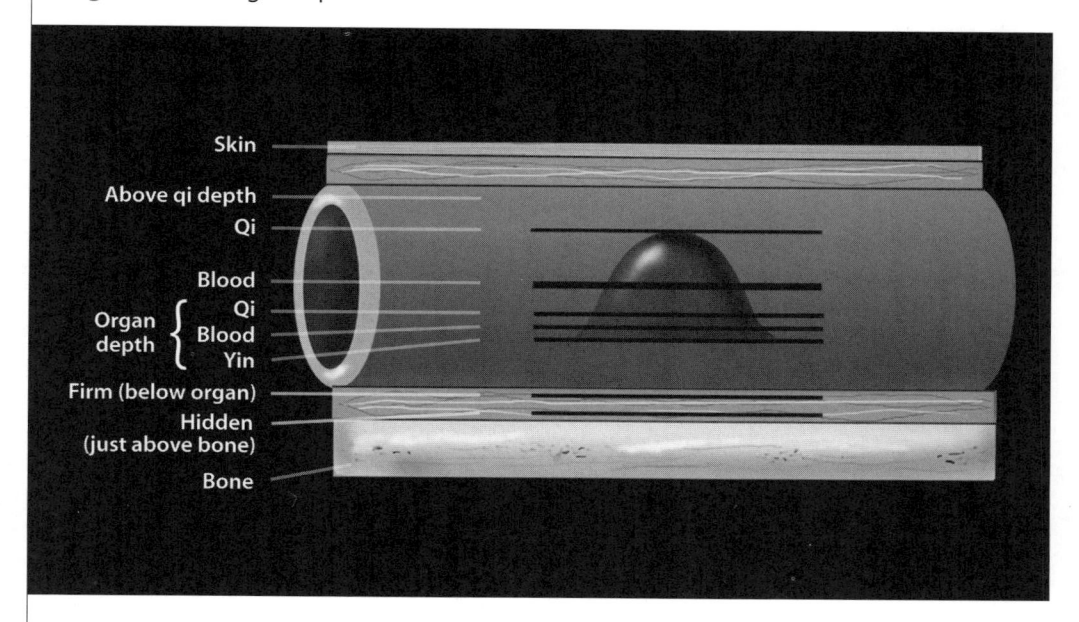

```
Skin
Above qi depth
Qi
Blood
Organ   { Qi
depth   { Blood
        { Yin
Firm (below organ)
Hidden (just above bone)
Bone
```

Ordinarily the organ depth is the widest and most tangibly substantial part of the pulse. As pressure is released on the pulse toward the surface, the pulse becomes less wide with less substance. The lightest sensation is closer to the surface at the qi depth, and the heaviest sensation is deeper at the organ depth.

The exact positions of the three depths are very subtle; they can only be demonstrated, and cannot be precisely conveyed by language alone. The distance between the depths is only about a tenth of a millimeter, and is accessed by very small increases or decreases in pressure from the wrists—and therefore the fingers—of the practitioner on the pulse. The movement is all in the wrists. The distance from the skin to the qi depth is about one-third greater than the distance from the qi to the blood depth, and the blood to the organ depth. The qi depth is below the surface at a precise point, and the organ depth is well above the bone at another precise point. The blood depth is half way between the two.

In other words, locating each depth depends upon the precise positioning of the practitioner's wrist, and not simply where the practitioner happens to first encounter the vessel. For example, by learning to 'calibrate' our wrist movements we can tell when a particular pulse quality is *absent* from the qi, blood, or organ depth. The entire system described in this book depends on mastering this tool, one which we carry with us wherever we go, and which opens up to us all the complexities which make taking the pulse such a valuable diagnostic skill.

Remember that the three depths—qi, blood, and organ—do not apply to the complementary positions or the distal positions. Although one can discern deeper and more superficial sensations in these positions, they do not correspond to the qi, blood, and organ depths.

Changes in Intensity or Qualities affect all of the depths that are present either over the entire pulse or at an individual position.

ABOVE THE QI DEPTH

The qualities found above the qi depth are Floating, Flooding Excess, Hollow Full-Overflowing, and, most often, Cotton.

QI DEPTH

All three positions are palpated with all three fingers, checking for the presence or absence of qualities at the qi depth. The most common qualities are Taut, Tense, Tight, Thin, Yielding, Diminished or Reduced Substance, Absent, Slippery, and Smooth Vibration.

BLOOD DEPTH

The blood depth is often indiscernible when it is free of problems. In palpating the blood depth, it is patterns of deficiency and excess that are being assessed. Deficiency is felt by gradually increasing pressure to the blood depth to observe if there is a Spreading quality, diminution, or absence of sensation. If the qi depth is intact and the blood depth separates or disappears under pressure, and the organ depth is clearly felt upon further pressure, this phenomenon is regarded as a Hollow quality. If the qi depth is present and the organ depth spreads apart under pressure, or is not clearly felt, the quality is Empty. If the qi depth is Absent and the blood depth is Spreading, there is deficiency of both qi and blood. If both the qi and blood depths are Absent and the organ depth is present, the qi and blood deficiency is even greater; a Thin quality indicates that the blood deficiency is greater still.

A pattern of excess in the blood is assessed by compressing the pulse to the organ depth to check for its presence and quality, and then gradually releasing toward the surface. Normally the pulse diminishes in size and strength as pressure is released. If the pulse fills out in the blood depth, and then diminishes at the qi depth, a disharmony (and pulse quality) such as Blood Unclear or Blood Heat is present. If the substance of the pulse does not diminish as pressure is released toward the qi depth, the condition (and pulse) is regarded as Blood Thick, and if the pulse increases in substance above the qi depth, the quality is Hollow Full-Overflowing. Other qualities which often accompany Blood Heat or Blood Thick are Slippery and Rough Vibration (see Chapter 13) at the blood depth.

ORGAN DEPTH

At the organ depth the pulse should normally have the greatest substance and present the greatest resistance. It represents the cardinal functional, and especially the material, aspect of the yin organs. It is explored for all of the qualities described in the section on organ depth in Chapter 13. The principal qualities found uniformly at the organ depth are Taut, Tense, Tight, Thin, Diffuse, Reduced Substance, Feeble-Absent, Slippery, Pounding, Rough Vibration, Separating, and Empty.

Within the organ depth, through a careful sense of touch, one can find a qi, blood, and more material yin layer, which I equate with the biomedical concept of parenchyma. Here, we are passing from the energetic to the material side of the equation. It is worth reiterating that qi, blood, and yin deficiency at the qi and blood depths are on a physiological continuum with the more profound organ deficiencies.

BELOW THE ORGAN DEPTH

While Dr. Shen limited his pulse model to what is found from under the skin to the organ depth, the literature mentions the Firm quality between what we call the organ depth and the bone, and a Hidden quality just above the bone. I felt the Hidden quality once in a person suffering from severe hypothermia, not commonly encountered nowadays in the average acupuncture practice. This subject is complicated by Dr. Shen's use in his book of the term Hidden for what we call Deep. (I have confirmed that this is what he meant.)

CLOSEST FOCUS

Principal and complementary individual positions

Having gained a sense of the larger picture, the individual positions are now palpated with the appropriate finger at all three depths, in the manner described above for the entire pulse. Accessing all three depths is more difficult in the confined distal positions, and irrelevant in all of the complementary positions, although the quality of each of these positions can vary with pressure (see Chapter 11).

Note: *in the illustrations that follow, heavy arrows indicate the correct finger for accessing the indicated position, and lighter arrows indicate the direction for rolling the finger.*

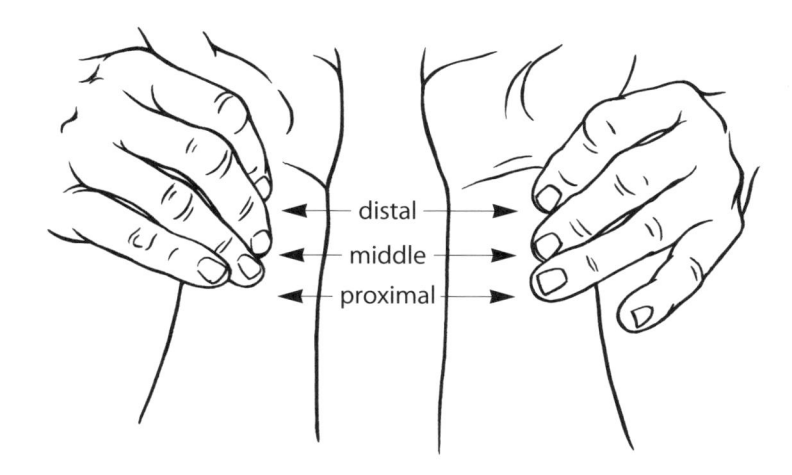

Fig. 4-4 Both hands

LEFT PRINCIPAL AND COMPLEMENTARY POSITIONS

Left Special Lung position

First to be palpated is the left Special Lung position, which is accessed with the flat pad of the right index finger, searching lightly for the unpredictable small branch of the radial artery; this branch is found medial to the radial artery, somewhere between LU-9 *(tai yuan)* and PC-7 *(da ling)*. The qualities found in this position are Tense, Tight, Wiry, Thin, Slippery, Vibration, Floating, Inflated, Muffled, Restricted, Change in Intensity, and Absent. The left Special Lung position reveals the status of the material right lung (and simultaneously the location of disharmony in the energetic right Lung) including the

Fig. 4-5 Left Special Lung position

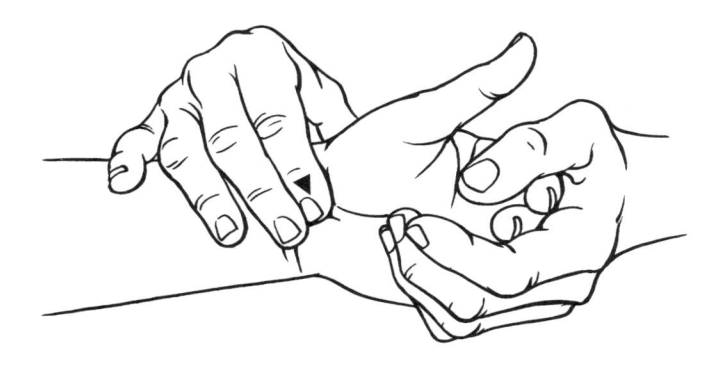

medial, lateral, upper, and lower aspects, each of which can be accessed by rolling the finger in the appropriate direction (see Fig. 2-2 in Chapter 2).

Left Neuro-psychological position

The left Neuro-psychological position is found in, on, or around a truncated depression located on the trapezium bone just distal to the principal left distal position. The qualities found in this position are usually either Vibration or an undifferentiated sensory presence which I call Doughy. The Vibration pulse is more often associated with fright and Heart shock, and the undifferentiated or Doughy quality with neurological problems, including headache. Change in Intensity, Tight, Muffled, and Choppy qualities have also been reported here. The qualities in this position are often ephemeral, will move from one to another part of the position, and are very subtle. Understanding the full significance of the qualities in this position requires considerably more investigation.

Fig. 4-6   Left Neuro-psychological position

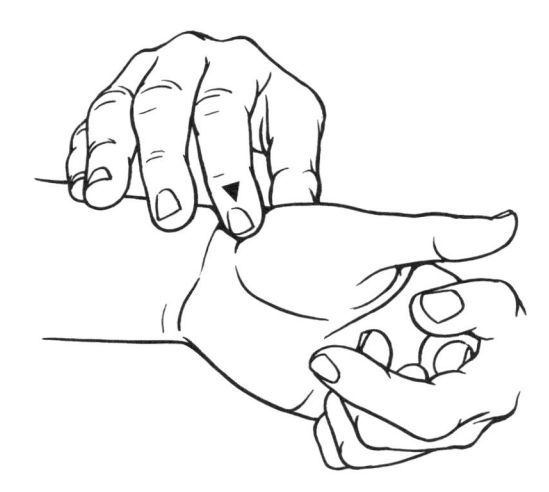

Left distal, Pericardium, and Large Vessel positions

Next, the left distal position is palpated by rolling the most proximal section of the radial side of the right index finger under the scaphoid bone. It is necessary to raise and rotate the entire right arm in order to get the index finger in the proper position to access the information emanating from under the scaphoid bone. Once in position, one must lighten the touch so as not to obliterate the pulse. Concentration is required to distinguish the different sensations arriving at each aspect of the finger. The goal is to distinguish the sensation coming to the radial side of the right index finger from the sensation coming from the proximal-to-distal direction. I have found it useful to facilitate access to the distal positions by holding the patient's hand with my free hand and slightly bending their wrist ventrally.

In order to avoid the sensory overlap of the middle burner into the distal aspects of the pulse, the distal positions are not accessed in the distal-proximal axis along the radial artery, as are the proximal and medial positions. Rather, they are accessed horizontally, along a radial-ulnar, medial-lateral axis just under the scaphoid bone, to which position one has rolled the radial edge of the index finger. Here we are not accessing the radial artery, but rather the fluid dynamics of its sudden breakdown into many smaller arteries, which sets up a wave informing us about the physiological integrity of the heart.

Fig. 4-7 Left distal position

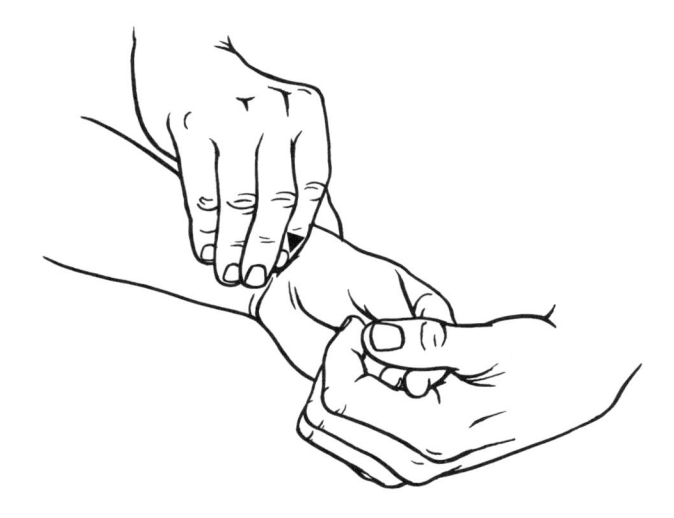

The qualities most often found at the left distal position are Tense, Tight, Thin, Flat, Inflated, Feeble-Absent, Vibration, Slippery, Muffled, as well as Change in Intensity, Change in Qualities, and Change in Amplitude. The Hollow Full-Overflowing, Floating, Wiry, and Choppy qualities are less commonly encountered.

While still in the left distal position, another distinct quality in the central Pericardium position is ascertained by rolling the edge of the index finger from the lateral to the medial aspect of the left distal position and back again, from medial to lateral. The Tight quality is by far the most commonly found in the Pericardium position, and is sometimes accompanied by Slipperiness.

The Large Vessel position is also accessed by rolling the index finger medially toward the ulna. At the intersection of the tendon of the flexor carpi radialis and the scaphoid bone is a hole or cave-like place that is palpated by the lateral distal edge of the index finger. This hole is sometimes occupied by either an Inflated (indicating aneurysm) or a Tense-Tight Hollow Full-Overflowing quality (indicating hypertension).

Fig. 4-8 Large Vessel position

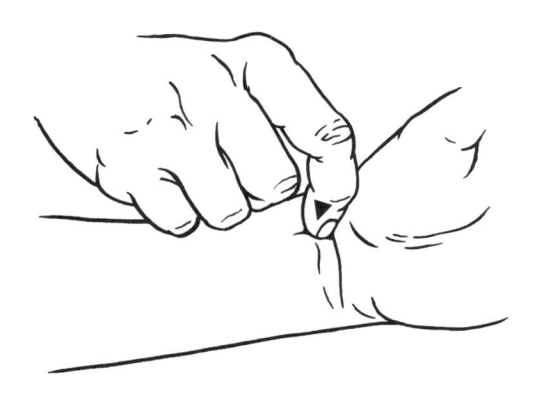

Mitral Valve position

With an especially light touch, the Mitral Valve is accessed laterally on the muscle-ligament connecting the styloid process and the scaphoid bone. The most common qualities found are Vibration and Slipperiness. Like the Neuro-psychological position, the qualities here are ephemeral, subtle, and sometimes moving around the position.

Fig. 4-9 Mitral Valve position

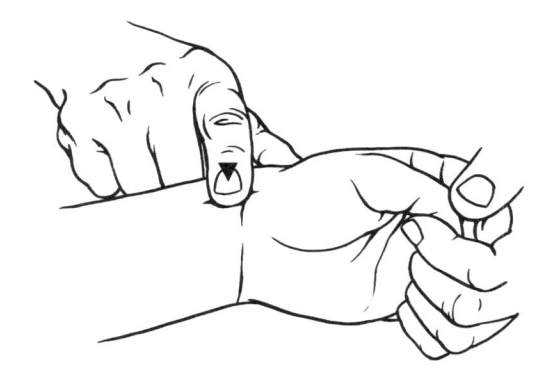

Left Diaphragm, Heart Enlarged, and distal Liver Engorgement positions

With a very light touch, the Diaphragm position is evaluated by rolling the index finger proximally toward the middle position, and then the middle finger from the middle position distally toward the distal position. The point here is to note whether or not the fingers sense an Inflated quality—as if the fingers are going uphill. If the Inflated quality is felt to come from both directions, qi stagnation is present in the left Diaphragm area.

Fig. 4-10 Heart Enlargement position

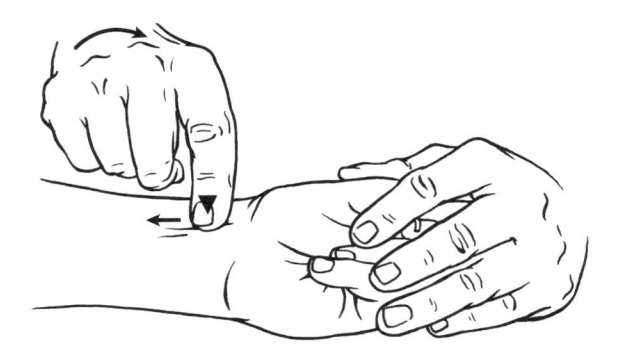

Fig. 4-11 Distal Liver Engorgement position

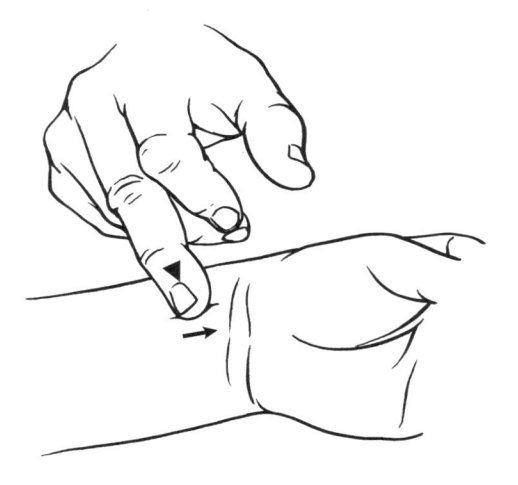

The presence of Heart Enlarged (the condition and its associated pulse) is discernible when the distal aspect of the left Diaphragm position is either more Inflated or Rougher than the proximal aspect.[11] The presence of distal engorgement of the Liver is discernable when the middle aspect of the left Diaphragm position is either more Inflated or Rougher than the distal aspect.

Left middle position

PRINCIPAL LEFT MIDDLE POSITION

With the right middle finger placed next to the index finger, the middle position is evaluated at all three depths. The most common qualities and conditions found here are Taut, Tense, Tight, Wiry, Thin, Pounding, Blood Unclear, Blood Heat, Blood Thick, Hollow Full-Overflowing, Deep, Feeble, Empty, Hollow, Slippery, Vibration, Diffuse, and Reduced Substance, as well as Changes in Qualities and Intensity.

Fig. 4-12   Left middle position

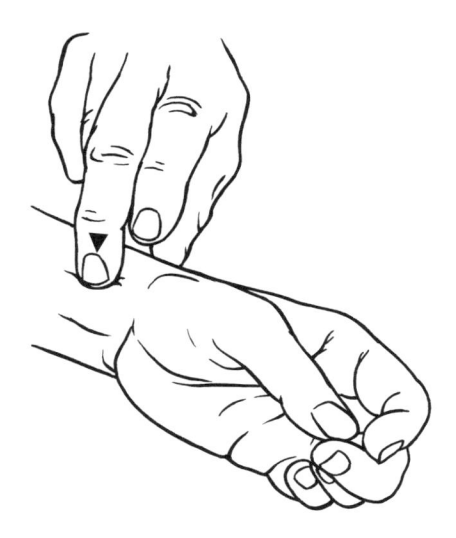

LATERAL AND MEDIAL ENGORGEMENT OF THE LIVER

Next, the fingers are rolled medially toward the ulna to palpate very superficially for medial Liver engorgement. This is felt superficially with the portion of the middle finger closest to the nail and is a very superficial Inflated quality between the artery and the flexor carpal radialis tendon.

Fig. 4-13   Liver Ulnar Engorgement position

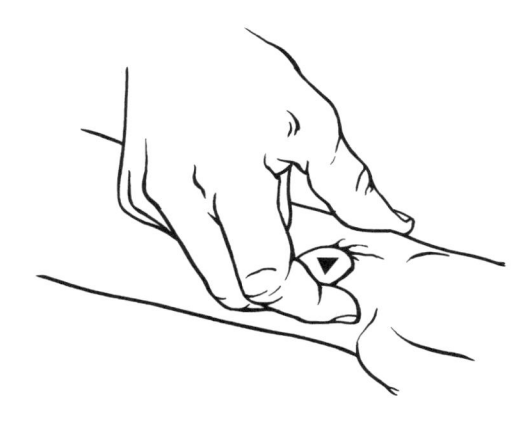

Thereafter, the middle finger is rolled laterally toward the radius to palpate for lateral engorgement of the Liver. This position is felt with the flat area of the middle finger between the end and the first distal interphalangeal joint of the finger. It is usually a thin, hard, or vibrating line, almost on the radial bone.

Fig. 4-14 Liver Radial Engorgement position

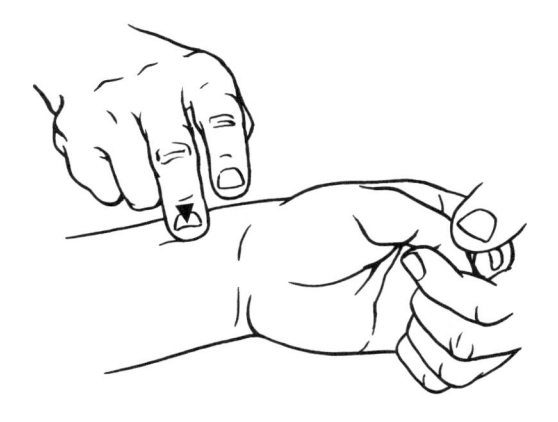

GALLBLADDER POSITION

Finally, the right middle finger is laid proximally from the left middle position along and on top of the artery seeking the Gallbladder position, with the ulnar (lateral) side of the middle finger around the first phalangeal distal joint. It is also sometimes necessary to roll the finger medially to find the Gallbladder position. The most common qualities here are Tense, Tight, Wiry, Inflated, Slippery, Choppy, Muffled, and Change in Intensity.

Fig. 4-15 Gallbladder position

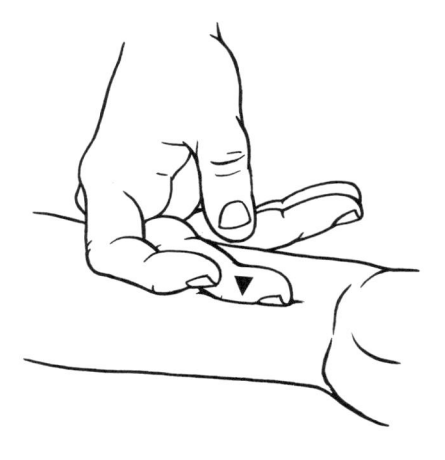

Left proximal position

The left proximal position is evaluated by placing the ring finger adjacent to the middle finger.

PRINCIPAL LEFT PROXIMAL POSITION

It is sometimes necessary to roll the fingers slightly medially to locate this position. Frequently found qualities here are Tense, Tight, Wiry, Reduced Substance, Deep, Feeble-

Absent, as well as Changes in Qualities, Amplitude, and Intensity. Less frequently encountered are Yielding Partially Hollow, Hollow, Hollow Full-Overflowing, Pounding, Flooding Excess, Slippery, and Choppy.

The harder qualities (e.g., Tight) suggest Kidney yin deficiency, while the more pliable ones (e.g., Feeble-Absent, and Changes in Qualities) suggest Kidney qi and yang deficiency. The harder qualities tend to override the pliable ones such that yin deficiency can mask concurrent qi and yang deficiency, though often one finds signs of both as the qualities shift back and forth. The excess qualities (e.g., Flooding Excess, Pounding) indicate fulminating acute infection of the intestines or pelvic organs. A Wiry quality can be a sign of severe pain, often menstrual, often in conjunction with the Choppy quality. The Wiry quality is also associated with early diabetes and/or hypertension.

Fig. 4-16 Left proximal position

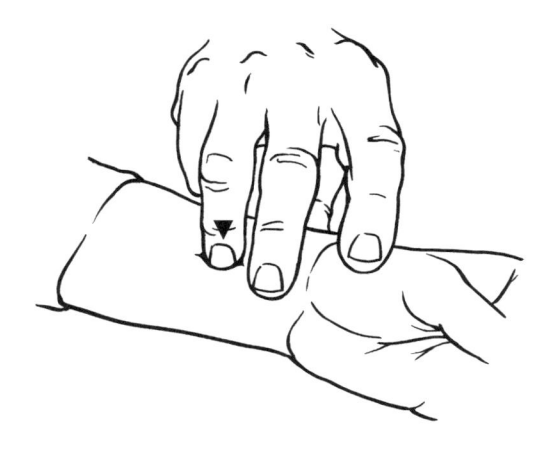

LARGE INTESTINE POSITION

The right ring finger is then rolled distally to find the Large Intestine position with the radial edge of the finger tip. The most frequent qualities encountered here are Tense, Tight, Slippery, Biting, and Muffled. Vibration, Changes in Intensity, and Choppy qualities are also occasionally found. Often the proximal positions are also Tense and Tight. To distinguish the presence of the Large Intestine, one's attention is drawn to the quality of Tenseness to note a subtle change, since a Tense or Tight quality can feel more focused, Robust, and Biting in an Intestinal position than in a proximal position.

Fig. 4-17 Large Intestine position

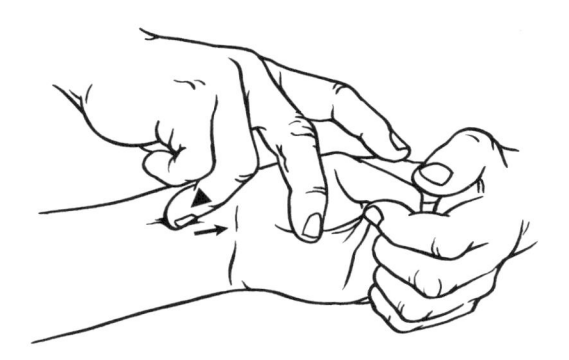

Left Pelvis/Lower Body position

The left Pelvis/Lower Body position is palpated by laying the right ring finger along the artery in a proximal and slightly medial direction; the area of the finger that is actually used is closer to the distal phalangeal joint. The qualities that are often found here are Tense, Tight, Slippery, Muffled, Choppy, and Change in Intensity.

Fig. 4-18   Left Pelvis/Lower Body position

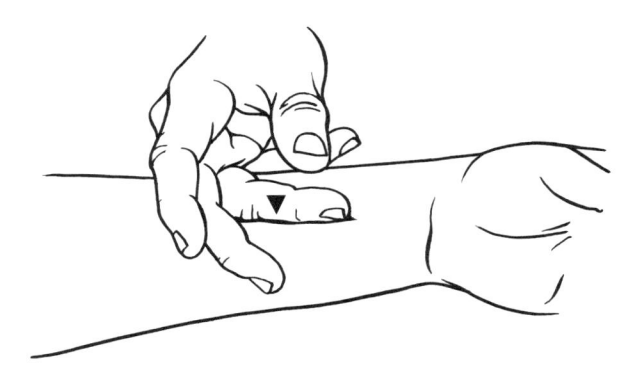

RIGHT PRINCIPAL AND COMPLEMENTARY POSITIONS

Right Special Lung position

On the right wrist, first to be palpated is the Special Lung position, which is found the same way as that on the left, but using the flat pad of the left index finger. The right Special Lung position reveals the status of the material left lung (and simultaneously the location of disharmony in the energetic left Lung), including the medial, lateral, upper, and lower aspects, each of which can be accessed by rolling the finger in the appropriate direction.

Fig. 4-19   Right Special Lung position

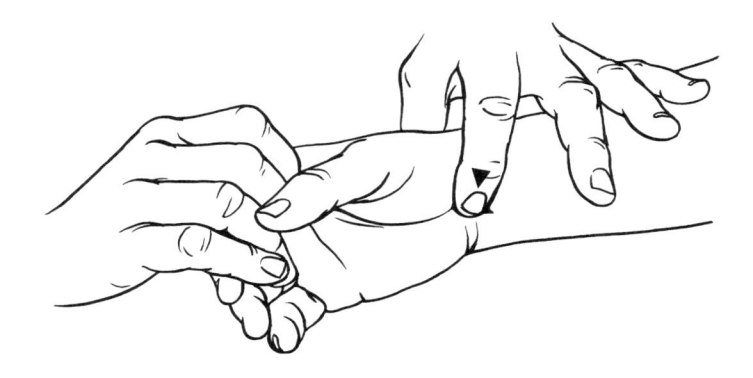

Right Neuro-psychological position

The right Neuro-psychological position is accessed in the same manner as the corresponding position on the left wrist, with the qualities and interpretation likewise being the same.

Fig. 4-20 Right Neuro-psychological position

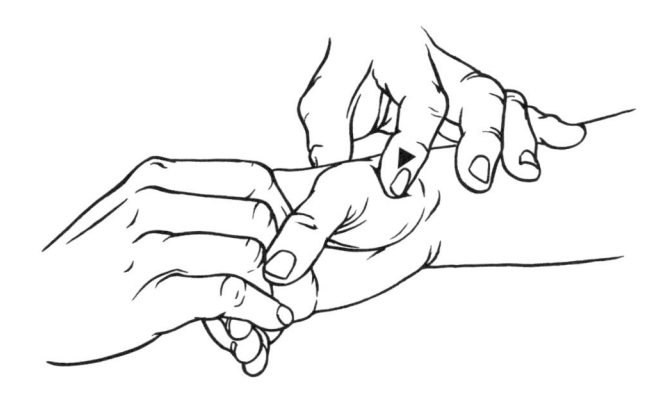

Right distal (regular Lung) position

To locate the right distal position, the entire left arm of the examiner must be raised, and the distal section of the left index finger rolled distally toward and slightly under the left scaphoid bone; the pulse is accessed with the radial side of the index finger, rather than the flat pad. Again, once in place, one must lighten the touch so as not to obliterate the pulse. I have found it useful to facilitate access to the distal positions by holding the patient's hand with my free hand and slightly bending their wrist ventrally.

As with the left distal position, in order to avoid the sensory overlap of the medial into the distal aspects of the pulse, the right distal position is not accessed in the distal-proximal axis along the radial artery, as are the proximal and medial positions. Rather, it is accessed horizontally, along a radial-ulnar, medial-lateral axis just under the scaphoid bone, to which position one has rolled the radial edge of the index finger. Here we are not accessing the radial artery, but rather the fluid dynamics of its sudden breakdown into many smaller arteries, which sets up a wave informing us about the physiological integrity of the Heart and Lungs.

Fig. 4-21 Right distal position

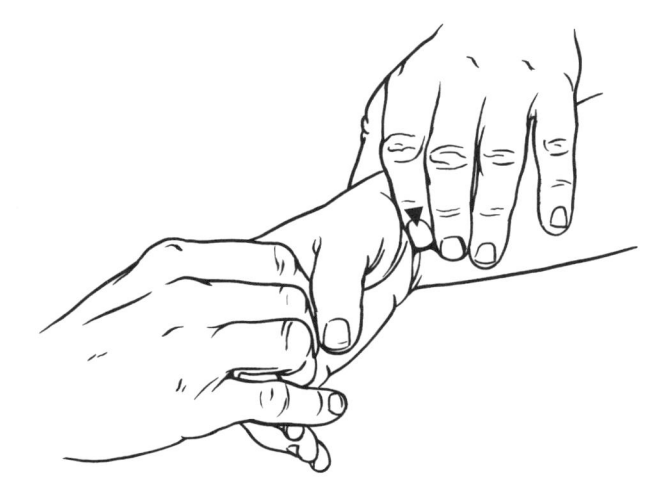

The most common qualities found in this position are Tense, Inflated, Tight, Wiry, Slippery, Vibration, Floating, Muffled, Feeble, Absent, and Change in Intensity. If the Dead quality is encountered, it is usually associated with cancer of the lung.

The right distal position can be used to locate the different lobes of the material left lung, and simultaneously the location of disharmony in the energetic left Lung. However, in my experience this is accomplished more readily and accurately using the Special Lung position, as shown in Figs. 2-2, 2-3, and 2-4 (Chapter 2).

Right Diaphragm, Pleura, and Esophagus positions

Again, with a light touch, the Diaphragm position is evaluated by rolling the index finger proximally toward the middle position, and then the middle finger distally toward the distal position. The goal is to determine whether or not the fingers sense an Inflated quality, as if the fingers are going uphill. If the Inflated quality is felt coming from both directions, qi stagnation is present in the right diaphragmatic area.

The presence of a pleural pathology is discernible when the distal aspect of the right Diaphragm position is either more Inflated or Rougher than the proximal aspect.

Fig. 4-22 Pleura position

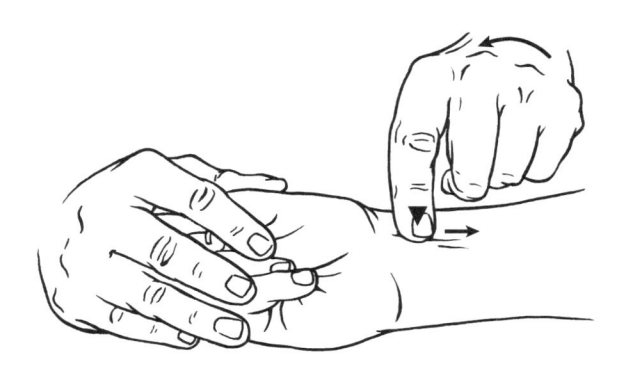

The presence of esophageal qi stagnation is discernible when the proximal aspect of the right Diaphragm position is either more Inflated or Rougher than the distal aspect. A Slippery quality instead of a Rough quality is a sign of esophageal food stagnation.

Fig. 4-23 Esophagus position

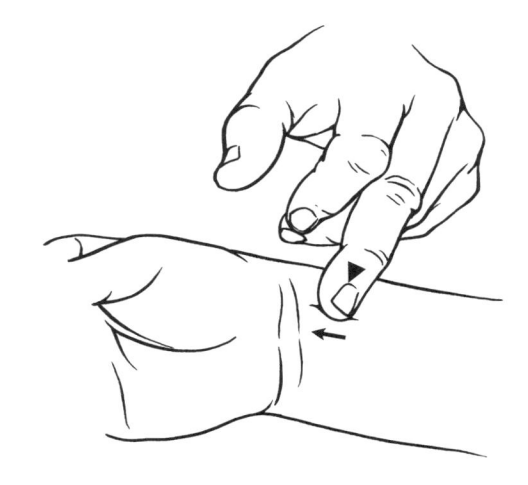

Right middle position

PRINCIPAL RIGHT MIDDLE POSITION

The harder qualities here, such as Tense and Tight, as well as Robust Pounding, are indications of Stomach heat from excess and deficiency, respectively. Another quality commonly found in the Stomach position is Inflated (indicating gas and qi stagnation), and rarely, Hollow and Slippery (both associated with gastritis and ulcers).

The more pliable qualities in this position, such as Spreading, Deep, Reduced Substance, Feeble-Absent, and Empty, are indications of Spleen qi deficiency. When Spleen qi deficiency and Stomach heat coexist, the Stomach heat impulse is felt more in the lateral-central part of the position, while Spleen qi deficiency is accessed on the more medial Spleen position, described below. Sometimes, simultaneous Spleen qi deficiency and Stomach heat are also indicated by a Change in Quality from Tense or Tight to Feeble, Absent, or Empty.

Fig. 4-24   Right middle position

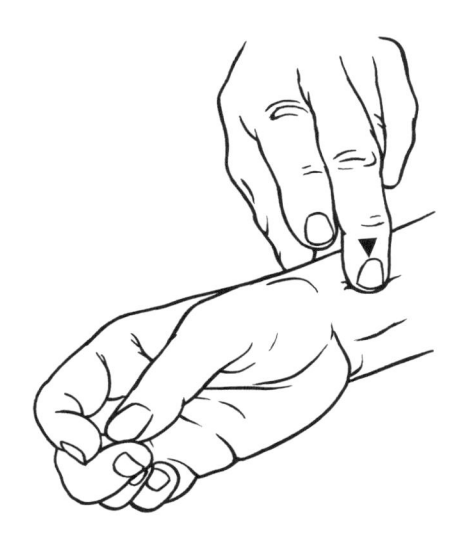

SPLEEN POSITION

On the right middle position, the middle finger is rolled medially and superficially toward the ulna to access the Spleen position, searching for a very superficial Inflated

Fig. 4-25   Spleen position

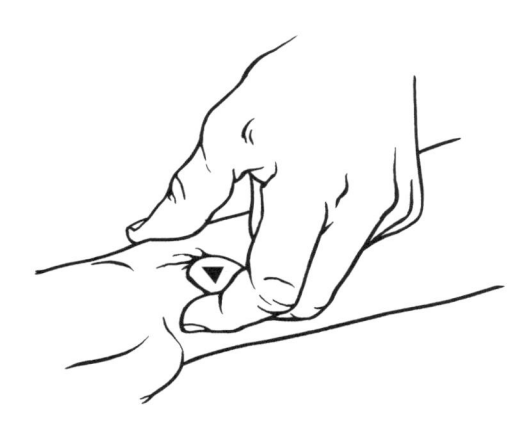

quality between the vessel and the flexor carpi radialis.

STOMACH-PYLORUS EXTENSION AND DUODENUM POSITIONS

The Stomach-Pylorus Extension position is palpated at approximately the first phalangeal joint by laying the left middle finger along the artery in the proximal direction from the right middle position, and rolling somewhat medially. In this position, the goal is to sense a change in quality from the principal position. Frequently found qualities are Inflated (with extreme Spleen qi deficiency), Tight, Choppy, Biting, and sometimes Hollow and Slippery, when an ulcer is present.

Fig. 4-26 Stomach-Pylorus Extension position

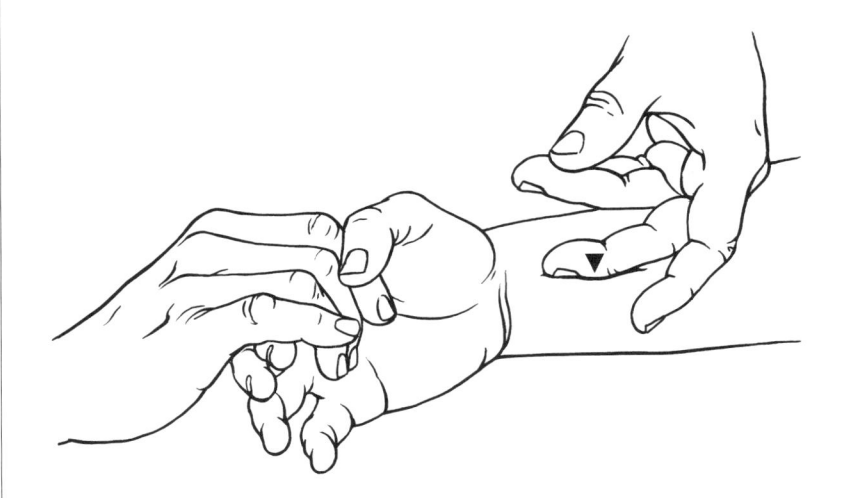

Pathology in the duodenum is reflected when the quality in the Stomach-Pylorus Extension position and in the Small Intestine position (see below) are the same, often Tight and/or Slippery, indicating a duodenal ulcer and/or energetic disharmony in this area. An Inflated quality here signifies a less severe energetic and physical pathology.

PERITONEAL POSITION

When both the Ulnar Engorgement position and Spleen positions are present, usually Inflated, it was Dr. Shen's contention that there was a problem in the abdominal, or more technically speaking, the peritoneal cavity. Most often this involved the pancreas, with either inflammation or tumor, less often with depleted enzymatic activity, and never involving its endocrine function (insulin). However, other kinds of tumors in the cavity (including the intestines), ascites, and more rarely trauma had to be considered.

Right proximal position

PRINCIPAL RIGHT PROXIMAL POSITION (BLADDER POSITION)

According to Dr. Shen, the health of the Bladder is reflected in the center of this position. I have found this to be true only when there is pathology in the Bladder, Small Intestine, or pelvic organs. Otherwise, I consider this position to represent Kidney yang, manifested by the more pliable qualities (Feeble-Absent or Changing). At the other end of the spectrum, severe Kidney yin deficiency can also manifest here, as on the left proximal position, with the harder qualities of Tight or Wiry, with Wiry indicative of pain, frequently menstrual.

The commonly found qualities in this position are Tense, Tight, Wiry, Deep, Reduced Substance, Feeble-Absent, as well as Changes in Qualities, Amplitude, and Intensity. The Pounding, Flooding-Excess, Slippery, and Choppy qualities are less frequently encountered. The qualities of excess (Flooding-Excess and Pounding) indicate acute and fulminating infection of the intestines or pelvic organs.

Fig. 4-27   Right proximal position

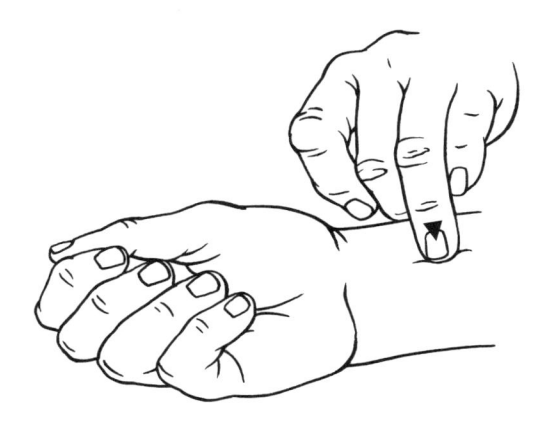

SMALL INTESTINE POSITION

The Small Intestine position is accessed on the right proximal position by rolling the ring finger distally toward the right middle position. The usual qualities found here are Tense, Tight, Biting, Slippery, and Muffled. Vibration and Choppy qualities are also sometimes encountered.

Fig. 4-28   Small Intestine position

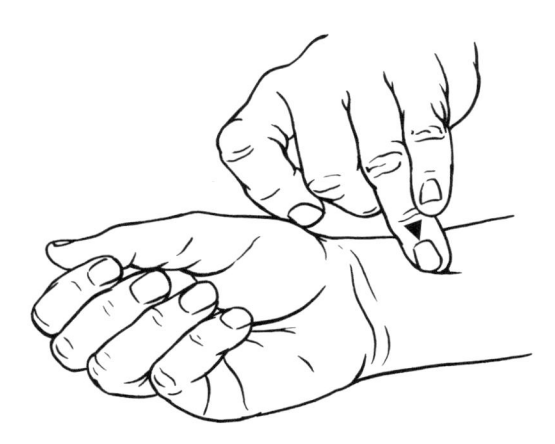

Right Pelvis/Lower Body position

The right Pelvis/Lower Body position is palpated in the same way as the corresponding position on the left side, except that the practitioner uses the left ring finger. As on the left wrist, qualities frequently found here are Tense, Tight, Slippery, Muffled, Change in Intensity, and Choppy.

Fig. 4-29 Right Pelvis/Lower Body position

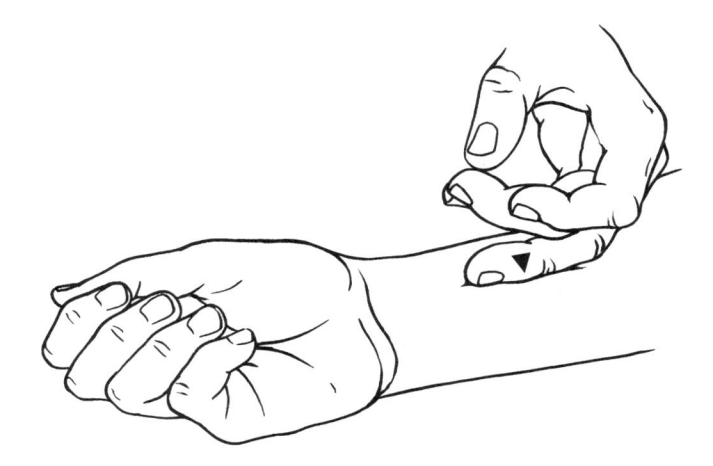

SIMILAR QUALITIES FOUND BILATERALLY AT THE SAME POSITION (BURNER)

The simultaneous appearance of the same quality at one position (burner) on both sides has a special significance, detailed in Chapter 14 and in Table 14-1. Some of the more common qualities found bilaterally are Floating, Cotton, Hollow Full-Overflowing, Inflated, Flat, Tense, Tight, Wiry, Slippery, Thin, Feeble-Absent, Empty, Hollow, and Vibration.

MUSCULOSKELETAL POSITIONS

I have observed that the Contemporary Chinese Pulse Diagnosis system emphasizes the organs. However, by rolling the fingers to the radial side of the area between the burners, one can detect musculoskeletal disorders. I have tended to ignore these positions while teaching, since patients usually tell the practitioner if something hurts.

The pulse is usually very Tight when there is musculoskeletal pathology. The Tight quality in these positions is also a sign of pain. Above the radial to the distal positions we can access the neck. Radial to the area between the distal and middle positions we can access the shoulder girdle. Radial to the area between the middle and proximal positions we access the hip, and radial to the area between the proximal and Pelvis/Lower Body positions we can access the knees.

RATE ON EXERTION

At the end of the examination the patient is asked to rotate one arm at the shoulder vigorously, immediately after which one takes the rate for 10 seconds and then multiplies this figure by six to get the rate on exertion. It is necessary to do this for only 10 seconds because after this the pulse quickly returns to its normal rate. I sometimes have two people do this and take the average, because the measurement can so easily be off by one or two beats, which amounts to six to 12 beats per minute when multiplied by six.

A REMINDER

The information gathered from the larger picture is, with rare exception, the pattern that must be dealt with first in the course of treatment if the therapy is to have lasting significance. Again, this larger picture includes the rhythm and rate, the qualities that are common or uniform over the large segments, the three depths, and the question of balance and chaos. For the best therapeutic results, I cannot overemphasize the importance of training oneself to approach pulse diagnosis in this manner.

The Learning Process

Learning pulse diagnosis at this level of complexity and subtlety is a slow process. For the beginner in Chinese medicine, as well as the experienced practitioner, it involves a series of advances and "aha!" experiences, interspersed with deflation, as new perplexities and questions are encountered. This is the normal learning progression during which the skill and material are absorbed in an organic manner, and which later become an integral part of the practitioner. It is an analog and not a digital process.

For the experienced clinician, I advise studying this methodology slowly, so that the rhythm of a successful practice is not interrupted. This is best accomplished by setting aside time, either by oneself or with colleagues, to devote to study, and allowing the material to gradually enter the practice at its own pace.

CHAPTER 5

Classification and Nomenclature of Pulse Qualities

CONTENTS

The Normal Pulse, 89
    Category, 89
    Attributes of the Normal pulse, 90
        Rhythm, 90
        Stability, 90
        Rate, 90
        Wave forms, 90
        Volume, 90
        Buoyancy, 90
        Shape, 90
        Balance, 91
            Depth, 91
            Position, 91
        ■ Fig. 5-1: Normal pulse wave, 91
    Individual attributes of normalcy from the literature, 91
        Normal characteristics of the organ pulses: *Inner Classic* (*Nei Jing*), 91
        ■ Table 5-1: Characteristics of the Normal pulse, 92
    Normal characteristics related to qi, spirit, and essence, 93
        Stomach qi, 93
        Spirit, 93
        Essence ('root'), 94
    Seasonal variations, 94
    Gender variations, 95

Age, 95
Pregnancy, 95
Aberrations from the Normal pulse, 96
Classification and Nomenclature of Pulse Qualities, 96
    Orientation to the style used in the classification of qualities, 97
        Ted Kaptchuk, 97
        Li Shi-Zhen, 97
        Wu Shui-Wan, 98
        Manfred Porkert, 98
        R.B. Amber, 98
        John Shen, 98
    The nine principal qualities, 98
    Format for presentation and discussion of the qualities, 98
    ■ Table 5-2: Qualities classified according to sensation (Hammer), 100
    ■ Table 5-3: Qualities classified according to Chinese condition (Hammer), 102
    ■ Table 5-4: Nine principal categories of qualities, 105

CHAPTER 5

Classification and Nomenclature of Pulse Qualities

This chapter is concerned with the style and format of the classification and nomenclature of the pulse qualities, which are described in detail in Chapters 6 through 11. We begin with a discussion of the Normal quality, from which all others are a departure.

The Normal Pulse

Why is it important to define the Normal pulse? The Normal pulse gives us a sensitive, precise, and measurable standard of health. It enables us to detect early deviations from health, and thereby provides us with a preventive medicine. All of these capabilities are wanting in our modern health care system.

Increasingly, people are acknowledging the failure of modern medicine to provide affordable healthcare. Therefore, the thrust is toward finding medical systems that emphasize the cheapest, most effective medicine—prevention. This growing recognition of the importance of what is missing renders pulse diagnosis, and our understanding of the Normal pulse, the most significant single body of current medical knowledge relevant to the development of an efficient preventive medical system. Pulse diagnosis, however, is only as useful as the proficiency with which it is practiced.

CATEGORY

In discussions of the pulse, many qualities have been associated with normal including moderate,[1] leisurely,[2] relaxed,[3] and long.[4] All of these sources state that the qualities associated with a Normal pulse can also be found with damp disorders if accompanied by signs of dampness. The exception is the Long pulse, which may be associated with heat if the pulse is a little Tense. My own opinion is that the Normal pulse cannot be defined as having any abnormal qualities if it is to serve as a baseline for health and a preventive medicine.[5]

It is important to say at the outset that pulse qualities that are abnormal for most people can, in rare instances, be normal in some individuals. Porkert[6] refers to something akin to this:

If on a very active individual all six sites uniformly show flooding or uniformly show large pulses—and, after very careful diagnosis, the total absence of any other pathological symptoms—such pulses must be considered to be normal pulses for this individual. Similar conclusions obtain for sanguine or phlegmatic types, if on such individuals at all sites of the pulse languid or minute pulses can be determined.

ATTRIBUTES OF THE NORMAL PULSE

In my experience, a Normal, healthy pulse must have all of the attributes listed below.

Rhythm

Consistently regular.

Stability

The amplitude and intensity are steady overall and in each position. The qualities, intensity, and amplitude are consistent over time and in each position.

Rate

Consistent with age (see Chapter 7). The pulses of women and children tend to be more Rapid than those of men. Athletes generally have Slower pulses.

There is some controversy about whether the rate is to be measured against the patient's or the practitioner's respiration. Because respiration can be very inconsistent in both, I don't consider either to be an effective gauge of rate.

A digital watch tends to interfere with an accurate count because each beat of a digital time piece has an arresting, spasmodic quality that distracts the pulse taker from measuring the pulse beats of the subject. During our seminars, it is my impression that more patients whose pulses were taken by students using digital watches were found with rates of 60 than was statistically justifiable. I use a 'kinetic' self-winding watch with a second hand.

Wave forms

The Normal wave is a sine curve that begins at the organ depth and gradually rises to the qi depth, then subsides again to the organ depth (Fig. 5-1). Unusual wave forms include the Hesitant, Hollow Full-Overflowing, Flooding-Excess, Flooding-Deficient, and Suppressed.

Volume

Moderate strength with spirit, depending on body build.

Buoyancy

Resilient, compressible, elastic, and with Robust Substance (intensity). The Normal pulse in a child (and a vegetarian) tends to be more Yielding, in a woman more Thin, and in a man more Wide.

Shape

Long and continuous, flowing smoothly with no turbulence. Pregnant women usually have more Slippery and more Rapid pulses.

Balance

DEPTH

Depth is balanced between superficial, middle, and deep. If the pulse has root, there is strength in the deep position. The qi depth is the lightest, increasing in breadth and strength as the organ depth is approached. Heavy people have Deeper pulses, and thin people more Superficial. The *Classic of Difficulties (Nan jing)* explains, "'At the surface' [superficial] [means that] the movement in the vessels occurs above the flesh."[7] In other words, "above the flesh," or above the qi depth, there should be no impulse or sensation. If a sensation is felt here, it means there is pathology.

POSITION

The relationship of one position to another is even and balanced. Normally, the qualities of the middle position tend to overflow into the other positions, thus occupying the most space. The proximal position occupies the second most space, and the distal position is the most confined.

Fig. 5-1 Normal pulse wave

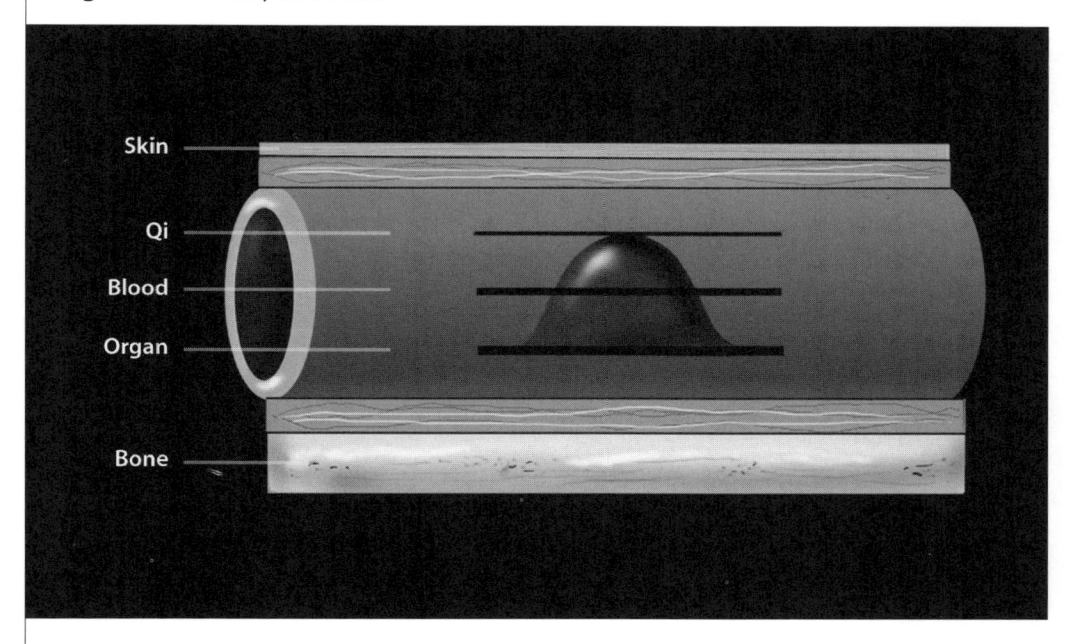

INDIVIDUAL ATTRIBUTES OF NORMALCY FROM THE LITERATURE

Normal characteristics of the organ pulses: *Inner Classic (Nei Jing)*

Here is a passage from the *Inner Classic* which describes the Normal pulses of the different organs:

> The five pulses should correctly appear in the following ways: The pulse of the liver should sound like the strings of a musical instrument; the pulse of the heart should sound like the blows of a hammer (continuous); the pulse of the spleen should be intermittent and irregular; the pulse of the lungs should be (soft) like hair (and feathers); the pulse of the kidneys should sound like a stone.[8]

Table 5-1 Characteristics of the Normal pulse

Following are some characteristics of the Normal pulse, which serves as a baseline and standard for health.

1. **Rhythm**
   Consistently regular

2. **Stability**
   The qualities, amplitude, and intensity are currently steady overall and in each position and over time

3. **Rate**
   Consistent with age

   Age and rate according to Dr. Shen:

AGE	RATE (per min.)
Birth → 4	90
4 → 10	84
10 → 15	78–80
16 → 40	76
41 → 50	72
51 → 70	66–68

4. **Wave**
   Sine curve

5. **Volume**
   Moderate strength and spirit, depending on body build

6. **Buoyancy**
   Resilient, compressible, elastic, with Robust Substance

7. **Shape**
   Long and continuous with no turbulence

8. **Balance**

   DEPTH

   - Balanced among superficial, middle, and deep
   - Qi depth is lightest, increasing in substance until the organ depth, which is greatest in substance and therefore has 'root'
   - Deeper in heavy people and more superficial in thin people

   POSITION

   - Middle position overflows into distal and proximal positions
   - Distal position most confined
   - Middle position least confined
   - Proximal position moderately confined

While the language of this passage is beautiful, even inspiring, I have not found one practitioner who has actually been able to use this material in the assessment of a pulse. In their time these metaphors likely had a concrete meaning to practitioners, which is incomprehensible to most of us in the context of our own times. Perhaps the reason these subtleties are lost to most of us today is because, regrettably, the pathology of our patients is more profound and complex than that of ancient agricultural societies. Pulse diagnosis in our time calls for more recognizable descriptions of qualities appropriate to the physiological depredations of the technological age, which this book attempts to realize.

NORMAL CHARACTERISTICS RELATED TO QI, SPIRIT, AND ESSENCE

Stomach qi

Contemporary Chinese Pulse Diagnosis

The concept of 'Stomach qi' is not used per se in this system of pulse diagnosis. Instead we find the terms *balance, stability, intensity,* and *moderation* to be more accessible. We assess the Stomach ('earth') at the right middle position and its associated complementary positions (see Chapters 4 and 12). We also look at the uniform qualities and the volume on the right side or 'digestive system' (see Chapter 14).

This ubiquitous aspect of the earth on the pulse and in the organism is mediated through the 'internal duct' of the Triple Burner, evaluated on the pulse by the balance of individual qualities among the burners and the individual positions (see Chapter 12).[9]

During life the earth feeds all of the organ systems. The integrity of the Spleen, Stomach, and Triple Burner qi is essential to the digestion, assimilation, transportation, and storage of all the organism's qi, blood, yin, and essence, apart from what is inherited from the ancestral qi. 'Stomach qi' is the term used by some for this earth energy. Because of its centrality to all functions, it is said to be reflected not only in the right middle position, but at all positions on the pulse.

Literature

This quality is defined in numerous ways. According to Porkert, it is the "force of the active and spontaneous maintenance of a harmonious balance, and of the distribution of all strains, stresses and disturbances."[10] Porkert defines the palpatory experience of 'Stomach qi' in two ways. One is that the pulse evens out, that is to say, if one position is too superficial, another will be relatively deep so that the sum of the depths of all the pulse positions will be a middle level pulse. In addition, the rate will be even and have an identical rhythm at all positions.

The mainstream modern Chinese approach, as described by Bensky, is that 'Stomach qi' in the pulse is characterized by moderation in speed, depth, and strength.[11] Deng agrees when he says that "A pulse with stomach qi is calm, even, moderate and the rhythm is regular."[12] Van Buren believes that a pulse has 'Stomach qi' if it "is not floating or deep and is regular and even."[13] Townsend and DeDonna access it at the middle depth where it is reflected in a smoothness and regularity of the pulse,[14] as does Dale.[15] Finally, Mann believes that it manifests in the "slowed-down" quality.[16]

Spirit

Contemporary Chinese Pulse Diagnosis

Spirit, in our model, is measured by the amplitude of the pulse, and is a function of the volume or yang force of the impulse.

Literature

As recorded by Bensky, spirit also relates to moderation, but here it refers to moderation in the shape or strength of the pulse. For example, a "weak pulse with spirit has a core of strength. A strong pulse with spirit has a feeling of elasticity."[17] Porkert refers to this as configurative force.[18] Van Buren believes that spirit "means moderation, not weak and draggy or excessively strong or tight or pushy."[19] Townsend and DeDonna also consider spirit to be felt as a quality of underlying strength, with slight elasticity.[20] Deng characterizes a pulse without spirit as one which, upon pressing, is "scattered or chaotic."[21] He does not, however, carry this forward to the concept of 'qi wild.'

Essence ('root')

Contemporary Chinese Pulse Diagnosis

Essence or 'root' is associated with Kidney qi. As explained in Chapter 2, there is both yin and yang essence. Deficiency of yin-essence is marked by a Wiry pulse, usually in the proximal positions, and yang-essence deficiency by an Absent or Empty quality in the proximal positions, and possibly a Doughy quality at the Neuro-psychological positions, a subject of continuing investigation.

Literature

To most modern Chinese, as noted by Bensky, root refers to an underlying strength in the Kidney position. Porkert says that its presence is a marker for a relatively good prognosis,[22] an opinion shared by Deng.[23] To Van Buren, root can either be the Kidney position or the deep depths in general. In both cases it is a marker for good Kidney energy.[24] To Townsend and DeDonna, the root refers to the deep level of the pulse at the proximal position. If the root is in good position, the pulse here will be

> clean and reasonably forceful, with a feeling of intrinsic strength and slight elasticity. The pulse should disappear slowly as pressure is increased, with a hint of pulse still present even at very deep pressure. If the pulse cuts off sharply on deepening pressure or weakens and fades very significantly, this indicates a weakness of the root.[25]

These authors are obviously pressing more deeply—probably to the bone—than our organ depth if "the pulse should disappear" with pressure. By contrast, we find that the strength of the pulse normally increases with pressure through the three depths, and is most robust at the organ depth.

SEASONAL VARIATIONS

Contemporary Chinese Pulse Diagnosis

I have found seasonal variations in those rare instances when I have taken the pulse of a person with little disharmony. Dr. Shen does not mention them. Subtle seasonal changes are lost in the overpowering presence of pulse patterns and qualities representing severe disharmonies and pathologies that I have found in my patients over the years.

Literature

In the *Inner Classic* there are several references relating the sensation or sound of the pulse and the seasons. Among these, Amber notes the following:

> [In the spring] the pulse of the stomach should be fine and delicate, like the strings of a musical instrument.... [In the summer] the pulse beats should be like the beats of a fine hammer.... During the long summer, the pulse should be soft and feeble... [In the autumn] the pulse is small and rough.... [In the winter] the pulse is small and hard, like a stone.[26]

GENDER VARIATIONS

Van Buren taught that yang cosmic qi enters the body on the right side, and yin cosmic energy on the left side. However, in its infinite wisdom, nature, needing to maintain balance, reverses this so that man and the cosmos balance each other. Therefore, the left side contains the male (yang) energy and the right side the female (yin) energy. For men to achieve balance, the yin channels are treated on the right and the yang channels on the left. The opposite holds true in the treatment of women.[27] He also believed that the left pulse was the most important side for diagnosing men, while the right was more important in women. Townsend and DeDonna state that while women's pulses are usually slightly faster than men's, there are no significant side-to-side differences.[28] Porkert agrees, at least for Indo-Europeans.[29] My own experience indicates that the pulse is normally somewhat stronger on the right side in women, and on the left side in men. While this was Worsley's original position, in the early 1980s he insisted that the left side should normally be more robust in everyone.

AGE

Contemporary Chinese Pulse Diagnosis

I have found that before the age of about eighteen, we can find extraordinary qualities indicative of severe disharmony and chaos, which are actually signs of rapid physiological growth and change, and not of pathology. In approaching the young this must be kept in mind. I have also found that the pulse tends to be more pliable in the young than in older patients.

Literature

Porkert observes:

> During infancy, as Chinese medical theory has it, an individual is 'entirely made up of yang.' Hence, at this age, good health is usually accompanied by rather superficial or accelerated pulses, compared with those of the adult. A consequence of this statement is that the appearance of true adult pulses such as a submerged or a slowed-down pulse, indicate a more critical situation than would be the case in an adult. During old age, all pulses, in particular those at the pedal sites, show a tendency toward infirmity [infirm pulses], i.e. yielding, narrow and submerged pulses.[30]

PREGNANCY

Contemporary Chinese Pulse Diagnosis

According to Dr. Shen, "If a woman's left chih [proximal] pulse is slippery (and both chih and ts'un [distal] pulses are a little tight, and in addition she has missed her menstruation), it is a sign of pregnancy."[31] I have found that from about three days to three months during a pregnancy, the entire pulse is Slippery.

The fetus is a boy, according to Dr. Shen, if there is a very Tense left distal position; if the fetus is a girl, there is no special change. Van Buren believes that the fetus is a boy if the left proximal position is very Tight, and a girl if the right proximal position is very Tight.[32] I have found the latter to be ninety percent accurate. According to Dr. Shen, a miscarriage is heralded by a suddenly Rapid rate, with either a Feeble-Absent or very Tight left proximal position; this is accompanied by dark lines on the tongue, and pain in the low back and abdomen.[33]

ABERRATIONS FROM THE NORMAL PULSE

The Normal pulse is rarely observed since the enormous stresses of modern life render all but the most enlightened dysfunctional. Still, the pulse remains a sensitive barometer of even these pressures, and is useful in guiding the practitioner to an accurate assessment of those aspects which need to be addressed by the patient for a return to harmony.

It should also be noted that medications often render the pulse uniform, obliterating both gross and subtle messages. To the uninitiated, the uniformity can be mistaken for normalcy, but the more experienced hand will recognize that the top of the Normal pulse wave has been flattened (Suppressed).

Some of the abnormal but uniform pulse qualities mentioned in Chapter 4 can appear to be Normal due to their uniformity. Commonly, these are the uniformly Tense pulses associated with what Dr. Shen terms the 'nervous system tense' condition, or the Hollow Full-Overflowing pulse associated with heat from excess in the blood. These are discussed at greater length in Chapters 10, 11, 13, and 14.

Uniformity can also be a sign of pretense during which, for a short period, a person can obliterate the subtleties of the pulse to protect themselves from detection of hidden problems and perceived weaknesses.

Classification and Nomenclature of Pulse Qualities

The differences in Chinese medical terminology are exemplified in the variety of terms adopted by various writers to describe the qualities of the pulse (see Table 1-1 in Chapter 1). In this book I have compared the pulse classifications and nomenclature of several prominent sources (Li Shi-Zhen, Wu Shui-Wan, John Shen, Ted Kaptchuk, Manfred Porkert, R.B. Amber) with my own terminology, which represents a distillation of these other systems as well as my own clinical experience. In addition, the reader is referred to the bibliography at the back of this book.

As explained in the introduction, the classification of pulses can be made on the basis of sensation or interpretation. In writing this book, I decided to organize the qualities by sensation. Table 5-2 at the end of this chapter summarizes the interpretation of qualities classified according to sensation which I have identified over the years. A detailed discussion of each of these qualities is the principal subject of this book. These qualities can potentially associate endlessly with each other. Yet, reassuringly, they form only a limited number of clinically significant combinations, each of which is explored in later chapters.

The discussion that fills the remainder of this book is not intended to be the final word on this thorny and involved discipline; it is clearly open to debate. The process of classification is one of continuing refinement.

Apart from the historical precedent of classification by sensation, I believe that the felt message from patient to clinician is the one that is most immediate and relevant to diagnosis. It is more instructive, more certain, and simpler to use the three-step method of identifying the sensation, adding a label, and then attaching meaning later. Only with experience can one automatically flash, for example, from a Hard sensation to the concept of yin deficiency. Furthermore, before we make the diagnostic leap and attach final meaning to what we feel, we must usually consult other signs such as the tongue, eyes, and color, as well as the overall symptom picture.

At first glance, my classification scheme appears more complicated than other systems. However, it is actually simpler because it corresponds to what one *senses* at one's finger tips, especially in relation to the presenting clinical condition. Our senses, and the sense of touch in particular, are much less developed than our intellectual faculties.

Feeling varying grades of hardness on the pulse is an exercise for which we are less prepared by education and acculturation, which overemphasizes the mental process of incorporating information. Still, for the sake of completeness, I have also classified the qualities according to condition in a general hierarchy of increasing seriousness for those who find both systems to be useful. (See Table 5-3 at end of chapter.)

Orientation to the style used in the classification of qualities

The style used in this book for the written expression of the qualities and their combinations requires some explanation. Take, for example, the combination Yielding Empty Thread-like. One might ask why the serial comma is not used to separate these three characteristics, as in Yielding, Empty, and Thread-like. To begin with, there are actually two rather than three qualities: Yielding is one quality, and Empty and Thread-like is the second. The practitioner senses the Tight and Empty qualities simultaneously, accompanied by a thin thread on the surface. (There are other Empty qualities that lack the Thread-like characteristic.)

As a general rule, I tend to avoid use of the serial comma in combinations of qualities because these terms are meant to express qualities that flow and cascade into each another, where they are experienced simultaneously as a single entity. They are felt sensations, and felt sensations have no grammar. In other words, I have written them the way they are felt and experienced on the pulse so that they have the same impact on the reader. Therefore, we have Yielding Empty Thread-like.

The exception to this rule are the qualities which define rate: Rapid and Slow. These are set off from other qualities by the word 'and' or 'with,' for example, Yielding Hollow Full-Overflowing and Slow. This is done to emphasize the importance of the rate in the overall pulse picture. In this example a Rapid rate with these other qualities has a totally different etiology from that of a Slow rate with the same qualities. The rate should be accessed separately and deliberately from the reading of the other qualities, with a watch or according to the number of beats per breath.

A few qualities are hyphenated. For example, the hyphenation of Full-Overflowing stems from the use by Dr. Shen of the term Overflowing for the sensation called Full in the literature. I put the two together since they feel the same and convey to those readers who are familiar with the literature what Dr. Shen is describing. The terms Feeble and Absent have been hyphenated as Feeble-Absent because they are so similar in sensation and interpretation that separating the two seemed redundant.

TED KAPTCHUK

In order to minimize the confusion that already exists regarding pulse terminology, I use the Kaptchuk system, which is largely based on that of Li Shi-Zhen, as a starting point from which to elaborate the enormous richness that pulse diagnosis offers (see Table 1-1 in Chapter 1).

LI SHI-ZHEN

There are few people today (I am certainly not one of them) who can compare their understanding of the pulse with that of Li Shi-Zhen. I therefore assume that it is because of my own shortcomings that I cannot understand certain aspects of his system. For example, I do not understand why he describes the Full pulse as being Deep, or why the Slippery and Tight pulses are always thought to be Rapid. Nor have I always found the Choppy and Arrhythmic pulses to be Slow.[34] The reader is again referred back to Table 1-1 for a complete list of his pulse classifications.

WU SHUI-WAN

Wu Shui-Wan's classification of pulse qualities (Table 1-1) largely follows that of Li Shi-Zhen, except for some significant differences set forth in Wu's book *The Chinese Pulse Diagnosis*.

MANFRED PORKERT

The qualities listed in Porkert's book are included in Table 1-1 since I refer frequently to his work in the detailed discussion of each quality later in this book. I have turned to Porkert as a reference because I find that his interpretations and descriptions vary refreshingly from other lists that have been monotonously handed down century after century without significant creative input.

R.B. AMBER

Amber's system of pulse classification is discussed here less for its immediate usefulness than for its historical importance. His book, *The Pulse in Occident and Orient,* is the only single-volume work which describes four major traditions of pulse diagnosis. Furthermore, it is the first book of which I am aware that was written specifically on this subject in English. Lastly, it is mentioned as a small tribute to a pioneer who, like Wilhelm Reich, literally paid with his life for practicing a medicine that deviated from the accepted norm of an intolerant medical establishment, which hounded him into jail and to an untimely death in a veteran's hospital. For specific interpretations of the conditions, readers are referred to his book.

JOHN H.F. SHEN

It is unfortunate that, over the course of his life, Dr. Shen wrote less than twenty pages about a subject to which he dedicated over six decades years of study and practice, and in which, from my own long years of close association, I can say that he was a true master.

Dr. Shen stated that the twenty-eight principal pulse qualities can be reduced to nineteen in practice. This belies the extraordinary number of qualities that I have recorded during the years in which I followed him. He has indicated that he simplified his message so as not to discourage students from pursuing this complex discipline. I see my function differently from his. My purpose is to chronicle the subject in all of its intricacy and let future generations choose for themselves. Having stretched the frontiers himself, Dr. Shen's work must be seen by others as a stepping stone to further knowledge, and not as the final word on the subject.

The nine principal qualities

Table 5-4 at the end of this chapter illustrates the nine principal categories of qualities, of which the other qualities are subsidiaries. In the table they are presented in very general synchronization with the eight principles of traditional Chinese medicine.

Format for presentation and discussion of the qualities

Except for the rate and rhythm, the outline presented below will be used as the basis for discussing the pulse qualities in later chapters. The substance of the information is drawn from Dr. Shen, from my own experience, and from the sources listed in the bibliography.

Category places the quality within the larger context of the classification according to the various sources.

The actual **feeling sensation** is described according to my own and other sources.

The **general interpretation** includes Dr. Shen's, my own, and others. It describes the quality in general, particularly when it is found over the entire pulse. Sections entitled 'Contemporary Chinese Pulse Diagnosis' provide this system's view of a particular quality, while other sources are cited in the endnotes.

Under **combinations** are interpretations of some of the common and important combinations of qualities.

Positions list the areas where a pulse quality commonly appears, with the relevant interpretations. In some cases it is more useful to organize the positions according to sensation, and in others, by condition. Under either arrangement, both will be discussed.

Information under the subheading of **bilaterally at same position** discusses similar qualities that frequently occur together at the same burner or among the burners at the distal, middle, and proximal positions, as well as between principal positions.

Under the subheading of **each side**, the significance of a quality that is present at all the positions on one wrist is addressed.

Interpretations of the qualities at **individual positions** are considered next. These include the various principal and complementary positions.

The remainder of this book discusses the pulse in detail. In this chapter we have looked at the pulse in its entirety, with an initial investigation of the Normal pulse, our baseline for health. Next discussed are the rate and rhythm, being the two most significant and critical diagnostic indicators. Each quality is then explored in terms of sensation and interpretation, and each position is discussed in a separate chapter. Then, vertically, the three depths—qi, blood, and organ—are examined. This is followed by a discussion of the uniformity of a quality over the entire pulse, and on the right and left sides, and then on the three horizontal positions, or three burners. The final chapters are devoted to a discussion of the psychological disharmonies associated with the pulses, prognostication, and interpretation.

Table 5-2 Qualities classified according to sensation (Hammer)

Normal quality
    Moderate
    Languid
    Leisurely-relaxed
    Slowed down
    Long
    Wide Moderate

Rhythm
    At rest:
        Rate measurable without missed beat
            Change in Rate at Rest
                Occasional
                      Small
                      Large
                Constant
                    Small
                    Large
        Rate measurable with missed beat
            Intermittent
                Constantly Intermittent
                    Frequently missed beats
                    Infrequently missed beats
                Inconsistently Intermittent
            Interrupted
        Rate not measurable
            Interrupted
                Constant
                Occasional
                Sudden Transient
                Literature:
                    'hurried'
                    'knotted'
    On exertion:
        Large increase in rate
            Constant
            Occasional
        Small increase, no change, or decrease in rate
            Small increase
            Same rate or decrease

Pseudo-Arrhythmia
    Hesitant Wave
    Large Change in Amplitude and Intensity
    Unstable

Stability
    Qi:
        Entire pulse
            Circulation
                Occasional Change in Intensity
            'Qi wild'
                Burners and positions vary greatly in qualities
                Empty
                Empty Thread-like
                Leather
                Minute
                Change in Quality
                Qualities Shifting from Side to Side
                Scattered
                Yielding Hollow Full-Overflowing and Slow
                Yielding Hollow Full-Overflowing and Rapid
                Sides vary greatly in substance
                Muffled
                Empty Interrupted-Intermittent
                Yielding Hollow and Interrupted-Intermittent
                Very high fever and very low rate
                Very low fever and very high rate
        Single position
            Extreme Qi, Yin, Blood & Essence
            Deficiency of a Yin Organ
                Empty
                Change in Quality
                Change in Intensity
                Change in Amplitude
                Unstable
                Nonhomogeneous
    Blood:
        Circulation out of control at individual positions
            Leather-like Hollow
            Rapid
            Slow
        Out of control over entire pulse
            Very Tense or Tight Hollow Full-Overflowing
        Circulation erratic over entire pulse
            Constant Change in Intensity
            Change in Intensity shifting from side to side

Rate
    Rapid:
        Bounding
    Slow:
        Mildly slow
        Moderately slow
        Very Slow
    Right and left side:
        Pulses vary in rate

Volume
    Robust:

    Hollow Full-Overflowing
    Robust Pounding
    Flooding Excess
    Inflated
        Inflated Yielding
        Inflated Moderately Tense
        Inflated Very Tense
Reduced:
    Suppressed Wave at qi depth
    Suppressed Pounding
    Yielding at qi depth
    Feeble at qi depth
        Absent at qi depth
        Spreading at blood depth
        Yielding Partially Hollow at blood depth
        Flooding Deficient (Retarded, 'push pulse')
        Diffuse
        Reduced Substance
        Reduced Pounding
        Deep
        Flat
        Feeble
        Absent
        Muffled
        Dead

Depth
    Superficial:
        Floating
            Yielding
            Tense
            Tight
        Cotton
        Empty
        Yielding Empty Thread-like (soggy, soft)
        Leather (drum-like)
        Minute
        Scattered
        Hollow
            Yielding Partially Hollow
            Leather-like Hollow
            Hollow Full-Overflowing
            Hollow Interrupted-Intermittent
    Submerged:
        Deep
        Hidden (primarily in literature)
            Hidden Tense
            Hidden Yielding
        Firm (primarily in literature)
            Firm Tense
            Firm Yielding

Width
    Wide:

        Blood
            Excess (entire pulse)
                Least Wide
                    Blood Unclear
                Less Wide
                    Blood Heat
                Moderately Wide
                    Blood Thick
                Extremely Wide
                    Tense Hollow Full-Overflowing
            Deficient (individual position)
                Leather-like Hollow
                    Sudden severe hemorrhage
                        Rapid rate: imminent
                        Slow rate: recent
        Organ
            Excess (usually one position)
                Extremely Wide
                    Flooding Excess
            Deficient
                Less Wide
                    Diffuse
                Moderately Wide
                    Yielding Hollow Full-Overflowing
                    Yielding Ropy
    Narrow:
        Thin
            Thin Tight
            Thin Yielding
        Yielding Empty Thread-like
        Restricted

Length
    Extended
        Long
            Long Robust Pounding
    Diminished:
        Restricted
        Short 'brief'
            Short Yielding
            Short Tense
        Bean (Spinning)

Shape
    Fluid:
        Slippery
    Non-fluid:
        Hard
            Taut
            Tense
            Tight

Wiry
Ropy
    Ropy Yielding
    Ropy Tense
    Ropy Tight
Uneven
    Choppy
    Vibration
        Smooth
        Rough
    Nonhomogeneous
    Doughy

Modifiers
Reduced or Robust
Rough
Smooth
Subtle
Biting

Ephemeral
Separating

Wave
Normal
Hollow Full-Overflowing
Flooding
    Excess
    Deficient
Hesitant

Anomalous
Three Yin or Hidden Left Side (*san yin mai*)
Transposed (*fan quan mai*)
Ganglion
Local trauma
Split vessel
Multiple radial arteries

Table 5-3 Qualities classified according to Chinese condition (Hammer). Qualities under each heading are generally listed in order of increasing seriousness.

1. Normal
    Moderate
    Languid
    Leisurely-relaxed
    Slowed down
    Long
    Wide Moderate

2. Deficiency
    A. Qi and yang
        Yielding at qi depth
        Feeble-Absent at qi depth
        Spreading at blood depth
        Flooding Deficient Wave
        Diffuse
        Reduced Pounding
        Reduced Substance
        Deep
        Flat
        Feeble
        Absent
        Firm Deficient
        Hidden Deficient
        Short Yielding
        Muffled
        Dead
    B. Parenchymal damage
        Nonhomogeneous
        Restricted
        Rough Vibration
        Muffled
        Dead
        Bean (Spinning)
    C. Blood deficiency
        General
            Spreading
            Yielding Partially Hollow
            Thin
                Thin Yielding (blood and qi deficiency)
                Thin Tight (blood and yin deficiency)
            Deep
            Leather
        Heart blood deficiency
            Rate Increases Excessively on Exertion
    D. Yin (heat from deficiency)
        General
            Tight
            Wiry
            Ropy Tight
            Very Tight (Hollow) Full-Overflowing
        Heart
            Hesitant Wave
            Tight at Pericardium or left distal position
    E. Essence
        Leather
        Wiry
        Doughy at Neuro-psychological positions

F. Internal wind
　　Floating Tight (blood and yin deficiency)

3. Stability
　A. Heart qi agitation (entire pulse)
　　i. Mild Heart qi agitation
　　　　Smooth Vibration
　　ii. Moderate Heart qi agitation
　　　　Occasional Change in Rate at Rest
　　iii. Severe Heart qi agitation
　　　　Constant Change in Rate at Rest
　　　　Occasionally Intermittent/Interrupted
　　iv. Severe heart shock
　　　　Rough Vibration and Tight over entire pulse
　　　　Bean (Spinning) at distal (positions)
　　v. Heart qi and blood deficiency
　　　a. Change in Rate
　　　　　Change in Rate on Exertion
　　　　　　Heart blood deficiency
　　　　　　　Large increase
　　　　　　Slight Heart qi deficiency
　　　　　　　Very small increase
　　　　　　Heart qi deficiency
　　　　　　　Stays the same
　　　　　　Heart yang deficiency
　　　　　　　Decrease
　　　　　Constant Change in Rate at Rest
　　　　　　Moderate Heart qi deficiency
　　　b. Change in Intensity over entire pulse
　　　　　Moderate Heart qi deficiency
　　　c. Rough Vibration at left distal position
　　　　　Heart qi deficiency and parenchymal damage
　　vi. Heart yang deficiency
　　　　Moderate
　　　　　Heart Large
　　　　Severe
　　　　　Rate stays same or decreases on exertion
　　　　Very Severe
　　　　　Intermittent/Interrupted Yielding Hollow
　B. 'Qi wild' (entire pulse)
　　Burners and positions vary greatly in qualities
　　Change in Amplitude
　　Empty
　　Yielding Empty Thread-like (yin and yang deficient)
　　Leather (essence, yin, blood)
　　Minute (yang, qi, blood)
　　Change in Qualities
　　Change in Qualities and/or Substance from side-to-side
　　Muffled
　　Scattered (exhaustion of yang)
　　Yielding Hollow Full-Overflowing
　　　Rapid
　　　Slow
　　　Yielding Hollow and Interrupted/Intermittent
　C. Separation of Yin and Yang (individual positions)
　　Nonhomogeneous
　　Unstable
　　Empty
　　Change in Amplitude
　　Change in Intensity
　　Change in Quality
　D. Fear/terror
　　Bean (Spinning)

4. Stagnation
　A. Qi
　　i. External
　　　Wind
　　　　Floating Tense
　　　Wind-cold
　　　　Floating Tense and Slow
　　　Wind-heat
　　　　Floating Yielding and Rapid
　　　Wind-damp
　　　　Floating Slippery
　　　Cotton
　　ii. Internal
　　　Medications
　　　　Suppressed
　　　Liver qi stagnation
　　　　Taut
　　　　Occasional Change in Intensity
　　　Liver qi stagnation and heat from excess
　　　　Tense
　　　Qi trapped in organ
　　　　Inflated Yielding Tense
　　　Qi trapped outside of organ
　　　　Flat
　　　Qi very stagnant (obstructed) within organ
　　　　Restricted
　　　Liver wind
　　　　Tight Floating
　　　Qi unable to circulate between organs or burners
　　　　Short (excess and deficient)
　　　Stagnation in hollow organ due to obstruction or in any organ due to trauma or shock
　　　　Bean (Spinning)
　　　Stagnation at cellular-molecular-chromosomal level (absolute yin)
　　　　Muffled
　　　　Dead
　B. Blood and circulation
　　i. Blood out of control (Hollow [scallion])
　　　Leather-like Hollow
　　　　Hemorrhage from yin organ

Very Tense/Tight Hollow Full-Overflowing
    Potential brain hemorrhage (stroke)
Yielding Partially Hollow
    Gradual slow hemorrhage
ii. Blood stagnation
    Tissues
        Choppy
        Liver Engorgement positions present
        Inflated Very Tense
    Vessels
        Slippery at blood depth
        Rough Vibration at blood depth
        Ropy Tense
    Cellular–Molecular Level
        Muffled
        Dead
iii. Circulatory system
    Heart qi agitation and heat from excess
        Too Rapid
    General qi or Heart qi deficiency
        Too Slow
    Blood toxicity
        Deep and very Slow
        Blood Unclear
    Heat from excess and turbid blood
        Robust Pounding at blood depth
        Wide Excess
            Blood Heat
            Blood Thick
        Tense Hollow Full-Overflowing
        Slippery at blood depth
    Vessel walls damaged
        Separation of yin-yang in vessels
            Ropy Yielding
            Ropy Tense
        Rough Vibration at blood depth
C. Essence
    Proximal positions very Taut
D. Heat from excess
    External
        Floating Yielding and Slow
    Internal
        Very Long
        Inflated Moderately Tense
        Tense
        Pounding with Force
        Flooding Excess Wave
        Ropy Tense
        Very Tense Hollow Full-Overflowing
E. Damp
    Slippery
F. Cold
    i. External
        Floating Tense and Slow
    ii. Internal
        Very Tight/Wiry
        Firm Excess
        Hidden Excess
        Short Excess
G. Wind
    External
        Floating Tense
    Internal
        Floating Tight (heat from excess)
H. Food
    Esophagus position: Slippery
    Short Excess
    Bean (Spinning): intestinal obstruction w/severe pain
I. Parenchymal damage
    Rough Vibration at individual positions

5. Systems
A. 'Nervous system'
    i. Tense
        Entire pulse Tense (consistently)
            Constitutional
                Slow rate
            Non-constitutional
                Normal or Rapid rate
    ii. Weak
        Early
            Yielding Floating and Rapid
            Smooth Vibration
        Middle
            Tight and Pounding just above organ depth
            Rapid
        Late
            Feeble-Absent
B. 'Circulatory system'
    Very Slow rate
    Consistent Change in Intensity
C. 'Digestive system'
    Eating too rapidly
        Right side
            Very Tight at surface of pulse
    Eating irregularly
        Right side
            Reduced Substance → Feeble-Absent
D. 'Organ system'
    Entire left side
        Deep Feeble-Absent → Absent

6. Pain
Early: Tight-Wiry and Rapid
Profound with fear: Bean (Spinning)
With blood stasis: Choppy Wiry

Table 5-4 Nine principal categories of qualities

Quality	Function	Sensation	Tongue	Pathology
1. RHYTHM	Most critical measure of Heart function	Regular	Normal	Heart and circulation normal
				Heart qi relatively strong
	Pivotal quality since Heart is 'emperor'	Arrhythmic	Pale	Heart relatively weak
			Red purple	Blood Stagnation
		Arrhythmic Hollow	Pale	'Qi wild'
2. STABILITY	Balance and/or contact between yin and yang in either the entire organism or within one organ system	Yielding Hollow Full-Overflowing over entire pulse	Pale, swollen, wet	'Qi wild'
		Change in Qualities/Amplitude over entire pulse		
	Stability is necessary for even minimal function	Inconsistent Change in Intensity over entire pulse	Red, dry	Qi Stagnation, 'nervous system' imbalance
	Instability indicates severe dysfunction	Consistent Change in Intensity over entire pulse	Red purple pale, wet	Blood circulation function of Heart impaired
		Change in Intensity, Qualities, or Amplitude at one position	Depends on yin organ system	Severe organ, qi, blood, yin deficiency ('qi wild')
		Unstable impulse changing position	Depends on yin organ system	Very severe organ, qi, blood, yin deficiency ('qi wild')
		Leather-like Hollow	Variable	Blood out of control, hemorrhage
3. RATE	Activity of Heart and circulation	1. Rapid: Heart shock 2. Slow: Heart qi deficiency	1. Coat thin, yellow red tip; vertical line 2. Pale underneath; vertical line	1. Increased activity of Heart/circulation 2. Decreased activity of Heart/circulation

	Heat and cold
	1. Heat
		1. Rapid, Robust Pounding
		  a. Very Rapid
		  b. Slightly Rapid
			1. Coating thick yellow, body very red
			2. Coating thin yellow, patchy, dry; body thin, red
				1. Heat from excess
				2. Heat from deficiency

	2. Cold	2. Slow
		  a. Acute: slightly Slow
		  b. Chronic: very Slow
			1. Coating thin white, body normal
			2. Coating white and wet, body pale and swollen
				1. Acute, external pathogenic factor
				2. Chronic qi-deficient cold

Quality	Function	Sensation	Tongue	Pathology
4. VOLUME	Spirit Functional heat Yang force	Amplitude 1. Robust a. Excess i. Full-Overflowing ii. Flooding Excess iii. Pounding .... b. Moderately Inflated .... 2. Reduced: a. Flooding Deficient .... b. Feeble Deep c. Absent	Red body " " " " Normal, slightly red and swollen in one area .... Coating thin white, body pale .... Coating thin white, body swollen, wet	Excess yang Excess heat in qi & blood " Excess heat in yin organs " .... Heat or qi trapped in organ or area .... Overwork: moderate qi deficiency .... b. Severe qi deficiency c. More severe qi deficiency
5. DEPTH	Location and stage of disease process	1. Superficial a. Floating: stagnant qi b. Cotton: stagnant qi .... 2. Deeper a. Deficient qi i. Deep: mild ii. Hidden: very deficient .... b. Excess qi Hidden Excess	Coating thin, patchy, white, normal .... Coating and body depend on type and degree of deficiency .... Coating/body depend on nature of excess	a. External pathogenic factor b. Superficial qi stagnation due to trauma, resignation .... Disease is deeper, internal, and/or later-stage chronic deficient .... Stagnation due to sudden severe excess
6. WIDTH	Activity & condition of substance: primarily blood (some qi) i. Excess a. Toxicity .... b. Heat .... c., d. Heat and viscosity .... ii. Deficiency	Intensity a. Slightly Wide .... b. Moderately Wide .... c., d. Very Wide .... Thin	 Normal .... Body red .... Body red .... Body pale	 a. Blood unclear .... b. Blood heat .... c. Blood thick .... Blood deficient
7. LENGTH	Condition of qi and circulation of qi between organs and burners Type and degree of disease activity	1. Long .... Long Robust Pounding .... 2. Short: a. Excess .... b. Deficiency	Normal .... Body slightly red Depends on type of stagnation .... Body pale	Normal .... Heat from excess .... a. Stagnation of qi, phlegm, food, blood .... b. Qi deficiency

Quality	Function	Sensation	Tongue	Pathology
8. WAVE	Variable	1. Normal 2. (Hollow) Full Overflowing 3. Flooding Excess 4. Flooding Deficient 5. Hesitant	1. Normal 2. Body red and dry 3. Body very red and thick, coating w/raised papillae 4. Pale, swollen, wet 5. Dry, bright red & shiny, raised red on end	1. None 2. Heat from excess and deficiency in the blood 3. Heat from excess in organ 4. Qi deficiency 5. Obsessive, mono-maniacal

9. SHAPE	Elasticity
	1. Fluid (yielding): excess yin
	2. Static (hard)
	a. Excess:
	  Qi
	  Qi and heat
	  Blood
	  Heat in blood vessels
	....
	b. Deficiency:
	  Yin
	  Yin-essence
	
	....
	Qi
	
	c. Parenchymal damage
		Slippery
		
		Taut
		Tense
		Choppy
		Ropy
		....
		
		Tight
		Wiry, Leather
		
		....
		Diffuse Feeble-Absent
		....
		Empty Thread-like
		Scattered
		Minute
		....
		Rough Vibration
		Nonhomogeneous
		Muffled
			Coating wet
			
			Normal
			Body slightly to very red
			Red-purple
			Red, dry
			....
			
			Coating dry, red patchy
			Very dry, red, thin to no coating
			....
			Pale, swollen, wet
				Damp stagnation
				
				Qi stagnation
				Qi stagnation and heat
				Blood stagnation
				Heat: vessels lose elasticity
				....
				
				Heat from deficiency
				Heat from extreme deficiency
				
				....
				Deficiency of qi-yang
				....
				Instability
				Separation of yin/yang
				
				....
				Parenchymal damage

CHAPTER 6

Rhythm and Stability

CONTENTS

Rhythm, 113
    Classification of arrhythmias, 114
    ■ Table 6-1: Classification of arrhythmias, 114
    Changes in rhythm and rate at rest, 114
        Rate measurable without missed beats, 114
            Change in Rate at Rest, 115
                Occasional Change in Rate at Rest, 115
                    Small, 115
                    Large, 116
                Constant Change in Rate at Rest, 117
                    Mild Heart qi deficiency ('Heart disease'), 117
        Rate measurable with missed beats, 118
        Intermittent, 119
            Constantly Intermittent, 119
                Frequently missed beats, 119
                Infrequently missed beats, 120
            Inconsistently Intermittent, 120
        Interrupted, 121
        Rate not measurable, 121
        Interrupted, 121
            Constantly Interrupted, 121
                Conditions associated with the Constantly Interrupted quality, 121
                    Heart qi and yang deficiency, 121
                    Heart blood stagnation ('Heart small'), 122
                    Phlegm confusing the Heart orifice, 122
                    Phlegm fire disturbs the Heart orifice, 122

Phlegm obstructs the Heart orifice, 123
Occasionally Interrupted, 124
Sudden Transient Interrupted, 124
Changes in rate on exertion, 124
Constant Large Increase in Rate on Exertion, 125
Occasional Large Increases in Rate on Exertion, 125
Decrease in Rate on Exertion, 125
Pseudo-arrhythmias, 125
- Fig. 6-1: Hesitant Wave, 126
Hesitant Wave, 126
Stability, 127
'Qi wild' condition, 128
Qualities associated with the 'qi wild' condition, 128
Related signs and symptoms, 129
Etiology, 129
Severe early environmental deprivation, including food and shelter, 129
Overwork during childhood, 129
Exercise beyond one's energy in early life, 129
Protracted menorrhagia in girls, 130
Sudden cessation of intense, prolonged exercise, 130
Sudden extraordinary episode of lifting, 131
Substance abuse, 131
'Qi wild' qualities with regular rate, 131
Empty types of 'qi wild' qualities, 131
Empty, 132
Leather, 132
Empty Thread-like (soggy, soft), 132
Scattered, 132
Minute, 133
Yielding Hollow types of 'qi wild' qualities: Yielding Hollow Full-Overflowing and Slow, 133
Yielding Ropy Hollow, 133
Qi wild qualities characterized by change, 133
Change In Qualities, 133
- Fig. 6-2: Change in qualities, 134
Change in qualities over the entire pulse, 134
Change in qualities in one position, 134
Change in qualities bilaterally in one burner, 134
'Qi wild' with irregular rate, 135
Empty or Yielding Hollow Interrupted or Intermittent (Constant), 135
Recapitulation of the 'qi wild' quality, 135
Instability related to Heart and circulation, but unrelated to rhythm and rate, 136
Entire pulse, 136
Change in Intensity, 136
- Fig. 6-3: Change in Intensity, 136
Change in Intensity: constant over time, 136
Etiologies, 137
Circulation affects the Heart, 137
Emotional trauma, 137
Physical trauma, 137
Hypothermia, 137

Heart affects the circulation, 137
Change in Intensity: inconstant over time, 137
Change in Intensity undulating from one position to another, 138
Change in Intensity undulating from one wrist to another, 138
Change in Intensity affecting only one wrist, 138
Change in Amplitude over the entire pulse, 138
    Fig. 6-4: Change in Amplitude, 139
Individual positions, 139
    Principal individual positions, 139
    Complementary individual positions, 139
Distinguishing Change in Intensity and Amplitude from Change in Qualities, 139
Distinguishing Change in Intensity and Amplitude from Arrhythmia, 139
One side robust and other side reduced, 139
Separation of yin and yang at individual positions, 140
Nonhomogeneous, 140
Unstable, 140
    Positions, 140
        Bilateral at specific positions, 140
        Each wrist, 141
        Individual positions, 141
'Blood out of control' (reckless blood), 141
    Hemorrhage rapid, 142
        Leather-like Hollow, 142
        Very Tense-Tight Hollow Full-Overflowing, 142
    Hemorrhage gradual, 142
        Yielding Partially Hollow and Slow (Full-Overflowing when very serious), 142
    Fig. 6-5a: Rhythm flowchart, 143
    Fig. 6-5b: Rhythm flowchart (detail), 144
    Fig. 6-6: Stability flowchart, 145

CHAPTER 6

Rhythm and Stability

This chapter is concerned with rhythm and stability and includes qualities that can be found either over the entire pulse or just at individual positions. Those qualities classified under the heading of rhythm (see Fig. 6-5 at end of chapter) occur over the entire pulse at all three positions on both wrists. Those classified under the heading of stability (Fig. 6-6) may involve either the entire pulse or just one position.

Rhythm and stability are closely associated with mind and emotion. Amber believes that the pulse is "under direct control of the nervous system."[1] It is important to remember that Chinese medicine attributes the mind-controlling function to the Heart; all problems with rhythm therefore concern Heart function. The dynamic interrelationships among the Heart, mind, and 'nervous system' with rhythm and stability make up the picture that follows.

Rhythm

The integrity of the rhythm is the single most important facet of pulse diagnosis. Rhythm primarily, and rate secondarily, are reflections of cardiac function. Since the Heart is the emperor, with rare exceptions, the rhythm and the rate are the overriding considerations in diagnosis and treatment, and overshadow the significance of all other findings. While arrhythmias by themselves are not 'qi wild' qualities, some combinations of other qualities with arrhythmias are forms of the 'qi wild' disorder (see glossary).

The following arrhythmias described by Dr. Shen involve Heart function and often manifest simultaneously with abnormal qualities on the left distal position and Heart complementary positions. While I have retained his terminology, I have also attempted to translate it into terms familiar to students of traditional Chinese medicine, or into new terms that I find closer to our concepts of physiology and pathology. For example, I use the term Heart qi agitation to convey the meaning of Dr. Shen's 'Heart nervous.'

A few points should be noted. One is that all shock, especially emotional, affects the Heart. A second is that, with Heart shock, there is usually disharmony between the Kidney and Heart. The third is that one Heart condition can lead to another. For example, prolonged but mild heat in the Heart ('Heart tight') can cause Heart qi agitation

114 ❖ Rhythm and Stability

('Heart nervous'), and either of them can, over a period of time, lead to more serious Heart disorders, such as Heart blood deficiency ('Heart weak') or Heart qi deficiency ('Heart disease').

CLASSIFICATION OF ARRHYTHMIAS

In terms of classification, the standard format described in Chapter 5 for discussing pulse qualities is not helpful to our discussion of rhythm or rate. Instead, I have devised a different model that is more appropriate to this subject. Arrhythmias—or changes in rhythm—are classified in accordance with the parameters in Table 6-1. These six parameters of arrhythmias form a natural system of classification. They also allow for a detailed consideration of this subject.

Table 6-1 Classification of arrhythmias

Arrhythmias are classified by the following parameters:

1. Does the change in rhythm occur at rest or on exertion?

2. Is the rate measurable?

3. If measurable, are there missed beats (Arrhythmic)?

4. If there are missed beats, do they occur consistently after the same number of beats (Intermittent) or inconsistently (Interrupted)?

5. How often does the irregularity occur?

6. If there are no missed beats, is the change in rate occasional or constant, large or small?

CHANGES IN RHYTHM AND RATE AT REST

Rate measurable without missed beats

In this category of qualities there is a change in pulse rate at rest without missed beats; it may occur occasionally or continually, and may be small or large. During palpation, the pulse alternately speeds up and slows down. The patterns associated with the Occasional Change in Rate at Rest and Hesitant qualities are variations on what Dr. Shen refers to as 'Heart nervous' (Heart qi agitation).[2] I refer to the condition associated with Occasional Change in Rate at Rest as Heart qi agitation, and to the Hesitant quality as one manifestation of early and minimal Heart yin deficiency.

According to Dr. Shen, all changes in rate, which always involve the Heart, are intimately intertwined with the 'nervous system,' each affecting the other. An unstable 'nervous system' destabilizes the Heart, which controls the mind, and this loss of stability in the Heart causes the 'nervous system' to become unbalanced. Mood and qi are constantly changing, one moment up and the next moment down, ultimately affecting the entire body.

As the condition associated with Change in Rate at Rest progresses, the symptoms of emotional instability remain, but increase in frequency and intensity. Consistent Change in Rate at Rest are a sign of Heart qi deficiency ('Heart disease'), while Change in Rate on Exertion are a reflection of either Heart blood deficiency ('Heart weak') or Heart qi deficiency, depending on the degree and direction of change (see below).[3]

The precipitating events leading to these patterns usually occur before the age of twenty. With Heart qi agitation ('Heart nervous'), the more consistent the rate change, the earlier or greater the triggering incident or incidents. The degree of rate change depends on the etiology, with worry causing the least, and shock the greatest, change. Constitutional Heart qi deficiency predisposes an individual to all arrhythmias.

With Heart qi agitation ('Heart nervous') the rate is always Rapid, especially when shock is the etiology. When the true qi is deficient the rate will be more Rapid immediately after a shock and during the early stages, than when the true qi is strong. If the Heart is constitutionally vulnerable, or the process continues for a long time, the Rapid rate weakens the Heart and the rate slows, except in times of stress when it may become temporarily elevated. The rate tends to be closer to normal and more stable when the true qi is stronger.

Change in Rate at Rest

Change in Rate at Rest is a quality based on the sensation it describes, independently of qualifying conditions. This quality feels as if it is continuously speeding up and slowing down. Originally characterized by Dr. Shen as involving emotional instability, over the years differences in associated symptoms insisted on a further delineation between frequent or occasional and small or large changes in each category, with which Dr. Shen concurred. Occasional and constant, small and large, are subsidiary to the basic quality, involving the basic sensation but qualifying it. Therefore, they are all related yet independent subqualities.

Occasional Change in Rate at Rest

This quality manifests as a Change in Rate at Rest one day, followed by no Change in Rate at Rest the next. This condition is less serious than when there is Constant Change in Rate at Rest (see below).

The subject of agitated Heart qi ('Heart nervous'), with which this quality is associated, is discussed in Chapters 12 and 15. The concept of *shen* or spirit disturbance covers a much more ambiguous scope of mental, emotional, and spiritual disturbance. That is why I have chosen the term Heart qi agitation to describe a specific emotional state. Treatment for the 'internal demons' is appropriate for this condition, especially when the changes are large.

Small

Sensation

If worry is the etiology, the rate is generally more stable, changing less often than when the etiology is shock, wherein the pattern is different (see below). The entire pulse can be slightly Tight, especially the left distal position and the central Pericardium position, if the body condition is good. With shock, the entire pulse is also Rapid. If the body condition is weak, the left distal position can be more Feeble, and the entire pulse less Rapid.

Diagnostic process and etiology

There are two sources of agitated Heart qi, heat from excess and heat from yin deficiency and mild shock (see also Chapters 12 and 15).

Heat from excess A small change in rate due to excessive tension or long-term mild heat in the Heart ('Heart tight') due to heat from excess rather than deficiency is usually more Rapid than would be the case if the heat were from deficiency. If all of the yin organ systems are equally strong, this tension affects the Liver first, causing excess Liver heat. Since the Liver nourishes the peripheral nervous system, tension causes hyperactivity of the nerves, which leads to Liver heat. Also, if the Liver's attempt to overcome the stagnation and eliminate the heat does not succeed through normal channels (e.g., the bile) the Liver will discharge the excess qi and heat to the most vulnerable organ. In particular, with a Heart whose function is already vulnerable due to constitution or life factors (or both), a Heart qi agitation ('Heart nervous') *shen* disturbance can develop. If the Stomach is the most vulnerable organ, the result can be gastritis, and if it is the Intestine, colitis can ensue.

Heat from yin deficiency A mild case of Heart qi agitation ('Heart nervous') can be thought of as an intermediate stage of Heart yin deficiency in which the diminished yin causes the nerves of the Heart to become slightly dry, easily excited, agitated, and thus unstable. I classify this pulse as agitated Heart qi since the yin deficiency aspect is not entirely clear. Although generalized yin deficiency is associated with agitation, as with Kidney yin deficiency, it is only with Heart yin deficiency that we have a pulse with Changes in Rate at Rest. With this process the rate is not as Rapid as when the heat is associated with excess.

One source of this condition is often a mild emotional shock to the Heart, which causes a sudden yin deficiency of the Heart as profound as the degree of shock. Another cause is prolonged heat from excess in the Heart, especially that which is due to constant tension, as described above. (The yin is depleted in its effort to balance the heat.) A third cause is constant, long-term worry in which case a Smooth Vibration is found along with the Changes in Rate at Rest (see Chapter 11 on the Vibration quality, and Chapter 15).

Symptoms

The most prominent symptom associated with this pulse is a mild roller coaster feeling, in which the mind races out of control as if it cannot be stopped, with alternating high and low moods and some difficulty in focusing thoughts and actions; there will also be constant self-doubt, and thus indecisiveness.[4] Other symptoms include nervousness and agitation with moderate to intense stress; fatigue after strenuous exertion; mild sporadic palpitations upon heavy exertion, which do not persist; sleeping lightly and waking easily after only a mild disturbance, then quickly returning to sleep, thus tending to be up and down all night; occasional tiredness in the morning.

Signs

The tongue and eyes are normal.

Large

This pattern is unstable such that the entire pulse feels as if it is beating with a slightly syncopated irregularity. The difference between this pulse and an irregular Interrupted quality is that there are no truly missed beats, and the rate is usually discernible. Other characteristics are that the left distal position is extremely Tight and may have a fine superficial Vibration. The left proximal position is Tight to Wiry and Deep. The entire pulse can be Tight.

In more severe cases, the left distal and proximal positions are somewhat Feeble, while the average rate is slightly Rapid. There may also be some slight Changes in Rate on Exertion.

Diagnosis	This is the more severe form of Heart qi agitation ('Heart nervous'). Even with this more severe pattern, there is a hierarchy of severity. The less dangerous form is seen in younger persons, and the more serious form occurs in individuals in whom the Heart qi agitation has been deteriorating for a long period of time into Heart blood deficiency ('Heart weak'). Advanced Heart qi agitation conditions are often seen, although not exclusively, in borderline psychological states.
Etiology	A moderately large change in rate results from shock due to a sudden moderate to large fright, or due to major physical trauma involving fright between the ages of fifteen and twenty. With these etiologies, constitutional Heart qi deficiency, and working beyond one's energy for a long period of time, results in a larger change in rate. These events involving shock usually affect the Heart directly, in addition to whatever other organ system is susceptible.
Symptoms	Individuals presenting with this pulse are constantly changing their minds, and have severe mood swings. They experience a more persistent roller coaster feeling. This is accompanied by considerable difficulty in focusing thoughts and actions, and constant self-doubt and indecisiveness, especially in those individuals whose eyebrows are continuous from one side to the other. Their lives are characterized by impotence, turmoil, and disarray. Moreover, these individuals are easily frightened, and are always worried, nervous, and insecure. They suffer persistent moderate to severe palpitations upon light exertion. They wake easily and frequently throughout the night due to very light sleep, although they quickly return to sleep; thus, they are tired in the morning. Infants are up and down all night if shock occurs from around birth through the first few months. Greater fatigue is present after moderate exertion in these individuals than in those with mild Heart qi agitation, although fatigue is less of a concern to people with this condition than is anxiety.
Signs	The tongue shape is normal or slightly thin. A shallow, central furrow may be present. The body is slightly red, especially at the tip; a bright red color might shine through. The coating is thin, dry, and yellow. In severe cases there can be a patchy loss of tongue coating, with a dark red body in the denuded areas. The eyes often show a confluence of blood vessels under the eyelid. If shock occurred in early childhood, a bluish hue may be evident over the entire or some part of the face.

Constant Change in Rate at Rest

This quality consistently speeds up and slows down without missing a beat, and is a sign of mild Heart qi deficiency ('Heart disease'). A small change signifies a less serious condition, and a large change a more serious one. However, the general condition that this pulse reflects is not as dangerous as when the qualities are Interrupted or Intermittent.

Mild Heart qi deficiency ('heart disease')

The entire pulse exhibits constant Changes in Rate at Rest. The left distal position can show any or all of the following: Changes in Intensity or Qualities, constant Deepness, Rough Vibration, or Slipperiness.

Diagnosis	All of the etiologies listed below lead to a gradual and, much later, extreme weakening of Heart qi and yang until the Heart qi can no longer control the circulation. With Constant Changes at Rest the process has reached only to the point of mild Heart qi

deficiency, if the changes are small or moderate, and moderate Heart qi deficiency if the changes are large. Small Constant Changes at Rest are also a sign of severe Heart qi agitation.

Etiology

Associated predisposing conditions may include prolonged Heart qi agitation, Heart blood deficiency ('Heart weak'), Heart stagnation ('Heart closed'), and trapped qi in the Heart ('Heart full'). The causes are inherited predisposition; congenital Heart qi deficiency; physical work beyond one's energy as a child and pre-adolescent; malnourishment as a child; unresolved shock to the Heart and circulation early in life due to severe emotional trauma; excessive and prolonged abuse of alcohol, drugs, and nicotine. Repressed and profound anger exacerbates all of the above.

Symptoms

Individuals with this type of pulse can suffer mild chest pain, and mild fatigue and shortness of breath upon exertion. They experience increasing coldness in the body, especially in the limbs, and can have very mild pitting, dependent edema. Other symptoms include a mild oppressive sensation in the chest such that the patient must sleep in a slightly raised position; palpitations, even upon moderate exertion; numbness of the upper limbs; and occasional spontaneous cold perspiration during the day upon minimal exertion. These individuals are often anxious and vulnerable during their entire lives, have poor concentration, and are forgetful. They may also experience the same lack of focus found with Occasional Changes in Rate at Rest.

Signs

The tongue shows a deep, central furrow, and is pale, swollen along the furrow, and wet; the tip is red. The insides of the lower eyelids are pale and show confluence rather than distinctness of the blood vessels. The face is pale, especially the forehead; a green-bluish hue may be present on the chin or around the mouth if the cause is constitutional or congenital. The nails may be concave, and the ends of the fingers may be clubbed, in the most serious cases.

Rate measurable with missed beats

Three pulses are usually described in the literature under this classification: Intermittent, Hurried, and Knotted. With the Intermittent pulse, the missed beats have a regular cadence, and the rate is usually measurable; here, it is classified with those arrhythmias that have a measurable rate. Dr. Shen refers to the Intermittent quality as the "pulse that stops suddenly."[5] With the Hurried and Knotted pulses, the rate is usually not measurable since they are irregularly irregular. Despite the fact that the rate of irregularly–irregular pulses is a matter of impression, the Hurried and Knotted qualities are actually traditionally classified according to whether the rate is Rapid or Slow.

However, in keeping with the principle of classification by sensation, I differentiate among these pulse qualities with missed beats based on whether the rate is measurable, rather than on the speed of the rate. This is because, in spite of beats being missed, the most immediate message to the fingers beyond the irregularity is whether or not the rate can be measured, and not whether it is Rapid or Slow.

I also find the classification according to the speed of the pulse—under which Hurried and Knotted appear—to be flawed, since it omits the entire (and important) Interrupted quality, which misses beats irregularly, and which feels neither Slow nor Rapid. Therefore, in this book the Hurried and Knotted pulses are classified as Interrupted qualities, which are distinguished from the Intermittent pulse by their irregularly-irregular aspect and by the practitioner's consequent inability to determine their exact rate. I have found impressions of Rapid or Slow associated with the Interrupted quality to be highly misleading.

Furthermore, the etiologies found in the literature associated with the Hurried and

Knotted qualities—heat and cold from excess, 'heat agitating qi and blood,' 'perverse fire penetrating the zang,' 'ulcers and abscesses,' 'heat penetrating the muscles,' or 'insufficient blood to fill and move within the blood pathways'—are rarely encountered in the modern clinic. The relevant etiologies in our time seem more closely associated with Heart function.

Considered separately from other concurrent complications, the Interrupted quality, in which the rate cannot be assessed, is the most serious. The Intermittent quality which frequently misses beats is slightly less serious than this Interrupted quality, but more serious than the Interrupted quality in which the rate can be assessed and the Intermittent quality which misses less often; all are more serious than the pulse that Changes Rate at Rest, but which does not miss any beats. Dr. Shen observed that individuals with these pulse qualities are highly vulnerable to emotional shock.

The usual variable in determining the presence or absence of the Intermittent and Interrupted pulse qualities is the condition of the upright, true, or Stomach qi. The stronger the true qi, the less likely these qualities are encountered. All of them are signs of significant danger.

Intermittent

This pulse stops on a regular basis after the same number of beats, and can also be described as delayed or syncopated. The interruption may be frequent, after every two beats, or infrequent, after every ten beats. Another term used to describe this pulse is "replacement."[6]

Constantly Intermittent

Frequently missed beats

This quality misses beats regularly, from every two beats in the most serious cases, to more than every ten beats in slightly less serious ones. The greater the interval between beats, the better the prognosis. In following patients with an Intermittent pulse, I have observed that the period between missed beats increases as the condition improves. Another characteristic of this pulse is that the left distal position is Feeble–Absent. The entire pulse can also be Hollow in the most serious cases.

Diagnosis

This type of pulse reflects Heart qi, blood, and yang deficiency.

Etiology and interpretation

Dr. Shen and I found that the etiology begins usually before the age of five to ten years, and includes Heart qi deficiency (often congenital or rheumatic in origin), collapse of all yin organs, pregnancy with toxemia, and severe childhood malnutrition. If this pulse appears in a person over the age of seventy, Dr. Shen claimed that it is of no consequence. However, this does not concur with my experience as a practitioner of biomedicine, since I would first attempt to rule out serious illness before drawing and acting on such a conclusion. Dr. Shen also stated that this pulse can be a normal quality during pregnancy, which again, if I were to find it, I would wish to explore more fully.

Kaptchuk notes that this pulse is "often associated with the Heart, signifying a serious disharmony, or it can signal an exhausted state of all the Organs."[7] He indicates that some of the associated conditions include exhaustion of all the yin organs, patterns of Heart qi deficiency with palpitation and pain, and cold from deficiency of the middle burner with vomiting.[8] If it occurs suddenly it may be due to temporary obstruction of qi in a wind pattern, pain, great emotional stress, or trauma. He says that, in certain situations when this pulse is congenital, it is "not necessarily a sign of disharmony,"[9] an assertion I would not make without prior exhaustive investigation.[10]

Symptoms	Symptoms associated with this pulse can include severe chest pain (angina), extreme fatigue, and shortness of breath upon exertion. Patients also experience coldness in the body, especially in the limbs, and have pitting, dependent edema. There is an oppressive sensation in the chest, causing a need to sleep in a sitting position. Other symptoms include palpitations even on mild exertion, and excessive spontaneous perspiration during the day, with beady and oily sweat. These individuals are often anxious and vulnerable throughout their lives.
Signs	The tongue usually shows a deep central furrow, especially if the cause originates primarily from life experience. A shallower furrow is more common if constitution is the more important etiology. Swelling is also apparent on either side of the furrow. The tongue body is pale, swollen, and wet. The insides of the lower eyelids are pale, the lips are blue, and the nails pale blue. The distal phalange of the thumb may be abnormally short, which is a sign of a constitutional disposition toward serious Heart disease as well as its current or imminent presence. The nails are often concave, and the tips of the fingers are clubbed, in severe cases.

Combinations with other qualities

Infrequently missed beats	This pulse is characterized by a regular interruption, from once every eleven beats to once every sixty beats. The less frequently it misses, the less serious the problem. After sixty beats it is difficult to track the regularity, and if followed carefully will probably prove to be an Interrupted pulse.
Diagnosis	This quality reflects less serious Heart qi and yang deficiency than with the more frequent interruptions.
Etiology and interpretation	The etiologies and interpretations listed above under the Frequently Intermittent quality apply to this pulse, including the complications of pregnancy, albeit to a considerably less degree of severity.
Symptoms	The following symptoms of Heart qi deficiency are less probable, and certainly less severe, and are likely to become less and less apparent as the frequency of missed beats declines: fatigue, angina, shortness of breath and palpitations upon exertion, oppressive sensation in the chest, excessive spontaneous perspiration upon exertion during the day.
Signs	The tongue shows a shallow central furrow which deepens as the condition becomes more serious. The tongue body is swollen, pale, and wet, the lips are purple, and the nails are pale blue. The more frequent the missed beats, the deeper the central furrow, and the deeper the color.

Inconsistently Intermittent

Sensation	This pulse misses a beat at regular intervals, but this occurs only during some examinations and not others.
Etiology and interpretation	The usual condition is serious Heart qi agitation ('Heart nervous') and/or Heart blood deficiency ('Heart weak') due to shock or trauma which has rendered the nerves of the heart unstable. However, it is less serious than a regularly missed beat each time the pulse is taken. See above for a description of the signs and symptoms of Heart qi agitation and below for Heart blood deficiency.

Interrupted

Sensation

This pulse misses beats irregularly, but one is still able to accurately assess the rate. The Interrupted quality in which the rate *can* be assessed is a sign of moderate Heart qi deficiency, with a milder form of some of the associated disharmonies listed below for the Interrupted quality with a rate that *cannot* be accurately measured. If this occurs occasionally, it is a sign of moderate Heart qi agitation and mild Heart qi deficiency. If it is constant, it is a sign of moderate Heart qi deficiency.

Rate not measurable

Interrupted

Sensation

The Interrupted quality misses beats with no fixed cadence and no reliably assessable rate.

Interpretation

I have found that in any of the disorders associated with this pulse, the rate may seem to be Rapid, Slow, or Normal and totally unpredictable from person to person, or from time to time in the same person. For this reason, and others mentioned above, I do not subscribe to the notion that the Hurried or the Knotted pulses are always supposed to be, respectively, Rapid and Slow.[11]

As already mentioned, and in keeping with the principle of classification by sensation, I differentiate these pulse qualities with missed beats on the basis of whether their rate is measurable rather than on the basis of speed.[12]

Constantly Interrupted

Beats are missed constantly and irregularly such that the rate is difficult to determine accurately, and changes from examination to examination. All of the patterns described below involve a serious Heart disharmony and should be considered as urgent or emergent unless proven otherwise.

Dr. Shen and I found that the Yielding Hollow Intermittent combination is a sign of the most severe form of Heart qi-yang deficiency ('Heart disease').[13]

CONDITIONS ASSOCIATED WITH THE CONSTANTLY INTERRUPTED QUALITY

The following conditions often, but not always, accompany the Interrupted quality.

Heart qi and yang deficiency

Sensation

The quality associated with this pattern is Interrupted over the entire pulse. The rate is difficult to measure, and is neither Rapid nor Slow. The left distal position is Thin and Feeble-Absent, often with Rough Vibration, Slipperiness, and Change in Qualities and Intensity.

Combinations and interpretation

Less serious: Empty Interrupted. With this form of 'qi wild' (separation of yin and yang) the qi and circulation are out of control throughout the body and in the yin organs. The patient experiences a sensation of no control over their own body, and has feelings of depersonalization and anxiety as well as fatigue. A severe disease (from a biomedical perspective) is possible within six months.

More serious: Yielding Hollow Interrupted. This is a more severe form of 'qi wild' and 'circulation out of control' in that the instability is not only in many of the yin organs, especially the Heart, but also the blood and circulation. The Constantly Interrupted quality, especially in combination with these qualities, is evidence of very severe heart organ damage; of all the qualities mentioned in this book, it is a sign of the most serious life-threatening illness. The presence or imminence of severe disease is great. The prognosis for longevity is poor.

Remember that the Interrupted and Intermittent qualities by themselves are not evidence of 'qi wild'; only in combination with the Empty and Hollow qualities are they signs of severe 'qi wild.'

Etiology

The events leading to this pulse picture begin before the age of ten, although the etiology of the more serious type probably begins before the age of five. The greater the irregularity, the earlier the onset or the more profound the cause. The origin can be early shock, congenital heart disease, rheumatic fever and heart disease, relentless overwork beyond one's energy (child labor), extraordinary and prolonged emotional stress beginning at a young and vulnerable age, and environmental deprivation including food, shelter, and clothing.

Symptoms

Individuals with this pulse often suffer congestive heart failure with edema, must sleep in a sitting position, exhaustive fatigue, severe palpitations, shortness of breath, faintness, and weakness that worsens upon even the slightest exertion. Other symptoms may include frequent episodes of sudden excessive cold perspiration during the day with oily body sweat, cold limbs, moderate angina, and an oppressive sensation in the chest such that the individual cannot lie flat. Mental instability occurs, especially with a vulnerable 'nervous system.'

Signs

The tongue is swollen, pale, and wet, and has a deep central furrow with a large swelling on either side. The insides of the lower eyelids are pale. The face, lips, and nails are dusky pale to cyanotic. The face is ashen gray.

Heart blood stagnation ('Heart small')

The entire pulse is Interrupted. The left distal position can be extremely Flat in the early stages, and in the later stages the left distal position (according to Dr. Shen) becomes very Deep, Thin, and Feeble, with a Normal, slightly Slow, or slightly Rapid rate.

My own experience with advanced Heart blood stagnation is different from Dr. Shen's. The pulse is Deep, Thin, and Feeble, but accompanied by Rough Vibration (similar to Choppy), Slipperiness, and is sometimes either Nonhomogeneous or Unstable, and Interrupted or Intermittent. The rate is Normal, slightly Rapid, or slightly Slow. Less often, I have observed a Choppy quality accompanying this condition.

Etiology

Diminished circulation of blood to and through the Heart due to Heart qi and yang deficiency; Liver qi stagnation from emotional repression leading to heat that reaches the Heart causing blood stagnation; 'blood thick' with phlegm and blood stasis and accumulation in the arteries and chest, which is the Chinese medical equivalent of atherosclerosis and coronary occlusion.

Symptoms

Palpitations with activity, severe intermittent angina with pain radiating down the left arm, oppressive sensation in the chest, and cold hands and feet.

Signs	The tongue is scarlet, dry, with a deep central furrow, red tip, and scanty coating. The face is dusky, and the lips and nails are cyanotic.

Phlegm confuses the Heart orifice

The entire pulse is Interrupted, and generally Tense. The left distal position is very Slippery and sometimes Muffled or (rarely) Inflated with this condition.

Etiology — One common scenario is stagnant Liver qi attacking and invading the Spleen, interfering with its function of transporting the fluids. The latter transform into phlegm, which travels to the Heart where it clouds the Heart's orifice. Excessive heat may stimulate the Gallbladder to produce dampness to counteract the heat. Together, the dampness and heat produce phlegm.

Symptoms — In severe cases there is mental confusion, clouding of consciousness, psycho-motor withdrawal, severe depression that is sometimes interrupted by manic behavior with poor reality testing; catatonia and paranoia; epileptic seizures. Biomedical diagnosis includes bipolar disease (depressed phase), schizophrenia of the catatonic type, and epileptic equivalents such as petit mal and psychomotor epilepsy.

In less severe cases there is the wide range of emotional disorders we classify generally as neurosis. Experience has led me to successfully treat all mental-emotional states, both serious and relatively benign, as phlegm 'misting' the Heart orifice.

Signs — The tongue has a white, greasy coating.

Phlegm-fire disturbs the Heart orifice

The entire pulse is Interrupted, Pounding, and Tight. The left distal position is Slippery, Robust Pounding, and Tight to Wiry.

Etiology — Liver qi stagnation leads to fire, which attacks the Heart. Dampness accumulates in the Heart because of impaired Spleen function, one reason for which might be the Liver qi attacking the Spleen, or dampness from the Gallbladder trying to balance the heat. The result is phlegm-fire in the Heart.

Symptoms — May include irritability, palpitations, bitter taste in the mouth, insomnia, excessive dreaming, easily startled; incoherent, rapid, loud, and rambling speech. Biomedical diagnosis includes bipolar disease, more often in the manic than in the depressed phase, with poor reality testing; schizophrenia of the hebephrenic type; and epilepsy.

Signs — The tongue has a red tip, and a thick, yellow, greasy coating.

Phlegm obstructs the Heart orifice

The pulse associated with this condition is Slippery and Wiry, or Hollow Full-Overflowing, and is usually Rapid. Its rate is difficult to determine.

Diagnosis — This pattern includes all three types of stroke: yang obstruction, yin obstruction, and exhaustion syndrome.

Etiology — The primary cause is Liver yang transforming into Liver wind, which generates heat and combines with pre-existing phlegm.

Symptoms   *Yang obstruction:* sudden collapse with loss of consciousness, lockjaw, trismus, clenched fists, retention of urine and feces, stiffness and spasm of limbs, redness of the face, and restlessness.

Yin obstruction: same as yang obstruction except that the face is pale, the limbs are cold, and there is no restlessness.

Exhaustion syndrome: mouth is open, hands relaxed, and eyes closed; there is oily perspiration and incontinence of urine and stool.

Signs   *Yang obstruction:* tongue is red and has a yellow, greasy coating; the eyes are congested.

Yin obstruction: tongue is less red and has a white, greasy coating. With both patterns the tongue may be twisted and tremble considerably.

Exhaustion syndrome: tongue is pale, swollen, and flaccid.

Interpretation   I have not found the Rapid aspect of the Interrupted pulse quality to be reliably associated with any of the etiologies mentioned here in which the pulse is Interrupted, with the possible exception of phlegm–fire disturbing the Heart orifice. The interpretation of this pulse by others appears to be that heat diminishes yin, which becomes denser and more difficult to move, thereby impairing circulation and leading to arrhythmias.

Occasionally Interrupted

This means that an Interrupted pulse is felt only occasionally. The more often it appears, the more serious the condition.

Etiology   Shock to the Heart, overwork and/or overexercise between ages fifteen and twenty, or prolonged mild heat in the Heart ('Heart tight') can lead to this pulse.

Diagnosis   This pulse reflects a severe form of Heart qi agitation ('Heart nervous').

Symptoms   Fatigue, joint pain of increasing severity which moves from joint to joint; anxiety, depersonalization, and dissociation and detachment.

Signs   The tongue is initially bright red, and later turns pale. The vertical blood vessels under the lower eyelids are also red at first and later turn pale. The sclera is injected during the early stage and later becomes less injected.

Sudden Transient Interrupted

This quality can appear with very high temperature (especially in children), extraordinary fatigue, severe physical trauma, and severe emotional shock. Often the Heart qi will already be deficient, although not enough to cause symptoms.

CHANGES IN RATE ON EXERTION

The pulse rate should normally increase about eight to twelve beats per minute with vigorous exertion, i.e., shaking the arms about ten times. With Heart blood deficiency, the Change in Rate on Exertion is greater. In more advanced stages it is often detectable after the patient walks in from the waiting room, or even as the patient extends their arm to have the pulse taken. Should the rate go up only a few beats per minute, stay the same, or be less than at rest, there is Heart qi-yang deficiency.

Constant Large Increase in Rate on Exertion

Diagnosis

This is Heart blood deficiency ('Heart weak'), which is primarily a pattern of deficiency of blood, and to a lesser extent of qi. As the Heart blood and qi deficiency ('Heart weak') progresses, the rate becomes slower at rest. The weaker the Heart blood, the more easily a rate change will occur on exertion. Even such slight movement as rolling over in bed can effect a change in rate by as much as twenty beats per minute. Usually the left distal position is Thin or Feeble-Absent in this pattern.

If the etiology is due to non-constitutional systemic factors based on life experiences, the entire pulse is Feeble-Absent, and the left distal and proximal positions somewhat more so. The degree of Feeble-Absentness depends on the duration of the condition. If the etiology is primarily constitutional Heart deficiency, the left distal and proximal positions are Feeble-Absent, but the remainder of the pulse is normal.

Etiology

Over time, unresolved Heart qi agitation ('Heart nervous') will evolve into Heart blood deficiency ('Heart weak'). In fact, over a long period *any* chronic Heart condition weakens the Heart blood and qi. Other causes are constitutional Heart qi deficiency; shock during early life, often before, at, or shortly after birth; and prolonged excessive work beyond one's energy level.

Symptoms

The principal symptoms of this condition, even without much exertion, are a feeling of weakness and cold along with fatigue to the point of exhaustion. Other symptoms include steady sleep for a few hours followed by early morning waking and some difficulty returning to sleep; poor concentration and forgetfulness; tiredness in the morning; memory and concentration difficulties; palpitations upon mild to moderate exertion due to insufficient blood circulating to the Heart; and slight cold and numbness in the extremities due to reduced circulation.

Signs

The tongue may show a central furrow, the depth of which correlates with the length of time the condition has existed. If the etiology is primarily constitutional, the furrow is shallower than when the etiology is due to life experience, or a combination of both. The insides of the lower eyelids are pale.

Occasional Large Increase in Rate on Exertion

The clinical picture is essentially the same, but significantly less serious than when the change in rate is constant.

Decrease in Rate on Exertion

On exertion the rate should increase at least eight to twelve beats per minute. When the rate increases less than eight beats, this is a sign of Heart qi deficiency. The lower the increase, the greater the deficiency. If the rate stays the same or decreases on exertion, this is a sign of Heart yang deficiency.

Pseudo-arrhythmias

Certain qualities and wave forms mimic arrhythmias. Examples include Changes in Intensity and Amplitude, and the Unstable quality, which are discussed below in the section on stability. Another is the Hesitant Wave quality, which will be discussed first.

Fig. 6-1 Hesitant Wave

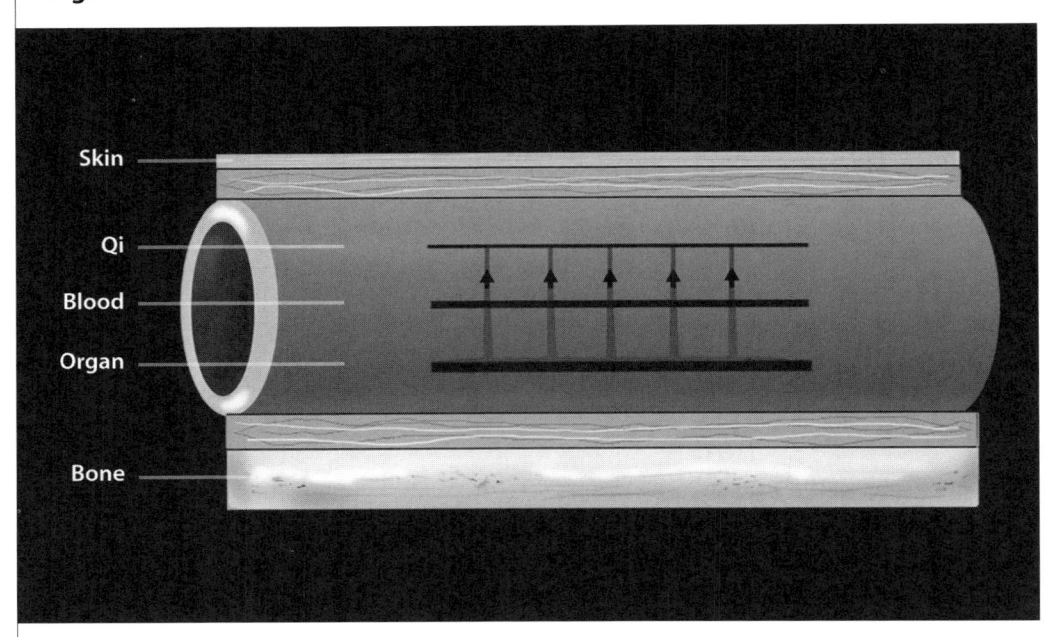

Hesitant Wave

This is a quality (Fig. 6-1) which I have observed with Dr. Shen and in my own practice, and which students have reported, but it has not been described (to my knowledge) in the literature. It is associated with mild Heart yin deficiency.

This quality is more correctly categorized as an abnormal wave pattern, and is actually characterized by the absence of a wave. It is included here with rhythms because it *seems* to be missing a beat. While there is no true loss of beat, the Hesitant quality gives that impression because there is an apparent space between impulses due to the loss of a sine wave and the abruptness of the beat. It is also included here because, like the arrhythmias, the Hesitant quality is a sign of a Heart disharmony.

Sensation This quality occurs only over the entire pulse as the Hesitant Wave. Descriptively, the pulse wave has lost its normal sine wave form, whereby the flow to and from the wave peak becomes sharp and abrupt, instead of being a gradual rise and fall. The term Hesitant is used because some people experience this quality as faltering or balking, yet not missing a beat.

Interpretation I have found that this quality occurs when an individual has a tendency to ruminate or think incessantly about one subject. (This is distinguished from a general tendency to worry about almost anything real or imaginary, which is expressed over the entire pulse as a superficial Smooth Vibration at all depths.) In the early stages, except for the symptom of worry or difficulty in falling asleep, there are no other related signs or symptoms. Later, the individual will seek help because of a strong sense of malaise and a feeling that they cannot keep up the pace that they have set for themselves. Individuals with this pulse quality often collapse suddenly, physically and/or emotionally.

The worst case scenario is a monomaniacal obsessive preoccupation with some aspect of life, usually work or health, in which the person's mind never ceases to rest even when asleep. Originally, I found this pulse in stockbrokers who could never stop thinking about money, and later in high level government political appointees who have no civil service safety net and are extraordinarily exploited by their political masters. Recently, however, I even found this pulse in acupuncturists.

The Hesitant quality is a form of the "push pulse" in which persons push themselves mentally, in contrast to that associated with the Flooding-Deficient quality, in which individuals push themselves more physically. Since mental "pushing" seems to precede the physical exhaustion, it is my impression that with similar etiologies, and a vulnerable Heart, the Hesitant quality precedes the Flooding-Deficient quality.

In traditional Chinese medical terms, the Hesitant quality is closest to mild Heart yin deficiency. Treatment for the 'internal demons' or 'possession' is appropriate for this condition.

Combinations

The Hesitant pulse can occur in combinations too numerous to catalog here as special or frequent.

Stability

The concepts of 'qi wild' and 'blood circulation out of control' are not included in the conventional Chinese medicine curriculum. Along with other aspects of Chinese medicine that do not conform to the modern dogma, they are rejected outright by some practitioners. Except for Manfred Porkert, Li Shi-Zhen, Jiang Jing, and the *Inner Classic*, discussed below, I have found no reference to these concepts in the English language literature. Nevertheless, they are among the most important aspects of Chinese pathology because they involve an entire range of disharmony and pathology rampant in our time for which many practitioners are unprepared to diagnose and treat.[14] (See Fig. 6-6 at the end of this chapter.)

What is frightening is the frequency that one encounters the most serious forms of instability—such as Change in Qualities, Intensity, Amplitude, and Rhythm of the pulse—in people who are on medication or with histories of substance abuse. Even more alarming is the fact that the 'qi wild' condition is occurring with increasing frequency in young people, particularly during the past decade.

With regard to sensation, Changes in Amplitude, Intensity, and Qualities, as well as the Flooding-Deficient wave itself, are frequently confused with one another. The differences among them are significant and require hands-on experience in order to distinguish their individual properties. Deeper, constant, and pervasive Changes in Qualities are the most serious signs of dysfunction in this group, while the Flooding-Deficient wave is generally a sign of the least disharmony.

According to Dr. Shen, all changes in the stability of the pulse, including rate, rhythm, amplitude, intensity, and quality, are intimately intertwined with the 'nervous system.' An unstable 'nervous system' causes the 'circulatory system'—involved with rate and rhythm—to become unstable, and the loss of stability of the 'circulatory system' in turn causes the 'nervous system' to become unbalanced. In the 'qi wild' conditions described below, the emotional and mental symptoms are more severe if the 'nervous system' is already tense or weak.[15]

All of the pulse qualities associated with 'qi wild' are accompanied by anxiety, confusion to some extent, as well as emotional fragility and a tendency to become easily fatigued. The lives of patients so affected are marked by chaos that may be more or less frantic depending on other factors. The pulse qualities associated with 'qi wild' include the Empty family of qualities, Yielding Hollow Full-Overflowing, Change in Qualities, Empty Interrupted, Interrupted Yielding Hollow, and Intermittent Yielding Hollow. The pulse rate is usually Slow.

'QI WILD' CONDITION

'Qi wild' (sān mài 散脈), literally 'scattered pulse,' is a condition of extreme functional weakness in which, for one reason or another, the yin and yang have separated—lost operative contact—and are thus unable to support each other. This term has been likened to "sand running out of one's hand" or "dispersing like a piece of bread that is crumbling." Dr. Shen believes that the term connotes the 'danger pulse': the immune system is injured and the body therefore has little power to resist disease, which will, he states, occur within six months unless intervention occurs.

One way of thinking of yin, the material energy of the universe, is as a gravitational force that holds or grasps the more effervescent yang energies. Should the yin become drained, however, it can no longer hold the yang. Instead, the lighter yang energies wander aimlessly to all parts of the organism, unable to function effectively without the organizing force of the yin. The result is physiological disarray in which the orderly circulation of yang to the channels and the organs is disrupted, impairing their ability to function.

'Qi wild' is thus a condition characterized by chaos, representing the most serious physiological disruption and disorganization. The 'qi wild' patient is highly vulnerable to serious and fast-spreading, even life-threatening, disease within a very short time, including cancer, auto-immune, or degenerative central nervous system disease. Mental illness is another form of this chaos. It is especially disruptive to the 'nervous system' which depends on the organized integrity of the lighter, fast-moving qi energies.

Dr. Shen points out that, except for two combinations of pulse qualities—Empty Interrupted, and Hollow Interrupted, both of which involve the Heart—the pulses associated with this extremely chaotic state of the true qi do not implicate any particular organ. They do, however, indicate that the individual will be highly susceptible to disease in any organ.[16]

Qualities associated with the 'qi wild' condition

The 'qi wild' condition affects the entire organism, and the pulse qualities associated with this condition must, in turn, affect the entire pulse (all three positions on both wrists) or they are not pathognomonic of the 'qi wild' state. These qualities include the Empty Interrupted-Intermittent, Yielding Hollow Interrupted-Intermittent, Empty, Yielding Hollow Full-Overflowing, Leather, Empty Thread-like, Scattered, Minute, and Changes in Qualities.

Another, less obvious, sign of a 'qi wild' disorder is when the pulse qualities at the burners and individual positions vary greatly. This is a sign of a serious disruption of the harmonizing function of the Triple Burner, including that between the right and left brain (corpus collosum), leading to physiological anarchy and serious disease. In my experience I have come to associate this sign with auto-immune diseases.

Still another rare 'qi wild' sign is a Change in Qualities from side to side, also observed with chronic auto-immune disorder. The qualities on the left and right sides periodically change places.

While all these qualities are signs of serious current or impending illness, the Empty Interrupted or Empty Intermittent and Yielding Hollow Interrupted or Yielding Hollow Intermittent are probably the most serious. One other combination of qualities—Rough Vibration and/or Change in Intensity over the entire pulse with a Feeble or Absent left distal position (Heart)—is a sign of Heart yang-qi deficiency ('Heart disease') with a less though similarly disorganizing effect on the entire organism, as is indicated by the Interrupted or Intermittent qualities just mentioned. (We will not discuss the Rough Vibration quality here, but in a different context in Chapter 11.)

Related signs and symptoms

Dr. Shen notes that the tongue associated with a condition of 'qi wild' is only slightly pale, and that with the collapse of the yin organ system, the tongue is very pale. With some 'qi wild' pulses I have observed, the patients' tongues seemed to have a flabby, milky-white appearance with loss of balanced or coherent shape, usually together with extreme fatigue and enfeeblement, even in young people.

Etiology

Most of the associated pulse qualities, discussed more fully in Chapter 9, are linked to problems that begin in early life. These include environmental deprivation (food, shelter, clothing), overwork, overexercise, excessive lifting, sudden stoppage of extreme exercise, extreme and prolonged emotional and physical abuse, or substance abuse. The more serious the pulse quality, the earlier the etiology.

SEVERE EARLY ENVIRONMENTAL DEPRIVATION, INCLUDING FOOD AND SHELTER

Apart from a profound constitutional or congenital insult, the most serious form of 'qi wild' is caused by an environment in early life marked by severe nutritional deprivation and inadequate shelter from the elements. We would expect to find this ubiquitously today in Third World countries racked by war and starvation, especially in Africa. But many children throughout the world—including the United States—are hungry. The signs and symptoms will vary widely depending on the severity of the living conditions, the age at onset, time elapsed, and subsequent remediation.

The pathogenesis of this 'qi wild' state is that the yin organs, which are severely depleted by conditions of deprivation, cannot support the qi, yin, and blood. In each affected yin organ system, the yin and yang separate due to this deprivation. Gradually this process expands to the entire organism until the 'qi wild' state is prevalent. The associated physiological aberrations result in severe and unpredictable forms of disease such as cancer, auto-immune disease, and profound mental illness. Without correction, the prognosis for a long life is poor. The associated pulse quality is Hollow Interrupted or Intermittent.

OVERWORK DURING CHILDHOOD

If the qi and blood are depleted by too much physical work before puberty, the yin organ systems will also be dangerously weakened. This type of pulse is found in individuals who are overworked at an extremely young age, such as child laborers forced to work in factories and mines before the age of ten. Furthermore, emotional shock combined with prolonged work and exercise beyond one's energy at an early age can also precipitate or exacerbate a 'qi wild' state.

The physiological consequences are similar to those of environmental deprivation, described above. This hazard to vulnerable, immature children can lead to developmental defects that manifest grossly as, for example, heart valve defects, or subtly as minimal brain dysfunction and learning disabilities.

The associated pulse quality is Interrupted or Intermittent at an early age (between five and ten years) or Yielding Hollow Full-Overflowing and Slow between the ages of ten to fifteen years.

EXERCISE BEYOND ONE'S ENERGY IN EARLY LIFE

Another cause of the 'qi wild' disorder is excessive exercise far beyond one's energy at a young age during the critical years of development. This is often seen in youth who, during puberty and before, are involved in the adolescent athletic frenzy and are pushed by adults to become superstars. These well-meaning adults, including parents and coaches, do not realize that everyone is *not* born with the same level of energy. The quality associated with this 'qi wild' disorder is Yielding Hollow Full-Overflowing and Slow between the ages of ten to fifteen years, and Empty and Slow between the ages of sixteen to twenty.

The long-range effect of exercise beyond one's energy is the diminishment of circulation, deleteriously affecting the Heart, which in Chinese medicine controls the mind. The resulting symptoms, including reduced attention and concentration, anxiety, excitability, restlessness, and a tendency to become easily exhausted, are signs of disorder in what Dr. Shen calls the 'circulatory system' affecting the 'nervous system' (see glossary).

From my perspective, an insidious cause of the 'qi wild' condition which affects people of all ages is the attempt to slow the Heart rate through aerobic exercise, under the assumption that this will strengthen the heart muscle. Running is a particular form of this exercise to which people become addicted. Those who feel better after this form of extreme exercise are those who begin with poor circulation and varying degrees of malaise. Circulation increases as a response of the Heart to the demand to work harder and push more blood through the system, and the malaise consequently is relieved, leading even to a mild 'high.' However, pushing the blood requires more Heart qi, which in turn weakens the Heart, requiring even greater exercise to get the same circulatory result. Over time the Heart becomes weaker, the rate becomes slower, and eventually the Heart cannot even supply enough blood to the coronary arteries. This leads to a variety of illnesses including coronary occlusion and arrhythmias.

In girls another long-term effect of overexercise can be blood stagnation in the lower burner, and severe, lifelong menstrual problems. In addition, the circulatory problem will frequently lead to pseudoarthritic migrating pain, whereby pain is experienced upon waking and then dissipates when activity begins. Biomedically, this is a misunderstood condition, and often results in mistaken interventions with powerful medications that can cause their own form of iatrogenic suffering.

PROTRACTED MENORRHAGIA IN GIRLS

Similar pulse qualities will be found with prolonged menorrhagia in pubescent and adolescent girls, in which case we have both the 'qi wild' and 'blood out of control' (reckless) states simultaneously. The long-term effect of prolonged menorrhagia is fatigue, myalgias, and depression. The pulse quality associated with this disorder is Empty Thread-like or Leather. Heavy exercise is a common etiology to which the body responds by closing down the menstrual cycle until the overexercise stops.

SUDDEN CESSATION OF INTENSE, PROLONGED EXERCISE

Conversely, the sudden cessation of extreme exercise, especially when young, is another etiology of the 'qi wild' condition. Because this is a more acute situation, it can lead to more profound symptoms than those linked to overexercise or overwork. The pulse quality associated with this condition is Yielding Hollow Full-Overflowing and Rapid over the entire pulse.

The pathogenesis is that exercise causes the vascular system to expand in order to accommodate the increased volume of blood which is necessary to satisfy the nutritional requirements of heavy exercise; the blood vessels are therefore more dilated than normal. When the exercise is abruptly stopped, the amount of blood in the vascular system likewise suddenly decreases, but the vessels themselves tend to remain expanded. This division between the two, that is, decreased blood volume and the still expanded vessels, leaves a gap that is reflected in the pulse as a Hollow quality.

In Chinese medical terms, the yin has lost control of the yang. Blood, as a form of heavier yin energy, and qi, as a form of lighter yang energy, flow contiguously in the blood vessels. The blood (yin) inclines logically to the center, and the qi (yang) to the periphery of the vessels. Yang is expansive and is held in check only by the centripetal force of the more substantial yin energies. When the yin, as here, is markedly and suddenly diminished, the yang loses its grounding and moves out of control, and thus, the 'qi is wild.' The resulting physiological chaos disrupts the orderly circulation of yang to the channels and organs, impairing their function. This chaos is especially disruptive to the 'nervous system,' which depends on the organized integrity of the lighter, fast-moving qi energies.

This scenario of suddenly stopping exercise is seen frequently among young people who excel in athletics during high school, but do not succeed at the more competitive college level. There is thus a sharp reduction in physical activity. The ensuing symptoms include vague complaints of tiredness, migrating pain, labile emotions, severe anxiety, explosive anger, feelings of dissociation and detachment (being 'spaced out'), and losing one's mind. Sometimes, especially when lying down, there is a sensation that the body and arms are floating away, that the body is not real— a sensation that causes profound terror. Such mental and emotional symptoms are particularly severe if the 'nervous system' is already tense or weak. Often, these young people are seen by psychiatrists who render a diagnosis of anxiety neurosis or panic attacks, demonstrating that the 'qi wild' disorder is totally misunderstood in the biomedical world. Lifelong emotional problems can develop, which are compounded by biomedical treatment in the form of drugs and shock therapy.

SUDDEN EXTRAORDINARY EPISODE OF LIFTING

More rarely, an instance during which an individual is called upon to suddenly lift a weight far beyond his or her capacity can also cause a Yielding Hollow Full-Overflowing Rapid quality and a 'qi wild' state. This phenomenon occurs, for example, in emergencies when a person summons hidden strength to lift an object that is crushing themselves or another person.

SUBSTANCE ABUSE

Increasingly in our time, another origin of the 'qi wild' disorder is substance abuse over many years, and the ubiquitous use of prescription pharmaceuticals. The exact mechanism by which the 'qi wild' state develops with substance abuse is unclear. Probably the yin organs, especially the Liver, Heart, and Kidneys, are exhausted, with sequential loss of control over and contact with the yang energies, which, as described above, wander aimlessly and without functional organization. In following long-term heavy (and even casual) users of marijuana, I have consistently found the Empty quality, especially in the left middle position (Liver).

'Qi wild' qualities with Regular rate

EMPTY TYPES OF 'QI WILD' QUALITIES

These are presented in approximate order of increasing severity. For more detail, see Chapter 9.

Empty

The Empty quality is palpable only at the most superficial qi depth; no pulse quality (or just a Separating quality) is felt at the blood and organ depths. This form of the Empty quality is mildly Tense, but more Yielding and pliable compared to the harder sensation found with the Leather quality, and harder than the very pliable sensations of the Empty Thread-like (soggy, soft) quality, the Scattered quality, and the Minute quality.

This quality occurs most often in the yin stages of the six stages of disease, and especially the lesser yin and terminal yin stages of the disease process. With the exception of transient mental illness, wherever it is found—upper, middle, or lower burner, over the entire pulse, or in one position—the Empty quality is usually a sign of advanced qi deficiency and of potentially serious illness within months. Age at onset of this etiology is usually between fifteen and twenty.

To repeat, the 'qi wild' disorder is signified by chaos. It represents a very serious disorganization and disruption of overall physiology. Mental illness is one form of that chaos, with the Empty quality being a marker for the anarchy of severe neurosis and psychosis. I once took the pulse of a child and his mother and found it to be transiently completely Empty in all three positions on both wrists. I was at first alarmed at the implications of extensive qi deficiency, and treated them accordingly, which changed nothing. I learned quickly that I was dealing with an Empty quality that was unrelated to its classical interpretation. In this type of case, the Empty quality was transient, lasting only a few weeks, and was a sign that these individuals had lost their center and were floating aimlessly, with extreme anxiety and somatic manifestations, as a result of a sudden and very stressful life situation, a form of the post-traumatic syndrome.

Leather

The Leather quality is similar to the Empty quality, except that the former is much harder at the surface and represents a more serious deficiency of essence, yin, or blood. The nature of the 'qi wild' disorder is more advanced in this case than when it is associated with an Empty pulse.

Empty Thread-like (soggy, soft)

The Empty Thread-like (soggy or soft) pulse is "like a strand of cotton floating on the water"[17] at the qi depth, and disappears on pressure. It is a sign of extreme deficiency of blood, essence, and yang.

Scattered

As one rolls the finger from distal to proximal position, the Scattered quality is broken into fragments, as if pieces of the pulse were missing, on and off. This pulse is a sign of a more extreme form of 'qi wild' and signifies a grave disintegration in the circulation of energy within and among yin and yang and blood, which is caused by profound deficiency. The damaging events usually occur before the age of ten and often involve excessive deprivation of some sort. The prognosis is poor for individuals who present with this pulse. Indeed, I have been told that this quality is characteristic of AIDS patients. My informants who treat AIDS patients tell me that the Scattered quality is referred to as the 'ceiling dripping' pulse. It is one of the traditional 'eight pulses of death,' characteristic of either the terminal yin cold or terminal yin heat patterns.

Minute

This quality is Thin and Feeble, and is found only in the middle depth. It shows little resistance to pressure and resembles the Scattered pulse in its lack of longitudinal continuity. This quality is a sign of extensive qi and yang deficiency in a person who is seriously ill. I view it as a stage in the development of a 'qi wild' disorder that is even beyond that represented by the Scattered quality, and in which there is not enough yang left to rise to the surface. With the same clinical manifestations associated with the Scattered quality (including AIDS), the Minute pulse is among the most serious, and can also indicate impending death.

YIELDING HOLLOW TYPES OF 'QI WILD' QUALITIES

We have already discussed the Yielding Hollow Full-Overflowing and Rapid quality under the aegis of etiology. This quality is most specifically associated with the condition that results from the sudden cessation of extensive and prolonged exercise. Another pulse that may also indicate 'qi wild' is the Yielding Hollow Full-Overflowing and Slow quality. While still a very serious sign, in terms of overall body condition this quality is a less profound sign of the 'qi wild' state than the Yielding Hollow Intermittent or Yielding Hollow Interrupted pulses, which also involve Heart function. Etiologic events, particularly occurring between the ages of eight and fifteen, such as environmental deprivation, overwork, and overexercise, can also give rise to this pulse.

The Empty and Hollow qualities are frequently confused with each other. The Hollow quality is palpable on the surface at the qi depth, is separating or missing in the blood depth, and is felt again in the organ depth, whereas the Empty quality is felt only at the surface qi depth, and often separating rather than Absent at the other depths. The Yielding Hollow quality informs us that the yin has even less control of the yang, and that the qi is even 'wilder,' than with the Empty quality. (Other types of Hollow pulses are discussed in Chapters 9 and 13.)

Yielding Ropy Hollow

The Yielding Ropy Hollow quality can also be found after inordinately excessive exercise or very hard physical work beyond one's energy over an extended period of time, or in an environment characterized by significant deprivation of food, clothing, or shelter before the age of fifteen.

Again, the yin blood and the more yang vessel wall become functionally dissociated. This can happen gradually where the blood vessel is of normal diameter, but because of nutritional deprivation or working beyond one's energy the volume of blood is reduced. Such nutritional deprivation causes a drying out of the intima of the vessel walls over a long period of time. This process is signified on the pulse by the Yielding Ropy quality.

QI WILD QUALITIES CHARACTERIZED BY CHANGE

Change in Qualities

An important issue in terms of qualities is the attribute of change. A Change in Qualities of the pulse is only slightly less serious than the Scattered pulse, the Yielding Hollow pulse, and pulses with rhythm disturbances such as the Yielding Hollow Interrupted or Yielding Hollow Intermittent.

Change in Qualities (Fig. 6-2) can occur over the entire pulse or in one or more positions. When found over the entire pulse the diagnosis is 'qi wild.' When found in just one position it represents the loss of contact between yin and yang and significant yin organ disease. Additionally, one interpretation that applies to both is that a Change in Qualities is a sign that the body or yin organ system is in a state of transition, and that the condition is either deteriorating or improving.[18]

Fig. 6-2 Change in Qualities

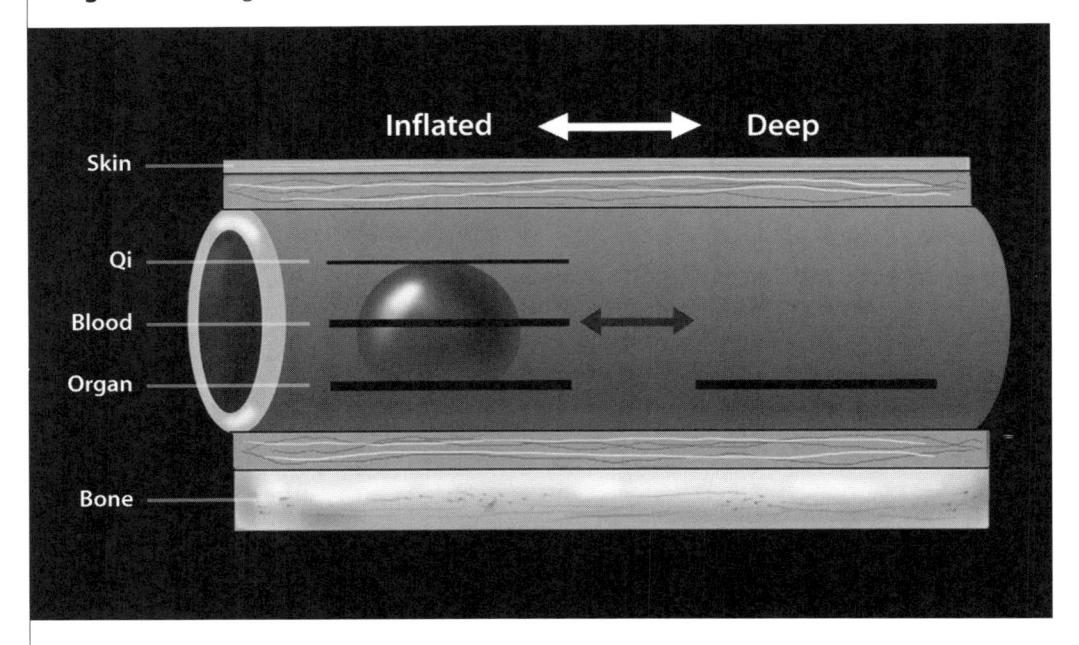

CHANGE IN QUALITIES OVER THE ENTIRE PULSE

This pulse instability is associated with an extreme imbalance in which function is seriously impaired. In many individual principal positions the quality keeps changing: one moment the quality is Tense, the next it is Empty, and thereafter again Tense, which shift continues indefinitely. This is a sign of a serious 'qi wild' condition in which the patient is at great risk. This type of pulse occurs in individuals who, for a long time, have been continually pushing themselves beyond their level of energy. I have also found this quality to be closely associated with individuals who use powerful chemical medications, with auto-immune diseases, or who live in geographic areas of chaotic energy.[19]

CHANGE IN QUALITIES IN ONE POSITION

This is a sign of extreme dysfunction in the yin organ associated with that position, signifying that the yin and yang have separated in that particular yin organ system. For example, Change in Qualities at the left distal position representing the Heart is a sign of serious instability of Heart qi, even in the presence of a normal rhythm and rate.

CHANGE IN QUALITIES BILATERALLY IN ONE BURNER

Pulse qualities can change in the same bilateral position. Thus, it is necessary to judge which position changes most in order to assess which of the yin organ systems is affecting the other. For example, in the middle burner, are the qualities changing most in the left middle position such that the Liver qi is the primary deficiency, and is affecting the Spleen? Or are the qualities changing more in the right middle position, such that the Spleen qi is the primary deficiency, and is affecting the Liver? Successful treatment strategy depends on a correct analysis.

In addition, however, qualities that are bilaterally in the same position can also point to a problem in the area unrelated to the associated yin organs. For example, Change in Qualities in both distal positions can signify physiological chaos in the upper burner, as with a mediastinal tumor or with breast cancer.

'Qi wild' qualities with Arrhythmic rate

The process leading to these qualities usually begins before the age of ten, and often before five. Unless very strong intervention is taken, all the qualities are pathognomonic of a very short life because of severely compromised Kidney qi and essence.

Empty or Yielding Hollow Interrupted or Intermittent (constant)

An Empty or Yielding Hollow Interrupted (or Intermittent) quality is technically a 'qi wild' pulse. The Interrupted (or Intermittent) quality alone, without the Hollow combination, is also a sign of severe instability affecting the entire organism, although more particularly only of Heart function. Therefore, while heart organ disease is ordinarily not technically a 'qi wild' condition (but is a sign of chaos in the Heart), where the pulse is Hollow Interrupted it should be considered as such, and as an extreme outcome of advanced Heart qi and yang deficiency and exhaustion. As 'emperor,' disease in the Heart has more far-reaching and serious consequences for the entire organism. This combination of qualities is a sign of the most serious life-threatening illness. The prognosis is poor for longevity.

Recapitulation of the 'qi wild' quality

One way of viewing deficiency is to distinguish between the kind that occurs with yin and yang in contact, and the more serious variety, in which yin and yang are separated. The qualities of both kinds of deficiency can occur over the entire pulse or in just one position.

Examples of qualities in which yin and yang are still in contact are the Feeble-Absent and Deep pulses. They are signs of significant deficiency of qi and blood wherever they are found, whether in one position or over the entire pulse, and a prognosticator of serious illness within three to five years.

On the other hand, a quality in which the yin and yang are separated is the Empty pulse. When this quality occurs in only one position the yin and yang of the organ represented by that position are out of contact, and it is a sign of extreme dysfunction in that organ. The separation of yin and yang in one organ, if not corrected, will ultimately generate 'qi wild' chaos throughout the organism.

When the Empty quality is found over the entire pulse, this means that the yin and yang have separated in the entire organism, and that the qi is 'wild.' When this occurs the person is at great risk for serious debilitating diseases such as cancer, auto-immune or degenerative diseases of the central nervous system.

INSTABILITY RELATED TO HEART AND CIRCULATION, BUT UNRELATED TO RHYTHM AND RATE

In terms of sensation, Changes in Intensity and Amplitude are sometimes indistinguishable and are occurring simultaneously. Therefore, for practical purposes, I have included them together in this section.

Entire pulse

Change in Intensity

Although this quality (Fig. 6-3) is a sign of physiological instability, technically it does not signify a 'qi wild' condition because it is more a reflection of the Heart and circulation than of the true qi of the entire organism. It is a sign of Heart qi or yang deficiency, the difference depending upon accompanying qualities.

In terms of physiology, the intensity is the substance, buoyancy, and resilience of the pulse wave, and reflects the condition of the qi, blood, yin, and essence of the organism. I have found Changes in Intensity over the entire pulse, in one position, or over the entire pulse in an undulating manner from one position to another, and from one wrist to another.

Fig. 6-3 Change in Intensity

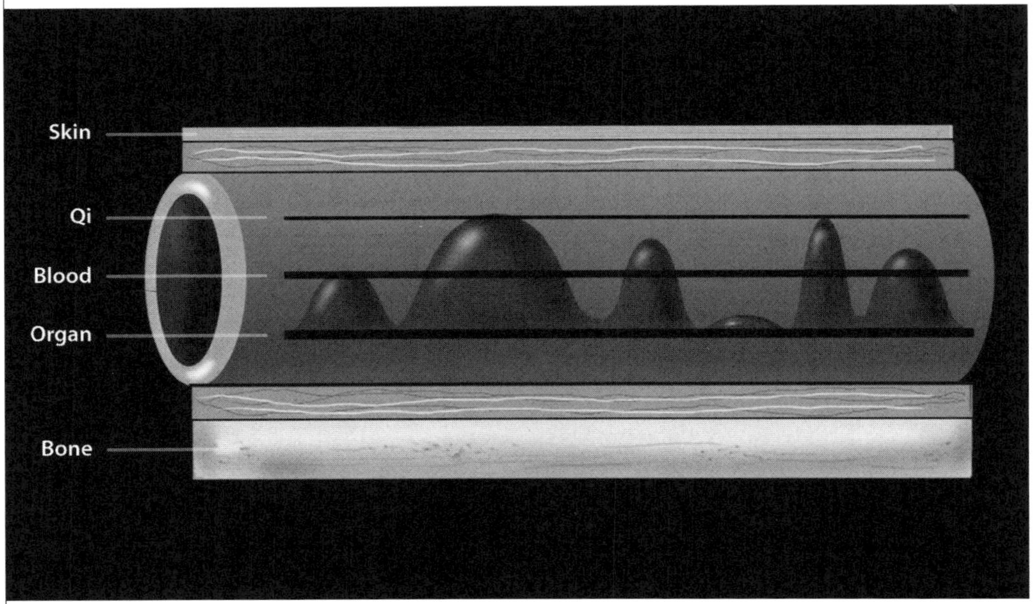

CHANGE IN INTENSITY: CONSTANT OVER TIME

In this case, the Change in Intensity over the entire pulse is constant and independent of when the pulse is taken. This quality signifies that it is the blood circulation that is affected. Symptoms include circulatory disorders such as cold hands and feet, migrating pain, a Heart spirit disturbance (Heart qi agitation), anxiety, and emotional instability if the Change in Intensity is small, and Heart qi deficiency if the change is large.

Etiologies

Constant Change in Intensity can have two etiologies, both of which involve the circulation and Heart energy. Since the change is undeviating, the circulation that is affected is more blood than qi. The relationship between the Heart and circulation is complex. Over time the pulse pictures tend to merge.

Circulation affects the Heart

When the circulation affects the Heart due to trauma, both physical and mental, the pulse at first will be Tight and Rapid. There will be a Change in Intensity over the entire pulse.

Emotional trauma

We know that emotional shock at any time in life drains Heart yin. At this point the face is red, especially around M-HN-3 *(yin tang)*, and the hands are more pale. On the pulse, the left distal position, especially the Pericardium, will be Tight, the entire position possibly Slippery, and the Diaphragm position may be Inflated. It the physical condition is good, the left distal position may be Inflated; if poor, it will be Flat. There will be Change in Intensity and Rough Vibration over the entire pulse.

In the beginning the rate is Rapid. However, over a long period of time the rate decreases to very Slow (about 50-60 beats per minute) and the left distal position becomes Feeble.

Physical trauma

Depending on the severity of the trauma, the pulse becomes very Tight and Rapid. In the affected area the pulse will be Inflated in a person of relatively robust health, and Flat in a person with reduced qi. There will be Change in Intensity over the entire pulse, but no Rough Vibration. The left distal position will be unremarkable.

Again, over a long period of time the rate will decrease to very Slow (50-60 beats per minute) and the left distal position will be unremarkable unless there are other factors affecting the Heart.

Hypothermia

The pulse is Firm or Hidden and very Slow, altogether too deep to show a Change in Intensity.

Heart affects the circulation

This is usually a manifestation of Heart qi deficiency being unable to move the circulation, typically a manifestation of a constitutional deficit, disease (rheumatic), overwork, overexercise, generally poor physical condition (Spleen qi failing to produce blood), or a long-term mental and emotional drain (worry, obsession).

The entire pulse will eventually reflect a Change in Intensity and Rough Vibration. The rate will be Slow, in the low 60s, except in those who do aerobic exercise, when it will be lower still. The left distal position will show varying degrees of deficiency or separation of yin and yang, from Feeble-Absent to Change in Qualities. Eventually the left distal position will be Slippery and show Rough Vibration and a greater Change in Intensity than the rest of the pulse. If the cause is constitutional, the proximal positions will be Feeble; if from chronic debilitation, the entire pulse might be Reduced, but less than in the left distal position. If there is an obsessional factor, the wave will be Hesitant; if there is long-term worry, the Vibration will be Smooth at first, then later moving to Rough. Since the issue here is the overworking of the mind, the proximal positions, especially the left, will be Tight.

CHANGE IN INTENSITY: INCONSTANT OVER TIME

When the Change in Intensity does not occur each time the pulse is taken, the cause is usually stress affecting the Liver. In Dr. Shen's view, the stress in men is due to overwork, and the stress in women is due to emotion. Qi is more ephemeral and dependent on diurnal energy levels that rise and fall for many reasons, and on stresses on the Liver, which also tend to fluctuate. When energy is reduced or stress elevated, the Change in Intensity is more obvious. Since it is one of the functions of the Liver to move the kinetic qi through the body, the circulation of qi and these changes in intensity and amplitude are tied to the vicissitudes of this yin organ system.

Change in Intensity undulating from one position to another

The intensity of this pulse waxes and wanes from one position to another. Some positions have a strong intensity, others diminished; some positions that are, for example, Robust, become diminished, and those that are Reduced become Robust. There is no regular pattern to this phenomenon.

I have found this condition in a few patients who experienced sexual abuse from infancy through childhood, involving both parents. My impression is that this is a form of chaos in the 'nervous system,' and especially the nervous innervation of the heart organ.

Change in Intensity undulating from one wrist to another

In this pulse, the strength of the intensity shifts from one wrist to another. At first, for example, the left may be Robust and the right Reduced, followed by the right being Robust and the left Reduced. This shifting is constant.

Most often associated with this pulse is a current and powerful interpersonal conflict, and less often, a recent episode in which the individual has exerted him- or herself considerably beyond their normal strength.

Change in Intensity affecting only one wrist

When the Change in Intensity occurs on only one wrist and the other wrist is relatively normal, one cause is trauma to the side of the body on which the Change in Intensity is occurring. Without a history of trauma, if it occurs only on the right side, the pathology is in the 'digestive system.' If it occurs only on the left, the 'organ system' is affected.

Change in Amplitude over the entire pulse

Amplitude is the height to which the pulse is generated from organ to qi depth or beyond (Fig. 6-4). Ordinarily it is considered to be a measure of the yang force, the basal metabolic functional heat and spirit of the organism. High amplitude reflects a strong yang force, and low amplitude is a mark of diminished yang force and basal metabolic heat.[20]

My experience, however, is that sometimes these changes seem to be taking place in the context of a Change in Intensity, and that they therefore reflect a similar interpretation of Heart qi and perhaps Heart yang deficiency. Some practitioners report that a Change in Amplitude over the entire pulse can be palpated on individuals with mitral valve prolapse.

Fig. 6-4 Change in Amplitude

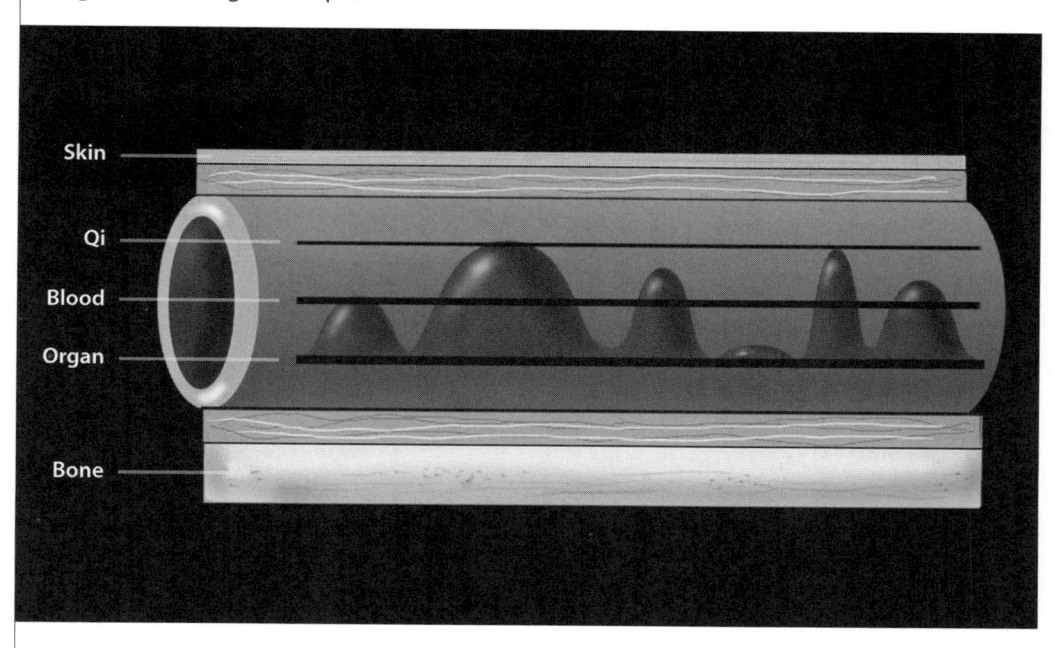

INDIVIDUAL POSITIONS

Principal individual positions

A Change in Intensity and Amplitude at individual positions on the pulse reflects significant deficiency of qi, blood, and yang, and of a separation of yin and yang, in the yin organ system associated with that position. A Change in Intensity at any one position indicates a transition in function, usually from better to worse. Thus, it is a signal to pay close attention to the performance of the yin organ represented by that position.

Complementary individual positions

A Change in Intensity and/or Amplitude in the complementary individual positions is a sign of impaired function in the associated organ or area.

DISTINGUISHING CHANGE IN INTENSITY AND AMPLITUDE FROM CHANGE IN QUALITIES

With Change in Qualities, the change is sudden from one quality to another, whereas with Change in Intensity, the change can be followed almost continuously as the pulse becomes more or less Robust.

DISTINGUISHING CHANGE IN INTENSITY AND AMPLITUDE FROM ARRHYTHMIA

When the Change in Intensity is considerable the pulse may simulate a Change in Rate at Rest, or even an Interrupted quality where the beats seem to be missing. Careful and patient observation and experience are necessary to make the proper distinction.

ONE SIDE ROBUST AND OTHER SIDE REDUCED

Discussed more completely in Chapter 14, this is a form of 'husband-wife' instability, which I associate with considerable chaos and physiological instability.

SEPARATION OF YIN AND YANG AT INDIVIDUAL POSITIONS

A less severe form of instability is when the 'qi wild' qualities described above (except for Yielding Hollow Interrupted-Intermittent) are found at only one position. The physiological functioning of the associated organs is in a state of chaos and requires urgent intervention. We have mentioned this in passing with regard to Change in Intensity and the Empty qualities in our recapitulation of the 'qi wild' qualities. There we said that the separation of yin and yang in a single organ is a potential threat to the entire organism over time unless the condition is corrected. Qualities that signify the separation of yin and yang and which appear only at individual positions and never over the entire pulse, are the Unstable and Nonhomogeneous, which we will discuss here.

Nonhomogeneous

This quality signifies such extreme stagnation, probably involving all the substance of an individual organ, that it represents the separation of yin and yang in that organ and the resultant physiological anarchy. It is discussed in Chapter 11.

Unstable

The Unstable quality is one that has an irregular nature on smaller segments of the pulse, such as at one position, or simultaneously at both positions (wrists) at one burner.

With regard to sensation, this pulse seems to rebound off the finger tremulously and erratically. It is like a pulsating point that moves from one part of the finger to another with a quick, jerky, and constantly changing movement. The sense under the finger at that position is of total chaos.[21] This is why some observers in the past have mistakenly attributed this phenomenon to a true arrhythmia. However, a true arrhythmia appears over the entire pulse at all positions.

Interpretation   The Unstable quality appears when the qi, blood, and yang of a yin organ, and especially the parenchymal material represented by that position, is significantly injured. When this quality is found, the patient's condition should be viewed as very serious until further investigation proves otherwise.[22]

Positions

To distinguish among the several possible pathologies at any one position, other modalities of Chinese and biomedical diagnosis are needed. Thus, it is inappropriate to make such distinctions here. Suffice it to say that anywhere this quality is found, it should be considered a sign of serious disharmony in the yin organ system which that position represents.

BILATERALLY AT SPECIFIC POSITIONS

I have found the Unstable quality bilaterally most often in the upper burner. When palpated in both distal positions, the problem could be in the chest, such as the long-term result of severe trauma with greatly impaired function of the chest organs, or a mediastinal tumor interfering with the functions of the Lungs, Heart, esophagus, or trachea. It could also represent serious dysfunction of both the Heart and Lungs simultaneously after a long period of cardiopulmonary illness.

In the middle positions this quality can signify severe dysfunction of the abdominal organs, possibly due to a tumor, abscess, ascites, or infection. Severe impairment of more than one individual organ, such as the Liver and Spleen simultaneously, is also a possibility, or with pancreatitis or a lymphoma.

In the proximal positions, severe chronic pelvic inflammatory disease, an expanding tumor, kidney failure, or severe impairment of several of the organs simultaneously in this area could account for this quality.

EACH WRIST

I have not felt the Unstable quality simultaneously at all the positions on one side.

INDIVIDUAL POSITIONS

When found at an individual position, the Unstable pulse is a sign of serious pathology. In all positions other than the left distal, the Unstable quality can be a sign of a neoplasm.

Left distal The Unstable quality here has been found with current or past major infarction of the left ventricle of the heart. In one instance where biomedical testing was unremarkable, treatment with Korean and American ginseng and placenta had a powerful effect on the patient's well-being physically, and especially emotionally. The same finding and treatment in the daughter led to the same result.

Right distal The Unstable quality here has been found with lung tumors, uncontrollable asthma, bronchiestasis, and the interstitial lung disorders, such as sarcoidosis and occupational lung diseases.

Left middle An Unstable quality here usually indicates lymphoma or other severe primary pathology, such as chronic hepatitis in the Liver or secondary metastasis from a tumor in another location.

Right middle The pattern that gives rise to an Unstable quality in this position is severe qi, phlegm, or food stagnation, as might occur with a tumor, probably malignant.

Left proximal An Unstable quality in this position can once again indicate serious gross pathology. Since the Kidneys are the foundation energy of the organism upon which all other energies depend, this sign here is especially portentous of a dangerously ill person. Addison's disease is one syndrome that comes to mind; another is the loss of function in one or both kidneys, requiring dialysis. With simultaneous symptoms of Heart dysfunction, the Unstable quality at this position indicates a more serious condition due to the Kidneys' inability to relieve the accumulation of fluid in the body. And again, the Unstable quality at this position can be a sign of a tumor in the kidneys or large intestine, probably malignant.

Right proximal Severe weakness of Kidney yang, Bladder, or Small Intestine disease should be considered when an Unstable quality is found here. It may also be a sign of a malignant kidney tumor.

'BLOOD OUT OF CONTROL' (RECKLESS BLOOD)

All of the qualities that indicate 'blood out of control' are under the Hollow category. Two of the three types of Hollow qualities signify blood out of control, and one, as we have already observed, is a sign of 'qi wild.' (Further differentiation among the three Hollow qualities is found in Chapters 9 and 13.)

The category of qualities subsumed under blood out of control does not appear in any source known to me other than Dr. Shen, and has been derived from clinical observation and discussions with him, rather than from anything he has written or spoken in public.

Hemorrhage rapid

Leather-like Hollow

With this pulse, the qi depth is very Hard and organ depth somewhat Tense, and the blood depth is completely absent of quality (Absent).

The Leather-like Hollow quality over the entire pulse is usually a sign of notable and even massive hemorrhage such as might occur with an aneurism, gastric ulcer, or sudden lifting beyond one's strength leading to the rupture of an artery: the lack of control over the blood occurs suddenly. This situation is life-threatening due to shock, which frequently accompanies sudden hemorrhage. More often, this quality appears in one position when a single organ can no longer control its blood, for example, the Stomach with a bleeding ulcer, or the uterus with menometrorrhagia. This quality is always serious whenever it is encountered, and calls for emergency measures. When the rate is Rapid the hemorrhage is imminent, and when Slow the hemorrhage is of recent occurrence.

Very Tense-Tight Hollow Full-Overflowing

The very Tense-Tight Hollow Full-Overflowing quality rises above the qi depth, separates or is completely Absent at the blood depth, and is very Tense at the organ depth.

The uniform appearance over the entire pulse or on either side of a very Tense-Tight Hollow Full-Overflowing quality can signify hypertension. In insulin-dependent diabetes, this combination of pulse qualities is more confined in location to the middle and especially proximal positions. Additionally, with the very Tense-Tight Hollow Full-Overflowing pulse the potential for cerebral bleeding (stroke) is always present, and is therefore classified as a form of 'blood out of control.' Since this is often due to blood heat, the term 'reckless blood' is appropriate here.

Hemorrhage gradual

Yielding Partially Hollow and Slow (Full-Overflowing when very serious)

With the Yielding Partially Hollow and Slow pulse, the qi depth is pliable and gives way lightly under pressure, the blood depth separates with pressure, and the organ depth is Normal or slightly Diminished.

In contradistinction to the Leather-like Hollow quality, the Yielding Partially Hollow pulse can, among other signs, be an indication of more gradual bleeding, which can also lead slowly to a chronic severe drain of qi that manifests as a secondary 'qi wild' condition as well as 'blood out of control.' Examples of such bleeding are moderately heavy menstrual bleeding over time, or repeated abortions or deliveries with blood loss. Over a long period of time, all of the symptoms of blood deficiency in the extreme, and of 'qi wild,' manifest with this process.

Fig. 6-5a   Rhythm

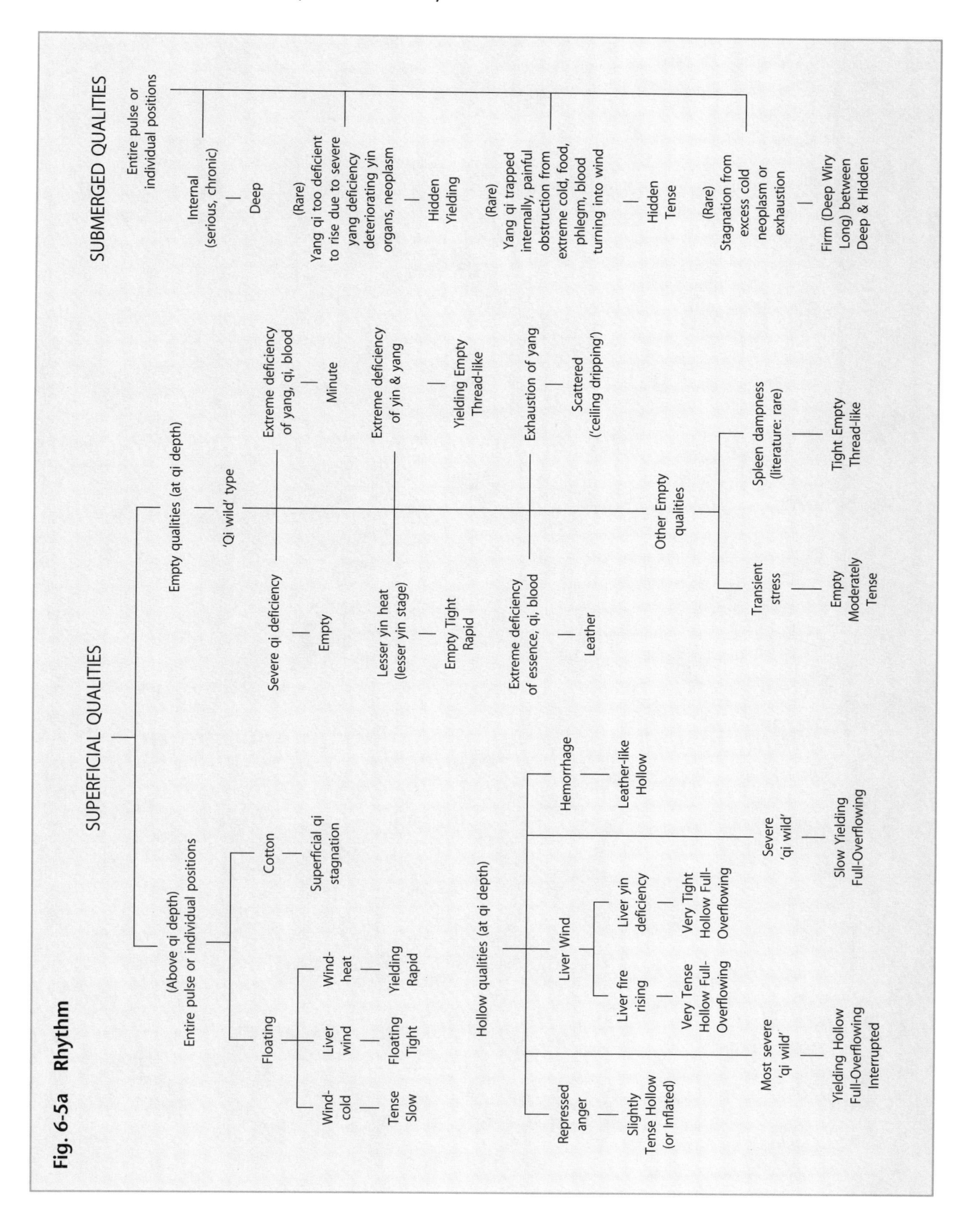

SUPERFICIAL QUALITIES
(Above qi depth)
Entire pulse or individual positions

- Floating
  - Wind-cold — Tense Slow
  - Liver wind — Floating Tight
  - Wind-heat — Yielding Rapid
- Cotton
  - Superficial qi stagnation

Empty qualities (at qi depth)
'Qi wild' type

- Severe qi deficiency — Empty
- Extreme deficiency of yang, qi, blood — Minute
- Lesser yin heat (lesser yin stage) — Empty Tight Rapid
- Extreme deficiency of yin & yang — Yielding Empty Thread-like
- Exhaustion of yang — Scattered ('ceiling dripping')
- Extreme deficiency of essence, qi, blood — Leather

Other Empty qualities
- Spleen dampness (literature: rare) — Tight Empty Thread-like
- Transient stress — Empty Moderately Tense

Hollow qualities (at qi depth)
- Hemorrhage — Leather-like Hollow
- Liver Wind
  - Liver yin deficiency — Very Tight Hollow Full-Overflowing
  - Liver fire rising — Very Tense Hollow Full-Overflowing
- Repressed anger — Slightly Tense Hollow (or Inflated)
- Most severe 'qi wild' — Yielding Hollow Full-Overflowing Interrupted
- Severe 'qi wild' — Slow Yielding Full-Overflowing

SUBMERGED QUALITIES
Entire pulse or individual positions

- Internal (serious, chronic) — Deep
- (Rare) Yang qi too deficient to rise due to severe yang deficiency deteriorating yin organs, neoplasm — Hidden Yielding
- (Rare) Yang qi trapped internally, painful obstruction from extreme cold, food, phlegm, blood turning into wind — Hidden Tense
- (Rare) Stagnation from excess cold neoplasm or exhaustion — Firm (Deep Wiry Long) between Deep & Hidden

Fig. 6-5b Rhythm (detail)

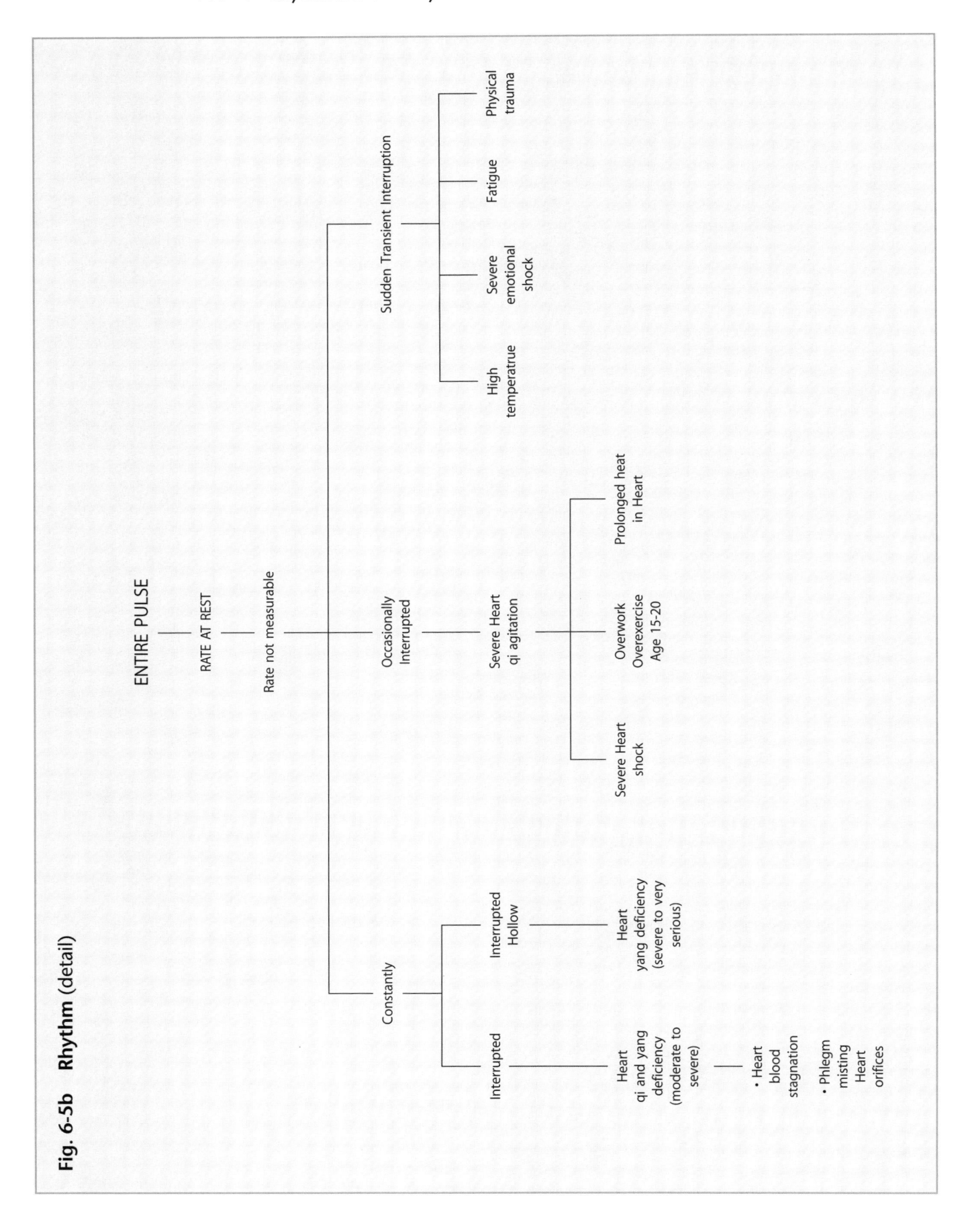

ENTIRE PULSE — RATE AT REST

- Rate not measurable
  - Constantly
    - Interrupted
      - Heart qi and yang deficiency (moderate to severe)
        - Heart blood stagnation
        - Phlegm misting Heart orifices
    - Interrupted Hollow
      - Heart yang deficiency (severe to very serious)
  - Occasionally Interrupted
    - Severe Heart shock
    - Severe Heart qi agitation
      - Overwork Overexercise Age 15-20
      - Prolonged heat in Heart
  - Sudden Transient Interruption
    - High temperatrue
    - Severe emotional shock
    - Fatigue
    - Physical trauma

Fig. 6-6 Stability

STABILITY

'QI WILD' (ENTIRE PULSE)

- Yielding Hollow with Rapid or Normal rate
- Yielding Hollow with Slow rate
- Empty (see depth)
  - Empty — Serious qi deficiency
  - Empty Thread-like — Extreme yin and yang deficiency
  - Leather — Extreme deficiency of essence, yin and blood
  - Minute — Extreme deficiency of yang, qi and blood
  - Scattered — Exhaustion of yang
- Changing
  - Quality Shifting from Side to Side
  - Change in Quality

COMBINED 'QI WILD' AND BLOOD OUT OF CONTROL (ENTIRE PULSE)

- Intermittent and Hollow — Profound physiological and metabolic dysfunction

Instability related to Heart & circulation
- Entire pulse
  - Inconstant Change in Intensity — Liver qi stagnation
  - Constant Change in Intensity — Heart qi & yang deficiency

YIN AND YANG SEPARATING AT INDIVIDUAL POSITIONS

- Empty
- Change in Qualities, Intensity, or Amplitude
- Unstable
- Nonhomogenous

Profound physiological and metabolic dysfunction

Blood Out of Control Hemorrhage
- Gradual — Yielding Partially Hollow
- Sudden
  - Entire pulse — Tense-Tight Hollow Full-Overflowing
  - One position
    - Recent — Leather-like Hollow with Slow rate
    - Imminent — Leather-like Hollow with Rapid rate

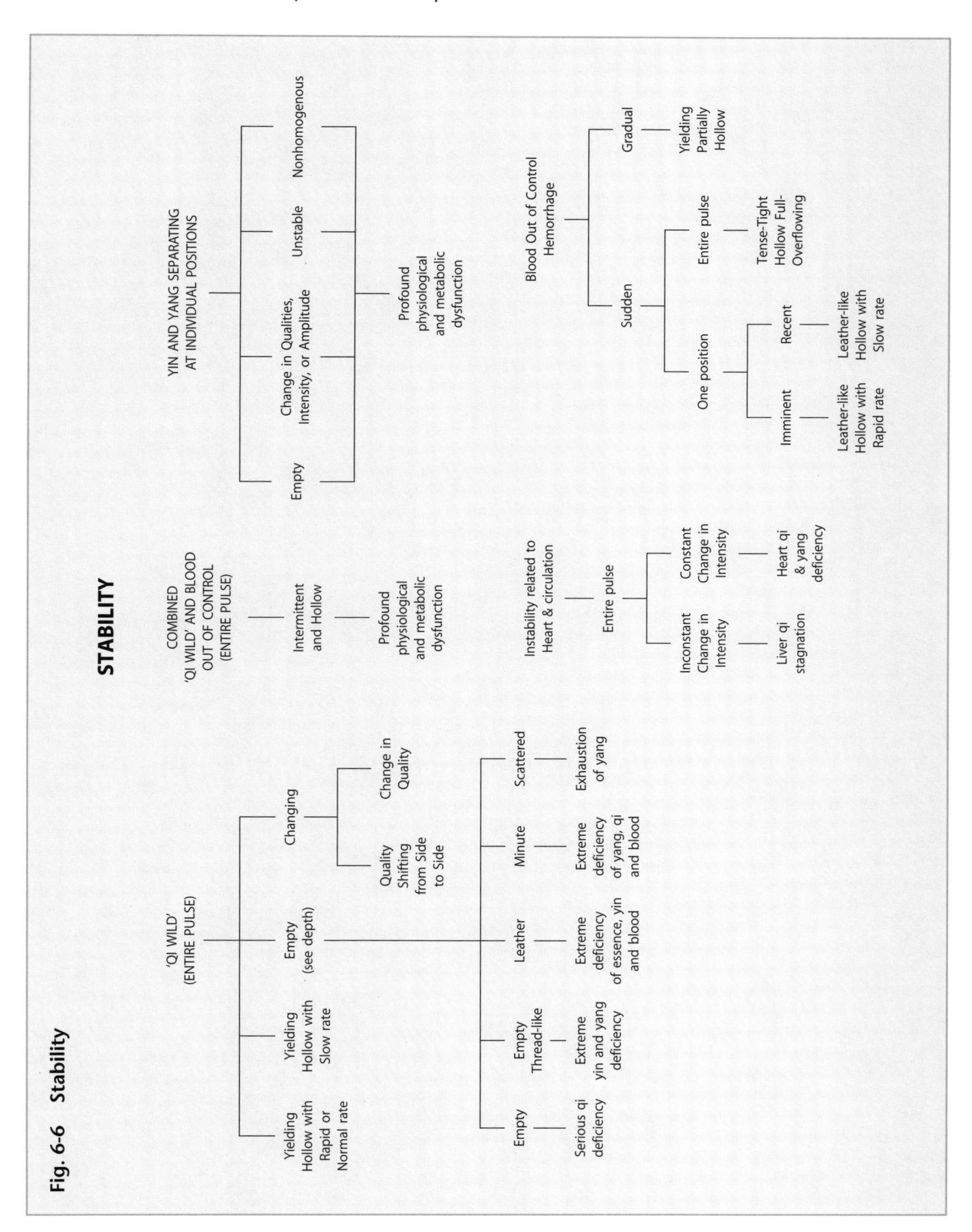

145 ❖ Rhythm and Stability

CHAPTER 7

Rate

CONTENTS

The Normal Rate According to Age, 152
The Rapid Rate, 153
    Rapid, 153
    Bounding, 153
    Rapid pulses categorized according to etiology, 153
        External etiology, 153
            External heat in the protective level, 153
            Heat stroke, 153
            Trauma (shock), 154
                Physical trauma, 154
                Emotional trauma, 154
                Condition of the true qi, 154
                Time elapsed since trauma, 155
            Seasonal variations, 155
        Internal-external etiology, 155
            The Heart, 156
                Emotional symptoms predominate, 156
                    Very mild Heart qi agitation, 156
                    Mild heat from excess, 156
                    Moderate to severe Heart qi agitation, 156
                    Heart qi stagnation, 156
                Physical symptoms predominate, 156
                    Trapped qi in the Heart, 156
                    Heart blood stagnation (mild-moderate and severe), 156
        Internal etiology, 156
            Heat from excess, 156

                Heat in the qi level, 156
                Heat in the blood, 157
                    'Blood heat', 157
                    'Blood thick', 157
                    'Nervous system tense', 158
                Heat from deficiency, 159
                    Entire pulse, 159
                    Individual positions, 160
                Internal etiology other than heat, 160
                    Imminent hemorrhage, 160
                    Pain, 160
                    Acute phase of chronic illness, 161
                    Lesser yin heat pattern, 161
            Sudden cessation of exercise or heavy work, 161
        Combinations, 162
The Slow Rate, 162
    Slow, 162
        Slow pulses categorized according to etiology, 162
            Common causes in contemporary society, 163
                External, 163
                    Cold from external excess, 163
                Internal, 163
                    Cold from deficiency (qi and yang deficiency), 163
                    Heart qi and yang deficiency, 163
                    Aerobic exercise, 163
            Less common causes, 163
                Liver qi stagnation and qi deficiency, 163
                Internal heat from excess: late stage 'blood thick' (middle stage arteriosclerosis), 164
                Yin deficiency (late stage arteriosclerosis), 164
                Poisoning, 164
                Medications, 164
                Heart qi and yang deficiency, 164
                Shock, 164
            Uncommon causes, 164
                Cold from internal excess, 164
                Internal heat pernicious influence, 165
                Damp-heat and phlegm-dampness, 165
                Heat exhaustion, 165
        Classification according to degree of slowness, 165
            Sixty-eight to seventy-two beats, 165
                Qi deficiency before age fifty, 165
                Liver qi stagnation and deficiency, 166
                Cold from excess at any age, 166
                    External cold, 166
                    Internal cold from excess, 166
            Sixty-four to sixty-eight beats, 166
            Sixty to sixty-four beats, 167
                Deficiency, 167
                    Cold from deficiency: qi and yang deficiency, 167
                    Yin deficiency, 167

                    Excess, 167
                        Cold, 167
                        Heat, 167
                Between forty and sixty beats, 168
                    Aerobic exercise, 168
                    Poisoning, 169
                    Deficient qi and yang affecting circulation of qi and blood, 169
                    Heart qi and yang deficiency, 169
                    Medications, 169
            Combinations, 170
Changes in Rate, 170
Rate Variations between Wrists, 170
    Etiology, 170
        Congenital anomaly, 170
        Shock during pregnancy, 170
        Heart qi deficiency, 170
        Trauma and/or heavy lifting, 170
        Habit, 170
        Digestive and organ system imbalance, 171
        ▪ Fig. 7-1: Rapid flowchart, 172
        ▪ Fig. 7-1b: Rapid flowchart detail, 173
        ▪ Fig. 7-2: Slow flowchart, 174

CHAPTER 7

Rate

Traditionally, the rate of the pulse has been associated with conditions of either cold or heat.[1] In my own experience, however, I have found that in our time the rate more commonly involves factors that affect Heart function and circulation, such as shock, overexercise, and overwork. Since the Heart is the 'emperor,' the rate and its regularity are, in my opinion, the qualities that supersede all other considerations in the interpretation of the pulse and in the therapeutic regimen that follows.[2]

The rate always involves the entire pulse (all three positions on both wrists) rather than an individual position or combination of positions.[3] I have never observed a rate at one position that differed from the overall rate. I have palpated the Unstable quality, which does give the impression of being more Rapid in one position, but actually reflects a condition of serious disorganization in the energetic and even parenchymal integrity of the yin organ represented by that position (see Chapter 6).

Dr. Shen describes situations in which the rate at first appears to be Normal, but is actually abnormal because various factors will balance each other. An example is a pulse that is Rapid because of nervous tension, but is also Slow because the individual runs regularly. The outcome is a false Normal rate, because overwork of the mind in the short term affects the 'nervous system' and causes the pulse to be more Rapid, while physical overwork or overexercise in the long term affects qi and causes the pulse to be Slow.

In this book, the rate as described is measured by a non-digital watch rather than by the breath. This is because of the contradictory methods of using the breath to appraise the rate. Some say that it is the breath of the practitioner, others the breath of the patient, that should be used. In addition, I have observed considerable variation in breathing rates from one practitioner to another, and even with the same practitioner. Thus, this is one of the few instances in which I accept, with measurable lament, the convenience of technology. The movement of digital timepieces, however, is distracting and interferes with an accurate reading of the rate.

Finally, a reminder to re-check the rate on exertion by taking the pulse again after the examination, for example, asking the patient to rotate their arm ten times at the shoulder (see Chapter 4).

As with rhythm, in discussing the rate we depart from the regular format, as set forth in Chapter 5, for reasons already explained there. Combinations of other qualities with a Rapid or Slow rate are described in detail later under each of the other qualities.

The Normal Rate According to Age

Included here are two views of the Normal rate based on the factor of age. Here is Dr. Shen's view:[4]

Age:	Rate:
Birth to 4 years	84-90/min
4-10 years	78-84/min
10-15 years	78-80/min
16-40 years	72-78/min
40-50 years	72/min
50+ years	66-72/min

Amber[5] offers a somewhat different list:

Age:	Rate:
In embryo	150-160/min
Upon birth	130-140/min
First year	115-130/min
Second year	100-115/min
Third year	90-100/min
Age 4-7	85-90/min
Age 8-14	80-85/min
Adolescence	85-90/min
Adulthood	75-80/min
Old age	60-75/min
Decrepitude	75-80

The Rapid Rate

Rapid

While attention, for the most part, is focused in this chapter on the variety of Rapid pulses based on etiology, it is relevant to first say a word about the effect of a Rapid pulse on an organism. A Rapid pulse over any length of time weakens the qi, yin, and blood of the Heart. Therefore, whatever the cause, it is expedient to return the rate to the age–normal range as quickly as safety allows. Over time the weakened Heart causes the rate to Slow. However, if after the initial shock, which affects the Heart, the individual's life is stressful, the combination of the shock to the Heart (manifested in a blue facial color), and the stress that affects the 'nervous system,' causes a more Rapid rate. Also, although a Slow rate is generally associated with conditions of severe deficiency, it is important to remember that the pulse can sometimes become very Rapid temporarily when the organism is under stress. This results when the deficiency leads to instability of the qi, particularly the qi of the Heart, and occurs especially upon exertion.

In terms of category and sensation, the Rapid quality (see Fig. 7-1 at end of chapter) involves the pulse as a whole rather than as an individual or combination of individual positions. Li Shi-Zhen classifies a Rapid pulse as six beats per respiration, a very Rapid pulse as seven beats, a Speeding pulse as eight beats, and a Collapsed pulse as nine beats.[6] I classify the Rapid pulse according to etiology and interpretation, as described below. In the literature, Running, Quick,[7] Accelerated, and Racing[8] are synonymous with Rapid.

Interpretation — Conventional wisdom and tradition associate a Rapid pulse with heat, both heat from excess as related to yang excess and acute infectious diseases, and deficient-type heat from constraint associated with yin deficiency and chronic disease. (In our times, I have found deficient-type heat from constraint present most often in persons with long-term or constitutional 'nervous tension.') My experience, however, has revealed that a Rapid pulse more often involves the effects of shock of one kind or another on the Heart and circulation. Furthermore, a Rapid pulse occurs in circumstances of great deficiency of qi during the lesser yin and terminal yin stages of disease, when the yin is too weak to grasp the yang, which, as it slips out of control, causes the pulse rate to increase.[9]

Bounding

A Bounding quality is one in which the pulse feels as if it is running away faster than the actual rate may be, for example, it feels like 120 beats/minute but is really only 100 beats/minute. This sensation is usually associated with severe anxiety and panic, high fever in a weak person, heat prostration and shock, and sometimes with pain or trauma. Cases have been reported of a Bounding quality associated with qi trapped in the chest (Inflated quality).

RAPID PULSES CATEGORIZED ACCORDING TO ETIOLOGY

External etiology

EXTERNAL HEAT IN THE PROTECTIVE LEVEL

This pattern's pulse is slightly Rapid. It is Floating and more Yielding than with wind-cold, especially in the right distal position; is more Reduced in a deficient condition; and is more Robust in a condition of excess.

Etiology — Wind-heat pernicious influence, i.e., a summer cold, is usually the cause of this pulse. The increase in pulse rate is due to a rise in body temperature resulting from increased activity of the body's protective qi in defense of the organism.

Symptoms — Individuals affected by this pattern experience a sudden onset of the condition, accompanied by such symptoms as high fever, headache, sensation of heat, aversion to heat, perspiration (less with an excess condition, more with a deficient condition). Other symptoms include thirst, cough, yellow and thick nasal discharge, yellow sputum, and generalized pain.

Other signs — The tongue is slightly dry and moderately red, and has a thin yellow coating. The eyes have red rims and the sclera are congested.

HEAT STROKE

The pulse is very Rapid (140-160 beats per minute) and is very Tense and Full-Overflowing, or Collapsing to Empty when 'shock' ensues.

Etiology — This pattern arises due to failure or inadequacy of heat loss often associated with heat in the blood and dehydration after overexposure to the sun.

Symptoms — Headache, weakness, sudden loss of consciousness, hot, red, and dry skin, and slight perspiration.

Other signs — The tongue is red and dry. The pulse is Rapid, Tense, and Hollow Full-Overflowing.

TRAUMA (SHOCK)

The pulse is determined by the type (physical or emotional), size, and extent of the trauma. Other factors include whether the trauma is general or local, the time elapsed since the trauma, the patient's true qi at the time of the trauma and since the incident, based on lifestyle. True qi refers to whether a person's general energy or energy in a specific area of the body is weak or strong. As later described, this is one important determinant of the pulse quality associated with trauma. Facial color differentiates the shock due to physical trauma from that caused by emotional trauma. With physical trauma, the face is often grey. In particular, serious and extensive trauma that is accompanied by pain causes the face to become darker. With mild and local trauma, the facial color is not significant.

Emotional trauma often leads to a blue-green color around the mouth, chin, or entire face when the trauma occurs at birth and during early infancy. Emotional trauma that occurs during adulthood results in a blue-green color around the nose, and between the eyes or temples.

Physical trauma

Extensive physical trauma causes the entire pulse to be very Rapid, Bounding, Tight to Wiry (with pain), Inflated, or Flat. The tongue body has a purple hue; ecchymosis or a large purple blister is present on the area of the tongue corresponding to the trauma site on the body. On the side of the trauma, a thick horizontal blood vessel is evident on the mucosa of the lower eyelid where the blood vessels are usually vertical.

Local physical trauma causes the pulse to be less Rapid than that of extensive physical trauma. It is Tight to Wiry in the position corresponding to the area of the body affected by pain. A Wiry quality is associated with greater pain, and a Tight quality with less pain. (See Chapter 4 and the discussion of musculoskeletal positions.)

The tongue has a small purple blister in the area and side of the tongue corresponding to the area of the local trauma. On the side of the trauma there is a horizontal blood vessel on the mucosa of the lower eyelid that is thinner and less obvious than that present with extensive physical trauma.

Emotional trauma

Great emotional trauma leads to a very Rapid Bounding pulse with a very Tight quality over the entire pulse, especially affecting the Pericardium position at first, and later the entire left distal position. Change in Intensity and Rough Vibration may occur over the entire pulse. The tongue and eyes are normal.

Minor emotional trauma causes the pulse to be slightly Rapid, and Tight at the Pericardium position. The tongue and eyes are normal.

Condition of the true qi

Trauma is a shock to the circulation either locally or generally, depending on the nature and extent of the trauma. Circulation into and out of an area is diminished. Apart from Tenseness, a quality that indicates circulatory stagnation and developing heat, the pulse is either Inflated or Flat. The Inflated pulse indicates that an area has abundant energy that cannot get out. The Flat pulse represents an area in which there is little energy, and outside energy cannot get in due to the diminished circulation.

From the moment of the trauma and shock to the circulation, an organism tries to overcome the resulting stagnation. Energy supplied by the body, or from an outside source such as herbs and acupuncture, is sometimes required to overcome this stagnation both locally and generally. If the stagnation endures for a long time without outside intervention, energy is gradually depleted and the pulse becomes increasingly Reduced.

After the trauma, if the individual has a strong body or a healthy lifestyle, the pulse will be Rapid and Inflated. When the trauma is physical, the color of the tongue body will be normal; there will be a purple blister on the same side of the tongue that corresponds to the side of the body on which the trauma occurred. The tongue will be normal when the trauma is emotional.

If the individual has a weak body or the health deteriorates, the pulse will be Rapid and Flat. When the trauma is physical, the tongue will be pale due to the deficient condition; there will be a purple blister on the same side of the tongue that corresponds to the side of the body on which the trauma occurred. The tongue will be normal, changing over time to bright red when the trauma is emotional.

Time elapsed since trauma

When the pulse is taken a short time after the trauma, it will be Rapid and Tight, as well as Inflated or Flat. When the trauma is physical, the tongue will have a purple hue; ecchymosis and/or a purple blister will be evident on the same side corresponding to the side of the body on which the trauma occurred. Over time the tongue will change from normal to bright red when the trauma is emotional. A thick horizontal blood vessel will be present on the mucosa of the lower eyelid when the trauma is physical. The eyes will be normal when the trauma is emotional. The facial color will be light grey with physical trauma, and greenish blue around the nose, between the eyes, and on the temples with emotional trauma.

If a long period has passed after the trauma without any resolution of the resulting conditions, the pulse due to physical trauma will be Feeble-Absent in the position corresponding to the body site affected by trauma. For example, if the trauma is in the chest, the distal positions will be Feeble-Absent. If the trauma is in the abdomen, the middle positions will be Feeble-Absent. The rate will be less Rapid (or even Slow) than with a more recent trauma. The tongue body will be pale, and the purple blister, though present, will have faded. The horizontal blood vessel on the mucosa of the lower eyelid, though present, will also have faded, and the vertical blood vessels will be pale. The face will be dark grey.

When the pulse is taken a long time after an emotional trauma, it will be Feeble-Absent in the left distal position, with the remaining positions being Normal. Change in Intensity and Rough Vibration will continue over the entire pulse. The tongue will be normal and the face will be pale.

SEASONAL VARIATIONS

According to Li Shi-Zhen, Lung yin deficiency conditions are aggravated by the natural dryness of autumn and lead to excess internal fire burning the Lung yin, as well as a Rapid pulse. He goes on to say that this type of problem is difficult to treat.[10]

Changes in the pulse with the seasons are minor considerations in the context of the major disharmonies and pathologies I find on the pulses of patients. However, independent of the pulse, each season does bring with it certain stresses which are important to susceptible individuals, as indicated by Li Shi-Zhen.

Internal-external etiology

Internal-external etiology refers to causes that are external, such as stress, which lead to an internal pathology. In Chinese medicine, birth trauma is always regarded as an emotional shock to the Heart. This is discussed in greater detail in the section on the left distal position in Chapter 12.

THE HEART

Emotional symptoms predominate

Very mild Heart qi agitation

This condition is characterized on the pulse by a Superficial Vibration. The individual is worried about some event in their life.

Mild heat from excess

The principal early sign of this condition is a Tight quality at the Pericardium position. The individual has been worrying for a relatively long period of time, such as several years.

Moderate to severe Heart qi agitation

This condition is marked by an occasional large Change in Rate at Rest. The individual feels as if they are out of control. Their emotions and life are on a rollercoaster, and they find it very difficult to focus and ground themselves.

Heart qi stagnation

The Flat wave at the left distal position is usually caused by early emotional loss with a lifelong tendency to vengefulness and spitefulness. Another common cause is birth with the cord around the neck. The qi is unable to easily enter the Heart.

Physical symptoms predominate

Trapped qi in the Heart

The left (and sometimes right) distal position is Inflated. It is difficult for qi to exit the Heart. A breech birth is a common cause. The individual tends to become easily angered, exhalation is difficult, the body feels uncomfortable, and there is fatigue. Much later the pulse becomes Deep, Thin, and Tight.

Heart blood stagnation (mild-moderate and severe)

With mild-moderate Heart blood stagnation the pulse is very Flat at first, then much later, with severe Heart blood stagnation, the pulse becomes Deep, Thin, and Feeble. Such individuals are fearful their entire lives, have difficulty inhaling, and experience varying degrees of angina.

Internal Etiology

Heat from excess

With heat from excess the pulse is usually very Tense.

Heat in the qi level

The pulse associated with this pattern is Rapid, Flooding Excess, and Tense and Slippery at the organ depth.

Etiology

The increase in pulse rate is due to a rise in body temperature resulting from increased activity of the protective and nutritive qi in defense of the organism. Infection or inflammation of an organ is usually the source and is located by searching for the Tightest position on the pulse. The symptoms of the pattern described below are partly characteristic of the yang brightness stage of the six stages of disease, with elements of the qi, nutritive, and blood levels of disease according to the later nosology of the four levels of disease.

Symptoms

Individuals with this pattern are affected by acute high fever, sensation of heat, aversion to heat, thirst with a preference for cold beverages, profuse sweating, severe pain, cough with yellow sputum, either constipation with small hard feces or diarrhea with a burning sensation and tenesmus, bloody or purulent dysentery, abdominal pain, nausea and vomiting, dysuria, yellow and scanty urine, irritability and restlessness, and dizziness. In more serious cases, delirium or coma may ensue.

Other signs

The tongue is red and dry with a thick yellow coating. The sclera are red and the face is flushed.

Heat in the blood

'BLOOD HEAT'

This heat syndrome can be either from excess or deficiency, depending on the etiology. When palpating the pulse of this pattern, the rate is slightly Rapid, the blood depth is expanded as finger pressure is released from the organ depth, and may be Slippery (see Chapter 13).

Etiology

This pattern is often due to over-indulgence in foods that give rise to heat from excess. These include wine, shellfish, coffee, fried foods, salted nuts, chili, and venison, among others.

Heat from deficiency can arise from overwork of the 'nervous system,' and especially from emotional stress causing Liver qi stagnation and the depletion of yin as the body tries to mitigate the heat and return to homeostasis.

Symptoms

Sore throat, sore tongue, canker sores, bleeding gums, hot face, headache, excitability, dark yellow urine, and hard stools.

Other signs

The tongue becomes dark red and has a thick yellow coating. The sclera are congested, and the vertical blood vessels on the mucosa of the lower eyelid are engorged.

'BLOOD THICK'

With this pattern, the blood depth is greatly expanded to the qi depth as finger pressure is reduced. If the condition is not corrected, the pulse may later become Full-Overflowing, Robust Pounding, Rapid and Bounding, and Tight (see Chapter 13).

Etiology

The cause of this pattern is often heat from excess due to a diet of excessive sugar and fat, or to nervous tension and stress, creating stagnation, rebellious Liver qi, and heat in the Liver; the rebellious Liver qi then transversely attacks the Spleen-Stomach-Intestine system. (Since the Liver stores the blood, heat in the Liver will transfer to the blood. When rebellious Liver qi attacks the Spleen-Stomach-Intestines, the latter systems' activity increases, creating heat in the Spleen-Stomach-Intestines. As the Spleen-Stomach is the source of the blood, this heat is also transferred to the blood.)

The picture described below is one in which heat in the blood has invaded the qi, and in which the blood has become more viscous due to excessive lipids. However, when chronic Liver qi stagnation is involved, strong signs of heat from excess are mixed with those of heat from deficiency due to Liver yin deficiency. The final stage of this process is arteriosclerosis and a Ropy, cord-like pulse.

Symptoms

The early-stage symptom is often acne, especially in young people. Late-stage symptoms include acute onset of such disturbances as severe headache, vertigo, parasthesia, tinnitus that is not relieved by pressure over the ear, irascibility, hypertension due to Spleen dampness, and Liver heat transforming into wind and stroke.

Other signs

The tongue is dark red and slightly swollen, and has a thick yellow and greasy coating. The sclera are very congested, and the vertical blood vessels on the mucosa of the lower eyelid are engorged. The face is flushed.

'NERVOUS SYSTEM TENSE'[11]

When Tension is found uniformly over the entire pulse, I refer to it as the 'vigilance pulse' because it appears constitutionally in certain ethnic, religious, or national groups whose survival through the centuries has required extraordinary vigilance. A similar quality can be found today in almost anyone living in a large city, or living with the constant need to be vigilant. Therefore, one must differentiate diagnostically between a constitutional 'nervous system tense,' and an acquired one which is due to ongoing chronic stress. This distinction is important since individuals whose tension arises from life experiences can alter their lifestyles as part of treatment. On the other hand, telling those who are *constitutionally* 'nervous system tense' that they will feel less tense if they alter their environment is only an exercise in frustration for them, and will reduce the chances that they might accept treatment that could otherwise help relieve some of the tension, and thereby avoid the illness in other vulnerable systems that will ultimately follow. I consider this quality to be a sign of vigorous essence, but in the long run, constant vigilance depletes the essence, and profound fear becomes its inevitable companion.

One way of diagnosing the constitutional pattern is to observe whether the patient's distress decreases after a few treatments, with the pulse remaining the same. Another is that, with the constitutional etiology, the pulse is Slower than that caused by daily stress. However, the principal distinction between a constitutional and acquired pattern is made through facial diagnosis and color. When the etiology is constitutional, the eyebrows are extraordinarily thick, such that the root of the individual hairs cannot be seen, and the color around the chin and mouth is blue-green. When the etiology is acquired, the roots of the eyebrow hairs are easily distinguished, and facial color is normal around the chin or mouth, unless there are other pathologies (e.g., this area will appear yellowish when the 'digestive system' is very deficient).

Etiology

CONSTITUTIONAL

As mentioned above, I have found this pulse most often in people whose background is one in which they have been subjected to centuries of oppression and unexpected danger. In my own practice, this pulse appears frequently in Jews and Israelis. It is the pulse and condition of 'vigilance' which, as the former German Jews know, is not something that one gives up without risk. In a sense, it seems to document the process of the survival of the fittest, and the fittest were those most vigilant to external danger.

The specific qualities of this pulse are that the rate is Slow, Normal, or slightly Rapid, mildly Robust Pounding, and uniformly Tense. This uniformity is enduring even when other problems such as overwork, trauma, and the like complicate the clinical picture. Some changes toward yin deficiency can be anticipated, especially as a Tight quality in the proximal positions, if the intervening events are prolonged and severe. If the circulatory system is vulnerable, some form of heat in the blood is possible.

Symptoms

The principal symptom is an ongoing tension that may or may not be unrelated to any particular life stress. This tension can be in the family over several generations.

Accompanying symptoms depend on the vulnerability of other organ systems that are affected by the excess, and especially deficiency-type heat from constraint, which can be a consequence of this condition when it persists over a long period.

Other signs

The tongue and eyes are normal. The eyebrows are thicker than normal—increasing in thickness with the increasing degree of inherited tension in the nervous system; the individual eyebrow hairs are indistinguishable. There are vertical lines (furrows) between the eyes: two if the problem is profound, and one if it is less serious. The color of the face is generally darker, and the color around the chin and mouth is blue-green.

DAILY STRESS

Stress-induced tension, frustration, and anxiety over a long period can cause a condition of qi stagnation in the Liver and mild heat from excess. The concept is that the superficial protective qi is moving too fast, thus giving rise to heat, and that the body is mobilizing metabolic heat to overcome the stagnation in the Liver. If the circulatory system is vulnerable, the heat readily affects the blood vessels and the blood.

In terms of the pulse, it is Tense and essentially the same as that of the constitutional etiology, except that it may be more Rapid. If the condition is mild and in its early stages, the Tension can feel stronger at the qi depth. As the condition progresses, the Tense quality will be felt more at the blood depth, and later it will be strongest at the organ depth when the condition has persisted for a long time. In contrast to the constitutional quality, the pulse becomes less Tense with treatment, as the patient's distress is relieved.

Symptoms

Individuals with this pattern are usually tense, but only since living under conditions that promote stress. Other symptoms include mild flushing of the face, intolerance to heat, mild headache, dryness of the eyes, thirst that is easily quenched, tendency toward constipation, difficulty getting to sleep, propensity to perspire, and eczema.

Other signs

One of the differences between the constitutional and acquired etiologies is that with the latter, over time the tongue and eyes show more signs of heat. The tongue is thin, bright red, and dry with a patchy coating or an absence of coating. The eyes are red and dry, and confluent under the eyelid (the vertical blood vessels on the mucosa of the lower eyelid lose their integrity and appear to flow into one another). The eyebrows are normal in thickness, and there are no furrows between the eyes. Facial color is normal.

Heat from deficiency

With heat from deficiency the pulse is usually Tight and less Rapid than with heat from excess.

Entire pulse

WITHOUT INTERNAL WIND

If the condition has lasted only a short time, then the entire pulse is slightly Rapid. It is also somewhat Tight due to reduced yin-fluids, and slightly Thin due to blood deficiency, which usually accompanies yin deficiency.

If the condition has lasted for a longer period, usually due to prolonged tension in the 'nervous system,' the pulse is slightly Rapid, and Tighter to Wiry, due to increased heat and reduced fluids. It is also Thinner owing to the developing blood deficiency. In general, the Tightest position indicates the principal source of the drain on the yin. (If the pulse is uniformly Tight and the face is dark, pain can be considered as a source of the Tightness.)

WITH INTERNAL WIND

Mild internal wind (Liver wind) is characterized by a Floating Tight quality and wind in the channels (paresthesias and 'little strokes'). Severe internal wind is signaled by a very Tight Hollow Full-Overflowing quality associated with an impending major stroke.

Etiology — Protracted overwork of the 'nervous system' and a lengthy condition of heat from excess (e.g., hepatitis) deplete the body of yin. The result is that the yang, which may be thought of as metabolic heat, is not balanced by the yin, and is therefore in relative, not absolute, excess.

Symptoms — Onset of symptoms is slow and includes hot flashes, night sweats,[12] fever in the afternoon and early evening, flushed face in the afternoon, thirst unquenched by fluids, sore throat, heat in the palms and soles, chronic irritability, insomnia, heightened libido, tinnitus, headache, dizziness, deafness, floaters in the eyes, dry stools and constipation, and scanty and dark yellow urine.

Other signs — The tongue is dry, and bright red at first, then turns scarlet as the condition progresses; the coating is patchy and yellow, or there is an absence of coating. The vertical blood vessels on the mucosa of the lower eyelid are confluent.

Individual positions

Heat from deficiency is the condition that follows a deficiency of yin. This is manifested on the pulse in a hardening sensation which is called Tight when it is not so hard, and Wiry when it is very hard. Heat from deficiency in a yin organ will therefore usually be accompanied by a Tight to Wiry pulse quality in the position which represents that organ. When the condition is chronic, the proximal position on the left (Kidney yin position) will also usually be Tight to Wiry, since Kidney yin is the source of yin for all of the other organ systems. Excluding other variables, the pulse will usually be slightly Rapid. Combinations of the Tight and Wiry qualities with the Rapid are discussed in Chapter 11.

Internal etiology other than heat

Imminent hemorrhage

The pulse of this pattern is Rapid and Leather-like Hollow.

Other signs — The tongue is extremely scarlet and dry. With hemorrhage and threatened miscarriage, the tongue also shows black stripes.

Pain

The following rate varies according to the degree and duration of pain. Over time there are increasing signs and symptoms of deficiency in addition to the initial diagnostic picture of excess.

The pulse is Rapid (90 to 106 beats per minute); there is Biting Wiriness in one or many pulse positions, especially during acute pain. The pulse is less Rapid during chronic pain, and even Slow with eventual qi depletion over a long period of time.

Symptoms — In addition to pain, the other symptoms include fatigue, irritability, and depression.

Other signs — The tongue shows ecchymosis and a purple blister only if the pain is from trauma. There is likewise a horizontal blood vessel on the mucosa of the lower eyelid only if the pain is from trauma. The face is dark grey if the pain is chronic or severe, and light grey if the pain is of recent origin or is mild.

Acute phase of chronic illness

While chronic illness is generally associated with a Slow rate, the appearance of a Rapid rate in chronic disease reflects either an acute exacerbation of symptoms, or the ability of the organism to mobilize—even for a short term—self-healing, by increasing circulation. This phenomenon often occurs in the autoimmune diseases such as systemic lupus erythematosus.

Lesser yin heat pattern

During the lesser yin and terminal yin stages of the six stages of disease, Kidney yin is depleted due to the chronicity of the overriding yang deficiency condition (lesser yin cold), which is characteristic of this stage. Yang can no longer push the yin, which in turn is unable to nourish the yang; thus, they are effectively separated. This means that the yin has become so deficient that it has lost control of the yang. With this separation of yin and yang, yang rises to the surface, creating the sensation of heat and hence a Rapid pulse. This is a form of 'qi wild.' The result is a paradoxical condition with a Rapid pulse and sometimes a low temperature. Some attribute these signs of heat from deficiency to Liver heat.[13] The pulse is Rapid—over 120 beats per minute. Li Shi-Zhen calls this a Collapsed pulse.[14]

With the lesser yin cold condition the pulse should be, and usually is, Slow. Here the condition and the pulse are congruous, which is a more favorable sign than with a lesser yin heat pattern in which the condition and the pulse are at odds with each other.

Symptoms Severe deficiency and debilitation, fever in the afternoon and early evening, flushed face in the afternoon, thirst unquenched by fluids, sore throat, hot palms and soles, chronic irritability, insomnia, tinnitus, headache, dizziness, deafness, floaters in the eyes, dry stools and constipation, and scanty and dark yellow urine. Serious cases may present with delirium and loss of consciousness.

Other signs The tongue is dry and without coating; the tongue body may be either thin and red, or later scarlet. The eyes are spiritless, and under the eyelids one finds a confluence of the vertical blood vessels on the mucosa of the lower eyelids.

SUDDEN CESSATION OF EXERCISE OR HEAVY WORK

The pulse is Normal to Rapid Yielding Hollow Full-Overflowing.

Etiology Circulation is impaired when one who has exercised a great deal suddenly stops. Consistent exercise causes blood volume to increase and the vessels to expand. With a precipitous cessation of exercise, blood volume decreases faster than blood vessel contraction, thus creating a break between yin (blood) and yang (qi). (Normally, the yang-qi circulates on the outer edge of the vessel and the yin-blood toward the center; yang-qi and yin-blood are thus in contact. Under circumstances as just described, in which the yin-blood diminishes rapidly, contact with the yang-qi circulating on the periphery of the vessels is broken.) This is one form of 'qi wild.' Sudden lifting far beyond one's ability, as in emergencies when individuals lift a heavy object to free themselves or others, can give rise to the same condition.

Symptoms Most of the symptoms of this condition fall into the category of 'qi wild' and occur acutely with this etiology. Since impaired circulation significantly affects Heart function, which in Chinese medicine controls the mind, the common symptoms include profound anxiety, labile emotions, fatigue, 'spaced out' feeling, and depersonalization. There is also a sense of loss of control over body and mind, during which parts of the body no longer feel connected to the rest of the body, especially when lying down, resulting in a feeling of drifting away. Severe migrating joint pain is another common complaint.

Other signs

Tongue and eyes are normal.

COMBINATIONS

My own interpretation of the Rapid pulse with other qualities is explained under individual pulse qualities in later chapters.[15]

The Slow Rate

Slow

While a Slow pulse is ordinarily associated with conditions of severe deficiency, it is important to remember that deficiency can also cause a very Rapid pulse, especially upon exertion, due to the instability of the qi, particularly the qi of the Heart.

The Slow quality (see Fig. 7-2 at end of chapter) involves the entire pulse and reflects the functioning of the entire organism. According to Dr. Shen, it is "any pulse that is four counts lower than the normal rate [for a person of that age], unless the individual is born with a slower rate."[16] Even if an individual appears to be well, once the circulation is slowed for any reason, they are vulnerable to disease.

In terms of sensation, Li Shi-Zhen noted that a Slow pulse is one "which beats only three times per respiration."[17] I have also heard it described as delayed, as if it is unable to catch up. For reasons explained under the Rapid quality, measuring rate by respiration is unreliable and a non-digital timepiece is recommended.

Interpretation

In my experience, by far the most common cause of the Slow quality is circulatory deficiency due to either energy depletion, the long-term effects of shock, or overexercise and overwork, all of which affect or are affected by the Heart.

Dr. Shen expressed his view in the following passage:[18]

> Since the pulse rate is based upon the working of the Heart, it is the best instrument for measuring how well the blood circulates. The rate of the blood Circulation has a great impact on an individual's health. So if the blood Circulation is too fast or too slow, it indicates an imbalance in the individual's body.... The slow pulse indicates the malfunctioning of the patient's blood Circulation. Slow pulses are indicative of han [cold] illness. This is not just the coldness of the weather, but a coldness within the body due to the malfunctioning of the internal organs. Excessive exercises [especially running] would also lead to a slowing down of Circulation, and a slow pulse would emerge.... Slow pulses are more related to the body as a whole, not individual organs. They tell about han illnesses: hsu-han [cold from deficiency] or shih-han [cold from excess], and whether the bad Circulation is related to the internal organs or the blood vessels. If the bad blood Circulation is due to weak internal organs, then it must be found out which organ is weakest.

SLOW PULSES CATEGORIZED ACCORDING TO ETIOLOGY

To identify the cause of a Slow pulse, one must determine whether it is qi or blood deficiency and the poor functioning of the organs that is slowing the circulation of qi and blood, or whether that circulation was first impaired by shock and trauma, which then affected the organs and finally the overall body energy (true qi). Deficiency is the primary cause, and less commonly, excess.

The following is a simple list of the origins of a Slow pulse. The differentiation and elaboration of each cause is provided further on in the section "Classification According to Degree of Slowness."

Common causes in contemporary society

EXTERNAL

Cold from external excess

Here, the Slow pulse is due to stagnation of the protective and nutritive qi caused by a cold external pathogenic influence. The pulse is Floating, Tense and Slow.

INTERNAL

Cold from deficiency (qi and yang deficiency)

Longstanding internal disease, overwork, overexercise, sex beyond one's energy, and protracted emotional strain can cause qi and yang deficiency. Since the qi is the motivating force underlying the circulation, the lack of qi results in a diminished circulation. The generic pulse is Feeble-Absent and Deep, but there is a wide range of qualities of increasing qi deficiency and 'qi wild' qualities which are described, especially in Chapters 8 and 9, including the Empty-type qualities. Others, such as Yielding Hollow Full-Overflowing and Slow, Change in Qualities, and Yielding Ropy, are described in Chapters 6, 15, and 11 respectively (all of those qualities in which the yin and yang of the vessels separate with consequential severe mental and emotional disability). I am finding this in younger people due to extraordinary emphasis on athletic training in children and adolescents.

Heart qi and yang deficiency

A qi and yang deficient Heart is unable to circulate qi and blood, which leads to a slowing of the pulse. If the cause occurs after birth, the entire pulse is Feeble and the left distal position is more Feeble or Absent than the rest of the pulse. If the cause is constitutional, only the left distal and proximal positions are Feeble-Absent; the other positions are Normal.

Aerobic exercise

A Slow pulse associated with aerobic exercise, including running, is usually somewhat Robust Pounding. The exact rate of the pulse depends on how far and fast the individual runs, how long he or she has been running, and the condition of the body.

Less common causes

LIVER QI STAGNATION AND QI DEFICIENCY

Liver qi stagnation and deficiency diminishes peripheral circulation and, while relatively rare, slows the pulse rate by depriving the circulation of the impetus that it normally supplies in moving the blood and qi through the vessels and channels. The pulse is Slow and Tense.

INTERNAL HEAT FROM EXCESS: LATE-STAGE 'BLOOD THICK' (MIDDLE-STAGE ARTERIOSCLEROSIS)

The circulation is slowed and the pulse is turning Ropy and Tense due to increased viscosity of the blood. The latter is caused by the accumulation of lipids, plaque formation, and heat in the blood over a long period of time. By this stage the slowing process due to the viscosity outweighs the accelerating process associated with the initial etiology, heat from excess.

YIN DEFICIENCY (LATE-STAGE ARTERIOSCLEROSIS)

In advanced yin deficiency the pulse will be very Tight Hollow Full-Overflowing and Slow, and when the vessels lose their elasticity and the pulse becomes Ropy and Tight, circulation decreases even more than in the 'blood thick' pattern.

POISONING

Over a long period of time, poisoning gives rise to a very Slow and Deep pulse. The rate is usually under fifty. I have observed this in artists and in industrial workers such as welders after many years of exposure to toxic solvents. Frequently, they also show a 'blood unclear' condition.

MEDICATIONS

The beta-blocker class of medications cause the pulse to become very Slow. The wave is suppressed. Unfortunately, this etiology is increasing.

SHOCK

Unresolved physical or emotional shock (trauma) initially inhibits the circulation of qi and blood causing the Heart to work harder and the rate to increase. Over a long period of time, in the attempt to open circulation of qi and blood, the organism becomes depleted and the pulse becomes Slow. Physical shock, due to trauma or exposure to extremes of weather, is associated with pain, and pain is associated with a Tight quality. Therefore, the pulse is Slow and Tight. The middle or blood depth can be Thin. Emotional shock is marked by a Tight Rough Vibration over the entire pulse, which becomes Slow over time.

Uncommon causes

COLD FROM INTERNAL EXCESS

Internal cold arises when cold foods and beverages are consumed from an early age; from excessive use of cold applications in the treatment of pain; or from frequent bathing in very cold water. Inadequate heating and attire during the winter because of poverty is unfortunately still more common than one cares to believe, and leaves its mark on children for their entire lives. The pulse associated with this pattern is Slow and Tight. Internal cold can lead to blood stagnation, which is reflected as a Choppy quality in deficient areas of the body, such as the Pelvis/Lower Body position.

The term Tight in this context requires some explanation. I have found that there is a hierarchy of diminishing flexibility and increasing hardness—a distinction lacking in the traditional literature—from Normal to Taut to Tense to Tight to Wiry, and that each of these qualities conveys different information (see Chapter 11). With moderate internal cold the pulse has a sensation which I call Tight. With extreme pain it is Wiry, which is to say, very hard like a metal wire.

Li Shi-Zhen[19] describes the Tight pulse as being "like a tightly stretched rope and feels twisted"; it "vibrates to the left and right." However, in the hierarchy of diminishing flexibility described above, I find that a Tight pulse feels thinner and harder than a stretched rope, a quality which I call Tense; moreover, it does not feel twisted. Only in extreme cases of life-threatening cold, such as hypothermia, do I find a pulse which we call Hidden Excess (Tense) at the level of the bone; it is this quality that feels like a "tightly stretched rope" and "twisted," and that "vibrates to the left and right." The Vibration aspect is akin to the Rough Vibration quality, which is associated with parenchymal damage, or what Dr. Shen calls 'organ dead.' Closely allied to this is the Choppy quality associated with blood stagnation, which, at the Hidden position, represents the congealing of blood in the vessels and impending death.

INTERNAL HEAT PERNICIOUS INFLUENCE

Kaptchuk refers to a rare heat condition related to a Slow pulse. If it is Tense, the cause may be "a Heat Pernicious Influence getting stuck," which he associates with "acute Heat patterns with abdominal distention or constipation."[20] This pulse is also often Pounding.

DAMP-HEAT AND PHLEGM-DAMPNESS

Kaptchuk[21] and Li Shi-Zhen[22] refer to dampness, the former to damp-heat and the latter to dampness and phlegm with Spleen yang deficiency. I assume, though they do not so indicate, that the pulse is also Tense (due to heat) and Slippery (due to phlegm-dampness). In my experience, a Slow pulse with Slipperiness only at the qi depth can be due to consumption of too much sugar over a long time.

HEAT EXHAUSTION

Heat exhaustion is due to excessive fluid loss. The pulse is Slow and Feeble. Other symptoms include low blood pressure, cold, pale, and clammy skin, and in extreme cases, disorientation and sudden loss of consciousness. There may also be extreme perspiration with fatigue, weakness, and anxiety.

CLASSIFICATION ACCORDING TO DEGREE OF SLOWNESS

The following etiologies are presented in the order of the frequency with which they are encountered in the Western clinic, with the most common listed first and the least common last.

Sixty-eight to seventy-two beats

This moderately Slow rate can be normal after age fifty when it occurs without other grossly abnormal pulse qualities, and without symptoms or other signs of disharmony.

QI DEFICIENCY BEFORE AGE FIFTY

With this pulse, the qi depth is Yielding or Feeble-Absent. The rate is determined by age (older = Slower), physical conditioning (weaker = Slower), and degree of overwork, overexercise, or chronic emotional stress (greater = Slower).

Etiology — The cause of this pattern is moderate overwork, moderate overexercise, emotional stress over time, or chronic illness.

Symptoms — Mild to moderate fatigue is the primary symptom.

Other signs — The tongue color is normal to slightly pale, and the tongue body is slightly swollen or has slight teeth marks. The eyes are normal.

LIVER QI STAGNATION AND DEFICIENCY

Symptoms of cold hands and feet accompany this form of stagnation, which is described above and is easily identified on the pulse by a Tense left middle position. With Liver qi deficiency, the left middle position has Reduced Substance, or is Empty (Tense only at the qi depth).

COLD FROM EXCESS AT ANY AGE

External cold

The pulse is Floating, Tense and Slow.

Symptoms — Typical symptoms include the common cold or flu.

Other signs — The tongue has a thin white coating. The eyes are normal to slightly congested.

Internal cold from excess

The pulse is Slow and Tight at the positions that correspond to the sites where cold has invaded (e.g., Stomach, Intestines, Uterus). Pain often accompanies internal cold, in which case the pulse could become Wiry. While the cold makes the pulse Slow, pain might increase it slightly. Internal cold will lead to blood stagnation, especially in dependent areas, which is often reflected at the Pelvis/Lower Body position.

Symptoms — Individuals with this pattern are affected by pain where cold has invaded, such as menstrual cramps. Over time, stagnating cold in the gastrointestinal tract drains Spleen qi and yang, with attendant consequences.

Other signs — The tongue coating is thick and white, and later is swollen with teeth marks. The eyes are normal.

Sixty-four to sixty-eight beats

The pulse is Slow and is Deeper and Wider (Diffuse) than the sixty-eight to seventy-two pulse. It also separates under pressure at the qi and blood depths (Spreading quality).

Etiology — This pulse can appear at any age, but is a sign of a more serious disorder when it is found in patients under the age of fifty. The cause is protracted overwork, overexercise, excessive sex, emotional stress over a long period, or prolonged illness.

Symptoms — Primarily increasing fatigue and vulnerability to disease in areas that are already deficient.

Other signs — The tongue is pale, slightly swollen with teeth marks; there is a thin white coating. The inside of the lower eyelids are normal to somewhat pale.

Sixty to sixty-four beats

DEFICIENCY

Cold from deficiency: qi and yang deficiency

The pulse associated with this pattern is Deep, Thin, Feeble-Absent or Empty, and Slow.

Etiology — The cause of this pattern is the same as that of the sixty-four to sixty-eight pulse, except the events are either more extreme, occur over a longer period of time or in a more deficient person, or a combination of the two.

Symptoms — May include sensation of cold, increasingly easily fatigued, shortness of breath, excessive perspiration, and disease in the most vulnerable organs.

Other signs — The tongue is pale and swollen with teeth marks, and has a white coating. There is pallor inside the lower eyelids.

Yin deficiency

This pattern is discussed above under the Rapid quality. However, in considering the Slow quality, the following should be noted about yin deficiency.

Overwork of the 'nervous system' over a long period of time usually leads to Heart and Liver yin deficiency, and ultimately Kidney yin deficiency. The heat from deficiency tends to cause a slight increase in rate, but the loss of yin in the vessel walls causes them to lose elasticity over time, thereby interfering with circulation and depleting Heart qi. Furthermore, prolonged yin deficiency leads to yang deficiency because the yin cannot nourish the yang. Both will cause a Slower rate. The pulse can be Ropy and Slow in the later stage of arteriosclerosis, and after a mild stroke. (After a major stroke the pulse is more often Slow and Feeble, but this is still the ultimate consequence of a process involving heat from excess and deficiency.)

EXCESS

Cold

See discussion above under the sixty-eight to seventy-two rate.

Heat

The pulse is very Tight Hollow Full-Overflowing, Ropy, and Slow.

Etiology — Heat from excess and the attendant thickening of the blood ('blood thick'), while initially causing an increase in rate, will over a long time interfere with circulation, slowing the pulse and leading to a Ropy quality. Associated syndromes are arteriosclerosis, chronic hypertension, and post-stroke sequelae. Just prior to stroke the rate will suddenly accelerate. A condition of excess with a Slow pulse is paradoxical, relatively uncommon, and suggests a very chronic and dangerous state.

Symptoms — Symptoms associated with this pattern include headache, epistaxis, parathesia, numbness, disturbances of cognition and speech, and paralysis.

Other signs — The tongue is red and swollen, and has a thick greasy coating. The sclera are injected, and there is extreme redness inside the lower eyelid.

Between forty and sixty beats

AEROBIC EXERCISE

The pulse is Slow and Yielding Hollow Full-Overflowing.

Etiology

The Slow pulse associated with aerobic exercise, especially running, is today the most common cause of a pulse rate under sixty. The exact rate is determined by the distance and speed that the individual runs, the length of time he or she has been running, and the quality of physical conditioning. Without symptoms and other signs from the pulse, tongue, and eyes, Chinese medicine can only deduce that such a Slow pulse is derived from deficient circulation of qi and blood, and that the organism is vulnerable to disease even without an obvious disorder of a yin organ. In biomedical terms, such individuals are especially prone to disorders like chronic fatigue syndrome, arthritis, circulatory diseases, anxiety and panic, sleep disorders, and cancer.

When the pulse rate moves below fifty-five, a zone of danger is being entered, suggesting that the person is exercising excessively beyond his or her energy level. A rate below fifty is a clear sign that circulation is significantly impaired. While this rate is not uncommon in competition athletes who are constitutionally strong, and is ordinarily not a source of concern, it is my impression—albeit unsubstantiated by statistics, but amply supported by clinical experience—that after these individuals reach middle age they are less healthy than their appropriately active peers.

Previously, this phenomenon occurred more often in men, but with the growing participation of women in sports and aerobics at very young ages, their vulnerability to the eventual symptoms described below has increased. Puberty is a period of rapid growth and change when individuals, especially girls during menarche, require all their reserves to achieve maturity. When aerobic exercises are performed at an especially dangerous level, that is, beyond the individual's energy level, osteoporosis and other gynecological symptoms such as menorrhagia, dysmenorrhea, and later amenorrhea are common and serious.

Here, perhaps, a word or two is in order with regard to misconceptions about aerobic exercise. Such exercise that is performed beyond one's energy level is an increasingly important health issue in the West. The popular myth is that a lower pulse rate strengthens the heart and spares it, since it is pumping less often. Exercise, especially running, tends to increase circulation and enkephalins, creating a temporary good feeling, which makes it addictive. Exercise, however, requires energy, which in turn is not available for circulation. Thus, in order to obtain the same circulation and good feeling, the exerciser must run or exercise a little longer than the previous session. But at the same time, energy is further diminished by the activity. This is a vicious cycle that has caused people to exercise well beyond their energy levels while their circulation and energy continue to decrease. The result, which I have seen innumerable times with runners, weight lifters, gymnasts, and students of the martial arts, are signs and symptoms of osteoporosis, chronic fatigue syndrome, and immune deficiency, with all of the 'qi wild' mental and emotional manifestations described here and in other sections. Many of the people who ignored my advice to stop running developed serious heart disease with all of the biomedical sequella, pacemakers, bypass surgery, etc.

Symptoms

Symptoms of this pattern, which is essentially a 'qi wild' state, develop gradually with this etiology. They include vague complaints of being easily fatigued and tired, migrating joint and muscle pain, insomnia, labile emotions, propensity toward anger, and feelings of being 'spaced out' and in some ways out of control. Sometimes, especially when lying down, there is a sensation of the body and arms floating away—the body is not real. Such feelings of profound depersonalization create severe anxiety and often terror. These individuals are often seen by psychiatrists and receive diagnoses of anxiety neurosis, panic attacks, and even schizophrenia. This disorder of chaotic qi, which is totally invisible to the biomedical world, leads to lifelong emotional problems that are compounded by treatments offered in the form of drugs and shock therapy.

Chronic fatigue syndrome, fibromyelgia, auto-immune disease, and chronic neurological disease are associated with this condition.

Other signs — The tongue is pale, wet, and swollen with teeth marks, and can be losing shape. The blood vessels of the mucosa inside the lower eyelids are pale.

POISONING

The pulse is very Slow, very Deep or Hidden, and Blood Unclear.

Etiology — Refer to the discussion of poisoning in the etiology section of the Slow pulse above.

Symptoms — Severe malaise, headache, skin rashes, and extreme fatigue. Over time the Liver and Kidneys can be fatally affected.

Other signs — The tongue is red and dry, and has black cracks. The sclera are injected.

DEFICIENT QI AND YANG AFFECTING CIRCULATION OF QI AND BLOOD

The pulse is very Slow, Deep, Flooding Deficient, Feeble or Absent; in later stages it turns Empty and Scattered.

Etiology — The cause of this pattern can be excessive exercise—especially running—beyond one's energy level, and in particular between the ages of ten to twenty; overwork, especially before age fifteen; chronic illness; emotional stress over a long period; excessive sex beyond one's energy level over a protracted period; and old age.

Symptoms — Fatigue, malaise, general weakness, migrating pain, coldness in the bones and extremities, anxiety, clouding of sensorium memory, attention deficits, and confusion. All of the chronic diseases are potential associated conditions.

Other signs — The tongue is pale, swollen, wet, and flabby. The blood vessels of the mucosa inside the lower eyelids are pale.

HEART QI AND YANG DEFICIENCY

The pulse is Slow, Deep, Feeble-Absent or Empty, and Thin.

Etiology — This pattern is associated with heart failure, bradycardia, or bundle branch block.

Symptoms — Symptoms include dependent pitting edema, oily sweat, coldness throughout the body and extremities, weakness, fatigue, shortness of breath, and cardiac asthma.

Other signs — The tongue is pale, swollen, and wet. There is pallor inside the lower eyelids.

MEDICATIONS

Beta-blockers and other heart medications are increasingly the cause of very Slow rates.

COMBINATIONS

My own interpretation of the Slow pulse with other qualities is explained under individual pulse qualities in later chapters.[23]

Changes in Rate

For a discussion of rate changes at rest and upon exertion, see Chapter 6.

Rate Variations between Wrists

Variations in pulse rate between the two wrists are very rare. The significant features to look at are the extent of difference in rate between the two wrists, the general quality of the wave on each wrist, and the quality at specific individual positions. With regard to the amount, a difference of two beats is small, four moderate, eight large, and beyond that very serious. If the difference between the two sides is very great, the person is in critical condition and could die.

Etiology

CONGENITAL ANOMALY

A significant congenital blockage of the large vessels on either side of the body can cause a differential in rate between the two wrists. An aneurysm is an example of such an anomaly. The Large Vessel position on the left distal position is Inflated with an aneurysm of the large blood vessels such as the aorta (coarctation).

SHOCK DURING PREGNANCY

If the client's mother suffered a great shock during pregnancy, this will sometimes cause an imbalance in rate between the two wrists of the child. The proximal positions, especially the left, are Feeble-Absent, and the left distal position may also be Feeble-Absent, reflecting impairment of constitutional energy.

HEART QI DEFICIENCY

Though even rarer, if Heart energy is deficient enough, there can be a difference of approximately four beats per minute between the two wrists. In this instance, the pulse on both sides is Feeble-Absent, with the left distal position being the most Feeble-Absent.

TRAUMA AND/OR HEAVY LIFTING

If the rate differential between the two wrists is due to an accident or sudden lifting of a weight considerably beyond one's energy, the pulse wave tends to be more Robust overall.

HABIT

In people who consistently use one side of the body more than the other, the pulse of the wrist that is more often used may be two beats more Rapid than the other.

DIGESTIVE AND ORGAN SYSTEM IMBALANCE

Very rarely, if the pulse on one wrist is slightly more Rapid and its wave is of a better quality than the other wrist, the problem will be on the side that is Slower. For example, the right side represents the 'digestive system' and the left side the 'organ system,' according to Dr. Shen (see glossary). If the rate is slightly more Rapid and the wave is better on the right than on the left, the indication is that the 'digestive system' is functioning well, but the 'organ system' is not.

Fig. 7-1a Rapid rate

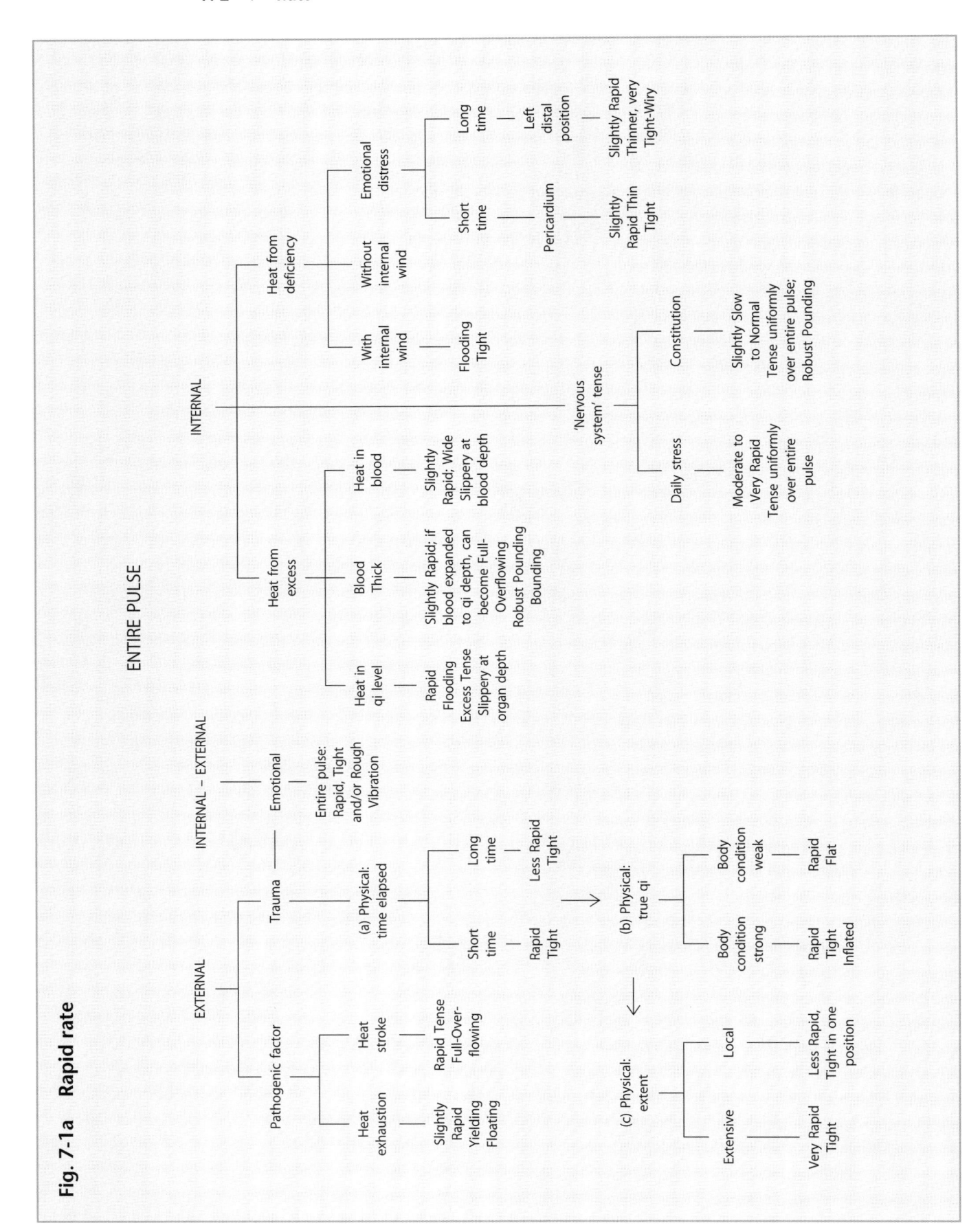

ENTIRE PULSE

- **EXTERNAL**
  - **Pathogenic factor**
    - Heat exhaustion — Slightly Rapid Yielding Floating
    - Heat stroke — Rapid Tense Full-Overflowing

- **INTERNAL – EXTERNAL**
  - **Trauma**
    - Emotional — Entire pulse: Rapid, Tight and/or Rough Vibration
    - (a) Physical: time elapsed
      - Short time — Rapid Tight
      - Long time — Less Rapid Tight
      → (b) Physical: true qi
        - Body condition strong — Rapid Tight Inflated
        - Body condition weak — Rapid Flat
      → (c) Physical: extent
        - Extensive — Very Rapid Tight
        - Local — Less Rapid, Tight in one position

- **INTERNAL**
  - **Heat from excess**
    - Heat in qi level — Rapid Flooding Excess Tense Slippery at organ depth
    - Blood Thick — Slightly Rapid; if blood expanded to qi depth, can become Full-Overflowing Robust Pounding Bounding
    - Heat in blood — Slightly Rapid; Wide Slippery at blood depth
  - **Heat from deficiency**
    - With internal wind — Flooding Tight
    - Without internal wind — Emotional distress
      - Short time — Pericardium — Slightly Rapid Thin Tight
      - Long time — Left distal position — Slightly Rapid Thinner, very Tight-Wiry
  - **'Nervous system' tense**
    - Constitution — Slightly Slow to Normal Tense uniformly over entire pulse; Robust Pounding
    - Daily stress — Moderate to Very Rapid Tense uniformly over entire pulse

Fig. 7-1b Rapid rate (detail)

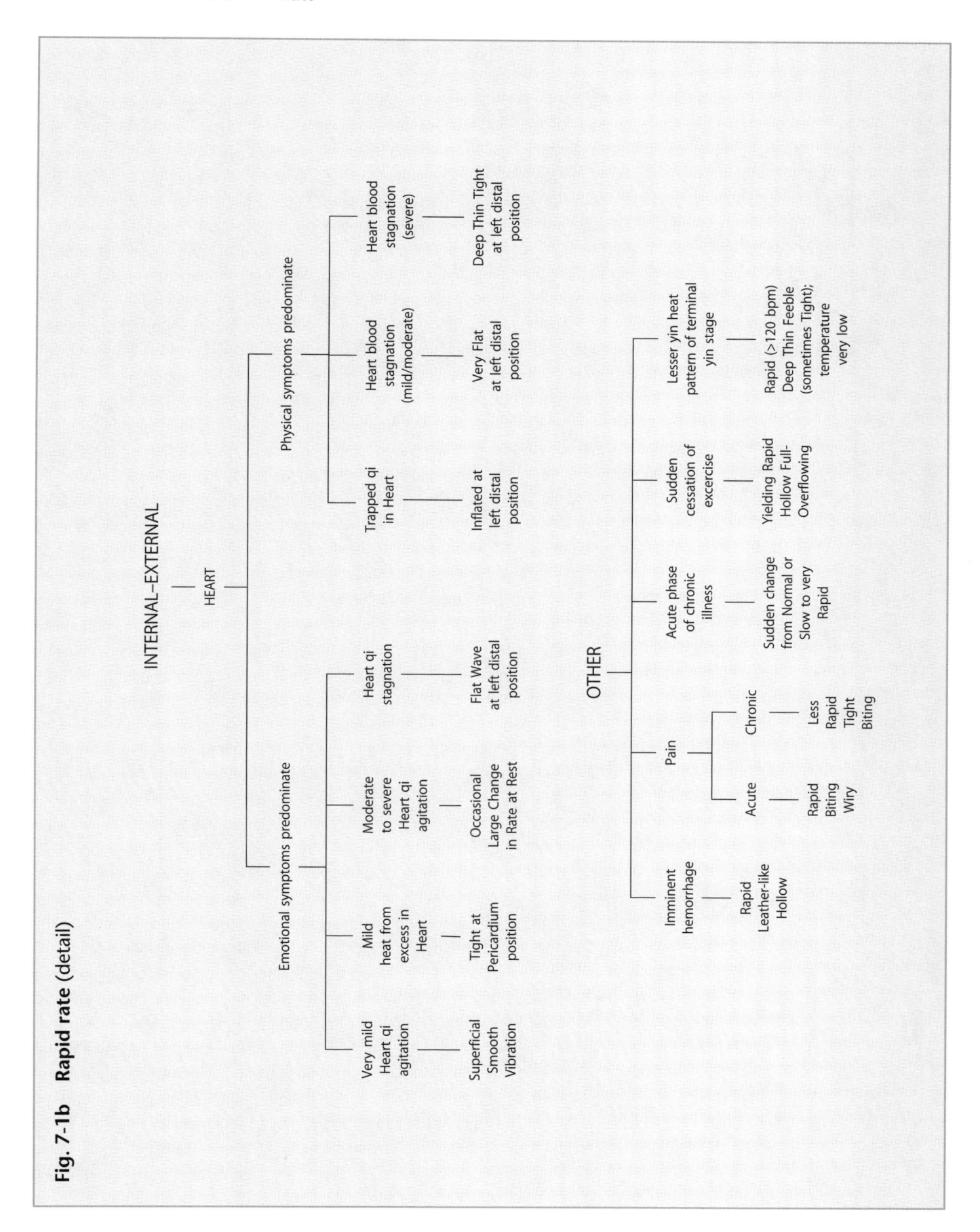

INTERNAL–EXTERNAL

HEART
- Emotional symptoms predominate
  - Very mild Heart qi agitation
    - Superficial Smooth Vibration
  - Mild heat from excess in Heart
    - Tight at Pericardium position
  - Moderate to severe Heart qi agitation
    - Occasional Large Change in Rate at Rest
  - Heart qi stagnation
    - Flat Wave at left distal position
- Physical symptoms predominate
  - Trapped qi in Heart
    - Inflated at left distal position
  - Heart blood stagnation (mild/moderate)
    - Very Flat at left distal position
  - Heart blood stagnation (severe)
    - Deep Thin Tight at left distal position

OTHER
- Imminent hemorrhage
  - Rapid Leather-like Hollow
- Pain
  - Acute
    - Rapid Biting Wiry
  - Chronic
    - Less Rapid Tight Biting
- Acute phase of chronic illness
  - Sudden change from Normal or Slow to very Rapid
- Sudden cessation of excercise
  - Yielding Rapid Hollow Full-Overflowing
- Lesser yin heat pattern of terminal yin stage
  - Rapid (>120 bpm) Deep Thin Feeble (sometimes Tight); temperature very low

174 ❖ Rate

Fig. 7-2 Slow rate

```
COMMON ETIOLOGY
├── External
│   └── Cold from excess
│       └── Slow, Floating, Tight
└── Internal
    ├── Qi & yang deficiency (overwork and/or over-exercise)
    │   ├── Under 20 years
    │   │   • Interrupted
    │   │   • Very Slow
    │   │   • Yielding Hollow
    │   │   • Full-Overflowing
    │   │   • Empty
    │   └── Over 20 years
    │       └── Slow, Feeble-Absent
    ├── Aerobic exercise
    │   └── Slow, Robust ──> Reduced Pounding
    └── Heart qi & yang deficiency
        ├── Constitution
        │   └── Slow; left distal & proximal positions Feeble-Absent
        └── Life experience
            └── Slow Entire pulse Feeble; left distal most Feeble

LESS COMMON ETIOLOGY
├── Liver qi stagnation
│   └── Slow, Taut-Tense
├── Internal heat from excess
│   └── Ropy, Tense
├── Yin deficiency (advanced)
│   └── Ropy, Tight
├── Poisons
│   └── Very Slow Blood Unclear very Deep
├── Medications
│   └── Slow Suppressed
└── Shock
    ├── Physical
    │   └── Slow Tight
    └── Emotional
        └── Rough Vibration over entire pulse

UNCOMMON ETIOLOGY
├── Cold from internal excess
│   • Slow
│   • Tight
│   • Firm
│   • Hidden Tense
├── Internal heat pernicious influence
│   └── Slow Tense Slight Robust Pounding
└── Damp-heat Phlegm-dampness
    └── Slow Tense Slippery

OTHER
├── Change in Rate
│   ├── At rest
│   └── On exertion
├── Congenital anomaly
├── Shock during pregnancy
├── Heart qi deficiency
├── Trauma & heavy lifting
├── Habit
└── Rate variations between wrists
    └── 'Digestive' or 'organ system' imbalance

Classification According to Degree of Slowness
├── 68-72 beats/min.
├── 64-68 beats/min.
├── 60-64 beats/min.
└── 40-60 beats/min.
```

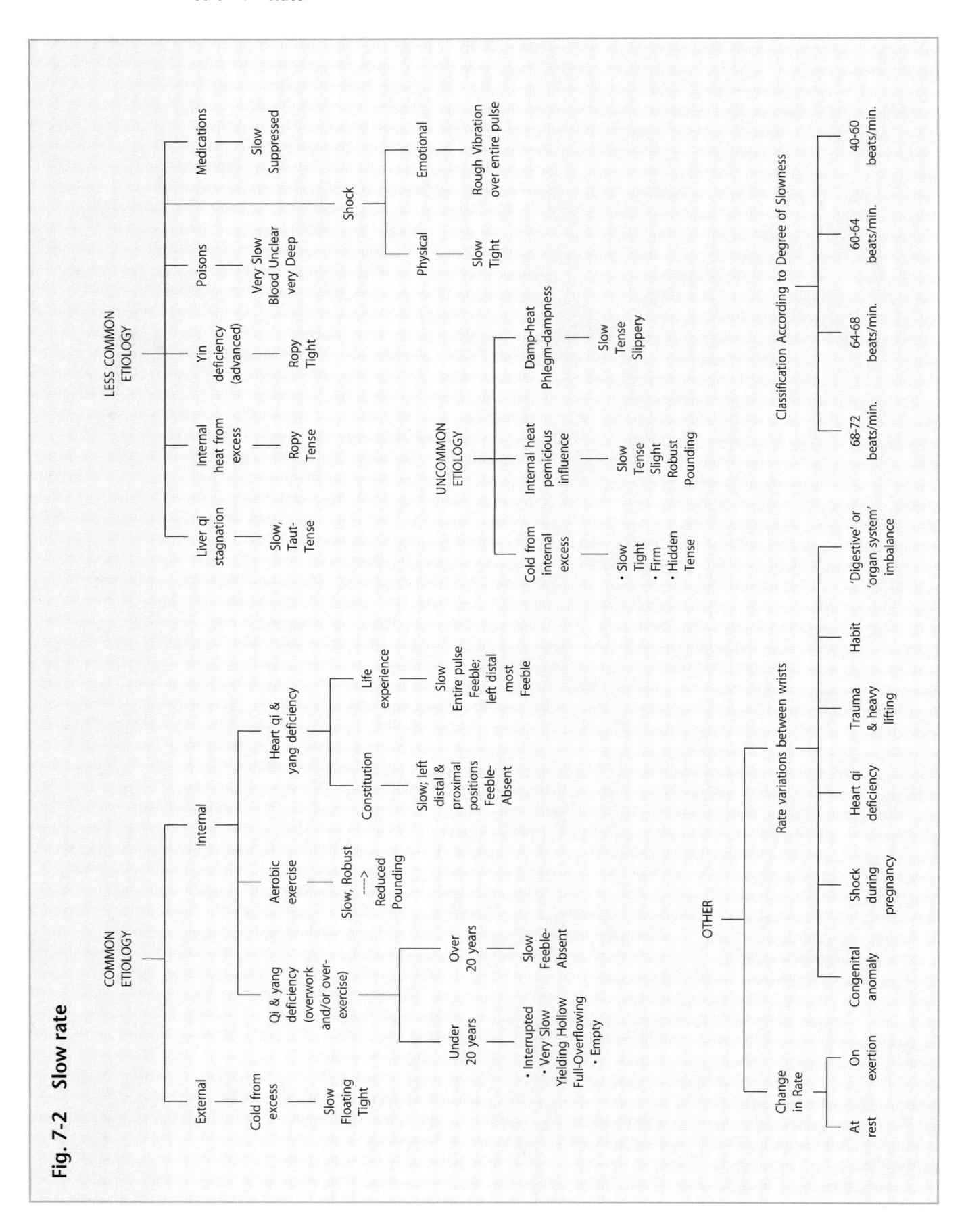

CHAPTER 8

Volume

CONTENTS

Robust qualities, 179
    Hollow Full-Overflowing, 179
        Fig. 8-1: Hollow Full-Overflowing quality, 180
        Types, 181
            Tense Hollow Full-Overflowing, 181
            Yielding Hollow Full-Overflowing, 181
        General interpretation, 181
            Conditions associated with the Tense Hollow Full-Overflowing quality, 182
                Hypertension, 182
                    Fixed ('true') hypertension, 182
                        Heat from excess, 182
                        Heat from excess in the blood, 183
                            Liver disharmony, 183
                            Heart and Liver disharmony, 183
                            Spleen disharmony, 183
                      Heat from yin deficiency, 184
                        Tight to Wiry Hollow Full-Overflowing, 184
                            Diabetes and Liver cirrhosis, 184
                      Heat from both excess and deficiency, 184
                      Heat from excess followed by heat from yin deficiency, 184
                      Qi and/or yang deficiency (heart and kidney qi/yang deficient hypertension), 185
                Labile ('not true') hypertension, 185
                Recapitulation of labile and fixed hypertension, 186
            Conditions associated with the Yielding Hollow Full-Overflowing Reduced Pounding quality, 186

Combinations, 187
- **Yielding Hollow Full-Overflowing and Slow**, 187
- **Yielding Hollow Full-Overflowing and Rapid**, 187
- **Hollow Full-Overflowing Leather-like Hollow and Rapid**, 187
- **Hollow Full-Overflowing Leather-like Hollow and Slow**, 187
- **Hollow Full-Overflowing Slippery over the entire pulse at all depths**, 187
- **Hollow Full-Overflowing Slippery and very Rapid**, 188
- **Hollow Full-Overflowing Tense Hollow and Slippery at the blood depth**, 188
- **Hollow Full-Overflowing Robust Pounding Bounding and Rapid**, 188
- **Hollow Full-Overflowing Reduced Pounding**, 188
  - Normal rate (although it feels rapid), 188
  - Slow, 188
- **Hollow Full-Overflowing Tight or Wiry**, 188
  - Later hypertension or diabetes, 188
- **Hollow Full-Overflowing Tight or Wiry and Slippery**, 188
  - Blood infection, 188

Positions, 189
- Bilaterally at same position, 189
- Sides, 189
- Individual positions, 189

Robust Pounding, 190
- **Robust Pounding and Flooding Excess**, 190
- **Robust Pounding and Full-Overflowing**, 190
- Combinations and positions, 190

Flooding Excess, 190
- Fig. 8-2: Flooding Excess quality, 191
- Positions, 192
  - Bilaterally at same position, 192
  - Sides, 192
  - Individual positions, 192

Inflated, 193
- Fig. 8-3: Inflated quality, 193
- Types, 194
  - **Inflated Yielding**, 194
  - **Inflated Tense**, 194
  - **Very Tense Inflated**, 195
- Combinations, 196
  - **Inflated and Yielding**, 196
  - **Inflated and Tense**, 196
  - **Inflated Yielding-Floating and slightly Rapid**, 196
  - **Inflated Tense-Floating and slightly Slow**, 196
  - **Inflated and very Tense**, 196
- Positions, 196
  - Bilaterally at same position, 196
    - Distal, 196
      - Yielding Inflated, 196
      - Tense Inflated, 196
      - Mildly Tense Inflated, 196
      - Moderately Tense Inflated, 197
      - Tense Inflated Floating, 197

Very Tense Inflated, 197
  Middle, 197
  Proximal, 197
 Sides, 198
 Individual positions, 198
  Between distal and middle positions (diaphragm position), 200
   Heart enlarged and distal Liver engorgement, 200
   Pleural and esophageal positions, 201
Suppressed, 201
 ▪ Fig. 8-4: Suppressed quality, 201
Reduced Qualities, 202
 Excess and deficiency, 202
 Qi depth, 203
 ▪ Fig. 8-5: Yielding at qi depth quality, 203
  Yielding at qi depth, 203
  Diminished or Absent at qi depth, 204
   ▪ Fig. 8-6: Diminished at qi depth quality, 204
   ▪ Fig. 8-7: Absent at qi depth quality, 205
 Blood depth, 205
  Spreading; Yielding partially Hollow; Diminished at blood depth, 205
  Flooding Deficient Wave, 205
   ▪ Fig. 8-8: Spreading quality, 206
   ▪ Fig. 8-9: Yielding partially Hollow quality, 206
   ▪ Fig. 8-10: Diminished at blood depth quality, 207
   ▪ Fig. 8-11: Flooding Deficient Wave quality, 207
Reduced Pounding, 208
Diffuse, 209
 ▪ Fig. 8-12: Diffuse quality, 209
Reduced Substance, 209
 ▪ Fig. 8-13: Reduced Substance quality, 210
Flat, 210
 ▪ Fig. 8-14: Flat quality, 211
  Combinations, 212
   Flat Tight and Rapid, 213
    Physical trauma, 213
    Emotional Trauma, 213
   Flat Tense, 213
  Positions, 213
   Bilaterally at same position, 213
   Between distal and middle positions, 215
   Individual positions, 215
Deep, 216
Feeble-Absent, 216
 ▪ Fig. 8-15a: Feeble (early stage) quality, 216
 ▪ Fig. 8-15b: Feeble (later stage) quality, 217
 ▪ Fig. 8-16: Absent quality, 217
  Contemporary Chinese Pulse Diagnosis, 218
  Combinations, 221
   Feeble-Absent Deep Choppy, 221
   Feeble-Absent Deep Slippery, 221
   Feeble-Absent Deep and Slow, 221

Feeble-Absent Deep and Rapid, 221
  Positions, 221
    Bilaterally at same position, 221
    Sides, 223
    Individual positions, 224
Muffled, 226
  Fig. 8-17: Muffled quality, 226
Dead, 227
Fig. 8-18: Volume flowchart, 228

CHAPTER 8

Volume

Volume is a reflection of the force of the functional basal metabolic yang heat of the body and is evaluated to a large extent by the amplitude of the pulse wave. Amplitude is the height to which the pulse is generated from organ to qi depth or beyond, and intensity is the measure of its fullness. A high amplitude reflects a strong yang force and a low amplitude is a mark of diminished yang force. The subject has been generally organized by distinguishing the Robust from the Reduced pulse qualities.[1]

Robust qualities

Hollow Full-Overflowing

With this quality we reach the crisis in terminology which I warned of in the first chapter. The reader's indulgence will be tested, but rewarded, I hope, by careful attention to what follows.

Category

The Full quality described by Li Shi-Zhen[2] is similar in sensation and interpretation to the Overflowing quality described by Dr. Shen and Wu Shui-Wan.[3] The principal distinction is that Dr. Shen finds this quality to almost always have a concomitant Hollow aspect, except sometimes in the combination Tight to Wiry Hollow Full-Overflowing. But the overlap is too great and there is not enough fundamental difference between Full and Overflowing to warrant the classification of separate qualities.

As we will see below, while holding to the essential interpretation of "accumulation of yang perverse heat" for the Tense Overflowing quality, Dr. Shen goes on to elaborate upon the sensation and interpretation of what Li Shi-Zhen calls the Full quality by discerning variations of sensation which I call Yielding and Tight Overflowing qualities. Therefore, I refer to this quality—variously called Full, Overflowing, and Huge—as Full-Overflowing, adding Dr. Shen's Hollow component, which I always find to be an accompanying aspect. This is my compromise with the present and the past.

To further complicate and stretch our rhetorical capacity, Dr. Shen does use the term Full to describe an entirely different sensation which I call Inflated, since Dr. Shen's Full quality feels like an inflated balloon. Therefore, in order to accommodate the fact that Dr. Shen and Wu Shui-Wan use the term Full to describe an entirely different quality from the Full quality of Li Shi-Zhen, we will identify two qualities in this book. The first is called Hollow Full-Overflowing, described here. The second is called Inflated, which accommodates the sensation that most closely fits that which Dr. Shen and Wu Shui-Wan describe as Full. This quality is discussed later in the chapter.

Dr. Shen describes three kinds of Full-Overflowing pulse: Yielding, Tense, and Tight. He also asserts that the Full-Overflowing pulse is always Hollow. Therefore in the ensuing discussion readers should bear in mind that, with the occasional exception of the Tight to Wiry Full-Overflowing pulse, each of the qualities includes the Hollow as an integral factor.

The reason that the Hollow quality accompanies the Tense Full-Overflowing quality is that heat from excess in the blood damages the intima of the vessels; this weakens the walls, which expand, and the blood in the vessels thus has less contact with the vessel walls. Later, as heat from yin deficiency becomes predominant, the lack of yin nourishment makes the intima of the blood vessels inflexible and harder to the touch; they lose the Hollow feeling and become more Tight to Wiry. Rigid vessel walls break easily and hemorrhage under stress, causing stroke.

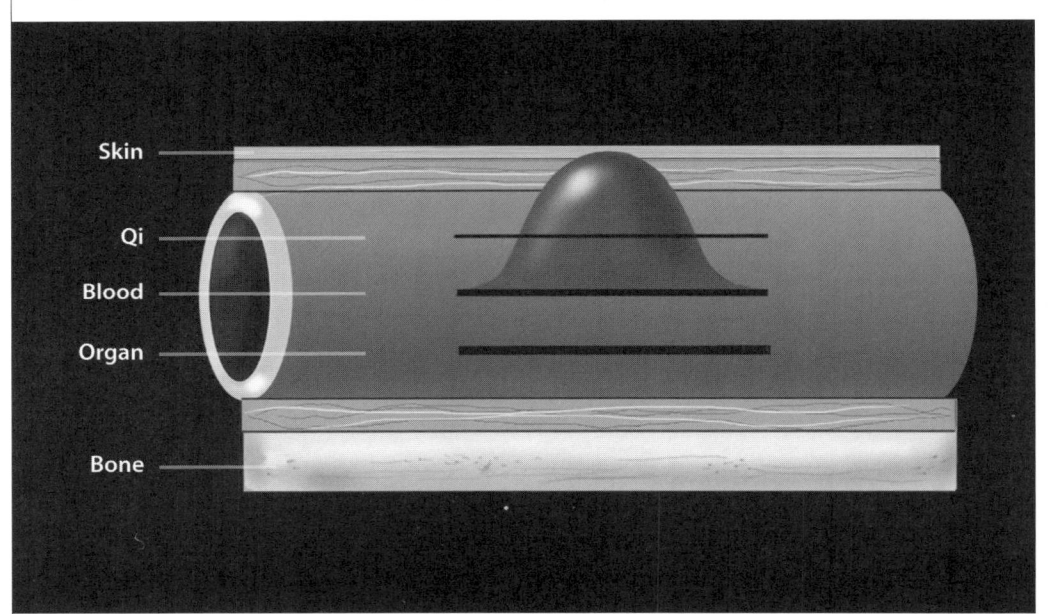

Fig. 8-1 Hollow Full-Overflowing quality

Sensation

As previously mentioned, two of the three types of Full-Overflowing pulse mentioned by Dr. Shen are somewhat Hollow. In terms of perception, the Hollow quality by definition implies that there is no sensation between the qi and organ depths. This is true, in fact, only of the Leather-like Hollow quality. With all other Hollow qualities the sensation seems to yield and separate between the qi and organ depths, but not disappear entirely.

The Full-Overflowing quality has the normal sine curve, comes from the blood depth, and rises above the qi depth. The Tense Tight Hollow Full-Overflowing pulse is especially felt coming from the blood depth, and the Yielding Full-Overflowing quality is felt slightly more superficially. The quality usually involves the entire pulse, but the Tense-Tight Hollow Full-Overflowing quality is often felt most prominently in the middle positions, especially the left middle. This is because the quality represents heat in the blood, and the blood is stored in the Liver.

Types

Tense Hollow Full-Overflowing

The Tense Hollow Full-Overflowing quality feels strong, forceful, swollen, blown-up, rising powerfully from the blood depth, both wide and expansive. The expansiveness felt at the middle blood depth moves vigorously and superficially to and past the qi depth, where the finger feels as if it is being pushed away from the wrist. I have heard this pulse described "like the roaring waves of the sea." It is classified under volume because its force is more obvious than it's superficiality. (Had that characteristic been more pronounced, it would have been classified with the qualities under the heading of depth.) However, even the Tense Hollow Full-Overflowing quality is more Yielding, and will separate more readily under pressure, than the Tense Inflated or any other Tense quality.

When the Hollow Full-Overflowing pulse has a pounding or thumping beat we refer to it as Robust Pounding and Hollow Full-Overflowing. The Robust Pounding quality tends to obscure the other qualities and must be reduced before we can reliably access them. The Hollow Full-Overflowing Bounding pulse has all of the attributes above, but seems at the same time to be running away. It may or may not actually be Rapid.

The Flooding Excess pulse has a stronger base at the organ depth. It begins feeling like a Full-Overflowing Pounding pulse but recedes rapidly as it reaches its apogee, lacking the last part of the curve of the normal wave. It is neither Yielding nor Hollow.

Yielding Hollow Full-Overflowing

The Yielding Hollow Full-Overflowing pulse has the same surge above the qi depth as the Tense Hollow Full-Overflowing quality—"like the roaring waves of the sea"—except that it separates even more easily under pressure than the Tense Hollow Full-Overflowing quality.

General interpretation

Our discussion is based on three etiologies: heat from excess, heat from deficiency, and 'qi wild.' Heat from yin deficiency is included here for the purposes of comparing the hypertension associated with the Tight-Wiry quality with that associated with the Tense Hollow Full-Overflowing quality.

In the literature, the Full-Overflowing quality is generally associated with heat from excess. Li Shi-Zhen[4] states that "The Full pulse occurs when perverse qi is strong," and "when excess perverse heat accumulates in the three heaters." Kaptchuk[5] says that "a full pulse is most often felt at the onset of an Excess/Heat disorder, but it can be part of any Excess pattern."

However, in my experience, and in our time, the deficient Yielding Hollow Full-Overflowing quality, pathognomonic of a 'qi wild' condition, is encountered with increasing frequency. I see massive qi deficiency more and more, and in younger and younger people. Kaptchuk[6] acknowledges that "Clinically, it is possible for a full pulse to be part of a Deficiency pattern if all the other elements of a configuration indicate Deficiency."

Whatever the etiology, whether it be heat from excess or deficiency, or qi and yang deficiency, it is Dr. Shen's basic premise that only a susceptible, vulnerable circulatory system will be involved in the pathologic process which leads to the creation of a Full-Overflowing pulse quality.[7] By 'circulatory system' he is generally thinking of the peripheral circulation, the integrity of the muscular structure of arteries, veins, arterioles, and capillaries.

CONDITIONS ASSOCIATED WITH THE TENSE HOLLOW FULL-OVERFLOWING QUALITY

Hypertension

It is important to mention that if the 'circulatory system' and the 'organ system' are strong, the progression to hypertension will not occur. The 'circulatory system' can be weakened primarily by excess-type heat from Liver qi or digestive stagnation, prolonged exercise and work beyond one's energy, the shock from trauma, the sudden cessation of prolonged, strenuous exercise, and by extreme weather conditions such as occur with hypo- or hyperthermia.

Fixed ('true') hypertension

Hypertension is a condition which is readily revealed by pulse diagnosis. Amber compares the Oriental and the Western approaches to the diagnosis of this disease.[8]

The pulse signs in the early and even later stages of most hypertensive states involve the left proximal and left middle positions of the Kidney and Liver respectively. Here we will find a progression from Tense to Tight-Wiry to Tense Hollow Full-Overflowing to Tight to Wiry Full-Overflowing. Only in one kind of hypertension with a relatively higher diastolic pressure is the Heart more involved, where we find a Feeble-Absent quality in the left distal positions, or the Hollow Full-Overflowing quality in the middle and distal positions.

HEAT FROM EXCESS

One important implication of a Tense Hollow Full-Overflowing quality is heat from excess. Simply stated by Kaptchuk,[9] it is "a sign of excess and is classified as Yang." The other implication, not clearly stated in the literature, is that this heat is from the blood. It is not from an organ, as is the case with heat from excess associated with a Flooding Excess quality. I classify it as one form of blood stagnation (see Chapter 14).

The Tense Hollow Full-Overflowing quality indicates that the heat at the blood depth or the fire in the Liver, which stores the blood, is expanding into the qi channels of energy. This quality is a sign that the organism is trying to eliminate the heat from the blood and the body by expanding the circulatory system and by a general acceleration of function.

The presence of this excess-type heat in the blood vessels for any length of time damages the intima of the vessels and weakens the vessel walls; as explained above, this accounts for the Hollow quality here. The Hollow Tense Full-Overflowing quality over the entire pulse is a sign of severe hypertension and of a dangerous, even fatal, stroke.

Also implied by a Hollow Tense Full-Overflowing quality is that, if the body can create this kind of heat, it must have sufficient strength to make the effort. Therefore, a Tense Hollow Full-Overflowing pulse usually implies true heat in the context of a strong body, as well as a strong disease state.

Etiology and pathogenesis

This heat may come from eating foods rich in lipids (cholesterol and triglycerides) or simple sugars (glucose, fructose, sucrose) over a long period of time, from alcohol, and from excessive intake of hot-type foods (spices, shellfish, lamb). Spleen qi deficiency and dampness can also contribute to heat, as explained below.

A common etiology is the continuous repression of emotion, such as anger, which develops from stress over a long period of time; this creates stagnation, primarily in the Liver. Heart dysfunction due to shock or prolonged worry and anxiety, and affecting the mental faculties, can also contribute to this process. With both there are two stages, one involving heat from excess and the other from deficiency.

Another source of heat in the Liver, according to Dr. Shen, is physical overwork, including excessive exercise. People who work long hours drive the Liver into a state of exhaustion because the Liver has the function of restoring the energy and giving us a second wind.

An increasingly familiar source of the Tense Hollow Full-Overflowing Robust Pounding quality is modern pharmaceuticals. When medications cause this quality, the distinguishing sensory factor is that the very top of the wave feels curtailed or suppressed. In the light of our discussion of the physiologic meaning of this quality we have some insight into the long-term effects of these medications on the integrity of the blood vessels.

HEAT FROM EXCESS IN THE BLOOD

Liver disharmony   Regarding the source of the heat from excess, overexertion and overcoming stagnation requires work. This work is driven by the healthy heat of the qi of the Liver and of the entire organism. We reach the condition known as Liver fire when the heat accumulates at a rate faster than it can be normally released. At this point the Liver fire will rise to other vulnerable parts of the body, such as the head where it causes headaches, or to the Heart where we call it Heart fire.

Since the Liver stores the blood, this heat is eventually absorbed by the stored blood. As the heat from excess in the blood increases, the arteries expand in an attempt by the body to rid itself of the heat. Furthermore, if heavy labor or exercise is a factor, the blood vessels expand faster than blood is available to fill them. At this point, the pulse will be Tense Hollow Full-Overflowing, and the blood depth will reflect the quality and condition which Dr. Shen calls 'blood thick.' When Liver fire and heat in the blood is involved, the systolic blood pressure is high.

When the Heart becomes stressed by this expanded circulatory system and by the need to release its own fire, it has to work harder. The Hollow Full-Overflowing pulse will then take on the quality of Robust Pounding, as described above. The beat is stronger. Other Heart disharmonies, such as the conditions described by Dr. Shen,[10] can contribute to this process. (The Robust Pounding quality, incidentally, is frequently found in coffee drinkers.)

As the heat and the Heart's work increase, the Heart Full-Overflowing pulse not only beats harder and pounds, its rate also increases. The pulse may feel as if it is running away, which we call Bounding, though the Bounding sensation sometimes occurs with a Normal rate. As the Heart becomes involved, the diastolic blood pressure tends to increase.

Heart and Liver disharmony   My own conception of another process involving the Liver and Heart, beginning with the Heart, is as a two-fold vicious cycle. The Heart controls the mind. When the Heart is in a state of disharmony for any reason, this discord in turn begets a more vulnerable, easily affected 'nervous system,' as defined by Dr. Shen.[11] Since the Liver nourishes the peripheral 'nervous system,' ligaments, and tendons, it is overburdened by maintaining the neuro-musculoskeletal manifestations of a dysfunctional mental apparatus. This overwork creates heat, which is eventually picked up by the blood and engenders the Tense Hollow Full-Overflowing Robust Pounding quality. This is especially true if the Liver is already burdened by the stress and tension mentioned above. Eventually, Liver heat will reach the vulnerable Heart, where it engenders more instability and overwork by the Heart, and the cycle will escalate as the excess-type heat enters the blood and 'circulatory system.' Liver cirrhosis is another etiology manifested in a Wiry left middle position.

Spleen disharmony   A damp condition in the Spleen can exacerbate all of the above. Usually this person is overweight, lethargic, and emotionally disturbed due to the phlegm reaching the Heart, where it obstructs or clouds the 'orifices' and blocks the clear Spleen qi from rising to the brain. The eyes lose their brightness *(ming)* and there is frontal headache. The blood depth is Slippery, the right side Tight, the Stomach pulse (right middle position) is Pounding, and the eyes are very red. Dampness in the blood increases resistance to flow, requiring more work, and thus excess-type heat.

HEAT FROM YIN DEFICIENCY

Tight to Wiry Hollow Full-Overflowing

As the vessels move to a state of yin deficiency, the pulse becomes harder, more Tight to Wiry in the extreme, and often loses the Hollow quality associated with the Tense and Yielding Full-Overflowing qualities.

Etiology and pathogenesis

The stagnation associated with repressed emotions simultaneously creates another heat-producing pathological process. As previously noted, heat from excess results from the effort of an 'irresistible force' to overcome an 'immovable object,' a process which occurs with Liver qi stagnation; this weakens the blood vessels by causing them to dilate. The body attempts to balance this heat with yin fluid. Eventually we have a deficient rather an excessive disorder—yin deficiency—affecting primarily the Heart, Liver, and later the Kidneys.

Heat from deficiency 'dries out' the nerves and makes them more irritable. It also eventually dries out the muscular wall of the blood vessels, making them brittle and fragile, and causing them to weaken and expand. This process takes us through the progression of the Taut, Tense, Tight, and Wiry pulse qualities. Thus, over a long period of time, a tense 'nervous system' can cause the pulse to become Tight to Wiry, especially at the left distal, middle, and left proximal positions, and a little Rapid. The tongue becomes bright red and dry, with a patchy coating.

Diabetes and Liver cirrhosis   The same progression of pulse qualities, from Wiry to Wiry Full-Overflowing, can be found in both early and late insulin-dependent diabetes. With diabetes the Tight to Wiry Full-Overflowing pulse is mostly on both the left middle, and especially the left proximal, positions.

Sometimes the etiology of a Wiry left middle position associated with 'true' hypertension is due only to the Liver cirrhosis and portal vein congestion caused by abuse of alcohol and other toxins, leading to a Wiry Liver (left middle position) pulse. Here the systolic blood pressure is elevated.

HEAT FROM BOTH EXCESS AND DEFICIENCY

During the ensuing discussion keep in mind that heat from excess weakens blood vessels by causing them to dilate and expand, while heat from yin deficiency damages the blood vessels by causing them to become dry, brittle, and fragile. It is always important to remember that whatever the etiology, a damaged 'circulatory system' is a prerequisite to the development of hypertension.

HEAT FROM EXCESS FOLLOWED BY HEAT FROM YIN DEFICIENCY

When the etiology is associated with a rich diet, repressed emotion affecting the Liver, a Tense 'nervous system,' physical overwork, and medication, the result is excess-type heat in the blood with a Tense Hollow Full-Overflowing quality. When heat from yin deficiency is the strongest pathogenic factor, we move from the Tense Hollow Full-Overflowing quality—a sign of heat from excess in the blood type of hypertension—to a Tight-Wiry Hollow Full-Overflowing quality. This can occur at a stage in the process when the body is less capable of generating yin.

As the yin is further depleted in its effort to balance the heat from excess, the vessel walls are deprived of nourishment and fluid. The vessel walls eventually dry out and harden, lose their flexibility, and become a foci for minerals and lipids in the blood. We call this condition athero-arteriosclerosis when the Tight (Hollow) Full-Overflowing pulse is replaced by a cord-like Tense Ropy quality.

QI AND/OR YANG DEFICIENCY (HEART AND KIDNEY QI/YANG DEFICIENT HYPERTENSION)

We can also get 'true' hypertension from either Heart or Kidney qi/yang deficiency, or both together. When the Heart, Kidney, or the large vessels (e.g., aorta) are involved, the diastolic pressure is relatively higher than the systolic. The process often progresses from yin to yang deficiency for both the Heart and Kidney.

When the Heart is yin deficient and the condition and quality is one of Heart qi agitation, the blood pressure is still labile. However, when the Heart is qi deficient and cannot push or control the circulation, the diastolic pressure stays high. The Heart pulse (left distal position) is Feeble-Absent at this point. With the same etiologies and a strong Heart, only the large vessels will be involved. With a strong Heart and a condition of heat from excess in the blood, the pulse quality at the Large Vessel position is Tense Hollow Full-Overflowing, and the diastolic blood pressure would show the biggest elevation.

Heart involvement is due to heavy work without rest, and to severe emotional problems where the Heart is already constitutionally vulnerable, or weakened from an experience such as a shock due to sudden fear. Examples of Heart conditions that lead to hypertension include Heart yin deficiency, Heart blood stagnation ('Heart small'), Heart qi stagnation ('Heart closed'), Heart trapped qi ('Heart full'), and Heart qi and blood deficiency ('Heart large').[12]

Kidney yang deficiency can also be associated with hypertension. The greater the deficiency, the higher the diastolic pressure. More commonly the origin is a constitutional, chronic debilitating disease, and less often, very protracted Kidney yin deficiency. A tense 'nervous system' can affect the 'organ system' by driving the yin organs until they become yin-deficient and dry, and function poorly. This process affects the Kidneys in particular, which supply yin to the entire organism, leading to Kidney-related 'true' hypertension. Ultimately, the yin deficiency turns to yang deficiency. The left proximal position moves from a Tight to a Feeble-Absent quality.

For another explanation we can turn to Western physiology where the substance renin is the kidney factor associated with high blood pressure. A poorly functioning Kidney in the Chinese sense would of course affect the production of renin as well as the steroids in the adrenal cortex and the epinephrine in the adrenal medulla, all of which can affect the blood pressure. The blood deficiency could also be related to another substance recently found in kidney tissue called the hemopoietic factor, which is associated with the function of bone marrow production of red blood cells.

With Heart and Kidney qi/yang deficiency as the source of hypertension, the Heart and Kidney pulses are Feeble-Absent by the time that the diastolic has risen to abnormal heights. When both Heart and Kidney qi/yang deficiency and heat in the blood vessels are involved simultaneously, both diastolic and systolic pressures are high.

Labile ('not true') hypertension

With the labile or 'not true' hypertension there is no true yin organ blood or circulatory pathology, the Heart and circulatory system are strong, and the blood pressure varies considerably from day to day, especially the systolic, increasing with nervous strain and decreasing when relaxed. Both a constitutionally tense 'nervous system' making one vulnerable to these fluctuations as well as a lifestyle which involves consistent and prolonged nervous strain or deep worries and concerns about life situations, put a similar strain on the nervous system. This can sometimes occur with only a Tense quality when a tense 'nervous system' directly affects a vulnerable 'circulatory system.' The greater the 'nervous system' problem, the larger the swing in pressure. A classic example is 'white coat hypertension' which occurs in a person whose blood pressure rises in a doctor's office and then falls at home.

When Liver qi stagnation is due to continuously repressed anger and frustration we can have a Taut to Tense quality at the left middle position, and later over the entire pulse. Sometimes there is inconsistent Change in Intensity over the entire pulse. The tongue and eyes are relatively clear at this early stage of the process. Qi stagnation by itself can be attended by labile hypertension when constrained qi is released, which Dr. Shen calls 'not true' hypertension. Here the systolic pressure is more elevated than the diastolic, and there is fluctuation, with stress increasing and relaxation decreasing the blood pressure.

Recapitulation of labile and fixed hypertension

With prolonged Liver qi stagnation, heat from excess develops that enters the blood and gradually affects the vessels and circulation, leading to the Tense Hollow Full-Overflowing type of 'fixed' hypertension. The overworked nervous system depletes yin and leads to the Tight to Wiry (Hollow) Full-Overflowing type of 'fixed' hypertension. Therefore, what Dr. Shen calls 'not true' hypertension (labile) can become 'true' hypertension (permanently elevated).

It is important to reiterate that if the 'circulatory system' is strong, the progression to hypertension will not occur.

While labile hypertension is related only to constrained qi escaping, or to 'tightness' of the 'nervous system' and blood vessels, fixed hypertension always involves either heat in the blood vessels, a profound depletion of yin causing heat from yin deficiency, or a Heart-Kidney qi/yang deficiency. With 'fixed' hypertension that is not labile, the body feels tight and uncomfortable.

With heat in the blood and the Tense Hollow Full-Overflowing quality, the degree of elevation of the systolic blood pressure will be greater than the diastolic blood pressure. With fixed hypertension due to Heart/Kidney qi deficiency, and to a lesser extent with heat from yin deficiency, the diastolic rises relatively more than the systolic.

If the etiology is primarily heat from excess the treatment of hypertension is easier than when the primary etiology is heat from yin deficiency, which is more difficult to treat. With either etiology, an increase in rate will presage a stroke.

Dr. Shen believes that one can have hypertension with a Normal pulse. He regards this as a constitutional issue, and suggests that the elevated pressure in this instance is not pathological. In fact, with a constitutionally normal elevated blood pressure, when the blood pressure falls toward what would be normal in the larger population, the patient becomes ill.

CONDITIONS ASSOCIATED WITH THE YIELDING HOLLOW FULL-OVERFLOWING REDUCED POUNDING QUALITY

These conditions include chronic fatigue syndrome and auto-immune disorders. The Yielding Hollow Full-Overflowing Reduced Pounding pulse is not a sign of excess. This pulse may represent a defective organism in which the Hollow Full-Overflowing and Reduced Pounding quality represents a compensatory effort to rise to the energic demands of life. It is as if the organism is making a final attempt to mobilize itself. It is more Yielding than the Tense Hollow Full-Overflowing Pounding pulse, and with a Slower rate, except in the terminal stages of the process, when the rate can be more

Rapid and/or the rhythm is Arrhythmic.

Under these circumstances the Yielding Hollow Full-Overflowing Reduced Pounding pulse, as in any situation in which there is a disparity between signs and symptoms, is considered to be a more serious sign. To the uninitiated, the pulse appears to be a sign of excess while the person is extremely weak. According to Wu Shui-Wan,[13] and in my own experience, this pulse can be found in people who have been seriously ill for an extended period with extreme loss of qi, blood, and fluid. Kaptchuk[14] states that this pulse is "illusionary and thought to be a sign that the prognosis is poor".

The Yielding Hollow Full-Overflowing Reduced Pounding quality can be found in children who are constitutionally deficient of true qi. From the beginning of their lives they are unable to keep up with other children, and tend to be energetically impaired throughout life. Under these circumstances the pulse is even more Yielding.

A Yielding Hollow Full-Overflowing Reduced Pounding and Rapid pulse also occurs when a person who is overworking or exercising heavily suddenly stops. This pulse, described in our discussion of 'qi wild' in Chapter 6, can represent the irrevocable separation of yin from yang.

Combinations

All of the following Full-Overflowing qualities are also Hollow, unless otherwise specified.

Yielding Hollow Full-Overflowing and Slow

Described above, this is a 'qi-wild' sign due to gradual depletion of qi from overexercise and overwork over a long period of time.

Yielding Hollow Full-Overflowing and Rapid

Described above, this is a 'qi-wild' sign due to the sudden cessation of extreme physical activity such as exercise or work.

Hollow Full-Overflowing Leather-like and Rapid

This is a serious sign of imminent bleeding and stroke. There is absolutely no sensation felt between the qi and organ levels.

Hollow Full-Overflowing Leather-like and Slow

This indicates recent bleeding, probably associated with stroke. The Hollow aspect of the pulse is complete. There is no sensation felt between the qi and organ levels.

Hollow Full-Overflowing Slippery over the entire pulse at all depths

This indicates a pregnancy which has reached full term and will deliver within one week.

Hollow Full-Overflowing Slippery and very Rapid

If this combination appears before the baby is due, a miscarriage may occur. Check for vertical black lines on the tongue.

Hollow Full-Overflowing Tense and Slippery at the blood depth

This combination can be a sign of 'blood thick' with excess lipids such as cholesterol.

Hollow Full-Overflowing Robust Pounding Bounding and Rapid

In acute febrile illnesses such as heatstroke, the rate is very Rapid as long as the temperature is elevated; the tongue will have a yellow coating, and the sclera of the eyes and vertical lines under the lower eyelid will be injected and red.

Acute anxiety states can be differentiated from acute febrile illness based on the temperature, tongue, eyes, and pulse rate. With anxiety the tongue and eyes are normal, and the rate is more Rapid only during the height of the acute attack.

Hollow Full-Overflowing Reduced Pounding

Normal rate (although it feels Rapid)

This quality can occur in a strong person whose body has been overworking for a long period of time to reopen circulation constricted by the shock of a major trauma.

When the Reduced Pounding is due to exercise or work beyond one's energy for a moderate period of time, the rate may be Normal. This pulse does not have the powerful Full-Overflowing quality that one finds with heat in the blood. It is more even at all depths, and is very Yielding at the surface.

Slow

With a Slow rate, this combination occurs when the amount of exercise or work beyond one's energy is even greater, or sustained for a longer period of time, than that above. The quality is mildly Full-Overflowing, Yielding, Reduced Pounding, and Slow.

Hollow Full-Overflowing Tight or Wiry

Later hypertension or diabetes

Indicates a combination of heat from both excess and deficiency. This pulse is found in hypertension and sometimes in diabetes. Classically, it is associated with concomitant Liver fire and Liver/Kidney yin deficiency.

Hollow Full-Overflowing Tight or Wiry and Slippery

Blood infection

This pulse may be found with septicemia or massive infection in the blood. There is considerable fever and some pain, and there are signs of infection on the tongue and in the eyes. The pulse is Slippery at all depths.

Positions

BILATERALLY AT SAME POSITION

Distal — I have observed this once in a person with severe headache due to hypertension. The pulse at the middle and lower burner positions was Feeble or Absent.[15]

Middle — Hypertension and diabetes must be considered here.[16]

Proximal — Hypertension and diabetes must also be considered here.[17]

SIDES

Left — The Yielding Hollow Full-Overflowing quality over the entire left side is associated with a person who is easily angered and provoked into outbursts of impotent rage.

While the Tense Full-Overflowing Hollow quality is rarely found over the entire left side, it can occur with hypertension and diabetes, as explained above. This portends a stroke on the left side of the body.

Right — The Yielding Hollow Full-Overflowing quality here can indicate qi deficiency and stagnation in the digestive system. The Tense Hollow Full-Overflowing quality portends a stroke on the right side of the body.

Both — If both sides have a very Tight-Wiry Hollow Full-Overflowing Rapid pulse, there is imminent danger of a serious, life-threatening cerebrovascular accident.

INDIVIDUAL POSITIONS

Except in the left middle position, it is rare to find a Full-Overflowing quality at an individual position alone, and almost never at the right side individual positions.

Left distal — The Tense Hollow Full-Overflowing pulse here is rare. It may denote Heart fire and elevated blood pressure, often associated with severe headache. Dr. Shen says that one "must beware of the heart dilating or the hardening of the blood vessels of the heart."[18]

A Tight Full-Overflowing pulse at the Large Vessel position of the left distal position can occur with elevated blood pressure. The Large Vessel position develops this sign under circumstances which lead to hypertension when the Heart itself is functioning well.

Right distal — I have never found this quality alone at the right distal or at the Special Lung positions.

Left middle — Any process which leads to heat in the Liver and blood—such as prolonged stress due to frustration and anger, or foods rich in lipids and simple carbohydrates (sugars)—may produce the Tense Hollow Full-Overflowing quality in this position. This is because the quality represents heat in the blood, and the Liver stores the blood. Hypertension and diabetes must be considered, especially if this quality also appears at the left proximal position.

Right middle — This quality is rarely found alone at this position, and is here often mistaken for the Inflated quality.

Left proximal — The Tense Hollow or Tight Full-Overflowing quality at the left proximal position is found with both hypertension and diabetes, especially if the quality simultaneously appears at the left middle position. With diabetes the pulse is usually Tighter than with hypertension, and often Wiry.

Right proximal | The Full-Overflowing quality is rarely found alone at this position, and is sometimes mistaken for the Flooding Excess quality.

Robust Pounding

This quality is associated with heat from excess. It tends to obscure other pulse qualities, and must itself be muted before we can reliably access the other qualities. (For the Reduced Pounding quality, see the Reduced qualities in the latter part of this chapter.)

Category | There is no category in the literature called Pounding. Kaptchuk is the only one to use the term in connection with his description of the big pulse.

Sensation | Pounding means to beat heavily or throb. Force means strength, energy, vigor, and power, referring especially to the intensity of the power or impetus. When the pulse pounds with force the palpating fingers feel as if they are being blown away from the wrist.

Interpretation | Robust Pounding usually reflects an attempt by the body to expel heat from excess through the circulation. However, Robust Pounding is also associated with acute anxiety, when the cause is agitated Heart qi, in which case the rate is often very Rapid, but the tongue and eyes are normal.

Robust Pounding and Flooding Excess

The strongest Robust Pounding is associated with a febrile illness such as hepatitis, where the pulse is often Flooding Excess either over the entire pulse or at one position, and the rate is Rapid; the tongue and eyes are red. The Pounding quality here is an expression of the body's attempt to eliminate heat from one or more of the yin organs.

Robust Pounding and Hollow Full-Overflowing

When the Full-Overflowing Hollow pulse has a pounding, thumping beat it is referred to as Hollow Full-Overflowing Robust Pounding. The Pounding quality reflects the body's attempt to eliminate heat from the blood. The rate will be less Rapid than with the Flooding Excess pulse, and the eyes and the tongue will be less red.

Combinations and positions

For other combinations and positions, consult the other qualities which the Robust Pounding quality modifies. Robust Pounding is generally found over the entire pulse, and somewhat less often at individual positions; however, should it so appear, it would have the same interpretation.

Flooding Excess

Category | The Hollow Full-Overflowing and the Flooding Excess qualities are often confused with each other because both are found above the qi depth, and both are often associated with the Rapid and Robust Pounding qualities. Furthermore, both involve heat from excess.

The distinction between them can be found in both the sensation and the interpretation. The Flooding Excess pulse is a sign of acute heat from excess in an organ, while Hollow Full-Overflowing is a sign of chronic heat from excess or deficiency (Tense or Tight) in the blood. And while they are both found above the qi depth, the Hollow Full-Overflowing quality has a complete sine curve, while the Flooding Excess pulse reaches the apogee of the sine curve and falls away precipitously.

There are two kinds of Flooding pulse. The one described in the literature, which is related to heat from either excess or deficiency, I call Flooding Excess. The other is Flooding Deficient, which, in my own and Dr. Shen's experience, is a sign of yin organ qi deficiency; Dr. Shen refers to it as a 'push pulse.' (There is further elaboration of this pulse under the heading of reduced volume.) Li Shi-Zhen[19] also refers to "the flooding pulse with deficient symptoms," and Kaptchuk[20] describes a Flooding pulse which "is then considered a sign of Deficiency." I disagree with Li Shi-Zhen,[21] who classifies the Flooding pulse as one of the seven types of Floating pulses, by which he means Superficial, since a true Floating pulse has no wave form (see Chapter 9). 'Big' is a confusing surrogate term he uses for Flooding.[22]

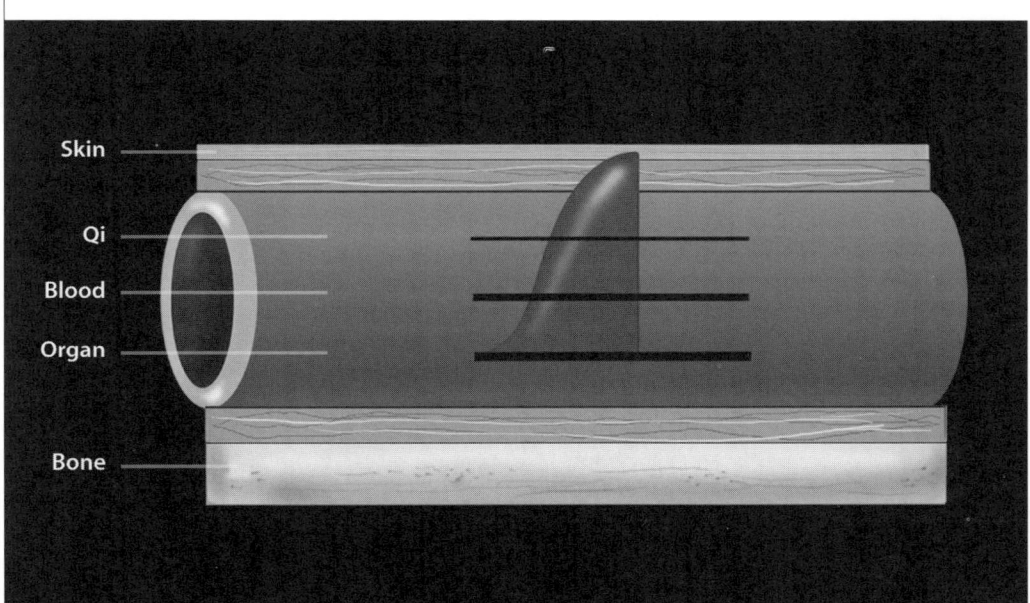

Fig. 8-2 Flooding Excess quality

Sensation

The Flooding Excess quality (Fig. 8-2) begins feeling like a Hollow Full-Overflowing Robust Pounding quality, with the first part of the normal sine curve above the qi depth, but recedes rapidly as it reaches its apogee, lacking the last part of the curve of the normal wave. It has a stronger base at the organ depth than the Hollow Full-Overflowing quality, and is also not Yielding or Hollow. It was described to me as feeling "big as it strikes the finger, and weak and long when leaving." Dr. Shen does not mention this in his book, although he consistently confirmed it over the years in private communication. This pulse does not give way to pressure as easily as the Hollow Full-Overflowing pulse, suggesting that the rising heat comes from the yin organs rather than from the blood, which is considered the source of the Tense Hollow Full-Overflowing quality.[23]

General interpretation

I find that this pulse primarily represents acute heat from excess in the yin organs, usually of an infectious nature. The Flooding Excess quality is characteristic, for example, of acute hepatitis, of the yang brightness phase of the six stages (appendicitis, bacillary dysentery), and of episodes of mania in bipolar disease. Secondarily, one can find, when the conditions creating this quality have acutely recurred over time, simultaneous signs and symptoms of yin deficiency. The interpretation of heat from excess in the yin organs applies both when the Flooding Excess quality is found over the entire pulse, and at just one position.[24,25]

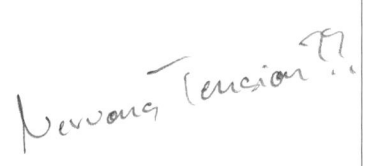

Positions

The Flooding Excess quality is found most often at individual positions, or over the entire pulse, and rarely bilaterally or on just one side.

BILATERALLY AT SAME POSITION

Distal

This quality may accompany acute fulminating myocarditis or pericarditis.

Middle

Here the quality is associated with acute infection in a yin organ, such as pancreatitis or hepatitis, and peritonitis. Li Shi-Zhen[26] observes that "when excessive liver yang damages the jin [fluids] in the stomach and spleen, both guan [middle] pulses become flooding."

PROXIMAL POSITION

The possibility of acute fulminating prostatitis and pelvic inflammatory disease should be entertained if a Flooding Excess quality at this position is accompanied by pain and urinary difficulty. Less often, in my experience, this pulse may reflect an acute overwhelming ulcerative colitis or regional ileitis.

LEFT SIDE

A Flooding Excess pulse on only the left side is rare, and can be found with fulminating hepatitis, cholecystitis, or myocarditis. In my experience with these conditions, the entire pulse is more likely to reflect this quality.

RIGHT SIDE

A Flooding Excess pulse on only the right side is rare with a fulminating peritonitis, appendicitis, or pancreatitis, which more often manifests over the entire pulse.

LEFT DISTAL POSITION

Rarely, Heart fire rising with dry and sore throat, mouth and tongue ulcers, irritability, bitter taste, insomnia, and a flushed face can be accompanied by a Flooding Excess pulse.[27] It is found with acute myocarditis. It can also occur with Liver fire rising to become Heart fire, and is associated with Grave's disease, mania, and the early stages of cocaine addiction.

RIGHT DISTAL POSITION

The Flooding Excess quality can appear here with fire in the Lungs, usually due to infection such as pneumonia or bronchitis. Li Shi-Zhen[28] also speaks of "excessive fire in the lung" causing "symptoms of coughing, asthma, pain in the chest and coughing blood." Worsley refers to "heat at lungs; coughing; sputum."[29]

LEFT MIDDLE POSITION

As noted above, Li Shi-Zhen[30] observes that "when excessive liver yang damages the jin [fluids] in the stomach and spleen, both guan [middle] pulses become flooding." Excessive Liver fire can also produce this pulse at the left middle position alone. Worsley mentions "heat at liver; vexation; hot limbs."[31] This quality at the left middle position is most often associated with acute hepatitis and fulminating Gallbladder infection.

RIGHT MIDDLE POSITION

Li Shi-Zhen,[32] with whom I concur, associates this pulse with "abundant heat stasis in the stomach, causing swelling, fullness, upset stomach and vomiting." Worsley writes "gastritis; vomiting; thirst."[33] Peritonitis, pancreatitis, and appendicitis are the most common conditions.

LEFT PROXIMAL POSITION

I have found the Flooding Excess quality with fulminating colitis, pelvic inflammatory disease, and prostatitis. Worsley correctly mentions "heat at bladder."[34]

RIGHT PROXIMAL POSITION

I have found this pulse in connection with the same conditions listed for the left proximal position, including acute bladder infection. Worsley alludes to "tympanitis; constipation or bleeding."[35]

Inflated

Fig. 8-3 Inflated quality

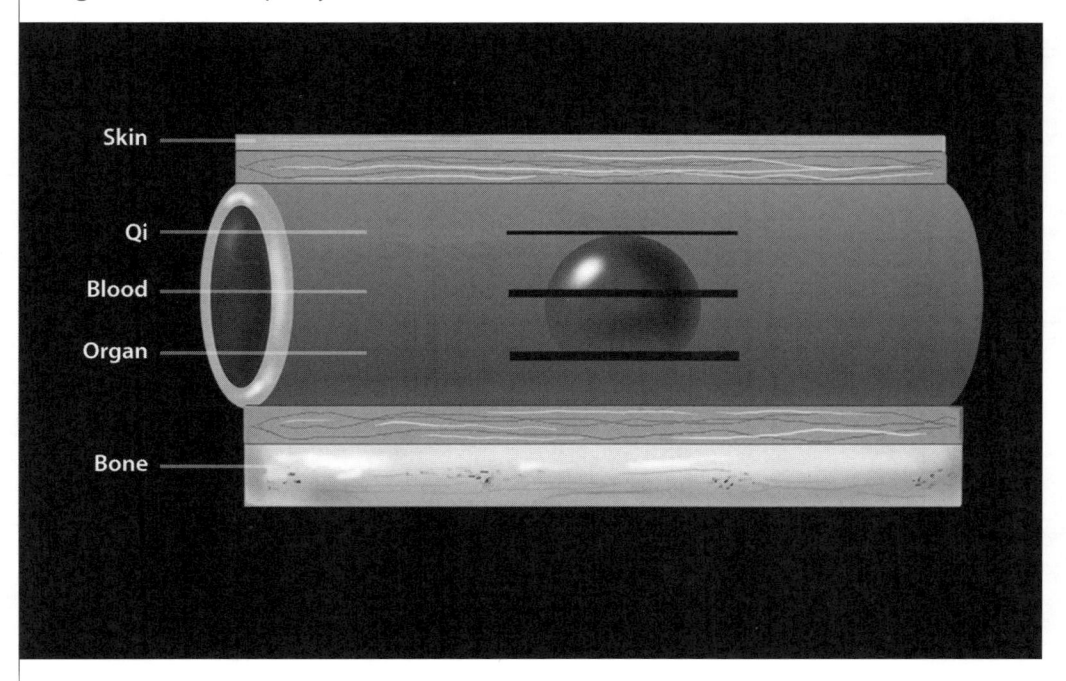

Category

As previously mentioned, Dr. Shen calls this pulse Full, and Wu Shui-Wan uses the term Full as distinguished from Overflowing, but compares it to a long rather than a round balloon (as we describe it). We are avoiding the use of the term Full for this quality to prevent confusion, since it has an entirely different interpretation and sensation in Li Shi-Zhen's and Ted Kaptchuk's conceptions. Porkert[36] describes a pulse quality which he calls 'Replete' which has some of the characteristics of the Inflated quality.

There are two main subcategories of this quality, Inflated Tense and Inflated Yielding. It is important to remember that with the Inflated quality, qi has difficulty getting out of an organ or area in which it is trapped due to the suppression of the circulation of qi and heat. It is also important to bear in mind that an individual in whom this quality appears was relatively strong when the events occurred which caused the circulation to decrease. A rare variant of this pulse is the Very Tense Inflated quality.

Sensation

The Inflated quality (Fig. 8-3) feels like an inflated balloon. It gives a round ball-like impression in which there is a constant level of tension which resists giving way under pressure. It stays within the three depths (though it conveys the sense that it will keep expanding) and tends to be equal at all of them. Porkert[37] describes his Replete quality as a "strong pulse manifesting itself on any of the three levels [depths]. Usually it can already be detected under slight pressure, and even heavy pressure will not make it disappear."

General interpretation

There are two principal (and one rare) causes for the Inflated quality. The principal causes are accumulated heat and qi trapped in an organ or area of the body. Porkert[38] observes it when "active energy is mobilized massively, thus producing a jam in the conduits [channels]." It is found in a person whose true qi was strong at the time of the precipitating event.

The Inflated quality must be distinguished from the Taut-Tense, Hollow, and Flat qualities. The Flat quality is a sign of a condition in which qi cannot get into an organ. With a Taut-Tense quality, the qi stagnation occurs due to conflicting forces within an organ, such as repressed emotion in the Liver; here, the qi cannot move within the organ. By contrast, with an Inflated quality the qi is unable to get out of an organ. Given the same precipitating event, such as trauma, the Inflated quality will more likely be found in a strong person, and a Flat quality in a more deficient person.

A rare variation of the Inflated Tense quality is the Very Tense Inflated quality, which is caused by trapped blood.

Types

Inflated Yielding

Sensation

The sensation is as described above, except that with trapped qi, the quality is more Yielding.

Interpretation

This quality is associated with trapped qi. The causes are mild trauma, the abuse of qi (as with singers and meditators who use wrong breathing techniques), wind-cold, sudden lifting beyond one's energy, excessive rumination, and separation in which tender feelings are repressed and replaced by anger, especially while eating.

Inflated Tense

Anger (and lifting) that is very strong, sudden, and unexpressed is reflected in the Inflated quality at the distal positions. Separation, in which tender feelings are repressed and replaced by anger, is attended by a Tense Inflated quality at the Diaphragm positions. Also, anger (and lifting) that is chronic and repeated will cause Inflation in the

Diaphragm positions if they involve restricted breathing. Chronic repressed emotion, especially anger, representing an internal conflict is usually signalled by a very Tense left middle position, but has been found in people with chronic anger who sometimes lose control. An important cause occurs at birth during a long delivery, when the infant's head is detained in the birth canal, as with a breech presentation.

Each of these etiologies will affect different pulse positions, delineated below. When the Inflated pulse is due to lifting, the pulse tends to be slower than if qi is trapped by sudden emotion, anger, fright, or shock.

Sensation

With the Inflated Tense quality the tension of the "inflated balloon" is more resistant to pressure than with the Inflated Yielding quality.

Interpretation

This quality is associated with trapped heat. Any of the factors giving rise to a Yielding Inflated pulse—associated with trapped qi—can, over time, produce heat from excess due to the work required to overcome the stagnation caused by diminished circulation. The pulse is seen most often when the body fails to repulse pathogenic cold,[39] which then penetrates a yin organ and subsequently transforms into heat. The yin organ is usually the Lungs; this pulse is thus often felt at the right distal position and sometimes the Special Lung position. It has been clinically associated with chronic inhalant allergies, emphysema, breast pathology, some types of asthma, and the excessive use of antibiotics for repeated upper respiratory infections over a long time, especially in childhood.

One explanation for the latter instance is that, while antibiotics may inhibit a virus, kill bacteria, and reduce symptoms, they do not remove the cold. Initially, the cold causes stagnation of qi circulation. The body's effort to overcome the stagnation requires work, which is accomplished by mobilizing good (non-pathogenic) heat. If the stagnation is not overcome, however, the heat will remain trapped in the yin organ, usually the Lungs. This will be reflected in the right distal position of the pulse, the Special Lung position, or more rarely, bilaterally in the upper burner position. Until the heat is dissipated, the heat will continue to manifest as an Inflated Tense pulse.

Gradually, this process depletes energy, leading in a vicious cycle to more stagnation, increased heat, and finally depletion of qi and yin, which is reflected in a different pulse quality.

In the early and middle stages of infection in an organ or area, one may sometimes feel an Inflated and Robust Pounding pulse, as, for example, with pancreatitis or peritonitis in the middle positions, if qi is trapped in an organ or area in association with the result and/or attempt to repel the pathogenic factor. Sudden, unexpressed anger, trauma, and a single major episode of heavy lifting are also associated with the Inflated Tense quality.

Very Tense Inflated

A rare variation of the Tense Inflated quality occurs with trapped blood, in which case the Inflated quality is very Tense at the surface. Of all the Inflated qualities, that due to trapped blood is most resistant to pressure.

The primary cause is extravasated blood due to severe trauma, or an episode of extraordinary lifting, which ruptures blood vessels and capillaries. The quality will be found weeks after the event in the position associated with the site of the trauma. Just prior to acute hemorrhage the pulse can be Leather-like Hollow and Rapid, and just after it is Leather-like Hollow and Slow. Blood stagnation which has developed slowly over time in a particular area or organ will produce a Choppy quality in the associated aspect of the pulse. One area where this frequently occurs is the Pelvis/Lower Body.

Combinations

Inflated Yielding

Qi cannot escape from an organ or area of the body.

Inflated Tense

Heat is trapped in an organ or area of the body.

Inflated Yielding-Floating and slightly Rapid

Attributable to a recent attack of wind-heat with internal retention of heat. The pulse is Yielding above the qi depth and slightly Tense at the qi, blood, and organ depths.

Inflated Tense-Floating and slightly Slow

Attributable to a recent attack of wind-cold with internal retention of heat.

Inflated and very Tense

Blood is trapped in an organ or area of the body.

Positions

BILATERALLY AT SAME POSITION

Distal

Yielding Inflated

People who talk or sing using the breath incorrectly may present with a Yielding Inflated quality bilaterally at the distal position. This often occurs, especially with singers, but also with teachers and those who use erroneous breathing techniques during meditation. A Yielding Inflated quality bilaterally in the distal position has been found with unresolved grief over a long period of time.

Tense Inflated

A Tense Inflated quality can occur with trauma, chest surgery, and a single major episode of lifting beyond one's energy. With the latter etiology one observes the Inflated quality in either the left distal position, the right distal position, or bilaterally at this position. Repeated episodes are more often reflected in stagnation between burners.

Mildly Tense Inflated

This is found at the distal position with a breech birth presentation. When the head of the fetus is in the birth canal too long, this pulse may then appear bilaterally in the distal position, although more often with this etiology the quality is found only at the left distal position.[40]

Moderately Tense Inflated

One major episode of sudden, extraordinary, unexpressed anger with Liver qi 'attacking upward,' as well as breast pathology, are associated with this quality bilaterally at the distal positions. Emphysema and invading cold turning to internal heat are also found with this quality.

Tense Inflated Floating

Inflation with a Floating quality can be a sign of acute wind-heat or wind-cold.

Very Tense Inflated

This is a sign of extravasated blood in the chest area which is found very rarely in an acupuncture practice (hopefully).

Middle

Spleen qi deficiency followed by qi stagnation due to deficiency can lead to abdominal distention with accumulated gas; the pulse will show an Inflated Yielding quality bilaterally in the middle position. While this can occur bilaterally with this etiology, it actually occurs more often only at the right middle position. It is often found in those who ruminate while they eat.

Liver qi stagnation, causing Spleen and Stomach qi stagnation, will interfere with the movement of qi in the gastro-intestinal system. This can cause abdominal distention, gas, and an Inflated Yielding to Tense Inflated pulse bilaterally at the middle position more quickly and acutely than will simple Spleen qi deficiency. Both sides will reflect this quality, as each is highly susceptible to qi disharmonies in the other.

If the Liver is the source of the stagnant qi it is usually due to repressed emotion, especially anger and frustration. Stomach qi stagnation is often attributable to resuming work too soon or overworking after meals. With Liver qi stagnation the pulse also tends to be more Tense to Tight than with Stomach qi stagnation.

Frequent lifting of heavy objects or overworking after meals by a strong person will cause the pulse to be Inflated bilaterally in the middle position. This pulse is firmer and less elastic. Similarly, trauma to the abdomen in a strong person can cause this quality bilaterally in this position. In addition, the quality may occur with obsessive rumination, especially while eating, in a relatively strong person.

If, as one rolls the finger medially over both middle positions, they both feel Inflated and Robust Pounding, this can indicate chronic pancreatitis, peritonitis, or some other chronic inflammatory disorder in the middle burner. Acute inflammatory disorders are accompanied by the Flooding Excess quality and a Rapid rate.

Proximal

An Inflated pulse in the lower burner is rare. One cause for this pulse bilaterally in the proximal position is excessive gas in the small and large intestine due to partial obstruction or retarded peristalsis. Here the pulse is Inflated and Slow. Complete obstruction has been accompanied by a Bean (Spinning) pulse.

SIDES

Left

An Inflated quality over the entire left side occurs rarely, and is primarily associated with qi stagnation in the Liver from a sudden unexpressed anger while inactive. Once again, the sensation of Liver excess will tend to be experienced as spreading to all three burners.

Right

An Inflated quality over the entire right side occurs, in my experience, when there is considerable qi stagnation and gas accumulation in the gastro-intestinal tract. Actually, the Inflation is primarily in the middle burner. Excess in the middle burner often gives the false sensory impression of excess in all three burners. It also occurs, less frequently, in the earlier stages of heat from excess in the yang brightness stage of illness. Under these circumstances, the more common quality is Flooding Excess and Robust Pounding.

When people eat too fast, Stomach heat will spread to and affect the entire 'digestive system,' as defined by Dr. Shen.[41] If there is enough qi stagnation, an Inflated quality may appear, although I would tend to describe the pulse as more generally Tense, and Tight at the qi depth.

INDIVIDUAL POSITIONS

Left distal

An Inflated quality over the entire left distal position is found in conditions in which qi, heat, or blood is trapped inside the Heart. A Yielding Inflated quality is found with Trapped qi, which Dr. Shen calls 'Heart full.' A Tense Inflated quality is found with Trapped heat, and a very Tense Inflated quality with Trapped blood (very rare).

Qi or heat trapped in the Heart is often attributable, in my experience, to a lengthy delivery in which the head remains inside the birth canal too long (mildly Tense Inflated); unresolved grief (Yielding Inflated, more often bilaterally at the right distal position); and violent, unexpressed anger while active (moderately Tense Inflated). More rarely, it is due to a single major episode of lifting beyond one's energy, or to trauma to the left side of the chest (Tense Inflated). An Inflated pulse associated with anger, lifting, and trauma is not a serious sign, since with these causes the Inflated quality infers that the individual's general energy is strong, probably enough to release the qi or heat in the Heart naturally, or that they will respond to therapy if treated within a reasonable time.

On the other hand, if the etiology is prolonged delivery with the head inside the birth canal too long, the Mildly Tense Inflated quality can be a sign of qi dilation of the Heart, which is usually associated with a breech presentation. With this cause I find the condition to be more serious symptomatically, with graver consequences in terms of ultimate Heart qi deficiency, which is more difficult to treat, especially since it has usually persisted for a long time, since birth.

Dr. Shen refers to the Inflated quality at the left distal position due to trapped qi as 'Heart full.'[42] According to him, but unobserved by me, there is a progression in pulse qualities associated with 'Heart full,' from Inflated and sometimes a little Hollow to Deep (Sinking), Thin, Tight, and very Rapid. The latter indicates a more advanced stage which can develop into severe Heart qi deficiency ('Heart large')—a more serious functional disorder which is identical to the biomedical concept of an enlarged heart—and further to heart failure or Heart yang deficiency, in Chinese terms. Unless treated early and well, this condition may lead to these grave consequences later in life (see Chapter 12).

Similarly, the Inflated quality in the left distal position has also been associated with a disturbed and confused Heart orifice, although Slippery is more commonly found with this condition.[43] Rarely encountered in this position, especially in an acupuncture practice, is the very Tense Inflated quality associated with cardic tamponade.

Large Vessel	An Inflated Tense quality in the upper medial section of the left distal position indicates pathology in the large vessels, such as the vena cava, or, more often, the aorta (aneurism). Each of the five times it has been felt by me, or even more often reported by associates, an aortic aneurism has been diagnosed biomedically. I consider this a medical emergency.
Right distal	With the Tense Inflated Floating quality we have a recent wind-cold or wind-heat disorder. If it is also Slippery, phlegm-dampness in the Lungs is indicated. The moderately Tense Inflated pulse may also occur in emphysema, in which there is qi and air stagnation in enlarged alveoli. Unless there is also infection, the pulse is Slower than with either a wind-heat or wind-cold disorder.
Left middle	An Inflated pulse at this position means that qi and/or heat (or rarely blood) is trapped inside the organ. The pulse is more Yielding with trapped qi, and more Tense with trapped heat; it is very Tense with trapped blood, which is rare. (Trapped blood is most often associated with trauma to the Liver or to the right upper quadrant of the abdomen and right lower thorax. Stagnant Liver blood is more often represented on the pulse by the presence of the Liver Engorged complementary position, and much less often by a Choppy quality.) Trapped qi can occur for several reasons, the most common being sudden, temporary, unexpressed anger, which occurs when a person is relatively inactive. Here the pulse is often moderately Tense and slightly Rapid. Lifting a weight beyond one's energy, especially after eating, and returning to work too quickly after eating, will infrequently cause a Tense Inflated quality at only this position; more often, it will lead to Inflation bilaterally at the middle burner. The Inflated pulse is usually Slower than that generated by sudden anger.
Ulnar Liver Engorgement	The fingers are rolled medially toward the ulna to palpate an Ulnar Engorgement of the Liver by seeking a Change in Quality from that on the principal part of the middle position. This change is felt very superficially with the portion of the middle finger closest to the nail; it is an Inflated quality between the artery and the flexor carpal radialis tendon. This is a sign that the Liver is stagnant with congealed blood.
Right middle	An Inflated Yielding quality at the right middle position is a sign of stagnation of qi with gas distention due to mild or moderate Spleen qi deficiency, Liver qi stagnation, and Stomach heat. With Spleen qi deficiency, the Spleen position might also be Inflated. An Inflated quality here is also associated with a person who ruminates obsessively while eating, who overeats, or who eats food that is difficult to digest. An Inflated Tense quality can accompany Stomach heat (gastritis). This pulse is more Rapid and Tense than the Inflated quality associated with Spleen qi deficiency, and is accompanied by more acute pain and discomfort, as well as other signs and symptoms of heat.
Spleen	On the right middle position the middle finger is rolled medially toward the ulna to access the Spleen position; one is searching for a change in quality from the principal part of the right middle position. This change is felt very superficially with the portion of the middle finger closest to the nail; it is an Inflated quality between the artery and the flexor carpal radialis tendon. This is a sign of Spleen qi deficiency, often from an underlying Kidney qi deficiency, and represents a vulnerability that requires the individual to eat more slowly and regularly, and to eat easily digested foods in order to avoid gastrointestinal problems.
Stomach-Pylorus Extension	If, as one rolls the finger to the most proximal and medial part of the right middle position, the Stomach-Pylorus Extension position, one finds a Change in Quality to a

Yielding Inflated pulse, one is probably dealing with a prolapsed stomach. The prolapse is likely to be indiscernible by x-ray or ultrasound, but the person will have abdominal discomfort several hours after eating, insomnia after the evening meal, and will be fatigued in the morning.

Left proximal

An Inflated pulse confined to the left proximal position is relatively rare, in my experience. Dr. Shen reports finding it with dysmenorrhea, where I have consistently found a Choppy pulse instead. He also reports it with qi in the Large Intestine and with constipation, neither of which I have observed over the entire left proximal pulse. I have felt Inflation on the upper or distal part of the left proximal pulse, designated by Dr. Shen as the Large Intestine position, sometimes accompanying constipation.

Right proximal

An Inflated pulse in this position is rare, in my experience. Dr. Shen reports finding it with inflammation of the prostate, which I cannot corroborate.

Pelvis/Lower Body

I have never found an Inflated quality at this position.

BETWEEN DISTAL AND MIDDLE POSITIONS (DIAPHRAGM POSITION)

A common etiology when this quality is found between the positions is an interpersonal crisis involving separation, or a breach in a strong interpersonal attachment, such as a divorce. While the separation can be attended by strong hostility and resentment, the quality is, I believe, caused as much by a need to suppress the inevitable love and tender feeling that had to exist for the relationship to start, but with whose awareness it would be impossible to end, and carry through the separation. The appearance at the Diaphragm positions is due to the control of feeling through the control of breathing.

This is found more often on the left side, although it often appears bilaterally. The degree of Inflation depends on two factors. One is the length of time between the episode and the examination of the pulse, with the Inflation diminishing over time. The other is the importance of the separation to the person; the Inflation increases proportionately to the importance of the relationship. For this reason, the Inflated quality diminishes over time, but in my experience will usually last even as a small Inflation for up to ten years.

At a conference where I was demonstrating pulse diagnosis, a woman had a very prominently Inflated left Diaphragm position. She and others asked me what it meant, and I said that one of the possibilities was a recent separation or divorce. She began to cry almost uncontrollably, and whispered that she was in the midst of a very difficult and painful divorce.

Another cause for an Inflated quality between these positions in the Diaphragm position are repeated episodes of lifting beyond one's energy. The Inflated quality associated with this etiology appears between the positions more often on the right than the left side, although sometimes on both sides if the event was extreme. When it is found with this etiology between the distal and middle positions, the person has lifted with the upper part of the body. With lifting the pulse tends to be Slower than with emotional stress.

Very large Inflation at this position is associated with diaphragmatic hernia. Very small or absent Inflation has been found in the pulses of withdrawn people who have few or no intimate interpersonal relationships.

Heart Enlarged and distal Liver Engorgement

The presence of a Heart enlarged condition is discernible when the distal aspect of the left Diaphragm positions is either more Inflated or Rougher than the proximal aspect. The presence of a distal engorgement of the Liver is discernible when the middle aspect of the left Diaphragm positions is either more Inflated or Rougher than the distal aspect.

Pleural and Esophageal positions

The presence of a pleural pathology is discernible when the distal aspect of the right Diaphragm positions is either more Inflated or Rougher than the proximal aspect. The presence of esophageal qi stagnation is discernible when the middle aspect of the right Diaphragm positions is either more Inflated or Rougher than the distal aspect. A Slippery quality instead of the Rough quality is a sign of esophageal food stagnation. Reflux is associated with all three qualities.

Suppressed

Category

This is another entirely new category which is primarily associated with the recent presence in the human body of powerful synthetic chemical substances whose cataclysmic effects on human physiology is well catalogued in the warnings, side effects, and adverse reactions listed by the pharmaceutical companies which manufacture them.

Sensation

In the Suppressed quality (Fig. 8-4), the sine wave of the Normal pulse is cut off at the apex.

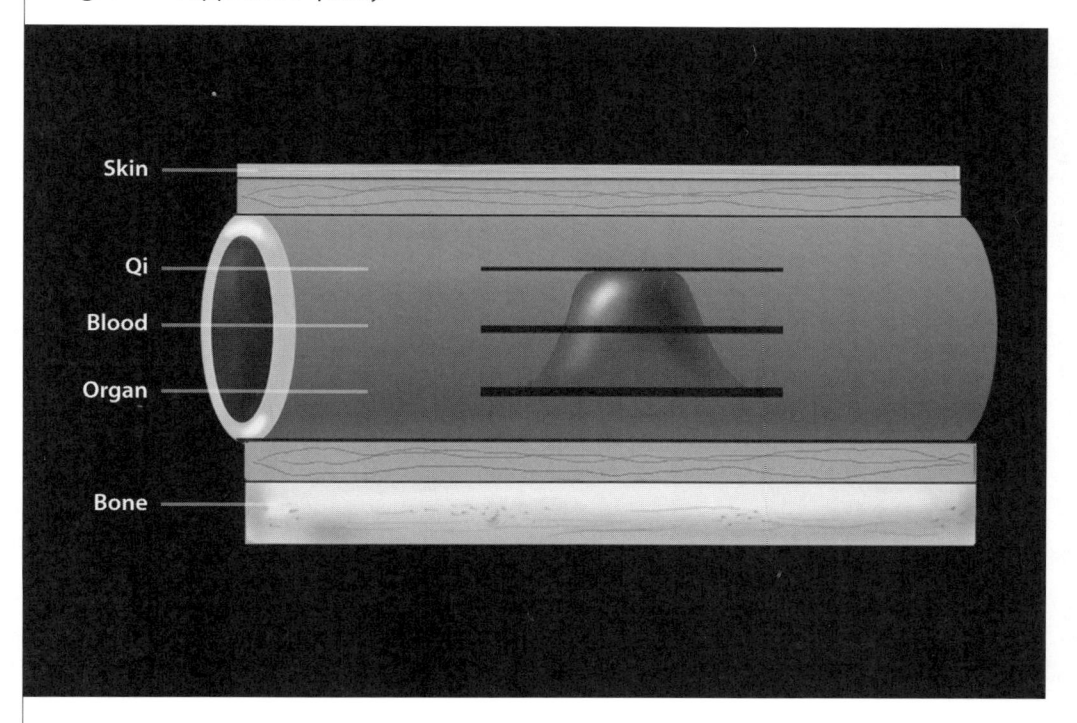

Fig. 8-4 Suppressed quality

General interpretation

This is a sign that the physiology of the circulation of qi and blood is impeded by synthetic materials foreign and toxic to human ecology, usually hypertensive and the monoamine oxidase inhibitors, tricyclic, and serotonin uptake inhibitor antidepressants. However, I have encountered patients with this wave who are not on medications, or only small amounts, who are aware that they are suppressing their feelings of resentment. Unlike the Cotton quality, these people are not resigned to living with these feelings, but they do not verbalize them directly to the person they resent. Rather they vent to others indirectly through cloaked humor or veiled allusions to their resentment, which is very difficult, but not impossible to confront.

From my discussions with James Ramholz, a master of the Korean Dong Han Pulse School, I am beginning to see a continuum with the Flat pulse, which is usually felt at the organ depth and whose emotional component is usually unconscious. This is in keeping with the increasing unawareness of emotions in the Korean system as the associated qualities appear deeper in the pulse.

Reduced qualities

EXCESS AND DEFICIENCY

As mentioned in Chapters 3 and 8, many of the pulse qualities described here, e.g., Empty and others that I classify according to sensation as Reduced qualities, are discussed in the literature according to their underlying condition; in that context, it is correctly noted that signs of deficiency can be due to an underlying excess.[44] While I would agree that Deep means 'interior' in terms of disease location, and while it could theoretically be due to excess, in our times the ancient causes of excess, such as interior cold from excess, are rare. With this caveat, I have chosen to confine my interpretations to the principal clinical realities in my own experience and that of others, including Dr. Shen. Yet the possibility of excess being associated with these qualities should still be considered, especially if there are other strong signs of excess, such as a very Rapid rate, high temperature, and acute pain.

Introduction

The classification of the Reduced pulse is baffling. What follows is an attempt to minimize the confusion by eliminating the use of overlapping terms, and introducing new terms for qualities that are more descriptive of sensation. This reorganization is essential, as elsewhere, to convey the finer clinical distinctions which enrich our diagnostic and treatment intervention. They are especially relevant to sharpening our prognostic skills in terms of defining where we are in the process of a disease.

Category

There is first of all the term 'weak.' This word has been used to cover several qualities, including one where only a little is felt on palpation to one where nothing is felt. In order to clarify this overlapping of sensations between the presence of some sensation to the absence of any, new terms are required to identify each separately. These terms come partially from requests by students.

Where little is felt on the pulse, we will use the term Feeble. Frail is a synonym in the literature for Feeble, which suggests a diagnostic judgment, and does not in my opinion convey as clearly as Feeble the actual sensation. When nothing is felt, we will use the term Absent.

Dr. Shen[45] describes three Feeble pulses (which he calls 'Weak'), one at the qi depth involving qi, one at the blood depth involving blood, and one at the organ depth involving the yin organs. I shall depart from this nomenclature—which classifies the Feeble pulse as Feeble-Floating, Feeble-Deep, and Feeble-Middle—for reasons explained below in the discussion of the Feeble-Absent quality.

In the literature there are two types of Feeble ('Weak') pulse. One is a Floating Feeble ('Weak') pulse, for which there are many terms now extant, and the other is a Deep Feeble ('Weak') pulse, for which the language is hardly less chaotic.

The term Weak-Floating pulse is used by Wu Shui-Wan,[46] Mann,[47] and Maciocia, who also equates it with soft.[48] It is known as soggy by Kaptchuk,[49] soft by Li Shi-Zhen,[50] and frail by Porkert.[51]

The Weak-Deep pulse is referred to by Kaptchuk as frail.[52] Porkert, on the other hand, uses the appellation infirm for the Weak-Deep pulse.[53] Li Shi-Zhen refers to the Weak-Deep pulse as simply weak,[54] with which Maciocia[55] and Worsley[56] agree.

Sensation and general interpretation

Reduced pulse qualities are those whose impulse and pulse wave lack intensity and force. There is a progression in the development of qi and blood deficiency leading to the Reduced pulses, just as there is for yin deficiency, which we discuss in Chapter 11. An understanding of the process which leads to increasing qi deficiency bears reiteration here.

At first the qi depth becomes Yielding on pressure, then Diminished, and then it disappears. As the process of qi depletion continues, it begins to separate on pressure at the blood depth, which we call Spreading. As the qi becomes more deficient, we have the Flooding Deficient Wave, the Diffuse and Reduced Substance qualities, and in the next stage both the qi and blood depths disappear, which we call Deep. Gradually, the pulse becomes less substantial, at which time we refer to it as Feeble. The Feeble pulse is felt progressively deeper, and then it disappears, at which time it is called Absent. (See Figs. 8-9 to 8-16.)

With increasing deficiency of qi, the yin and yang separate and the yang floats to the surface; we then have the Empty quality, which is a sign of 'qi wild.' The stages which follow the Empty pulse are further in the direction of 'qi wild,' or the extremes of deficiency and the separation of yin and yang. This progression to severe qi and blood deficiency can occur simultaneously with all of the other aspects of the pulse based on sensation, rhythm, rate, depth, size, width, length, and shape (see Chapter 9).

The standard format used to describe other qualities will be suspended for all of the Reduced qualities, except with regard to sensation and general interpretation. Combinations and positions will appear in conjunction with other pulse qualities as they occur elsewhere in the text. The reason is that the clinical insignificance of combinations for the Yielding, Qi Depth Diminished, Spreading, Flooding Deficient, Muffled, and Dead qualities do not warrant the space. The interpretation of each individual or large segment position is essentially the same as for the appearance of the quality over the entire pulse. In fact, all but the Muffled and Dead qualities are usually only found over the entire pulse. The exceptions are the Flat and Feeble-Absent qualities, which are discussed using the conventional format.

QI DEPTH

Yielding at qi depth

Fig. 8-5 Yielding at qi depth quality

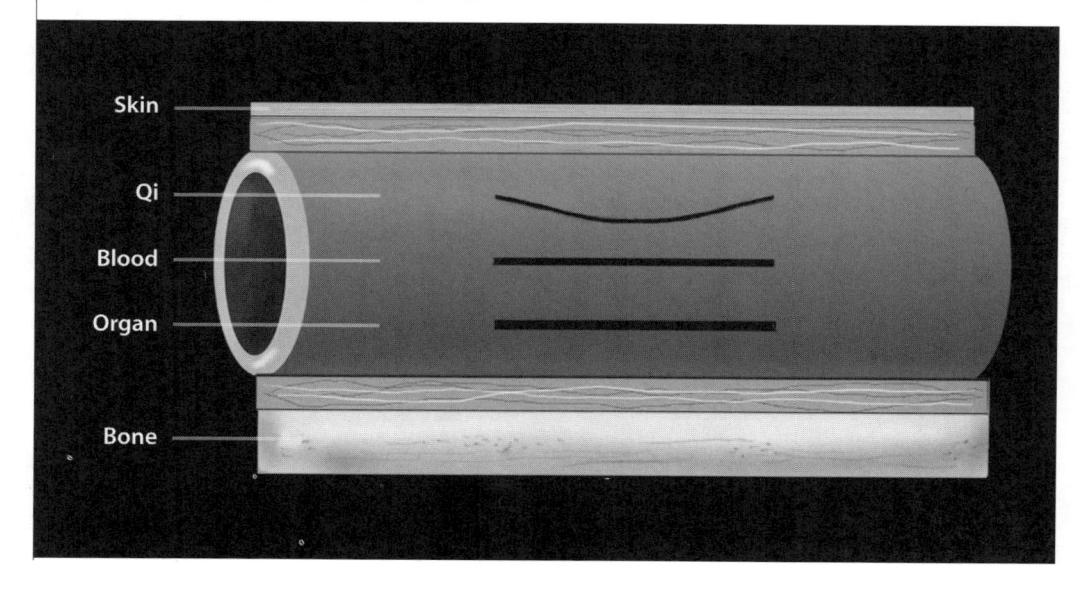

Category

This is a new category of a subtle deviation from normal which, in my experience, is of clinical and prognostic significance.

Sensation

The qi depth becomes more pliable or slightly softer on gentle pressure (Fig. 8-5). The word 'soft' is not used here in the classification because it has very specific meaning in the literature, explained below in our discussion of the Empty Thread-like (soggy) pulse quality.

General interpretation

This is the earliest sign of qi depletion and is associated with either working beyond one's energy, minor illness, or sometimes insomnia. It can also be an early sign of minimal menorrhagia or incomplete recovery from pregnancy and delivery, or a minor invasive medical procedure. Recognition of this subtle change enables the practitioner to address (and arrest) the process at this point, thereby preventing more serious illness.

Diminished or Absent at qi depth

Category

This is also a new category which documents the subtle progression of qi deficiency. It identifies yet another degree in this progression, and signals the need for slightly stronger tonification and circulation of qi. This quality is distinguished by the diminishment or absence of a pulse at the qi depth (Figs. 8-6 and 8-7).

General interpretation

This quality is associated with overwork beyond one's energy, either generally or in some smaller segment of physiology. This second pulse sign of qi deficiency, associated as it is with overwork, is an ubiquitous finding in a society which does nothing but work beyond its energy.

    A teacher, for example, with constitutionally deficient Lungs who speaks eight hours a day in a classroom will eventually lose the qi depth on the right distal position. An intern who works one-hundred twenty hours a week (as I did) and rarely sleeps more than a few hours or finishes a meal, sooner or later develops some degree of qi deficiency and reduction of the qi depth over the entire pulse.

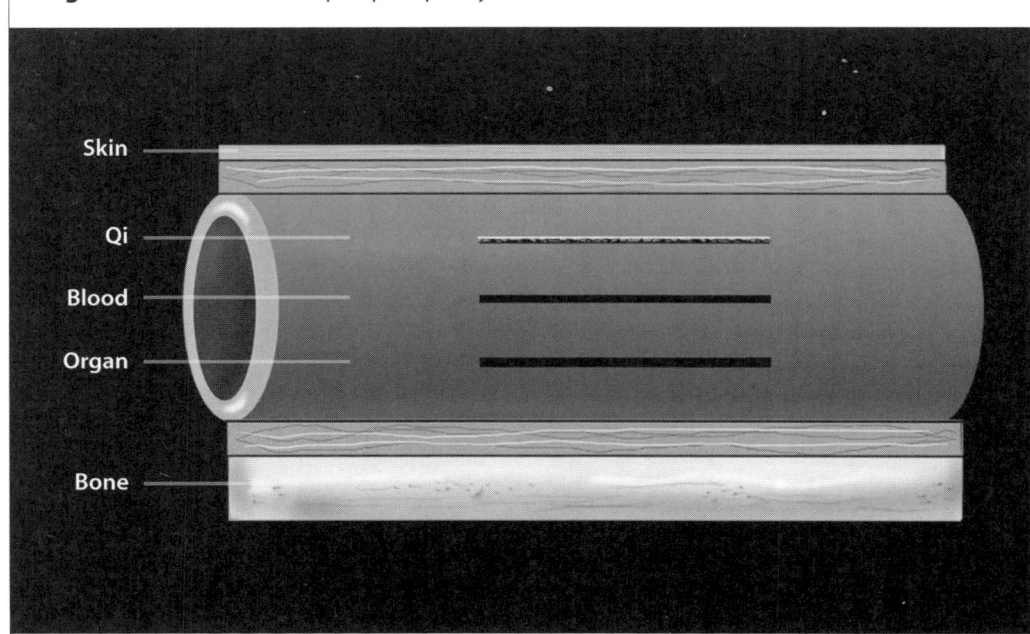

Fig. 8-6   Diminished at qi depth quality

Fig. 8-7 Absent at qi depth quality

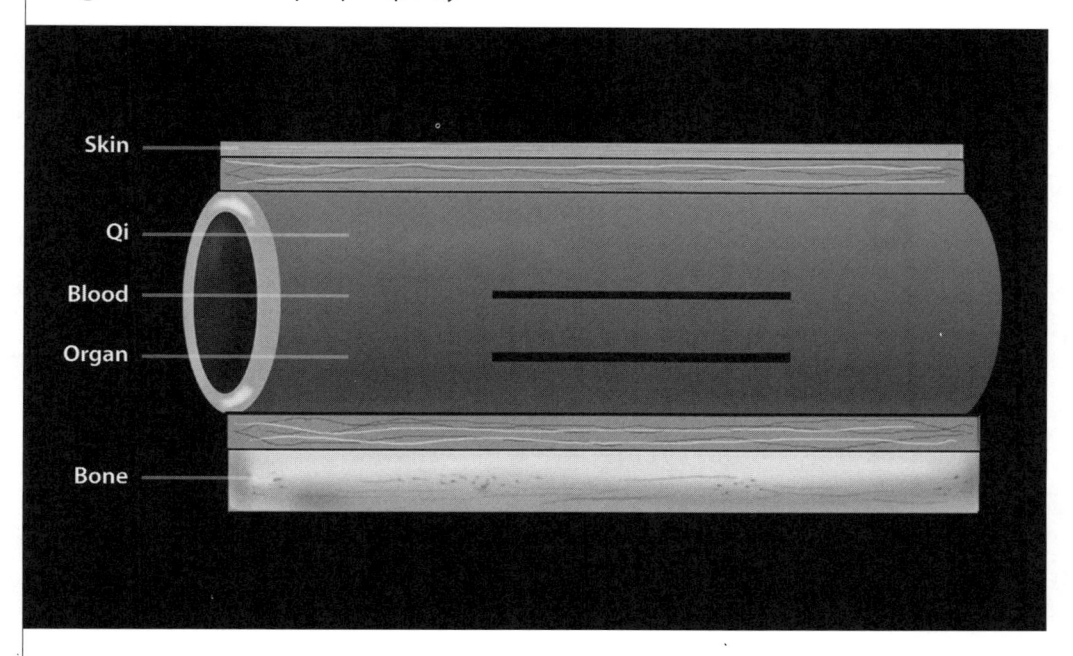

BLOOD DEPTH

Spreading; Yielding partially Hollow; Diminished at blood depth

Sensation

The Spreading quality (Fig. 8-8) is Yielding or Absent at the qi depth, and separating at the blood depth. The Yielding Partially Hollow quality (Fig. 8-9) is present at the qi depth and separating at the blood depth. With a Diminished quality at the blood depth (Fig. 8-10) there is no qi depth and the blood depth is barely palpable.

General interpretation

The etiology of the Spreading quality is similar to that of the Yielding and Absent at the qi depth qualities, except that the process has lasted for a longer time, or the person has become depleted of qi and blood for some other reason. The Yielding Partially Hollow and Diminished qualities at the blood depth are signs that the reduction of qi and blood has proceeded even further. All three qualities represent a gradual depletion of qi, and now blood, due to overwork without sufficient rest. This I have observed especially in medical students, interns, residents, and doctors who characteristically have that lifestyle for much of their adult years. More recently, I have felt these qualities in acupuncture students who study, work, and raise a family all at the same time.

Women, especially in the West, with multiple pregnancies, abortions, and miscarriages, who do not rest and recover their qi and blood sufficiently after delivery, also frequently show these qualities on their pulse while they are quite young. (In China, assistance in the home and with the new baby, as well as herbs, are ideally provided for a woman after delivery for at least one month.)

Flooding Deficient Wave

Category and sensation

The Flooding Deficient Wave quality (Fig. 8-11) is usually associated with mild to moderate qi deficiency.

Fig. 8-8 Spreading quality

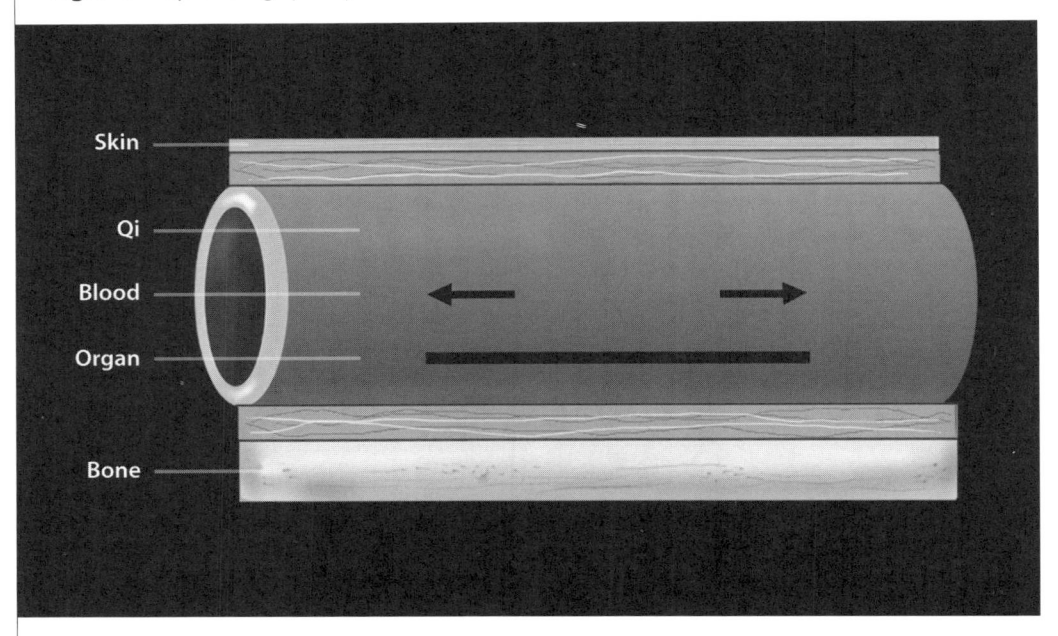

Fig. 8-9 Yielding partially Hollow quality

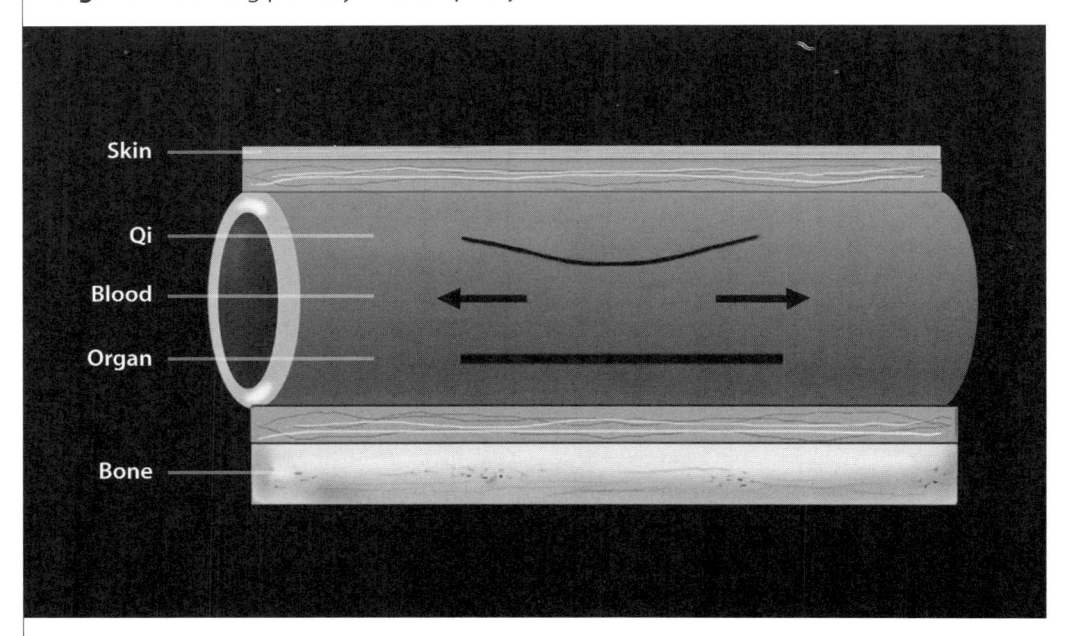

Fig. 8-10 Diminished at blood depth quality

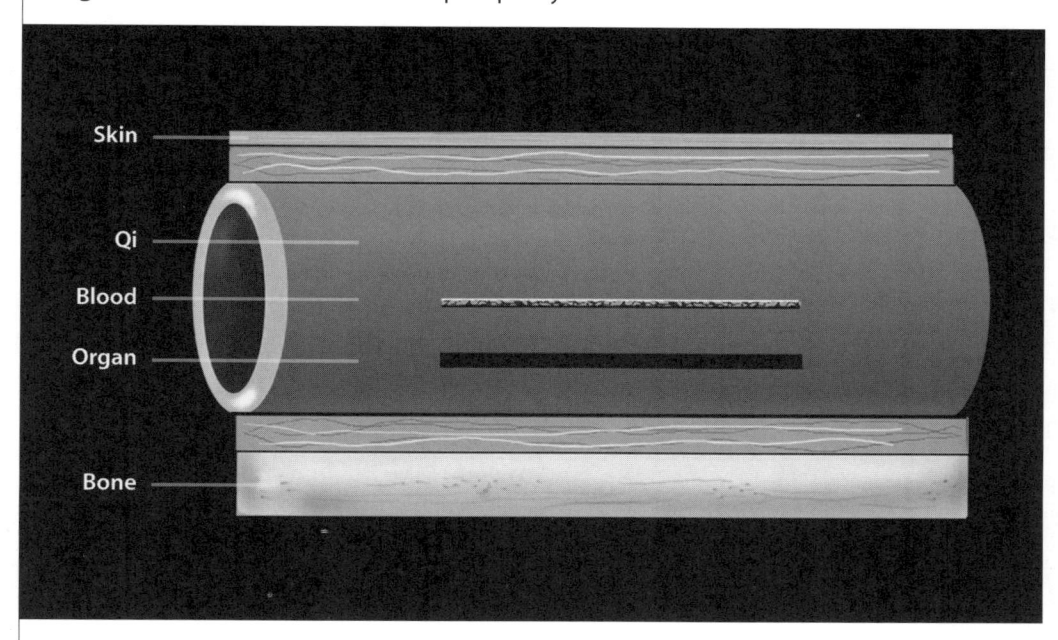

Fig. 8-11 Flooding Deficient Wave quality

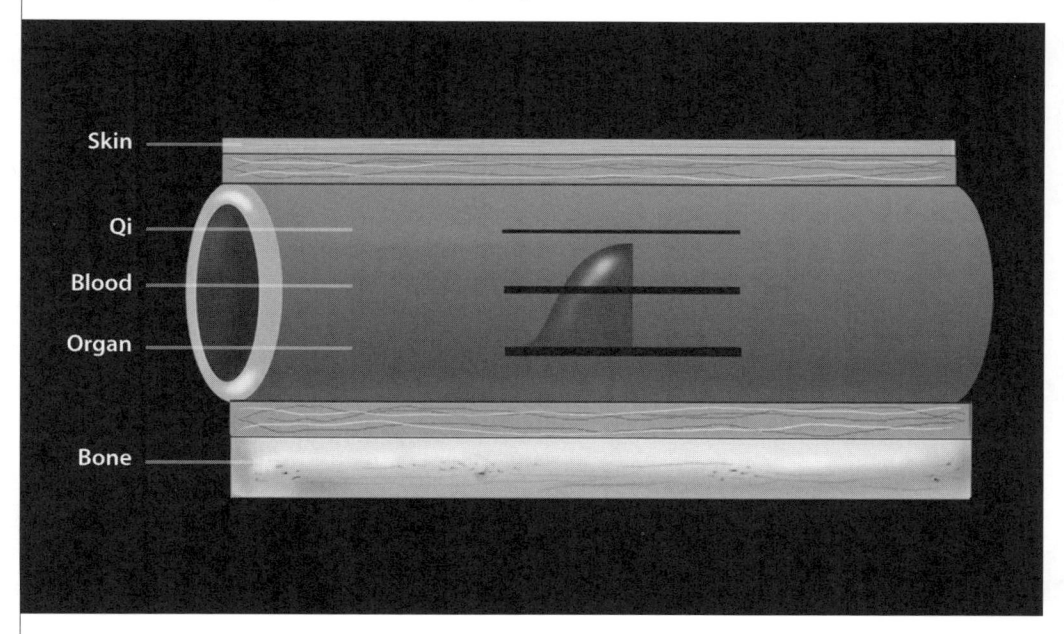

My own observation, which is confirmed by Dr. Shen, is that there is a pulse quality whose wave pattern is similar to the Flooding Excess quality, which normally rises to the surface (or just below) and suddenly drops away, but which lacks the force of the Flooding Excess pulse, which rises above the qi depth. I have classified it as the Flooding Deficient pulse, while Dr. Shen calls it the 'push pulse.'

General interpretation

Etiologically, the Flooding Deficient quality represents another step up the ladder of deficiency. In addition to overwork, this quality is associated with a ceaseless, obsessive drive to push oneself day and night. The individual's mind never ceases to rest even when asleep. Many of the people who were treated by Dr. Shen and I were stockbrokers who worked fourteen hours a day, seven days a week, traveled constantly across time zones, and slept poorly a few hours a night. This quality represents a degree of qi deficiency just short of that represented by the Deep quality. Individuals with this pulse tend to collapse suddenly.

The other quality which I find associated with this lifestyle is the Hesitant pulse, which is associated more with an incessant working of a mind obsessed with usually one preoccupation. It is my impression that with similar etiologies, and a vulnerable Heart, the Hesitant quality will precede the Flooding Deficient quality, although we often find the Flooding Deficient quality in transition to the Hesitant.[57]

Reduced Pounding

Category

There is no category in the literature called Pounding. Wu Shui-Wan refers to this quality as "Empty Big Pulse."[58] Kaptchuk, the only one to use the term pounding, states in his discussion of the full quality: "Clinically, it is possible for a full pulse to be part of a deficiency pattern if all the other elements of a configuration indicate deficiency. Such a full pulse is illusionary and is thought to be a sign that the prognosis is poor."[59]

Sensation

The pulse begins with a sensation of force and power, but does not sustain this vigor. It hits the finger more weakly than one would expect from the force at the beginning of the impulse.

Interpretation

Reduced Pounding is associated with qi deficiency and is a sign that the body is struggling, and barely able to maintain function. While it can be caused by any activity which drains qi, in our culture it is most often caused by work or exercise beyond one's energy. Often the pulse has Reduced Substance or is Feeble, the rate is Slow, and the tongue and eyes are probably a little pale.

Less often it is found in a person whose qi has been depleted over a long period by an attempt to overcome stagnation related to physical trauma. With trauma the pulse is often Tight with a normal rate, and one finds the characteristic signs on the tongue and eyes described elsewhere.

Sometimes the organ depth shows Robust Pounding, and little or no Pounding is found at the blood and qi depths. I have seen this with biomedical medications, such as anti-hypertensives.

Combinations and positions

For combinations, refer to the other qualities which the Pounding quality modifies. Reduced Pounding is generally found over the entire pulse, and frequently at individual positions; when it is, however, it would bear the same interpretation.

Diffuse

Category
There is no system of classification that I have reviewed which describes this quality.

Sensation
The sensation of the Diffuse quality (Fig. 8-12) in a principal position is one of a partially defined quality in the center of the position—such as Tense, Thin, or Tight—with the sense of another wider presence on either side of the main quality into which the principal quality merges without clearly defined borders, and which in itself is less defined; it has the sensation of cheese cloth or a moth-eaten fabric.

Interpretation
The Diffuse quality is a sign of moderate qi deficiency. Combined with the Thin Tight quality, it is a sign of combined qi, blood, and yin deficiency.

Position
While the Diffuse quality can be found at any position, I have found it most often at the left middle position, and somewhat less often at the left proximal and right middle positions.

Fig. 8-12 Diffuse quality (longitudinal cross section of radial artery)

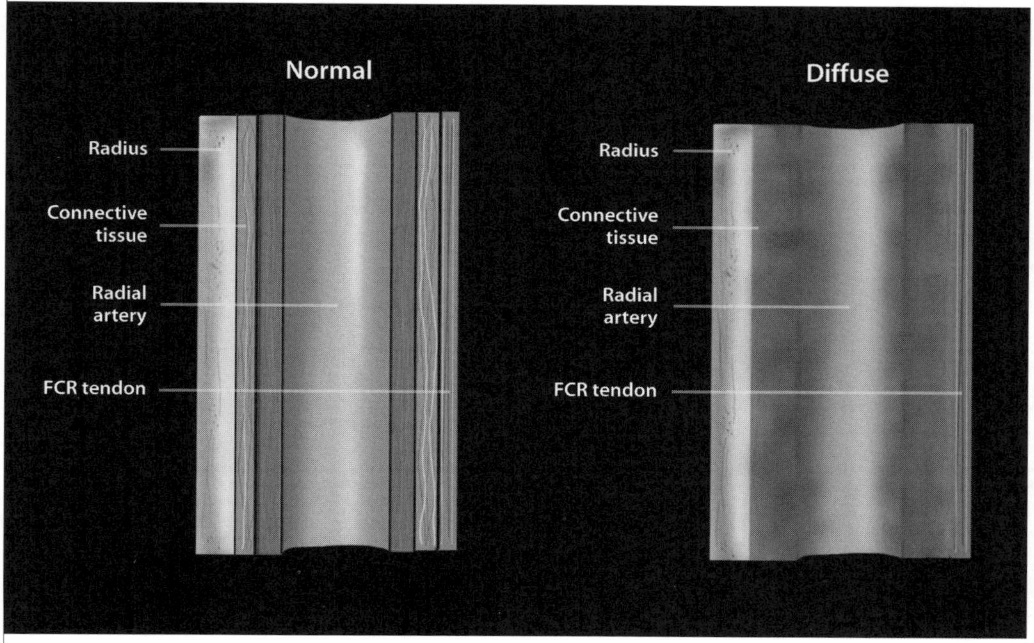

Reduced Substance

Category
Substance refers to the intensity, elasticity, buoyancy, and resilience of a pulse quality. It is a term which modifies the description of other qualities. A quality that is said to have Reduced Substance is a sensation somewhere between Normal and Feeble; this modifier serves to describe a pulse whose intensity and resilience is somewhere between the two.

Sensation
A quality that is said to have Robust Substance has form and feels buoyant, elastic, and resilient, and is experienced as alive and healthy. One that has Reduced Substance (Fig. 8-13) is one which lacks form and these attributes and is sometimes likened to a sweater whose cloth is becoming threadbare.

Fig. 8-13 Reduced Substance quality

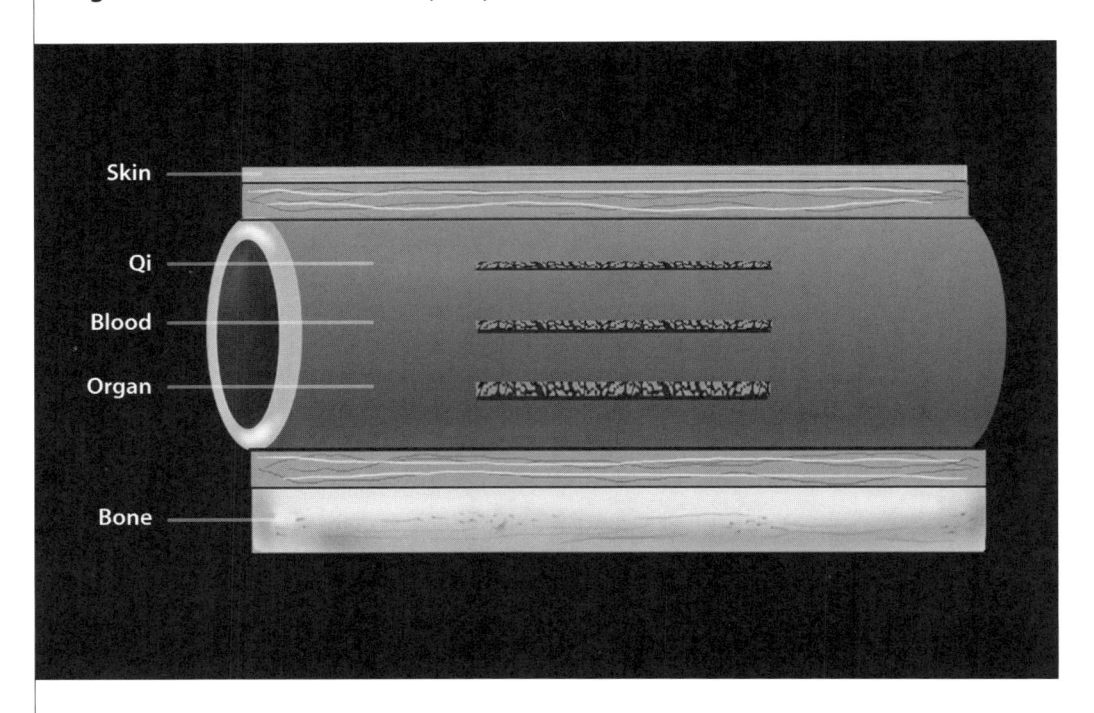

Interpretation

A pulse with Robust Substance is a Normal pulse, and one with Reduced Substance is only relatively less qi-deficient than the Feeble quality. For example, a Thin pulse with Reduced Substance is *mildly* blood- and qi-deficient, whereas a Thin Feeble pulse is *very* blood- and qi-deficient.

Position and combinations

The Reduced Substance quality can modify any other quality, in any and all combinations of positions, and can appear at any position.

Flat

Category

In terms of sensation, this quality could be classified in several categories including Submerged, since it is most often accessed at a deep position, and Shape, because of its loss of a complete wave. It is classified among those with Reduced volume because, like others in this classification, it is always a sign of deficiency as well as stagnation.

Issues in categorization

Dr. Shen calls this the 'stagnant pulse.' I use the term Flat instead because it aptly describes the sensation we are considering, and because Dr. Shen has delineated several other types of stagnant qualities in addition to Flat.

We have already discussed the Inflated quality, which is a sign of qi and/or heat trapped in a place where the qi is initially Robust. The stagnant condition for which the Taut and Tense qualities are signs is one in which there are two opposing and usually strong forces. The classic example is Liver qi stagnation, in which the qi is inclined to move about but is opposed and restrained by repressive emotional forces. The stagnant condition associated with the Flat pulse is one in which qi is unable to reach a place where the qi is deficient. The Flat and Inflated qualities can have similar etiologies, but with very different body conditions. An a priori condition of the Flat quality is deficient qi, and the a priori condition of the Inflated quality is robust qi.

Fig. 8-14 Flat quality

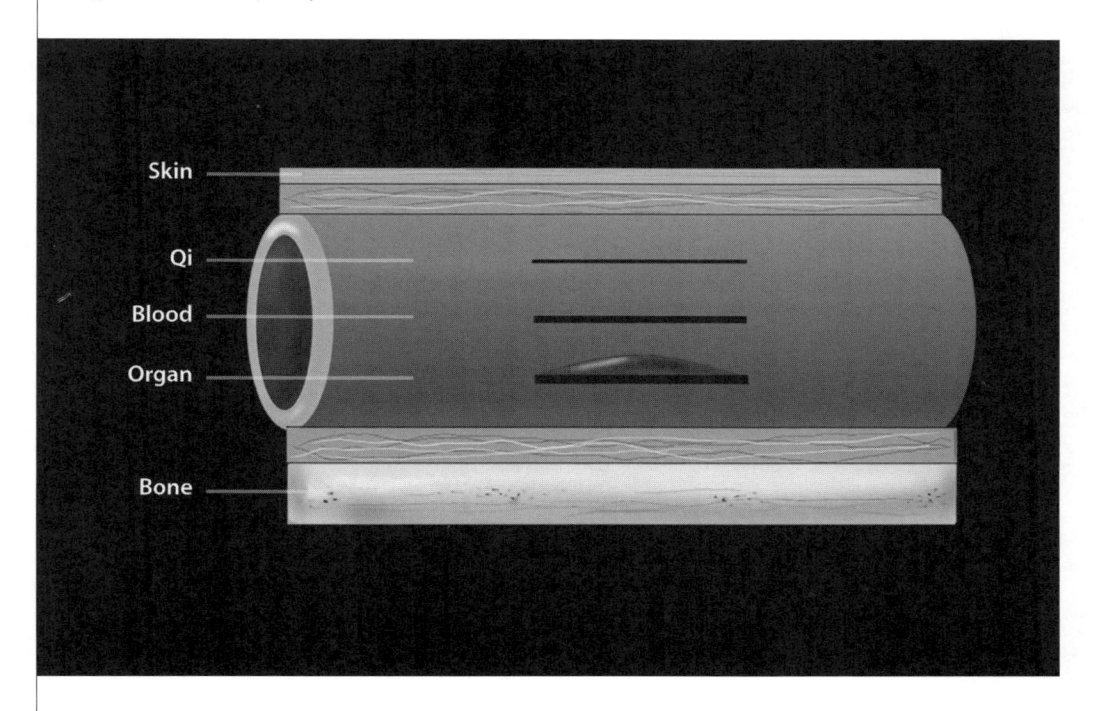

Initially I questioned whether this pulse might be the same as the Firm quality. Whereas I originally classified them together, the etiologies and interpretations given to me by Dr. Shen for the Flat ('stagnant') quality varied so much from those associated with the Firm quality in the literature, that I decided to separate them. Furthermore, the Flat quality has a distinctly suppressed wave form, which is not specifically mentioned elsewhere as being associated with the Firm quality, which is much deeper, below rather than above the organ depth. Another reason to distinguish the Flat from the Firm quality is that the Flat quality, even as a sign of stagnation, is always associated with deficiency, while the Firm quality can be associated with excess as well as deficiency. Therefore, I have placed the Flat quality with the Reduced volume pulses, and the Firm quality under Submerged depth.

Sensation

The Flat quality (Fig. 8-14) is palpable as a diminished stifled wave, usually at the organ depth. While other Deep pulses, once accessed, impinge upon the fingers with some energy, the Flat quality seems compressed and unable to come up to the finger through its own force. Dr. Shen[60] says that it is "suppressed and cannot last." In my experience, it is found only at individual positions. Most often these are the distal positions, but it can also be felt less often at the middle, Large and Small Intestine, and Bladder positions. It differs from the Suppressed quality in which the wave is cut off only at its peak, and which is felt most often over the entire pulse.

General interpretation

Discussion of this topic in Dr. Shen's book[61] is more limited than what he said about it in his clinical practice. He writes that this quality is "a result of emotional trauma; the individual has pent-up feelings and suffers from depression. After a prolonged period, the qi of certain organs is not regulated properly and so the stagnant pulse appears."

The following additional information is based on material shared by Dr. Shen during our eight intensive years together, and confirmed in the clinic during the ensuing eighteen years.

Generally, as a result of a shock to the circulation, the Flat quality is a sign that qi cannot reach an area or organ that is relatively deficient in qi. It occurs in a person whose energy is already deficient prior to the precipitating event. Since there was little qi there to begin with, there is less to be trapped when the circulation is impaired; or, in Dr. Shen's words, "Qi is stagnant and does not move well." The body attempts to restore homeostasis by bringing qi into the area. But under circumstances where qi is already deficient, it cannot overcome the closure of circulation caused by the shock. In fact, the effort to surmount the stagnation will itself further deplete the system. For this reason, the Flat pulse will ultimately become Feeble or Absent.

The Flat and Inflated qualities bear comparison. Each indicates that qi is blocked due to interference with the circulation of qi. If an individual suffers a major physical trauma such as an automobile accident, and their physical condition is otherwise good, the pulse will likely be Inflated. An Inflated quality is a sign that the qi is trapped in a part of the body and cannot get out. But the very fact that it is trapped indicates that the body had sufficient qi available to be trapped. On the other hand, if the physical condition was already compromised before the trauma, meaning that there was insufficient qi to begin with, the pulse is more likely to be Flat. Furthermore, the long range consequences associated with the Flat quality are more grave than those associated with the Inflated quality. These qualities are direct sensory representations of the underlying physiology.

As we said, the Flat pulse usually appears as the result of an event which the organism experiences as a shock. This quality, and the stagnation of which it is a sign, can result from emotional trauma, physical trauma such as an accident, lifting beyond one's energy, and, less often, from overwork. A common precipitating event occurs at delivery when the umbilical cord is wrapped around the infant's neck. Dr. Shen notes that, over time, when the shock is due to emotion the pulse is more Rapid, and when due to lifting or trauma, it is Slower.

This pulse can also develop more slowly in the middle position with people who sit bent over for long periods of time, such as secretaries and others who work in offices. I have found it in the proximal position with people who stand or walk for long periods as part of their employment, and with long-standing intestinal stagnation such as impaction. Again, whatever the cause, the Flat quality always appears in an individual who was deficient prior to the precipitating event.

When the shock is emotional, the Heart and sometimes Lungs are usually affected, and the pulse may initially be Rapid. With an accident there will be pain, a horizontal line under the lower eyelid, and possibly a small purple blister on the side of the tongue corresponding to the side of the body that was injured. If there is an emotional shock while eating, or an episode of lifting beyond one's energy after eating, the stagnation may appear between the right distal and right middle positions. Recall that with these etiologies the result could be an Inflated pulse at these positions if the physical condition was good at the time of the precipitating event.

With neoplasms in the Liver and the Lung, on a number of occasions I have observed a very Flat pulse. Especially in instances of Liver malignancy, this sign has appeared several years prior to symptomatology or a positive biomedical diagnostic test, which was undertaken as a result of finding a Flat quality at the left middle position.

According to Dr. Shen, but outside of my own experience, emotional stress and overwork with lack of rest over a long period of time in a person with deficient qi can also result in a Flat quality over the entire pulse.

Combinations

For the purpose of emphasis, I reiterate that all of the disorders associated with the Flat pulse below occur in individuals with insufficient qi.

Flat Tight and Rapid

PHYSICAL TRAUMA

This Flat pulse occurs in a deficient person immediately after sustaining physical trauma, and is usually accompanied by pain. Later the rate is Slower. The face has a darker hue than with emotional shock.

EMOTIONAL TRAUMA

This combination also reflects the initial response to emotional trauma in a deficient person. The greater the shock, the more Rapid the rate. The rate tends to stay Rapid longer than with physical trauma. The face has a greenish-blue color, and there is no physical pain.

Flat Tense

This combination occurs where there is accumulated heat from excess and the qi is unable to reach an organ or area of the body.

Positions

BILATERALLY AT SAME POSITION

Distal

Over a long period of time, the qi in the area associated with this position can become very deficient and lead to such serious disorders as cancer in the mediastinum. For this reason, a Flat pulse at this position is considerably more serious than, say, an Inflated pulse. This represents the relative closure of qi (and sometimes blood) circulation, meaning that the qi cannot reach the area.

Sudden emotional trauma

This pulse is found with a severe, relatively sudden disappointment such as the loss of a parent early in life, especially before the energic systems have reached full strength and mature stability. A young person's inexperience with grief, hurt, anger, and other emotions will force them to repress the outward expression or even inner awareness of such needs as to cry, scream, or shout. They control these emotions by holding the breath, which creates stagnation of qi in the chest, Lungs, Heart, and diaphragm.

The Flat quality at the distal positions is frequently found in adults who had such emotional experiences when they were very young, and which have long since been forgotten. Unfortunately, the energy systems remember, and the effect of stagnation on the circulation can have long-term, widespread pathological and disharmonious ramifications. These include unexplained depressions, profound unexplained fear, arthritic conditions, difficulty in healing, and ultimately even neoplasms.

With this etiology the pulse is slightly more Rapid than with those listed below.

Umbilical cord around infant's neck at delivery

Almost as frequently, the Flat pulse can occur bilaterally at this position when the umbilical cord is wrapped around the infant's neck during delivery.

Physical trauma and lifting

Trauma, such as a blow to the chest in a weak person, or a sudden and extreme episode of lifting beyond one's energy, will create stagnation and pain. The other eye and tongue signs described above in the general interpretation are found following trauma. According to Dr. Shen, if, over a long period of time, the stagnation is not corrected, this pulse may portend a carcinoma in the mediastinum or breasts.

Misuse of voice or breathing

This pulse may also appear in a deficient person who repeatedly overuses their voice, or engages in improper breathing habits.

Middle

The Flat pulse bilaterally at the middle position implies that qi is unable to enter the area. This is usually and eventually accompanied by swelling in the area of the diaphragm due to an accumulation of qi which cannot descend. This is sometimes diagnosed as a diaphragmatic hernia.

Bending

Those who work at a keyboard or typewriter and others whose work involves bending forward in a seated position for extended periods of time, and whose middle burner is qi-deficient beforehand, will develop a Flat pulse in the middle positions. Slowly developing stomach and intestinal disorders are frequently found in this group of people. It is recommended that they break up their routine by standing and moving about frequently.

Trauma

This quality may also be found following trauma in a person whose general energy (or energy in this region) was not strong beforehand. Usually the patient will complain of pain in the area fairly soon after the event, which can be attributed to qi being trapped, unable to descend, and accumulating in the diaphragm.

Lifting

Frequent lifting beyond one's energy using the abdominal muscles, especially just after eating, can produce a Flat quality in the middle positions over time. It may be accompanied by pain soon after the event, although usually the pain is more gradual in onset.

Proximal

Prolonged standing on hard surfaces

Standing or sitting in one place for a long period of time may give rise to this pulse in a relatively deficient person. Soldiers standing motionless on guard duty, policemen who regulate traffic, and taxi drivers, are three examples. The result is often intestinal stagnation leading to constipation, fecal impaction, and hemorrhoids. Should impaction occur over a period of time, there may be diarrhea from leakage around the impaction.

Walking on hard surfaces

People who walk on hard surfaces for long periods of time may show this pulse, with the same pathological consequences as standing on hard surfaces. This was common among policeman who used to "walk the beat" before the advent of squad cars.

Another possible consequence of standing or walking for long periods on a hard surface is blood stagnation. The clinical consequences are prostatic hypertrophy and related urinary complications, varicose veins, and hemorrhoids. One would expect to find a Choppy pulse under these circumstances at the Pelvis/Lower Body position.

BETWEEN DISTAL AND MIDDLE POSITIONS

Lifting

While rare, the Flat quality in this position can be found due to repeated lifting of a very heavy object beyond one's energy, in a deficient person. It is often accompanied by some discomfort. The usual quality found under these circumstances is Inflated at the right Diaphragm position.

INDIVIDUAL POSITIONS

Left distal

Emotional shock

This pulse reflects a pattern of Heart qi stagnation ('Heart closed'), often associated with the repression of emotional pain, usually early in life, from the loss of a parent, for example. The Flat wave is a sign that the Heart qi was deficient or immature at the time of the incident, as would be the case in childhood. This sign means that qi is unable to enter the Heart. Sudden rejection by a loved one in adulthood can also bring on this pulse, although it tends to be transient, lasting only until the emotional wound is healed. With the earlier etiology, the individual may suffer from lifelong vengefulness and spite.

An extremely Flat wave is also found in early stages or mild cases of Heart blood stagnation, when the heart muscles are tense, the coronary arteries are in spasm but not yet blocked, there is transient angina, and inhalation is difficult. Dr. Shen would say that the Heart is "suffocating." Ultimately, if uncorrected, the Flat wave will lead to the occlusion of the coronary arteries (heart attack).

Umbilical cord

The Flat quality at this position may also reflect the umbilical cord having been wrapped around the neck of an infant during delivery. Unless corrected, this sign may last a lifetime, and the clinical consequences may evolve into severe pathology in the upper burner, including emotional problems associated with Heart qi stagnation or Heart blood stagnation. With the former, there may be lifelong vengefulness and spite, and with the latter, lifelong unexplained fear. Dr. Shen states that the later stages of Heart blood stagnation is accompanied by a Deep, Thin, Feeble pulse. I cannot corroborate this.

Right distal

I have observed the Flat pulse in this position with carcinoma of the lung. Dr. Shen reports this pulse when "worries have hurt the Lungs."

Left middle

Here the Flat pulse is associated with overwork and insufficient rest, repressed anger in a deficient person, and, in my experience, with primary carcinoma of the bile duct.

Right middle

Dr. Shen reports this pulse with "an individual who thinks too much during eating."

Left proximal

The Flat quality in this position is rare. Conceivably, trauma to the left lower part of the body, or especially a large tumor here, could be responsible.

Right proximal

The Flat quality in this position is also very rare. Conceivably, trauma to the right lower part of the body, or a large tumor here, could be responsible.

Between left distal and left middle (left Diaphragm)

Very rarely, the wave is somewhat Flat at this position in a deficient person, with unresolved emotions concerning a separation in the context of an important relationship such as marriage. Far more commonly, and also in a stronger person, the pulse would be Inflated.

Between right distal and right middle (right Diaphragm)

Very rarely, the Flat quality is found here, usually due to repeated episodes of heavy lifting beyond one's energy in a very deficient person, which has caused qi stagnation in the diaphragm. Very rarely is it caused by repression of tender emotions, in which case it is also found at the left Diaphragm position.

Deep

Depth is the subject of the next major classification of pulse qualities, and is dealt with more fully in Chapter 9. It is mentioned here without elaboration to indicate its place as a pulse sign in the progression of increasing qi depletion.

Feeble-Absent

Category

Dr. Shen described three Feeble-Absent (Weak) pulses: overflowing, middle, and deep. He said that they are all related to "qi illness," except that "if the middle depth on the pulses is weak, then it is blood Xu [deficient]." Blood, he said, is a heavier form of qi.

'Overflowing and weak'

The Feeble-Absent (Weak) quality that is described by Dr. Shen as "overflowing and weak" and "qi Xu [deficient]"[62] is essentially the same as the Empty quality described in Chapter 9. In personal communications over the years, Dr. Shen described the Empty quality as a sign of 'qi wild' when found over the entire pulse. He consistently stated that a 'qi wild' quality is distinct from, and a sign of much greater deficiency than, a Feeble-Absent (Weak) quality, suggesting a more immediate onset of severe illness.

Furthermore, although the term Empty frequently entered our discussions, it is not included in the classification of pulse qualities in Dr. Shen's book. The confusion here is one of language. When Dr. Shen uses the term 'overflowing and weak' he is referring to

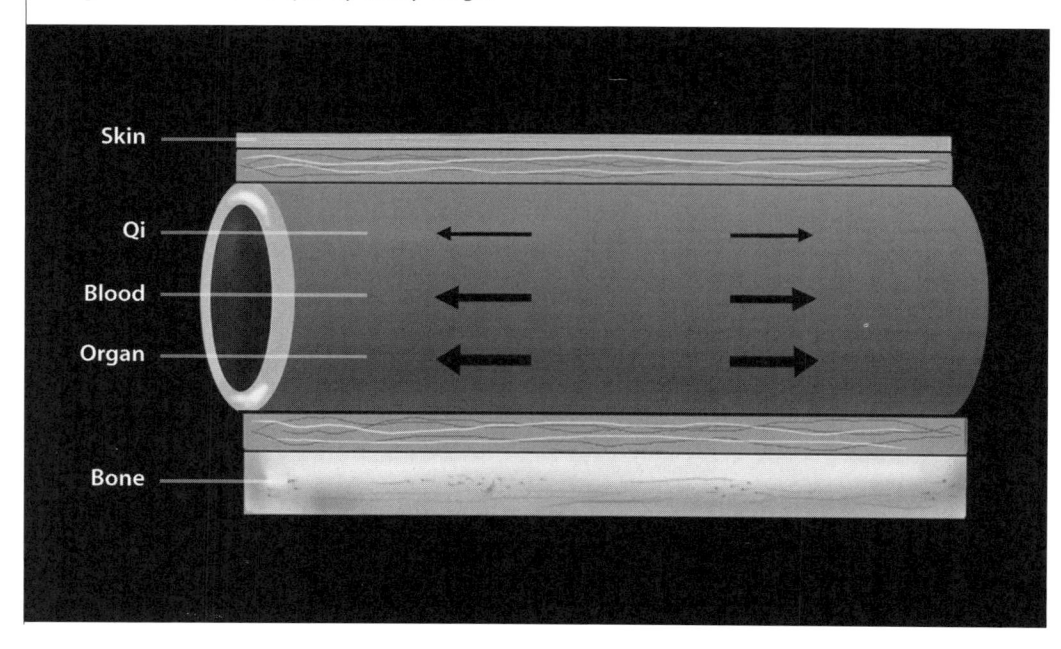

Fig. 8-15a Feeble quality (early stage)

Figs. 8-15b   Feeble quality (later stage)

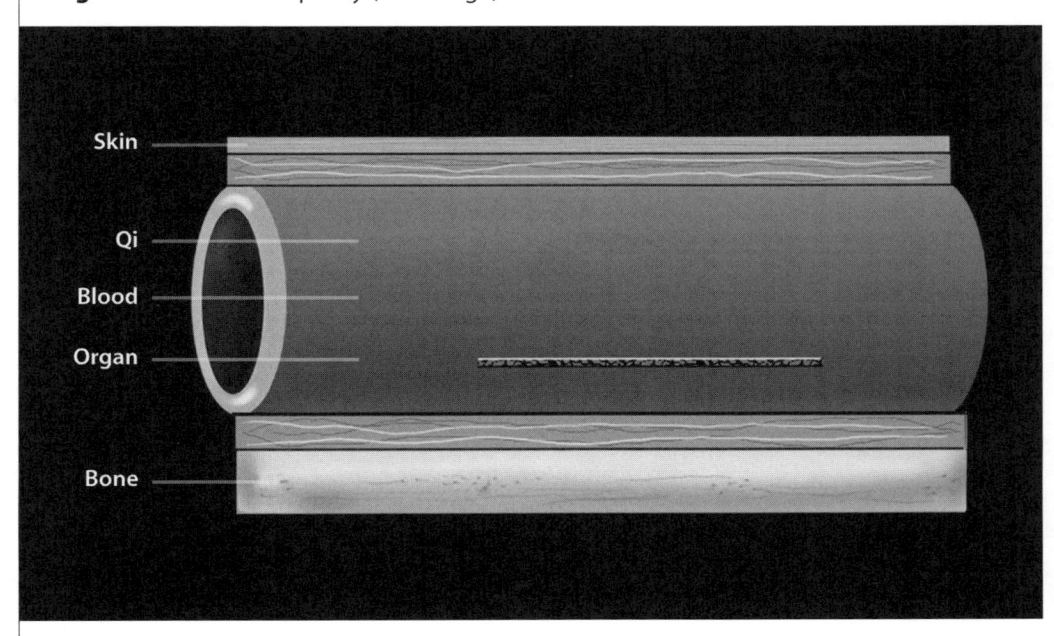

Figs. 8-16   Absent quality

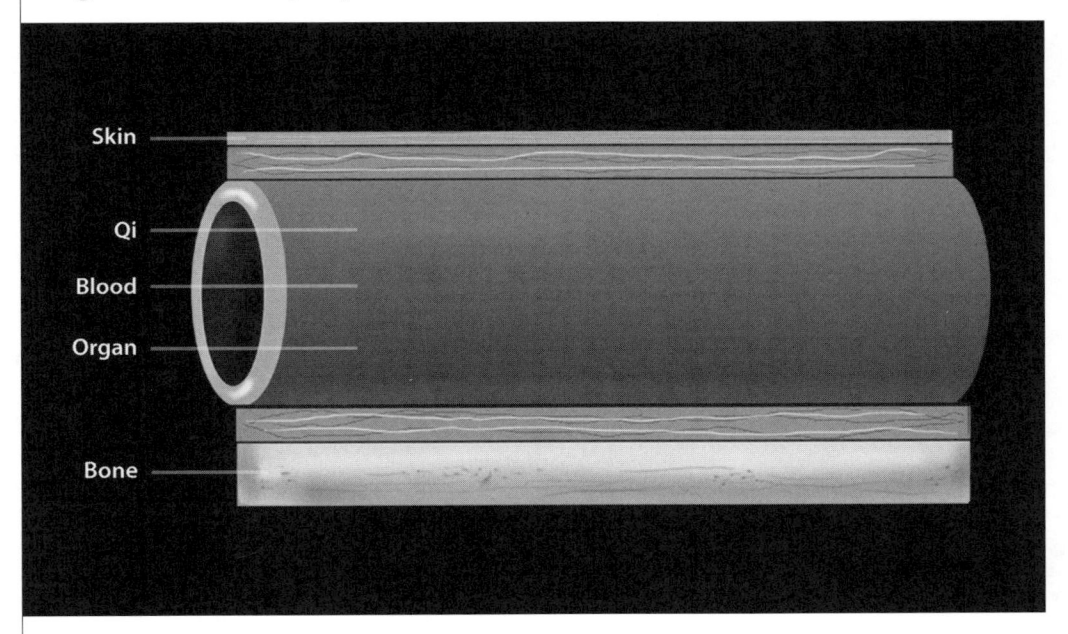

the Empty qualities, in particular the one discussed later, Empty Thread-like (soggy, soft). Felix Mann[63] also refers to this type of Empty quality as Weak-Floating.

The Feeble-Absent Deep quality represents a condition which is a less serious stage in the disease process just preceding the physiological state represented by the Empty pulse. (I have heard the Empty pulse referred to as one of the "eight pulses to death.")

'Middle weak'

Feeble-Absent (Weak) in the middle depth is, according to Dr. Shen, a sign of "blood Xu [deficient]." However everyone, including Dr. Shen, agrees that a pulse which is diminished at the blood depth is usually referred to as a Hollow or Scallion pulse. As mentioned above, Dr. Shen thinks of blood as a heavier form of qi: diminished blood always means diminished qi.

'Deep weak'

Of the three types of Weak pulse, the only one mentioned by Dr. Shen which bears elaboration here is the Feeble-Absent type. It alone refers directly to what is more widely regarded as a Weak pulse, for which I have substituted the term Feeble-Absent, as explained below.

CONTEMPORARY CHINESE PULSE DIAGNOSIS

Reconsideration of terminology

In reviewing this classification, I realized that the term Weak was being used for two separate feeling sensations. The first is one where something, however insubstantial, is palpable, and the second is where nothing at all is palpable. In other words, the same word, Weak, is being used to describe two different qualities.

In addition, in my classes students have been unclear when we discussed the pulse quality Weak, confusing it with the pathological condition of weakness. Finding terminology suitable to make this distinction seemed desirable. Another purpose in creating a new classification is to unify the terminology which uses so many different terms for the same quality, such as Frail, Infirm, and Deficient, as well as Weak.

Feeble versus Absent

Categories in this book are based on the sensation of touch. The following discussion is an attempt to nosologically distinguish the quality in which something insubstantial is palpated from the quality in which nothing is palpated.

Feeble seems the best choice for a perception which conveys an insubstantial sensory impression. Absent seems the clearest to communicate the complete absence of palpable impulse. These terms were drawn from the recommendations of students and from my own sensory impressions of these qualities.

The Feeble and Absent qualities, while distinct perceptually, are classified together because their clinical implications differ only slightly in degree.

Depth

The Feeble-Absent quality can occur at any depth. In the literature it is more commonly considered only in the deep position, but in my opinion, this is incorrect. The following is a quick review of the Feeble-Absent quality at the three depths.

QI DEPTH

The conception of the Feeble-Absent quality at the qi and blood depths in this book is totally different from Dr. Shen's reference to these two depths, discussed just above. At the qi depth, I refer to the quality as Yielding or Diminished.

BLOOD DEPTH

When the qi depth is Absent and the pulse separates under pressure at the blood depth, I refer to this as the Spreading quality, since the sensation is that the substance of the pulse is moving to the sides. Both qualities are discussed earlier in this chapter under the heading of volume, as prior stages in the continuum of increasing qi deficiency and diminished intensity.

ORGAN DEPTH

The majority of sources consider the Feeble-Absent quality to be accessible specifically and only at the organ depth. The following discussion will concern itself primarily with the Feeble-Absent Deep pulse.

Sensation

The Feeble Deep pulse is barely palpable, a step beyond Reduced Substance, and the Absent Deep quality is literally missing, at the yin organ depth. When it is there at all (Feeble), it separates and disperses easily under pressure. It is also unevenly distributed throughout the position.

In my experience, the Feeble pulse may be either broad or thin, which differs from the account in some of the other sources. Both qi and blood deficiency are always involved with this quality at the yin organ depth. When it is broader—which is far more common—we are dealing more with qi deficiency, and when it is thin, more with blood deficiency.

General interpretation

This quality can occur over the entire pulse, or at any single position or combination thereof. At the qi depth the Feeble quality is a sign of slightly less, and the Absent quality of slightly greater, qi deficiency. Found deeper, at the blood and organ depths, it is a sign of significant qi and blood deficiency.

ENTIRE PULSE

As previously mentioned, the Feeble-Absent quality at the qi depth over the entire pulse indicates deficiency of protective qi, and deficiency at the qi level of energy. It is an early sign of working beyond one's energy. If the pulse appears only occasionally it may just indicate a lack of sleep. But insufficient sleep is a form of working beyond one's energy, since one is presumably engaging in some energy-depleting endeavor when one is not sleeping. Even people who lie awake worrying are overworking, in this instance with their mind, which actually consumes more glucose than the physical body per unit of work. And of course the lack of rest obviates energy renewal, which means that the energy drain is double that of any other kind of activity.

The pulse which is uniformly Feeble-Absent and deep in all positions reflects primarily a deficiency of true qi, and a deficiency of qi and blood in all of the related yin organs.

INDIVIDUAL POSITIONS

The Feeble-Absent Deep quality at individual positions is a sign of qi and blood deficiency in the yin organ associated with that position on the pulse. In terms of deficiency the meaning is the same, but the consequences will vary from position to position, and from one combination of positions and qualities to another.

VULNERABILITY

According to Dr. Shen, the Feeble-Absent quality is a sign of vulnerability to disease, rather than the presence of disease. He observes that without contemporaneous symptoms or other signs of illness, the individual will become ill within one year unless there is intervention. (I find the time frame to be between one and three years.)

While I have frequently corroborated Dr. Shen's observation, I have often found this pulse quality to be a sign of extreme deficiency short of the 'danger' or 'dispersed' pulse qualities (previously discussed) associated with the 'qi wild' condition, in which yin and yang have lost functional contact.

It is my impression that people with strong constitutions who abuse their energy are more likely, given the same degree of abuse, to have a Feeble-Absent pulse than those with less robust constitutions, who are more likely to present with one of the qualities associated with 'qi wild,' such as an Empty pulse.

SERIOUSNESS OF CONDITION

All of my sources concur that when this pulse appears in a young person it is a cause of concern that there may be a dangerous illness. However, a word of caution. Developing and maturing children and adolescents frequently show serious signs that are only transient, and are merely indicative of transitory stages of growth. In the elderly it is a less serious sign, more often a common result of the depletion of Kidney essence which accompanies aging. Likewise, in chronic illness, it is a natural sign of qi depletion resulting from the organism's efforts to heal the affliction.

CHRONIC ILLNESS AND ENERGY DRAIN

In my own experience, the Feeble-Absent Deep quality usually represents a chronic process such as a prolonged illness, aging, or a lifetime of exceeding one's energy with work, exercise, or sex. This quality is also associated with an impaired immune system from a variety of causes, including improper or excessive medication. It is present in some individuals suffering from chronic fatigue syndrome.

The Feeble-Absent pulse is a common finding in women with prolonged menorrhagia, or who have given birth to children beyond their ability, especially with excessive blood loss. Other slow and mild internal bleeding over a long period of time, as with frequent and small nosebleeds and bleeding hemorrhoids, is attended by this pulse. All blood loss is accompanied by a loss of qi; thus with blood loss, the Feeble quality will also be Thin.

According to Dr. Shen, where the bleeding is attended by a Leather-like Hollow pulse, it is always associated with a yin organ, and the bleeding is always a very serious, sudden hemorrhage. Where this quality is absent, the loss of blood will be from other than a yin organ. (Menorrhagia from the uterus would be an example of bleeding from other than a yin organ.)

'NERVOUS SYSTEM WEAK'

Another condition, termed by Dr. Shen 'nervous system weak,'[64] is one which I have observed frequently. This occurs in a person with a constitutionally determined, lifelong history of neurasthenia, one whose symptoms are always changing. This individual is highly vulnerable, unstable, and easily disturbed or stressed, and subject, for example, to constantly fluctuating food and inhalant allergies. The pulse goes through a series of stages, eventually ending in a generally Feeble-Absent Deep pulse with a Tight quality at the surface of the pulse, which does not represent a current illness as much as a constant vulnerability to illness. Consistent with Dr. Shen's notion that the pulse in this instance represents a constitutional Kidney essence deficiency is Li Shi-Zhen's statement[65] that the quality is "usually caused by damage and deficiency of yin jing [essence] with failure of yang qi."[66]

RECAPITULATION

It has already been mentioned, but bears repeating, that the Feeble-Absent Deep pulse does not in itself necessarily represent a state of disease, but is more an indication of a general deficient condition in the yin organs (immune deficiency) which sets the stage for disease. In fact, the point was repeatedly made by Dr. Shen that a Feeble-Absent quality over the entire pulse is less a sign of present danger than a pulse which is out of balance and has many different qualities distributed throughout the various positions.

Combinations

While the Feeble-Absent Deep quality may occur with other qualities, it is difficult to clearly discern other qualities since the pulse is so slight. In assessing the meaning of these combinations, we begin by assuming a significant deficiency of qi and blood, and then add the meaning of the other quality.

Feeble-Absent Deep Choppy

A Feeble-Absent Choppy quality would indicate deficiency of qi and blood and resultant blood stagnation, possibly more the result of the deficiency than, for example, the result of Liver qi stagnation or heat. This is felt primarily in the proximal and Pelvis/Lower Body positions.

Feeble-Absent Deep Slippery

A Feeble-Absent Slippery pulse would signify that there is qi and blood deficiency with an accumulation of dampness, mucus, and phlegm. The latter would probably be due to deficient qi unable to move fluids, rather than to some other cause such as qi stagnation.

Feeble-Absent Deep and Slow

An accompanying Slow quality indicates that the deficiency associated with the Feeble-Absent quality has caused a circulatory deficit. Together, these qualities are signs of greater qi deficiency than either quality alone.

Feeble-Absent Deep and Rapid

An accompanying Rapid quality may indicate simultaneous qi and blood deficiency and the result of shock to the Heart, and less often to heat. The heat could be either from excess or deficiency, which other signs and symptoms would help differentiate.

When there is severe deficiency—for which a Feeble-Absent pulse is a reliable sign—it is important to remember that the pulse can sometimes be very Rapid, especially with exertion or stress, due to the instability of the qi, particularly the Heart qi.

In the lesser and absolute yin stage of disease, a paradoxical Feeble-Absent Deep Rapid pulse may be present due to the separation of yin from yang as a result of extreme yin and yang deficiency, with the yang rising to the surface causing heat stasis and the Rapid rate. An Empty quality is even more likely under these circumstances.

Positions

BILATERALLY AT SAME POSITION

Distal

At this position bilaterally, the Feeble-Absent quality may indicate qi deficiency of the Heart, Lungs, and chest.

Early emotional shock

This may be due to a long delayed and slowly developing reaction to a severe emotional shock during childhood, which caused a closure of qi circulation in the chest area due to suppression of the associated disappointment, sadness, hurt, loss, and trauma with which young children are not emotionally equipped to deal. In adulthood these events are largely forgotten, and the related emotions are beyond awareness. Posture is often marked by a collapse on the chest due to unconscious sadness. This causes further stagnation of qi in the area, which aggravates the sadness and qi deficiency due to a mind-body feedback mechanism involving inefficient air and qi exchange.

Initially the pulse can be Inflated or Flat, becoming Feeble-Absent over time as the energy in the area is exhausted trying to break through the stifled circulation.

Physical trauma

Trauma to the chest in a person who is already weak, or trauma that occurred in the long distant past but was not treated, may manifest with this pulse. Again, the energy in the area is exhausted trying to break through the stifled circulation.

Overwork of Lungs

This pulse is found in those, such as professional teachers or singers with Lung qi deficiency, who use the qi of the Lungs and chest beyond their capacity over a long period of time.

Middle

At an earlier stage, when stagnation of qi is the more central process, Inflation or Flatness will precede the Feeble-Absent Deep quality. The latter pulse will appear after an unsuccessful attempt by local and general energies to overcome the obstructed circulation in the area.

Gastrointestinal difficulties, depending partly on other variables such as constitution, are the usual consequence. This will vary from gas, distention, pain, and reflux to gastritis, ulcer, severe diarrhea or constipation, and even cancer over a long period of time.

Spleen and Stomach qi deficiency

Deficiency of Spleen and Stomach qi resulting from either poor nutrition or irregular eating habits in childhood, adolescence, or middle life, including anorexia and bulimia, may be reflected in a Feeble-Absent Deep pulse. Ultimately, the Liver-Gallbladder will be affected, probably due to dampness resulting from the Spleen qi deficiency.

Bending

Another cause is sitting in a bent position for long periods of time and over many years, as with secretarial work or taxi driving, or due to sadness. Some depressed people tend to sit bent over, holding their head with their hands. This posture is especially injurious during mealtime. Again, stagnation of qi is the initial response with the Inflated or Flat qualities, followed by Feeble-Absent much later due to the exhaustion of qi from its efforts to reopen circulation in the area.

Poor eating habits

A Feeble-Absent Deep and Slow pulse is found in an individual who, over a long period of time, resumes work too soon after meals. In the shorter term the pulse is Feeble-Absent or Separating at the qi depth, and the rate is closer to Normal.

Parasites

Over a considerable period of time the chronic energy drain caused by gastrointestinal and liver parasites can lead to a Feeble-Absent quality bilaterally in the middle burner.

Proximal

Deficiency in the lower burner is something that I have encountered more frequently in recent years, and in younger and younger people, implying that even at the very beginning of life there are serious insults to the genetic organism. This is probably due to the remarkable proliferation of environmental toxins, as well as individual toxicities from drugs, alcohol, or nutritional deficits to which our essence is exposed as we grow to child-bearing age, and to which women are subject during pregnancy. This is complicated by the traumatic delivery techniques of the past sixty years, including drug induction, forceps, and unnecessary caesarean sections, often for the convenience of the gynecologist. Recent reports even implicate the loss of the ozone layer in immune deficiency.

Constitutional Kidney deficiency

Except in the elderly, a Feeble-Absent Deep quality at this position is usually a reflection of constitutionally deficient Kidney qi, essence, or yang. Since this is the foundation of original and stored qi and essence for the entire organism, an individual with this pulse is vulnerable to many disorders. These might include problems of menstruation, low back and hernia, heart, respiration (e.g., childhood asthma), and digestion, since Kidney yang and qi support the digestive aspects of Spleen qi and yang, and help the Lungs move the qi downward.

An entire array of mental and emotional problems are also related to constitutionally deficient Kidney qi and essence. These include endogenous depression and schizophrenia, as well as severe genetic neurological deficits like retardation. Kidney yin and yang essence is responsible for the development and maintenance of the central nervous system. Kidney yin and yang deficiency is associated with endocrine problems, especially in women.

Excessive sex

Another cause of deficiency in the lower burner may be long-term excessive sexual activity in a person of normal energy, or an inappropriate level of sexual activity in a person whose energy was more compromised to begin with.

Menorrhagia and chronic colitis

Likewise, any continuous drain on qi, yin, blood, and essence such as excessive menstruation, chronic colitis, or diarrhea over a very long period of time may be signaled by a Feeble-Absent Deep pulse at the proximal position.

SIDES

The Feeble-Absent and very Slow quality occurs after a stroke on the side of the body which is paralyzed. If, however, it should appear over the entire pulse after a stroke, this suggests a more serious situation.

Left

A Feeble-Absent pulse over the entire left side is a sign of severe deficiency in what Dr. Shen refers to as the 'organ system.' This includes the Heart, Liver, and Kidney energies, and through these, all of the other yin and yang organ functions. Apart from being easily fatigued and other symptoms of general and severe deficiency, the individual is often in a chronically depressed state, which can be reversed only by restoring these energies.

Constitution, overwork, and excessive sex

There are several possible causes of a Feeble-Absent pulse over the entire left side. One is constitutional Kidney deficiency. Another is overwork beyond one's energy over a long period of time. Still another is long-term excessive sexual activity beyond one's original energic endowment. A strong constitution takes longer to develop the same level of deficiency.

Nervous system affects organ system

Finally, there is the effect on the organ system of prolonged stress on the nervous system.[67] Although yin deficiency is the first consequence of this protracted tension, it will eventually deplete the remaining substances of the organism which is supporting it.

Here the pulse would be moderately Deep, Feeble, a little Wider than one would otherwise expect, with a Normal or Slightly Rapid rate, and most importantly, with a Thin Tight line palpable just above the organ depth. The Tightness is a sign that the nervous innervation of the organs is depleted of yin due to overwork, and is more dry and therefore even more excitable. The latter sign may take some skill to palpate, and is accessed by resting one's fingers very lightly on the pulse. This pulse picture is similar to the combination attending the 'nervous system weak' condition, described above, except that the rate is Slow.

Right

The right side represents what Dr. Shen refers to as the 'digestive system.' He notes that the Lungs digest mucus, the Spleen digests food, and the Kidneys digest water. Symptoms include a changing appetite, a vague feeling of discomfort, and irregular bowel movements. The latter change from soft to hard, constipation to loose, from day to day and week to week, with no explanation based on life experience or eating habits. The principal cause is ignoring the messages which announce bodily needs. Here the cause is irregular eating habits. One eats when one is not hungry, and does not eat when one is hungry, because other needs—such as work—take precedence. Gradually, the Spleen is injured, leading to dampness and yang deficiency of the Spleen, which impairs the overall functioning of the Triple Burner.

INDIVIDUAL POSITIONS

Left distal

The Feeble-Absent Deep quality at this position is associated with some or all the signs of Heart qi and blood deficiency. These include loss of mental clarity, memory impairment, sleep and dream disturbance, palpitations, depression, and fatigue in the morning.

The Feeble-Absent Deep pulse at this position indicates Heart qi/yang deficiency, which may be associated with high diastolic hypertension. Any factor in life or heredity which deprives the Heart of its full vigor will lead to Heart qi/yang deficiency. This is discussed elsewhere in more detail.[68]

Right distal

All of the signs of Lung qi deficiency are associated with the pulse at this position. These would include shortness of breath, spontaneous sweating, susceptibility to external pathogenic factors, deficient asthma, cough, and inhalant allergies.

Tuberculosis

Dr. Shen mentioned a Feeble-Absent quality at the right distal (Lung) position with a Floating Slippery quality at the Special Lung position as a sign of tuberculosis.

Left middle

Fatigue, especially after work or later in the day, with difficulty recovering and getting one's second wind, is one symptom associated with the Feeble-Absent Deep pulse at this position. It is also associated with lassitude and depression due to a lack of what Porkert calls 'active' moving energy. Other symptoms may include such musculoskeletal problems as spasms, being easily injured, and difficulty recovering from injuries and fibromyalgia. Menstrual problems with delayed or missed periods, sensitivity to light and other eye problems, and digestive difficulties such as stagnant gas and distention, may also result from deficiency in this position.

I have found the Feeble-Absent pulse at this position to be increasing in tandem with the proliferation of drug use, especially marijuana, and with what seems to be an epidemic of mononucleosis and hepatitis. The danger of primary liver cancer and lymphomas with this pulse is also increasing.

Right middle

The Feeble-Absent pulse at this position is indicative of digestive problems, including deficient stagnation of food with gas, severe constipation, severe diarrhea (with dampness), and all of the problems associated with a condition of Spleen qi deficiency and dampness. If the Spleen qi deficiency is accompanied by dampness, there may be disturbances of the sensorium (concentration and attention), with a spacy feeling, heaviness, lassitude, and headaches. Spleen qi deficiency may also be partially implicated with fibromyalgia. Problems with prolapse, being easily bruised, and bleeding under the skin can also occur.

Left proximal

At this position, the Feeble-Absent pulse is associated with all of the consequences of deficient Kidney qi and essence. This includes sexual disturbances such as impotence and premature ejaculation, spermatorrhea, tinnitus, night sweats, cocks-crow diarrhea, an empty feeling in the head, and degenerative central nervous system diseases. Dr. Shen refers to lifelong sadness—what I call endogenous depression— as another associated condition. This pulse may be caused by excessive sex and heavy physical work with Kidneys that are already vulnerable for other reasons, including constitutional.

A Feeble-Absent Deep quality in this position, indicating Kidney qi/yang deficiency, may be associated with hypertension when the left distal position is also Feeble-Absent. With this type of hypertension, the greater the deficiency, the higher the diastolic pressure.

As previously mentioned, over a long period of time, a tense 'nervous system' can affect the 'organ system' by pushing the yin organs until they become yin deficient, dry, and poorly functioning. This process in particular affects the Kidneys, which supply yin to the entire body, leading to Kidney related 'true hypertension.' Ultimately, over a very long time, the yin deficiency transforms into qi/yang deficiency, and the pulse evolves from Tight to Feeble-Absent.

Right proximal

Since a Feeble-Absent Deep quality at this position is a sign of Kidney qi/yang deficiency, all of the Kidney qi-deficient symptoms mentioned above may be present, accompanied by an ongoing feeling of internal cold independent of the weather or climate.

Complementary

Feeble qualities at the Special Lung, Pelvis/Lower Body, Gallbladder, Stomach-Pylorus Extension, and Intestine positions are clearly signs of deficiency. The Heart Enlarged, Pleura, Distal Liver Engorgement, and Esophageal positions are all part of the Diaphragm area where Feeble and Absent are not relevant.

Originally, Dr. Shen said that the complementary positions would have no qualities (Absent) if they were normal. But, as previously noted, I have found this to be true for some and not for others, and about one I am uncertain. With regard to the Large Vessel position, it is clearly best if there are no qualities and it feels like an empty hole. This is also true for the Mitral Valve, Diaphragm, Ulnar and Radial Engorged, and Spleen positions. The one position about which I am unsure is the Neuro-psychological position. In my experience an Absent quality at the Special Lung position is a sign of grave danger, a finding with which other observers have found exception.

Muffled

Category

This quality was not mentioned by Dr. Shen or in the literature by either name or description. It is, however, a sensation which I encounter frequently and have attempted to define over time through clinical information associated with it. The Muffled pulse has become one of the most important qualities because it is perhaps the most reliable sign of serious illness, often unrecognized at the time of examination. Describing the sensation to Dr. Shen, he recognized the Muffled quality as within his own experience, carrying with it the same sense of urgency. He referred to it only as a form of "stagnant" pulse during our discussion, and never gave it a Chinese name.

Sensation

One can palpate a distinct quality, but the sensation is slightly muted and unclear, as if a towel or blanket separated one's fingers from the pulse (Fig. 8-17). It differs from the Flat quality, which has a clear, distinct, but compressed wave shape, and the Cotton quality, which appears above the qi depth only, has no shape, and gives a sensation of spongy resistance.

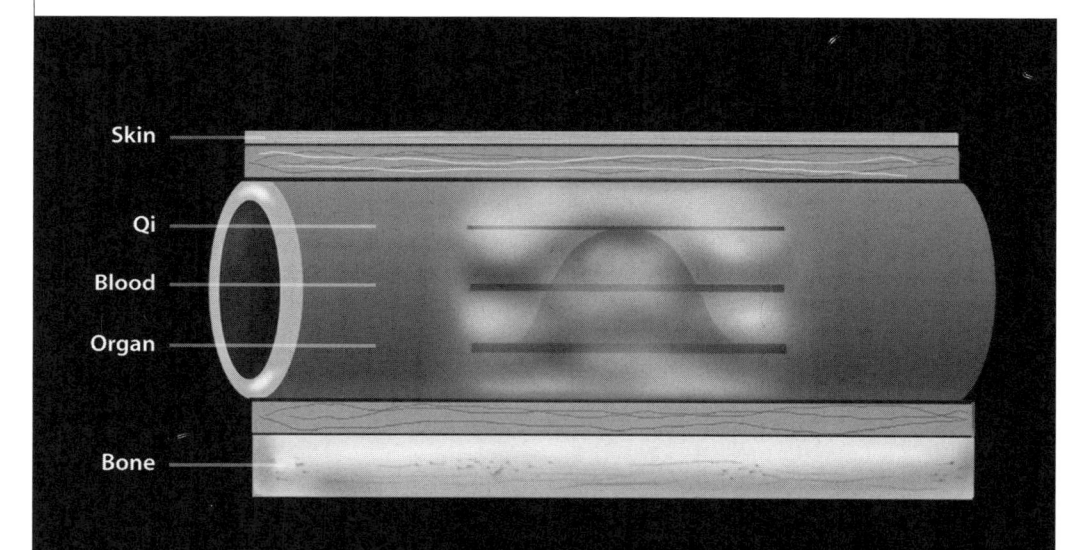

Fig. 8-17 Muffled quality

General interpretation and position

The Muffled quality mostly appears wherever coherent active qi function is impaired at the cellular-molecular level by extraordinary stagnation or physiological chaos equivalent to a profound separation of yin and yang, which we call 'qi wild.' This stagnation and chaos is most often associated with tumors, often malignant. I first identified this quality in the right distal and the Special Lung positions in the presence of lung cancer. As I became more familiar with the sensation, I was able to find it in all of the positions, almost always associated with severe disease. Finally, I came to identify the quality over the entire pulse, again always associated with advanced pathology. More recently I have come to distinguish the qualitative aspects of the Muffled pulse and have found that, when classified as a one on a scale of one to five over the entire pulse, the person might be depressed. With proper treatment the Muffled quality associated with depression is rather quickly reduced. When, however, the cause is a more serious disease, the Muffled quality will persist.

In the left distal position this quality is usually a sign of the Heart type of depression, featuring a lack of joy. It is also found with a thickening of the Pericardium (usually with an accompanying arrhythmia) and/or an occlusion of the coronary arteries. In the right distal and Special Lung positions it is associated with tumors of the lung and breast. Bilaterally in the upper burner it is a sign of tumors, most often malignant, in the breast and mediastinum.

I have found the Muffled quality at the Gallbladder position when there are many gallstones, severe infection, and, especially, when the gallbladder is necrotic or close to being so. I can recall one case of cancer of the bile ducts when it was also found on the left middle position.

I have found this pulse in the Large Intestine and Small Intestine complementary positions, with some degree of fecal impaction and loss of peristaltic activity. I have also found it in the Pelvis/Lower Body position as a sign of extreme stagnation of blood and qi, with uterine and ovarian tumors, with quiescent pelvic inflammatory disease, following surgery, and with chronic quiescent venereal disease.

Although Dr. Shen never formulated a term for this quality, when questioned he associated it with profound deficiency of qi and blood in a yin organ. He observed that if the rate is Slow the etiology can be traced to overwork, and if the rate is Normal the etiology is associated with having been upset for one's entire life. Another observer's explanation for the Muffled quality in its association with neoplasms is that it represents fragility of the blood vessels and easier metastasis.

Dead

Category

This quality is not described anywhere in the literature, and although the term was used frequently by Dr. Shen in conversations associated with clinical examinations of the pulse, it is not mentioned in his book.

Sensation

There is a sense of a presence which is not moving. It feels literally like putting ones fingers on a dead animal. There is substance without movement. By contrast, with an Absent quality there is no discernible substance, with a Flat quality there is a slight wave, and with a Muffled quality there is a muted, unclear sensation.

Interpretation

Each time I felt this quality it was associated with an advanced malignant neoplastic condition. I have felt it at the right distal, left middle, and Pelvis/Lower Body positions.

Fig. 8-18 Volume

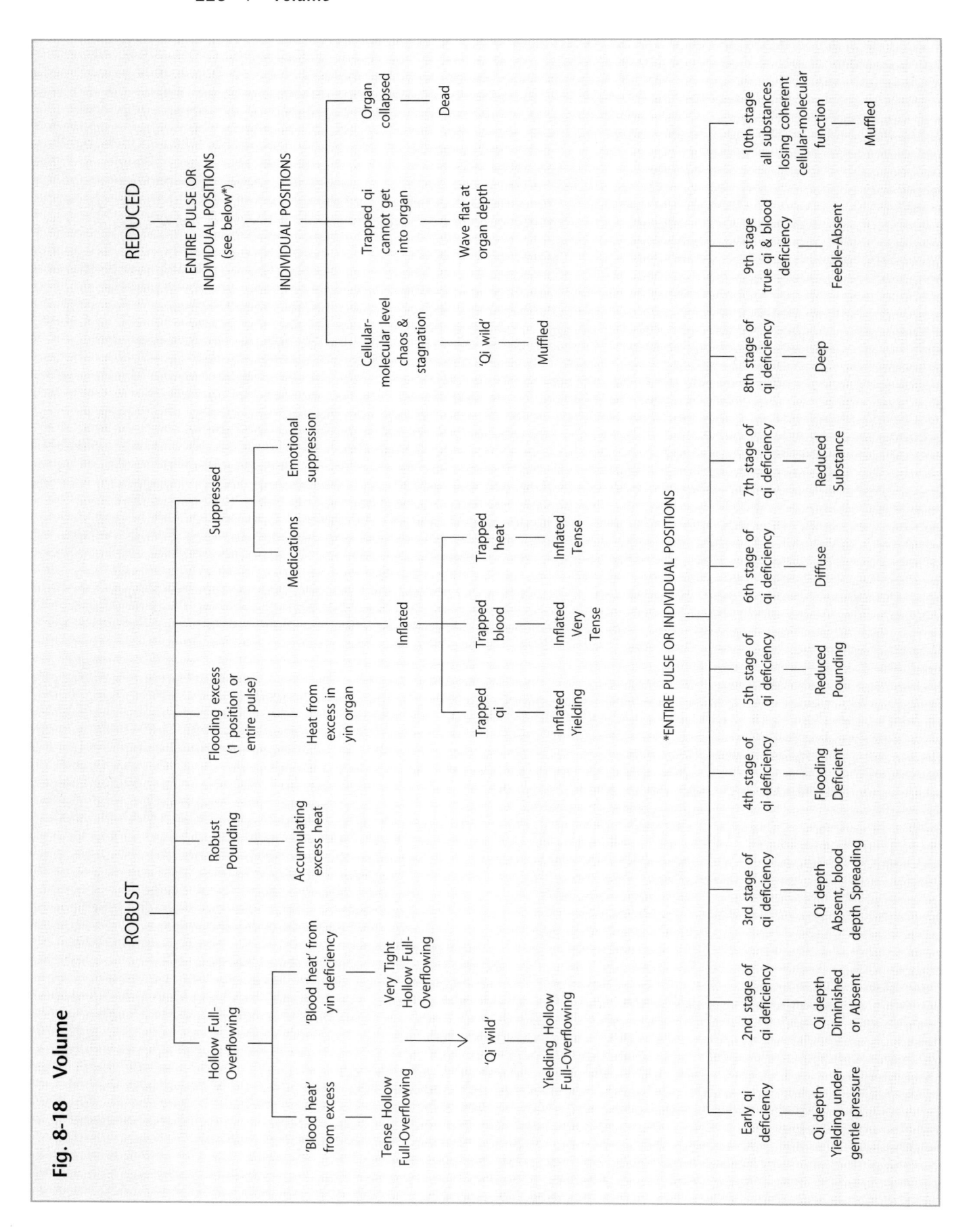

ROBUST
- Hollow Full-Overflowing
  - 'Blood heat' from excess → Tense Hollow Full-Overflowing
  - 'Blood heat' from yin deficiency → Very Tight Hollow Full-Overflowing
  - 'Qi wild' → Yielding Hollow Full-Overflowing
- Robust Pounding
  - Accumulating excess heat
- Flooding excess (1 position or entire pulse)
  - Heat from excess in yin organ
- Inflated
  - Trapped qi → Inflated Yielding
  - Trapped blood → Inflated Very Tense
  - Trapped heat → Inflated Tense
- Suppressed
  - Medications
  - Emotional suppression

REDUCED — ENTIRE PULSE OR INDIVIDUAL POSITIONS (see below*)

INDIVIDUAL POSITIONS
- Cellular-molecular level chaos & stagnation
  - 'Qi wild' → Muffled
- Trapped qi cannot get into organ
  - Wave flat at organ depth
- Organ collapsed → Dead

*ENTIRE PULSE OR INDIVIDUAL POSITIONS

Early qi deficiency	2nd stage of qi deficiency	3rd stage of qi deficiency	4th stage of qi deficiency	5th stage of qi deficiency	6th stage of qi deficiency	7th stage of qi deficiency	8th stage of qi deficiency	9th stage true qi & blood deficiency	10th stage all substances losing coherent cellular-molecular function
Qi depth Yielding under gentle pressure	Qi depth Diminished or Absent	Qi depth Absent, blood depth Spreading	Flooding Deficient	Reduced Pounding	Diffuse	Reduced Substance	Deep	Feeble-Absent	Muffled

CHAPTER 9

Depth

CONTENTS

Excess and Deficiency, 235
Superficial Pulse Qualities, 235
    Cotton, 236
    ■ Fig. 9-1: Cotton, 236
        Positions, 238
            Bilaterally at same position, 238
            Sides, 238
            Individual positions, 239
    Floating, 239
    ■ Fig. 9-2: Floating, 240
        Differentiating Floating from other qualities, 240
            Floating and Empty, 240
            Floating and 'Weak Floating', 241
            Floating and Inflated, 242
            Floating and Cotton, 242
            Floating and Hollow Full-Overflowing, 242
            Floating and Flooding Excess, 242
        External disharmony, 242
            Floating Tense and Slow, 243
            Floating Yielding and slightly Rapid, 243
            Floating Yielding with Normal rate, 243
        Internal disharmony, 244
            Liver wind, 244
                Floating Tight, 244
        Combinations, 244
        Positions, 244

                Bilaterally at same position, 244
                    Floating Tense and Slow, 244
                    Floating Tense with Normal or slightly Rapid rate, 244
                    Floating Yielding and Rapid, 245
                Sides, 245
                Individual positions, 245
Empty, 245
- Fig. 9-3a: Empty (early stage), 248
- Fig. 9-3b: Empty (middle stage), 248
- Fig. 9-3c: Empty (later stage), 249
        Combinations, 249
            Frequent combinations, 249
                Empty Yielding and Slow, 249
                Empty Tight and Rapid, 249
                Empty Moderately Tense, 249
            Less frequent combinations, 250
                Empty Interrupted-Intermittent, 250
                Empty at proximal and middle positions, 250
        Positions, 250
            Bilaterally at same position, 250
            Sides, 252
            Individual positions, 252
Yielding Empty Thread-like, 253
- Fig. 9-4a: Yielding Empty Thread-like (early stage), 254
- Fig. 9-4a: Yielding Empty Thread-like (later stage), 254
Leather, 255
- Fig. 9-5a: Leather (early stage), 255
- Fig. 9-5b: Leather (later stage), 255
Scattered, 256
- Fig. 9-6: Scattered, 257
Minute, 258
- Fig. 9-7: Minute, 258
Hollow, 259
        Types of Hollow qualities, 260
            Entire pulse, 260
                Yielding Partially Hollow, 260
                Yielding Hollow Full-Overflowing, 261
                Yielding Hollow Full-Overflowing and Slow, 261
                Slightly Yielding Hollow Full-Overflowing and Normal to slightly Rapid, 261
                Yielding Hollow Full-Overflowing and Interrupted-Intermittent, 261
                Yielding Hollow Ropy, 262
            Individual positions, 262
                Yielding Hollow Full-Overflowing, 262
                Yielding Partially Hollow, 262
                Tense Hollow Slippery and Rapid, 262
                Leather-like Hollow and either Rapid or Slow, 262
                    - Fig. 9-8: Leather-like Hollow, 263
                Tense Hollow, 263
                Tense and very Tense Hollow Full-Overflowing, 263
                Tight and very Tight Hollow Full-Overflowing, 264

              Combinations, 264
              Positions, 264
                    Bilaterally at the same position, 264
                        Distal, 264
                            Leather-like Hollow, 264
                            Yielding Hollow Full-Overflowing, 264
                        Middle, 264
                            Leather-like Hollow, 264
                            Yielding Partially Hollow, 265
                            Tense Hollow, 265
                            Yielding Hollow Full-Overflowing, 265
                            Tight and very Tight Hollow Full-Overflowing, 265
                        Proximal, 265
                            Yielding Hollow Full-Overflowing and Slow, 265
                            Leather-like Hollow, 265
                            Tight and very Tight Hollow Full-Overflowing, 265
                    Sides, 265
                        Left, 265
                            Yielding Hollow Full-Overflowing and Slow, 265
                            Tight and very Tight Hollow Full-Overflowing, 266
                        Right, 266
                            Yielding Hollow Full-Overflowing, 266
                            Tight and very Tight Hollow Full-Overflowing, 266
                    Individual positions, 266
                        Left distal, 266
                            Tense-Tight Hollow Full-Overflowing, 266
                            Leather-like Hollow, 266
                        Left middle, 266
                            Leather-like Hollow, 266
                            Tense Hollow, 267
                            Yielding Partially Hollow, 267
                            Yielding Hollow Full-Overflowing and Slow, 267
                            Tight and very Tight-Wiry Hollow Full-Overflowing, 267
                        Left proximal, 267
                            Leather-like Hollow, 267
                            Yielding Hollow Full-Overflowing, 267
                        Right distal, 267
                            Leather-like Hollow, 267
                            Yielding Hollow Full-Overflowing, 267
                        Right middle and Stomach-Pylorus Extension, 268
                            Leather-like Hollow, 268
                            Tight-Wiry Hollow Slippery, 268
                        Right proximal, 268
                            Yielding Hollow Full-Overflowing, 268
                            Slightly Tight Hollow Full-Overflowing, 268
                            Tight and very Tight Hollow Full-Overflowing, 268
Submerged Pulse qualities, 268
    Deep, 268
        Fig. 9-9: Deep quality, 269
            Combinations, 270
                Deep Diffuse, Deep Reduced Substance, or Deep Feeble-Absent, 270

		Deep Tight, 270
		Deep Wiry, 271
		Deep Flat, 271
		Deep Slippery, 271
		Deep and Slow, 271
		Deep and Rapid, 272
		Deep Thin, 272
		Deep Wide, 273
		Deep Choppy, 273
	Positions, 273
		Bilaterally at same position, 273
			Distal, 273
				Deep Flat, 273
				Deep Feeble, 274
				Deep Slippery, 274
				Deep Thin Tight, 274
				Deep and very Tight or Wiry, 274
				Deep Tight-Wiry and very Rapid, 275
			Middle, 275
				Deep Flat, 275
				Deep Tight, 275
				Deep Feeble-Absent, 275
				Deep Slippery, 275
				Deep Wiry, 276
				Deep Thin, 276
			Proximal, 276
				Deep Flat, 276
				Deep Wiry, 276
				Deep Feeble, 276
				Deep Slippery, 276
		Sides, 277
			Left, 277
				Deep Feeble, 277
				Deep Tight, 277
			Right, 277
				Deep Feeble, 277
				Deep Tight, 277
		Individual positions, 277
			Left distal, 277
				Deep Feeble with Increase in Rate on Exertion <8 beats/min, 278
				Deep Feeble with large Increase in Rate on Exertion, 278
				Deep Flat and slightly Rapid or Slow, 278
				Deep Thin Feeble with Normal or slightly Rapid rate, 278
				Deep Thin Tight and very Rapid, 278
				Deep Slippery, 278
			Right distal, 278
				Deep Feeble, 279
				Deep Thin Tight and Rapid, 279
				Deep Tense to Tight with Normal rate, 279
			Left middle, 279
				Deep Feeble, 279

                    Deep Slippery, 279
                Right middle, 279
                    Deep Feeble, 279
                    Deep Slippery, 279
                    Deep Thin Tight to Wiry Hollow, 279
                Left proximal, 279
                    Deep Feeble and Slow, 280
                    Deep Tight, 280
                    Deep Slippery Tense, 280
                    Deep Slippery Wiry and Rapid, 280
                    Deep Slippery Feeble, 280
                Right proximal, 280
                    Deep Feeble, 281
                    Deep Slippery Tight and Rapid, 281
                    Deep Slippery Feeble and Slow, 281
                Large and Small Intestine, 281
    Firm, 281
    ▪ Fig. 9-10: Firm quality, 282
    Hidden, 282
    ▪ Fig. 9-11a: Hidden Excess quality, 283
    ▪ Fig. 9-11b: Hidden Deficient quality, 283
        Types of Hidden qualities, 284
            Hidden Deficient, 284
            Hidden Excess, 284
            Hidden Normal, 285
▪ Fig. 9-12: Depth flowchart, 286

CHAPTER 9

Depth

Depth informs us of two important diagnostic parameters: the duration and the location of the disease process. Generally, superficial pulses are associated with acute disease processes involving the surface protective qi and qi energies, while deeper pulses are identified with more profound chronic illness located in the yin organs. A uniformly Deep pulse without other signs or symptoms indicates a significant potential for disease, such as an impaired immune system. Generally, the deeper the pulse, the more serious the illness. Exceptions are mentioned in the discussion of individual qualities. It should be noted that the pulses of heavy or obese individuals are normally deeper than those of thinner individuals.

The organization of pulse depth in this chapter is by qualities that appear superficially, and those that are submerged.

Excess and Deficiency

As mentioned in Chapter 3, many of the pulse qualities described here—Feeble-Absent, Empty, Deep, and others which I classify according to sensation as Reduced qualities—are discussed in the literature according to their associated conditions. In that context, it is correctly observed that false signs of deficiency can be due to underlying excess. While both views would agree that Deep means 'interior' in terms of the disease location, and while I will accept that, theoretically, it could be due to excess, in our times the ancient causes of excess (e.g., interior cold from excess) are rare. With this caveat, I have chosen to confine my interpretations to the principal clinical reality in my own experience and that of others, including Dr. Shen. However, the possibility that these qualities might be associated with excess should always be kept in mind, especially if there are other strong signs of excess, such as a very Rapid rate, high temperature, and acute pain.

Superficial Pulse Qualities

Floating is the term used in the literature for the pulse that we call superficial. Under our methodology the Floating quality is just one of the pulses in the superficial category, with its own characteristics and meaning. Superficial is the broader, more inclusive category of pulses felt only at or above the qi depth. Thus, superficial would include the Floating as well as the Cotton qualities, which are palpated above the qi depth. These qualities, unlike the Full-Overflowing and the Flooding Excess qualities, do not have a wave form.

The superficial qualities are arranged here in order of increasing deficiency of qi, essence, yin, and yang. The least deficient quality is the Cotton, and the most deficient the Yielding Hollow Full-Overflowing pulse. Except for the Floating and Cotton qualities, the superficial pulses are felt primarily at the qi depth and are subsumed within the 'qi wild' category.

The Hollow Full-Overflowing and Flooding Excess qualities are also superficial pulses whose sensory experience is, however, perceived more by the vigor with which they push upward against the fingers, and their strong base at the blood and organ depths respectively, than by their superficiality. For this reason, and despite their superficial nature, in a nosology based on sensation, they are more appropriately classified under Robust volume (see Chapter 8).

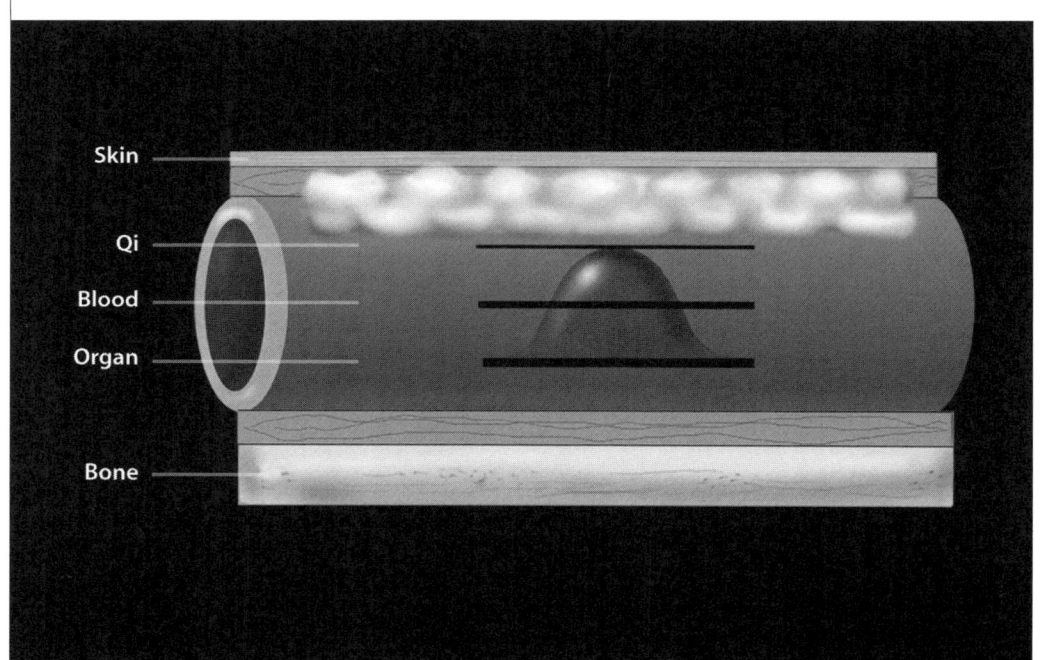

Fig. 9-1 Cotton quality

Cotton

Category

The Cotton quality is not described in any text with which I am familiar, and has been demonstrated to me clinically only by Dr. Shen. It is a pulse that I have palpated hundreds of times once I could identify it, and it has always proven to be an accurate sign of the disharmony that Dr. Shen ascribes to it.

The term Cotton is often confused with Soggy, Soft, and sometimes Slippery, all of which represent totally different sensations and pathologies. For example, Li Shi-Zhen compares the Soft pulse to a piece of cotton;[1] Kaptchuk calls it Soggy.[2]

Since the Cotton quality is felt only above the qi depth and to the depth at which the other qualities are first accessed, I have classified it with the superficial pulses.

Sensation

The Cotton quality (Fig. 9-1) conveys a spongy, amorphous, formless resistance that is without structure and wave form. As gentle pressure is exerted from the surface to the qi depth, this shapeless entity feels exactly like pushing one's finger through cotton. All other qualities accessed above the qi depth—the Floating, Full-Overflowing, and Flooding Excess—have a shape, and the latter two have a clear wave form. Furthermore, once the finger is through this nebulous superficial zone, the pulse reveals itself without hindrance at the qi, organ, and blood depths with the remainder of its message about the pulse and the person. When the qi depth is absent, the Cotton quality is felt to the blood depth, and to the organ depth when the pulse is absent of other qualities at the other depths.

Although the Empty Thread-like quality is felt at the qi depth, and is somewhat indistinct compared to other qualities, its thin, thread-like sensation is much more definite in shape than the Cotton quality. Unlike the Cotton pulse, with continued pressure the Empty Thread-like quality is Empty beneath the surface. There is also none of the horizontal swishing movement in one direction under the finger with the Cotton quality that is clearly felt with the Slippery quality, with which it is also sometimes confused.

Obesity, characterized by a thickening of the connective tissue, can be differentiated from the Cotton quality by a hardness which is not characteristic of a purely Cotton quality.

Interpretation

The Cotton quality is a sign of superficial qi stagnation, which reduces the circulation of qi wherever the stagnation occurs. The organism attempts to reopen the circulation by calling forth local and general body energies. Over time, this effort depletes the body, especially when it is not strong, or when the cause of the stagnation is ongoing, or when the initial stagnation is too great. Eventually, since the qi moves the blood, the circulation of blood as well as the functions of the yin and yang organ systems will also suffer.

The primary cause of the qi stagnation that leads to the Cotton quality is emotional suppression, and, less commonly, physical trauma. Both etiologies can occur simultaneously, and are differentiated primarily by history and the darker facial color which appears with extensive physical trauma.

EMOTIONAL SUPPRESSION AND RESIGNATION

According to Dr. Shen, this pulse is known in China as the 'sad' pulse. In my experience, it reflects a sense of oppression, resignation, and hopelessness based on the felt inability to change specific onerous conditions of one's life. They feel 'stuck.' One example is an unhappy marriage which the individual cannot leave even when it is clear that the commitment to make it work is not there. This feeling is expressed in Thoreau's famous passage, "The mass of men lead lives of quiet desperation."[3] I have found that individuals with a thick, heavy Cotton quality over the entire pulse tend to blame others rather than take responsibility to extricate themselves from their predicaments. They thereby suppress or blunt the emotional pain associated with both the feeling of, and the cause for, the sadness. Consciousness of the provocative life events and the associated emotions, however stifled, remain in subdued yet easily aroused awareness. The adaptive restorative mechanism is suppression rather than the more profoundly unconscious repression, and resignation rather than resolution.

The oppression extends across the physical and emotional spectrum, and often life is on hold due to the unsettled nature of the individual's feelings. Just beneath consciousness there is an awareness of protracted sluggishness of function, both mentally and physically. Depression and some slowing of psychomotor function is possible depending on the degree and the duration of the condition. While many people can mask their true feelings, when the pulse quality is presented to them in these terms, they are usually more inclined to verbalize their physical and mental complaints and their sense of helplessness, hopelessness, and resignation than are those with other qualities representing emotional problems.

In an adult this sadness, associated with the Cotton quality, does not usually come from childhood, but is of relatively recent origin. Where it is found on the pulse tells us generally about the duration. It usually begins at the left distal position and spreads with time down the left side, and eventually over the entire pulse. The thicker and heavier the Cotton quality, the deeper the oppression and sadness.

TRAUMA

A major physical trauma is a shock to the circulation of qi in the channels. As a result, the free flow of qi is inhibited at the surface of the body. The Cotton quality can reflect this stagnation from trauma; when pain is a factor, the qualities at the qi, blood, and organ depths are Tight. The facial color is darker. Inside the lower eyelids there may be a horizontal red line, and on the tongue a purple blister.

Prognosis

The long-term consequences of the qi stagnation associated with the Cotton quality depend on its location. Generally, the sequelae after many years are serious and include tumors and severe depression. It has been noted that the Cotton quality disappears quickly with the use of seratonin uptake inhibitors such as Prozac, and more slowly with superficial and deeper qi-moving herbs. Since herbs that tonify the Kidney yang help to dissipate the Cotton quality in some people, it may be fair to attribute some of the resignation mentioned above to the loss of will associated with Kidney qi-yang deficiency.

Combinations

The Cotton quality can be found simultaneously with any other quality or combination of qualities. In such combinations the Cotton quality continues to retain its significance as a sign of stagnation of qi due to emotional suppression or trauma. Likewise, the significance of each of the other qualities is not altered by the presence of the Cotton pulse. Although stagnation above the qi depth affects the function of the entire organism, the different pulse qualities can coexist as separate signals.

Positions

BILATERALLY AT SAME POSITION

When found bilaterally at one of the three burners, the Cotton quality indicates that the qi stagnation in that area is due to physical or emotional trauma. In the upper burner the cause is a minor trauma to the chest or a recent or ongoing emotional conflict in which the person is stifled and cannot act upon or verbalize their feelings. In the middle burner the causes are emotional conflict of the same nature which occurs while eating, ruminating while eating, sitting in one position for long periods of time, resuming work too soon after eating, and minor trauma to the abdomen. In the lower burner it can be attributed to the presence of mild Kidney qi deficiency or minor trauma to the lower burner.

SIDES

When found only on the right side, this quality is a sign that the individual worries and is emotionally upset during mealtimes, and that the digestive system is deficient, or that there has been mild trauma to the right side. When found only on the left side, it is a sign of a relatively early stage of emotional trauma or mild physical trauma to the left side.

INDIVIDUAL POSITIONS

It is rare for the Cotton quality to appear only at an individual position, except possibly at the left distal position. It is a sign of qi deficiency in the yin organ represented by that position, resulting from stagnation.

Sadness or severe emotional trauma

Appearing only at the left distal position, the Cotton quality indicates an episode that has caused sadness for about one year; at the left distal and middle pulses, for up to three years; and over the entire left side, for five years. When the entire pulse (all three positions on both wrists) presents with the Cotton quality, the condition has persisted for at least ten years and has probably had a notable effect on the entire physiology.

Local trauma

When it appears at only one position, the Cotton quality in one position can be a sign of a minor local trauma, although this usually expresses itself as a bilateral pulse sign. For example, a blow to the chest ordinarily affects both distal positions similarly in terms of pulse quality. With trauma the qualities at the qi, blood, and organ depths are much Tighter than ordinary, usually the result of pain.

Left distal — Without other indications of emotional suppression or local trauma, the Cotton quality at this position alone can be a sign of mild Heart qi and/or blood deficiency.

Right distal — The Cotton quality at this position alone can signify mild Lung qi deficiency.

Left middle — The Cotton quality at this position alone is a sign of Liver qi deficiency which may indicate that the person has worked long hours beyond their level of energy.

Right middle

ULCER AND GASTRITIS

When accompanied by pain and other signs of Stomach heat, the Cotton quality at the right middle position is sometimes a sign of excess stomach acid. Often the eyes show a yellowish tissue medial to the eyeball.

EATING HABITS

The Cotton quality at this position alone can also be a sign of mild Spleen qi deficiency due to habitual failure to pay attention to one's food, with irregular eating patterns, or being upset during mealtimes. The pulse also tends to show Reduced Substance or be Feeble or even Empty. More often these etiologies, which initially cause stagnation and then deficiency, show the Cotton quality over the entire right side or 'digestive system.'

Left proximal — According to Dr. Shen, but outside of my own experience, the Cotton quality at this position alone can be a sign of protracted grief.

Right proximal — According to Dr. Shen, but again outside of my own experience, the Cotton quality at this position alone can be a sign that Small Intestine function is poor.

Floating

Category — The Floating quality is a superficial pulse. The classification of this quality is perhaps more bewildering than any other pulse. One of the main problems in pulse diagnosis,

Fig. 9-2 Floating quality

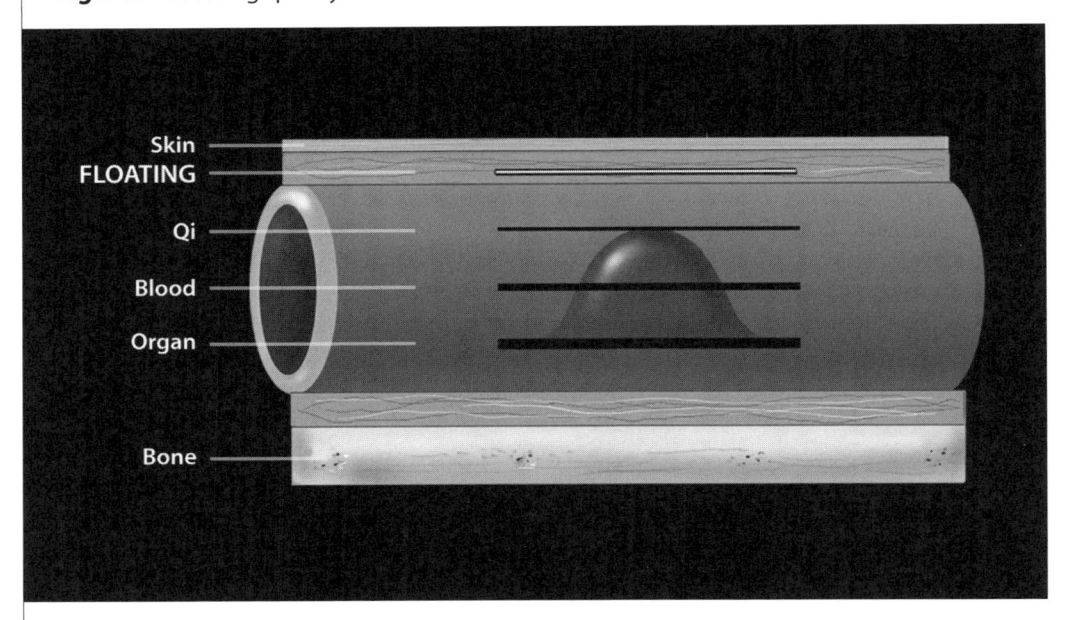

and with the Floating quality in particular, is that many practitioners forget or do not know that the depths are at very specific pressures of the fingers, and not wherever the pulse wave is first accessed. Many practitioners are under the impression that a pulse may be called Floating simply because it is not deep. The qi depth is at a very specific elevation below the skin and above the bone, with some allowance for differences in individual weight, and the Floating quality appears *above* the qi depth, not *at* the qi depth. The source of this confusion is the literature itself, wherein the term Floating can mean any pulse quality that is found only superficially, and not just above the qi depth.

Sensation

The Floating quality (Fig. 9-2) is specifically felt superficial to the qi depth, and has density throughout all depths. Although, as explained below, other pulse qualities may also have a Floating aspect, they can be distinguished from the Floating pulse by other, more enduring characteristics.

The Floating quality is accessed by placing the fingers lightly on the skin, without any pressure, at the proper position above the radial artery. The pulse wave is felt superficially to the qi depth as an outward extension of the qi, or most superficial level of energy. This quality lingers above the qi depth such that the normal sine curve wave is not as apparent until the fingers access the qi depth. The sensation of this quality can be Tense, Tight, or Yielding.[4]

Differentiating Floating from other qualities

Unless one is trained to read the subtleties, the Floating pulse is a quality that is easily confused with other expansive qualities, chiefly the Empty, Inflated, Hollow Full-Overflowing, and Flooding Excess qualities.

FLOATING AND EMPTY

The Floating quality is perhaps more often confused with the Empty quality than any other. The Empty quality is a sign that yin and yang have separated and that yang has lost its anchoring, organizing ground in the yin. By contrast, with one exception (Floating Tight), the Floating quality is a sign of an external pathogenic factor.

The nosological difficulty begins here. Li Shi-Zhen observes, "A pulse which feels strong under slight pressure, but loses its strength when pressure is increased, is classed as a floating pulse."[5] To this, Porkert adds, "As pressure is released the pulse regains its full strength."[6] Thus, the inference is that whenever the Floating quality is encountered, the pulse below the surface lacks strength and is deficient.

Yet this is simply not supported by clinical experience. For example, a condition of wind-heat is usually accompanied by a Floating Yielding quality, and the pulse usually has more strength at the inner depths than above the surface. In other words, the Floating quality does not, as a part of its defining sensation, necessarily lose strength when pressure is increased. Li Shi-Zhen's statement, apparently repeated by rote by those who have followed,[7] has led to the mistaken identification of the Floating with the Empty quality, which by definition *does* lose strength as pressure is increased.

Continuing, it is generally acknowledged that when an attack of wind-cold occurs, the surface of the pulse is Tense, while the deeper aspects appear to be relatively Empty. But this does not mean that the pulse is actually Empty. Rather, it means that below the Tense Floating aspect of the pulse, the quality is essentially normal (unless there is other disharmony) when the qi, blood, and organ depths are all intact. In other words, the loss of strength below is only relative, not absolute. This mistake is even easier to make under conditions of generalized deficiency, where the pulse is naturally less substantial at the qi, blood, and organ depths.

I was taught by Dr. Shen that a pulse which, in the words of Li Shi-Zhen, "feels strong under slight pressure, but loses its strength when pressure is increased,"[8] is actually Empty, not Floating. Substantiating this position, Cheung and Belluomini describe the Floating pulse as follows: "To light palpation, this pulse has more than the normal amount of strength; to heavy palpation, it has less than the normal amount of strength, but does not feel Empty and still responds to the fingers."[9] By contrast, they call the Empty pulse "deficient," noting that the pulse "feels floating, big, slow and soft and is perceptible to light pressure, and feels Empty to increased pressure."[10]

Under our pulse methodology, there may be a Floating aspect accompanying such 'qi wild' pulses as Empty, Leather, Empty Thread-like (soggy), Minute, Hollow, and Scattered. Most of these 'qi wild' qualities are those which are usually accessed at the qi depth, and diminish markedly or even disappear on pressure. The Yielding Hollow Full-Overflowing pulse (also reported below) diminishes or disappears only at the middle depth, and is felt again at the yin organ depth. This might suggest that the degree of disengagement between yin and yang is greater when these qualities are accompanied by a Floating aspect. Or that the 'qi wild' disorder is accompanied by one of the conditions associated with the Floating quality—for example, wind-cold or wind-heat—since one can have a 'qi wild' disorder and still "catch cold."

In the face of this complexity, I reiterate that, in practice, the Floating pulse is a discrete clinical entity from the Empty pulse qualities.

FLOATING AND 'WEAK FLOATING'

Another quality that incorporates the word Floating, thereby adding to the confusion, is the Weak Floating pulse. As used by Mann,[11] Maciocia,[12] and Wu Shui-Wan,[13] it is the same as what we call the Empty Thread-like pulse, and what still others refer to as Soggy or Soft.[14]

The interpretive dilemma continues when the Floating pulse is weak. Kaptchuk[15] and Li Shi-Zhen[16] refer to it as a sign of yin deficiency "because the pulse is active or 'dancing,' a sign of relative Excess Yang and therefore of Deficient Yin."[17] But whereas the disengagement between yin and yang may be attributable to deficient yin, it can occur more often for other reasons, including yang deficiency. Li Shi-Zhen refers to a situation in which blood deficiency is unable to support the qi, which "jumps" to the exterior of the body.[18] Again, the confusion is with the Empty 'qi wild' qualities.

FLOATING AND INFLATED

Trapped or stagnant qi, sometimes in the form of gas in the gastrointestinal tract, is expressed as an Inflated quality on the pulse, commonly misread as Floating because of its round, full, balloon-like sensation. However, by definition, the Inflated quality does not rise above the qi depth. Another example is trapped qi and heat in the Lungs and Heart. Although it is actually Inflated, this can also feel expansive and Floating if one is not correctly accessing the qi depth. With the Inflated quality the stagnation is internal, while with the Floating quality it is external.

FLOATING AND COTTON

The Cotton quality appears above the qi depth. It is completely amorphous, with no shape except for a spongy, formless sense of resistance as the finger moves back and forth from the surface of the skin to the qi depth. This distinguishes it from the Floating quality, which has shape such as Tension.

FLOATING AND HOLLOW FULL-OVERFLOWING

Excessive blood heat and 'blood thick' in the general circulation, and especially in the Liver, is identified by the Tense Hollow Full-Overflowing pulse. This quality is often associated with hypertension, and less often with summerheat. Like the Floating quality, the Tense Hollow Full-Overflowing pulse is palpated above the qi depth, but is always Hollow below, and is usually Pounding. There is also a Yielding Hollow Full-Overflowing quality associated with extreme qi deficiency or separation of yin and yang. In contrast to the Floating quality, which has no wave pattern, both of these other qualities have a full sine curve wave above the qi depth.

FLOATING AND FLOODING EXCESS

While the Flooding Excess quality appears above the qi depth, it is usually Pounding; and instead of having no wave, like the Floating quality, it has a sine curve that falls off suddenly at the apex. Li Shi-Zhen identifies the Floating quality with the Flooding quality if it has "strong beats."[19] The Flooding Excess quality is a sign of heat from excess in the yin organs.

Etiology, pathogenesis and interpretation

In general, the Floating quality is a sign of increased activity of the superficial, quicker energies of the body. These energies are called upon to either defend against or rid the body of external pathogenic factors. In the case of the former, the associated pulse is the true Floating quality, which indicates disharmony at the body surface. In the case of the latter, depending on the pathogenic factor, the Floating quality is differentiated by the tenseness or pliability and the rate of the pulse. Li Shi-Zhen notes, which I cannot corroborate, that "When felt during autumn, the floating pulse is an indication of health."[20] Interpretations of specific Floating qualities are described below.

External disharmony

External pathogenic factors stimulate the body to mobilize the protective qi at the surface of the body. The indication is that the true qi, of which the protective qi is a manifestation, is strong, and that the subject can resist disease. It should also be mentioned that when external pathogenic factors invade internally, especially into the lesser yang stage of the six stages, chronic respiratory disorders such as allergies and asthma may result. The Floating quality can appear over the entire pulse (all positions on both wrists) or be confined to the distal positions and the Special Lung positions in the acute stages. In the later stages the Floating quality is usually found at the right distal and Special Lung positions.

External pathogenic factor: early stage

When an external pathogenic factor such as wind, wind-cold, or wind-heat attacks, the pulse will be Floating. With wind-cold, there will also be slight Tension, and with heat, a Yielding quality.

External pathogenic factor: later stage

When an external pathogenic factor invades the Lungs and reaches the lesser yang (six divisions) or qi level (four levels) in such disorders as allergies, asthma, bronchitis, and pneumonia, the right distal position can still be slightly Floating, Flooding Excess, Pounding Inflated Tense. The Special Lung position is Floating Pounding Slippery Tight. (For a complete discussion of these signs, see right distal position in Chapter 10.)

Wind-cold

Floating Tense and slightly Slow

The pulse is Floating Tense and slightly Slow; this may include the entire pulse or be confined to the distal, especially the right distal, and to the Special Lung positions. Symptoms of this pattern include chills, aversion to cold, muscular aches and pains, cough, headache, stuffy nose, mild fever, and mild sweating (when deficiency is also present). The tongue is slightly moist and has a thin white coating.

Wind-heat

Floating Yielding and slightly Rapid

The pulse is Floating Yielding and slightly Rapid; this may include the entire pulse or be confined to the distal, especially the right distal, and to the Special Lung positions. The symptoms are the same as those of the wind-cold pattern, except that the chills and aversion to cold are less severe, the fever is higher, and the thirst more severe. The tongue has a thin, white, and dry coating.

Wind

Floating Yielding with Normal rate

The pulse is more Floating and Yielding, the rate Normal, and the signs and symptoms are the same—but less severe and more transient—than those associated with the wind-cold and wind-heat patterns.

Phlegm with wind-cold or wind-heat

When dampness (and the resultant phlegm) accompanies a wind-cold or wind-heat pattern, the Floating quality is attended by the Slippery quality. This quality, also known as wind-water, is a sign of stagnation of qi (wind-cold) or agitation of qi (wind-heat), which interferes with the movement of fluids at the surface of the body. The Floating Slippery quality is sometimes associated with hives.

Internal Disharmony

LIVER WIND

Floating Tight

The Floating Tight quality is a sign of Liver wind and is usually found initially at the left middle position. Later, as the condition becomes more serious, the Floating Tight quality can appear over the entire pulse. This quality is an internally-generated precursor to stroke, preceded or accompanied by wind in the channels, characterized by transient neurological symptoms such as numbness, tingling, other parasthesias, and transient aschemic attacks (TIA). Prior to a major stroke it may evolve, without correction, into the very Tight Full-Overflowing quality.

Combinations

The Floating quality can appear with almost any other quality. For example, an individual with an internally-generated disorder may, at the same time, catch a cold or the flu, in which case the pulse will become transiently Floating, in addition to its other qualities.[21]

In the literature, the Floating quality may also be associated with interior deficiency. But I have rarely found this to be the case. Rather, most of these so-called deficient Floating pulses are actually Empty pulses. This is because the Empty quality is felt only at the qi depth, and is often wrongly perceived as Floating.

Here is a list of combinations that I have identified with this pulse.

- Floating Tense and Slow: wind-cold in the channels and collaterals
- Floating Yielding and slightly Rapid: wind-heat
- Floating Tense Rapid: external cold becoming internalized and transforming into heat
- Floating Yielding and Slow: prolonged and unresolved external pathogenic factor in an individual whose qi is becoming depleted
- Floating Flooding Excess, or Hollow Full-Overflowing Wide: invasion of summerheat
- Floating Slippery: wind-water
- Floating Tight: internal Liver wind[22]

Positions

BILATERALLY AT SAME POSITION

As previously noted, the Floating quality is, with one exception, a sign of invasion by an external pathogenic factor.

Distal position

Floating Tense and Slow

This is a sign of current wind-cold with symptoms of upper respiratory infection. The tongue is moist with a thin white coating.

Floating Tense with Normal or slightly Rapid rate

This is a sign of unresolved external cold. The indication here is that cold has entered the deeper channels, the chest, or the Lungs, creating qi stagnation. To overcome the stagnation, the body brings heat to the area, which gradually accumulates if the stagnation is not resolved. This pulse is more likely to occur in a stronger person whose body is capable of mobilizing the heat.

Floating Yielding and Rapid

This is a sign of a current invasion by wind-heat.

SIDES

Again, with one exception, the pulses attributed to the Floating quality on one or the other wrist are not truly Floating. Rather, the Tense, Pounding, and Flooding Excess pulses, as well as the Hollow Full-Overflowing pulse, are often confused with the Floating quality on the left side. But on the left side, there is occasionally a Floating Tight quality. On the right, the Inflated quality is mistakenly called Floating. To reiterate, the Floating quality appears only above the qi depth, and shows no special wave characteristics; both of these attributes distinguish this quality from the others mentioned here.

INDIVIDUAL POSITIONS

With one exception, the true Floating quality is found only over the entire pulse, bilaterally at the distal positions, especially the right distal, and only when external pathogenic factors are present. If found at other individual positions, the Floating quality is only apparent, and not real, except the Floating Tight quality, which is found mostly as the left middle position.

Left distal — At the left distal and the Large Vessel positions, the Tense Hollow Full-Overflowing and Pounding pulse, and the Inflated pulse, can be mistaken for the Floating pulse, which is rarely found here alone.

Right distal and Special Lung — The Empty and Inflated qualities are the two pulses most commonly mistaken for the Floating pulse in these positions. When found only in these positions, the Floating quality is an early sign of an external pathogenic factor.

Left middle — At this position the qualities mistaken for Floating include the Empty, Hollow Full-Overflowing, and the Flooding Excess Pounding. A Floating Tight quality is found at this position with Liver wind.

Right middle and Stomach-Pylorus Extension — Qualities mistaken for Floating at the right middle position are the Inflated, Empty, and Hollow Full-Overflowing.

Proximal — Generally, the pulse in the proximal positions tends to be deeper than in the other positions. Therefore, an apparent Floating quality in the proximal positions is even rarer than in the other positions. The Flooding Excess and the Empty Tense Hollow Full-Overflowing qualities have been mistaken for the Floating quality in the proximal positions.

Empty

Category — Although not mentioned in his book, Dr. Shen frequently referred to the Empty quality during our years together in the clinic. This quality is classified as superficial because, as

Dr. Shen uses the term, it is felt only at the qi depth. It is actually not Floating, which in our system is a quality that is palpated superficial to the qi depth.

The sensation of the Empty quality is often confused with, and must be differentiated from, the Hollow pulse. The Empty quality and certain kinds of Hollow qualities are signs of dangerous disharmonies. The Yielding Hollow Full-Overflowing pulses are associated with a 'qi wild' disorder of distinctly different etiology, and signal a much more serious pathology.[23]

The term Empty in the Chinese medical literature has come to have two meanings: symptoms of deficiency (as opposed to excess), and the discrete pulse quality referred to as Empty by almost all sources. The distinction between Empty symptoms and the Empty pulse quality has become muddled over the centuries, even in works by the most capable writers.

Sensation

The Empty quality (Figs. 9-3a~c) is superficial and is accessed at the qi depth. The Empty quality separates and diminishes significantly, or even disappears, as pressure increases to the blood and organ depths. It can also feel Tight, Tense, or Yielding at the surface depending on the associated disorder. (Very rarely is the Empty quality accessed above the qi depth; when it is, it is a sign of even greater physiological chaos.)[24]

Differentiating the Empty and Floating qualities

As emphasized earlier in this chapter in our discussion of the Floating quality, the Empty and Floating qualities are overwhelmingly confused in the literature. They are two separate and distinct qualities, both in sensation and meaning. The Floating pulse is not Empty. The only defining sensation of the Floating quality is that it is specifically felt superficial to the qi depth and has no wave form.

Interpretation

In the opinion of Dr. Shen, which is supported by my own experience, this quality, when found over the entire pulse, is usually a serious—although the least dangerous—sign of a 'qi wild' disorder. At first, only the qi and blood are affected, and not the organs. The patient looks healthy, but feels extremely tired and has no energy. In the long run, however, it may affect the organs. Dr. Shen believes that, if not already ill, a person with an Empty pulse that is also Yielding will become clinically ill within six months. With the Feeble-Absent quality, Dr. Shen says that it will take longer—more like a year—to become ill.

The key to understanding the Empty quality is that the ineluctable physiologic relationship between the expansive yang (qi) and the centripetal, sinking, and heavier yin aspects (fluids and blood) has been injured. The yin serves as a centripetal organizing matrix for the yang. The yang is expansive and is held in check only by the centripetal force of the more substantial yin energies. While Dr. Shen, in our discussions, attributed this condition to extremely deficient yang alone, I believe that anything that causes the yin and yang to lose this functional affiliation, which is essential to health and harmony, will do so. If the yin is sufficiently depleted and is unable to nourish the yang, the yang floats away aimlessly to the surface; communication is then broken, the qi becomes 'wild,' and the Empty pulse quality results. If the yang is deficient and is unable to move the yin, the result is the same. Kaptchuk refers to this as "Qi not governing or 'wrapping' the blood."[25]

The 'qi wild' condition is characterized by chaos. It represents the most serious disorganization and disruption of overall physiology. Cancer is, by definition, physiology that is chaotic, that has become 'wild.' Occurrence of the Empty pulse can be an early sign of an impending neoplastic process. Mental illness is also a form of chaos. In certain situations the Empty quality is a marker for the anarchy of severe neurosis and psychosis.

By way of example, I once examined on separate occasions two patients, one an adult, the other an only child, each of whose pulse was completely Empty but more Tense than usual. At first I was alarmed at the significance of the extensive qi deficiency in each, and treated them for this, which changed nothing. I learned quickly that I was dealing with an Empty quality that was unrelated to its classical interpretation. It was a sign instead that the individual had lost his center and was literally floating aimlessly, with extreme anxiety and related somatic manifestations.

Also, those whose adaptation to socialization or to anxiety is to become extroverted can present with a transient Empty quality initially as an energetic expression of this exuberance. Under the circumstances of a lengthy pulse examination the Empty quality quickly disappears and the enduring, valid pulse picture emerges.

Entire pulse

Over the entire pulse the Empty quality is usually a sign that the body's true qi has reached a critical state of deficiency in which the yin and yang have separated. This is the 'qi wild' condition or 'danger pulse' which, Dr. Shen warns, presages imminent major illness. He indicates a time frame of six months, although I believe that the range is more like three months to three years, if corrective measures are not taken.

Individual position

At an individual position the Empty quality is largely a sign that yin and yang have separated at the organ represented by that position, which is probably also extremely deficient. This is similar to the 'qi wild' condition, where the yin and yang are separated, except that here the chaos and deficiency is limited to one organ. Although outside my experience, the Empty quality is also reported to have been found at the position representing an organ which has been surgically removed, such as the gallbladder or uterus.

Etiology

The causes that lead to this quality are usually a combination of impoverished environment, including inadequate nutrition, shelter, and clothing; work beyond one's energy; drug abuse; premature or excessive sex; or constitutional deficiency. Especially when these factors occur between the ages of fifteen and twenty, the quality that develops is the Empty pulse.

In terms of overwork beyond one's energy, this can also include physical exercise. I have seen this increasingly, especially among young people who are being pushed to exercise harder and harder at younger and younger ages. Particularly with girls and young women, overexercise is becoming the most common source of a completely Empty pulse. (Another complication, discussed below with the Hollow pulse qualities, occurs upon the sudden cessation of exercise.) Exercise causes the blood vessels to expand beyond their normal size. Individuals who persistently exercise beyond their level of energy cannot generate sufficient blood to fill the expanded vessels. The consequence, in Chinese medical terms, is a functional disengagement of the heavier yin energy from the lighter yang energy. Cheung and Belluomini note, in connection with this pulse, that "the vessel is dilated and thus is heart and nervous system regulated. There is weak tonus of the arterial wall, and insufficient filling of blood in the vessel."[26]

The symptoms that can result include fatigue and migrating joint pain accompanied by severe anxiety and panic attacks, which are only partially attributable to experiences of dissociation and depersonalization. Patients report feeling as if parts of their body were floating away, especially their arms and legs when they lie down. This is the consequence of dysfunctional yang qi energy which is no longer grounded or nourished by the yin.

The other increasingly important causes of this pulse quality are the use of recreational drugs, especially among the young, and, to a slightly lesser extent, liver infection. Sometimes alone and sometimes accompanying the abuse of drugs is a history of either mononucleosis or hepatitis. With these etiologies the Empty quality is usually confined to the left middle (Liver) position.

When this pulse is the result of a lifetime of physical or emotional insults, the condition is serious, and the treatment prolonged and difficult. If the Empty pulse occurs in the course of a serious illness, it may indicate impending death, as one of the eight pulses that portend death.[27]

Figs. 9-3a Empty quality (early stage)

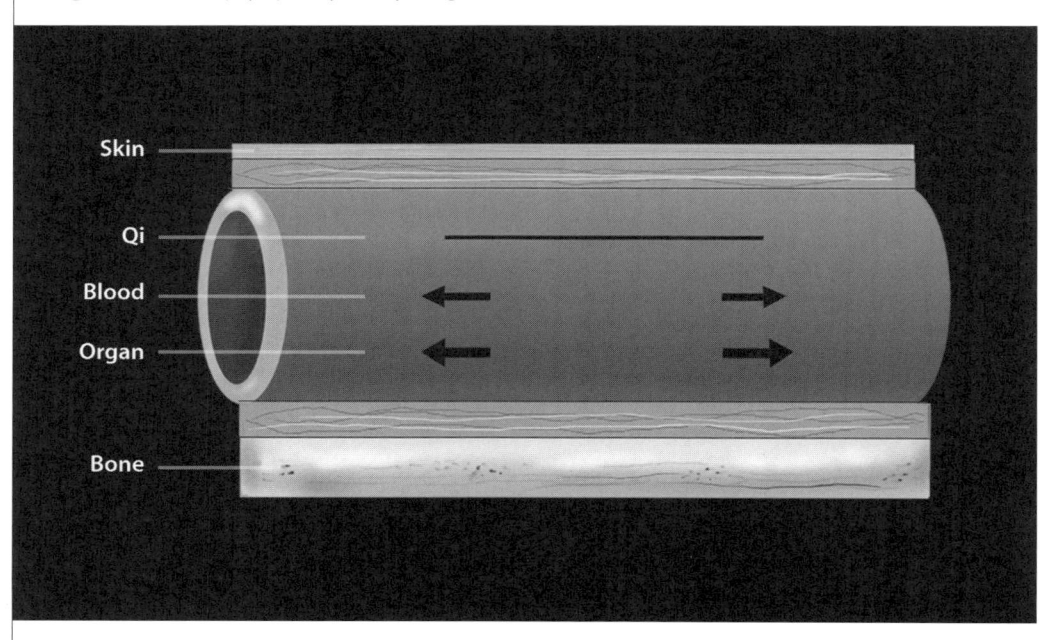

Figs. 9-3b Empty quality (middle stage)

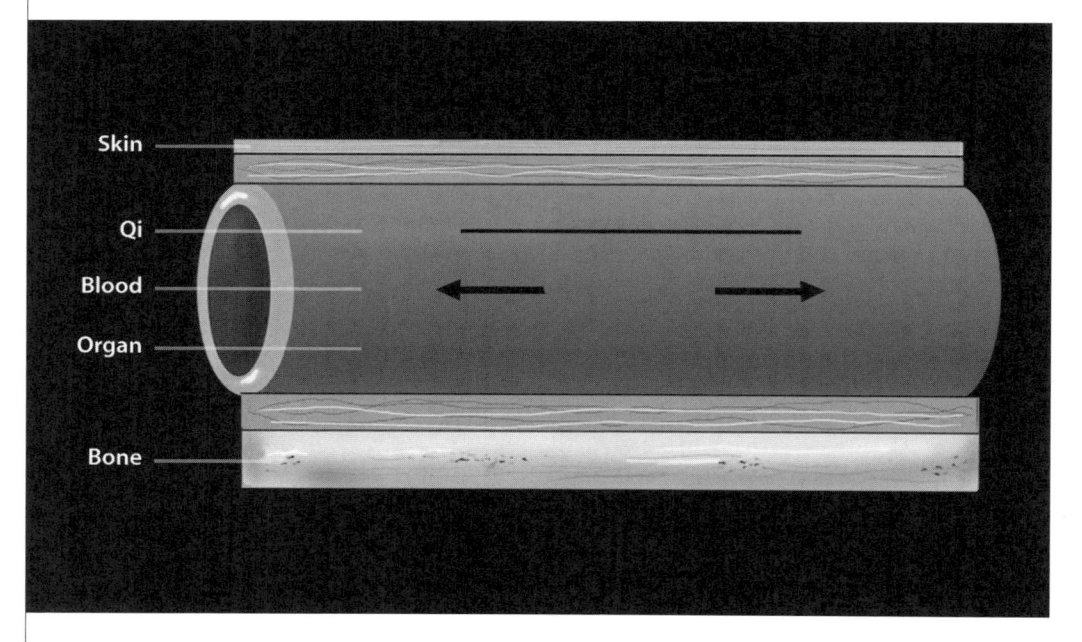

Figs. 9-3c Empty quality (later stage)

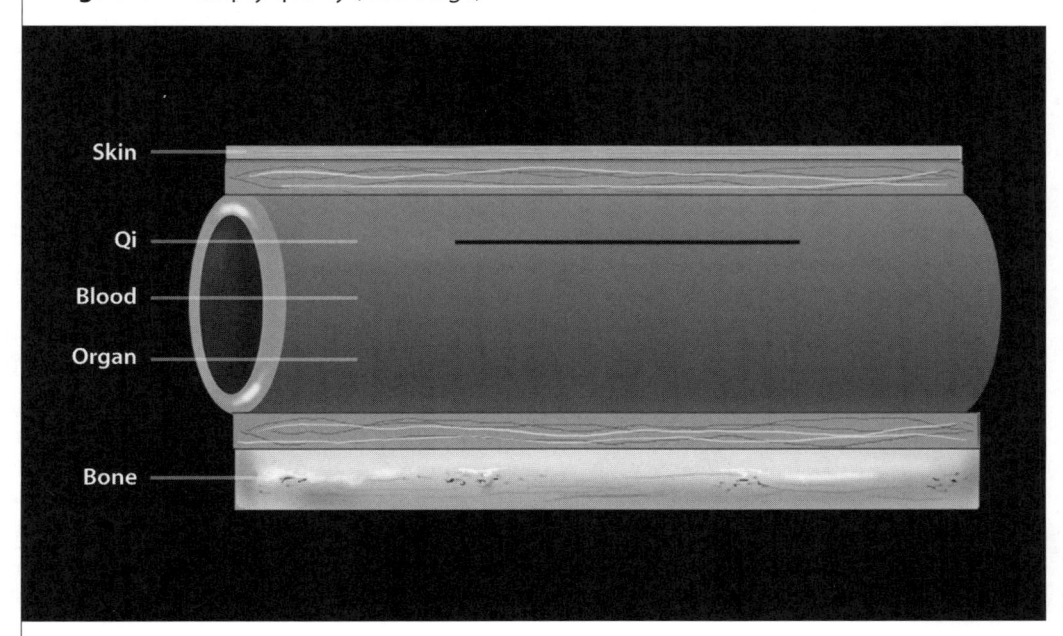

- Skin
- Qi
- Blood
- Organ
- Bone

Combinations

FREQUENT COMBINATIONS

The following are the most common and important types of Empty pulses.[28]

Empty Yielding and Slow

The Empty Yielding pulse with a Slow rate that appears simultaneously in all six positions signifies extreme deficiency of true qi, even more so than the Feeble-Absent quality. This qi deficiency deprives the organ systems of nourishment and diminishes their effectiveness, and leads to the separation of yin and yang and the chaotic 'qi wild' condition. When found at an individual position, the yin organ represented by that position is severely qi deficient, and the yin and yang have separated.

Empty Tight and Rapid

One scenario associated with this form of 'qi wild' is the lesser yin heat stage of the lesser yin or absolute yin stages of disease. Here, the entire body energy—yin and yang—is depleted, and yang escapes to the surface. The accompanying symptoms are those associated with heat: elevated temperature, irritability, restlessness, flushed face, and insomnia. In this connection, Li Shi-Zhen observes, "Internal heat is caused by yin deficiency—the yin is unable to nourish the yang. To treat, nourish the yin and the heat will decrease."[29]

Empty Moderately Tense

I have observed this combination with post-traumatic stress syndrome, as a phenomenon in extremely tense people who have been under unusual stress to which they have not successfully adapted. It is a sign that they have lost their centers and that their spirits are dispersed. Li Shi-Zhen states that this pulse appears "after palpitations caused by heart blood deficiency, or after fear or fright caused by heart shen [spirit] deficiency."[30] I have found this pulse quality at the special Lung position in persons who are grieving the recent loss of someone to whom they were very close.

LESS FREQUENT COMBINATIONS

Empty Interrupted-Intermittent

With this combination the instability is already in the yin organs, especially the Heart. Severe disease is present or imminent. Here, the Empty quality signifies that the yang is no longer balanced by yin and is out of control, and that the qi is 'wild.' The Intermittent and Interrupted qualities are signs that the Heart qi is out of control. While separately each is a sign of serious physiologic dysfunction, the combination of 'qi wild' and Heart qi out of control is one of the most profound 'qi wild' pulse combinations in Chinese medicine. The significance of this combination is that the problem began very early in life, at least before the age of five, and possibly at birth or even during pregnancy. Usually, the weaker the left distal (Kidney) position, the earlier the etiology began.

Empty at proximal and middle positions

When both the proximal (Kidney root) and right middle positions are Empty, the primary source of the problem is the Kidneys, which is linked to severe deprivation before the age of fifteen, or to constitutional deficiency. Spleen qi and yang depend on the Kidney yang fire ('fire of the gate of vitality'), which some equate with the function of the thyroid gland in driving the metabolism.

Positions

The following refers only to the Yielding or slightly Taut (Long) type of Empty quality. While the etiologies are similar to lesser degrees of deficiency and chaos, either the person was more deficient at the outset, or the events occurred over a much longer time or were of a greater degree.

BILATERALLY AT SAME POSITION

Distal

The Empty quality is rare at the distal positions. When found, it can be due to the following causes.

Overwork of chest and Lungs

Work beyond one's energy involving the upper burner, such as singing, talking, or playing a wind instrument, especially in a person who was initially deficient, can, over a long period of time, result in the Empty Yielding quality at this position.

Physical trauma

Unresolved circulatory stagnation due to trauma to the chest area in a very deficient person can give rise to the Empty Yielding quality at this position over a long period of time. The progression of pulse qualities would be first the Inflated, then the Flat, followed by the Feeble-Absent, and finally the Empty Yielding pulse.

Middle

Emotional trauma

A profound loss or disappointment experienced by a very deficient person, especially in childhood, can lead to this pulse quality in late adulthood. Again, the Empty pulse will be preceded by the Flat and then the Feeble-Absent qualities.[31]

Grief

Grief for the recent loss of a loved one, found more often at the Special Lung positions.

Impoverishment

Impoverishment due to inadequate nutrition, especially during childhood and adolescence, can give rise to the Empty quality at the middle position bilaterally.

Sitting bent over

Depressed individuals suffering sadness can develop this quality when they persistently sit in a hunched-over position, with head in hands. Likewise, those who sit hunched over as part of their work can, over a long period of time, develop the Empty quality at this position. Initially there is qi stagnation, followed by food stagnation, with gradual depletion in the gastrointestinal system leading to an Empty quality at the middle positions.

Rumination

An Empty quality across the middle position can develop when an individual habitually ruminates while eating. Excessive thinking drains the Spleen qi, particularly when this qi is simultaneously required for digestion. This quality represents severe Spleen qi deficiency, which has caused the Liver energy to overwork in a compensatory effort to move the qi in the digestive system.

Resuming work too soon after eating

Returning to work too soon after eating can, over a long period of time, lead to the Empty Yielding and Slow quality, especially when the work is physical.

Physical trauma

Trauma in a very weak person, or circulatory shock that remains unresolved for a long period of time, can induce the Empty quality at the middle position.

Liver attacking the Spleen

Both middle positions will be Empty when the Liver attacks the Spleen over a long period of time. On the surface, the Liver pulse in the left middle position is usually slightly Tight Empty, and the right middle Stomach/Spleen more Empty Yielding. Digestive symptoms such as belching, distention, and hypochondria pain are typically present.

Anorexia and bulimia

I have also observed the Empty quality bilaterally at the middle position with advanced anorexia or bulimia, although with the latter it is more Tight, and with the former more Yielding. Also, a diet of foods that are difficult to digest—such as brown rice—can, over time, lead to severe digestive problems attended by the Empty quality. This signifies exhaustion of Spleen qi due to the energy expended by the digestive organs in trying to digest and assimilate undigestable food.

Chronic parasites

Chronic parasites drain Liver and Spleen qi which, over time, can manifest as an Empty quality bilaterally at the middle positions.

Pancreatic failure

Severe pancreatic insufficiency has been attended by an Empty quality bilaterally at the middle positions.[32]

Proximal

The Empty quality, representing Kidney yang deficiency, is rare at this position. If it does occur, the cause may be constitutional deficiency, excessive sexual activity, severe and prolonged menorrhagia or colitis, or any long-term behavior that abuses and drains an organ; the Kidneys will compensate for any deficiency with their own stored essence. Other causes are chronic menorrhagia and subclinical colitis.[33]

SIDES

Left

The Empty quality over just the entire left side is a sign that the yin organ system is profoundly deficient and chaotic, usually attended by severe fatigue. According to Dr. Shen, if, at the same time, the entire right side of the pulse is more or less normal, this means that the 'digestive system' is trying to compensate for the deficiency in the 'organ system,' and is capable of doing so.

Right

The Empty quality over the entire right side signifies a seriously deficient and chaotic 'digestive system.' If the left side of the pulse is simultaneously normal, the yin 'organ system' is still intact.

INDIVIDUAL POSITIONS

The Empty quality at a single position represents the separation of yin and yang associated with severe qi, yin, and blood deficiency in the organ represented by that position. While outside my own experience, others have found this quality at one position to correspond to an organ that had been removed.

Left distal

The Empty quality at this position is rare, but can appear with severe Heart qi or yang deficiency leading to a separation of Heart yin and yang.

Right distal

The Empty quality at this position indicates severe qi deficiency of the Lungs leading to the separation of Lung yin and yang. Kaptchuk associates this sign with "spontaneous sweating," which I interpret as indicating severe qi deficiency, especially protective qi.[34]

Left middle

The Empty quality at this position represents the separation of Liver yin and yang associated with severe Liver qi-yang deficiency. Long-term consequences are lymphomas and other cancers of the liver. I have often found this quality in persons who have substantial past or current histories of marijuana, LSD, and heroine use. Mononucleosis, subacute or chronic hepatitis, and parasitosis can often lead to the Empty quality at this position. Extreme overwork beyond one's energy over a long period of time is another etiology.

Kaptchuk indicates that the Empty quality at this position is due to the "blood [being] unable to nourish [the] tendons," which suggests Liver blood deficiency secondary to Liver qi deficiency.[35] Worsley mentions "paralysis, anaemia, [and] shortness of Chi" as symptoms.[36]

Right middle	The Empty quality at this position is a sign of the separation of Spleen yin and yang associated with severe Spleen qi-yang deficiency. The accompanying symptoms of Spleen qi deficiency include lassitude, sallow complexion, loss of appetite, and either diarrhea or constipation.[37] The separation of Spleen yin and yang lends itself to the development of stomach and pancreatic neoplasms and lymphomas.
Left proximal	The Empty pulse at this position is a sign of Kidney qi or yang deficiency leading to the separation of Kidney yin and yang. Although this interpretation is linked to the appearance of the Empty quality at this position alone, it is often accompanied by an Empty quality at the right proximal position as well. And in conjunction with an Empty quality at the left middle position, it is a sign of a very deficient 'organ system.' In younger persons, the presence of this quality at the left proximal position is a sign that the deficiency is of constitutional or congenital origin. When the proximal pulses are Empty, the 'root' energy of the *ming men* (gate of vitality) in particular is depleted.[38]
Right proximal	The Empty quality at the right proximal position is also a sign of Kidney qi or yang deficiency leading to the separation of yin and yang. In my experience, it is rare to have an Empty quality at the right proximal position without the left proximal position also being Empty. Dr. Shen reported that the Empty quality at this position indicates inflammation of the prostate, which I have never personally observed. Kaptchuk mentions "dark urine [and] constipation,"[39] and Worsley "cold pain [in the] belly, diarrhea, [and] sore joints."[40]

Yielding Empty Thread-like

Category	Although this quality can be classified with the reduced-volume pulses, I have placed it here with the superficial pulses, for that is the only depth at which the Yielding Empty Thread-like quality is felt.[41]
Sensation	The terms Soggy and Soft, used elsewhere in the literature, do not convey the true sensation since the pulse does not, overall, actually feel soggy or soft. Yielding Empty Thread-like (Figs. 9-4a and 9-4b) is a more accurate and less confusing description of what is really felt, which is like a thread floating on water at the qi depth. Like the Empty quality, the Yielding Empty Thread-like quality separates or disappears under pressure.[42]
Interpretation	Yielding Empty Thread-like is a rare pulse quality which I have found to be a sign of extreme deficiency of yin and yang. It is found primarily in persons who are in the terminal stages of disease, and is a more severe sign of a 'qi wild' condition than the Empty pulse.[43]
Combinations	I have no experience with combinations involving this pulse.
Positions	I am familiar with this quality only when it appears simultaneously over the entire pulse at all positions, as a sign of a 'qi wild' disorder. The patient is almost always in the latter stages of a terminal illness. Yet in our time it is rare for a practitioner of Chinese medicine to pre-empt biomedicine in treating patients at this stage of an illness. Accordingly, I have no experience with this pulse and its associated symptoms at individual pulse positions.[44] This quality has been reported to me by students who are nurses in intensive care facilities or who treat AIDS patients.

Fig. 9-4a Yielding Empty Thread-like quality (early stage)

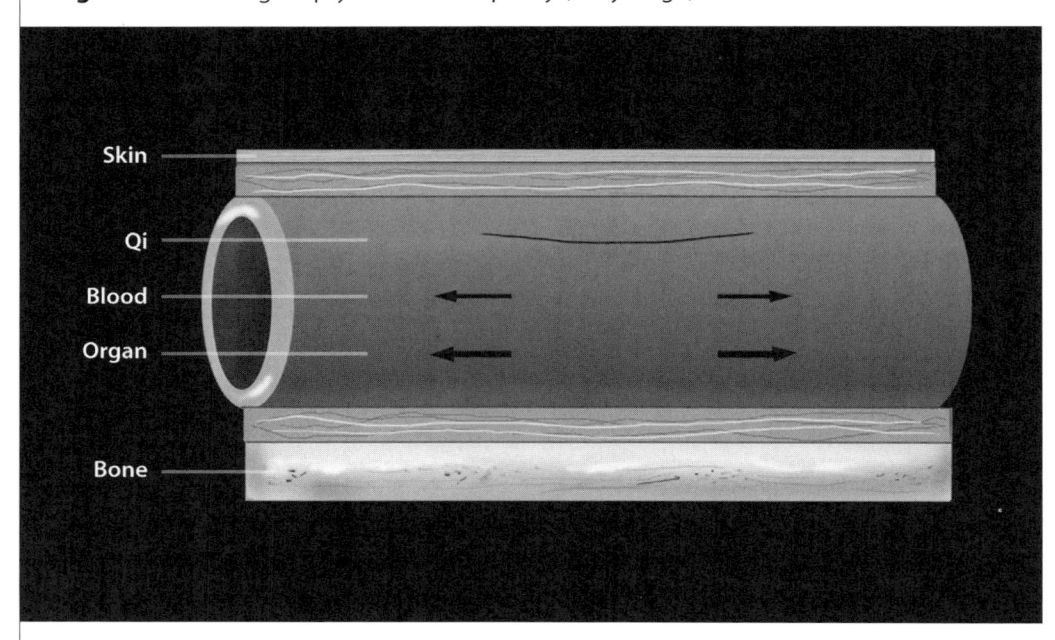

Fig. 9-4b Yielding Empty Thread-like quality (later stage)

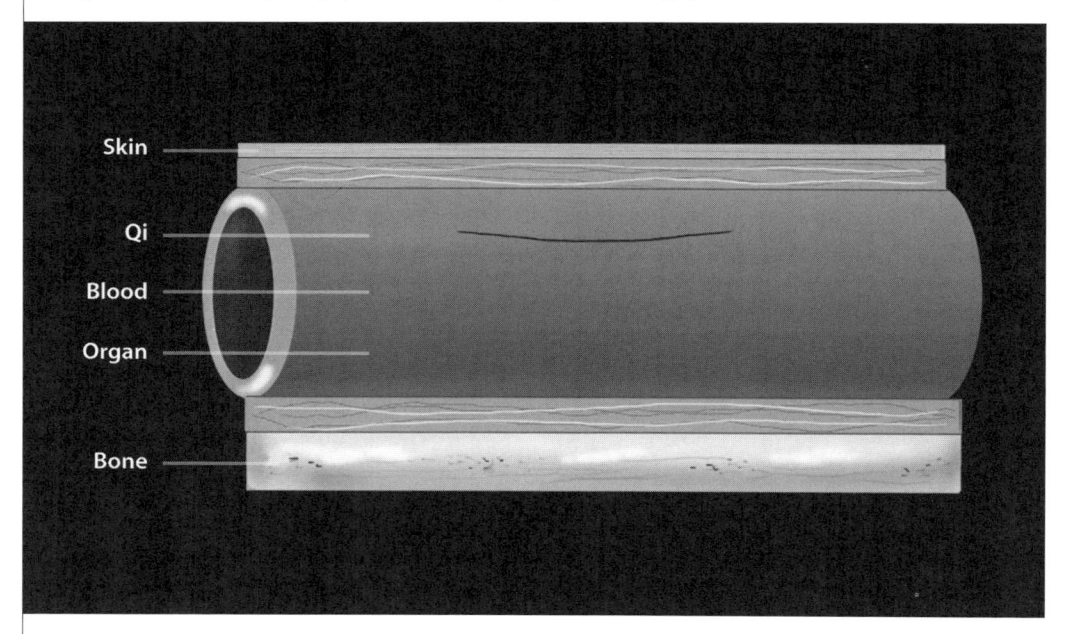

Category

Leather

The Leather quality is rare. In the literature it is always classified as a Floating pulse, which is why I place it with the superficial pulses. However, as explained earlier, like most other superficial pulses, it does not meet the criteria of a Floating quality because it is not found above the qi depth. The Leather quality is called drum-like by Worsley,[45] and tympanic by Porkert.[46] It is not mentioned by Dr. Shen.

Fig. 9-5a Leather quality (early stage)

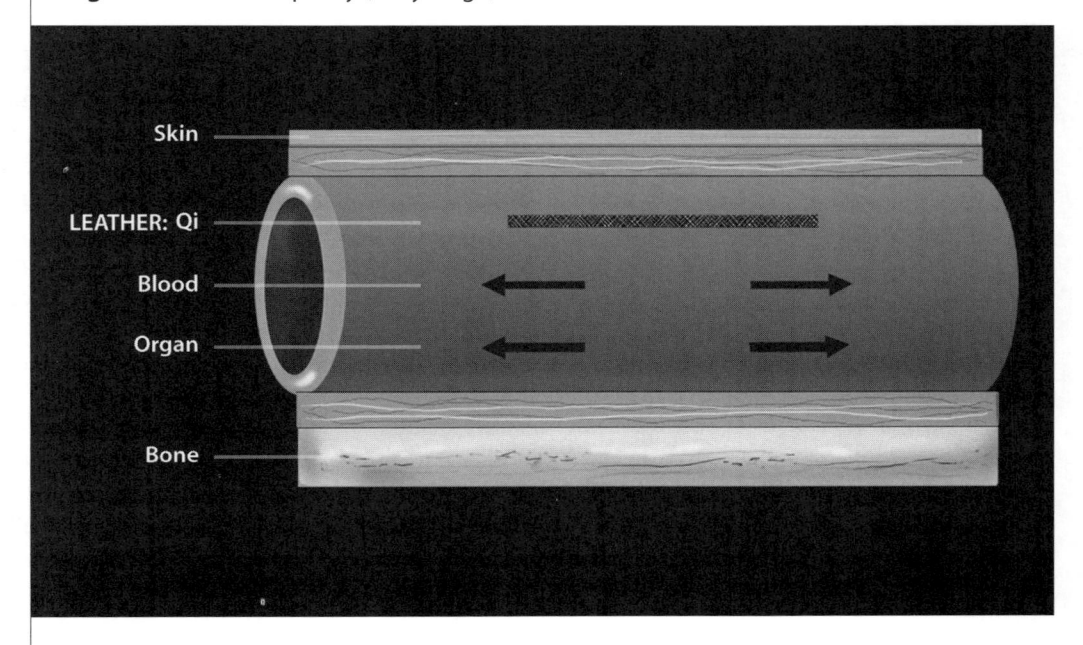

Fig. 9-5b Leather quality (later stage)

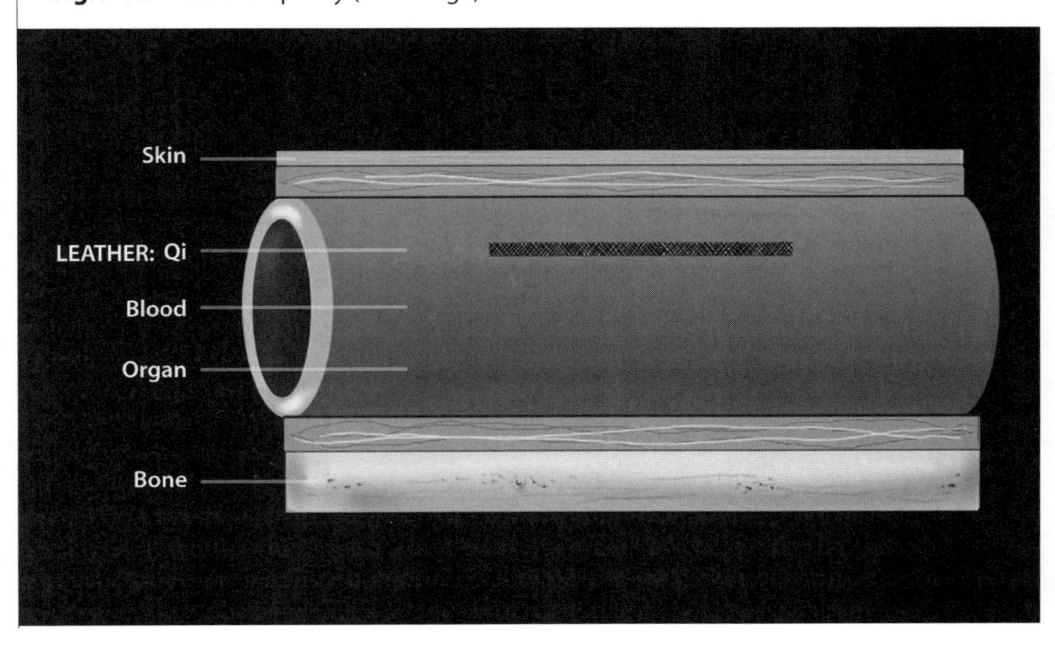

Sensation

Amber sums up my experience, as well as the descriptions in other sources, when he says that the Leather pulse is "like touching the surface of a drum."[47] Kaptchuk speaks of this quality as "a combination of the Wiry and Floating pulses, with aspects of the Empty pulse."[48] Li Shi-Zhen adds that it "feels wiry, almost rapid and without substance in its center" and "is a combination of hollow and wiry."[49] (See Figs. 9-5a and 9-5b.)

The dilemma in the literature centers around whether the pulse is Empty or Hollow. The diagrams found in the sources, including Li Shi-Zhen,[50] Kaptchuk,[51] and Cheung and Belluomini,[52] display the Empty pulse. My experience is that the quality is Empty.

All of the traditional interpretations of the Leather-like Hollow pulse (discussed in Chapter 13) mention *acute* blood loss, while interpretations of the Leather, Soggy, and Empty qualities are associated with the *gradual* loss of substances such as qi, yin, blood, or essence.

Interpretation

The Leather quality is a sign of extreme essence, yin, and especially blood depletion. It is another rare pulse which, in my opinion, is similar in meaning to the Empty pulse in terms of its association with the separation of yin and yang in a 'qi wild' disorder. The relative hardness at the surface indicates that there is greater yin, essence, and blood depletion than with the Empty quality. Another explanation is that the separation of yin from yang which occurs with both qualities is greater with the Leather quality, because the heat from deficiency that accompanies the expanding and escaping yang as it rises to the surface tends to give the pulse a greater sensation of density.[53]

Combinations

I have no experience with combinations involving this pulse.[54]

Positions

Although the Leather quality is usually found over the entire pulse, it can theoretically appear at an individual position alone, or at any combination of positions. No matter the pulse scenario, this quality has the same meaning and must always be viewed as serious. I have never encountered it bilaterally at the same position, nor on one side alone, nor at an individual position. Otherwise, I have encountered this quality only rarely.

Scattered

Category

This is one of the most serious of the Empty qualities, falling into the category of 'qi wild'.[55] A pulse term that has recently come into prominence, and which underlines the seriousness of this quality, is "ceiling dripping," found frequently in AIDS patients.

Sensation

The Scattered quality (Fig. 9-6) is felt only at the qi depth where it is more indistinct than the Empty quality. Instead of feeling continuous, it disperses on pressure into separate pieces, as if divided. This is especially true when the fingers are rolled proximally and distally along the radial artery. With light pressure the quality gradually disappears and is totally indiscernible at the deeper aspects.

My favorite description of this quality is "superficial pulse, like willow flowers scattering in the wind." This is one of the few classical metaphors which translate into a recognizable sensation after one has learned it in a clinical context. I have also heard it called "broken," another appropriate term. Because of its broken, discontinuous sensation, some practitioners mistake this quality for the Interrupted pulse, where the rhythm is discontinuous. What is a disturbance in the continuity of substance feels like a disturbance in the continuity of cadence.

Dr. Shen writes that this quality "fluctuates between being strong and weak. Sometimes it can be felt, sometimes not."[56]

Fig. 9-6 Scattered quality

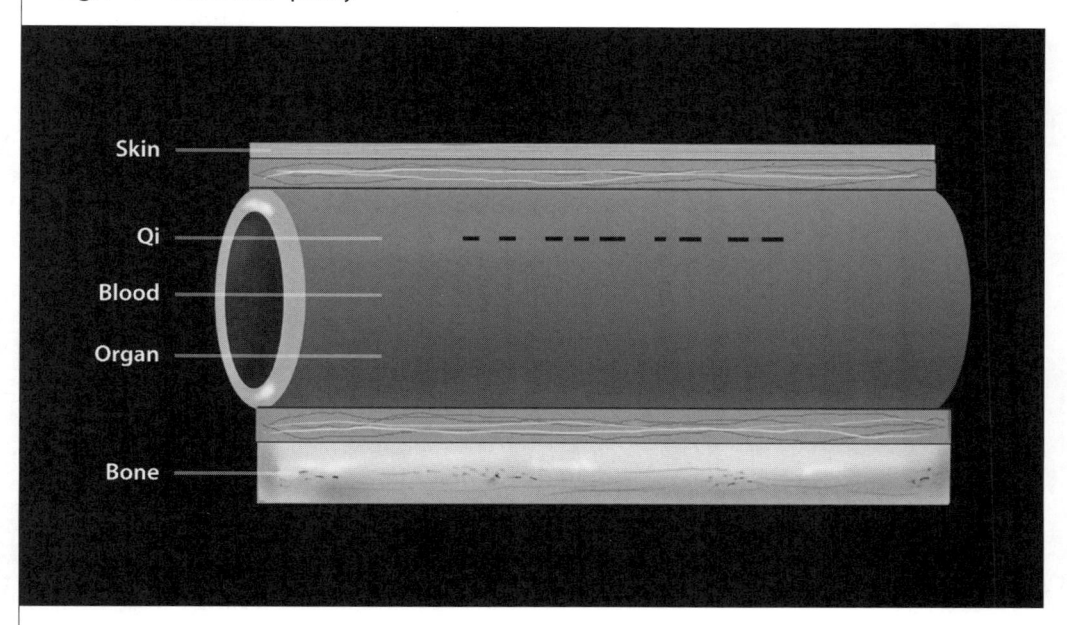

Interpretation

The Scattered quality occurs with profound deficiency of qi, blood, and yang—especially Kidney yang—and is a sign of extreme 'qi wild.' Along with pulses that reflect a disturbance in rhythm, such as the Frequently Intermittent, the Intermittent Hollow, and the Wildly Interrupted with unobtainable rate, this is the most serious of all qualities in terms of prognosis. As previously mentioned, it is the pulse quality associated most frequently with AIDS.

Apart from other symptoms, this pulse signifies extraordinary vulnerability. Dr. Shen indicates that if "the symptoms are fatigue and weakness, and if it is not treated in time, the individual will not live long," and when found "during a serious illness, it indicates imminent death." He also says that if this quality appears "in a healthy person, it is due to overwork before puberty, since the qi and blood have deteriorated." Other etiologies suggested by Dr. Shen include the sudden loss of blood, resuming normal activities too soon after a serious illness or surgery, and excessive sex or work in a deficient individual. He appears to regard this more as a matter of blood than qi deficiency.[57]

Combinations

I am in complete agreement with Kaptchuk, who says that the seriousness of this pulse remains regardless of whatever other quality accompanies it.[58] With this in mind, listing combinations is superfluous.

Positions

Although generally accessed over the entire pulse, some exceptions are reported in the literature. When found at an individual position, the Scattered pulse is probably being mistaken for the Unstable pulse. But with either quality, the implication of a very severe dysfunction or chaos in a yin organ is present.

Bilaterally at same position

The Scattered quality does not appear bilaterally.

Sides

Left

The Scattered quality on this side indicates that the yin organs, or what Dr. Shen calls the 'organ system,' are severely damaged.

Right

Should the Scattered quality be found on this side, the entire 'digestive system' is severely compromised.

Individual positions

As mentioned above, the Scattered quality in my experience does not appear in an individual position, only over the entire pulse or one side. When one thinks it can be felt at an individual position, one is actually feeling the Unstable quality.[59]

Fig. 9-7 Minute quality

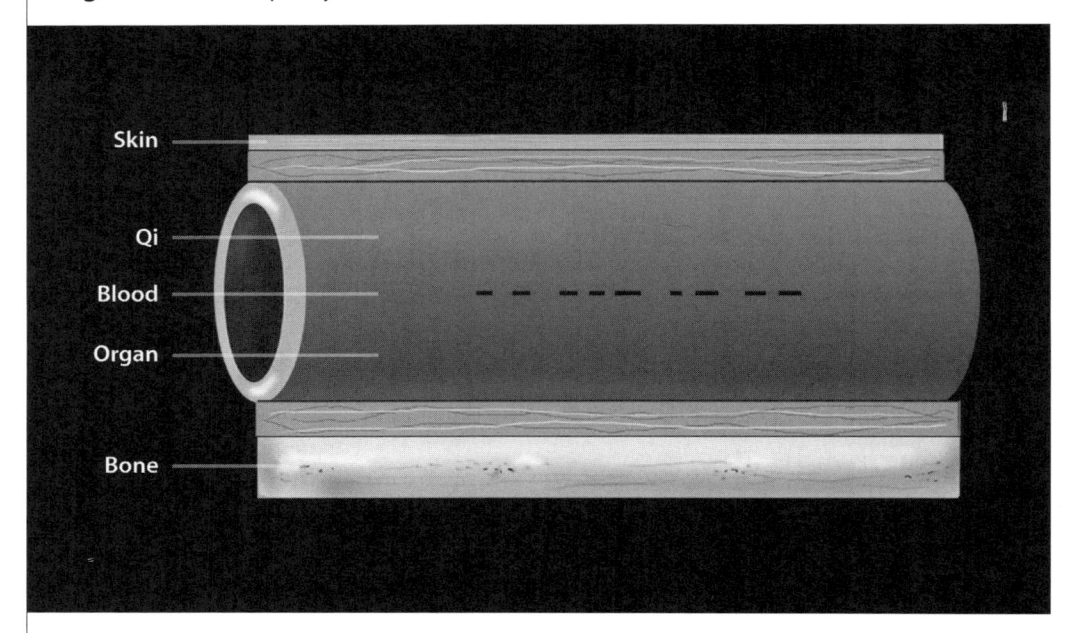

Minute

Category

The Minute quality is found only at the middle blood depth, a view shared by Kaptchuk,[60] Cheung and Belluomini,[61] and Li Shi-Zhen.[62]

While the Minute pulse is also narrow in shape, I believe that it is more appropriate to place the Minute pulse with the Empty and Scattered qualities, whose distinguishing sensation is the absence or relative diminishment of the pulse at its deeper aspects, rather than its presence at the blood depth. The interpretation of this pulse is also much closer in the literature to the severe general depletion associated with the Empty and Scattered 'qi wild' qualities than to the moderate blood depletion associated with the Thin quality.

Sensation

The principal characteristics of the Minute quality (Fig. 9-7) are that it is found at the blood depth, is Thin but ill-defined ("blurry"), gives way under pressure like an Empty quality with nothing below, and is not continuous as the fingers are rolled from the proximal to the distal position, as with the Scattered quality. It is Yielding and disappears and reappears sporadically as the fingers are rolled horizontally along the radial artery from distal to proximal position. In this respect, it most closely resembles the Scattered quality, which is found only at the qi depth. The Thin quality, on the other hand, does not disappear under pressure and does not disperse as the fingers are rolled in the distal-proximal directions.[63]

Interpretation | The Minute pulse can signify a deficiency of yang, qi, or blood. It is especially a sign of extensive qi and yang deficiency in one who is seriously ill. Some experienced practitioners refer to it as the classic pulse quality (also called Scattered) of AIDS. I see it as a 'qi wild' stage beyond that of the Empty and Scattered qualities, in which there is not enough yang left to rise to the surface. The Minute quality is distinguished from the Thin in that the latter more often represents blood deficiency alone, while the Minute is more often a sign of extreme qi and especially yang deficiency in the terminal stages of illness.[64]

Combinations | I have no experience with the combinations associated with this pulse.[65]

Positions | I have found this quality rarely, and then only simultaneously at all pulse positions.[66]

Hollow

Category | Porkert (who calls it Onionstalk[67]) and I classify this pulse with the superficial qualities because it is accessed at the qi depth and organ depth, and is either diminished, separating, or absent at the blood depth. Li Shi-Zhen[68] and Wu Shui-Wan[69] classify it with the Floating pulses.

The Hollow quality is a sign of a serious disorder in most of its manifestations. It is one of those qualities whose description is muddled because it is confused with the Empty quality. Distinguishing between the two is extremely important.

The Hollow quality is often accompanied by the Full-Overflowing pulse and vice versa. While the Hollow quality is most often associated with deficiency, and the Full-Overflowing quality with heat in the blood, the predominance of one or the other is determined by the hardness of the pulse, together with signs on the tongue and eyes. With deficiency, the pulse is Yielding Hollow and the tongue is pale with a thin white coating. With excess-type heat in the blood, the pulse quality is more Tense, the tongue and sclera of the eyes are injected, and there is a thick, dry tongue coating. With heat from deficiency the pulse quality is harder, Tight to Wiry, the tongue is bright red and dry with little coating, and the sclera is less injected.

Sensation | The Hollow pulse is felt with a light touch superficially at the qi depth. As pressure is increased, the pulse diminishes, feels pushed to the sides (separates), or disappears altogether until the organ depth is reached, where the pulse returns.

While the literature is clear that with the Hollow quality there is no sensation between the qi and organ depths, this is true only of the Leather-like Hollow quality when sudden hemorrhage is the cause. With all other Hollow qualities the sensation seems to yield and separate between the qi and organ depths, but does not disappear entirely.

According to Dr. Shen, with the few exceptions mentioned in the following discussion, the Hollow pulse is closely associated with the Full-Overflowing quality. I have recorded seven types of Hollow pulse during my years with Dr. Shen, each with a distinctly different meaning. These Hollow pulses include Yielding Hollow Full-Overflowing, Yielding Partially Hollow, slightly Tense Hollow Full-Overflowing, Leather-like Hollow, Tense and very Tense Hollow Full-Overflowing, Tight and very Tight Hollow Full-Overflowing, Yielding Hollow Ropy, and Hollow Interrupted-Intermittent.

With the Yielding Hollow Full-Overflowing pulse, the Full-Overflowing quality is found primarily at the superficial end of the pulse. With the very Tense Hollow Full-Overflowing pulse, the Full-Overflowing quality extends throughout the qi and blood depths.

While the Hollow quality is most often found with the Full-Overflowing pulse, in the following pages where the two are mentioned together, the Full-Overflowing aspect is not necessarily—though almost always is—a part of the picture. Only with the Yielding, Tense, and very Tense Hollow qualities—the former associated with a 'qi wild' condition, and the latter two with diabetes and hypertension—is the Full-Overflowing aspect always an integral part of the quality. With the Leather-like Hollow quality there is never a Full-Overflowing component, and with the very Tight Hollow Full-Overflowing quality, only sometimes is the Hollow quality present.

In terms of differentiation, it is clearly important to distinguish this pulse from the Empty quality. While both can be palpated at the qi depth, and both often separate at the blood depth, unlike the Empty quality the Hollow pulse feels as though it has a bottom as pressure is applied from the qi through the blood to the organ depth.

The Hollow quality is sometimes mistaken for the Slippery quality because, at the blood depth, the pulse separates. To some, this separating movement of the substance of the pulse feels like Slipperiness. However, the distinction is that a Slippery quality moves on its own in only one direction, while a Hollow quality separates and moves both proximally and distally only with pressure.[70]

The Hollow quality is also often confused with the Yielding Inflated quality. The Inflated quality is like a compressible balloon and sometimes gives the impression of hollowness. However, unlike the Hollow quality, it does not separate at the blood depth with pressure, and when pressure is released, the Inflated quality fills out and follows one's finger to the qi depth. Though it does not expand beyond the qi depth, it feels as if it will. The Hollow quality separates or disappears at the blood depth, and has much less sense of filling out with the release of pressure.

Interpretation The Hollow pulse is associated with disorders of both the blood as well as the qi. Dr. Shen has described seven types of Hollow pulse, one or more related to heat from excess, heat from deficiency, trapped qi, 'qi wild,' severe qi and yang deficiency, blood deficiency, and hemorrhaging. The pathogenesis can be, respectively, heat from excess causing a very Tense Full-Overflowing Hollow quality; yin deficiency causing heat from deficiency leading to a very Tight Full-Overflowing Hollow pulse; sudden cessation of long-term and excessive exercise, resulting in a Yielding Hollow Full-Overflowing quality with a Normal or Rapid rate; deficiency of qi and yang leading to a Yielding Full-Overflowing Hollow quality with a Slow rate; imminent or recent blood loss, where the pulse is Leather-like Hollow and not Full-Overflowing; exercise beyond one's energy over a long period with separation of yin and yang, and hardening of the arteries without heat, causing the Yielding Hollow Ropy quality; and, according to Dr. Shen, a Yielding Partially Hollow quality (without Full-Overflowing), a sign of mild blood deficiency.

Almost every Hollow quality is an indication that the blood vessel wall and the blood itself is sufficiently out of contact that there is notable functional disengagement of yin and yang. The Yielding Hollow Full-Overflowing quality over the entire pulse is a sign of 'qi wild.' The other forms are signs that 'blood is out of control.'

Types of Hollow qualities[71]

ENTIRE PULSE

Yielding Partially Hollow

This is a sign of mild general blood deficiency, less than with a Thin quality, but more than with a Spreading quality. The pulse separates at the blood depth but does not disappear. (See Fig. 8-9 in Chapter 8.)

Yielding Hollow Full-Overflowing

This quality can be found over the entire pulse or at any single position. When found over the entire pulse the Yielding Hollow Full-Overflowing quality signifies one of the most severe types of the 'qi wild' disorder; it indicates considerably greater qi deficiency than the Empty quality. Usually, the individual has very deficient true qi.

Generally, the causes of this pulse occur in younger (between the ages of ten and fifteen), immature individuals who are less able to adapt to certain stresses than are older, more mature individuals. The etiologies are as follows.

Yielding Hollow Full-Overflowing and Slow (excessive exercise, hard labor, deprivation, or gradual bleeding)

The Yielding Hollow Full-Overflowing quality with a Slow rate can be found after inordinately excessive exercise or hard physical labor beyond one's energy, especially in childhood. An environment characterized by significant deprivation of food, clothing, or shelter in childhood can also lead to this quality. The pathogenesis is that the yin blood and the yang vessel walls become functionally dissociated. This can happen gradually whereby the blood vessels are of normal diameter, but because of nutritional deprivation or working beyond one's energy, the volume of blood is reduced. With this etiology the rate is usually Slow and the symptoms of extreme fatigue, anxiety, cold extremities, and migrating joint pain develop slowly.

Gradual but excessive loss of blood—as with menorrhagia—over a long period of time can also give rise to the Yielding Hollow Full-Overflowing Slow quality. With mild bleeding the pulse tends to be Thinner and ultimately Feeble-Absent.

Slightly Yielding Hollow Full-Overflowing and Normal to slightly Rapid (sudden cessation of excessive exercise)

Another etiology, increasing in frequency, is the sudden cessation of activity by young persons who have been exercising beyond their energy for a long time. The younger the individual is when this pulse is discovered, the more severe the condition. Here, the pathogenesis of the functional disjunction of yin and yang is that the diameter of the blood vessels becomes greater than the diameter of the blood itself. The reason is that, when exercise is abruptly stopped, the blood volume contracts more rapidly than the blood vessel, which has been greatly expanded to accommodate the increase in blood volume required by the exercise. The yin blood and the yang vessel walls become functionally dissociated. With this quality the pulse is frequently more Rapid and slightly less Yielding, and the symptoms—severe fatigue, severe anxiety, panic, dissociation and depersonalization, explosive anger, cold extremities, and migrating joint pain—develop quickly.

Yielding Hollow Full-Overflowing Intermittent or Interrupted

This is a severe form of 'qi wild' in that the instability is already in the yin organs, especially the Heart, which is the 'emperor.' Here we have the combination of general yin organ and circulatory chaos. The presence or imminence of serious disease and death is great.

Yielding Hollow Ropy

This quality has been found in those who have exercised considerably beyond their energy for many years, causing a separation of yin and yang in the form of decreased blood volume relative to the diameter of the vessels, which remains constant. The inability of this reduced blood volume to nourish the vessel walls deprives them of adequate fluids (yin) and hardens them, which eventually leads to the Ropy quality. This is a very different process from the one leading to a Tense Ropy quality, which always involves heat.[72] While previously found only among the elderly, I now find it in younger people, probably associated with the inadvisable excesses of exercise in young maturing children. While generally found over the entire pulse, it is rarely found alone at the left middle position.

INDIVIDUAL POSITIONS

Yielding Hollow Full-Overflowing

Though rarely found at an individual position, the Yielding Hollow quality is always a sign of qi deficiency and the separation of yin and yang. It is a more serious sign of this separation than is the Empty quality.

Yielding Partially Hollow

Especially at the left middle position, this is a sign of mild blood deficiency, less than with a Thin quality, but more than with a Spreading quality.

Tense Hollow Slippery and Rapid

This combination of qualities is a sign of infection or inflammation in the organ or area represented by the pulse position. I have found it only at the right middle position and Stomach-Pylorus Extension position when there was gastritis or ulcer, and the pulse was more Tight-Wiry.

Leather-like Hollow and either Rapid or Slow

The Leather-like Hollow quality (Fig. 9-8) is distinguished from all other Hollow qualities by three characteristics. First, it is never Full-Overflowing. Second, and more importantly, the blood depth is absolutely absent. And third, the qi depth is hard and thick like leather. While with other Hollow qualities the blood depth more often separates upon finger pressure rather than completely disappearing, with the Leather-like Hollow quality the blood depth is entirely absent. The experience of palpating this pulse is unforgettable.

The Leather-like Hollow quality is a sign of imminent or past sudden hemorrhage. When the pulse is Rapid, the hemorrhage is imminent; when Slow, the hemorrhage has just occurred. This quality can be found over the entire pulse, which indicates massive bleeding from many sources, as with massive trauma. It can be found bilaterally at the distal, middle, or proximal positions, on one side or the other, or at only one position if the bleeding is confined to one area or one organ, as, for example, at the right middle position when there is bleeding from a stomach ulcer. According to Dr. Shen, bleeding accompanied by the Leather-like Hollow quality is always from a yin organ, and bleeding unaccompanied by this quality is from other than a yin organ. Menorrhagia from the uterus is an example of bleeding from other than a yin organ; it will appear as a Yielding Partially Hollow or Thin quality.

Fig. 9-8 Leather-like Hollow quality

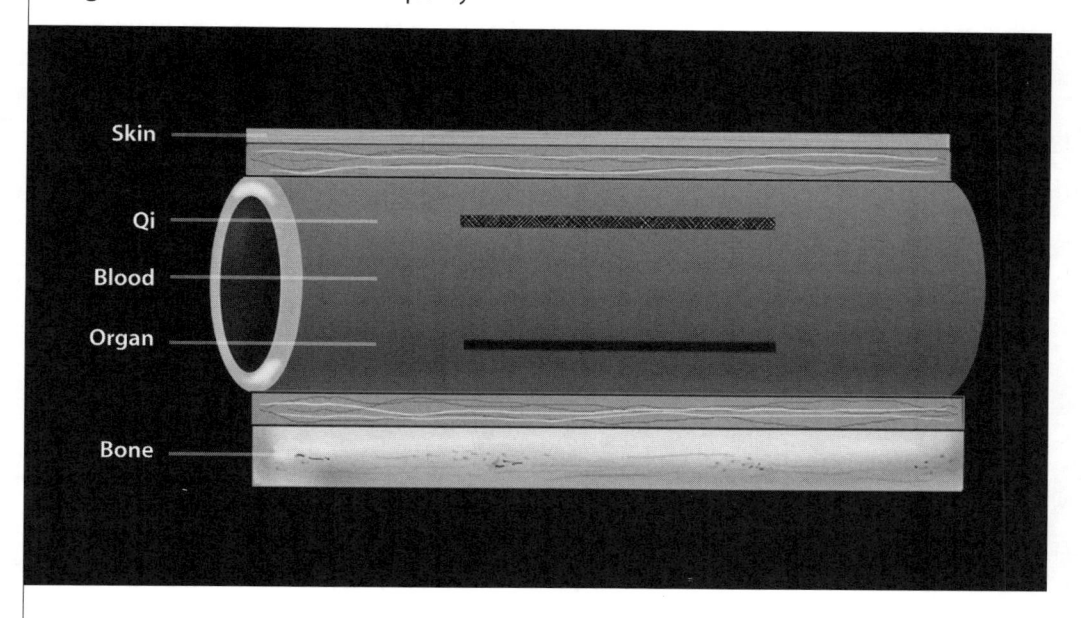

This quality should always be viewed as a serious sign requiring emergency and preventive measures. The possible exception is the left proximal position where it can be a sign of excessive loss of sperm. In his book, Dr. Shen specifically mentions the Lung, Stomach, Liver, and Intestine positions as the more common locations for this quality. Sudden lifting causing a "vein to be broken" is one etiology; trauma and internal disharmony is another, as with a sudden acute hemorrhaging of a duodenal ulcer.[73]

The Hollowness associated with this quality is attributable to a contraction of blood volume from the blood vessels. Dr. Shen believes that as the organ is attempting to contain and prevent the loss of blood by astringing and constricting itself, this leads to a form of stagnation which is perceived as the Leather-like Hollow quality. A Rapid quality is a reaction of the Heart to the crisis in another organ, since the Heart senses that it is losing control of one of its main functions, to control circulation.

Tense Hollow

Especially at the left middle position, this is a rare sign of repressed anger over a long period of time. With this condition I find the pulse to be more often Tense Inflated.

Tense and very Tense Hollow Full-Overflowing

This quality at the left middle and distal positions is associated with the Liver fire type of hypertension that causes elevated diastolic blood pressure. At the left middle and proximal positions, it is a sign of either hypertension with an elevated systolic pressure and/or diabetes.

Tight and very Tight Hollow Full-Overflowing

The very Tight Hollow Full-Overflowing pulse is a sign of heat from extreme yin deficiency, which has dried out and weakened the blood vessel walls. The excessive heat produced must be offset by an increase of yin; this gradually depletes the Kidney yin and the yin of the vessel walls. The vessels lose their flexibility, cannot contract and expand, and are less able to accommodate changes in blood volume. The hardened walls increase circulatory turbulence and blood stagnation, which attracts minerals and lipids to the walls, leading to an atherosclerotic process. Without flexibility of the vessels, and with increased resistance of the blood stagnation and atherosclerosis, the heart has to work harder to increase the diastolic pressure.

This pulse quality mainly reflects primary hypertension or secondary hypertension associated with insulin-dependent diabetes. Due to the fragility of the blood vessels, the very Tight Hollow Full-Overflowing quality can also be a precursor sign of hemorrhaging leading to stroke.

Combinations

See discussion under types of Hollow pulses above.

Positions

BILATERALLY AT SAME POSITION

It is very rare to find the Hollow quality bilaterally. In brief review, with a Yielding Hollow Full-Overflowing quality the qi is more 'wild' than with an Empty quality. When the pulse is Leather-like Hollow, it is always a sign of bleeding, indicating a serious situation that must be attended to immediately as a matter of life and death. When the rate is Rapid, the bleeding is imminent; if Slow, the bleeding occurred recently.

The Tense, Tight, or very Tight Hollow quality is associated with the Full-Overflowing quality and is found with hypertension and heat in the blood from excess or deficiency.

Distal

Leather-like Hollow

This is a sign of trauma to the chest with possible hemorrhage.

Yielding Hollow Full-Overflowing

Though rare, lifting beyond one's energy, such as sudden lifting of a very heavy weight just one time, can cause this quality to appear at this position. More often, the quality is Inflated. Frequent lifting over time usually causes an Inflated quality at the Diaphragm position, especially on the right side.

Middle

Leather-like Hollow

Abdominal hemorrhage may be reflected in the pulse at this position.

Yielding Partially Hollow

This is a rare sign of mild Liver blood deficiency, less than with the Thin quality, but more than with the Spreading quality.

Tense Hollow

This is a sign of repressed anger over a long period of time. The Inflated quality here is more often associated with a sudden bout of repressed anger.

Yielding Hollow Full-Overflowing

This quality occurs either when a person habitually engages in physical labor too soon after eating, or sits for long periods of time and is chronically irritable. Hyperacidity ("sour stomach") is associated with this quality (often accompanied by a Slippery quality) and with these etiologies.

Tight and very Tight Hollow Full-Overflowing

Advanced hypertension and/or diabetes may be associated with this pulse bilaterally at the middle positions.

Proximal

Yielding Hollow Full-Overflowing and Slow

This quality may be due to gradual menstrual bleeding that is moderate in amount. Poor intestinal function due to heavy physical labor after eating, with alternating constipation and diarrhea, is another possible etiology.

Leather-like Hollow

If the rate is Rapid, this pulse is associated with imminent bleeding from the intestines or in the pelvis. A Slow rate indicates that bleeding recently occurred.

Tight and very Tight Hollow Full-Overflowing

This combination is a sign of advanced diabetes or hypertension.

SIDES

Dr. Shen notes that the Hollow quality over the entire left side is usually more serious than over the entire right side.

Left

Yielding Hollow Full-Overflowing and Slow

This quality, which is rarely found on only the left side, is a sign of severe deficiency of the 'organ system,' and is associated with chronic fatigue.

Tight and very Tight Hollow Full-Overflowing

This pulse is associated with potential cerebrovascular accident or paralytic stroke that affects the left side. It is due to hypertension, or, as Dr. Shen put it, "veins too tight." Diabetes should also be considered.

Right

Yielding Hollow Full-Overflowing

Over a long period of time, a person who eats irregularly, has a poor diet, or suffers from anorexia or bulimia may develop this quality over the entire right side. It is a sign of a seriously impaired 'digestive system.'

Tight and very Tight Full-Overflowing

As on the left wrist, this quality on the right side may indicate the same potential stroke condition, except that it is the right side of the body that is affected.

INDIVIDUAL POSITIONS

Below are some general comments about the types of Hollow qualities already described in connection with individual pulse positions.

The Leather-like Hollow quality at any position is a sign of either impending or recent hemorrhage. It should be managed as an emergency, usually requiring biomedical intervention.

The Yielding Hollow Full-Overflowing quality in one position is usually a sign of severe qi deficiency and the separation of yin and yang.

Left distal

Tense-Tight Hollow Full-Overflowing

Usually in association with the same quality at the left middle position, this is a sign of hypertension with an elevated diastolic pressure.

Leather-like Hollow

Acute bleeding from the Heart into the Pericardium would be accompanied by this quality.

Large Vessel

The Very Tight Hollow and Full-Overflowing quality at the Large Vessel position indicates that the large vessels have elevated blood pressure, especially the diastolic. In a person with competent cardiac function, portal hypertension and carotid artery blockage are the possible causes. (An Inflated quality here is associated with an aneurysm.)

Left middle

Leather-like Hollow

This quality may be associated with bleeding from the portal circulation, as in liver cirrhosis or trauma, and is a sign requiring emergency biomedical intervention.

Tense Hollow

The Tense Hollow quality at the left middle position is a rare sign of repressed anger over a long period of time.

Yielding Partially Hollow

This is a sign of mild Liver blood deficiency. More often, gradual blood deficiency in this position is manifested as a Thin quality.

Yielding Hollow Full-Overflowing and Slow

This quality at the left middle position is a sign of extreme Liver qi deficiency and the separation of Liver yin and yang.

Tight and very Tight-Wiry Hollow Full-Overflowing

Insulin-dependent diabetes or essential hypertension are the most likely causes when this quality is found here and at the left proximal position.

Left proximal

Leather-like Hollow

Associated with imminent, current, or recent bleeding from the kidneys, ureter, bladder, prostate, or urethra. Worsley mentions only the symptom of hematuria.[74]

Yielding Hollow Full-Overflowing

Associated with gradual uterine bleeding over a long period of time, as with a slow menorrhagia, or excessive loss of sperm.

Large Intestine

When palpated only at the Large Intestine position, the Leather-like Hollow quality is a sign of compromised intestinal function and possible bleeding from the intestines. This quality here is rare in clinical practice. Under the same circumstances I have found large Changes in Intensity.

Right distal

Leather-like Hollow

The Leather-like Hollow quality is rare at the right distal position. It is a sign of sudden severe hemorrhage in the Lung, imminent if Rapid, and just past if Slow.

Yielding Hollow Full-Overflowing

This is a rarely found quality at the right distal position, indicating great Lung qi deficiency and the separation of Lung yin and yang.

Right middle and Stomach-Pylorus Extension

Leather-like Hollow

Here, this quality is usually a sign of present or potential bleeding from a gastric and duodenal ulcer, again dictating emergency measures.

Tight-Wiry Hollow Slippery

This can be a sign of gastritis, accompanied by burning epigastric pain due to an early ulcer. If the quality is felt toward the middle part of this position, the ulcer is gastric, and if in the Stomach-Pylorus Extension position, duodenal or pyloric.

Right proximal

Yielding Hollow Full-Overflowing

Here this quality is regarded by Dr. Shen as a sign of severe Kidney qi deficiency and the separation of yin and yang. I have never palpated this quality at this position, although with severe Kidney qi and yang deficiency the usual quality is Feeble-Absent or, rarely, Empty.[75]

Slightly Tight Hollow Full-Overflowing

According to Dr. Shen this is a sign of back pain. I have never observed this association myself. With back pain I usually find a Tight-Wiry Biting and Choppy quality in the proximal and Pelvis/Lower Body positions.

Tight and very Tight Hollow Full-Overflowing

Dr. Shen says that this quality can be found here with diabetes or essential hypertension, although it is rare. He believes that with this condition, the same quality also appears at the left proximal position, and often the left middle positions.

Small Intestine

In my experience, whatever the rate, when the Leather-like Hollow quality is confined to the Small Intestine position, the indication is a potential hemorrhage in the Small Intestine.

Submerged Pulse Qualities

In contrast to the superficial qualities that are characteristically found at the surface of the pulse, we will now consider those qualities that occupy the deeper regions of the pulse.

Deep

Category

I have chosen the term Deep rather than Sinking because students find the latter term ambiguous and confusing. Sinking signifies a process rather than a constant, of something *going* down rather than something *already* down.

Sensation

The Deep quality (Fig. 9-9) can be felt only with considerable pressure. Nothing is felt at the qi or blood depths. The pulse is felt only at the organ depth, which normally is wider and has more substance than the qi and blood depths. With regard to sensation, it is opposite in feeling to the Floating quality. Except for the very rare Firm and Hidden qualities, it should be noted that if the fingers are pressed to the muscle, tendon, ligament, or bone, one is no longer accessing this model of the Chinese pulse, and, within this model, the information perceived cannot be related to Chinese medicine. The organ depth, or deepest location of the authentic Chinese pulse, is above these tissues.[76]

Fig. 9-9 Deep quality

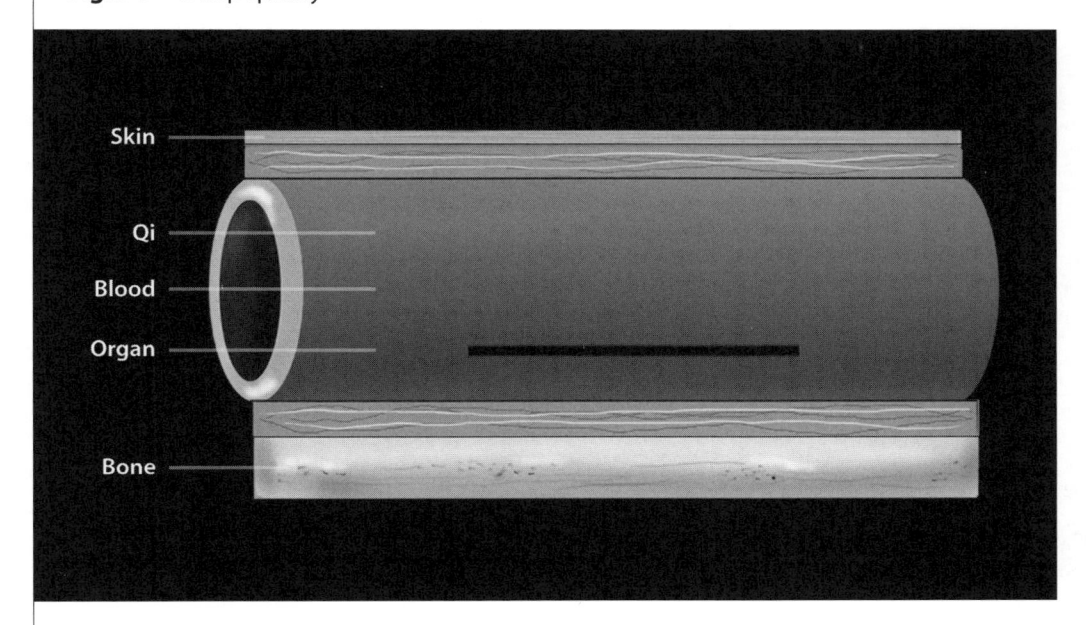

Interpretation

Traditionally, a Deep pulse is taken to mean a significant depletion of the true qi, either from an internal disease, disharmony of the yin organs, a chronic or serious illness, an illness that is more difficult to cure, or all of the above. The quality may appear over the entire pulse or at a single position. With these etiologies, the pulse is also frequently Feeble.

True qi is strongly linked with the yang basal metabolic heat, which drives the body and is based on the integrity of the Kidney yang. This heat gives the pulse expansiveness, force, and amplitude and shows itself more superficially. As this energetic heat is used up through work—either physical or mental—beyond a person's energy, or from poor eating habits like anorexia and bulimia, from lack of sleep, excessive sex, or illness, diminishment in the amplitude and superficiality of the pulse becomes evident. This diminishment can also be, in part, the consequence of constitutional Kidney yang deficiency. Since the Kidney energy supports almost every mental and physical function, and the Kidneys are the repository of stored energy, a Deep pulse can be associated with an appreciable deficiency of Kidney energy.

A far less common etiology in developed countries in this era is stagnation of qi due to cold from excess preventing the yang qi from rising. Usually this occurs with an external pathogenic factor when the yang qi is already deficient. On more rare occasions the pathogenic factor has entered so suddenly and forcefully that the yang qi has had no opportunity to respond. Other, less common etiologies are various kinds of stagnation or accumulation (congestion in a delimited area causing pain or pain on movement). With these origins the pulse is more likely to also be Tense or Tight.

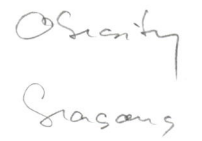

In an obese person a relatively Deeper pulse (all positions) may be normal. If the individual is obese and the pulse is not deep in proportion to weight, the indication is of a more serious problem. In a healthy person it is normal for the entire pulse to be slightly deeper in the winter, but this is barely discernible. With some individuals, though rare, constitutionally Deep qualities can exist for an entire lifetime without consequence. In a conversation with a physician who practices Korean constitutional medicine, he mentioned a constitutional Deep quality without the usual significance of an advancing disharmony. It is my experience that his is a valid impression.

On the positive side of this pulse quality is the inference that although true qi is depleted, yin organ energies are still more or less intact and functioning. I have found a transient Deep quality in very introverted people whose initial response to new social contact is to energetically withdraw, which, on prolonged examination, quickly reverts to the enduring and valid pulse picture. While the Deep quality is a sign of an intensifying disharmony, it is still far from the more serious signs of qi deficiency such as the Feeble-Absent quality, or of 'qi wild' conditions such as the Empty quality.

All sources agree with the above interpretations. Worsley[77] mentions additional symptoms such as "swelling in the chest and ribs [probably meaning distention], tumor, diarrhea, fainting, full of phlegm, cold in the stomach."

Combinations

Qualities that accompany the Deep quality range across the spectrum of classification. Interpretations from the literature are included with my own.

Deep Diffuse, Deep Reduced Substance, or Deep Feeble-Absent

These combinations signify chronic dissipation of the general qi, and of the yang of the yin organs, due to constitutional weakness, work, exercise beyond one's energy, old age, or after a long illness. Yin energy may still be intact. The depletion of qi in this instance occurs over a long period—longer if the energy is substantial in the beginning, and shorter if the original qi is insubstantial. In the latter case, the proximal positions diminish first. The important aspect of this pattern is the concept of going beyond one's energy. Overwork has become a common phenomenon in America. Indeed, this is increasingly a problem for women, who, in addition to a career, have responsibilities at home.

In terms of sensation, these combinations develop in stages, beginning with a diminution at the qi depth, then a gradual Spreading of the pulse at the blood depth that gives way on pressure to the Flooding Deficient wave, Diffuse, and Reduced Substance qualities, and eventually becomes Deeper and Feeble to Absent.[78]

Deep Tight

Yin deficiency

The Deep and Tight combination reflects chronic dissipation of the general qi, and of the yin of the yin organs. The yin deficiency is usually due to prolonged emotional stress and anxiety, which at first has brought stagnation, followed by heat from excess to overcome the stagnation, to the organ. To balance the heat, the yin of both these organs and of the Kidneys is consumed, resulting in heat from deficiency, especially of the Liver, Kidneys, and Heart. With regard to specific organs, chronic tension most affects the Liver; acute, shock-like emotional experiences affect the Heart; and fear and chronic depression affects the Kidneys.

External cold that leads to pain

Another etiology that can cause this pattern, although infrequently, is invasion of an external factor, especially cold, in a deficient person. This can be accompanied by pain due to stagnation caused by the cold, which the deficient organism cannot overcome. I have found that when one is affected by this type of pain, the Tightness is sharper (even Wiry) and more Biting than the Tight quality due to yin deficiency. If the pain is sufficiently severe or prolonged it will affect the entire body, and consequently the pulse, since as the body's general energy attempts to overcome the stagnation, the qi is depleted and the pulse becomes Deep Feeble-Absent.[79]

Deep Wiry

This combination is similar to the Deep and Tight quality except that the process of yin depletion has progressed further and is more serious. I have found this combination frequently in the left middle position in alcohol-dependent patients, and less often in those who do not drink, but whose mothers drank heavily during pregnancy. In particular, this quality is an early sign of hypertension and diabetes when found at the left middle and proximal positions. When the quality is also very Slow, chronic toxicity should be considered.

The Deep Wiry quality in the proximal positions is often a sign of severe lower abdominal, pelvic, or perineal pain, low back pain, or pain in the lower part of the body (legs, knees, ankles, and feet), or of Kidney stones with very severe pain. Frequently, there is a Choppy quality in the Pelvis/Lower Body positions indicating pain due to blood stagnation.[80]

Deep Flat

This combination reflects a chronic condition in which trauma, either physical or emotional, occurred when the individual was in a weakened or vulnerable state, especially during childhood when the body is immature. In addition to the chronicity indicated by the Deep quality, its Flat aspect means that qi is unable to enter the area or organs represented by the position where the pulse is Flat.

Deep Slippery

This combination can result from the accumulation of dampness or stagnant food, or phlegm, and often accompanies infection in the area represented by the position that is Slippery. The slipperiness can be due to the extensive qi stagnation or concomitant qi deficiency, which the Deep quality implies. Differentiation can also be made based on the pulse (Tense or Feeble), the tongue, and other symptoms. Dampness causes the tongue to be wet; food stagnation causes a thick, sticky coating; and phlegm is indicated by a thick coating and thread-like mucus in the mouth. When the tongue body is pale and slightly swollen, the cause is deficiency; a normal or red tongue together with a Deep pulse indicates stagnation.[81]

Deep and Slow

The Slow pulse is far more complex, involving the Heart and circulation more often than cold. Although the Deep and Slow quality usually indicates a chronic disease process, there are circumstances, e.g., in hypothermia, when this quality can be brought on sooner.

Heart and circulation

A Deep and Slow quality in our time is usually a sign of disharmony in the circulation or of the Heart. This may result from various kinds of shock to the circulation, such as severe trauma, toxicity, and hypothermia, that affect the Heart (pulse is Tighter), or the source may be Heart qi deficiency affecting the circulation (pulse is more Feeble).

Cold from excess or deficiency

Another, less common cause in our time involves cold from either excess (hypothermia) or deficiency (Kidney yang deficiency) affecting a person with qi and blood deficiency. With cold from excess the pulse tends to be Tight, and with cold from deficiency, more Feeble.[82]

Toxicity

A very Deep and very Slow pulse, under 50 beats/minute, should alert the practitioner to possible chronic toxicity (poisoning). The pulse can also be Thin and Wiry. Li Shi-Zhen[83] mentions a "sinking hidden pulse [that] occurs when yin poisoning and accumulation create severe vomiting and diarrhea." Dr. Shen describes a Deep and Slow pulse with a rate under fifty, which appears with chronic and severe poisoning. The blood may also be unclear.

Deep and Rapid

Shock

The Rapid pulse is much more involved with Heart shock than the literature would suggest. In our time the rate is associated more with Heart and circulatory disorders arising from emotional shock than with heat from excess or deficiency. When the heart is stressed, with Heart qi deficiency, the rate becomes Rapid. I once had a patient with a Deep and very Rapid pulse who was in congestive heart failure. The Heart qi is not strong enough to maintain cardiac homeostasis under stress, either physical or emotional. (See Chapter 7 for a discussion of the Rapid quality.)

Heat from excess and deficiency

When Heart and circulatory disorders are not present with this pulse combination, the other possible source is heat from excess or deficiency. While I have seen many chronic conditions due to heat from excess or deficiency, very few had a Rapid rate. Compared to our counterparts in the centuries before antibiotics, the modern practitioner of Chinese medicine sees relatively few acute disorders due to heat from excess. The pulse is more Rapid with heat from excess, and less Rapid when the heat is from deficiency.[84]

Deep Thin

This combination signifies depletion of qi and blood, the blood indicated by the Thin quality, and the qi by the Deep quality of the pulse.

Deep Wide

If the pulse is Deep, Wide, and without substance, this suggests that the qi deficiency is increasing. If on the other hand the pulse is Deep, Wide, and Tense, the probability is that there is blood heat and mild blood stagnation in the yin organ associated with the position where the pulse is Deep. If the blood stagnation becomes more profound, the quality could change to Deep, Tense, and Choppy. In this instance, the blood stagnation may be due to a combination of qi deficiency and heat from excess, rendering the organ unable to move the blood from within to the outside of the organ.

Deep Choppy

This combination is associated with simultaneous blood stagnation and qi deficiency. It is usually encountered in one position, especially the Pelvis/Lower Body and proximal positions, and rarely over the entire pulse.[85]

Positions

BILATERALLY AT SAME POSITION

Distal

Deep Flat

The Flat quality is usually Deep by the time a practitioner feels it. This is because a significant amount of time has passed since the quality first appeared in childhood. Flatness is associated with deficiency at the time of the causative event. In this case, the Flat quality is a reflection that qi is unable to enter an area, a form of qi stagnation. Over an extended period of time the effort to overcome the stagnation causes increasing deficiency, transforming the pulse quality from Flat to Deep and later to Feeble. If uncorrected, the consequence can be neoplasm, and in the short term, difficulty with inhaling, as reflected by the need to take many short breaths, and tightness and pain in the chest when fatigued.

Severe emotional shock during childhood

This type of shock, such as the loss of a parent at an early age when the child cannot cope emotionally with the loss, is not currently in the conscious mind, and causes stagnant qi in the chest. At this point the wave is Flat. Over a long period of time the stagnant qi evolves into qi deficiency in the chest, Heart, and Lungs, with difficulty in breathing deeply. By then the pulse has become Deep and then Feeble.

Fetus presents with cord around neck at birth

This is perhaps second in etiology only to emotional shock in childhood. A good birth history is helpful.

Physical trauma

A blow to the chest when the energy is not strong, or one sudden and extreme episode of lifting with the upper torso, may also lead to this pulse combination at this position. Again, the Flat quality indicates that qi is unable to get into the chest. Over the long term, the effort to overcome this stagnation depletes the qi, leading to a Deep and then Feeble pulse quality.

Deep Feeble

Bilaterally at the distal (upper burner) position, the Deep and Feeble quality is one step beyond the Deep and Flat quality. The body has exhausted its qi in the upper burner in an effort to move qi into the area from which it has been excluded. Here, this combination is associated with profound Heart qi deficiency, which slows the circulation of qi and blood in the Lungs, causing a suffocating sensation in the chest and depression. Symptoms such as palpitations, shortness of breath, excessive daytime perspiration, chills, and cold limbs are also present.

Dr. Shen describes a "deep, weak and slow" pulse bilaterally which indicates "a sickness of the upper torso" due to trauma or overwork in which "the chest may often feel stifled and a great many deep breaths are needed."[86] During my time with Dr. Shen, I recall feeling this pulse combination in recent Chinese immigrants who had to perform heavy labor.

Deep Slippery

Here, this combination indicates phlegm-dampness in the Heart, Lungs, or chest. If the Heart is more affected, emotional or neurological symptoms are more prominent; if it is the Lungs, asthma is more likely.[87]

Deep Thin Tight

This pulse combination is associated with qi, yin, and blood deficiency with symptoms of palpitations, irritability, easily startled, loss of concentration and memory, vertigo, insomnia, excessive dreaming, dry mouth and throat with unquenchable thirst, and other signs of rising heat from deficiency. The latter may include hot flashes, night sweats, tinnitus, generalized dryness, and heat in the palms, soles, and between the eyes. Asthma accompanied by an unproductive cough and afternoon fevers are also possible. The qi deficiency may cause lethargy, shortness of breath that worsens with exertion, spontaneous sweating, and an oppressive sensation in the chest.

One cause of this disorder is protracted, unresolved emotional shock with ongoing stress, worry, and anxiety which can lead to severe yin deficiency in the upper burner, Heart, and Lungs. If the pulse also changes with movement, there is Heart qi agitation, called 'Heart nervous' by Dr. Shen. Symptoms include fatigue, especially in the morning, frequent waking during the night, palpitations, mild irritability, mood swings, and a sense of being out of control.

Deep and very Tight or Wiry

Trauma and lifting, accompanied by pain

This pulse combination may be attributable to one sudden, catastrophic episode of lifting a heavy object using the upper part of the body, or trauma to the chest resulting in stagnation of qi and severe pain on movement.

Febrile illness

Severe and prolonged febrile illness in the upper burner that consumes Heart, Lung, and ultimately Kidney yin can also lead to this pulse combination. This includes tuberculosis.

Deep Tight or Wiry and very Rapid

If the rate is also very Rapid, cardiac asthma may be present.

Middle

Deep Flat

This pulse combination can be caused by sitting bent or hunched over for long periods of time, by trauma to the abdomen to a person with deficient qi in this area, or following an episode of lifting a heavy object by a person with deficient qi. Resuming work too soon after eating, and excessive rumination while eating, are other causes. All can impair the movement of qi into the middle burner.

Deep Tight

According to Dr. Shen, this pulse combination at the middle position results when "the qi has been damaged from sitting too long and the middle burner [is injured]."[88] In this instance, the Tight quality represents pain.

The Flat quality is associated with the same etiology when there is initial qi deficiency in the area, while the Tight quality appears when the initial qi is relatively normal. The pain is greater when the body has more energy to open the circulation closed by stagnation. Over the long term both qualities can evolve into a Deep and Feeble combination due to the exhaustion of the local qi trying to open the stagnation.

Deep Feeble-Absent

This combination at the middle position indicates qi and yang deficiency of the Liver and Spleen, or in that area. This may be attributable to several etiologies. One is poor nutrition or irregular eating habits from childhood, through adolescence and middle life. Bulimia and anorexia are increasingly common causes. Other etiologies in a continuum from the Flat and Tight qualities over time are sitting bent or hunched over for prolonged periods, either because of one's occupation or owing to profound sadness. Finally, this combination can also arise from continual resumption of work too soon after eating. The circulation of qi in the middle burner is disturbed, at first causing pain and later qi deficiency, at which point the pain becomes less severe. Dr. Shen associates this etiology with a "deep, weak and slow pulse due to bad circulation of the qi in the middle heater."[89]

Deep Slippery

This can be a sign of chronic infection in one or all of the organs in the area including Liver, Gallbladder, Spleen, Stomach, and pancreas. It may also be attributable to Spleen dampness affecting the Liver and Gallbladder and resulting in all the signs and symptoms of Spleen/Gallbladder damp-heat. Chronic hepatitis, candidiasis, and parasites should be considered.

Deep Wiry

This pulse combination at the middle position is often associated with a gastric or duodenal ulcer or neoplasm in this area (e.g., the pancreas), which is accompanied by deep pain. A Slippery Hollow quality also often attends the ulcer condition.

Deep Thin

This combination at the middle position is a sign of long-term qi and (especially) blood deficiency of the Liver, possibly attributable to the inability of a deficient Spleen to produce blood, or to chronic bleeding or the inability of the Liver to hold the blood. Usually the entire pulse will be Deep and Thin with this etiology.

Proximal

The pulse is normally deeper in the proximal position than in any other position.

Deep Flat

This combination indicates stagnation in the area that initially had deficient qi caused by standing for long stretches of time, or walking long distances. This can cause Intestinal qi stagnation, or stagnation that leads to enlargement of the prostate or hemorrhoids.

Deep Wiry

At the proximal position this pulse is associated with blood stagnation in the pelvis/lower body, or with kidney stones, usually accompanied by severe pain, in which case the pulse is often Choppy as well. It may also be attributable to early insulin-dependent diabetes or early hypertension.

Deep Feeble

This combination may indicate constitutionally deficient Kidney qi and yang associated with a lifelong propensity toward serious respiratory, neurologic, psychological, developmental, or cardiovascular illness. This quality can also arise from prolonged and excessive sexual activity beyond one's energy, or (rarely) chronic colitis or diarrhea in a subacute stage or in a very weak person, or any profound abuse of any of the organs for which Kidney qi, essence, yin, and yang are the foundation.

Dr. Shen states that "if both chi pulses are deep, fine and weak, the qi in the lower abdomen is stagnant as a result of overwork."[90]

Deep Slippery

This can be a sign of kidney stones accompanied by severe pain (in which case we also have a Wiry quality), or sometimes of chronic infection of the bladder, prostate, ovaries and uterus, or of the Intestines such as ulcerative colitis, regional enteritis, or Crohn's disease, in which cases the pain is less acute. With chronic low-grade intestinal diseases this quality is usually confined to the complementary individual position of the Large Intestine at the distal end of the proximal position. With prostate, uterus, and ovary disease the signs are usually at the Pelvis/Lower Body position, and bladder infections usually manifest at the right proximal position.[91]

SIDES

Left

Deep Feeble

This pulse over the entire left side indicates a generalized qi deficiency of the yin organ system—especially the Heart, Liver, and Kidneys—due to a fragile constitution, or prolonged serious illness, excessive sex, exercise, or work beyond one's energy. In the elderly, a general decline in health may also be reflected in this combination.

Deep Tight

When this pulse combination appears only at the surface of the Deep pulse, it indicates that in addition to qi deficiency, there is tension in the 'nervous system' which has caused heat in the qi function or nervous innervation of the yin organ system, especially the Heart, Liver, and Kidneys. If the Tightness pervades the entire Deep quality, this combination can be interpreted to mean combined yin and qi deficiency of these organs. The yin deficiency gives rise to heat, which further irritates the nerves and renders them even more excitable.

Right

Deep Feeble

This pulse combination over the entire right side indicates qi deficiency of the 'digestive system' due to irregular eating habits.

Deep Tight

This pulse over the entire right side indicates heat from deficiency in an already qi-deficient 'digestive system' caused by habitually eating too fast. If the cause is tension, the Tightness frequently appears primarily on the surface of the Deep quality. The left middle position can also be Tense or Tight when the tension is due to the Liver attacking the Stomach/Spleen.

INDIVIDUAL POSITIONS

A Deep quality at any individual position indicates deficiency but not exhaustion of qi in the organ represented by that position.

Left distal

Many of the following pulse combinations contain references to Dr. Shen's concept of the energetic pathology of the Heart.[92] The Deep quality automatically assumes Heart qi deficiency.

Deep Feeble with Increase in Rate on Exertion <8 beats/min

With this combination we have a condition of Heart qi deficiency. If the rate stays the same, the condition is more likely to be one of Heart yang deficiency.

Deep Feeble with large Increase in Rate on Exertion

Dr. Shen refers to this combination as Heart Weak, primarily due to Heart blood (and less to Heart qi) deficiency.

Deep Flat and slightly Rapid or Slow

These are signs of Heart qi stagnation ('Heart closed') or an earlier stage of Heart blood stagnation ('Heart small'). The Heart is said to be suffocating for lack of qi. Thus, the Heart muscle is tense because of sudden shock—such as birth trauma, or loss of a parent in childhood—such that breathing becomes difficult, and the individual often becomes depressed, fearful, or vengeful depending on whether the Heart is 'small' or 'closed.' Heart qi stagnation and Heart blood stagnation are mentioned together because the similarities in their pulses overlap in the early stage of Heart blood stagnation. Their etiologies are actually quite different, and the seriousness and outcome of each should be differentiated, as described in Chapter 12 and the glossary.

Deep Thin Feeble with Normal or slightly Rapid rate

This is a sign of a more advanced Heart blood stagnation ('Heart small') pattern in which lifelong fear is a major symptom.

Deep Thin Tight and very Rapid

These qualities are found at the left distal position in the later stage of either trapped qi in the Heart ('Heart full') or severe Heart qi deficiency ('Heart large'), conditions in which the Heart is dilated. In the early stages the pulse is Inflated. Patients are unable to sleep on their back or left side.

Deep Slippery

This is usually a sign of phlegm in the Heart orifice or in the Pericardium, which can be confirmed by the tongue and symptoms.[93]

Right distal The Deep quality here always represents a chronic Lung disorder. Its final significance depends on the accompanying qualities, and those found at the Special Lung position. Space does not allow for repetition of all these combinations here. Readers are referred to the discussion of the right distal position in Chapter 12.[94]

Left middle

Deep Feeble

This quality indicates Liver qi and yang deficiency pathognomonic of malfunction such that the individual does not recover easily from fatigue, and has difficulty gaining a "second wind." Liver cancer and lymphomas are long-term possibilities.

Deep Thin Tight and Rapid

This combination signifies chronic inflammation of the liver, with Liver qi, blood, and yin deficiency.

Deep Tense to Tight with Normal rate

At the left middle position this quality indicates protracted Liver qi stagnation that is exhausting the Liver qi and yin and causing heat from deficiency.

Deep Tight Slippery

This combination signifies chronic liver infection and is often associated with parasites.[95]

Right middle

Deep Feeble

This combination at the right middle position indicates Spleen and Stomach qi deficiency with attendant digestive problems.

Deep Slippery

This is a sign of Spleen dampness, which may involve diarrhea as a symptom. However, I have found that a true Slippery quality here is quite rare, and often mistaken for the Cotton or Separating qualities. According to Dr. Shen, and confirmed in my own experience, this quality can also indicate hyperacidity of the stomach. With this condition the Slippery quality is more often found at the Stomach-Pylorus Extension position.

Deep Thin Tight to Wiry Hollow

This combination, often accompanied by a Slippery quality, may indicate a gastric ulcer with pain or severe Stomach qi and yin deficiency.[96] It is more often found at the Stomach-Pylorus Extension position.

Stomach-Pylorus Extension

At this position the Deep Thin Slippery Hollow Rapid combination may indicate inflammation of the pylorus or duodenum, including duodenal ulcer. Pain is usually an accompanying symptom.

Left proximal

Generally speaking, both proximal positions are normally slightly deeper than the other positions. When the left proximal has a Deep quality, the indication is primarily chronic disharmony of the Kidneys. Since the Kidneys control the lower burner, all gynecologic, urinary, lower bowel, low back and knees, and sexual/genital functions can be affected. Differentiation depends on other signs and symptoms.

While the Large Intestine ordinarily occupies only the distal part of the left proximal position, its qualities can dominate the entire proximal area when the problem is fulminating colitis. Similarly, an overwhelming left pelvic/lower body pattern, such as pelvic inflammatory disease, can dominate the left proximal position. With these conditions the pulse is usually Flooding Excess at this position.

Deep Feeble and Slow

This combination indicates Kidney qi-yang deficiency, which includes a wide variety of symptoms involving growth and development, as well as lung, lower bowel, genital, and urinary functions. According to Dr. Shen, "Men will suffer from abdominal pains and impotence and lower back pains; women will have menstrual pains."[97] Other symptoms may include pain and coldness of the knees and low back pain, and in women, leukorrhea.

Deep Tight

The depth of the pulse indicates Kidney qi deficiency, and the Tightness of the pulse, Kidney yin deficiency.

Deep Slippery Tense

This combination may indicate developing kidney stones. With acute pain, the quality is more Tight to Wiry.

Deep Slippery Wiry and Rapid

This is a sign of the presence of kidney stones accompanied by severe pain and passage of stones.

Deep Slippery Feeble

This combination is a sign of Kidney qi deficiency, with the possibility of infection associated with the Slippery quality. The pattern can result from chronic parasitic infestation (in which case the left middle position is also Slippery), kidney infection, or other chronic infection in the lower burner.[98]

Right proximal

Dr. Shen identifies the principal position here with the Bladder. In my opinion, this position reflects Kidney yang function unless there is Bladder disharmony. In the latter case, the pulse qualities of the more acute Bladder patterns will override those that indicate the ongoing Kidney yang disorder.

Deep Feeble

With this combination, first consider Kidney yang deficiency with cold and lower burner symptoms. In addition, the Bladders qi is deficient, which impairs Bladder function with such symptoms as dribbling, incontinence, frequency, and urgency.

Deep Slippery Tight and Rapid

This combination indicates damp-heat and inflammation or infection in the Bladder with symptoms of urgency, frequency, and scanty hot urination. Other possible patterns are kidney stones, hematuria, phlegm-dampness accompanied by turbid urine, as well as subacute prostatitis, regional enteritis, and pelvic inflammatory disease.

Deep Slippery Feeble and Slow

Associated with a pattern of damp-cold affecting the Bladder. Symptoms include incontinence and incomplete urination.[99]

Large and Small Intestines

Here, the Deep Slippery Tight and Rapid combination reflects chronic heat in the Small Intestine with chronic inflammation, as in regional enteritis, or in the Large Intestine with chronic colitis. The Deep aspect indicates the chronicity and loss of qi in the organ.

Firm

The Firm quality is included in this book primarily because I originally classified it with the Flat or Stagnant quality described by Dr. Shen. By the time I realized that they were not the same, I had completed the following research which I have decided to publish for the sake of completeness rather than conviction. The distinction between this quality and the Hidden pulse seems academic, and I have serious misgivings about both.

The danger here is that the student will be misled from the basic principle of the specificity of the three depths and become accustomed to the already pervasive error of pressing too deeply. The Firm and Hidden qualities were probably more significant in places, usually in the distant past, when people were subjected to extreme cold, or died with overwhelming infections and extraordinarily high temperatures.

Category

The Firm quality is classified under the Submerged quality. Other terms used more or less synonymously with Firm are Fixed,[100] Confined,[101] Prison,[102] and Hard.[103] Li Shi-Zhen[104] catalogs it as one of the five Sinking pulses.

In the literature the descriptions of the Firm qualities are essentially synonymous with the Hidden quality, although Firm is described as being more Wiry.[105]

Originally I questioned whether this quality is the same as what Dr. Shen describes as Stagnant, or a pulse with a Flat wave. The Flat quality has a distinctly suppressed wave form that is not specifically mentioned in the literature associated with the Firm quality, except possibly by Worsley[106] who says, "When the fingers are pressed down the pulse does not seem to move."

Fig. 9-10 Firm quality

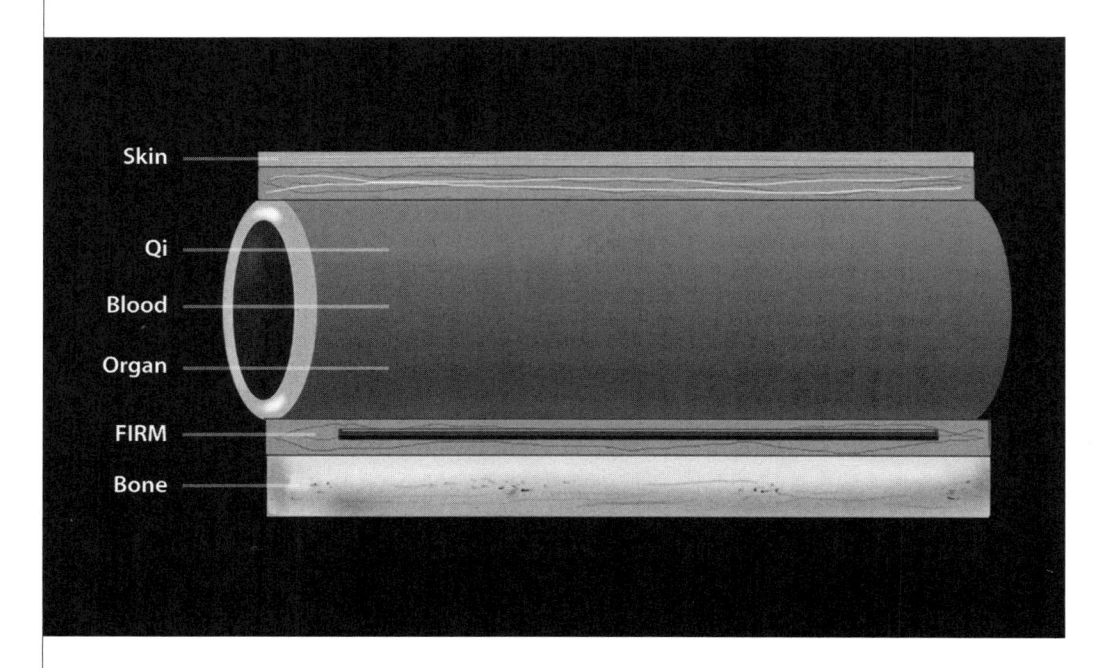

Labels on figure: Skin, Qi, Blood, Organ, FIRM, Bone

While I had initially classified the Flat and Firm qualities together, because the interpretations of the Flat quality provided to me by Dr. Shen varied from those in the literature, I decided to separate them. Thus, to emphasize the distinction, I have placed the Flat quality with the reduced volume pulses, and the Firm quality with those of submerged depth.

Sensation

The Firm quality (Fig. 9-10) is slightly deeper than the Deep quality, and slightly more superficial than the Hidden quality. It feels hard and unyielding to the touch, and, as Wu Shui-Wan[107] says, it "does not respond to the finger."

Interpretation

In the literature,[108] stagnation and serious interference with qi, blood, and fluid circulation by internal cold are the obvious reflections of this quality.

Combinations

I cannot recall any combination and none is listed, although it is conceivable that this pulse can coexist with the Choppy quality when the stagnation it represents includes blood.

Positions

At any position, this quality indicates severe stagnation of qi in the organ associated with that position, and must be viewed as a sign of serious illness until proven otherwise.[109]

Hidden

Category

Although Dr. Shen mentions this quality in his book,[110] he does not identify its depth. In personal communications he indicated that his use of the term Hidden is the same as my term Deep, and at the same time stated that a quality accessed below the organ depth cannot be interpreted in the framework of this pulse model.

Fig. 9-11a Hidden Excess quality

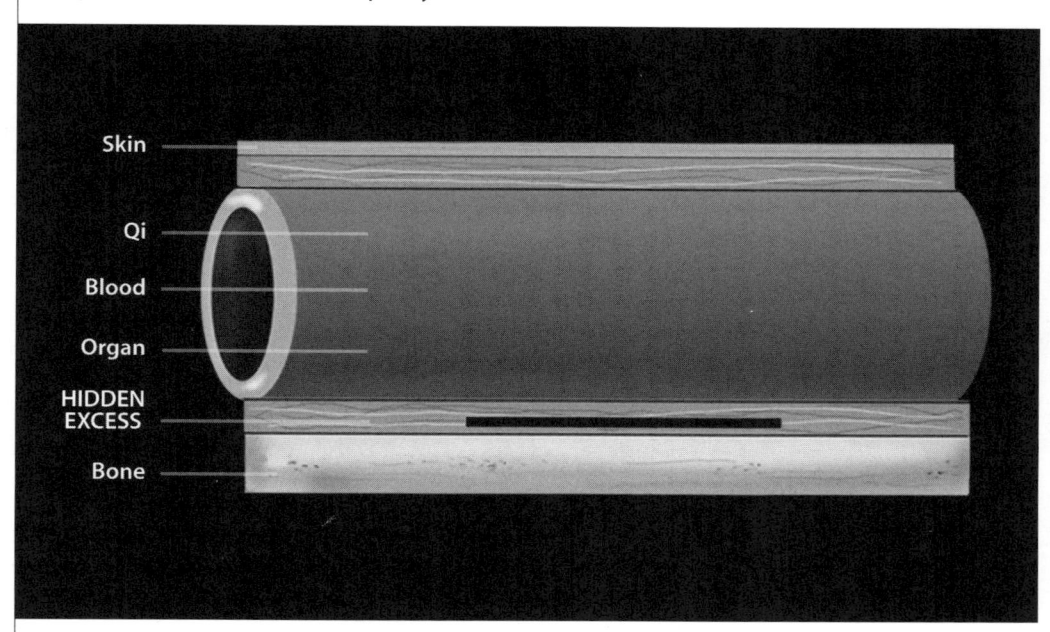

Fig. 9-11b Hidden Deficient quality

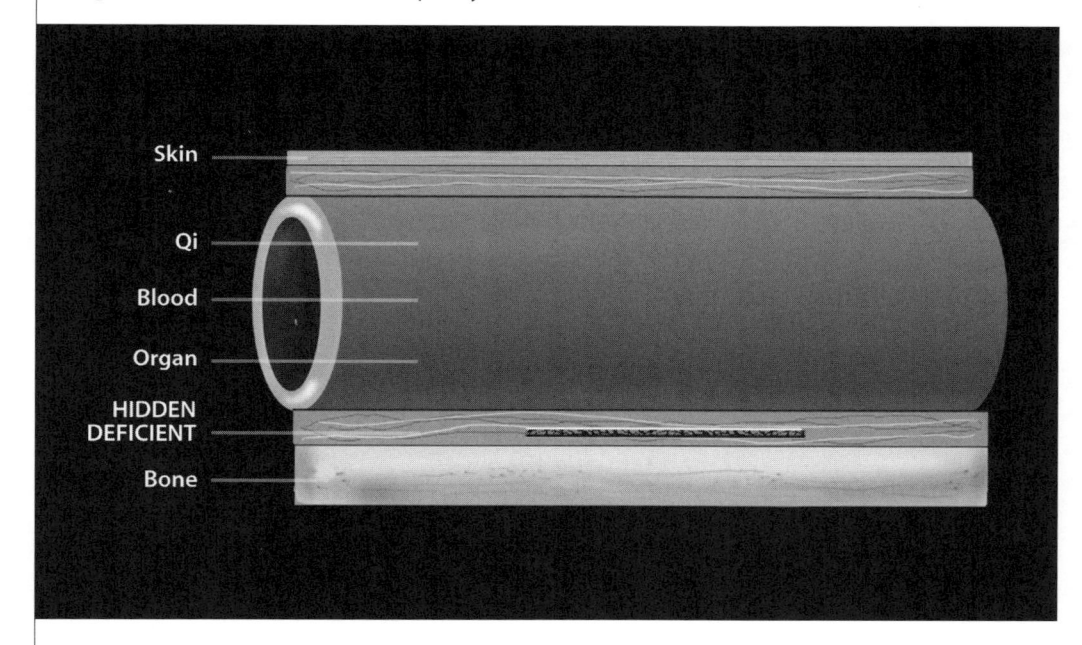

I have encountered the Hidden quality only once. However, pulses which fit this description have been reported to me by rescuers of people suffering from extreme hypothermia in the mountains and freezing lakes, where I now live, and the ocean, near where I lived for twenty years. That one case was a fisherman who had been frozen near the Yalu River in North Korea during the Korean War and who previously and subsequently fished in very cold waters. When he was brought to me he was totally paralyzed, but partially recovered with ginger baths, cupping, and moxa so that he could walk and use his limbs; but he was weak. I saw him only a few times but learned that he died in a veterans hospital at about the age of fifty-five from unknown causes.

I present this quality for that reason, and because it is reported in the literature, but I do so with hesitation for reasons explained in the previous section. The Hidden quality, when drawn to my attention by others, occurs either when the student has pressed too deeply or when it has been mistaken for the Dead or very Muffled qualities. As previously noted, the Hidden quality was probably of greater significance in the past.[111]

Sensation

The Hidden quality (Figs. 9-11a and 9-11b) is felt only with extreme pressure below the organ depth. It is accessed on or just above the radial bone, which curves under the radial artery. The Hidden Excess pulse has a hard Tense quality, and the Hidden Deficient pulse a more Pliable sensation.

Note: In learning this quality, there is a danger that students will mistakenly learn to exert excessive pressure when taking the pulse. In fact, as a general matter, the most common mistake in pulse-taking is the tendency to press too deeply, beyond the fine parameters of the Chinese pulse according to this model, and beyond the realm of its interpretive function. If the bone or tendon is reached, one has departed significantly from the scope of the physiologic value of pulse diagnosis. The boundaries of the pulse are extremely subtle.

Interpretation

Every source agrees that this pulse is usually a sign of serious illness in which the disease process has entered deeply into the yin organ system. Most agree that it is a sign that yang qi is unable to bring the pulse wave to the surface. What differentiates the Hidden Excess from the Hidden Deficient pulse is the factor which prevents the yang qi from rising.

I have found that the Hidden quality is often mistaken for the Dead or very Muffled qualities associated with neoplastic disease. I have seen this especially in cancer of the lung and liver. Dr. Shen has also related that this pulse is a sign of cancer. Among other sources, only Worsley[112] alludes to tumor as an associated quality at both proximal positions.

Types of Hidden qualities

Hidden Deficient

With the Hidden Deficient pulse the probable cause of the yang qi not rising is severe yang deficiency. The accompanying symptoms are severe shortness of breath, palpitations, anorexia, spontaneous sweating, nausea and vomiting, diarrhea, frequent urination, and severe fatigue.[113]

Dr. Shen believes that "it indicates that the internal organs' qi and blood are all used up" and that "deterioration of the internal organs" is evident. He asserts that this pulse is found in individuals who have had severe handicaps during the developmental years, such as malnutrition or overwork, and will not live long.[114]

Hidden Excess

This quality may reflect severe painful obstruction due to severe stagnant external cold (e.g., hypothermia) or internal cold which has transformed into heat, and from stagnation of food, phlegm, or blood, and also from extreme heat transforming into internal wind.[115]

> ### Hidden Normal
>
> Dr. Shen suggests that when the Hidden Normal pulse is found in a relatively healthy person, the quality may be a congenital anomaly. Kaptchuk[116] notes that this quality can be normal in pregnancy.
>
> I have chosen to omit a discussion of the combinations and positions of this pulse because I feel that the more accurate sensations are the Dead and very Muffled qualities (see Chapter 8) which may, by their stifled nature or lack of sensation, convey a sense of being palpated below the organ depth, and because Dr. Shen has always emphasized that sensations below the organ depth cannot be interpreted within the framework of Chinese medicine.

286 ❖ Depth

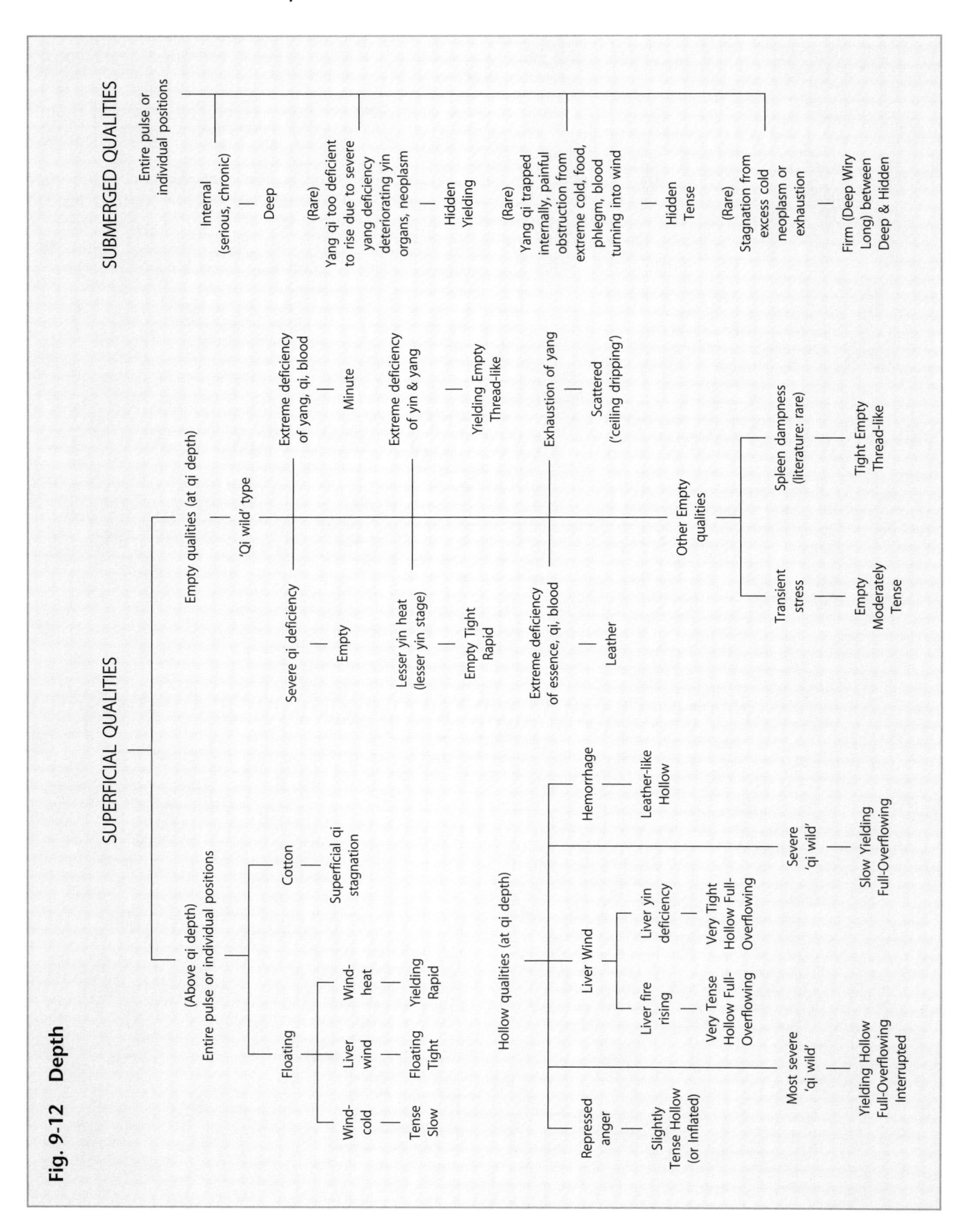

Fig. 9-12 Depth

SUPERFICIAL QUALITIES

(Above qi depth)
Entire pulse or individual positions

- Floating
  - Wind-cold — Tense Slow
  - Liver wind
  - Wind-heat — Floating Tight
  - Yielding Rapid
- Cotton
- Superficial qi stagnation

Empty qualities (at qi depth)

- 'Qi wild' type
- Severe qi deficiency — Empty
- Extreme deficiency of yang, qi, blood — Minute
- Lesser yin heat (lesser yin stage) — Empty Tight Rapid
- Extreme deficiency of yin & yang — Yielding Empty Thread-like
- Extreme deficiency of essence, qi, blood — Leather
- Exhaustion of yang — Scattered ('ceiling dripping')

Other Empty qualities
- Transient stress — Empty Moderately Tense
- Spleen dampness (literature: rare) — Tight Empty Thread-like

Hollow qualities (at qi depth)
- Hemorrhage — Leather-like Hollow
- Liver Wind
  - Liver fire rising — Very Tense Hollow Full-Overflowing
  - Liver yin deficiency — Very Tight Hollow Full-Overflowing
- Repressed anger — Slightly Tense Hollow (or Inflated)
- Most severe 'qi wild' — Yielding Hollow Full-Overflowing Interrupted
- Severe 'qi wild' — Slow Yielding Full-Overflowing

SUBMERGED QUALITIES

Entire pulse or individual positions

- Internal (serious, chronic) — Deep
- (Rare) Yang qi too deficient to rise due to severe yang deficiency deteriorating yin organs, neoplasm — Hidden Yielding
- (Rare) Yang qi trapped internally, painful obstruction from extreme cold, food, phlegm, blood turning into wind — Hidden Tense
- (Rare) Stagnation from excess cold neoplasm or exhaustion — Firm (Deep Wiry Long) between Deep & Hidden

CHAPTER 10

Size: Width and Length

CONTENTS

Width, 289
    Wide pulse group, 289
        Wide Excess qualities, 289
            Tense Hollow Full-Overflowing, 290
            Flooding Excess, 291
        Wide Moderate qualities, 292
            Blood Unclear, 292
            Leather-like Hollow, 292
            Tense Ropy, 293
        Wide Deficient qualities, 293
            Wide Yielding Hollow Full-Overflowing with Normal or slightly Rapid rate, 293
            Diffuse and Reduced Substance, 293
            Yielding Ropy, 294
    Narrow pulse group, 294
        Qi deficiency, 294
            Thin quality in young man, 294
        Yin-essence deficiency, 295
            Tight-Wiry, 295
        Blood deficiency, 295
            ■ Fig. 10-1: Thin quality, 295
            Thin, 295
            Types and combinations of the Thin quality, 296
                Pliable thin qualities, 296
                      Thin Yielding, 296
                      Thin Deep, 297
                      Thin Deep and very Feeble, 297

             Thin Minute, 297
          Hard thin qualities, 297
             Thin Tight-Wiry, 297
             Thin Tight and Rapid, 298
       Positions, 298
          Bilaterally at same position, 298
             Distal, 298
                Thin, 298
                Thin Deep Feeble, 298
                Thin Arrhythmic, 298
                Thin Tight, 299
                Thin Slippery, 299
             Middle, 299
                Thin Feeble, 299
             Proximal, 299
                Thin Tight and Rapid, 299
                Thin Deep Tight-Wiry and Slow, 299
                Thin Deep Feeble and Slow (sometimes Slippery), 299
          Sides, 300
          Individual positions, 300
             Left distal, 300
                Thin, 300
                Thin with Increase in Rate on Exertion, 300
                Thin Deep Feeble or Tight and Rapid, 300
             Severe yin and yang deficiency, 300
                Yielding Empty Thread-like, 301
             All substances, 301
                Restricted (width), 301
Length, 301
   Extended Length, 301
      Long, 301
         Fig. 10-2: Long quality, 301
   Diminished Length, 302
      Short (Abbreviated), 302
         Fig. 10-3: Short quality, 303
      Restricted (length), 303
         Fig. 10-4: Width flowchart, 304
         Fig. 10-5: Length flowchart, 305

CHAPTER 10

Size: Width and Length

Width

Width tells us primarily about the condition of the blood in terms of excess, toxicity, heat, viscosity, plasticity, and deficiency, and the qi in terms of mild deficiency. This is in contrast to spirit or volume, which tells us primarily about qi, and hardness, which tells us about yin.

The Wide pulses are generally associated with excess or heat, and with the more acute patterns.[1] The Narrow pulses are generally associated with deficiency, and with the more chronic patterns. There are, however, important exceptions to these rules, as we shall see below.

WIDE PULSE GROUP

There are three categories within the Wide group of pulses: Wide Excess, Wide Moderate, and Wide Deficient. In the category Wide Excess are the qualities Blood Heat, Blood Thick, Hollow Full-Overflowing, and Flooding Excess. The category Wide Moderate includes the qualities Blood Unclear, Leather-like Hollow, and Tense Ropy. The category Wide Deficient includes the qualities Yielding Hollow Full-Overflowing, Yielding Ropy, and Diffuse. Each of these pulses is discussed elsewhere in this book, especially in Chapters 8 and 9.

In the literature, the terms 'big' and 'large' are generally used for what I call the Wide pulse, as they are portrayed primarily in terms of their width.[2]

Wide Excess qualities

Category

The Wide Excess category encompasses pulse qualities which are wider than normal, primarily those that are caused by pathology of the blood. This includes the Blood Heat, Blood Thick, and Tense Full-Overflowing qualities, discussed at length in Chapters 8 and 13.[3]

Porkert, who refers to the Wide pulse as 'large,' captures the dilemma of defining this quality:

In the majority of Chinese texts on pulse diagnosis, the large pulse is usually taken as synonym for the flooding pulse, hence receives no separate treatment. Clinical experience, however, shows that it can and must indeed be distinguished from the flooding pulse.[4]

Sensation

A Wide Excess pulse has breadth and strength, which varies from mild with Blood Unclear to extreme with a Tense Hollow Full-Overflowing and Flooding Excess quality. It feels distinctly wide or thick in diameter at the blood depth with Tense Hollow Full-Overflowing, or at the organ depth with Flooding Excess, and "has a full quality beneath the fingers."[5] When placing one's finger on the pulse, a Wide pulse occupies more area from side to side than does a Normal pulse.[6]

General interpretation and qualities

The Wide Excess category by itself suggests heat, although in a large person with no other signs or symptoms, it could represent strength or health. However, in a small, thin person, and in women, it should be regarded with suspicion.

Wide Excess Moderate pulses imply pathology affecting the blood. They also may be a little Rapid. This is most easily detected by palpating the organ depth and releasing pressure gradually. If the pulse widens and fills out as one's finger pressure lightens, this is the Blood Heat quality, which is an indication of heat in the blood. If, as one releases finger pressure from the organ to the qi depth, the blood depth widens very slightly, we have a Blood Unclear condition associated with toxicity in the blood. If it widens moderately, we have Blood Heat.

Dr. Shen calls it Blood Thick if it becomes very Wide and continues to widen as one releases finger pressure to the qi depth. Sometimes this quality is associated with early stages of hypertension.

A Blood Thick pattern may be attended by the following signs and symptoms: the tongue and eyes are very red, and there may be skin rashes, mouth and tongue sores, bleeding gums, dark urine, hard stools, sore throat, and other signs of heat. The Blood Unclear, Blood Heat, and Blood Thick qualities and related disorders are discussed in Chapter 13, and the Hollow Full-Overflowing quality in Chapter 8. Our principal discussion will include the Tense Hollow Full-Overflowing quality, which is Wide at the blood depth, and the Flooding Excess quality, which is Wide at the organ depth. Both of these qualities are also classified as abnormal wave patterns (see Chapter 5).[7]

Tense Hollow Full-Overflowing

Sensation

The pulse seems to arise from the blood depth, where it is Wide, and expands to above the qi depth with force as one releases finger pressure. It has a sine curve wave. However, above the qi depth it is slightly Hollow to light pressure (see Chapter 8).

Interpretation

The Tense Hollow Full-Overflowing quality is a sign that the body is unable to efficiently release heat from excess through the normal channels: urine, bowel movement, and perspiration. The heat is accumulating in the vessels and seeking relief by expanding the circulation of blood.

Combinations

The Tense Hollow Full-Overflowing (and sometimes Rapid) combination accompanies the progression from Blood Heat to what Dr. Shen calls Blood Thick. Here the heat in the blood has increased, causing the arteries to dilate. The body is clearly trying to eliminate this heat, which is transforming into wind. The tongue and eyes are very red, and symptoms of extreme heat—headache, epistaxis, hematemesis, hypertension, stroke—are possible. Li Shi-Zhen notes that this combination "indicates excessive fire."[8]

Positions

BILATERALLY AT SAME POSITION

The Tense Hollow Full-Overflowing quality is found bilaterally at each of the three burners (see Chapter 13). At the upper burner position bilaterally, it is often a sign of headache associated with hypertension, and at the middle and lower burners, of hypertension or diabetes.

SIDES

Left

A Tense Hollow Full-Overflowing quality over just the left side can be a sign of an impending cerebrovascular accident involving paralysis on the left side of the body.

Right

Over the entire right side, this pulse could be a sign of an impending cerebrovascular accident involving paralysis on the right side of the body.

INDIVIDUAL POSITIONS

The Wide Excess category includes Blood Heat, Blood Thick, and Tense Hollow Full-Overflowing. For the most part these qualities are found over the entire pulse and rarely at individual positions. The following, therefore, includes information only from the literature for the sake of completion under the aegis of the 'big' pulse.

Left distal

The Hollow Full-Overflowing quality at this position is a sign of Heart related hypertension with a high diastolic.[9]

Left middle

The Hollow Full-Overflowing quality at the left middle position alone is associated with hypertension of the labile variety, with a high systolic.[10]

Left proximal

The Wide Excess category of qualities at the left proximal position is rare. The Tense Hollow Full-Overflowing quality at this position alone is rare. More often this constellation of qualities occurs over the entire pulse, or on one side or the other, at the left middle and proximal positions, or bilaterally at the same burner, as indicated above. It would be a sign of essential or fixed hypertension and/or diabetes.[11]

Right distal

I have not found the Hollow Full-Overflowing quality alone at this position.[12]

Right middle

I have not found the Hollow Full-Overflowing quality at this position alone. It is often confused with the Inflated quality, which does not rise above the qi depth and is common in this position.[13]

Right proximal

I have not found the Hollow Full-Overflowing quality alone at this position.[14]

Flooding Excess

Sensation

The Flooding Excess quality (see Chapter 9) begins with a wide base at the organ depth, rises with force to above the qi depth, and then falls off suddenly.

Interpretation

This is a sign of fulminating heat from excess in one or more of the yin organs. While it can be found at any position, I have found it most often at the middle and proximal positions. We rarely see the acute pneumonias in acupuncture clinics, when it would be found at the right distal position. The Flooding Excess Slippery Tight Rapid combination at the proximal position may signify acute damp-heat or inflammation of the Bladder or Kidneys, or a fulminating colitis. Acute inflammation of the prostate is another possible etiology, especially if there is underlying chronic prostatitis. Acute pelvic inflammatory disease can also present the same pulse picture when there is underlying chronic infection. At the left middle position the cause is most often acute hepatitis or gallbladder infection. Appendicitis, peritonitis, and pancreatitis are causes of the Flooding Excess Wave at the right middle position, or bilaterally at the middle position, and mania and Grave's disease at the left distal.

Wide Moderate qualities

Category

The Wide Moderate category includes the Blood Unclear, Leather-like Hollow, and Ropy qualities, which are discussed in Chapters 9 and 13.[15]

Blood Unclear

Dr. Shen calls Blood Unclear the quality (and associated conditions) in which the blood depth has just barely perceptibly increased in size rather than decreased as one raises one's finger from the organ depth toward the qi depth. Often the pulse is also slightly Slippery.

This sign of toxicity in the blood is usually accompanied by a slightly red tongue that may have a yellow moist coating. The eyes appear normal (without heat signs) and the symptoms often include fatigue and skin-related conditions such as eczema and psoriasis. Dr. Shen likens this condition to a glass of water in which dirt is suspended: the quality of the blood is not good.

The most common cause of this quality is exposure to environmental toxins. I first encountered it with artists using highly toxic solvents, often in poorly ventilated rooms, and with the use of acetylene torches in art and industry (welders).

Another related origin is a stagnant or deficient Liver that is not adequately detoxifying. In addition to storing the blood itself, the Liver also stores the blood toxins that are not metabolized by the Liver. These toxins contaminate the blood and ultimately the entire organism which it nourishes. Skin symptoms are one obvious attempt to discharge that toxicity.

Still another cause of this pattern is a qi-deficient Spleen which is not adequately building the blood due to poor absorption and digestion of food, especially protein. The protein is only partially digested into small chain polypeptides the size of viruses instead of being completely digested down to amino acids. The small chain polypeptides are absorbed and the body reacts to them as if they were viruses by inappropriately mobilizing the immune system. Eventually, autoimmune diseases develop.[16]

Leather-like Hollow

Sensation

The pulse is Wide, especially at the blood depth. It is Leather-like at the qi depth and completely Hollow (not separating) at the blood depth, and present at the organ depth.

General interpretation

The Leather-like Hollow quality is the only pulse which falls into this category. It is a sign of serious hemorrhage: to be anticipated if the rate is Rapid, or already past if the rate is Slow. While more often found at individual positions, it has more rarely been found over the entire pulse.[17]

Positions | A Leather-like Hollow quality can be felt at any position where acute hemorrhage is involved, as explained above under the general interpretation.

Tense Ropy

Sensation | The pulse is cord-like, big, hard, and round and is distinct from the surrounding anatomical structures, giving the impression that the vessel could be grasped like a rope, lifted, and moved. It is sometimes straight and sometimes a bit twisted, and it varies in degree of hardness and in size. It is always continuous through all positions.

Interpretation | The Tense Ropy quality is specifically a sign of chronic heat in the blood from excess and deficiency that has vulcanized the muscular walls of the vessels so that they have lost all flexibility and elasticity. The pulse is usually considered to be an indication of a widespread general athero-arteriosclerotic process, and is sometimes preceded or accompanied by hypertension. It is regarded as a pulse that is difficult to alter, and is usually treated at first by reducing heat, and then with yin-nourishing and blood-moving herbs.

While this quality is generally encountered in an older person with a lifelong 'nervous system tense' disorder, or one who has had a diet of excessively rich foods, Dr. Shen reports finding the Tense Ropy quality in a young person following a serious accident.

Position | Whereas the Tense Ropy quality is found in all six positions simultaneously, it is often most prominent at the left middle position. This is possibly because the Liver stores the blood and is therefore the organ which would most likely reflect the heat in the blood, which is one of the causes of the hardening process. I have never felt this quality completely alone in any one position, on just one side or the other, or bilaterally at just one level.

Wide Deficient qualities

This category includes the Yielding Hollow Full-Overflowing and the Diffuse Yielding Ropy qualities.

Wide Yielding Hollow Full-Overflowing with Normal or slightly Rapid rate

The Wide Yielding Hollow Full-Overflowing quality is a sign of a severe 'qi wild' disorder with symptoms of depersonalization, severe panic and anxiety, irritability, and extreme fatigue. It occurs in people who exercise excessively over long periods of time and then stop suddenly. This quality is only found over the entire pulse, and is discussed more fully in Chapters 6 and 8.[18]

Diffuse and Reduced Substance

Category | There is no other system of classification that I have reviewed which describes these qualities. It is discussed more fully in Chapter 9.

Sensation | The perception of the Diffuse quality is of a wide, nebulous piece of cheese cloth without definite boundaries surrounding the principal impulse, into which it blends imperceptibly. The Reduced Substance quality lacks form and feels like a thread-bare sweater.

Interpretation	The Diffuse and Reduced Substance qualities are signs of early qi deficiency, wherever it is found.
Position	While the Diffuse quality can be found at any position, I have found it most often at the left middle position, and somewhat less often at the left proximal and right middle positions.

Yielding Ropy

Sensation	Yielding Ropy, as described in Chapter 11, is cord-like, big, and round but yielding, and slightly hollow rather than hard. It is also distinct from the surrounding anatomical structures, giving the impression that the vessel could be grasped, lifted, and moved, but more like a soft flexible tube than a hard rope.
Interpretation	Dr. Shen attributes this quality to a situation in which a person has either been participating vigorously in sports, or has been exercising beyond their energy for a relatively long period of time. (This 'qi wild' condition is discussed in Chapter 9.) The drying out of the intima and media of the vessels occurs in this case due to lack of nourishment, rather than heat. The yin and yang in the blood vessels has separated. Exercising beyond one's energy for a long period of time causes the yin (nourishing blood and qi) flowing in the center of the vessel to diminish and then separate from the activating yang qi at the surface of the vessel, thus depriving the walls of the nourishment required to keep them flexible. Overexercise causes gradual shrinkage of yin-blood (due to using up more than can be replaced), while the heart pumps harder to maintain circulation, causing the walls to stay distended. I have now observed this quality combination several times in recent years, including a 60-year-old man who was subsequently diagnosed with Parkinson's disease. It is my speculation that this may involve impaired circulation to the brain related to alterations in the blood vessels indicated by the Yielding Ropy quality. I do not have enough clinical experience with this quality to cogently address the issue of associated medical syndromes.
Positions	This quality is found only over the entire pulse, although it may be more obvious at the left middle positions, as they represent the Liver which stores the blood and where blood and blood vessel disorders are most easily assessed.

NARROW PULSE GROUP

Qi deficiency

Thin quality in young man

A narrow Thin quality in a young man is associated more with severe qi deficiency attended by grave, chronic auto-immune disease than with the usual interpretation of blood deficiency. Naturally, both deficiencies exist simultaneously, but the qi deficiency seems more prominent. A typical example of the seriousness of the Thin quality in a young man was a recently examined 46-year-old man with systemic histoplasmosis, which has a ninety-percent fatality rate.

Yin-essence deficiency

Tight-Wiry

The Tight and Wiry qualities are both Thin, especially the Wiry quality. They are described more fully in Chapter 11.

Blood deficiency

Fig. 10-1 Thin quality

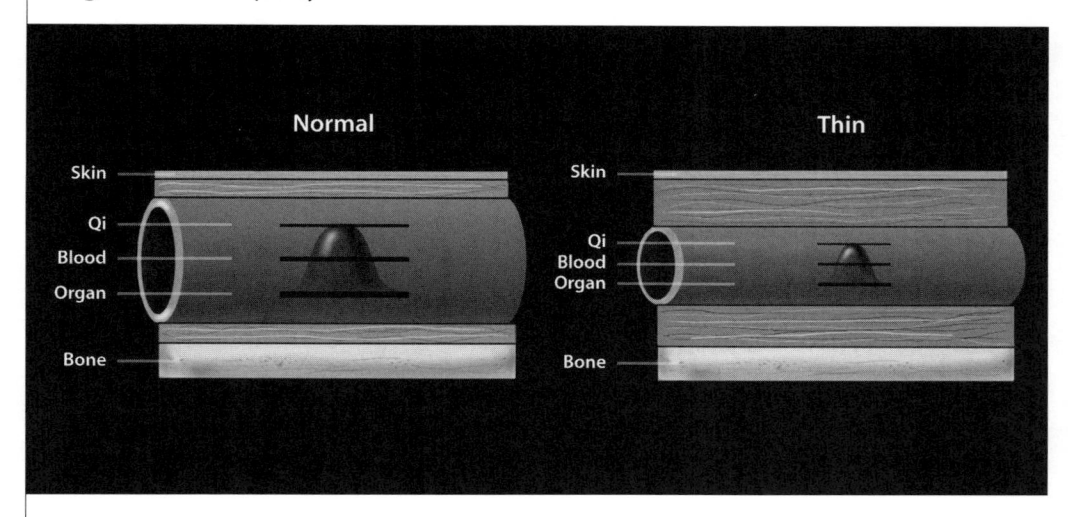

Thin

Category	Although perhaps not exactly the same, the terms Thin, Fine, Thready, and Small are used interchangeably throughout the literature. Even though Dr. Shen refers to this pulse as Fine, we shall refer to it as Thin, since it describes the feeling sensation unambiguously. It is clearly the logical antonym of the term Wide, and is therefore consistent with our terminology. There are two kinds of Thin pulse. One is Tight and is associated by me with blood and yin deficiency. The other is Yielding and is associated with blood and qi deficiency.
Sensation	The Thin quality (Fig. 10-1) is narrower than the width of the Normal pulse. Dr. Shen speaks of two kinds of Thin (Fine) pulse qualities, one that is "a little tight (or a little strong)" and another that is "weak."[19]
General interpretation	**SHEN** Most sources agree that this quality is a sign of both blood and qi deficiency; blood deficiency, however, is primary. According to Dr. Shen, "The deficiency of blood will result in a deficiency of qi."[20] **CONTEMPORARY CHINESE PULSE DIAGNOSIS** The Thin quality, especially at the organ depth, is a sign that there is blood deficiency in the yin organs, and not just in the circulating blood. The Thin quality at the blood depth alone is a less serious sign, and at the qi depth, even less serious. A Yielding Partially Hollow quality is an even less serious sign of blood deficiency, primarily in the

circulatory system, and the Spreading quality with an Absent qi depth and separation at the blood depth is primarily a sign of mild qi deficiency with some blood deficiency.

The term blood deficiency is confusing since it has been used to mean both anemia, a diminished number of circulating red blood cells in the Western biomedical tradition, and as dryness in the continuum of yin deficiency in the Chinese medical system. Since blood in the Western model includes a solid (red blood cells) and a liquid (serum) component, anemia, in my opinion, refers primarily to reduced red blood cells, and blood deficiency to a reduction in the serum component, with some overlap. Kaptchuk alludes to blood as a "liquid."[21]

Types and combinations of the Thin quality

There are two principal types of Thin pulse. One is pliable, or Thin Yielding, which indicates both blood and qi deficiency, and the other is hard, or Thin Tight, characteristic of blood and yin deficiency.

PLIABLE THIN QUALITIES

Thin Yielding

This quality represents the concomitant presence of blood and qi deficiency. There are three general etiologies. One is related to loss of blood, either rapid or gradual, due to hemorrhage or disease. The second is due to an insufficiency in the production of blood. The third is the result of stagnation, either qi stagnation or deficiency, blood stagnation, or even fluid stagnation.

Blood leads qi

When the cause is loss of blood, the most frequent etiology is excessive menstruation over a long period of time. The latter can be due to the Liver failing to fulfill its function of storing the blood, or the Spleen failing to govern the blood. Childbirth, abortion, miscarriage, hemorrhage due to trauma (including surgery), hemoptysis, epistaxis, hematemosis, and rectal bleeding are other causes.

Qi leads blood

With regard to a more gradual depletion, blood deficiency may also result from dehydration, which is often seen in old age or during a prolonged wasting illness. Dr. Shen notes that the Thin pulse "indicates that the individual's physical condition is weak."[22] He adds that if the problem occurs in middle age, then "the individual has overworked or overexercised between the ages of fifteen to twenty."[23] This combination usually accompanies a chronic condition, or is found in a weak individual.

Another cause of blood deficiency (just mentioned), which is more apparent than real, is deficient circulation, most often due to Heart qi deficiency. The amount of blood is sufficient, but the delivery is inadequate. This factor is often overlooked in menstrual, obstetrical (including infertility), and gynecological problems, and is frequently accompanied by lower burner blood stagnation for the same reason.

With regard to the insufficiency of production, blood has two sources. One is from the combination of nutrient (food) qi from the digestion of food, and qi from the air, both of which combine with clear fluids in the digestive tract. Blood deficiency, therefore, can result from the poor digestion of food by the Spleen qi, which produces too little nutrient qi, or from a disease of the Lungs, which interferes with the reception of cosmic qi. The other source of blood is the medulla (marrow), nurtured and controlled by Kidney essence. If the essence is deficient, this can impair the function of the medulla, and thereby cause blood deficiency. Dr. Shen comments that when the Thin and "weak" (Yielding) pulse is found in teenagers, "it is of congenital origin."[24]

Stagnation leads blood

Blood stagnation due to heat from excess, birth control devices, medications, or surgery can also lead to blood deficiency. This usually occurs in the other direction, however, with blood deficiency leading to blood stagnation.

The qi moves the blood. Anything which interferes with the circulation of qi can lead to blood deficiency, and thus a Thin pulse quality. Qi stagnation or deficiency may therefore be implicated in anything which interferes with the circulation of blood, and therefore causes de facto blood deficiency. There is enough blood, but it is not reaching the tissues. Li Shi-Zhen, in particular, emphasizes the role of circulation. He mentions a fundamental connection with "yang qi" and says that circulation should therefore be strong in the spring and summer; a young person with a Thin pulse at these times of year is at risk.[25] Similarly, a Thin pulse found in an elderly person during the fall and winter, when this energy is diminished, "does not indicate disease, but reflects a normal reaction to weather."[26]

Thin Deep

In the absence of pain, this pulse indicates deficiency of circulating qi and blood. Although it is outside of my own experience, the literature says that, with pain, it is a sign of "dampness obstructing qi and blood."[27]

Thin Deep and very Feeble

This combination signifies deficiency of blood, qi, and possibly yang in the yin organs.

Thin Minute

This combination is a sign of severely deficient yang, qi, and blood, which leads to a 'qi wild' separation of yin and yang.

HARD THIN QUALITIES

Thin Tight-Wiry

Blood deficiency and yin deficiency

According to Miles Roberts, the Japanese regard blood deficiency as the precursor or earlier manifestation of yin deficiency.[28] The Thin quality would precede the Tight quality if blood deficiency came first, and the Tight quality would precede the Thin quality if the etiology was yin deficiency. It is my opinion that either yin or blood deficiency can lead to the other.

The Thin Tight combination is usually associated with overwork of the mind and 'nervous system' due to emotional stress over a long period of time. It is often found only at the qi depth in the intermediate stages of this disorder, as the pulse qualities move from Tense to Tight. Cheung and Belluomini agree, noting that the Thin ('small') pulse quality "indicates both blood and yin deficiency."[29]

Thin Tight and Rapid

In the absence of pain, and with clear eyes and tongue, this combination, especially when found at the qi depth over the entire pulse, indicates a long-standing nervous condition equivalent to Dr. Shen's concept of an overworked 'nervous system.'

With pain due to trauma, there will likely be corresponding signs on the tongue and inside the lower eyelids that appear with trauma. A horizontal red line will appear on the inside of the lower eyelid on the side of the trauma. A purple blister will appear on the side of the tongue on the same side as the trauma. (See Chapter 7 for further discussion of eyelid diagnosis.)

Positions

BILATERALLY AT SAME POSITION

Distal

Thin

Here we have blood deficiency in the Heart, and perhaps consequently in the Lungs, with a pale and/or peach-colored tongue, pale under the eyelids, and symptoms which include impaired concentration and memory, palpitations, anxiety, insomnia, excessive dreaming, and dizziness. The thinner the pulse, the greater the blood deficiency.

Despite the absence of a specific Lung blood pattern in the available literature, logic would dictate that blood, which in Chinese medicine is said to flow through all of the channels, must also nourish the Lungs.

Larre and Rochat de la Vallée note that

> the transport and circulation of blood, although under the authority of the Breadths of the Heart, nevertheless need the Breadths of the Lung to be able to spread out everywhere with ease, and it is by connecting with the *mai* [vessels] of the Heart that they communicate freely everywhere in the whole body.[30]

Thin Deep Feeble

With this pulse combination one will find Heart and Lung qi and blood deficiency with such symptoms as shortness of breath on exertion, excessive sweating, fatigue, and a stifling sensation in the chest, problems with mentation, palpitations, anxiety and insomnia, and a tongue that is pale and somewhat flabby or a little swollen.

According to Li Shi-Zhen, but not observed by me, this combination may be attributable to deficiency of qi due to severe vomiting.[31] With Heart qi deficiency, the rate may decrease on exertion, or increase considerably with emotional stress.

Thin Arrhythmic

This is a sign of Heart blood and yang deficiency with such symptoms as shortness of breath, excessive spontaneous daytime sweating, fatigue, suffocating chest, chills, and cold, as well as memory and concentration problems, palpitations, anxiety, and insomnia.

Thin Tight

Heart and Lung yin and blood deficiency, with a peach-colored and red-tipped tongue. If there is more blood deficiency than yin deficiency, the pulse rate will probably be closer to Normal or a little Slow. Should there be a greater degree of yin deficiency and more heat from deficiency, the pulse will tend to be a little Rapid and perhaps more Tight, which is frequently found with yin-deficient asthma.

Thin Slippery

This pulse combination usually indicates Heart blood deficiency, with an accumulation of damp-phlegm in both the Heart and Lungs. If the phlegm is more in the Heart, the symptoms will be emotional or neurological; if the phlegm is more in the Lungs, the symptoms will be asthmatic.

Middle

Thin Feeble

Over a long period of time, deficient Spleen qi may cause blood deficiency affecting the blood of the Liver (as well as the Heart,) expressed as Thin and Feeble qualities bilaterally in the middle position.[32]

Proximal

Thin Tight and Rapid

The Thin Tight and slightly Rapid pulse bilaterally at the proximal position is most often a sign of Kidney yin deficiency. More rarely, it may accompany an acute though mild exacerbation of chronic dysentery, colitis, severe bladder or kidney infection, pelvic inflammatory disease, or prostatitis, especially if the pulse is very Rapid.

Thin Deep Tight-Wiry and Slow

This pulse quality, bilaterally at the proximal position, could be a sign of Kidney qi, essence, and yin deficiency due to constitutional deficiency, excessive sex or masturbation, or especially overworking of the nervous system. Here the Wiry quality can also be a sign of pain, of blood stagnation, and very early diabetes, determined by other pulse signs (such as Choppy in the Pelvis/Lower Body positions), symptoms, and the tongue, eyes, and color.

Thin Deep Feeble and Slow (sometimes Slippery)

This combination is associated with Kidney yang deficiency and/or sluggish bowel and lower abdominal stagnation (Slippery) from either Kidney qi deficiency due to constitution or excessive sex or masturbation, a long-term improper diet of refined foods lacking in fiber, or any abuse which drains qi from any yin organ, such as overwork draining the Liver qi.[33] Stagnant qi in the lower abdomen, leading to lower burner deficiency, may also be attributable to overuse of this area, as with sit-up exercises.

SIDES

Left — A Thin pulse restricted to the left side indicates a deficiency of qi and blood in the 'organ system,' and is a sign of potential or current severe weakness and illness.

Right — A Thin pulse restricted to the right side implies a relatively severe weakness of both qi and blood, in what Dr. Shen refers to as the 'digestive system.' This is reflected in symptoms of a fluctuating appetite, general abdominal discomfort, irregular bowel movements varying from loose to constipated, and mucus in the chest and throat.

INDIVIDUAL POSITIONS

Left distal

Thin

At this position, the Thin pulse signifies that the blood is not nourishing the Heart. Kaptchuk mentions "Heart palpitations; insomnia."[34] There is also impaired memory, concentration, and excessive dreaming.

Thin with Increase in Rate on Exertion

If, on mild exertion, the rate increases more than eight beats per minute, this is a greater sign of Heart blood deficiency ('Heart weak'). (See Chapter12 for an assessment of 'Heart weak.') The eyelids are pale and the tongue is pale or peach-colored. Mentation and sleep are even more impaired than with only a Thin quality at the left distal position.

Thin Deep Feeble or Tight and Rapid

If the combination is Thin Feeble with a Normal or slightly Rapid rate, the condition is one of severe Heart blood stagnation ('Heart small'). If the combination is Thin Deep Tight and very Rapid, it is trapped qi in the Heart ('Heart full'). The latter is one step away from an enlarged heart. These pulse findings are outside of my own experience.

Right distal — Lung qi deficiency is associated with this quality here.[35]

Left middle — Thin and Tight indicates Liver blood and yin deficiency. Thin and Yielding means Liver blood and qi deficiency.[36]

Left proximal — Kidney essence and yin is exhausted due to excessive sexual intercourse or masturbation, severe or prolonged diarrhea, or pituitary deficiency. Kaptchuk mentions "spermatorrhea; diarrhea,"[37] and Worsley, "cold at belly; diarrhoea; pollution."[38]

Constitutional weakness of original qi is also associated with the Thin quality at this position. It is my clinical impression that deficiencies of both Kidney yin and yang may be found at the left proximal position, with the former accompanied by a Tight, and the latter by a Feeble-Absent, quality. Depending on degree, if both yin and yang deficiency exist simultaneously, the harder Tight quality will more likely be palpated until the yang deficiency is very severe.

Right proximal — Kidney yang is depleted due to excessive sex or masturbation, severe or prolonged diarrhea, or constitutional deficiency of original qi.[39] Kidney yang deficiency is associated with thyroid deficiency.

Severe yin and yang deficiency

Yielding Empty Thread-like

This is a narrow pulse quality described more fully in Chapter 9, and mentioned briefly above under combinations of the Thin quality. It is a 'qi wild' quality due to extreme yin or yang deficiency.[40]

All substances

Restricted (width)

This very narrow quality has been observed only in the Special Lung position as a sign of pulmonary obstructive disease and cancer of the lung, chest, and breast. It seems to involve severe stagnation and deficiency of all substances. In this position, it has been mistaken for the Thin quality. This is a less serious sign than the Restricted (length) quality discussed below.

Length

Except for the Short quality with Absent distal and proximal positions and Robust middle positions, I have not found the Long or Short qualities to be clinically useful. They are included here only in the form of Figs. 10-2 and 10-3. An extended discussion of the Long quality has been placed in the endnotes.[41]

EXTENDED LENGTH

Long

Fig. 10-2 Long quality

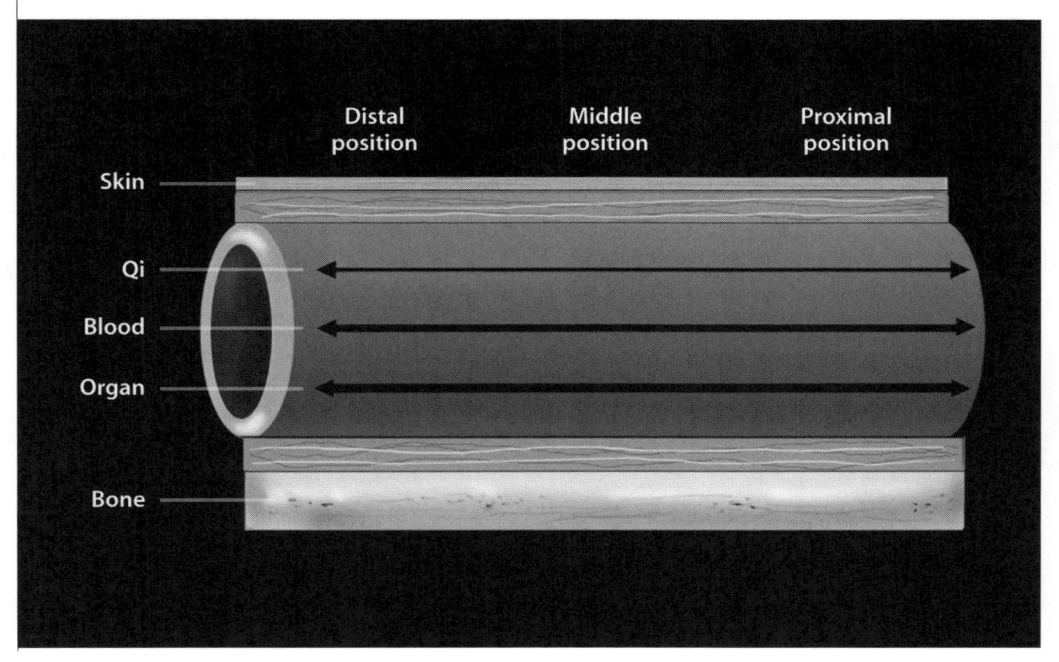

Category	The Long pulse is obviously categorized in terms of length. Li Shi-Zhen places this pulse with the Short and Wiry qualities. He considers the latter to be a quality partially defined by length because it is "stiff and tightly stretched."[42] It is also cataloged as a Normal pulse.
Sensation	The Long quality (Fig. 10-2) is continuous between the three principal positions and feels like an elongated stroke. It slightly exceeds the parameters of the Normal pulse beyond the distal and proximal positions in both directions. When it is a sign of health, it has all of the other characteristics of the Normal pulse.[43]
General interpretation	The normal moderately Long quality described above is a sign of strong qi, health, and the potential for a long life. When the Long pulse is combined with other qualities, as described in the endnotes, disease is indicated, most often involving heat from excess.

DIMINISHED LENGTH

Short (Abbreviated)

Category	As is self-evident, this pulse is classified by its diminished length. The Short quality is either Short Strong (stagnant) or Short Weak (deficient).[44]
Sensation	The literature says that the Short quality feels disconnected rather than continuous between the distal, middle, and proximal positions. Kaptchuk states that "sometimes a pulse is called short even when it is felt in all three positions but the beats touching the fingers feel too small in length."[45] This is, in fact, quite rare. Most practitioners are unaware of the Diaphragm positions between the upper and middle positions bilaterally, the Gallbladder position between the left middle and proximal positions, and the Stomach-Pylorus position between the right middle and proximal positions. In some descriptions of the Short quality, either the proximal or distal position is Absent. In practice, the interpretations of these pulse qualities do not match the classical interpretation discussed below, but have quite different meanings such as deficiency of the upper burner, Heart, and Lungs, or of the lower burner or Kidneys. The only configuration of the Short quality that I have encountered which matches the classical interpretation is illustrated in Fig. 10-3. Here the only palpable position is the middle one.[46]
General interpretation	According to most sources, the Short quality, and the stagnation between organs associated with it, is a sign of deficiency. What I have found in practice is that there appears to be a very Robust middle position, and Reduced or Absent upper and lower positions. This represents diminished circulation between the upper and lower burners through the middle burner. This is associated with either severe stagnation of substances in the middle burner; qi, blood, and food interfering with the passage of substances; or severe deficiency of qi in the upper and lower burners which is unable to move substances through the middle burner. The differentiation among etiologies is made by the response to treatment. If using the Girdle vessel releases the stagnation in the middle burner we know that the cause was one of excess. If the Girdle vessel does not change the configuration we must consider deficiency as the cause and especially treat the upper and lower burners to nourish the qi and blood, and only later move them.
Combinations and positions	I have no personal experience with combinations involving this pulse quality, or with positions beyond what I have already described.

Fig. 10-3 Short quality

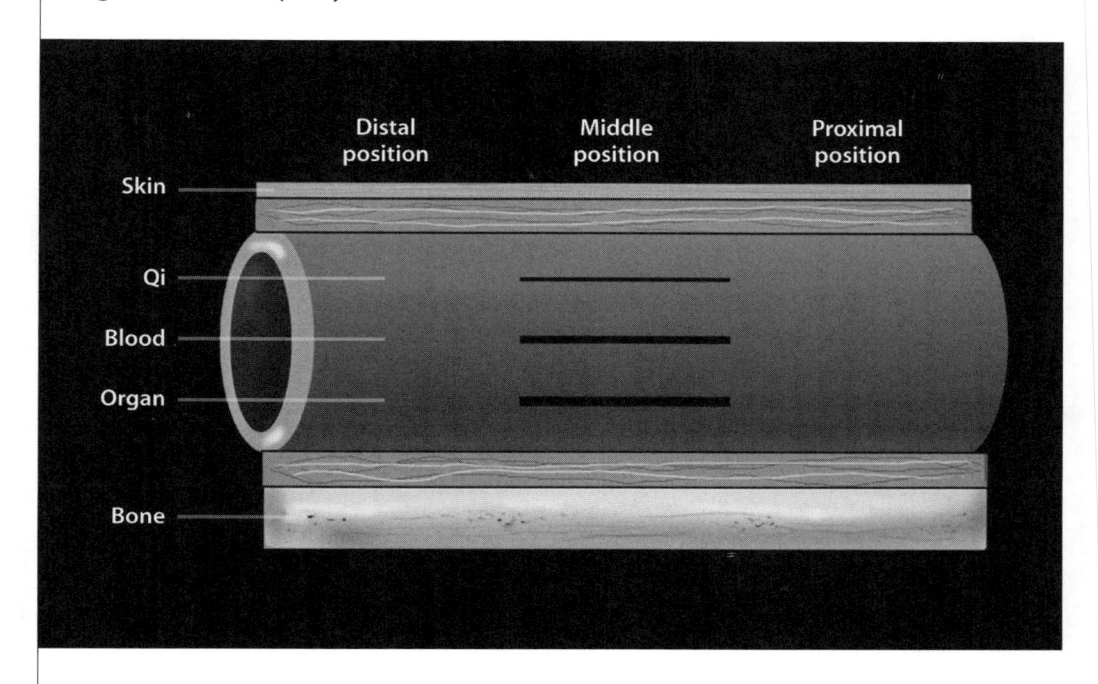

Restricted (length)

This very short quality, like Restricted (width), has been found only in the Special Lung position as a sign of pulmonary obstructive disease and cancer of the lung, chest, and breast. It seems to involve severe stagnation and deficiency of all substances, and signifies a more serious illness than the Restricted (width) quality.

Fig. 10-4 Width

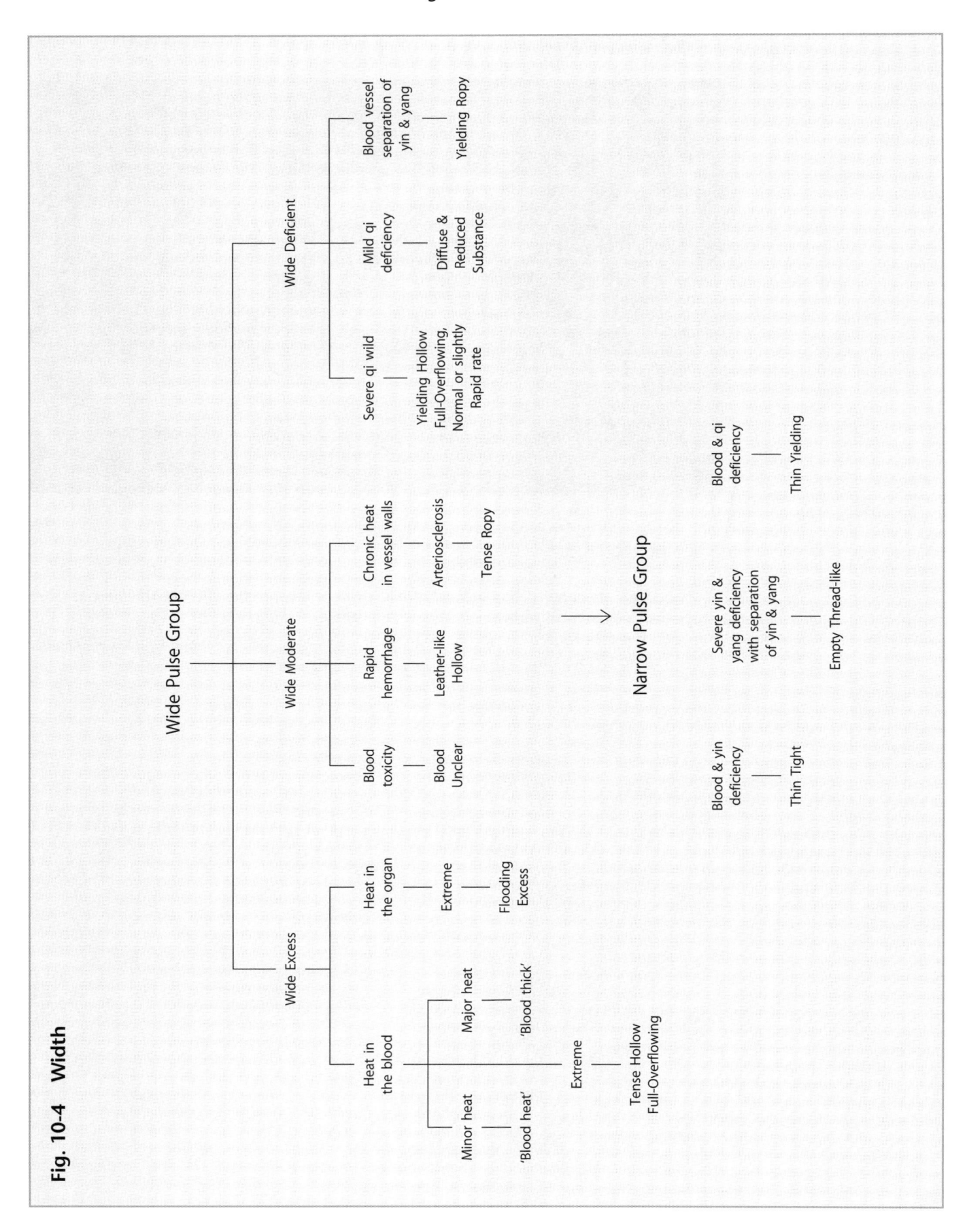

Wide Pulse Group

Wide Excess

- Heat in the blood
  - Minor heat — 'Blood heat'
  - Major heat — 'Blood thick'
  - Extreme — Tense Hollow Full-Overflowing
- Heat in the organ
  - Extreme — Flooding Excess

Wide Moderate

- Blood toxicity — Blood Unclear
- Rapid hemorrhage — Leather-like Hollow
- Chronic heat in vessel walls — Arteriosclerosis — Tense Ropy

Wide Deficient

- Severe qi wild — Yielding Hollow Full-Overflowing, Normal or slightly Rapid rate
- Mild qi deficiency — Diffuse & Reduced Substance
- Blood vessel separation of yin & yang — Yielding Ropy

→

Narrow Pulse Group

- Blood & yin deficiency — Thin Tight
- Severe yin & yang deficiency with separation of yin & yang — Empty Thread-like
- Blood & qi deficiency — Thin Yielding

Fig. 10-5 Length

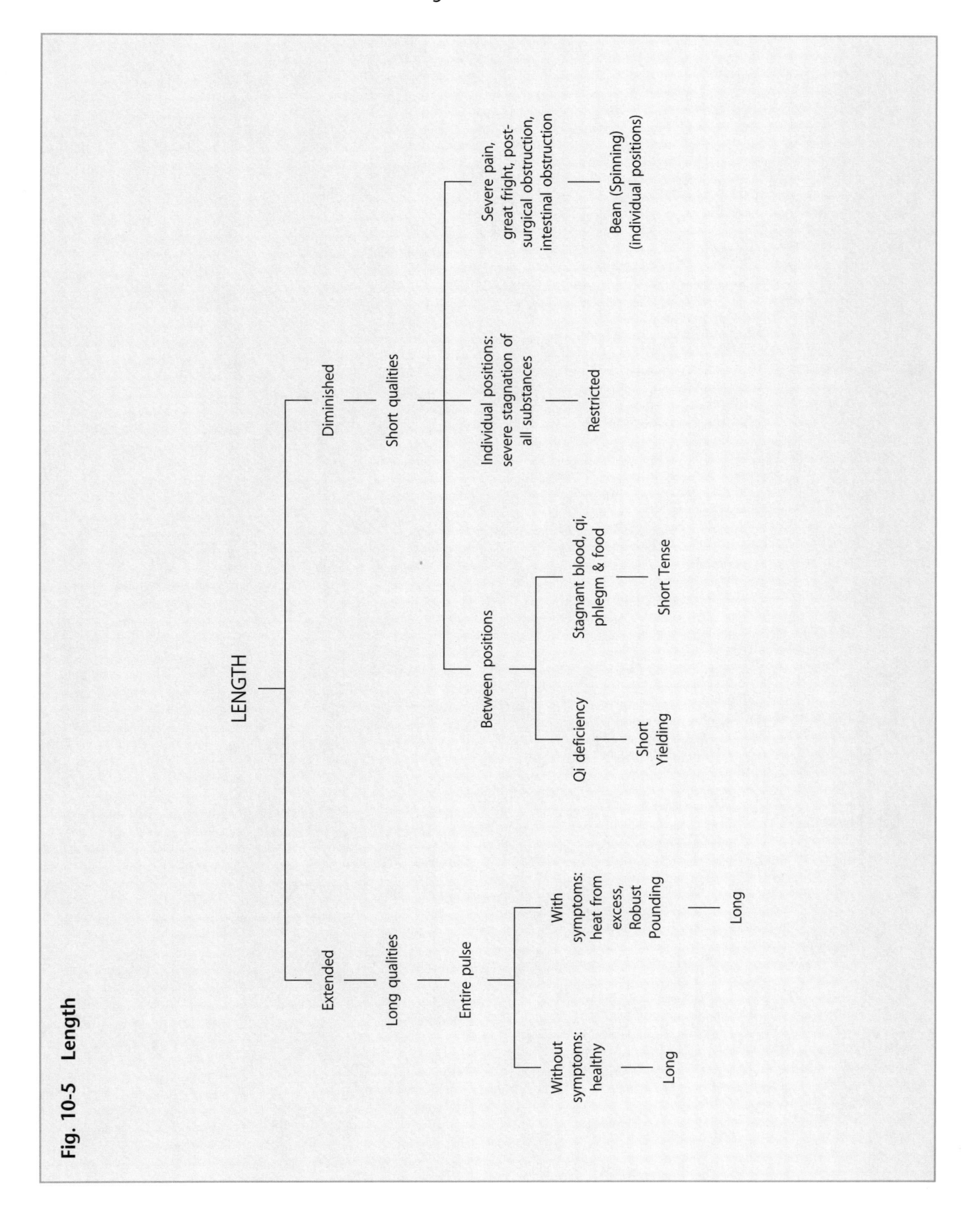

LENGTH

- **Extended**
  - Long qualities
    - Entire pulse
      - Without symptoms: healthy — Long
      - With symptoms: heat from excess, Robust Pounding — Long
- **Diminished**
  - Short qualities
    - Between positions
      - Qi deficiency — Short Yielding
      - Stagnant blood, qi, phlegm & food — Short Tense
    - Individual positions: severe stagnation of all substances
      - Restricted
      - Severe pain, great fright, post-surgical obstruction, intestinal obstruction — Bean (Spinning) (individual positions)

CHAPTER 11

Shape

CONTENTS

Fluid Qualities, 313
    Slippery, 313
        Fig. 11-1: Slippery quality, 314
        Depths, 314
             Entire pulse at all depths, 314
                  Slippery Tight Hollow Full-Overflowing and Rapid, 315
                  Slippery Feeble and Slow, 315
            Qi depth, 316
                  Tense Slippery with Normal or slightly Rapid rate, 316
                  Yielding Slippery and Slow, 316
                  Transiently Slippery, 316
            Blood depth, 316
                'Blood unclear,' 'blood heat,' blood thick', 316
                Heart qi deficiency, 317
            Organ depth, 317
            Individual positions at all depths, 317
        Combinations, 317
            Slippery and Slow, 318
            Slippery and Rapid, 318
            Slippery Transient above the qi depth, 318
        Positions, 318
             Bilaterally at same burner, 318
                  Distal, 318
                      Slippery Tense and Rapid, 318
                      Slippery Tight and slightly Rapid, 318
                      Slippery Tense and Slow, 318

Special Lung, 318
Middle, 319
Proximal, 319
Sides, 319
  Left, 319
    Slippery and Slow , 319
    Slippery Tense and Normal rate, 319
    Slippery Tense and Normal to slightly Rapid rate, 320
    Slippery Tense and very Rapid (possibly Flooding Excess Wave), 320
    Slippery and very Tight Hollow Full-Overflowing, 320
  Right, 320
    Slippery Tense at qi depth with Normal or slightly Rapid rate, 320
    Slippery Feeble and Slow, 320
    Slippery and very Tight Hollow Full-Overflowing, 320
    Slippery Tense at all depths, 320
Individual positions, 320
  Left distal, 320
    Slippery and Slow, 320
    Slippery Tense and slightly to very Rapid, 321
    Very Slippery Deep and very Rapid, 321
    Slippery and very Tight Hollow Full-Overflowing and Rapid, 321
    Slippery Feeble with Normal rate, 321
    Slippery and very Rapid with high fever, 321
    Slippery at Mitral Valve position, 321
  Right distal, 322
    Slippery, 322
    Slippery Tight Flooding Excess and Rapid, 322
    Slippery Tight and Slow, 322
    Slippery Feeble, 322
  Left middle, 322
    All depths, 322
      Slippery Feeble and Slow or Slippery Empty, 322
      Slippery Tense and slightly Rapid, 322
      Slippery Tight and Rapid, 322
      Slippery Tight Flooding Excess and Rapid, 322
      Slippery Tight and Slow, 323
    Qi depth, 323
      Mildly Slippery Yielding and Slow, 323
      Mildly Slippery Tense with Normal to slightly Rapid rate, 323
    Blood depth, 323
    Organ depth, 323
      Moderately to severely Slippery, 323
  Gallbladder, 323
    Slippery Tense, 323
    Slippery Tight-Wiry, and (rarely) Choppy or Muffled, 323
  Right middle, 323
    Slippery Tight and slightly Rapid, 324
    Slippery Feeble and Slow, 324
    Slippery Inflated, 324
    Slippery at Esophagus position, 324
    Slippery Tight (Hollow) at Stomach-Pylorus Extension position, 324

Rapid rate, 324
Slow rate, 324
Left proximal, 324
Slippery and Slow, 324
Slippery Tense and Slow, 324
Slippery Deep Feeble and Slow, 325
Slippery Deep Tight to Wiry and Rapid, 325
Slippery Tense Flooding Excess (and possibly Rapid), 325
Slippery only at organ depth, 325
Right proximal, 325
Slippery Tense, 325
Slippery Tight Flooding Excess and Rapid, 325
Slippery Deep Feeble, 325
Intestines, 325
Pelvis/Lower Body, 326

Nonfluid Qualities, 326
    Old classification of nonfluid qualities, 326
    New classification of nonfluid qualities, 327
        Pathogenesis, 327
        Sensation, 327
        ■ Fig. 11-2: Violin (nonfluid qualities: Taut, Tense, Tight, Wiry), 328
        Clinical significance, 328
        The relationship of the hard qualities to deficiency, 329
    Even nonfluid qualities, 329
        Taut, 329
            Combinations, 330
                Taut Floating, 330
                Taut and slightly Rapid, 330
                Taut Inflated, 330
                Taut Wide, 330
                Taut Choppy, 330
                Taut and Slow, 330
                Taut Slippery, 330
            Positions, 331
                Bilaterally at same burner, 331
                Sides, 331
                Individual positions, 331
        Tense, 332
            Combinations, 333
                Tense Floating, 333
                Tense Deep, 333
                Tense and Rapid, 333
                Tense and Slow, 333
                Tense Inflated, 334
                Tense Wide, 334
                Tense Hollow Full-Overflowing, 334
                Tense Choppy, 334
                Tense Slippery, 334
                Tense Slippery, Flooding Excess, Robust Pounding, 334
            Positions, 335
                Bilaterally at same position, 335
                Sides, 336

              Individual positions, 336
       Tight, 337
              Combinations, 338
                     Tight Floating, 338
                     Tight Deep, 338
                     Tight and Rapid, 338
                     Tight Thin, 338
                     Alternating from Tight to Yielding, 340
                     Tight Inflated, 340
                     Tight Choppy, 340
                     Tight Wide Slippery, 340
                     Tight Flooding Excess, 340
              Positions, 340
                     Bilaterally at same burner, 341
                     Sides, 343
                     Individual positions, 344
                            Left distal, 344
                                   Tight at Pericardium position, 344
                                   Tight over entire left distal position, 345
                                   Tight with Change in Rate at Rest, 345
                                   Tight Deep Thin and very Rapid, 345
                                   Tight Deep Thin Feeble and slightly Rapid, 345
                            Left middle, 346
                                   Tight Floating, 346
                                   Tight Thin, 346
                                   Tight Slippery Robust Pounding and Rapid, 347
                                   Tight, Flooding Excess, Robust Pounding, Slippery and Rapid, 347
                                   Tight Empty at qi depth, 347
                            Gallbladder, 347
                            Right middle, 347
                                   Tight only at qi depth, 347
                                   Tight at Esophagus position, 348
                                   Tight at Stomach-Pylorus Extension position, 348
                            Left proximal, 348
                                   Tight, 348
                                   Tight Robust Pounding and Rapid, 348
                                   Tight Thin, 348
                                   Tight Hollow Full-Overflowing, 348
                            Large Intestine, 348
                            Right proximal, 348
                                   Tight, 348
                                   Tight Deep, 349
                                   Tight, Flooding Excess, Robust Pounding and Rapid, 349
                            Small Intestine, 349
                            Left and right Pelvis/Lower Body, 349
       Wiry, 349
              Combinations, 351
                     Wiry Thin, 351
                     Wiry Deep, 351
                     Wiry and Rapid, 351
                     Wiry Slippery at Blood depth with Normal or slightly Rapid rate, 351

Wiry Slippery and very Rapid, 351
Wiry Robust Pounding and Rapid, 352
Wiry Empty and slightly Rapid, 352
Wiry Deep and Slow, 352
Wiry Inflated, 352
Wiry Choppy, 352
Positions, 352
Bilaterally at same burner, 352
Sides, 355
Individual positions, 356
Uneven nonfluid qualities, 360
Ropy, 360
Fig. 11-3: Ropy quality, 360
Tense Ropy, 360
Ropy Yielding Hollow, 361
Fig. 11-4: Choppy quality, 361
Choppy, 362
Combinations, 364
Choppy Tight or Wiry, 364
Positions, 364
Bilaterally at same position, 364
Sides, 365
Individual positions, 365
Vibration, 366
Fig. 11-5: Smooth and Rough Vibration qualities, 366
Types, 367
Smooth Vibration, 367
Rough Vibration, 367
Overall attributes, 367
Etiology, 367
Entire pulse, 367
Individual position, 367
Seriousness of condition, 367
Signs and tests of seriousness, 368
Individual attributes, 368
Consistency, 368
Time, 368
Degree of smoothness, 368
Depth, 369
Entire pulse, 369
Consistent Rough Vibration, 369
Smooth Vibration, 371
Combinations, 371
Positions, 371
Bilaterally at same position, 371
Neuro-psychological, 371
Distal, 371
Middle, 371
Proximal, 371
Sides, 372
Left, 372
Right, 372

      Individual positions, 372
       Left distal, 372
      Smooth Vibration, 372
        Superficial Smooth Vibration, 372
        Less superficial Smooth Vibration, 372
        Smooth Vibration both superficial and deep, 372
        Progression from left distal to other positions, 372
      Rough Vibration deeply or at all depths, 373
       Neuro-psychological, 373
       Mitral Valve, 373
       Right distal and Special Lung, 373
       Left middle, 373
       Gallbladder, 373
       Right middle, 373
       Esophagus, 373
       Stomach-Pylorus Extension, 373
       Proximal, 373
       Intestine, 373
       Pelvis/Lower Body, 373
Miscellaneous Shape Qualities, 374
  Nonhomogeneous, 374
  Bean (Spinning), 374
    Combinations, 375
      Bean (Spinning) Wiry, 375
      Bean (Spinning) Tight very Slippery and Rapid, 375
    Positions, 375
      Bilaterally at same position, 375
      Individual positions, 375
  Doughy, 375
Qualifying Terms, 376
  Biting, 376
  Rough, 376
  Smooth, 376
  Subtle (vague), 377
  Ephemeral (transient), 377
  Robust or reduced force, 377
  Robust (with) substance and reduced (without) substance, 377
  Separating, 378
Anomalous Qualities, 378
  Three yin *(san yin mai)* or hidden left pulse, 378
  Transposed pulse *(fan quan mai)*, 378
  Ganglion, 378
  Trauma, 378
Anomalous Vessels, 378
  Split vessels and multiple radial arteries, 378
    Multiple radial arteries, 379
    Split vessels, 379
  Summary, 379
▪ Fig. 11-6: Shape flowchart, 381
▪ Fig. 11-7: Qualifying terms and anomalous qualities flowchart, 382

CHAPTER 11

Shape

Classification by shape implies that the pulse quality is recognized more by shape than by other descriptive parameters such as depth, width, volume, length, rate, and rhythm. Shape may be subdivided into those qualities whose sensation is relatively unyielding and lacks fluidity, such as Taut, Tense, Tight, Wiry, Ropy, Leather, Choppy, and Vibration, and those which are fluid and more yielding, of which there is just one quality, Slippery. As far as I know there is no record of the subtle differentiations among the unyielding pulses, except for some distinctions noted by Dr. Shen:

> There are three kinds of Tight pulse distinguished by degrees of tightness: the shi-xian is the most tight—it is strong and firm; ping-xian is less tight; wen-xian, which is least tight.[1]

In my view it is more productive to separate these into Taut, Tense, and Tight than to refer to most, less, and least. I hope to demonstrate the clinical value of making these distinctions below.

Fluid Qualities

Slippery

Category

I classify the Slippery quality under the category of shape, and as a form of stagnation due to a wide variety of causes. This is similar to Kaptchuk[2] who takes this pulse to represent yang (excess) with yin (dampness), as do I.[3]

Sensation

With the Slippery quality (Fig. 11-1) the pulse slides rapidly under the fingers in one direction. The movement is independent of finger pressure.

This quality is most commonly confused with the Spreading, Empty (Separating in stage one and two) and Hollow qualities, where the separating movement is felt in two directions, distally and proximally, but not directly under the center of the finger, and where the sensation of separation increases with pressure. That shift gives the false impression of a flowing movement that can easily be confused with the Slippery quality, whose movement is also flowing, but is continuous independent of pressure, and remains under the center of the finger, always flowing in just one direction.[4] The confusion with the Spreading quality is most often when the sensation involves the entire pulse, and with the Empty and Hollow qualities at individual positions such as the right and left middle positions respectively.

General interpretation

Except in pregnancy, Dr. Shen regards the Slippery quality as always indicating a pattern of disharmony with impaired function. While the literature associates the Slippery quality with excessive fluid, closer examination reveals a much more complex situation.

Fig. 11-1 Slippery quality

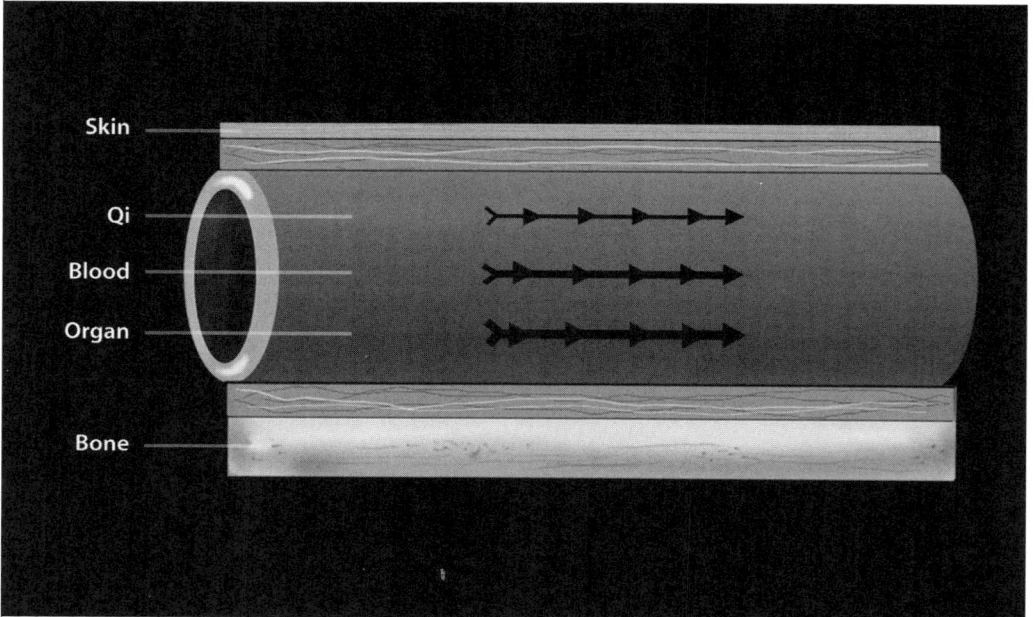

Depths

ENTIRE PULSE AT ALL DEPTHS

The interpretation of the Slippery quality over the entire pulse depends on the depth. Often when only one depth is Slippery, later in the pathological process it will become Slippery at all depths. While the particular combination of Slipperiness with other qualities helps point the way, the diagnosis should be confirmed by other diagnostic signs.

Pregnancy

The appearance of Slipperiness at all depths over the entire pulse may be a very early sign of pregnancy. Here it is interpreted as an excess of fluid in the form of blood necessary to sustain the fetus. A distinction may be made with some accuracy (ninety percent, in my own experience) between a male and a female fetus. If the left proximal position is stronger, a boy may be expected; and if the right proximal position is stronger, a girl may be expected. Dr. Shen also finds a more Robust left distal position and a generally more Rapid pulse with a male fetus, which I cannot confirm.

Elevated blood lipids and glucose

Slipperiness over the entire pulse at all three depths can also be a sign of highly increased blood viscosity for reasons other than dampness or pregnancy, as with increased serum lipids (cholesterol and triglycerides) and glucose. Slipperiness over the entire pulse for this reason, which is usually also Tense, is a sign that only blood turbulence and not the blood vessels are involved. When the blood vessels are damaged there is a Tight Rough Vibration at the blood depth. More often with elevated lipids the Slippery quality is found only at the blood depth.

Blood infection

If the rate is very Rapid, the quality is Tight-Tense, and the color under the eyelids is very red, we are dealing with systemic blood infection (heat or fire), a serious condition known in biomedicine as septicemia.

Systemic infection

With acute systemic infection one expects a very Rapid rate, a Tense Flooding Excess quality, and overwhelming debilitating symptoms, including a very high fever. With chronic systemic infection, such as parasites or hepatitis, the pulse is Slower and less Tense than it would be with elevated blood lipids and glucose.

Heart qi deficiency and shock to circulation

Severe Heart qi deficiency is another factor which can lead to the creation of extreme turbulence in the blood, causing a Slippery and Slow quality over the entire pulse at all three depths, rather than just the blood depth, where it could be found with less Heart qi deficiency. The Heart controls the circulation, which will decrease with any interference to Heart function, or from shock directly to the circulation, as with trauma. With Heart qi deficiency the left distal position, or even the entire pulse, will be Feeble. With trauma the pulse will be more Tight, with a horizontal red line on the inside of the lower eyelid and a purple blister on the tongue.

Hypertension

Slippery Tight Hollow Full-Overflowing and Rapid

This combination is found with impending stroke as an expression of Liver wind due to blood heat, and with phlegm clouding the orifices of the Heart.

Slippery Feeble and Slow

This combination over the entire pulse occurs shortly after a stroke.

Iatrogenic, blood dyscrasias, and auto-immune disease

Another scenario for this quality over the entire pulse at all three depths is the use of corticosteroids, which causes water retention; in such cases, the rate is Normal or slightly Slow. I have found this quality over the entire pulse at all depths with blood dyscrasias, such as sickle cell anemia and hemochromatosis, as well as with auto-immune diseases such as lupus.

QI DEPTH

Tense Slippery with Normal or slightly Rapid rate

If the pulse is Tense and Slippery at the qi depth, we must first consider excessive sugar in the blood.

Yielding Slippery and Slow

Less often, Slipperiness at the qi depth alone indicates that the qi is deficient. If the rhythm is unbalanced it is serious, but if the rhythm is Normal it is not serious. The deficiency of qi renders it less able to move fluids in the connective tissues, creating a superficial damp disorder with reduced perspiration in warm weather. This qi deficiency is often primarily of the Heart.

Transiently Slippery

Another, less common, cause of Slipperiness at the qi depth is accumulation of dampness in the protective qi level due to an attack by wind, or 'wind-water.'

BLOOD DEPTH

'Blood unclear,' 'blood heat,' blood thick'

I associate the Slippery quality at the blood depth with turbulence in blood flow due to any cause which increases viscosity, such as dampness and heat, elevated lipids, or infection. According to Dr. Shen, Spleen and Gallbladder damp-heat is the greatest source of the Slippery quality at the blood depth. The turbulence is an indication that the conditions for the laying down of plaque already exist and that arterio-atherosclerosis is well on its way. It can also be due to blood flowing in the wrong direction, as with an incompetent heart valve. Ultimately, turbulence in the blood from any cause will cause the Heart to overwork and become weakened.

Slipperiness in the entire blood depth, its more common location, often accompanies conditions (and pulse qualities) described by Dr. Shen as 'blood unclear' (impure blood), 'blood heat,' or 'blood thick.' In Western terms, this would be conceived as various stages of toxicity or increasing blood viscosity. If the entire pulse is Slippery and Tense at the blood depth, the cause is heat in the blood, and if the entire pulse is Rapid, Slippery, and Tight at the blood depth, the cause is infection in the blood.

The principal source of the 'blood unclear' disorder and associated pulse is environmental toxins. Solvents used in industrial processes or by artists is a common etiology. Dr. Shen associates a condition in which the entire pulse at the blood depth is a little Unclear, Tight, and Slippery with arthritis due to blood toxicity. The vertical lines inside of the lower eyelid are not straight and vary from light to dark.

Another source of the 'blood unclear' toxicity is poor digestion associated with the Spleen qi. This especially involves the incomplete digestion of protein into small polypeptide molecules the size of virus molecules rather than into amino acids. These small molecules are absorbed, circulate in the blood, and are reacted to by the immune system as if they are foreign bodies. This can lead to auto-immune disorders and food allergies.[5] Another source is inadequate metabolism by the Liver, which stores the blood. This can be due to longstanding qi stagnation, usually associated with stress and repressed emotions, and sometimes chronic parasites, impairing the Liver's ability to detoxify the blood.

'Blood heat' can be caused either by excessive hot and spicy foods or Liver qi stagnation and yin deficiency associated with a 'nervous system tense' condition over a long period of time. The 'blood thick' pattern is related to excessive fat and sugar consumption, or to Stomach fire due to Liver attacking the Stomach-Spleen over a prolonged period, or to spicy foods.

Pathological changes in the intima of the vessels, such as loss of elasticity, are involved in the early stages with Rough Vibration at the blood depth, and later when the pulses become Tense and Ropy.

Heart qi deficiency

Heart qi deficiency is another factor which can lead to the creation of turbulence in the blood and a Slippery quality at the blood depth. The Heart controls the circulation, which will diminish with any interference in Heart function or from shock directly to the circulation, as with trauma. Slipperiness appears only after the impairment has caused considerable turbulence.

ORGAN DEPTH

Slipperiness at the organ depth alone over the entire pulse is rare and is associated with severe systemic infection.[6] With the latter condition it appears more often at the organ depth on the left side or left middle position.

INDIVIDUAL POSITIONS AT ALL DEPTHS

Slipperiness can be found over an entire individual position, or at just the qi, blood, or organ depth. Especially at the organ depth, it is frequently a sign of infection in the associated organ, as in the Kidneys (stones) and Liver (parasites, hepatitis). At the qi depth it is often a sign of qi deficiency, and in the middle positions at this depth, a sign of excessive sugar in the blood.

Slipperiness can also have a more specific meaning, depending on the location. In some positions, such as the Esophagus and Stomach-Spleen, Slipperiness indicates food stagnation, gastric hyperacidity, or an ulcer. True Slipperiness over the entire middle position is rare. It is usually confused with the Cotton or Separating qualities. When it is really present, it indicates Spleen qi deficiency. Here it is associated with persistent dull headache, tinnitus (water sloshing), and vertigo (room swirling), as well as clouding of consciousness.

As the thickness of the retained fluids increases, with the simultaneous appearance of heat or cold from excess, it is designated as phlegm. This heat, paradoxically, can develop slowly because of the stagnation due to dampness. It may also come from another source, such as Liver fire (fire from excess) or yin deficiency (heat from deficiency) of the Kidneys, Liver, Heart, and Lungs, either alone or in combination. The cold can be attributed to an external pathogenic factor that has become internal, severe exposure, or the ingestion of very cold food and drink over time.

The dampness may be associated with the appearance of phlegm in the upper burner with sputum, pulmonary symptoms such as cough with bronchitis, or mental-emotional symptoms such as schizophrenia and epilepsy; in the middle burner with phlegm, indigestion, nausea, and undigested, stagnant food; and in the lower burner with damp-heat or damp-cold 'pouring' into the Bladder, Large Intestine, and uterus.[7]

Combinations

Many combinations have already been mentioned above.

Slippery and Slow

These qualities represent the presence of cold-phlegm.

Slippery and Rapid

This combination indicates the presence of hot-phlegm.

Slippery Transient above the qi depth

This combination of qualities represents a rare form of an external pathogenic factor, such as wind-cold or wind-heat, creating an excess of phlegm. With this etiology, the combination can appear over the entire pulse if the person is very weak, or if the pathogen is extremely virulent. It is more commonly restricted to the Lung and Special Lung pulses.

An attack of wind-dampness with signs of urticaria may also be accompanied by a Slippery Transient pulse. 'Wind-water' with edema of the face and eyes, cough, and shortness of breath caused when wind obstructs the dispersing and downward-directed actions of the Lung may also be attended by a Slippery quality above the qi depth

Other combinations are found in the literature, but are outside of my experience.[8]

Positions

BILATERALLY AT THE SAME BURNER

Distal

Slippery Tense and Rapid

Slipperiness at both distal positions simultaneously may be a sign of asthma due to a damp-heat pattern in the Lungs.

Slippery Tight and slightly Rapid

Phlegm-fire in the Heart is sometimes accompanied by Slipperiness at both distal positions at times, though it is usually greater at the left distal position. In this condition the orifices of the Heart are 'obstructed' or 'disturbed,' leading to neurosis and mental illness, such as mania or schizophrenia, or neurological illness, such as epilepsy (see Chapter 15). This indicates qi stagnation, phlegm, and heat in the entire chest, usually from long-standing Liver qi stagnation or food stagnation in the middle burner. This pulse may also be found in pre- and post-stroke victims, where phlegm as well as fire and wind are etiological factors.

Slippery Tense and Slow

This can be a sign of phlegm alone clouding the orifices of the Heart, which is usually accompanied by depression. While Spleen dampness is usually present, neither fire nor Liver qi stagnation is involved.[9]

Special Lung

Slipperiness at these positions alone indicates the presence of dampness in the Lungs from an earlier pathology.

Middle

Spleen dampness and Liver-Gallbladder damp-heat

Slipperiness and a Yielding and Slow quality bilaterally at both middle positions implies severe Spleen qi deficiency and dampness. As explained above, this pulse is rare and is confused with the Cotton and Separating qualities. A Slippery Tense and Rapid quality bilaterally involves damp-heat in the Liver-Gallbladder system, with signs of Liver-Gallbladder inflammation.

Peritonitis, pancreatitis, appendicitis, hepatitis

The Tight Slippery quality bilaterally in the middle position is a strong sign of infection in the peritoneal area. A very Rapid Flooding Excess pulse is a sign that the infection is acute, a Slow Tense pulse that it is chronic. Peritonitis, pancreatitis, appendicitis, and even hepatitis are associated with these pulse qualities.[10] Often with these conditions there is simultaneously present both the Spleen and Liver Engorged Ulnar positions.

Proximal

Kidney stones and infection

Slipperiness bilaterally at this position is associated with kidney stones, inflammation, and mucus in the intestines, such as in ulcerative colitis and regional enteritis, or pelvic inflammatory disease. Accompanied by a Tight to Wiry Rapid quality, there is the likelihood of sharp pain, usually associated with kidney stones. Colitis, regional enteritis, and pelvic inflammatory disease is usually attended by a Flooding Excess quality. The differentiation is made based on the symptoms. If, for example, it is accompanied by severe flank pain, it is usually a kidney stone. With regard to diabetes, the rare Slipperiness that I have observed here has always been at the blood depth, usually accompanying a Wiry quality, and less often a Tense-Tight Hollow Full-Overflowing quality.[11]

SIDES

Most often, Slipperiness at the qi depth on one side alone, with a Rapid rate, is a sign of excessive sugar. With a Slow rate, this pulse on the left side would indicate 'organ system' deficiency, and 'digestive system' deficiency on the right side. Slipperiness and a Normal or slightly Rapid rate confined to one side at the organ depth, or at all depths, could also be a sign of chronic infection in one or more of the yin organs represented on that side. Slipperiness on either side, accompanied by a Tight Rapid Hollow Full-Overflowing quality, may portend a stroke due to phlegm blocking the orifices of the Heart, 'blood heat,' or Liver wind. The stroke will occur on the side where these qualities are found. If this pulse is accompanied by a Feeble and Slow quality, the stroke may already have occurred.

Left

Slippery and Slow

This is a sign of qi deficiency in the 'organ system' involving a subtle deficiency of the Heart, Liver, and Kidneys.

Slippery Tense and Normal rate

This is a sign of excessive sugar and fat in the blood, especially if the blood depth is wide. The eyes are slightly injected, and the tongue has a moderately thick coating.

Slippery Tense and Normal to slightly Rapid rate

Especially if the Slipperiness is greater at the organ depth, this combination is a sign of chronic infection in the yin organs, particularly the Liver. Parasites and chronic hepatitis should be considered.

Slippery Tense and very Rapid rate, possibly with Flooding Excess Wave

This combination is a sign of acute infection in the yin organs, especially the Liver, involving hepatitis, mononucleosis, or even parasites.

Slippery and very Tight Hollow Full-Overflowing

This is a sign of impending stroke on the left side.

Right

Slippery Tense at qi depth with Normal or slightly Rapid rate

This is also a sign of mild excessive sugar in the blood. The eyes are injected.

Slippery Feeble and Slow

Slipperiness over the entire right side may indicate a severe damp-cold disorder, such as candidiasis, in the 'digestive system,' which would indicate a failure of water metabolism and regulation in the Spleen, Lungs, and Kidneys. In this situation the eyes would be clear.

Slippery and very Tight Hollow Full-Overflowing

This is a sign of impending stroke on the right side.

Slippery Tense at all depths

This combination may also indicate 'digestive system' damp-heat and infection developing in the culture medium which dampness creates. Bacterial infection *(B. Pygeum)* should be considered. Here the sclera of the eyes would be injected.

INDIVIDUAL POSITIONS

Left distal

The Slippery quality at this position is almost always accompanied by some form of emotional or neurological disturbance (see Chapter 15).

Slippery and Slow

With this combination one can find severe depression, mental confusion, delusions, clouding of consciousness, and talking to oneself. This pattern is usually associated with Liver qi invading the Spleen, impairing its capacity to transform and transport fluids.

Emotional stress causes the Liver qi stagnation. The phlegm is thought to be in the Pericardium, which covers and protects the Heart, but through which it must communicate. In the West we might identify this as a psychotic depression with psychomotor retardation.

Slippery Tense and slightly to very Rapid

The latter may evolve to phlegm-fire disturbing the Heart. The fire is generated from prolonged Liver qi stagnation leading to heat from excess in the Liver, which is balanced by fluids which accumulate in the Gallbladder and go to the Heart. The signs and symptoms are more closely identified in biomedicine with mania, schizophrenia, autistic behavior, or epilepsy, and in Chinese medicine with the 'utmost heat' of Liver wind: coma. The tongue is more red, especially the tip, and the tongue coating more greasy. The patient is more active, both physically and verbally.

Very Slippery Deep and very Rapid

According to Dr. Shen, this combination indicates serious impairment of the circulation of blood in the heart involving coronary artery occlusion. Probable symptoms are angina, palpitations, and shortness of breath.

Slippery and very Tight Hollow Full-Overflowing and Rapid

These could be signs of impending stroke, although usually the signs can be found over one entire side, or, in very severe cases, over both sides. Here we have phlegm obstructing the orifices of the Heart combined with Liver wind and 'blood heat.'

Slippery Feeble with Normal rate

Slipperiness over the entire left distal position without fever is a sign of phlegm obstructing the orifices of the Heart. This may be found with post-stroke patients, although often the Slippery Feeble quality is over the entire side of the stroke, or over the entire pulse if the stroke is severe. Other signs include a white, greasy tongue, a dull expression with a blank stare, loss of consciousness, phlegm in the throat with gurgling, aphasia, and paralysis.

Slippery and very Rapid with high fever

This combination may indicate fire toxin or an infection of the Pericardium, which is called myocarditis in biomedicine.

Mitral Valve

Slippery

Whereas a Vibration quality at this position is an indication of a mildly insufficient mitral valve, Slipperiness is a sign of a more serious prolapse of the valve,[12] associated in biopsychiatry with panic disorders.

Right distal

Slippery

Slipperiness in the right distal position is a sign of a currently active damp disorder in the Lungs. Often, with chronic dampness in the Lungs, Slipperiness is discovered only in the Special Lung position, rather than in the right distal position. This indicates that the problem began earlier in life and is now not clinically active. (For more detail, see the section on the right distal position in Chapter 12.)

Slippery Tight Flooding Excess and Rapid

A current infection may be indicated. The Tighter and more Rapid and Flooding Excess the pulse, the more profound the problem, from mild bronchitis to pneumonia.

Slippery Tight-Wiry and Slow

This pulse is associated with a chronic Lung affliction such as pneumonitis.

Slippery Feeble

This usually implies stagnant fluids accompanied by bronchial asthmatic symptoms due to Lung qi deficiency, or it may be a sign of pulmonary edema with more serious signs of cardiopulmonary failure.[13]

Left middle

Slipperiness at the organ depth is an indication that whatever the condition, the entire body may be affected. If it is found only at the blood and qi depths, the condition is restricted to the Liver.

All depths

Slippery Feeble and Slow or Slippery Empty

This is a sign of severe impairment of Liver qi affecting the function of the entire organism. We must be concerned with lymphomas or primary liver cancer.

Slippery Tense and slightly Rapid

This is a sign of Liver damp-heat and moderate chronic infection.

Slippery Tight and Rapid

The Rapid rate in this combination is a sign of a more active subacute disorder and can be present with symptoms of chills and fever and indigestion, as with acute mononucleosis. With right subcostal pain we may have acute gallbladder disease with stones.

Slippery Tight Flooding Excess and Rapid

If this combination is accompanied by fever and debility, there may be acute, fulminating hepatitis.

Slippery Tight and Slow

If there is low-grade fever with great fatigue and lymphadenopathy, there may be chronic mononucleosis or hepatitis.

Qi depth

Mildly Slippery Yielding and Slow

This combination here is interpreted as a sign of a slight impairment of Liver function due to mild overwork.

Mildly Slippery Tense with Normal to slightly Rapid rate

This is a sign of excessive sugar in the blood.

Blood depth

Slipperiness at this position is a sign of turbulence in the blood.

Organ depth

Moderately to severely Slippery

This is usually a sign of damp-heat in the Liver and infection with greater impairment of Liver function. The Slipperiness may sometimes be felt at the organ depth over the entire left side, or at least at the proximal and middle positions.[14] Parasites should be considered if the pulse rate is Normal or a little Rapid, and candidiasis if Slow.

Gallbladder

Slippery Tense

It is most common for this combination of qualities to appear in the Gallbladder position, usually without other symptoms. Here, these qualities are a marker for a developing damp-heat disorder, which should be considered in any preventive treatment program. Diet and stress associated with decisions are important etiological factors.

Slippery Tight-Wiry and (rarely) Choppy or Muffled

With this combination we have clear signs of advancing inflammation of the gallbladder and significant cholelithiasis. With Wiriness the process is probably symptomatic, with pain and indigestion. With Choppiness we may have necrosis of the gallbladder, while a Muffled quality here is a sign of more advanced necrosis and possible rupture. Black spots on the sclera confirm gallstones.

Right middle

The Slippery quality in the right middle position is reported far more often than it actually appears, and is frequently mistaken by practitioners for the Cotton and Separating qualities.

Slippery Tight and slightly Rapid

This pulse is found with mild gastric hyperacidity accompanied by abdominal discomfort. The Slipperiness is somewhat superficial at the qi depth. (A Hollow quality can also accompany a more severe gastric hyperacidity, or gastric ulcer.) Slipperiness at the organ depth is usually a sign of infection in the stomach *(H. Pylori)*.

Slippery Feeble and Slow

In the right middle position this combination would be more indicative of Spleen qi deficiency with dampness, especially if occurring with loss of appetite, fatigue, sallow complexion, and other signs of qi deficiency. Frequently, the complementary Spleen position is also Inflated. Chronic candidiasis is associated with these signs.

Slippery Inflated

This combination may indicate stagnant food if accompanied by signs of bloating, gas, fullness, reflux, and heartburn after eating. Since this pattern may also be accompanied by heat, the pulse may also be slightly Rapid.

Esophagus

Slippery

This is a sign of food stagnation.

Stomach-Pylorus Extension

Slippery Tight (Hollow)

RAPID RATE

This indicates inflammation (gastritis) in the lower Stomach, and if the Small Intestine position has the same qualities, it indicates the duodenum has ongoing inflammation or ulcer.

SLOW RATE

This indicates qi stagnation or an accumulation of hydrochloric acid, which will eventually lead to a 'cold' gastric or duodenal ulcer, due to qi deficiency.[15]

Left proximal

Slippery and Slow

This combination denotes dampness in the lower burner due to deficiency with signs of Kidney essence and qi deficiency, such as nocturnal spermatorrhea, cold limbs, pain in lumbar area and legs, and impotence.

Slippery Tense and Slow

Here, according to Richard van Buren,[16] there are dreams accompanying the nocturnal spermatorrhea, which is outside of my experience.

Slippery Deep Feeble and Slow

With this pulse, Van Buren[17] says that there are no dreams accompanying nocturnal spermatorrhea. (I have not seen this pulse.) More importantly, this sign is found with intestinal qi deficiency and intestinal disorders sometimes associated with Kidney essence and qi deficiency and/or Spleen qi deficiency. Here we have symptoms of chronic cold diarrhea, often with mucus (mucous colitis), and occurring on awakening (cock's crow diarrhea) with Kidney deficiency.

Slippery Deep Tight to Wiry and Rapid

When this combination is accompanied by severe flank or back pain, a kidney stone with kidney infection is probably the cause. Without acutely severe pain, one must consider a low level colitis, prostatitis, or pelvic inflammatory disease.

Slippery Flooding Excess Tense (and possibly Rapid)

This pulse may accompany a more acute and fulminating dysentery from poor digestion or parasites, and if the pulse is also Rapid, from bacterial infection, or a fulminating colitis, prostatitis, or pelvic inflammatory disease.

Slippery only at organ depth

Slipperiness at the organ depth at the proximal position is usually accompanied by Slipperiness at the same depth on the left middle position. This combination is a sign of a chronic infection, often systemic. If it is found only at the organ depth at the left proximal position, it is a sign of infection localized to the Kidneys.[18]

Right proximal

Slippery Tense

This pulse is often a sign of qi stagnation and damp-heat in the bladder and urinary tract.

Slippery Tight Flooding Excess and Rapid

With this pulse combination there can be Bladder infection, or damp-heat pouring down accompanied by pain. Acute flare-up of chronic pelvic inflammatory disease, colitis, or prostatitis can also be involved, differentiated by symptoms and history.

Slippery Deep Feeble

In this position this combination is a sign of qi deficiency in the Bladder with urinary frequency, dribbling, incontinence, and nocturia. This is usually found with Kidney qi or yang deficiency.[19]

Intestines

The Slippery quality in these positions is often a response to either heat from excess (Rapid rate) or cold stagnation (Slow rate) in the intestinal tract, almost always in association with an accumulation of mucus, often in the stool.

Pelvis/Lower Body — The Slippery quality in the Pelvis/Lower Body position is a sign of damp-heat (with a Rapid rate) or damp-cold stagnation in the pelvic and perineal area (Slow rate). An associated disorder is pelvic inflammatory disease, and symptoms of dampness such as leukorrhea may appear, yellow or thick with heat, and white and thin with cold. Often the Slippery and Choppy qualities appear simultaneously in this position, indicating stagnation of both dampness and blood. Endometriosis, cervical dysplasia, fibroids, and ovarian cysts occur with these signs.

Nonfluid Qualities

Sorting out the qualities in this area of pulse diagnosis is perhaps the most difficult challenge I have encountered. There is thus an unfortunate, yet necessary, repetition in this section. The system has evolved with its own internal logic in terms of sensation and interpretation, which is consistent with my clinical experience. My purpose here is to present a clear analysis of the hard, nonfluid qualities. Therefore, I have chosen, after much consideration, to exclude many possible references to the literature when discussing these qualities, where the Chinese terms have been variously and confusingly translated.

OLD CLASSIFICATION OF NONFLUID QUALITIES

The descriptive terms tight, wiry, bow-string, string-taut, threadlike, and stringy are often used synonymously in the literature to describe the hard, nonfluid qualities, without clear distinctions either in terms of sensation or interpretation.

Bow-string (string-taut or *xian*) is especially found in English language texts from China to cover a wide spectrum of qualities, including wiry, all of which tend to some hardness on the pulse. For example, *Essentials of Chinese Acupuncture*[20] says of the wiry pulse that it feels "as though pressing on the string of a bow." Although further sensory distinctions are made, the Tight pulse has been referred to by Kaptchuk as "like a taut rope,"[21] and the wiry quality similarly "has a taut feeling."[22] Porkert refers to what others call tight as tense,[23] and what others call wiry[24] as stringy, which he describes as being "sharp and taut."[25]

Furthermore, the classification in this area of pulse diagnosis often defines the meaning of qualities which do not reflect current clinical experience. I have no argument with the probable correctness of these interpretations, based as they are on another place and time long ago. For example, the Tight pulse, which in older sources is almost always associated with stagnation due to internal cold, in our times is much more often found with moderate heat from deficiency. And what is referred to as the wiry quality—which I call Tense, and which does *not* feel like a wire—is mentioned in the literature in connection with malaria, or more appropriately for our time, wind and pain; yet no mention at all is made of its current and most commonly associated pattern of qi stagnation and heat from excess. What I refer to as the Wiry quality—which *does* feel like a wire—is generally a sign of severe deficient yin-essence, or of pain.

I do feel that in our current practice in the West, the acute medical problems mentioned by these authors, such as malaria and internal cold obstruction, are not commonly seen by most practitioners. Today, in developed countries, acupuncturists are primarily engaged in treating chronic disease largely based on stress, either emotional, physical, chemical, or socioeconomic. The meanings of these qualities have changed as our society moved from acute to chronic phases of disharmony.

Basing treatment on interpretations of pulse qualities which do not comport with our contemporary environment is dangerous. Treating a Tight pulse as if there were cold stagnation when in fact there is heat from deficiency is obviously not in the best interest of the patient. This underscores the need to create separate categories for each of what are now overlapping qualities so as to reduce the confusion.

Reviewing the literature in English, and sifting through the confusion just mentioned, there are actually only two types of nonfluid, hard sensations recorded, the tight and the wiry qualities. Yet this is inconsistent with my clinical experience and with what I actually feel on the pulse under specific circumstances. Further distinctions in the classification of the hard pulse qualities in both sensation and interpretation are needed. These varying nomenclatures, none of which in my opinion reflects current clinical reality, get in the way of practice. Therefore I have felt compelled to create a new, more structured and integrated classification, as described below.

First and most importantly, I suggest that we redefine tight and wiry in keeping with current clinical observation. Second, I suggest that we rescue pulse diagnosis by discarding the terms bow-string, stringy, and string-bow. At least four categories of increasing hardness are required to accomplish this task. At one end of the spectrum is Taut, the least hard, followed by Tense, Tight, and finally Wiry, the most hard. With this arrangement of pulse qualities and interpretation, treatment, especially with herbs, becomes more logical and rational.

NEW CLASSIFICATION OF NONFLUID QUALITIES

Clinically we find that there is a gradual progression from Taut through Tense and Tight to Wiry. This is expressed on the pulse by mixed qualities such as Tense-Tight, which says that there is more heat from excess than from deficiency, but that the process is moving away from excess toward deficiency, yet both exist simultaneously in varying degrees. On the other hand, if the pulse already has more heat from deficiency than excess, the pulse would be more Tight than Tense, which we would notate as Tight-Tense. Likewise, the same principle would hold for the notation Tight-Wiry in terms of the progression from mostly yin-deficient toward essence-deficient.

Pathogenesis

I have reorganized the nonfluid and generally more rigid pulses according to a progression that I have observed in the clinic over the past three decades. The process is one which leads to yin (and often blood) deficiency, rather than to the qi deficiency which we observe in the progressions of those pulses with reduced volume. The concept of a progression of qi stagnation and developing heat from excess, and later deficiency, as I have formulated it here, is based originally on Dr. Shen's clinical teaching, but represents my own organization and development of the material.

The mechanism is one that leads from stagnation rather than depletion of qi, and almost always involves a lifetime of strain and stress in the 'nervous system.' The sequence of increasing hardness is one which reflects growing degrees of qi stagnation, to degrees of heat from excess due to the body's attempt to overcome the stagnation. Overworking of organ systems in the service of reducing stagnation and reopening qi circulation requires (and depletes) the yin to balance the heat. The diminishing yin leads to increasing intensity of heat from deficiency.[26]

Sensation

I have given each grade of increasing hardness its distinct term—Taut, Tense, Tight, and Wiry—rather than referring to them as degrees of tightness. The feeling sensations, interpretations, and clinical approach are all distinctly different and warrant a careful delineation.

There is some overlap in sensation between my nosology and the confusion of the past, which I mention only for completeness. What I call Tense roughly fits the older description of tight, and what I call Tight is slightly similar to descriptions of wiry in the literature, except for Porkert's. In terms of interpretation, there is almost no concurrence between my own observations and what I have read.

Classified by feeling sensation, we might compare the nonfluid pulses to the strings of a violin (Fig. 11-2): the most flexible G string would be like the Taut pulse, the slightly less flexible D string like the Tense pulse, the even less flexible A string like the Tight pulse, and the least flexible and most rigid E string would be like the Wiry pulse. This progression represents increasing stagnation and heat from excess from Taut to Tense, and increasing heat from deficiency from Tight to Wiry.

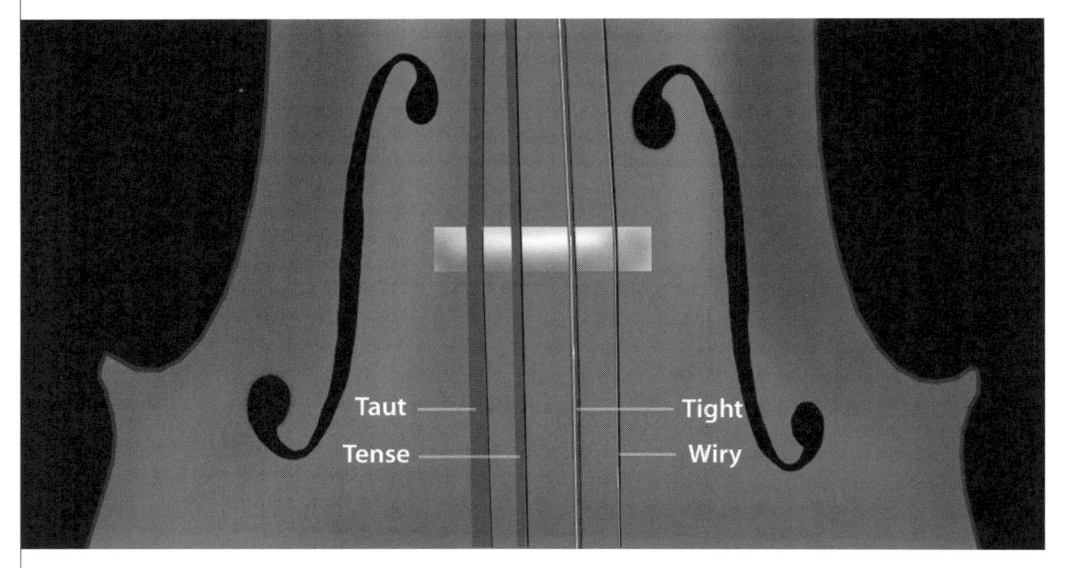

Fig. 11-2   Violin strings (nonfluid qualities: Taut, Tense, Tight, Wiry)

Clinical significance

To put these qualities in perspective, consider the following sequence of herbal formulas that might be prescribed for progressive Liver qi stagnation. Each of the formulas is appropriate for the pulse quality associated with a particular stage in the development of the disorder. *(Warning:* These formulas are chosen only for the purpose of illustration, and should not be prescribed without a complete diagnostic assessment.)

- The Taut quality represents mild qi stagnation and only minimal heat from excess. This would call for herbs that primarily move stagnation rather than remove heat from excess. Frigid Extremities Powder *(si ni san)* would be appropriate for this purpose.
- The Tense quality is associated with greater qi stagnation, increasing heat from excess, and also some heat from deficiency, since the pulse is becoming harder. A blend of herbs that have stronger qi-moving and excess heat-removing properties is indicated. Here, a formula like Minor Bupleurum Decoction *(xiao chai hu tang)* would be appropriate.
- With the Tight quality we must still deal with qi stagnation, but now the thrust is more toward building yin and blood. Six-Ingredient Pill with Rehmannia *(liu wei di huang wan)* and Rambling Powder *(xiao yao san)* might be considered at this stage.
- Once the pulse becomes Wiry our focus is almost entirely on building yin essence as quickly as possible. Formulas such as Lycium Fruit, Chrysanthemum, and Rehmannia Pill *(qi ju di huang wan)* or Restore the Left [Kidney] Decoction *(you gui yin)* would be appropriate.

This example illustrates the importance of making diagnostic distinctions, which is indispensable to proper treatment.

The relationship of the hard qualities to deficiency

In my experience the most common error in pulse diagnosis is mistaking the hard qualities for excess. In fact, the Tight and Wiry qualities signify deficiency, a very important deficiency of yin and yin-essence. This view is, I believe, supported by Jiang Jing[27] in his discussion of the string pulse, which he describes in much the same terms as I describe the Tight quality.

> [I]t may feel like putting your finger on a tight guitar string. The energy becomes tense and agitated, but in reality it is also a deficient, passive and negative pulse since it does not contain a normal level of energy, sometimes creating friction and tension which lead to heat. This is very similar to the concept of false fire.

Further on, he adds that the string pulse

> is just being very urgent and very desperate in its action to continue its activity or function. That is its present condition, so there is not much left, but it tries to continue with what it has left.... If the String pulse is found in the heart, the heart will be tense and deficient. It will not freely pump since there is not enough capacity; so it will tighten and palpitate faster, attempting to compensate.

The important message here is that a hard quality can just as easily be a sign of deficiency as it is of excess.

EVEN NONFLUID QUALITIES

Taut

The Taut and Tense qualities come closest to the description given to the wiry pulse in modern Chinese texts, one of which describes it as "taut and forceful, as though pressing on the string of a drawn bow."[28] But for anyone with archery experience, a drawn bow does not feel like a wire, which after all is metal, and as hard a substance as one is likely to encounter.

Sensation — This quality has the resilience and flexibility of a very wide rubber band that has been moderately stretched, but has considerable give on pressure. It may be likened to the widest and most supple of the strings on a violin, the G string.

General interpretation — I found this quality in the clinic, apart from other references. Since I find it necessary to a rational nosology, and to reduce confusion, there is no literature cited.

This quality represents the earliest sign and first stage of qi stagnation from causes other than shock. Whatever the cause, it is the mildest form of qi stagnation perceptible by pulse diagnosis in a person with a relatively good level of energy and of average constitution. (A weaker person might develop a Flat quality instead, in the incipient phase of qi stagnation.) By itself, it is the closest quality to Normal that any of us will ever see.

Etiology — The most common cause is the moderate repression of emotion on a daily basis, and the most common position at which it is found is the left middle position, which represents the Liver. When it is found uniformly over the entire pulse I refer to it as the 'vigilance' pulse. One should look for a moderate constitutional 'nervous system tense' or ongoing chronic stress, as explained in Chapter 13.

Other common etiologies are physical labor beyond one's energy, generalized but relatively mild chronic pain, and the chemical onslaught of pollution everywhere in our world. One important source of chemical stress is stimulants, especially coffee, and of course recreational stimulants such as cocaine and amphetamines.

Depending where on the pulse this quality is found, there may be other causes. A Taut pulse may occur in the right middle position with mild food stagnation, or cold from excess due to cold food and drink, and in the middle burner position bilaterally with mild trauma to the abdomen or emotional stress. All of these may be accompanied by mild pain. A Taut quality may appear in the right distal position with mild cold from excess associated with external pathogenic influences, and in the proximal position with sexual abstinence.

Combinations

Taut Floating

This represents an early stage in a mild attack of an external pathogenic influence, probably wind-cold.

Taut and slightly Rapid

One can find this combination when there is a 'nervous system tense' condition due to daily stress.

Taut Inflated

These are found together where there is stagnation due to trapped qi and mild heat from excess leading to distention and pain, usually at the right middle position.

Taut Wide

This combination is associated with heat in the blood, especially when found at the blood depth.

Taut Choppy

This indicates simultaneous blood and qi stagnation.

Taut and Slow

This represents qi stagnation interfering with circulation, possibly due to cold in the channels or Liver qi stagnation. If found over the entire pulse it is a sign of a constitutional 'nervous system tense' condition.

Taut Slippery

Theoretically, this combination can be found where there is stagnation of both qi and fluids. However, as mentioned in our discussion of the Slippery quality, the meaning of the Taut Slippery combination is complex. Depending on where it is found, it can signify infection, elevated blood sugar, qi deficiency, blood turbulence, or pregnancy. For example, this is sometimes found at the qi depth on the left middle position when, in addition to early Liver qi stagnation, there is excessive sugar in the blood. In the right middle position it is found with an acid stomach, and with ulcers.

Positions

BILATERAL AT SAME BURNER

Distal — A Taut pulse here may indicate stagnation of qi due to a mild or recent trauma to the chest; to mild lifting over time beyond one's energy; to an unresolved cold external pathogenic factor which has begun to internalize, creating stagnation and a little heat; and mild asthma associated with the latter etiology, or with Liver qi attacking the Lungs.

Middle — Mild pain with mild qi stagnation due to small and recent trauma to the abdomen; mild emotional stress affecting the Liver which is attacking the Stomach–Spleen; sitting in a bent-over posture for a short period of time; resuming work too soon after eating; pain associated with food stagnation or cold from either excess or deficiency of the Stomach; and occasional lifting beyond one's energy, especially after eating, using the stomach muscles.

Proximal — Mild pain from qi stagnation due to recent or mild pelvic trauma, or following light pelvic surgical intervention such as a laparoscopy or less invasive techniques including IUDs, or sexual abstinence.

SIDES

Left — When the entire left side of the pulse is Taut we have mild qi stagnation in the 'organ system,' which is probably due to the prolonged effect of tension in the 'nervous system' affecting the 'organ system,' or to trauma to the left side. Eye and tongue signs of trauma listed above would aid the differential diagnosis.

Right — When the entire right side is Taut we have qi stagnation with some distention in the 'digestive system' due to nervous tension and eating too quickly, or separately due to a mild trauma to the right side.

INDIVIDUAL POSITIONS

Left distal — A Taut quality here probably represents minimal qi stagnation in the Heart due to a recent mild emotional, heartfelt pain from disruption in an intimate relationship; or to a mild physical shock on the left side of the chest.

Right distal — I have observed the Taut quality at this position in people who have been smoking lightly or for a short period of time, after mild lifting, or from slight physical trauma to the right side of the chest.

Left middle — This pulse is most commonly associated with a recent, slowly developing rather than sudden, mild repressed emotion, principally mild resentment and anger. This quality tends over time to dominate the other qualities, and appears to characterize the entire pulse.

Right middle	The Taut quality at this position represents qi stagnation in the Stomach and Spleen of a mild degree, or for only a short period of time. This is probably due to an early stage of Liver qi stagnation affecting ('attacking') the Stomach-Spleen, or mild overeating (or eating a bit too rapidly) for a short time.
Left proximal, Large Intestine, and Pelvis/Lower Body	Tautness at these positions is an early sign of excess Kidney yang due to sexual abstinence, a quality, according to Dr. Shen, which was found so frequently among monks that it was called monk's or Buddha's pulse. With the Taut quality at the Large Intestine position, one should also consider the early stages of qi stagnation in the Intestines as a precursor to colitis, and to prostatic hypertrophy or prostatitis when the Taut quality is found at the Pelvis/Lower Body position.
Right proximal, Small Intestine, and Pelvis/Lower Body	Here the Tautness must be considered as qi stagnation in the Bladder, which may be a precursor to later inflammation in these organs. Check the Small Intestine position where the Taut quality may be a very early sign of qi stagnation as a precursor to inflammatory conditions such as regional enteritis. For the Pelvis/Lower Body, refer to the left proximal position.

Tense

Category	In our system, the Tense pulse is a Taut pulse which has moved one or more steps further along the path of qi stagnation, with signs of heat from excess developing as the body tries to overcome the stagnation. This heat is a challenge to the maintenance of temperature homeostasis requiring the mobilization of functions which remove heat or balance it with cold (yin).[29]
Sensation	The rubber band—which we described above in connection with the Taut quality as being wide—is somewhat narrower with the Tense quality, with less flexibility and resilience, and feels as if it has been more stiffly stretched. It therefore feels harder against one's fingers, though still more elastic than the Tight or Wiry qualities. It corresponds to the thinner though still relatively wide second (D) string on the violin. It may also be compared to a stretched rope or clothesline.
General interpretation	This is a delineation of pulse qualities which I have found in the clinic, apart from other references. Since I find it necessary to a rational nosology, and to reduce confusion, there is no literature cited. The Tense quality signifies increasing qi stagnation with the development of heat from excess. The slight narrowing of the pulse and hardening (relative to the Taut quality) are signs of heat.
Etiology	The etiologies of the Tense and Taut qualities are similar, but with the Tense pulse the condition is either more severe, or has lasted a somewhat longer time. The stagnation here is largely due to stress, primarily of repressed emotion; usually there is slowly growing anger and resentment involving an internal conflict in which two opposing forces create a stalemate. Constrained Liver qi is a classic example, with the irresistible force of the active energy of the body, which demands movement, at an impasse with the immovable object of repression, which opposes it. When this quality is found uniformly over the entire pulse I refer to it as the 'vigilance' pulse or condition, having found it constitutionally in ethnic groups whose survival through the centuries has required extraordinary vigilance. This is now true of anyone living in a large city. One must look to a moderate constitutional 'nervous system tense' or ongoing

chronic stress, as explained in Chapter 13. The rate is Normal with the constitutional etiology, but tends to be Rapid with tension associated with life. Furthermore, if, after several treatments, the patient's distress diminishes but the pulse stays the same, the etiology is constitutional.

One must also consider physical stress from work beyond one's energy, generalized but relatively mild chronic pain, and chemical stress from exposure to pollution, as well as the other factors discussed under the Taut quality. Stimulants, including coffee, cocaine, and amphetamines, are also a significant source of chemical stress.

I have also felt this pulse where infection or toxicity creates acute internal heat accompanied by one or more of the following: fever, thirst, sweating, and injected conjunctiva (bloodshot eyes). Hepatitis and an acute alcoholic episode come to mind as examples, although with acute hepatitis a Flooding Excess quality might dominate the pulse picture.

Combinations

Indications of the Tense quality in combination with other qualities are similar to those of the Taut quality combinations, except there is greater stagnation and heat from excess.

Tense Floating

This harder Floating pulse is associated with greater, or slightly longer term, stagnation in the channels due to wind-cold than is the case with the Taut Floating pulse. The cold has penetrated inside, leading to qi stagnation and diminished qi circulation, causing the body to mobilize heat to overcome the stagnation and reopen circulation.

Tense Deep

This combination is found in chronic conditions affecting the 'organ system' in which there is both qi deficiency (Deep) causing increasing qi stagnation, and simultaneously some qi stagnation and heat from excess in the yin organs attributable to another cause such as the 'nervous system.'

Tense and Rapid

This combination is associated with generalized qi stagnation due to nervous tension or an emotional shock with developing heat from excess. Tension with a Rapid rate is usually due to stressful life circumstances.

Tense and Slow

The Tense quality in this pulse combination is usually associated with a constitutional 'nervous system tense' disorder. Less often it may indicate interference with circulation as indicated by its Slow quality, conceivably due to cold in the channels; a previous trauma; or Liver qi stagnation. The developing heat, as reflected in the Tense quality, is the consequence of unsuccessful efforts by the general body energy to overcome the stagnation.

Tense Inflated

This combination is found with qi stagnation and increasing trapped qi and heat. Inflation means that qi is trapped in the organ and cannot get out (see Inflated quality in Chapter 8). With this interpretation, it can be found in the left distal (Heart), right distal (Lungs), left middle (Liver) with unexpressed anger, and right middle (Stomach) positions.

Tense Wide

Together, these qualities are a sign of increasing heat in the blood and of blood viscosity, at a stage which Dr. Shen describes as Blood Thick, its associated pulse quality. (See Chapter 13 for a discussion of the blood depth, including Blood Heat and Blood Thick.)

Tense Hollow Full-Overflowing

This combination indicates that the heat in the blood has expanded to invade the qi depth. It is often associated with a full-fledged hypertensive condition.

Tense Choppy

This combination reflects increasing qi stagnation and heat from excess, possibly causing blood stagnation (or, less likely, caused by it) as expressed by its Choppy quality.

Tense Slippery

At the blood depth over the entire pulse, with Normal or slightly Rapid rate

If this combination is found at the blood depth it may be a sign of a 'blood unclear,' 'blood heat,' or 'blood thick' condition mentioned above, with the Tense Wide combination.

Very Slippery at all depths (especially blood depth), Robust Pounding, and very Rapid

This combination is a sign of infection in the blood, a septicemia which may have originated in one organ and spread through the blood to the entire body. The higher the rate, the more serious the condition.

At all depths or just the organ depth

This is a sign of infection, or heat from excess, in an organ. This combination is most commonly found on the left middle (Liver) position with subclinical hepatitis and chronic parasitic infiltration of the liver.

Tense Slippery, Flooding Excess, Robust Pounding

This combination indicates an acute fulminating infection wherever it is found.

Positions

The following discussion of the Tense quality reflects its similarity to the Taut quality, except that there is increased qi stagnation and heat from excess.

BILATERALLY AT SAME POSITION

Distal

A Tense quality here may indicate stagnation of qi due to one of several causes.

Moderate or less recent trauma to the chest

It can occur in a relatively strong person who has unresolved qi stagnation due to chest trauma. In the short term, pain and restricted ability to take a deep breath are often the result. Mediastinal and breast tumors are possible in the long term.

Unresolved internalized cold

The external cold has internalized, creating stagnation and heat from excess associated with certain types of asthma.

Lifting beyond one's energy

A Tense quality at the distal positions can develop in an individual with normal qi, after a single extraordinary episode of lifting beyond one's energy. As with trauma (above), it signifies qi stagnation in the chest, which may cause symptoms of pain and restrict one's ability to take a deep breath. Even if asymptomatic, it may later develop into problems such as mediastinal and breast tumors.

Using the Lungs beyond one's energy

Excessive talking and singing, for a relatively short period of time, can lead to a Tense quality at these positions in a person with normal qi. This represents Lung qi stagnation with heat from excess.

Middle

The Tense pulse at this position is associated with the following causes.

Trauma

Trauma to the abdomen, including adhesions after surgery, causes moderate pain due to qi stagnation.

Emotional stress

Emotional stress causes qi stagnation in the Liver, which attacks the Stomach-Spleen.

Food stagnation or cold from either excess or deficiency in the Stomach

Food stagnation and cold in the Stomach for a moderate period of time in a relatively strong person can be signaled by a Tense quality bilaterally at the middle burner position.

Bending

Habitually bending over, especially after eating, can be signaled by a Tense quality at these positions. In a strong person this quality may develop after years of such behavior, and in a weaker person after a few months.

Resuming physical labor immediately after eating

Returning to work during or immediately after eating does not leave time for digestion, eventually causing qi stagnation and heat from excess, which is evidenced in a Tense quality at this position. This includes lifting beyond one's energy using the stomach muscles.

Proximal — Moderate pain, again due to qi stagnation, is associated with the following causes.

Trauma

Less recent or moderate pelvic trauma, or following moderate pelvic surgical intervention, probably with some scar tissue.

Overexposure of feet to heat

Walking barefoot on hot sand or rocks over the course of days to weeks or even months can lead to heat in the feet and lower extremities. Rashes in these areas of the body are a common manifestation of such heat, and the pulse is very Tense bilaterally.

Early inflammatory condition in lower burner

The Tense and Rapid quality is found with subacute pelvic inflammatory disease, colitis, and prostatitis. When the Flooding Excess quality is also present, the condition is acute and fulminating.

Monk's or Buddha's pulse

According to Dr. Shen, a very Tense quality in these positions and a Normal to Slower rate are associated with long-term sexual abstinence.

SIDES

Left — When the entire left side is Tense we have moderate qi stagnation and heat from excess in the 'organ system.' This is probably due to the effect on the organ system of prolonged tension in the 'nervous system.'

Right — When the entire right side is Tense we have qi stagnation and heat from excess with moderate distention in the 'digestive system,' usually due to nervous tension and eating too fast.

INDIVIDUAL POSITIONS

Left distal — A Tense pulse at this position probably represents a non-recent emotional or physical shock on the left chest, or suppression of 'heart' feelings over a period of time. There is qi stagnation and heat from excess in the Heart. The heat may also be due to rising fire from the Liver.

Right distal — I have observed the Tense quality at this position in people who have been smoking heavily or for a long time, and with one episode of extraordinary lifting or physical trauma to the right side of the chest. There is qi stagnation and heat from excess in the Lung.

Special Lung — Without signs of pathology at the right distal position, the Tense quality at the Special Lung positions is a sign of stagnant heat from excess in the Lungs, usually due to past cold which invaded the Lungs and evolved into heat due to the effort of the Lungs to expel the cold.

Left middle	The Tense quality here is due to a long-term, slowly developing (not sudden), moderately repressed emotion, usually resentment or anger. It represents qi stagnation and heat from excess in the Liver, when an irresistible force (emotion) meets the immovable object (repression). Over time this quality tends to dominate the qualities in the other positions and to characterize the entire pulse.
Right middle	The Tense quality in this position represents qi stagnation and heat from excess in the Stomach and Spleen of a moderate degree, or for a relatively long period of time. This is often due to Liver qi stagnation affecting ('attacking') the Stomach-Spleen, or eating foods that are rich in spices.
Left proximal, Large Intestine, and Pelvis/Lower Body	Tension here is a later sign of excessive Kidney yang, stagnant essence with heat from excess, due to sexual abstinence. (As previously noted, this pulse is associated with what is called monk's or Buddha's pulse.) At the Large Intestine position one should also consider the later stages of qi stagnation and heat from excess in the Intestines as an early sign of colitis. At the Pelvis/Lower Body positions one should consider prostatic hypertrophy, an early sign of prostatitis or pelvic qi stagnation and/or inflammatory disease.
Right proximal, Small Intestine, and Pelvis/Lower Body	Here the Tension must be interpreted to mean moderate qi stagnation in the Bladder. At the Small Intestine position it is a sign of heat from excess, which may be a precursor to an acute infection. With infection, the rate is more Rapid. With regard to the Pelvis/Lower Body position, see above under left proximal position.

Tight

Category	As a matter of interpretation, the Tight quality described here is a totally new category which most clearly corresponds with descriptions of the wiry quality in the literature.
Sensation	The Tight quality may be best identified as feeling like the next to thinnest A string on a violin. (The thinnest E string is descriptive of the Wiry pulse.) It is harder, less resilient and flexible, and usually thinner than the Tense quality. However, it still has both some flexibility and resilience, in contrast to the Wiry quality, which has neither. With pain the Tight quality often has a sharper, Biting sensation.[30]
General interpretation	### HEAT FROM YIN DEFICIENCY (AND SOME BLOOD DEFICIENCY) **Etiology and pathogenesis of heat from deficiency** In our times the Tight quality is associated primarily with heat from yin deficiency due mainly to stagnation from nervous tension. We are referring here to a 'nervous system' which is overworking for a longer period of time than with the Tense quality. This etiology will usually affect the entire pulse. If the source is constitutional, the rate will be Normal or Slow. If the source is due to life experiences, the rate may be slightly Rapid. A Tight quality that characterizes the entire pulse due to an uncomplicated yin deficiency is often slightly Rapid. According to Dr. Shen, the progression of yin deficiency on the pulse proceeds from Tightness at the qi depth with minimal yin deficiency, to Tightness at the blood depth, and finally at the organ depth, as it increases and persists. He has also said that Tightness at the qi depth represents heat from yin deficiency in the peripheral and autonomic nervous system, with increased agitation and hyperactivity of that system.

Yin and blood deficiency

The Thinness of a Tight quality implies concurrent blood deficiency. Yin and blood deficiency often occur simultaneously in clinical practice. However, it is the hardness that signals the yin deficiency, since it is possible to have a Thin blood-deficient pulse that is not hard. However, concurrent Thinness and Tightness at the qi depth is associated with an overworking 'nervous system.'

Heat from yin deficiency in one organ usually results from overworking that organ over a long period of time. Causes may include emotional stress, as is often observed at the left middle position; worry or emotional shock, at the left distal position; smoking, at the right distal position; and eating too rapidly, at the right middle position.

Heat from yin deficiency in the 'circulatory system' may be the end stage of heat from excess in the blood over a long period of time, as explained in the description of the Blood Thick quality in Chapter 13, and the Hollow Full-Overflowing quality in Chapter 8. Nervous tension is, again, one of the etiologies, along with a diet rich in spices, fat, and sugar, which can lead to heat in the blood.

The shift in feeling sensation from Tense to Tight is a reflection of the shift in the body from a predominance of stagnation and heat from excess in the early stages of the disease process, to that of consumption of yin and the concomitant development of heat from deficiency in the later, more chronic, stages of the disease process. With the Tight quality, heat from yin deficiency becomes the significant aspect of the disharmony and focus of treatment, although the stagnation and even the heat from excess may still be operative pathological factors.

In my experience the Tight quality most often and most importantly signifies deficiency of yin fluids. When heat from excess is generated by the body's attempt to overcome stagnation, the Kidneys and Triple Burner are called upon to mobilize fluids in order to maintain a thermo-homeostasis.

Hot flashes and night sweats

Hot flashes and night sweats are most often associated with female menopause, although there are, of course, other associated conditions. In the context of menopause, Chinese medicine generally attributes them to a yin-deficient condition often accompanied by a generally Tight pulse quality, although sometimes the Tightness is restricted to the proximal position. In such cases, formulas such as Two Immortals Decoction *(er xian tang)* are often prescribed.

In my own experience, however, more often than not the hot flashes are not due to yin deficiency, and they do not respond to Two Immortals Decoction. Formulas that treat qi stagnation, rising qi, and blood heat, such as Tang-kuei and Cyperus *(nu shen san)*, are more effective. The rising qi often occurs in situations where blood stagnation in the lower burner has caused the blood and qi to separate, and the qi to rise.

Night sweats are also usually associated with a yin-deficient condition and a Tight quality. However, the underlying problem is actually due to a separation of yin and yang, which can be due to deficiency of one or both.

During the day, the yang of the sun helps the deficient yang of the body control the loss of internal yin and yang. At night, however, when the yang of the sun is absent, yin rises to the surface and escapes in the form of perspiration, partly to balance escaping internal heat, and partly because of the disconnection between the yin and the yang, which is no longer in equilibrium.

At first the pulse is a little Rapid, a little Tight, and slightly Thin. Later it is a little Rapid, and Tighter to Wiry. One searches for the Tightest position—Kidney, Lung, Heart, and Liver—for the source of the problem. (The tongue is bright red at first and darker red later, with a dry, patchy, yellow coating, or no coating. The eyes have confluent vertical lines inside the lower eyelid.)

Pain, trauma, infection, inflammation, hyperactivity, and external cold

The Tight quality can appear with pain due to stagnation of qi, blood, fluids, cold, or food. Examples are qi stagnation from invading cold in the muscles, or with qi and blood stagnation due to trauma. The pain tends to make the pulse a little more Rapid at first, while the cold, for example, tends to slow the pulse; the two seem to balance each other, leaving a Normal rate. With chronic pain the facial color is often dark.

If the Tightness is a sign of inflammation and infection (fire toxin), the position which is most Tight is the location of the organ or area where the infection originated or is currently most active. With pain, the Tight quality often has a sharper, Biting sensation. In some positions, such as the Small and Large Intestines, the Tight quality can also represent bowel irritability as well as discomfort.

Combinations

Tight Floating

External pathogenic factor

This combination suggests a lingering, or very strong, acute cold external pathogenic factor with muscle and joint pain, headache, and slight fever, suggesting an internal invasion of cold. The Tight quality here is primarily associated with pain.

Liver Wind

With Liver wind the pulse is a little Tighter. This is more often found above the left middle position or above the entire left side.

Tight Deep

This is primarily a sign of heat from deficiency (Tight), and qi deficiency (Deep) in a yin organ.

Tight and Rapid

This is indicative of a yin deficiency of relatively recent origin, where the heat from deficiency can cause an increase in rate. These qualities may be associated with emotional stress over a very long period of time, with irritability. In the absence of pain, when the entire pulse is very Tight and Rapid, Dr. Shen attributes the combination to individuals who are experiencing extreme guilt, and fear in connection with the guilt, usually in my experience in combination with Rough Vibration. Dr. Shen states that Rough Vibration indicates concomitant Heart qi deficiency, which is not my impression.

Tight Thin

It has been mentioned that one way of differentiating Tight from Tense is that the Tight quality is Thinner than the Tense quality. The Thinness to which we refer here goes beyond that distinction in terms of the narrowness of the pulse.

Combined, these qualities are signs of both heat from deficiency and blood deficiency (referred to above in the discussion of yin and blood deficiency), which is commonly found in women who do not recover completely from childbirth, abortion, miscarriage, menorrhagia, or are in menopause. However, concurrent Thinness and Tightness at the qi depth is associated with an overworking 'nervous system' and a more advanced 'nervous system tense' condition.

Alternating from Tight to Yielding

Although apparently contradictory, I have found that this combination of qualities can be a sign of combined yin and qi or yang deficiency. This is a situation in which both the 'nervous system' has been tense for a long time, and one has worked physically beyond one's energy, with insufficient rest. A Change in Qualities is also a serious sign of the separation of yin and yang.

Tight Inflated

When this combination is found in one position it is a sign of trapped qi, heat from excess, and heat from deficiency in an organ. The Tightness here can also be a sign of pain. For example, a Tight and Inflated pulse at the right middle position indicates pain and distention in the gastrointestinal system, and possibly Stomach yin deficiency.

Tight Choppy

This combination indicates a condition of simultaneous heat from deficiency and blood stagnation, or pain and blood stagnation. The differentiation is made on the basis of the history, tongue, under the eyelid, and facial color.

Tight Wide Slippery

Although the Tight (hard) quality is usually also narrow (because it is a sign of yin and some blood deficiency), if there is a 'blood heat' or 'blood thick' condition, the associated pulse is Wide instead of Thin at the blood depth. The Slippery aspect, also at the blood depth, is a sign that the blood heat is creating turbulence in the blood. The Tight quality, signifying yin deficiency in this instance, would be found at the qi and organ depths.

Tight Flooding Excess

I have usually found the combination of Tight and Flooding Excess at the proximal positions in connection with fulminating colitis, prostatitis, or pelvic inflammatory disease, and at the left middle position with acute hepatitis,[31] in the context of a chronic yin-depleting condition, as with chronic colitis.

Positions

If the Tightness is a sign of infection, the position which is most Tight is the location of the organ or area where the infection originated, or is currently most active. With infection, the pulse is usually also Slippery.

If there is pain or a history of trauma, and with a horizontal line under the eyelid, possibly accompanied by a small purple blister on the side of the tongue, a Tight quality in any position may indicate pain associated with the trauma.

If the pulse is Tight at a single position only at the qi depth, this is an early sign of yin deficiency in the associated yin organ. The etiology is usually that the qi (nerves) of that organ has been agitated by some kind of stress, emotional, physical, or chemical. If the Tightness is at the organ depth the deficiency is more advanced.

BILATERALLY AT SAME BURNER

Distal

Cardiac asthma

If the rate is Rapid, cardiac asthma is a distinct possibility. One would look for other signs and symptoms of cardiac insufficiency (Heart qi or yang deficiency, see Chapter 12) and asthma. These would include an arrhythmia; Change in Intensity and/or Rough Vibration over the entire pulse; a left distal position which is Tight with Change in Intensity or Qualities (to Feeble); and a Tight right distal position with Rough Vibration and Special Lung positions that are Tight, Slippery, and with Rough Vibration.

Trauma

This would be trauma or shock to the chest, which occurred in a relatively strong person, neither very recently, nor in the too distant past. (See Chapter 13 for a discussion of trauma.)

Hypertension and headache

If the two distal positions are Tight, and the other positions are Feeble-Absent, rising fire associated with hypertension and bursting headache is possible if the insides of the lower eyelid and tongue are red. If neither is red, severe headache from rising qi is probably a principal cause.

Mania, cocaine abuse, and acute Grave's disease

A very Tight quality found bilaterally in only the distal positions can accompany mania and cocaine abuse, in which case the pulse is also Slippery and Rapid. With Grave's disease there is acute inflammation and enlargement of the thyroid gland, rendering the upper burner (especially the left distal positions) with a Tight Flooding Excess and Robust Pounding quality.

Pain with tumor

A very Tight quality found bilaterally in only the distal position can also be a sign of severe pain possibly due to a tumor in the chest. With a tumor the distal position might also be Muffled.

Febrile illness in the upper burner

Inflammation of the pleura or other infection in the chest area can give rise to these qualities. The pulse would also be Rapid, and the Pleura position would either be Inflated, Rough, or very Tight.

Special Lung

Tightness at these positions is a sign of lingering stagnation and heat from yin deficiency in the Lungs, usually of long duration, especially from premature birth (incubator), childhood, or even congenital. It is often associated with yin deficient asthma. If the right distal position is also abnormal, it may suggest a current as well as chronic illness, with progressive stagnation and increasing heat from yin deficiency. This can only be correctly evaluated when the right distal position returns to Normal.

Middle | ### Nervous tension

Heat from yin deficiency and dryness of the Liver and Stomach due to nervous tension is usually associated with Liver qi stagnation and the Liver attacking the Stomach-Spleen, with the progression from Taut to Tense to Tight over time. If the tension is constitutionally based, the rate is probably Normal; otherwise, the rate is probably a little Rapid.

Infection

A pulse that is Tight, Slippery, and Rapid, sometimes accompanied by fever, is a sign of an infection somewhere in the area or in one or all of the organs of the middle burner, including the pancreas, for which one must search further. In addition to pancreatitis, other possibilities are gastric ulcer, parasites, hepatitis, appendicitis, and gallbladder disease. Pancreatitis, ulcer, appendicitis, and gallbladder disease are frequently attended by pain; the Tight quality thus represents pain as well as inflammation.

Hypertension and/or diabetes

In the middle burner a very Tight quality may indicate a very early stage of an impending diabetic or a hypertensive condition, or a later stage if the pulse tends also to be Hollow Full-Overflowing.

Stomach-Liver yin deficiency and heat from deficiency

Lifting and bending right after eating, or eating too quickly or when tense, will, over a long period of time, cause a Tight quality in a person who is relatively strong. With trauma, lifting, and bending, the initial quality would be Taut. The body's effort to overcome the stagnation generates heat, leading to heat from excess and a Tense quality. Finally, in an attempt to balance the heat, the fluids (yin) will be depleted, which leads to yin deficiency and a Tight pulse.

Pain

Pain can be due to a tumor, infection (appendicitis), ulcer, or trauma, as well as long-term lifting and/or bending, especially after eating.

TRAUMA TO THE ABDOMEN

This usually involves qi and blood stagnation in a relatively strong person, in which the circulation of both blood and qi in the abdomen is impeded.

LIFTING

This quality is associated with persistently lifting things too soon after eating in a relatively strong person, which impedes the circulation of blood and qi in the abdomen.

BENDING

Relatively strong individuals who sit in a bent-over posture for long periods of time, over many years, such as a secretaries with poor posture, will experience qi stagnation in the middle, leading through the progression from Taut to Tense to Tight mentioned above.

Proximal | ### Heat from yin deficiency

Kidney yin deficiency is more often accompanied by a Tight quality at the left proximal position alone, but it can occur bilaterally if the condition is severe. More often than not, it is the later stage of a systemic yin-depleting process for which the kidneys can no longer compensate.

Diabetes

Early diabetes is a consideration when this quality appears bilaterally at this position. As the Tightness evolves toward a Wiry quality, and later a very Tight-Wiry Hollow Full-Overflowing quality, the illness is becoming more severe and the diagnosis is more likely, especially if it is also found at the left middle position.

Infection, inflammation, and irritability

Extreme Tightness alone at this position may indicate infection or inflammation in the associated areas or in organs such as the Kidney and Bladder, and more rarely in the Intestines or prostate. If the rate is Rapid there can sometimes be a mild acute flare-up of a chronic infection such as ulcerative colitis or enteritis, prostatic inflammation, oophoritis, salpingitis, nephrities, urethritis, or pelvic inflammatory disease. (A severe flare-up is usually accompanied by a Tight Flooding-Excess quality.) Check the associated Intestine and Pelvis/Lower Body positions where these qualities are more likely to be found.

Pain

KIDNEY STONES

While a Tight pulse bilaterally may occur with the severe stagnation associated with Kidney stones, or a bladder infection, the quality is usually Wiry when accompanied by severe pain. Often there is also some Slipperiness.

TRAUMA

Unresolved past trauma, including surgery, may eventually lead to this quality, especially if there is pain. The Choppy quality, a sign of blood stagnation, often accompanies the Tight quality here with trauma.

HERNIA

Pain associated with hernia can cause a Tight quality at this position.

SIDES

Left

'Nervous system' affects the 'organ system'

This can occur when, in Dr. Shen's terms, the 'nervous system' has created tension in the 'organ system.' The nerves or qi facet of energy in the yin organs are tense and contracted, creating stagnation which eventually leads to the heat from deficiency to which we have often alluded. Here the Tightness is felt at the most superficial level of the pulse. Even when the pulse is Deep, the Tightness is felt at the surface of the organ depth, which in itself theoretically has a qi, blood, and organ or more material yin aspect. Due to the limitations of human sensory perception, these subtle differentiations at the organ depth are accessible to relatively few.

Liver wind

The pulse is Tight Floating and is a moderate sign of incipient wind in the channels and stroke.

Hypertension

As an early sign of hypertension, usually of the labile type which increases with stress and decreases with relaxation, the entire left side can be Tight. This condition is a later stage or extension of the process described in the previous paragraph regarding the effect of the 'nervous system' on the 'organ system,' to a more severe Liver, Kidney, and Heart yin deficiency with heat from deficiency. It may ultimately lead to cerebrovascular accident with paralysis, probably on the left side.

Pain from trauma

One can find this quality over the entire left side of the pulse in conjunction with pain or trauma on the left side of the body. One would depend on history, a horizontal line under the eyelid, and a small purple blister on the left side of the tongue to determine whether trauma is the etiology.

Right

Eating habits

A Tight quality on the right side, especially on the surface of the pulse, can be a sign of heat from excess or deficiency in the 'digestive system' due to persistently eating too quickly.

Pain or trauma

Pain or trauma to the right side of the body can give rise to a Tight quality over the entire right side of the pulse. Again, check the history, under the eyelid, and the tongue.

INDIVIDUAL POSITIONS

Heat from deficiency follows yin deficiency. This is expressed on the pulse by a hardening sensation, which we have called Tight when it is less hard, and Wiry when it is very hard. Heat from deficiency in a yin organ will therefore usually be accompanied by a Tight to Wiry pulse in the position associated with that yin organ. When the condition is chronic, the proximal position on the left—the Kidney yin position—will usually also be Tight to Wiry, since Kidney yin is the source of yin for all of the other organs. Excluding other variables, the pulse will usually be a little Rapid. Wherever one finds Tightness, one must also inquire about pain.

Left distal

There are two types of Tightness at the left distal position. One can be found over the entire position, and the other just in the center of that position. Both are patterns associated with Dr. Shen's 'Heart tight' condition (see Chapter 12 and the glossary).

Tight at Pericardium position

Tightness in the center of the left distal position is somewhat different in sensation than in the other burners. Here it is narrow, sharp, and more focused, striking the finger like the point of a pencil, rather than feeling like a hard line. This kind of Tightness in the center with a slightly Rapid rate is a sign of heat in the Pericardium. This is usually heat from excess, most often from the Liver. However, the condition can also be heat from deficiency in the later stages. With heat from excess there is more Robust Pounding and a more Rapid rate, and with heat from deficiency, less Pounding and a less Rapid rate. Other signs are helpful in making the diagnosis. Heat in the Pericardium is associated with worry and anxiety, insomnia, and restlessness for a moderate period of time, from months to a few years. Myocarditis would have a Tense Pounding Flooding Excess quality over the entire distal pulse.

Tight over entire left distal position

Tightness over the entire position indicates heat from yin deficiency of the Heart. It is associated with agitated Heart qi due to worry, emotional shock, anxiety, insomnia, and restlessness for a relatively long period of time, over several years.

Tight with Change in Rate at Rest

A Tight left distal position with a pulse rate that changes moderately at rest is a sign of a more advanced stage of Heart qi agitation ('Heart nervous'). This is associated with an emotional shock to the Heart, usually earlier in life. Sexual abuse is among the many emotional assaults in life which could cause such a shock. A roller coaster feeling, and being easily fatigued, are common symptoms (see Chapter 12).

Tight Deep Thin and very Rapid

This combination at the left distal position indicates trapped qi in the Heart at an advanced stage, or 'Heart full' (see glossary). At an earlier stage of this condition, the Inflated quality is found at the left distal position. The trapped qi in the Heart is a precursor to an enlarged heart, a condition of severe Heart qi deficiency.

Tight Deep Thin Feeble and slightly Rapid

This combination indicates an advanced condition of Heart blood stagnation ('Heart small'). At an earlier stage the pulse at the left distal position is Deep and very Flat.

Right distal

I am including the Special Lung position in our discussion of this position. Tightness here is one of the more common findings, along with Slipperiness and Vibration. In this section it is more useful to classify by condition than sensation.

Qi stagnation from invading cold and heat from deficiency

If the right distal position shows no serious qualities such as Tight-Wiry, Slippery, Inflated, Rough Vibration, Change in Qualities, or Feeble-Absent, then the Tight quality at the Special Lung position is a sign of qi stagnation and Lung yin deficiency associated with a previous invasion of the Lungs by cold, and its sequelae, which has not fully resolved. The heat and stagnation remain, leaving the Lungs vulnerable, even though the symptoms have disappeared.

Tuberculosis

A very Tight quality at the Special Lung positions combined with a Normal rate and a Deep Thin quality at the right distal position indicates a history of tuberculosis, with continuing vulnerability. With current tuberculosis the right distal position is either Wiry, if the disease is an early to intermediate stage, or Feeble or Absent in the later stages, and the Special Lung position is Deep, Thin, and Tight-Wiry, Slippery, Change in Intensity with Rough Vibration, and the rate is paradoxically Slow.

Asthma

A yin-deficient, treatment-resistant type of asthma is found with a Tight right distal position, a very Tight yet Slippery Special Lung position with moderately Rough Vibration, and a slightly Rapid rate. The pulse is not as Deep as with tuberculosis. I have found this pulse and condition associated with premature birth and incubation.

Pneumonitis and obstructive lung disease

With this condition the right distal position is very Tight and Slippery with Rough Vibration, and the Special Lung position is Restricted, Muffled, very Tight and Slippery with Rough Vibration, and the rate is Slow. In one case I observed, the Special Lung position was Absent.

Acute bacterial infection

With an acute bacterial infection such as pneumonia, the pulse is usually very Rapid, the right distal position Tense, Robust Pounding, and Flooding Excess, and the Special Lung position Tight with Robust Pounding Vibration and Slipperiness, and is accompanied by high fever, upper respiratory symptoms, and debility.

Iatrogenic

The frequent use of antibiotics, antihistamines, steroids, and decongestants for Lung disorders often leads to depletion of yin, and to trapped heat and heat from deficiency in the Lungs. This will cause the right distal position to be Tight and a little Inflated, and the Special Lung position to be Tight.

Nicotine and other inhaled irritants

Tobacco smoke tends to dry the Lungs and deplete yin. The result is severe Lung yin deficiency with a Tight right distal position and a Tight to Wiry quality at the Special Lung position that is usually also Slippery with very Rough Vibration, Change in Intensity, and even Muffled.

Overwork of the Lungs

If the right distal position is Feeble, indicating Lung qi deficiency, and the rate is Normal to Slightly Rapid, Tightness in the Special Lung position is a sign of Lung yin deficiency, usually due to persistent overwork of the Lungs. I have felt this combination in people who use their Lungs beyond their energy level, such as singers and teachers.

Left middle

Tight Floating

This is a very early sign of incipient wind in the channels and stroke, usually the result of long-term heat from excess leading to Liver yin and blood deficiency, which in the extreme case becomes Liver wind.

Tight Thin

This is a sign of Liver blood and yin deficiency.

Tension and hypertension

The Tight-Wiry quality at this position usually reflects qi stagnation due to long-term emotional repression, which causes heat from yin deficiency in the Liver. This will sometimes lead to hypertension if the heat goes to the blood, which the Liver stores. With this condition the same quality can also appear at the left distal position. Later, the Tight quality can evolve into the very Tight Hollow Full-Overflowing quality, first at the left distal position, then the left side, and even over the entire pulse.

Diabetes

The Tight-Wiry quality at this position may signal an early diabetic condition, especially if it is also found at the left proximal position. Later, the Tight quality can evolve into the very Tight Hollow Full-Overflowing quality.

Chemical toxicity (including alcohol)

Exposure to chemical toxins either in a large quantity for a short time, or in small amounts over a long period of time, can give rise to a Tight quality at this position. Because of its role as a detoxifier, these substances concentrate in and cause the Liver to become dry. The single greatest source of this toxicity in my experience is alcohol. I have felt this quality in individuals whose mothers drank alcohol in quantity during pregnancy. The pulse is also usually Deep.

Tight Slippery Robust Pounding and Rapid

Here we may have a subacute developing damp-heat disorder in the Liver and Gallbladder, such as the first stage of acute hepatitis or mononucleosis.

Tight, Flooding Excess, Robust Pounding, Slippery and Rapid

This combination indicates a fully developed phlegm-fire condition in the Liver with Liver fire rising, probably signifying a fulminating hepatitis.

Tight Empty at qi depth

I have found this combination in a Liver that was damaged by previous hepatitis, with poor recovery. With a history of mononucleosis, the qi depth is less Tight than with a history of hepatitis.

Gallbladder

A Tight and Slippery pulse in the Gallbladder position is a sign of damp-heat in the Gallbladder, including gallstones, which may be painful. If the pulse is also Rapid, and the individual experiences alternating chills and fever, there may be acute infection in the Gallbladder.

Right middle

If in the center of the tongue the coating is thin, patchy, and dry with a bright red body, the condition is deficient-type heat from Stomach yin deficiency.

Tight only at qi depth

If the Tightness is only at the surface of the pulse, this indicates a condition of heat from yin deficiency in the Stomach due to habitually eating too fast.

Tight at Esophageal position

Qi stagnation in the esophagus, with pain.

Tight at Stomach-Pylorus Extension position

If the pulse becomes Tight as you roll one finger proximally to the Stomach-Pylorus Extension position, this indicates an inflammation of the stomach, pylorus, and possibly duodenum, including gastritis and ulcer. Other qualities that are frequently present with these disorders are Slippery and Hollow.

Left proximal

Tight

This is a sign of moderate Kidney yin deficiency due to the exhaustion of yin by the overworking of other organs or the nervous system.

Tight Robust Pounding and Rapid

This quality can appear with a moderate acute exacerbation of pelvic inflammatory disease, chronic prostatitis, or chronic colitis, if accompanied by the appropriate symptoms. The pulse can also be Rapid and Pounding with these conditions. A severe acute exacerbation of these disorders would be accompanied by a Tight Flooding Excess pulse. Check the Large Intestine and Pelvis/Lower Body positions where these conditions tend to be confined.

Tight Thin

This is a sign of a more advanced yin deficiency of the Kidneys. The Thin quality here is a sign of concomitant blood and qi deficiency, despite the absence in the literature of a Kidney blood deficiency syndrome.

Tight Hollow Full-Overflowing

This is a sign of diabetes or hypertension, especially if the same quality is found at the left middle position.

Large Intestine

Tightness in this position, when the left proximal position is Tight, is sharper and more focused. Tightness at the Large Intestine position can mean irritability, with an inflammation of the intestine, such as colitis or irritable bowel syndrome and diarrhea, but not as widespread and severe as those conditions described above when the quality is found over the entire left proximal position and is accompanied by Flooding Excess and a Rapid rate.

Right proximal

Tight

Tightness at this position can be a sign of bladder/ureter inflammation. When the Tightness is found bilaterally at the proximal positions, Kidney yin deficiency is the usual condition.

Tight Deep

This could be a sign of chronic Bladder inflammation and Kidney qi deficiency with bladder distention, some burning on urination, dribbling, incontinence, diminished stream force, frequency, and urgency.

Tight, Flooding Excess, Robust Pounding and Rapid

Most often this indicates a fulminating bladder infection, less often pelvic infection, acute prostatitis, or colitis, which conditions tend to be confined to the involved area and organs.

Small Intestine

Tightness in this position, accompanied by Tightness in the right proximal position, is sharper and more focused. Tightness at the Small Intestine position is a sign of irritability and inflammation in the Small Intestine, such as an ulcer or chronic regional enteritis. If it is also Slippery, we may have infection.

Left and right Pelvis/Lower Body

Signs in the Pelvis/Lower Body positions cannot be lateralized anatomically. A Tight quality here indicates mild to moderate stagnation of qi and possibly inflammation in either the prostate, pelvis, either ovary or uterus, an inguinal or scrotal hernia on either side with lower abdominal pain, or pain in the lower back or knees.

Wiry

Category

The term 'wiry' is perhaps the one most misapplied term in the entire lexicon of Chinese pulse diagnosis. In the current literature, the term is almost always associated with the descriptive expression 'taut.' The various sources use the term wiry to describe many sensations other than one which feels like a wire, and they do not agree on a uniform sensation for this pulse quality.

This is one of the many arguments, already discussed, for the need to describe four separate qualities within the traditional tight and wiry categories, so as to organize the overlapping, disparate descriptions and interpretations. In terms of sensation and interpretation, the term wiry has been used synonymously in the literature with what I have variously delineated above as the Taut, Tense, and Tight pulses. What I designate as the Wiry pulse is therefore a new quality, not new in sensation, only in description and interpretation.

Sensation

Calling to mind the hardness of a metal wire, one has the best sense of how it feels to palpate a Wiry pulse. With the slightest pressure it feels thin, hard, and cutting to the touch, long and continuous, and does not move away. Consider the sensation of palpating the E string, which is the narrowest on a violin.

In English, the term wiry unambiguously refers to a metallic substance which, next to diamonds, is the hardest material that we commonly encounter. When alluded to as Wiry, we would hope that we are describing the hardest, most rigid material. Anything less than the hardest and most rigid sensation does not justify the term Wiry.

General interpretation

EXTREME YIN-ESSENCE DEFICIENCY AND PAIN

While there is considerable overlap with the Tight quality, the Wiry quality represents the final, extreme stage in the depletion of yin. It is my opinion that it differs from the Tight pulse, which primarily reflects a deficiency of yin, in that the Wiry quality is a sign of deficient essence as well as yin. Heat from deficiency usually ensues from the effort of the body to overcome chronic and prolonged stagnation from any cause: overwork, nervous tension, cold, or dampness. In our time and place, emotional stress and overwork are the principal etiologies. The Wiry quality is also found with *very* severe acute or chronic pain.

Etiology

NERVOUS TENSION AND LIVER WIND

The hardest Wiry quality is associated with the most common etiology: persistent overwork of the 'nervous system.' This pulse is sometimes Floating and a little Rapid.

The restriction of qi circulation in the Liver-Gallbladder due to stress and nervous tension, and the accumulation of heat from excess generated by the body's effort to overcome the stagnation, depletes the yin and blood, creating Liver wind, for which a Wiry pulse quality is often a later sign. Because qualities in the middle positions tend to dominate the sensations of the other positions, an extreme Liver wind Wiry quality may often be felt over the entire left side, or even the entire pulse. Associated with a Liver wind Wiry quality are the early stages of diseases such as yin-essence deficient hypertension and diabetes.

CEREBROVASCULAR ACCIDENT

Wiriness over the entire pulse with elevated blood pressure is a sign of a potentially very severe and widespread stroke, the final sequelae of prolonged nervous tension. The pulse at this stage is usually Wiry Hollow Full-Overflowing, and often Slippery as well, when the etiology is also nutritional.

Quoting Dr. Shen, "If the six pulses are shi-xian [most tight] and quite rapid, the heat then lies in the blood. In this case, perhaps the sugar content in the blood is too high or the blood is too thick."[32] Elevated glucose, triglycerides, and cholesterol in blood chemistry are related to excessive intake of rich foods, and to the conditions of 'blood heat' or 'blood thick,' with a red tongue and injected eyes, and a tendency to hypertension associated with heat from excess.

PAIN AND COLD

The Wiry quality at one position may be a sign of often intractable pain in the associated area of the body, usually accompanied by muscular spasm and inflamed nerves. The Wiry quality over the entire pulse, especially in young people, could be the result of an invasion of cold throughout the body, which obstructs the qi and blood in muscles and in the nervous system. I often saw this when working with fishermen in East Hampton. Ginger baths were the most effective therapy. With chronic conditions, this pulse is Slower.

INFECTION

A Wiry Robust Pounding Rapid quality accompanied by a high fever in one position can indicate localized infection in a deficient person, for example, in the left middle position (Liver) with acute hepatitis. With this etiology the pulse is also often Flooding Excess in a stronger person.

CHEMICAL TOXICITY

Chemicals, including ethyl alcohol, have a drying effect, especially on the liver. The long-term effect is cirrhosis of the liver, although the drying affects the entire organism. The depletion of yin and essence leaves the pulse with a Wiry quality, especially in the left middle position.

Combinations

Wiry Thin

'Wiry Thin' is a bit redundant since the Wiry quality is always very Thin. However, the implication is that the combined hardness and thinness are signs of a combined heat from yin-essence and blood deficiency condition, especially Liver blood deficiency ('dried blood'). This is commonly found in women who do not recover their blood after multiple childbirths. Some of the symptoms of this deficiency are muscular spasms, numbness and tingling, blurred vision, light sensitivity, and painful or diminished menstruation. In the extreme case one arrives at the Leather quality (see Chapter 9).

Wiry Deep

This is a sign of heat from yin-essence deficiency in the yin organs, combined with qi deficiency. It is found in early yin-essence deficient hypertension, and with diabetes with qi deficiency.

Wiry and Rapid

If the rate is very Rapid with little Pounding, it may indicate very severe pain of recent onset. If the rate is slightly Rapid, the etiology is more likely less severe pain, localized infection, or generalized yin-essence deficiency. Wu Shui-Wan believes "that the disease is caused by 'wind and heat.' It means that the infection (or inflammation) is caused by germs or virus, etc., and high fever internally."[33]

Wiry and Slippery at blood depth with Normal or slightly Rapid rate

Over the entire pulse this is associated by Dr. Shen with the conditions 'blood heat' or 'blood thick,' which he interprets as excessive sugar or cholesterol in the blood. I interpret it to mean an extreme drying out of the vessels with turbulent blood.

Wiry Slippery and very Rapid

Slippery at the blood depth

This combination, especially the very Rapid rate, indicates infection in the blood (septicemia) with fever and excessive redness inside the lower eyelids.

Slippery at the organ or at all depths

This combination is a sign of a generalized chronic systemic infection with pain and/or severe depletion of yin-essence.

Wiry Robust Pounding and Rapid

Over large segments of the pulse

This combination over the entire pulse, or just the left side, in a more deficient person, can be a sign of moderate hypertension that is progressing in severity. In a stronger person the pulse would be more Hollow Full-Overflowing.

At individual positions

As mentioned above, this combination found at one position, when accompanied by a high fever, can indicate localized infection, especially in a deficient person. The Wiry Robust Pounding Rapid quality can be found in the left middle position (Liver) with acute hepatitis. The Flooding Excess quality is often present with fulminating infections in strong people.

Wiry Empty and slightly Rapid

This combination can be found in the lesser yin heat pattern of the lesser yin and terminal stages of the six stages. Here the extreme deficiency of yang has caused the yin and yang to separate, and the heat from deficiency to rise and become 'wild.'

Wiry Deep and Slow

This combination is found in either longstanding pain syndromes where circulation of qi and blood has diminished, or where the yin-essence and qi is very depleted.

Wiry Inflated

When this combination is found at one position, usually the right middle, it is a sign of very prolonged trapped qi in the associated organ or area of the body, often the gastrointestinal system. Pain and distention, sometimes due to intestinal obstruction, is severe. The Wiriness here is primarily a sign of the extreme pain.

Wiry Choppy

This combination, frequently associated at the proximal and Pelvis/Lower Body positions, indicates a condition of simultaneous severe heat from deficiency and blood stagnation, or more often, intense pain and blood stagnation. The differentiation is made by examining the tongue and under the eyelid, and by other symptomology.

Positions

BILATERALLY AT SAME BURNER

Distal

All of the following are etiologies of the Wiry quality bilaterally at the distal position, where this quality represents severity, and often severe pain.

Excess

QI AND BLOOD STAGNATION

At this position the Wiry quality is usually accompanied by severe chest pain and pressure and heavy breathing. Also, pain from severe headache without rising heat may be due to qi and blood stagnation, trauma, or tumor. The eyes and tongue are not red.

TRAUMA

The source may be recent severe trauma to the upper burner accompanied by intense pain, a horizontal line under the eyelid, and possibly a small purple blister on the side and toward the end of the tongue.

LIFTING

If the eye is normal, we may be dealing with qi and blood stagnation and severe pain for reasons other than trauma, such as the sudden lifting of a heavy object, far beyond one's energy, with the upper part of the body.

ASTHMA COMPLICATED BY MEDICATION

Wiriness bilaterally at the distal positions is sometimes a sign accompanying severe chronic asthma in which there has been excessive use of medication. With this condition the Wiry quality is usually also found at the Special Lung position.

Deficiency

ADVANCED YIN-ESSENCE DEFICIENT ASTHMA

The Wiry quality bilaterally in the distal position, accompanied by a Wiry, Slippery, very Rough Vibration quality at the Special Lung position, often attends a severe yin-essence deficient asthma.

COCAINE ABUSE

Although more often found at just the left distal position, the Wiry quality bilaterally at the distal positions is found in our times with long-term cocaine abuse, especially when inhaled. It is an example of severe depletion of yin due to Heart and Lung fire caused by the heat-producing action of cocaine.

YIN-ESSENCE DEPLETION OF HEART AND LUNGS

We may be dealing with a depletion of yin-essence in the upper part of the body due to long-term excessive emotional stress, especially prolonged excitement (mania), and anxiety. If the pulse is a little Rapid or lacking stability, there can be a history of emotional shock long in the past.

Rising heat

YIN AND QI DEFICIENCY WITH IMBALANCE

If the other positions are Feeble-Absent, Wiriness here can mean rising heat, especially Liver yang associated with Liver yin deficiency, with severe and unremitting throbbing headache as the principal symptom. Hypertension with bursting headache is possible if the insides of the lower eyelid and tongue are red. With hypertension, Wiriness will ordinarily also be found at the left middle and proximal positions.

FEBRILE DISEASE

A Wiry quality in the upper burner may also result from febrile disease in the Pericardium or Lungs consuming yin-essence, as in tuberculosis.

Middle

Severe pain

TRAUMA

Wiriness here can be due to trauma in the area of the middle burner, in which case there would be a history of trauma and the usual horizontal lines under the eyelid, and possibly a purple blister on the side of the tongue.

GASTRITIS OR ULCER

There is a possibility of painful gastritis or a gastric or duodenal ulcer. This could be due to Liver qi stagnation and the Liver 'attacking' the Stomach-Spleen over a considerable period of time. Hollowness and Slipperiness often accompany the Wiry quality with this condition, especially in the Stomach-Pylorus Extension position.

TUMOR

The severe pain may also be due to a neoplasm in a middle burner organ or in the peritoneal area.

INFECTION

A Wiry, Slippery, and Rapid pulse, at the organ or at all depths, with accompanying fever and severe pain, is a sign of an infection somewhere in the area or in one or all of the abdominal organs, for which one must search further. Pancreatitis, appendicitis, and peritonitis should be considered.

Eating habits

Eating too quickly over a very long period of time will produce a thin layer of Wiriness at the surface of the pulse, independent of the depth. There will be a Normal to slightly Rapid rate, and the center of the tongue will be bright red, dry, and with a patchy thin yellow coating.

Emotional stress

Wiriness uniformly found throughout the depths rather than just on the surface is often due to a social situation in which there is generally strong emotional stress during and after eating, over a very long period of time.

Where eating quickly is due to general tension over a long period of time, both the tongue and the eyes will tend to be more normal, at least in the early and middle stages of the process, and only at this stage—when the pulse becomes Wiry—will there begin to be other signs of yin deficiency.

Liver-Kidney hypertension or diabetes

The Wiry quality at this position can sometimes presage hypertension or diabetes, especially if the left distal or left proximal positions are also involved.

Proximal

Diabetes or hypertension

This can be a sign of incipient diabetes and should always be seen as a warning sign to check further into the possibility that the disease is already well underway. However, I have seen a number of patients who exhibited this pulse, and in whom there was a strong family history of diabetes, who had not yet developed the disease themselves, but were potentially vulnerable. With these conditions, the Wiry quality will eventually almost always be found at the middle positions as well, especially the left middle position.

Infection

Wiriness over the entire position with a very Rapid pulse, red eyes and tongue, can sometimes be associated with an acute flare-up of severe chronic prostatitis, colitis, or pelvic inflammatory disease in a deficient individual. In a stronger person, these conditions would more likely be accompanied by a Flooding Excess quality.

Pain and blood stagnation

A Wiry pulse at the proximal positions is sometimes associated with intractable menstrual pain, hernia, and kidney stones due to blood stagnation, even in the absence of a Choppy quality. This type of blood stagnation can also be due to cold from excess such as long-term ingestion of ice-cream and ice. If the pain is acute the pulse rate could be Rapid, but if the pain is chronic or from cold, the rate could be Slow.

Deficiency of essence

Wiriness in the proximal positions is also associated with deficiency of yin-essence, especially if the pulse is Deep and the rate is very Slow.

Intestines

If the Wiriness (here a sign of severe irritability and inflammation) is found only at the Intestine positions on both sides, the problem is less severe fulminating colitis or enteritis than if it is also found in the proximal positions.

Pelvis/Lower Body

Heat from excess (infection)

If the Wiry quality is found only at the Pelvis/ Lower Body positions, the problem, though still severe, is less severe prostatitis or pelvic inflammatory disease than if it is also found in the proximal positions.

Pain

When the Wiry pulse is found bilaterally at the Pelvis/Lower Body position, it is usually a sign of severe low back pain, provided the rate is not Rapid and the tongue and eyes are relatively normal. If the pain is due to trauma, the lower eyelid may show the horizontal line and the tongue a purple blister. Even in the absence of a Choppy quality, with which it is often found in the lower burner positions, it could here be a sign of blood stagnation, which is often a factor in intractable low back pain.

SIDES

Left

Pain

Wiriness can appear with severe pain over the entire left side of the pulse. If it is due to trauma, there is often a horizontal line under the left eyelid and/or a small purple blister on the left side of the tongue.

Emotional tension

Wiriness at the superficial aspect of the organ depth is a sign of the 'nervous system' overworking for a very long time, which eventually causes the qi or nervous innervation of the organ to become dry, tight, and contracted. The tongue and eyes are unremarkable.

Cerebrovascular accident

A Wiry quality and Rapid rate over the entire left side of the pulse with hypertension in a deficient person can be a sign of an imminent stroke on the left side of the body. The quality would be Hollow Full-Overflowing in a strong person. The tongue would be dry and patchy red with a yellow coating, and the vessels inside the lower eyelid would be confluent rather than separate.

Right

Eating habits

Wiriness here can be due to heat in the 'digestive system' due to eating too quickly over a long period of time.

Severe pain

Pain on the right side of the body can be accompanied by a Wiry quality on the right side of the pulse. If trauma to the right side of the body is suspected, one will search for the appropriate history, a horizontal line under the right eyelid or a small purple blister on the right side of the tongue. With a recent acute trauma the rate will be very Rapid, and with chronic pain, slightly Rapid.

Cerebrovascular accident

Wiriness over the entire right side of the pulse with a Rapid rate and elevated blood pressure is a dangerous sign of imminent stroke on the right side of the body, especially in a deficient person. A stronger person would have a Hollow Full-Overflowing pulse.

INDIVIDUAL POSITIONS

Wiriness at any single position, in addition to the other issues to be discussed, can mean severe pain in the corresponding area of the body or organ. Pain should therefore always be questioned when this quality is found at an individual position.

Left distal

Blood stagnation in the Heart

Severe angina-type pain, due to other causes such as blood stagnation, can account for the Wiry quality at this position. It can be oppressive, shooting (down the left arm), or needle-like.

Hypertension

The Wiry quality at this position can occur with hypertension in a deficient person, but almost always simultaneously with the Wiry quality at the left middle position. The quality is Hollow Full-Overflowing in a stronger person.

Hashimoto's disease and Grave's disease

With Hashimoto's and Grave's disease the Wiry quality is accompanied by a Flooding Excess Wave, Robust Pounding, and a Rapid rate in the early acute phase of the disease.

Cocaine abuse

With cocaine abuse the Wiry quality is found at a later stage in the disease process.

Pericardium

Wiriness, like Tightness, is sometimes a somewhat different sensation at the left distal position than in other positions. In such a small area it is difficult to differentiate from the similar Tight quality. It is sometimes shorter and even more focused in the center at the Pericardium position, and has a sharp, harder quality when it hits the finger, like the point of a pencil rather than a straight line. Found in this position, the Wiry quality is a sign of heat from excess changing to heat from deficiency. I have found it with a history of pericarditis.

Right distal

In my experience, a Wiry pulse has occurred at this position on only a few occasions, mostly in individuals with a long history of heavy tobacco smoking. However, the Wiry Deep quality in this position has long been associated with intermediate stage tuberculosis, and I have found it here and at the Special Lung position with severe yin-deficient asthma associated with premature birth and a long time in an incubator.

Special Lung

A Wiry pulse at this position is more common. If the regular Lung position is Normal, it represents some residual heat from deficiency and stagnation in the Lung from previous Lung illness, usually from early in life, or even congenital. Childhood asthma or allergies are common causes. As with any abnormal quality at the Special Lung position, the Lungs must always be considered vulnerable, even if the right distal position shows no abnormality.

Left middle

Acute infection of the Liver (hepatitis)

A Wiry quality may be present here in a deficient person with acute hepatitis and high fever and a very Rapid Robust Pounding and Bounding pulse. In a more robust individual, there would also be Flooding Excess.

SUBCLINICAL HEPATITIS

This quality can occur in subacute or chronic hepatitis, again due to severe yin depletion associated with a prolonged fever and low-grade infection.

Chronic advanced yin deficiency of the Liver

LONGSTANDING REPRESSED EMOTIONS

The cause is usually repressed emotions over a very long time, often leading to a drying of the liver and to early hypertension, which is commonly associated with this quality here due to the Liver wind generated from rising Liver yang and Liver blood deficiency. With hypertension, the Wiry quality is also often found simultaneously at either the left distal or left proximal position.

Diabetes

Wiriness also appears at this position with early diabetes, usually in conjunction with Wiriness at the left proximal position.

Chemical toxicity

Exposure to chemical toxins, either in a large quantity for a short period of time or in small amounts over a long period, can create a Wiry quality at this position. In my experience, the single greatest source of this toxicity is alcohol. I have felt the quality at this position in individuals whose mothers drank alcohol in quantity during pregnancy.

Gallbladder

The Wiry quality at the Gallbladder position usually accompanies pain with severe inflammation and infection within the gallbladder. Associated qualities with this condition are the Choppy and Muffled qualities when necrosis is an issue.

Right middle

Pain

ULCER

I have found Wiriness at this position with a gastric or duodenal ulcer, often accompanied by pain. Slipperiness and Hollowness often accompany this quality, especially at the Stomach-Pylorus Extension position.

STAGNANT FOOD

The pain can be due to stagnant food at the esophagus with regurgitation and cancer.

INTERNAL COLD FROM EXCESS

Pain here is often found in persons with a lifelong indulgence in cold foods, such as chewing on ice or ice cream. In women this often occurs simultaneously with severe menstrual pain.

Eating habits

If the Wiriness is found at the superficial aspect of the pulse, it may be due to eating too quickly over a very long period of time. Frequently this occurs over the entire right side of the pulse, implicating the entire 'digestive system.'

Emotional stress

Very long-term emotional stress can lead to extreme Liver yin and blood deficiency due to Liver qi stagnation generating heat, which consumes the yin of the Stomach.

Chemical toxicity

The ingestion of chemicals can deplete the yin of the Stomach. Alcohol is the most commonly associated etiology, but in my experience nicotine is also a major factor leading to stomach cancer.

Stomach-Pylorus Extension

A Wiry quality at the Stomach-Pylorus Extension position is often a sign of an ulcer in the pylorus or duodenum. It is frequently accompanied by a Hollow and Slippery quality with this disorder.

Left proximal

Severe yin deficiency

GENERAL CONDITION

Wiriness at the left proximal position reflects severe yin-essence deficiency. This is sometimes found in connection with a Tight or Wiry pulse in the left distal position (Kidney-Heart disharmony), the Special Lung position, and the left middle position, and less often in the right middle positions.

The meaning is simply that overwork of these systems, the Heart, Lungs, Liver, and Stomach, has exhausted the Kidneys' ability to provide the yin required to balance the heat from deficiency produced in those organs.

Severe essence deficiency, with all the attendant sexual and lower body dysfunction, can accompany a Wiry pulse at this position. However, essence deficiency can take many forms, among them genital, developmental, central nervous system, bone, and bone marrow (hemapoeitic) disorders.

SPECIFIC CONDITION

Perhaps the most extreme Wiry pulses I have ever felt were associated with the early stages of diabetes, in which the Wiriness frequently also appears on the left middle position. The next stage is the very Tight Hollow Full-Overflowing quality.

Wiriness at the left proximal position can also indicate the early stages of hypertension, although this is less common.

Pain, infection, or inflammation

INTESTINES, PROSTATE, AND PELVIS

I have also felt this quality in deficient individuals with fulminating severe chronic prostatitis, pelvic inflammatory disease, and severe chronic colitis, usually accompanied by pain and either urinary or intestinal symptoms. Again, in stronger individuals with these conditions the pulse is also Flooding Excess.

KIDNEY STONES

A Wiry quality can be a sign of kidney stones accompanied by severe pain.

Right and left Pelvis/Lower Body

Low back pain

A Wiry pulse at the Pelvis/Lower Body position may be present with severe low back pain.

Urogenital and gynecological disorders

The Wiry quality can sometimes be found here with uterine, ovarian, fallopian, and other pelvic and menstrual disorders, including endometriosis, and sometimes with less advanced prostatitis, especially with severe pain. When there is blood stagnation in this area, there is often an accompanying Choppy quality. With infection, the pulse is more Rapid in deficient individuals, and, rarely, Flooding Excess in stronger individuals.

Right proximal

Bladder position

I have often felt Wiriness over the entire right proximal position with painful chronic urinary infections, usually involving pain. In deficient individuals, it occurs here rarely with mild acute exacerbations of chronic prostatitis, pelvic inflammatory disease, colitis, or regional enteritis. Usually with this etiology the Wiry quality in deficient individuals is found bilaterally at the proximal position, or alone on the left proximal position.

Large and Small Intestine

Here the Wiry quality indicates inflammation and irritability of the Small (right side) or Large (left side) Intestine, including chronic regional enteritis or colitis respectively, usually accompanied by severe pain.

360 ❖ Shape

UNEVEN NONFLUID QUALITIES

Ropy

Category

There is no written record of this pulse quality in any book in English of which I am aware, except the brief excerpt from Amber quoted below. Dr. Shen is my principal source for the following information. I have placed this quality here under the general category of Shape, where it is a progression in the continuum of the pulses which range from stagnation to heat (Taut to Wiry). It is only found over the entire pulse in all positions simultaneously. (See Fig. 11-3.)

Tense Ropy

Sensation

The pulse is cord-like, big, hard, and round. It is distinct from the surrounding anatomical structures, giving the impression that the vessel could be grasped like a rope, lifted, and moved. It is sometimes straight and other times somewhat twisted. It varies in degree of hardness and in size, and is always continuous through all positions.

Amber[34] describes it as follows:

> Empty the vessel by pressure and roll it under the fingers, slipping the skin over the vessel. A Normal radial artery is scarcely to be felt except in a very thin wrist, but one that is sclerosed is firm, cord-like and perhaps tortuous. While it is empty, measure its size by running the finger along the vessel in order to detect calcareous beading or plates of lime salts.

General interpretation

The Tense Ropy quality is specifically a sign of chronic heat from excess and/or deficiency in the blood that has vulcanized the muscular walls of the vessels such that they have lost all flexibility and elasticity. The pulse is usually regarded as an indication of a widespread, general arteriosclerotic process, and is sometimes preceded or accompanied by hypertension. It is believed to be a pulse that is difficult to alter, usually treated at first by yin-nourishing and blood-moving herbs.

While this quality is generally encountered in older individuals with a lifelong 'nervous system tense' condition or history of excessive ingestion of rich foods, Dr. Shen reported having found the quality in a young person who had a severe accident.

Fig. 11-3 Ropy quality

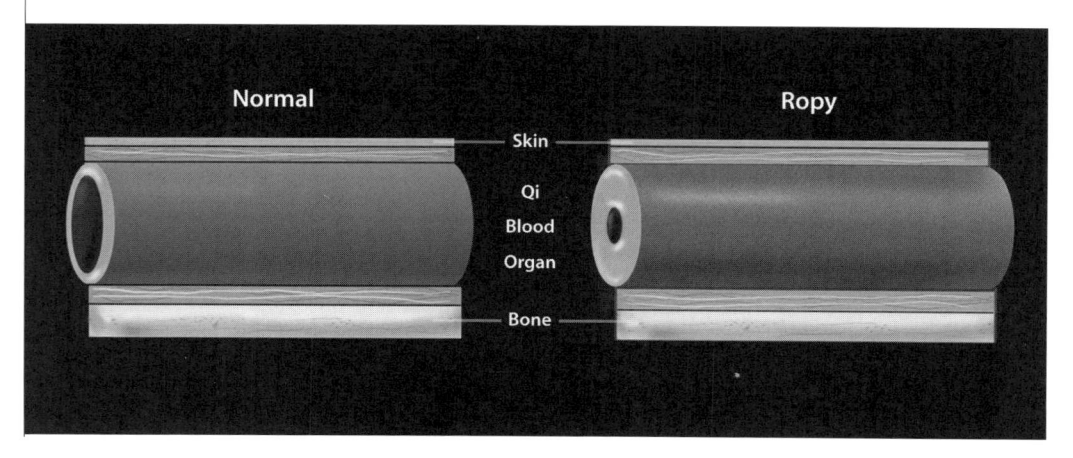

Ropy Yielding Hollow

Sensation

The pulse is cord-like, big, and round, but Yielding and Hollow rather than hard. It is also distinct from the surrounding anatomical structures, giving the impression that the vessel could be grasped, lifted, and moved, but more like a soft flexible tube than a hard rope.

General interpretation

Dr. Shen attributes this pulse to a situation in which the individual has been participating in vigorous sports, and especially one who has exercised beyond their energy, for a relatively long period of time. (This 'qi wild' condition is discussed in the section on the Hollow and Hollow Full-Overflowing qualities in Chapter 8.) The drying out of the intima and media of the vessels in this case is due to lack of nourishment, rather than heat.

Exercising beyond one's energy over a long period of time causes the yin (nourishing blood and qi) flowing in the center of the vessel to separate from the activating yang qi at the surface of the vessel, thereby depriving the vessel walls of the nourishment needed to maintain their flexibility. Overexercise causes gradual shrinking of yin-blood—using up more than can be replaced—while the heart pumps harder to maintain circulation, causing the walls to remain distended. I have observed this combination several times in recent years, and once found it in a 60-year-old marathon runner subsequently diagnosed with Parkinson's disease. I would speculate that this may involve impaired circulation to the brain related to the alterations in the blood vessels indicated by the Ropy and Yielding quality. However, I do not have enough clinical experience with this quality to cogently address the issue of associated syndromes.

Positions

While the Ropy pulse is found at all six positions simultaneously, it is usually most prominent in the left middle position. This is possibly because the Liver stores the blood and is therefore the organ which would most likely reflect heat in the blood, which is one of the causes of the hardening process. I have never felt this quality completely alone in any one position, or on just one side or the other, or bilaterally at just one level.

Fig. 11-4 Choppy quality

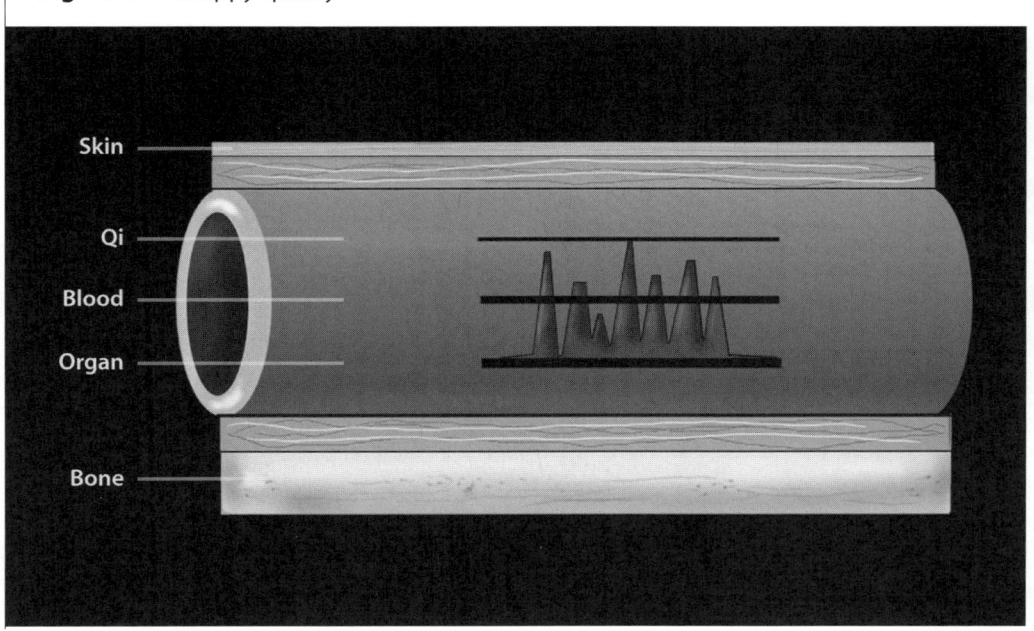

362 ❖ *Shape*

Choppy

Category

I classify the Choppy pulse under the heading of shape, as does Kaptchuk.[35] This means that it cannot be defined by depth, width (size), volume (strength), length, rhythm, or rate. It can only be delineated by its unique shape. The Choppy pulse is classified without elaboration by Li Shi-Zhen[36] as one of the Slow pulses.

Sensation

In order to access the Choppy quality (Fig. 11-4) one must roll one's finger across the position. I have found it to be uneven and grating to the finger, like rubbing it across a washboard. The degree of roughness varies with the position and the degree of associated stagnation. It is felt most often at the middle and organ depths, and less often at the qi depth.[37] The *Inner Classic (Nei jing)* alludes to it as 'scraping bamboo.'

As previously noted, no single contributor to the literature on pulse diagnosis is better known or has had a greater impact on pulse diagnosis than Wang Shu-He, author of *The Pulse Classic (Mai jing)* in the second century. Wang describes the Choppy pulse as follows:

> It is fine and slow, coming and going with difficulty and scattered or with an interruption, but has the ability to recover.[38]

These words have been repeated for nearly two millennia, and appear in the writings of Li Shi-Zhen (70), Kaptchuk (309), Wu Shui-Wan (20), and Deng (119-21), among others. Yet many different disorders will inevitably cause some blood stagnation. And so, as the contemporary scholar Lu Yubin (70) has noted, there should be *different* pulse qualities corresponding to each.

Indeed, there are a variety of qualities which signal one of the many disorders that can lead to blood stagnation, but they are not in themselves signs that blood stagnation has actually occurred. It would therefore be wrong to suggest that the appearance of these other qualities necessarily represents the presence of blood stagnation. Lu Yubin, who refers to the Choppy quality as "uneven," develops this argument as follows:[39]

> [A]lthough the uneven [Choppy] pulse is often seen together with the thready pulse, the slow pulse, the short pulse, the scattered pulse, etc. in the clinic, they are not the basic factors constituting the uneven pulse.
>
> Since the uneven pulse is felt unsmooth, some doctors in history have suggested that it has intermissions. But their suggestions are not accepted by most physicians, because the uneven pulse, unlike the pulses with intermissions such as the intermittent pulse, the running pulse and knotted pulse, has no abnormal intermission, although it is felt unsmooth.
>
> The uneven pulse is also different from the slow pulse. The slow pulse is marked by the slowing of the pulse rate, beating three to four times in one respiratory cycle; while the uneven pulse, although felt hesitant, has a normal pulse rate. As the uneven pulse is often seen in critical diseases marked by loss of Blood, consumption of Essence, stagnation of Qi and Blood stasis, it often occurs together with the thready pulse, the slow pulse, the scattered pulse or the short pulse. So, in history, many doctors advocated that the uneven pulse should have the changes of pulse like reduce or increase of the pulse size [intensity and amplitude], irregular changes of the pulse rhythm, or abnormal changes of the pulse rate. However, the uneven pulse is only defined based on changes of the pulse in its shape, or the unsmooth feeling on pulse-taking, *so an uneven pulse occurring together with other pulse conditions mentioned above only indicates coexistence of these pulses. In essence, the uneven pulse has not these additional conditions.* [emphasis added]

Lu Yubin thus recognizes the need for a more complete differentiation of qualities to obviate the use of one quality to describe several different conditions, as often occurred in the past. Apart from Choppy, all of the qualities described above appear frequently with no other clinical sign or symptom of blood stagnation, such as a purple tongue or intractable pain. Therefore, if we were to treat based on Wang's list of associated qualities, taking them all to be signs of blood stagnation, we could do irreparable harm.

CHOPPY AND VIBRATION

The sensation of the Choppy quality is sometimes confused with the Vibration quality. The former is a rougher sensation, the latter much finer. However, the sensation of the Choppy and very Rough Vibration qualities are at times difficult to distinguish. Whether I call the quality Choppy or Rough Vibration sometimes depends on the location and the depth.

However, even the roughest Vibration has a more delicate quality than the least coarse Choppy quality. While 'buzzing' is closer to the sensation of Vibration, 'grating' more aptly captures the feeling of a Choppy quality, which is the exact opposite of the smooth sensation associated with the Slippery quality.

While there are exceptions, an important distinction between palpating the Choppy quality on the one hand, and the Vibration and Slippery qualities on the other, is that to access the washboard sensation of the Choppy quality one has to roll one's finger along the position. With the Vibration and Slippery qualities, the movement occurs while one's finger is stationary on the position.

At the qi depth, I am more inclined to call this quality Rough Vibration, whatever its location. The sensation is most often found to be Choppy at the proximal and the Pelvis/Lower Body positions.

General Interpretation

The Choppy quality is always a sign of serious pathology.[40]

BLOOD STAGNATION

There are several types of blood stagnation classified by location and by etiology. None has the "fine and slow pulse, coming and going with difficulty and scattered or with an interruption" features associated by Wang Shu-He with the Choppy quality.

By location, there is blood stagnation in the tissue, which is almost always signaled by a Choppy ('scraping bamboo') quality. (Rarely, there is a very Tense Inflated quality associated with the extravasation of blood into a body cavity, as with a subdural hematoma, pericardial tamponade, or a significant hemorrhage into the intestinal or stomach cavity with colitis or an ulcer, respectively.)

Signs of blood stagnation in the blood include the qualities Blood Heat and Thick, Hollow Full-Overflowing, Ropy and Liver Engorgement (of the portal system). Classified by excess and deficiency, there are two kinds of blood stagnation recognized in the literature, that due to excess and that due to deficiency. Kaptchuk[41] writes:

> A choppy pulse can have aspects of either Deficiency or Excess. If a Choppy pulse is also weak or thin, it is a sign of insufficient Blood or Jing to fill the Blood Vessels. If it is strong, resisting the fingers, it is generally a sign of Congealed Blood Obstructing Movement.

My own clinical experience with the Choppy quality has confirmed the presence of blood stagnation in the tissue as the almost exclusive condition associated with this quality. The cause of the blood stagnation can be heat from excess or deficiency, qi deficiency, blood deficiency, cold from excess, neoplasm, or trauma. Blood stagnation in the blood is signaled by the Blood Unclear, Blood Heat, Blood Thick, Full-Overflowing, and Tense Ropy qualities.

This pulse is found most commonly in the left distal position in angina, the left middle position with 'dried blood,' the right middle position with cancer, or left proximal and Pelvis/Lower Body positions with dysmenorrhea, fibroids, endometriosis, and ovarian cysts.

Another situation associated with this pulse is imminent miscarriage, theoretically due to difficulty in nourishing the fetus.[42] Check the tongue for black lines lengthwise.

INFLAMMATION

The Choppy quality is sometimes found at the Gallbladder, Stomach-Pylorus Extension, and Intestine positions in conditions of extreme inflammation, and consequent ulceration and necrosis.

DIFFERENTIATING THE VIBRATION QUALITY

I have already made the sensory distinction between the Choppy and Vibration qualities. It is my contention, therefore, that Kaptchuk's and Porkert's 'choppy strong' pulse, by definition, is the same as my Choppy quality, and that their 'choppy weak' pulse is partially equivalent to my Vibration quality.

The contrast between the Choppy and Vibration qualities, in meaning as well as feeling sensation, more than warrants their division into two separate and distinct classifications. The Choppy quality is a sign of stagnation, primarily blood stagnation, and Rough Vibration, discussed later in this chapter, is often a sign of parenchymal damage and severe physiological disorganization of the organ in which it is found.

Combinations[43]

Choppy Tight or Wiry

Especially when found in the middle positions, the left distal, Pelvis/Lower Body, and left proximal positions, this combination implies blood stagnation and pain that is more profound than when the pulse is just Wiry. By definition, Tight and Wiry qualities also necessarily feel Thin.

Positions

BILATERALLY AT SAME POSITION

I have rarely observed Choppiness bilaterally, except in the Pelvis/Lower Body position. What is reported here includes a mixture of personal experience with information from the literature.[44]

Middle — The Choppy pulse across the entire middle position, although rare, has in my experience always been a sign of severe obstruction of both qi and blood in the entire area, or of one or more organs therein. The worst case scenario includes the possibility of either an ulcer which has bled, or cancer, especially in the stomach or duodenum.[45]

Proximal and Pelvis/Lower Body — I have found Choppiness at this position, especially bilaterally at the Pelvis/Lower Body position, primarily in women with endometriosis, fibroids, and ovarian cysts, and several times in chauffeurs and taxi drivers who suffered from hemorrhoids or chronic prostatitis. It is a sign of blood stagnation in the lower burner.[46]

SIDES

Choppiness confined to one side is extremely uncommon and is mentioned here only for purposes of completeness.

Left — Although rare, a Choppy quality on the left side of the pulse indicates long-past trauma to that side of the body, with significant residual blood stagnation. One would expect to find a horizontal line under the left eyelid, and, in more severe cases, some evidence of a purple blister on the left side of the tongue might linger.

Right — The same applies to the right side as to the left side, except that the trauma and auxiliary signs are on the right side. (On one occasion, this finding, without the line on the lower eyelid or purple blister on the tongue, seemed to be associated with a high level of blood cholesterol and potential stroke, presumably on the right side of the body.)

INDIVIDUAL POSITIONS

Left distal — Choppiness in the left distal position usually means that there is blood stagnation in the coronary arteries with chest pain and palpitations. The problem is with blood circulation in the Heart, usually due to tension and life's pressures, which, in Dr. Shen's words, make "the Heart nerves tight," and/or due to poor nutrition with resulting atherosclerotic coronary arteries. In a personal communication, Dr. Shen indicated that, with this quality in this position, a person could die at any time.[47]

Neuro-psychological — Choppiness here has been clearly associated with multiple past head traumas and chronic intractable headache, probably involving manifold micro loci of intracranial blood stagnation.

Left middle — I have found a Choppy and Thin quality in the left middle position in connection with the condition of 'dried blood' in the Liver. Here the Liver is unable to store blood, especially for the menstrual cycle, and the consequence may be amenorrhea as well as dizziness and blurring of vision.[48]

Gallbladder — Choppiness at the Gallbladder position is a sign of advancing necrosis of the gallbladder, the result of long-term severe chronic inflammation and infection.

Right middle and Stomach-Pylorus Extension — Choppiness in these positions is rare. It implies advanced stagnation with pain due to blood stagnation associated with a necrotic ulcer or cancer.[49] It occurs much more frequently at the Stomach-Pylorus Extension than at the right middle position.

Esophagus — Choppiness here, although rare, means stagnation in the esophagus of either food or qi. With the latter, there is discomfort only while eating, and with the former, the discomfort is more ongoing. The cause may be trauma or emotion, and this finding is often coincident with the diagnosis of hiatal hernia. More ominous is its association with regurgitation and cancer of the esophagus.

Left proximal and/or left Pelvis/Lower Body — A Choppy quality at these positions usually involves blood stagnation in the pelvic area, especially the uterus. It may accompany endometriosis and is almost always present with dysmenorrhea. A neoplasm, malignant or otherwise, must be considered. The precise diagnosis should be established by Western diagnostic techniques. The Pelvis/Lower Body position can, by itself, often be Choppy for the same reasons, and is especially identified with uterine fibroids.[50]

Right proximal and/or — Choppiness here usually means blood stagnation and poor function in the pelvic-per-

right Pelvis/Lower Body

oneal area, which must be further investigated with Western diagnostic techniques to rule out neoplasm. Often there can be urinary problems, including obstruction of the urethra and cancer of the urethra or bladder.[51]

Large Intestine

Although rare in my experience, Choppiness at the Large Intestine position may indicate chronic minor bleeding of mucosa made fragile by inflammation and irritation. Choppiness at this position has also been reported with hemorrhoids, and malignancy should be investigated.

Small Intestine

I have rarely encountered the Choppy quality in this position. It is a sign of extreme fragility in the lining of the intestine with bleeding and residual blood stagnation, as with regional enteritis.

Vibration

Category

The quality Vibration appears nowhere in the literature of pulse diagnosis. Nevertheless, it is a quality which was acknowledged by Dr. Shen in his clinical practice, in our recent discussions, and during the years of my apprenticeship. The quality is included in notes from some of his seminars in England, but does not appear in his book. It is a quality supported by my own clinical experience as conveying very important information.

There are several grades of Vibration, from very Smooth to very Rough. Rough Vibration in practice can be confused with the Choppy (Grating, Rough, Difficult) and Unstable qualities, from which the following discussion will, I hope, distinguish it both in feeling sensation and meaning. In the preceding discussion of the Choppy quality I identified Vibration partially with what Kaptchuk and others describe as 'choppy deficient.' The clinical material in the ensuing discussion will establish this quality as requiring the distinction which I have afforded it here.

Fig. 11-5 Smooth and Rough Vibration qualities

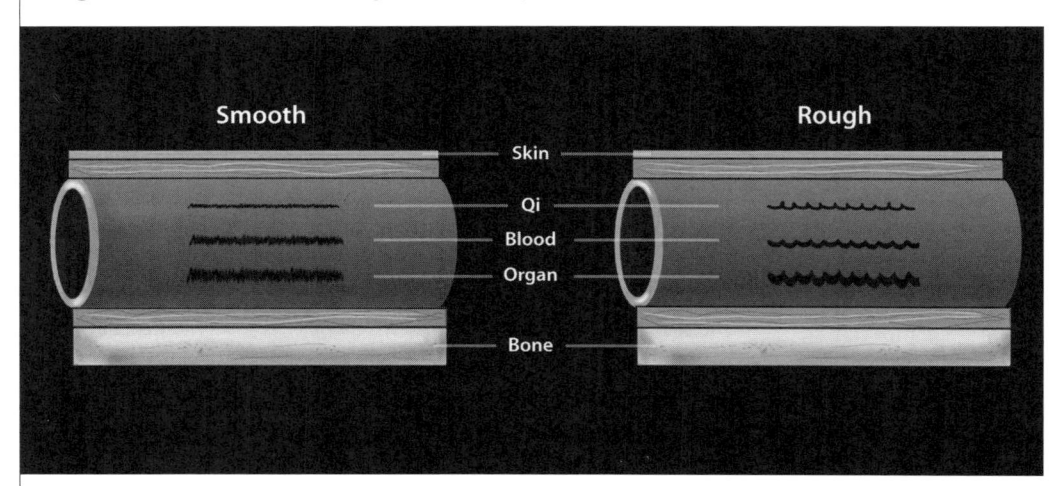

Sensation

The Choppy quality is sometimes confused with the Vibration quality. However, as previously noted, even the roughest Vibration has a more delicate quality than the least coarse Choppy quality. While 'buzzing' is closer to the sensation of Vibration, 'grating' more aptly captures the feeling of the Choppy quality. Another important distinction between them is that, to access the washboard sensation of the Choppy quality, one has to roll one's finger along the position. With the Vibration (and Slippery) qualities, the movement occurs while one's finger is stationery on the position.

Types

Smooth Vibration

Smooth Vibration is a fine buzzing sensation under the finger for which the terms shaking, trembling, tingling, reverberating, palpitating, shivering, wavering, quivering, vacillating, and oscillating are all useful synonyms. One student described it as 'seltzer bubbles' and another as 'sparkles.' This sensation varies from very smooth to slightly less smooth, each involving different meanings, which will be explained below.

Another sensation with which Vibration can be confused is the Unstable quality. This quality is always found at only one position. There it gives the sensation of rapidly hitting different parts of the pad of the finger with an irregular pattern (see Chapter 6).

Rough Vibration

With Rough Vibration the sensation under one's fingers is that of a very coarse buzzing.

General interpretation

OVERALL ATTRIBUTES

Vibration is a quality whose interpretation varies depending on the degree of its smoothness, consistency, position, depth, and response to treatment, as well as the time it has existed. Smooth Vibration is a benign sign of agitation of Heart qi. Rough Vibration is a serious sign of parenchymal damage and serious physiological dysfunction. According to Dr. Shen, all Vibrational qualities are associated with some kind of shock.

While we will attempt to discuss each variable separately for the sake of clarity, these variables are more often encountered in clinically significant combinations. As with all qualities, its interpretation also depends diagnostically on location, other signs and symptoms, and history.

Etiology

Entire pulse

Generally, the causes of Smooth Vibration over the entire pulse are current worry, a tendency to worry, and lack of sleep (Heart qi agitation). Rough Vibration is a sign of shock or terror when, according to Dr. Shen, there is also some Heart qi deficiency. Otherwise, with shock and without some Heart qi deficiency, he said that the pulse would only be very Tight and Rapid. (I cannot independently confirm this statement.) Over time, both Smooth and Rough Vibration with these etiologies will affect the 'nervous system,' as Dr. Shen defines that term.

Individual position

The only individual position in which Smooth Vibration is found by itself is the left distal position, where it is a sign of Heart qi agitation. Rough Vibration at any individual position is a sign of parenchymal damage.

Seriousness of condition

As a sign, Vibration varies in seriousness from benign to very serious. The deeper, more consistent, and ubiquitous its appearance, the longer it has persisted, and the rougher the Vibration, the more dangerous is the condition it represents.

If it is inconsistent, if it is more superficial, if it occupies fewer positions over a shorter time, and if it is very smooth, the problem is probably not as emergent. The number of positions involved is a less reliable sign of seriousness than the other variables. Serious or not, the appearance of Vibration should always be thoroughly investigated to confirm one's impression.

Signs and tests of seriousness

A test of seriousness suggested by Dr. Shen is to ask the patient to rest for a week and then check the pulse again. A similar trial of seriousness is the evaluation of change in the pulse after one or two treatments. With both tests, if the quality continues to exist as it was, it is an indication of more serious dysfunction.

If, after rest and a few treatments, the Vibration becomes less consistent, more superficial at fewer positions, and less Rough, the condition is less serious. For example, with regard to Heart function, the Vibration which becomes less Rough is then more a reflection of a condition related to transient worry or to a small emotional shock than it is to Heart qi deficiency and parenchymal damage. If under stress the Vibration reappears, then we can consider that organ vulnerable to functional damage.

INDIVIDUAL ATTRIBUTES

Consistency

As just mentioned, when Vibration appears inconsistently we are faced with a less serious condition, and when it is more persistent we are confronted with a more serious problem. Consistency, for example, is a more reliable sign of seriousness than the number of positions involved.

For example, Smooth Vibration found consistently over the entire pulse is a sign of prolonged obsessive worry. Such a person will find something to worry about even if there is nothing to worry about. On the other hand, inconsistent Vibration at the left distal position or over the entire pulse would be a sign of relatively innocuous, transient worry or mild emotional shock, or as a sign of a long-term tendency to worry only under moderate real stress. The Vibration disappears when the stress is resolved. If the Vibration persists, we must concern ourselves with the progression of these states to more serious Heart dysfunction.

Time

The longer Vibration persists, whether or not it is consistent, the more likely it will be a sign of a more grave condition. Unless the cause is corrected, over time it will tend to be less smooth, deeper, more consistent, and found in more positions.

If worry, for example, continues for a considerable period of time, the Vibration will spread down the left side from the left distal position first, then to the left middle position, then the entire left side, and finally down the right side from the right distal to right proximal position. Over a longer period of time, Heart qi and yang will be affected and the Vibration will also gradually increase in roughness.

Degree of smoothness

The smoothness or roughness of the Vibration will depend on the strength of the causative factor and the length of time it has existed. A transient or minor concern will manifest as Smooth Vibration. If, for example, the cause is worry, the greater the degree of worry and the longer it lasts, the rougher the Vibration and the greater the number of affected positions there will be.

Smooth Vibration is a sign of Heart qi agitation. If the Vibration is very Smooth to Smooth, this may be interpreted to mean that the individual has had a mild emotional shock or is very worried about something that is currently an issue, or that they are sleep deprived. I have observed this quality increasingly in seminars on the pulses of people suffering from a significant lack of sleep.

If the quality is slightly Rougher, or appears over the entire pulse at all depths, then the individual has a tendency to obsessive worry, and will find something to worry about even if there is no current cause. This sometimes is found concurrently with a Hesitant quality, which involves obsessive thinking, not necessarily worry.

On the other hand the Vibration caused by a severe shock is a Rougher Vibration than any Vibration caused by even the most profound worry. When this Rougher Vibration occurs at all depths over the entire pulse, the shock has affected the qi of the entire body, and is accordingly a serious disorder. When Rough Vibration is found at only one position, the function of the organ associated with that position is more compromised by parenchymal damage than when the quality of the Vibration is smoother.

Depth

According to Dr. Shen, Vibration can appear at all depths and depends on the health of the body, the strength of the pathogenic factor, and the length of time it has existed. If the body is strong, the pathogenic factor insubstantial, or the condition has existed for only a short time, it will most likely appear primarily at the qi depth. I allude to this as Heart qi agitation, especially when the Vibration is Smooth.

If the body is strong, the pathogenic process weak, or the Vibration has persisted for only a short time, the Vibration will first be felt at the qi depth. As the condition worsens, the Vibration will move from the qi to the blood depths, and finally to all three depths. With increasing depletion of qi, the qi and blood depths will disappear first, and Vibration will appear only at the organ depth.

When Vibration is superficial and appears inconsistently we are faced with a less serious condition than when the Vibration is either deep at the organ depth, or at all three depths, and is consistent. If, for example, the Vibration at the left distal position is superficial, it is a sign of transient worry in a reasonably healthy person for a relatively short time, creating some agitation in the Heart qi. Except for anxiety, mild fatigue, transient palpitations, and insomnia, there are no other signs or symptoms.

If the cause is a more serious Heart condition, such as trapped blood in the Heart in a more depleted person, for a longer period of time, the Vibration at the left distal position will either be deeper or more pervasive, with symptoms of fear, tension, breathing difficulty, and chest pain. The combination of increasing depth, roughness, and consistency is a sign of increasing pathology.

Vibration confined to the blood depth is a sign that the vessel walls are compromised by whatever process is occurring in the blood, such as 'blood heat' or 'blood thick.' It is also usually accompanied by the Slippery quality, a sign of concomitant turbulence in the blood.

ENTIRE PULSE

Consistent Rough Vibration

Differentiation of Vibration associated with shock, guilt, and fear

According to Dr. Shen, the consistent appearance of the Rough Vibration quality at all positions and all depths may be due to emotional shock, profound guilt, and fear only when there is Heart qi-yang deficiency. Otherwise, said Dr. Shen, we would find only a very Tight Rapid combination. In my own experience I have found that with shock, guilt, and fear the Rough Vibration quality can occur with a very Tight Rapid combination, especially at first, but not necessarily with concomitant Heart qi-yang deficiency.

They seem to be independent of each other, except that eventually, if uncorrected, this condition accompanied by these qualities will lead to Heart qi-yang deficiency.

With fear the entire face has a green color and constricted pupils; with shock the face is blue; with guilt the color is normal, but the *shen* or spirit in the eyes is dull, and according to Dr. Shen, the individual cannot look you directly in the eye. (I have not found the latter to be a consistently reliable behavior.) With both guilt and fear one would expect to find the face and eye signs simultaneously. With Heart qi-yang deficiency the face has an absence of color, the eyes are dull, the pupils a little wide, and the cheeks are sometimes red.

A distinction must be made between the Rough Vibration which appears in people whose guilt and fear concerns their own transgressions against others, and those cases where the Vibration appears in the victim of those transgressions.

Fear and guilt from transgressions against others

This is related, as far as I know, to some real, and not imagined, antisocial act perpetrated by the individual, with guilt and fear concerning a major transgression of societal rules and laws up to and including murder. Such individuals, said Dr. Shen, cannot look you directly in the eye, which he relied upon as a vital diagnostic sign of guilt. However, I have found people who, despite having this guilt and fear, are able to look others directly in the eye.

I have encountered this in only three people, two of whom had committed murder. One of the murderers had been severely sexually abused as a young child. The guilt and fear do not seem to be out of immediate and current concern with being caught for their crimes. One patient had murdered someone in North Africa some thirty years prior to his examination. The other had been involved in multiple murders of newborn infants in a satanic cult when she was a child. Neither was in any danger of being prosecuted for their crime.

While the committing of a major crime should be considered when a consistent Rough Vibration with a Tight Rapid pulse is found at most or all of the positions and depths, I believe that guilt and anxiety based on imagined rather than real acts is a possibility to be explored. My own experience here is too circumscribed to have a firm opinion. However, it is my strong hunch that such a pervasive appearance of this quality is more likely to reflect a real rather than imagined act.

Fear, guilt, and shock in the victims of transgressions

Recent experience indicates that consistent Rough Vibration over the entire pulse should be investigated in connection with rape, childhood sexual abuse, and multiple personality syndrome. With this etiology the Vibration often appears in a setting of a 'qi wild' disorder (Change in Qualities, Yielding Hollow, Empty) or where the Heart shows instability through the presence of a Change in Rate at Rest, or more seriously, Interrupted-Intermittent ('Heart nervous'), and more rarely with a Bean (Spinning) quality. Rough Vibration is also often present at the Neuro-psychological positions.

In a slightly different vein, recently a young woman who contracted HIV after sleeping with a transient lover one time showed most of the above mentioned qualities, including Rough Vibration over her entire pulse. She lived in constant terror of AIDS.

Shock

Rough Vibration over the entire pulse can be a sign of severe emotional shock, or a physical shock which has a strong emotional component. The pulse is generally Tight, the left distal position could be Inflated or Flat, and the rate tends to be Rapid and Change in Rate at Rest. The facial color is blue: over the entire face if the shock is very severe; around the chin and mouth if it is congenital, or from very early in life; and between the eyes and at the temples if later in life.

Smooth Vibration

Smooth Vibration over the entire pulse at all depths is, as already mentioned, a sign of a previous mild emotional shock and of anxiety for a very long time, at least ten years. The more consistent it is, the more serious the worry and its effect on physiology. However, beyond a sign of worry, this consistent Smooth Vibration over the entire pulse at all depths is even more a sign of an obsession with worry itself, that even if there were nothing to worry about, one would find something to worry about. I have also observed this quality increasingly in seminars on the pulses of people with significant lack of sleep.[52]

Combinations

I am unaware of combinations with other qualities which are of particular significance, except as mentioned above in the general interpretation.

Positions

BILATERALLY AT SAME POSITION

Neuro-psychological

A Smooth Vibration pulse at this position is associated with agitated qi of the Heart and anxiety. Sometimes this pulse is accompanied by Rough Vibration in most of the remainder of the pulse, with the same implications. One such young woman, mentioned above, who I met while teaching a seminar, had recently contracted HIV during a casual sexual encounter.

It is Dr. Shen's contention that Vibration in this position is always related to Heart function involving some degree of emotional instability. I see this in terms of the traditional relationship between the Heart and mind, wherein the Heart controls the mind.

A Rough Vibration quality at this position is more rarely encountered and questionably associated with central nervous system disease. However, although very infrequent, I have observed it in cases of multiple sclerosis, with a history of electric shock therapy, with intractable headache, and more recently with a history of severe childhood sexual abuse. Frequently with central nervous system disease, this quality coexists with the Rougher quality in the Neuro-psychological position, and less often is accompanied by an extreme Tightness in the most superficial part of the remainder of the pulse, or, in particular, at the surface of the organ depth on the left side. Also reported is extreme fear and terror.

Distal

If the Vibration is very Smooth to Smooth, comes and goes, and is superficial, this may be interpreted to mean that the individual is worried about something that is currently an issue. If the Vibration is at all depths, or just deep, and Rougher, the indication is a disease process that is serious and is affecting the mediastinal area due to trauma or tumor, or serious Heart and Lung (cardiopulmonary) disease.

Middle

The appearance of the Rough Vibration quality bilaterally at the middle position usually indicates either trauma or serious problems in the digestive system, including the Liver-Gallbladder component, suggesting Western diagnostic investigation.

Proximal

In this zone, Vibration is again a sign of trauma or parenchymal damage in the pelvis or any one of the organs in the area, including the entire urogenital system and lower bowel.

SIDES

Left

Smooth Vibration over the entire left side would suggest worry which has existed for a considerable period of time (at least five years, roughly speaking).

Right

According to Dr. Shen, this quality does not appear alone on the right side. It will always be accompanied by the same quality on the left side, as mentioned above in the general interpretation, but may not be clearly felt if the left side is very Reduced. If it is a continuation of the Smooth Vibration found over the entire left side, the worry associated with the quality has existed for at least ten years.

The Vibration, however, can occasionally be slightly stronger on the right side than on the left. When it is more prominent on the right side, and the Vibration is Rough, the cause may be habitually working during or immediately after eating. With this etiology, the individual will experience pain in the chest and abdomen, and the tongue will have a thick coating.

INDIVIDUAL POSITIONS

In any single position other than the left distal, the Rough Vibration quality is frequently a sign of significant dysfunction in the associated organ, which may be compromised on a material (parenchymal damage) as well as energic level of function. A Western medical evaluation of that organ should be considered, especially if the Vibration is deep at the organ depth, or at all three depths. However, if the Rough Vibration is found generally over the entire pulse, its appearance at an individual position is of no consequence unless the quantity is much greater at the individual position.

Left distal

Smooth Vibration

Smooth Vibration at this position must always be regarded in terms of that function of the Heart which controls the mind. It is seen as a less serious sign of the drain on the Heart by an overactive mind than is the Tight quality, in this or the Pericardium position.

Superficial Smooth Vibration

This indicates worry, which probably concerns something of recent origin and is not too serious.

Less superficial Smooth Vibration

This indicates longer-lasting worry of slightly more serious concern, which might interfere with sleep.

Smooth Vibration both superficial and deep

Smooth Vibration both superficial and deep is a sign that the agitation of qi excited in the Heart by the constant use of the mind and lack of good sleep is draining Heart qi. Fatigue in the morning would begin to be an issue.

Progression from left distal to other positions

Sudden worry in the form of a mild shock such as bad news is, for example, one important cause of Vibration. In its earliest phase the Vibration will occur first on the left distal position as a very superficial Smooth Vibration. If the worry continues for a considerable period of time, and the effect on the Heart is not corrected, the quality will spread.

Vibration will continue down the left side, first to the left middle and left proximal positions. If the worry is not alleviated, over time the Vibration will continue progressing to the right distal position and down the right side, finally reaching the right proximal position. However, consistent Smooth Vibration at all depths over the entire pulse can be a sign of obsessiveness, with the need to worry, in contrast to superficial Smooth Vibration, which would reflect only current worry.

Rough Vibration deeply or at all depths

Very Rough Vibration appearing deeply or at all depths can indicate parenchymal damage and possible Heart qi-yang deficiency that requires immediate further investigation and therapeutic intervention. If the pulse is also very Rapid, and the temperature is below normal, or there is an arrhythmia, the sign is extremely serious; even, according to Dr. Shen, to the point of impending death.

Neuro-psychological	See discussion under bilaterally at the Neuro-psychological position.
Mitral Valve	Vibration at this position is a sign of a mild incompetency of the mitral valve. This finding is sometimes accompanied by Slipperiness, which is a sign of a greater insufficiency and prolapse. The less Smooth the quality, and the greater the Slipperiness, the greater the defect. Both are signs of Heart qi deficiency, the Slippery quality being associated with greater Heart qi deficiency than is the Vibration.
Right distal and Special Lung	Vibration at these positions is a sign of Lung qi deficiency, and Rough Vibration is also a sign of impairment of alveolar function.
Left middle	With a Smooth Vibration at the qi depth in the left middle position, the person has been working beyond their energy, especially working too late. Rough Vibration is a sign of Liver qi deficiency and parenchymal damage. The rougher the Vibration, especially at the organ depth, the greater the deficiency and damage. Vibration confined to the blood depth at the left middle position is a sign of deterioration of the blood vessel walls.
Gallbladder	A Rough Vibration here could be a sign of gallstones and necrosis of the gallbladder wall. More often it is the Choppy quality that is found here with these conditions.
Right middle	Rough Vibration in this position is a possible sign of severe Spleen-Stomach dysfunction. The deeper and rougher the Vibration, the greater the parenchymal damage.
Esophagus	Rough Vibration in this position was rare in the past, but is recently increasing with a rise in the incidence of esophageal reflux. It is a sign of serious pathology, including Barrett's Syndrome and esophageal adencarcinoma.
Stomach-Pylorus Extension	Rough Vibration at this position is a possible sign of serious pathology (including carcinoma) either in the lower part of the stomach, the pylorus, or possibly the duodenum.
Proximal	Again, the deeper and rougher the Vibration, the greater the dysfunction. One must consider Kidney or adrenal failure, and carcinoma in the lower burner.
Intestines	Rough Vibration in these positions is possibly a serious sign of Intestinal dysfunction, including diseases such as regional enteritis, Crohn's disease, and carcinoma.
Pelvis/Lower Body	Rough Vibration in these positions is possibly a sign of serious pathology in the lower burner, including tumors or ectopic pregnancy.

Miscellaneous shape qualities

Nonhomogeneous

Category

There is no other system of classification that I have reviewed which describes this quality.

Sensation

The sensation is not accessed uniformly within the domain of a particular position. In some parts of the position there is consistently more substance to the pulse than in other parts. It therefore has a smooth, uneven, bumpy feeling as one's finger passes over the surface, in contrast to the Choppy quality, in which the unevenness and bumpy feeling is rough.

Interpretation

I consider this sensation to be a sign of stagnation of all substances if the position is Robust, and of deficiency of all substances if it is Reduced. In both instances, this quality is a sign that yin and yang have separated and that physiological function of the associated organ is very seriously impaired.

Position

This quality can be found at any position, although I have found it most often in the left distal position when it is Robust, and in the left proximal position when it is Reduced. (See below for a discussion of Robust and Reduced.)

Bean (Spinning)

Category

Of all the qualities this is the most problematic in terms of the disparity between my experience and the descriptions in the literature. The term itself is a partial anachronism since the 'bean' aspect has been far more prominent in my experience than the 'spinning.' I have therefore decided to compromise with tradition by emphasizing the Bean but continuing to use the term Spinning in parenthesis so that it will be recognizable to those more familiar with the original terminology.

Spinning Bean is a term used by Kaptchuk.[53] Mann,[54] Wu Shui-Wan,[55] and Li Shi-Zhen refer to it as 'moving.'[56] It is classified by Li Shi-Zhen[57] as one of the 'rapid' pulses, and is termed 'mobile' by Porkert,[58] 'agitated' by Cheung and Belluomini,[59] and 'unsteady' by Worsley.[60] Apart from its bean-like properties, I originally classified it with the Diminished Short qualities because it is found in one position quite separate and apart from the rest of the pulse. Li Shi-Zhen[61] uses 'short' in his description, as "rapid, tight, slippery and short with strong beats."

Sensation

While relatively rare, this quality is dramatic and unforgettable due to its unique sensation when compared to all of the other qualities. It cannot be overlooked. I have always found it to be very Tight to Wiry, with a sense of urgency, and often like a hard object such as a splinter sticking out from and counter to the longitudinal flow of the rest of the pulse. Tight, hard, short, and like a bean have been far closer to my experience than Slippery or Rapid. It is Short, meaning that it occupies only one position, and it is said to be without head or tail. However, the Short pulse lacks the strength of the Bean (Spinning) quality.[62]

For me this quality has almost always occurred partially between and partially on a position, rather than entirely on a position, which is what we find with all other qualities. I have felt this pulse on the lower portion of the right distal position, and overlapping the Diaphragm position on one occasion. Another time I found it on the lower border of the right middle position overlapping the Small Intestine position, and twice at the left proximal position.

General interpretation	In my experience this quality is associated with profound emergent and traumatic events. While pain, and severe fright or terror, are the two life experiences which I most commonly identify with this pulse, I have found it in other situations as well, always involving a profound disturbance to the physiology. (See, e.g., the description of the left proximal and right middle positions below.)

Combinations

Bean (Spinning) Wiry

This combination is more characteristic of the presence of severe and acute pain.

Bean (Spinning) Tight, very Slippery and Rapid

In my experience, this combination is found especially with fright.[63]

Positions

BILATERALLY AT SAME POSITION[64]

INDIVIDUAL POSITIONS

Left	In my experience, associated with extreme fright.[65]
Right	In my experience, associated with extreme fright.[66]
Left middle	This is outside of my experience.[67]
Right middle	In my experience, associated with extreme pain due to gastric ulcer.[68]
Left proximal	A Bean (Spinning) quality was reported to have been found by an advanced student of mine around the left proximal position in a man who had a recent and unexplained gastrointestinal blockage, relieved by nasopharyngeal suction. It occurred in the same position in another man where there was extreme exposure to toxins, with episodes of binding-up of his entire body and an enlarged prostate. In the latter case, I believe that there may have been underlying damage to his kidneys.[69]
Right proximal	This is outside of my experience.[70]

Doughy

Sensation	This is the most common quality found in the Neuro-psychological positions. It is an ill-defined, undifferentiated impulse that does not correspond in sensation to any of the other qualities described in this book. I would best offer to describe it as an amorphous glob of clay, whose shape is never the same and whose volume varies from very faint to moderately robust.
Interpretation	The Doughy quality has been found thus far only at the Neuro-psychological positions where it was originally associated during my years with Dr. Shen with chronic neurological disease, especially multiple sclerosis. Because of this association, and since the Kidney essence controls the central nervous system (marrow), I have tentatively identi-

fied the Doughy quality as a sign of Kidney essence deficiency. And because all of the patients in whom I found this quality were severely qi deficient, I would further postulate that it is a sign of Kidney yang essence deficiency. In this connection, I theorize that since yang is associated with the faster moving energies of the body, it is functionally associated with the myelin sheath where the central nervous system's most rapid electrical impulses occur, and where the lesions of multiple sclerosis occur. It would follow that Kidney yin essence is functionally associated with the substance of the central nervous system, whose excess or deficiency involves a different order of neurological disease.

However, it should be noted that the Doughy quality has been found frequently at this position with no clinical signs of such serious disease, and with intractable headaches and sometimes with a history of electro-shock therapy. The entire position is currently the subject of a database study to better correlate the findings with Chinese and biomedical diagnosis. The idea is being entertained that damage to the brain probably occurs at subtle levels in many if not most people, manifesting in varying degrees of subtle and often subclinical mental, emotional, endocrine, and neurological disorders.

Qualifying Terms

BITING

The Biting quality is a form of the Tight and Wiry qualities which, as its name implies, involves a nipping sensation on the finger like that made by a kitten or puppy. It is found almost exclusively at the Intestine positions and is a sign of discomfort and pain, usually in the abdominal area.

ROUGH

Category

The term Rough is a useful adjective for refining the description of other qualities. In the literature it is a term frequently used by Li Shi-Zhen, especially in connection with his characterization of the Choppy quality.[71] I have found the term to be useful in enhancing my depiction of the Vibration quality.

Sensation

Rough is partially defined by its opposite, Smooth. It feels grating and uneven.

Interpretation

With regard to Vibration, the rougher the sensation the more serious the implications of the Vibration (see discussion of Vibration above). The same is true for the Choppy sensation, which is by definition Rough. The Rough quality has the same meaning in all individual positions and combinations of positions.

SMOOTH

Category and sensation

Smooth is a term used to modify the sensation of the principal qualities in the direction of a more delicate sensation, as opposed to Rough. A Smooth quality has no roughness and feels more level, regular, uniform, unvarying, and homogenous than the Rough quality.

Interpretation

Smooth is associated with a less serious condition than is indicated by the quality Rough. For example, Smooth Vibration over the entire pulse is generally a sign of a more benign state, such as worry, than is Rough Vibration, which is a sign of parenchymal damage and possibly Heart qi deficiency. The meaning of the Smooth quality is the same in all individual positions and combinations of positions.

SUBTLE (VAGUE)

Category — The term Subtle is an adjective which further defines other qualities. I have not found it used in the literature.

Sensation — Subtle means that the pulse it qualifies requires a finer palpatory distinction to access, and is more elusive.

Interpretation — A Subtle quality is generally associated with less pathology than a quality that is not Subtle. The meaning of the Subtle quality is the same in all individual or combined positions.

EPHEMERAL (TRANSIENT)

Sensation — This is a quality that is transient and fleeting, appearing and disappearing at a particular position throughout the examination.

Interpretation — The Ephemeral quality modifies the meaning of the principal quality in the direction of a less disharmonious condition than when the same quality is more enduring at that position.

Positions — This quality occurs most often at the Neuro-psychological and Mitral Valve positions.

ROBUST OR REDUCED FORCE

Category — Pounding, Hollow Full-Overflowing, and Flooding are the qualities in the literature which are most commonly associated with a pulse that has force. 'Without strength' is an expression used by Li Shi-Zhen with regard to the Soft,[72] Scattered,[73] and Thin[74] qualities.

Sensation — Force is defined as strength, energy, vigor, and power, referring especially to the intensity of the power or impetus. A pulse quality can be Robust (with force or power) or Reduced (without force or power). The strength of the impulse is the measure of Robust or Reduced. (See also Robust and Reduced Pounding in Chapter 8.)

Interpretation — I use these terms most commonly to modify the depiction of the Pounding and Flooding qualities. A Reduced Pounding pulse (without force) hits the finger without the follow-through and impact of a pulse that has Robust Pounding (with force), beginning strong but losing momentum. It is a sign that a depleted body is attempting to compensate in order to function normally. A Robust Pounding quality (with force) is a sign that the body is attempting to rid itself of excess, usually heat.

Positions — This modifying quality can be accessed at any position or can be used to describe Pounding over the entire pulse.

ROBUST (WITH) SUBSTANCE AND REDUCED (WITHOUT) SUBSTANCE

See the discussion of this topic in Chapter 8.

SEPARATING

Category

This quality is not described in the literature. Separating is a modifying term, not a true quality, since it has no interpretation apart from other qualities.

Sensation

On pressure, the pulse moves in two directions, distally and proximally, at the same time.

Interpretation

This modifier helps define a sensation of the Empty, Hollow, and Spreading qualities. It is always associated with the early stages in the development of these qualities, and is independent of location.

Anomalous Qualities

THREE YIN (SAN YIN MAI) OR HIDDEN LEFT PULSE[75]

The entire pulse on the left side is Hidden. This is thought to be a congenital anomaly and both this characteristic and the qualities which can be discerned are of no clinical significance.

TRANSPOSED PULSE (FAN QUAN MAI)

This is a congenitally anomalous artery on the dorsal side of the arm which renders the pulse unavailable to the diagnostic process. It can occur on one or both sides.

GANGLION

A ganglion is a small synovial cyst which can form at any time over the radial artery for no clear reason, which again renders the pulse useless as a diagnostic tool.

TRAUMA

I have been puzzled and fooled by arteries which have been traumatized by intra-arterial tubes inserted for the emergency delivery of blood. I am both embarrassed and amused in retrospect by my diagnostic impressions before being informed of the trauma.

Anomalous Vessels

SPLIT VESSELS AND MULTIPLE RADIAL ARTERIES

A series of observations since 1995 involve anomalous vessels of the radial artery, including the superficial palmar artery, which has been associated with the Special Lung position. Most of the 'split vessels' have been at the left middle position, several at the right middle position, and one at both the left middle and proximal positions. One anomalous vessel with 'multiple radial arteries' involved three separate vessels on the left side and two on the right, and one involved two vessels on the left side. None of the latter which I examined had either a 'three yin' or 'transposed' pulse.

Multiple Radial Arteries

The most medial and thinnest of the three arteries on the patient with three vessels on the left wrist was considered by the practitioner to be the Special Lung pulse. The Special Lung position is found on the superficial palmar branch of the radial artery. This branch leaves the radial artery at about the level of the styloid process. From there it runs medially and upward toward the trapezium bone, which is part of the lower row of the carpus.

It is my contention that the most medial and thinnest of the three pulses in this patient is the superficial palmar branch of the radial artery, which has anomalously branched from the radial artery at a point very proximal to its ordinary departure, further up the arm. The other two vessels represent an almost equal split from the regular radial artery at some point.

The patient with two vessels on the left side had been seen a year before the second deep vessel was discovered. She had chronic sinusitis, and her pulses showed signs of heat for which treatment provided no relief. Upon discovering the second deeper vessel, which was considerably Reduced in Substance, she was treated with nourishing herbs and acupuncture, to which she responded. The practitioner feels, therefore, that the deeper vessel is the more valid of the two.

Split Vessels

Most of the 'split vessels' in the middle positions that I observed were associated with current malignancies and traumatic events, one in the right middle position in a 28-year-old woman who was abandoned at birth at a train station in Korea, and lived in an orphanage for nine months before being adopted by an American family in Seattle. She had a miscarriage several months prior to the examination, when she was four months pregnant. Another woman was attacked by a gang of young men at the age of sixteen, and was certain she would die. Still another had attempted suicide, with a history of heavy drug abuse.

Interpretations by practitioners varied. Two felt that those they examined were associated with 'near death experiences.' In one case with a split vessel found at the left middle position, they felt that the yin and yang (*po* and *hun*) had separated, and that the separation was associated with a compromised blood supply. In my opinion, the term 'near death experience' should not be considered in the literal sense in which it has entered the culture, in which a person almost dies and returns. Rather, the split vessels would seem to attend any experience which arouses the fear of the unknown. Prospective death, as with malignancy (with which it has been most commonly associated) or abandonment at an early age, or even adoption, can arouse in a child profound fear of the unknown. The most recent case of a split vessel that was brought to my attention was a child of holocaust survivors whose father told her and her siblings that when they opened the refrigerator, a Nazi was hiding inside and would jump out at them, or had poisoned the food.

SUMMARY

The question with all of these vessels, as with the 'three yin' and 'transposed' pulses, is whether the qualities felt therein are valid for interpretation within our system of pulse diagnosis. With the 'three yin' and 'transposed' pulses, Dr. Shen was very clear that they are not valid.

For example, the most medial thin vessel (superficial palmar branch of the radial artery) does travel in the direction of the Special Lung position and is the artery on which the Special Lung position is ordinarily found when it branches at its usual anatomical position. However, whether the qualities found on this vessel are valid when it branches considerably proximal to the usual place is highly questionable. I would not feel safe in using the qualities found on this or any other anomalous pulse until it was clearly demonstrated over time that these qualities are valid indicators of pathology within the framework of our pulse model.

I emphasize "within the framework of our pulse model" because the qualities felt there may still have some meaning not available in our system. It would take many cases and a great deal of investigation to establish whether the qualities felt on anomalous vessels are consistently useful in our system, and whether some other system could be devised if they were not. One practitioner found that the radial artery on a clearly 'transposed' pulse did help her with that patient, and another practitioner felt the same about a patient with the anomalous radial artery mentioned above.

It is my impression that the qualities found on anomalous vessels are as atypical as the vessels themselves. However, practitioners must decide for themselves when and how an anomalous vessel will be useful.

Fig. 11-6 Shape

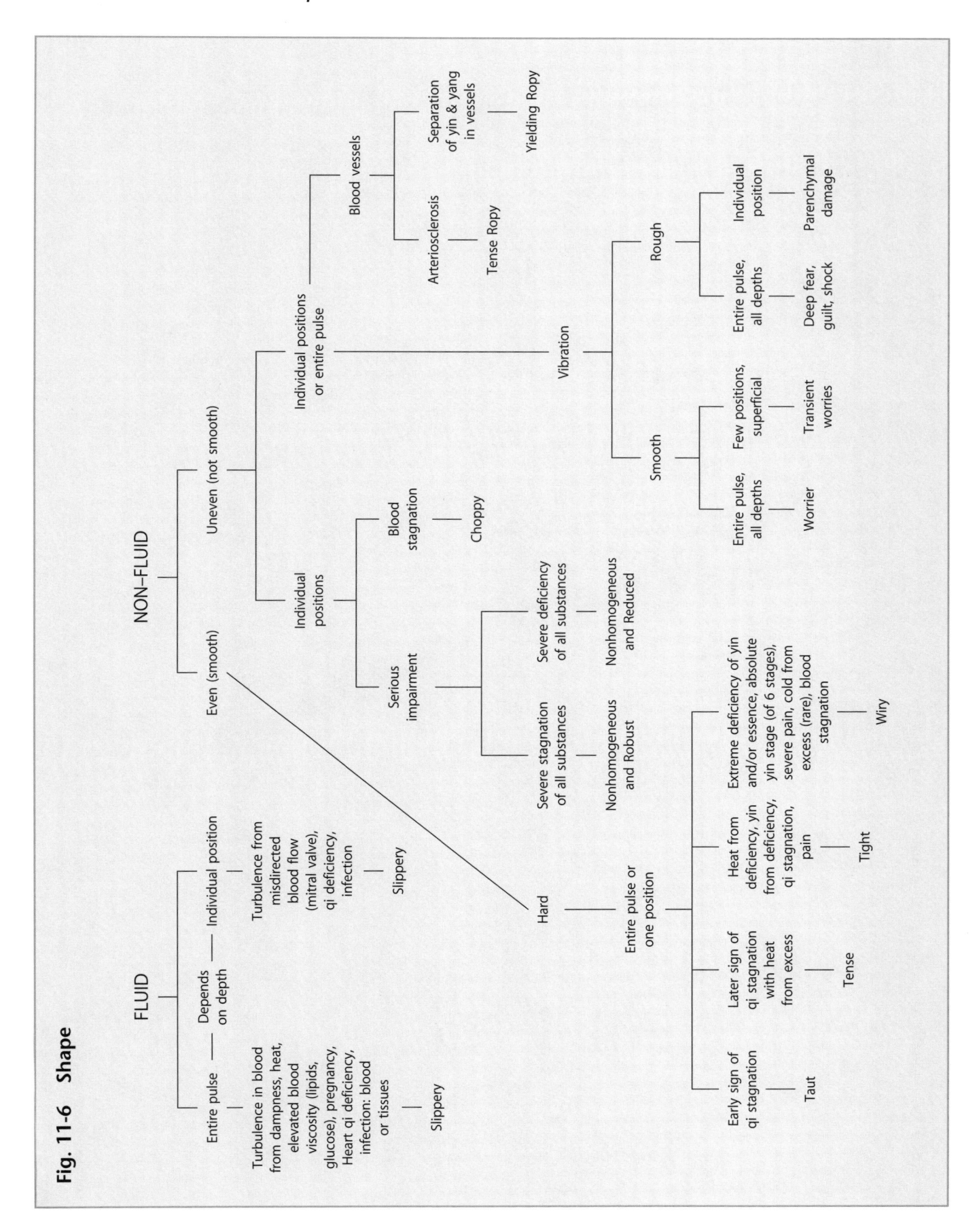

```
                                              Shape
                                                │
                        ┌─────────────────────┬─┴──────────────────────┐
                      FLUID                                         NON-FLUID
                        │                                               │
              ┌─────────┴─────────┐                         ┌───────────┴───────────┐
         Entire pulse      Depends on depth            Even (smooth)          Uneven (not smooth)
              │                   │                         │                       │
        Turbulence in       Individual position            Hard         ┌───────────┴───────────┐
        blood from                │                         │    Individual positions    Individual positions
        dampness, heat,    Turbulence from         Entire pulse      positions              or entire pulse
        elevated blood     misdirected blood       or one position        │                       │
        viscosity (lipids, flow (mitral valve),         │          ┌──────┴──────┐          Vibration
        glucose), pregnancy, qi deficiency,    ┌────┬──┴──┬─────┐  Serious    Blood               │
        Heart qi deficiency, infection         │    │     │     │  impairment stagnation   ┌──────┴──────┐
        infection: blood                       │    │     │     │     │          │       Smooth        Rough
        or tissues                             │    │     │     │  ┌──┴──┐     Choppy       │             │
              │                    │           │    │     │     │  Severe Severe       ┌────┴────┐   ┌────┴────┐
          Slippery             Slippery        │    │     │     │  stagn. deficiency   Few      Entire Entire  Individual
                                               │    │     │     │  of all  of all      positions, pulse, pulse,  position
                                          Early Later Heat Extreme substances substances superficial all     all
                                          sign  sign  from defic.   │         │            │    depths depths  │
                                          of qi of qi defic., yin    │         │        Transient │      │    Parenchymal
                                          stag- stag- yin   and/or   Nonhomo- Nonhomo-    worries Worrier Deep damage
                                          nation nation from essence, geneous  geneous                    fear,
                                                with  defic., yin stage and      and                      guilt,
                                                heat  qi     (of 6 stages), Robust Reduced                shock
                                                from  stag-  severe pain,
                                                excess nation, cold from
                                                      pain   excess (rare),
                                                             blood
                                                             stagnation
                                            │     │    │       │
                                          Taut  Tense Tight  Wiry

                              Blood vessels
                                   │
                        ┌──────────┴──────────┐
                   Arteriosclerosis      Separation of
                        │                yin & yang in vessels
                   Tense Ropy                 │
                                         Yielding Ropy
```

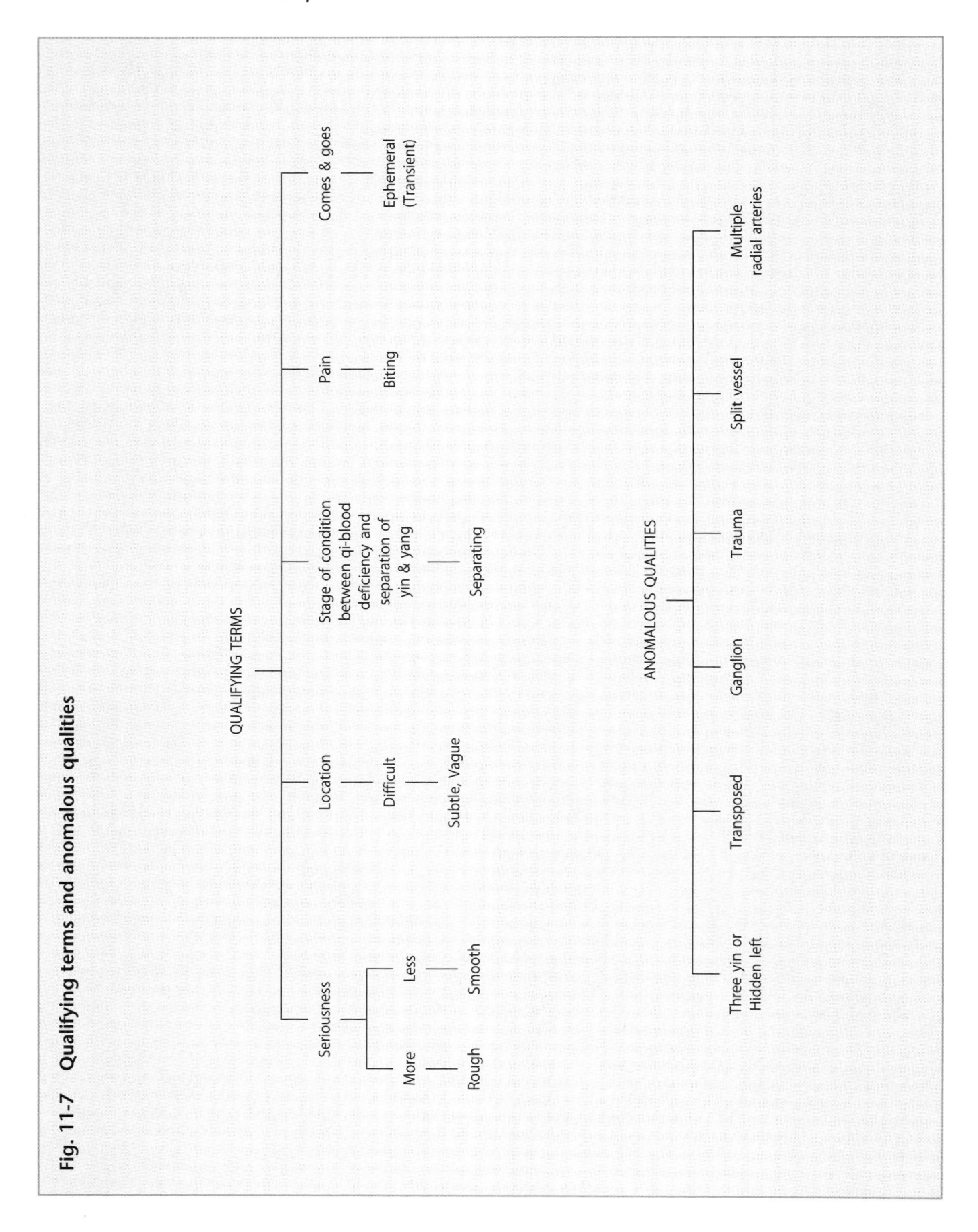

Fig. 11-7 Qualifying terms and anomalous qualities

QUALIFYING TERMS

- Seriousness
  - More — Rough
  - Less — Smooth
- Location
  - Difficult
    - Subtle, Vague
- Stage of condition between qi-blood deficiency and separation of yin & yang
  - Separating
- Pain
  - Biting
- Comes & goes
  - Ephemeral (Transient)

ANOMALOUS QUALITIES

- Three yin or Hidden left
- Transposed
- Ganglion
- Trauma
- Split vessel
- Multiple radial arteries

CHAPTER 12

Individual Positions

CONTENTS

Location of the Principal Impulse, 391
Three Yin *(San Yin)* and Transposed *(Fan Qua)* Pulses, 391
Relationships Among the Positions, 392
    Middle position overflows onto other positions, 392
    Proximal positions tend to be deeper, 392
    Qualities, 393
Complementary Positions, 393
Left Distal Position, 393
    Location, 394
    Depth, 394
    Qualities found at left distal position, 394
        Common qualities, 394
            Cotton, 394
            Tense, 394
            Tight in Pericardium position and moderately Rapid, 395
            Tight over entire position and slightly Rapid, 395
            Thin, 395
            Feeble-Absent, 395
            Feeble with Increase in Rate on Exertion <8 beats/minute, 395
            Superficial, Smooth, and Transitory Vibration, 395
        Less common qualities, 395
            Yielding Tense Inflated and slightly Rapid, 395
            Flat Wave, 396
            Slippery, 396
            Slippery with Normal rate, 396
            Slippery and Rapid, 396

    Slippery and very Rapid, 397
    Change in Intensity or Amplitude and Qualities, 397
    Rough Vibration, constant at left distal position at all depths or deep, 397
    Deep Thin Feeble-Absent and very Slow, 397
    Very Tense Hollow Full-Overflowing, 397
    Muffled, 397
   Uncommon qualities, 397
    Empty, 397
    Wiry, 397
   Rare qualities (usually associated with extreme illness), 398
    Choppy, 398
    Leather-like Hollow, 398
    Unstable, 398
    Deep Thin Feeble with Normal rate, slightly Rapid or Slow, 398
    Deep Thin Tight with rate >100 beats/minute, 398
    Yielding Hollow Full-Overflowing with rate >100 beats/minute, 398
    Robust Pounding Tight and slightly Inflated with Rapid rate, 398
    Very Tense Inflated, 398
    Bean (Spinning), 399
Complementary positions associated with left distal position, 399
  Pericardium position, 399
   Common quality, 399
    Tight, 399
   Uncommon qualities, 399
    Slippery, 399
    Inflated, 399
  Neuro-psychological position, 400
   Qualities, 400
    Smooth Vibration, 400
    Rough Vibration, 400
    Doughy, 401
    Choppy, 401
    Muffled, 401
    Other qualities, 401
  Mitral Valve complementary position, 401
   Qualities, 402
    Vibration, 402
    Slippery, 402
  Large Vessel complementary position, 402
   Qualities, 402
    Tense Inflated, 402
    Hollow Full-Overflowing (rare), 402
    Robust Pounding, Tight, and slightly Inflated (very rare), 403
  Heart Enlarged position, 403
Combinations of qualities at left distal and other positions, 403
  Left distal and right distal positions, 403
  Left distal and left middle positions, 403
   Similar qualities, 403
    Tense, 403
    Cotton, 404
    Slippery, 404

      Tense Hollow Full-Overflowing, 404
     Dissimilar qualities, 404
      Left distal Feeble-Absent and left middle very Tense Inflated or Hollow Full-Overflowing, 404
     Heart-Gallbladder qi deficiency, 404
   Left distal and right middle positions, 404
     Similar qualities, 404
      Thin Feeble Interrupted and Slow, 404
      Slippery, 404
   Left distal and left proximal positions, 405
     Kidney-Heart disharmony, 405
     Common combinations of qualities in the left distal and proximal positions, 405
      Feeble-Absent in both positions, 405
      Tight in both positions, 405
     Less common combinations with Kidney-Heart disharmony, 406
      Left distal Feeble-Absent and left proximal Tight, 406
      Left distal Tight and left proximal Feeble-Absent, 406
   Left distal and right proximal positions, 406
   Left distal and all other positions, 406
     Left distal and proximal positions Feeble-Absent, remainder Normal, 406
     Left distal and proximal Feeble-Absent and left middle Tense (Short Excess), 407
     Left distal Feeble-Absent and remainder Slippery at blood depth, 407
   Left distal position, rate and rhythm, 408
     Left distal Tight and Rapid, 408
     Left distal Tight and Slow, 408
     Left distal Feeble-Absent and Slow, 408
     Left distal Feeble-Absent and Rapid, 408
     Left distal with a Change in Rate at Rest, 408
      Occasional Change in Rate at Rest, 408
      Constant Change in Rate at Rest, 408
     Left distal Increase in Rate on Exertion >8-12 beats/min., 408
     Left distal and proximal Thin Feeble, entire pulse Interrupted or Intermittent, 409
     Left distal Tight with Hesitant Wave, 409
 Heart Conditions According to Dr. Shen, 409
   Mild Heart qi agitation: Heart Vibration, 409
    Heart Tight, 410
    Hesitant Wave ('push pulse'), 410
    Vibration at Neuro-psychological positions, 411
   Severe Heart qi agitation: Heart Nervous, 411
   Heart blood deficiency: Heart Weak, 412
   Heart qi stagnation: Heart Closed, 412
   Heart blood stagnation: Heart Small, 413
   Trapped qi in the Heart: Heart Full, 414
   Mild, moderate, and severe Heart qi deficiency: Heart Large, 414
   Heart yang deficiency: 'Heart disease', 415
   Summary of constitutional, congenital, and life-related conditions according to Dr. Shen, 415
   Heart and 'nervous system' affect each other, 417
     Heart qi-yang deficiency, 417
     Heart yin deficiency, 417

Heart and circulation, 418
    Circulation affects the Heart, 418
        Emotional trauma, 418
        Physical trauma, 418
        Hypothermia, 418
    Heart affects the circulation, 419
Right Distal, Special Lung, and Pleura Positions, 419
    Right distal position, 419
        Qualities found at right distal position, 420
            Floating, 420
            Tense, 420
            Tight, 420
            Wiry, 421
            Yielding Inflated, 421
            Tense Inflated, 421
            Flat, 421
            Reduced Substance, 422
            Feeble-Absent, 422
            Vibration, 422
            Deep, 422
            Empty, Change in Intensity and Qualities, 423
            Thin, 423
            Slippery, 423
            Muffled, 423
            Robust Pounding, 423
        Common conditions associated with right distal and Special Lung positions, 423
            Common cold, 423
            Influenza, 424
            Bronchitis, 424
            Pneumonia, 424
            Acute asthma, 424
            Chronic asthma, 424
                Qi deficiency, 424
                Yin deficiency, 424
            Emphysema, 424
            Tumor, 424
            Obstructive disorder, including smoker's or miner's lung, 424
        Combinations at right distal and other positions, 424
            Right and left distal positions, 424
            Right distal and left middle positions, 425
                Right distal Feeble-Absent, left middle Tense to Tight, 425
            Right distal and right middle positions, 425
                Floating Tense and Slow, 425
                Floating Yielding and Rapid, 425
                Tense, 425
                Slippery, 425
                Feeble-Absent, 425
                Tight, 425
            Right distal and left proximal positions, 426
                Feeble-Absent, 426
                Tight, 426

Right distal and right proximal positions, 426
        Feeble-Absent, 426
Special Lung position, 426
    Location, 426
    Palpation, 426
    Special Lung position qualities and the right distal position, 427
    Morphology, 427
    Specific qualities, 427
        Floating, 427
        Slippery, 428
        Tight or Wiry, 428
        Rough Vibration, 428
        Empty, 428
        Yielding Inflated, 428
        Tense-Tight Inflated at right distal and Special Lung positions, 429
        Restricted, 429
        Muffled, 429
Pleura position, 429
Left Middle Position, 430
    Common qualities at left middle position, 430
        Taut; Tense; Tight; Wiry; Thin, 430
        Blood Unclear; Blood Heat; Blood Thick; Tense Hollow Full-Overflowing, 430
        Slippery, 430
        Spreading, 431
        Reduced Substance, 431
        Yielding Partially Hollow, 431
        Tense Inflated, 431
        Empty, 431
    Less common qualities at left middle position, 431
        Change in Qualities and Intensity, 431
        Diffuse, 431
        Vibration and Choppy, 431
        Muffled and Dead, 432
        Flooding Excess and Robust Pounding, 432
        Floating Tight, 432
        Leather-like Hollow, 432
    Common combinations at the left middle and other positions, 432
        Left middle and left distal, 432
        Left middle and right distal, 432
        Left middle and right middle, 432
        Left middle and left proximal, 432
            Deep Wiry, 432
            Tense Hollow Full-Overflowing, 433
        Left middle with left distal and proximal, 433
        Left middle and right proximal, 433
Gallbladder position, 433
    Tense Slippery, 433
    Tight Slippery, 433
    Inflated, 433
    Muffled; Wiry; Change in Intensity; Choppy, 433
    Gallbladder-Heart deficiency, 434

Liver Engorgement positions, 434
    Distal Engorgement, 434
    Ulnar Engorgement, 434
    Radial Engorgement, 434
Liver qi 'attacks', 434

Right Middle Position, 434
- Yang organ (Stomach) occupies principal position, 434
- Stomach disorders and the right middle position, 435
  - 'Sour Stomach', 435
  - Stomach, pyloric, and duodenal ulcers, 435
  - Stomach fire, 436
  - Work habits, emotional disturbance, eating habits, and digestion, 436
    - **Reduced Substance**, 436
    - **Flat; Inflated; Deep; Feeble-Absent; Empty**, 436
    - **Tense-Tight**, 436
- Combinations of the right middle and other positions, 437
  - Right middle and left middle, 437
  - Right middle and left distal, 437
  - Right middle and right distal, 437
  - Right middle and left proximal, 437
    - **Deep; Feeble-Absent; Empty**, 437
    - **Tight**, 437
  - Right middle and right proximal (or distal), 437
    - **Feeble-Absent**, 437
    - **Tight**, 437
  - Right middle and over entire left side, 437
- Complementary positions of right middle position, 438
  - Esophagus position, 438
    - Qi stagnation, 438
    - Rebellious Stomach qi, 438
    - Food stagnation and regurgitation, 438
  - Spleen position, 438
  - Stomach-Pylorus Extension position, 439
  - Peritoneal Cavity (Pancreas) position, 439
  - Duodenum, 439

Proximal Positions, 439
- General information, 439
  - Depth and root, 439
  - Physiology, 440
  - Origin of disharmony, 440
- Left and right proximal positions, 441
  - Qualities commonly found at left proximal position, 442
    - **Tense**, 442
    - **Taut**, 442
    - **Tight-Wiry**, 442
    - **Reduced Substance**, 443
    - **Deep**, 443
    - **Feeble-Absent**, 443
  - Qualities less commonly found at left proximal position, 443
    - **Flooding Excess; Robust Pounding; Slippery; Tight-Wiry**, 443
    - **Empty**, 443

Individual Positions/Contents

     Change in Qualities and Intensity, 444
    Left proximal combined with other positions, 444
     Left proximal and left distal, 444
     Left proximal and left middle, 444
     Left proximal and right distal, 444
     Left proximal and right middle, 444
     Left proximal and right proximal, 444
    Large Intestine, prostate, and uterus, 444
  Right proximal position, 444
    Bladder position, 444
    Qualities commonly found at right proximal position, 445
     Tense, 445
     Flooding Excess; Robust Pounding; Slippery; Rapid, 445
     Tight-Wiry, 445
     Reduced Substance, 445
     Deep, 445
     Feeble-Absent, 445
    Right proximal combined with other positions, 446
     Right and left proximal, 446
     Right proximal and left distal, 446
     Right proximal and right distal, 446
     Right proximal and left middle, 446
     Right proximal and right middle and distal (entire right side), 446
      Feeble-Absent, 446
      Tight, 446
    Small Intestine, prostate, and uterus, 446
 Large and Small Intestine Complementary Positions, 446
  Location, 446
  Qualities commonly found at Large and Small Intestine positions, 447
   Tense, 447
   Tight, 447
   Biting, 447
   Slippery, 447
   Rough Vibration, 447
   Choppy, 448
   Change in Intensity, 448
   Robust Pounding, 448
   Inflated, 448
   Muffled, 448
Pelvis/Lower Body position, 448
Triple Burner position, 449
Gate of Vitality *(ming men)* position, 449
Other Complementary Positions, 450
  Diaphragm position, 450
  Musculoskeletal positions, 451

CHAPTER 12

Individual Positions

In order to avoid unnecessary repetition, the reader is referred to prior chapters for details concerning the specific qualities relevant to each position. The one exception is the left distal position, which represents the Heart; of all positions, this is the one for which Dr. Shen has provided the largest volume of information.

Location of the Principal Impulse

The single most important exercise in taking the pulse is locating the principal impulse. The principal vessel must be palpated directly in the middle of its path in order to communicate messages which are reproducible by another practitioner and which can be meaningfully compared.

The principal impulse is located where one accesses the strongest impulse. If one palpates to one side or the other of the vessel, the qualities will vary considerably from those at the center. This accounts for most of the differences between myself and students when we compare findings on the same pulse. The two radial arteries can be entirely medial, central, or lateral. Or one side may vary from the other, and even some positions vary from others. One must take the time to find the strongest impulse in each position.

Three Yin *(San Yin)* and Transposed *(Fan Quan)* Pulses

A word of caution. These anomalous qualities (see Chapter 11), as well as ganglia and local trauma, can obscure or obliterate the pulse, reducing its usefulness as a diagnostic tool within the parameters of this pulse system. This is important to bear in mind because one frequently encounters them in practice. Treatment based on such unreliable readings is unlikely to be effective.

Relationships Among the Positions

MIDDLE POSITIONS OVERFLOW ONTO OTHER POSITIONS

The pulse qualities of the middle burner (middle positions) tend to dominate and overflow onto the other positions, especially the distal positions. This is partly due to anatomical considerations. The abdominal area, represented by the middle positions, is much less confined than the chest (distal positions), and somewhat less confined than the pelvis (proximal positions). The qi in the middle burner is therefore anatomically more free to expand. The overflow from the middle positions to the distal positions is partly due to the nature of the qi and blood in the middle burner organs.

According to Dr. Shen, the qi in the middle right position and gas in the digestive lumen are equivalent. Gas, he says, is the qi in the Stomach. Because qi is yang energy, it is expansive by nature. This natural tendency is exaggerated when the qi in the Stomach and Intestines is stagnant or expands further when there is excessive heat in this system. (The Inflated quality is identified with this process.) This expansiveness is represented on the pulse by the appearance at the conventional right distal position of qualities similar to those found at the right middle position, often Inflated.

The middle position on the left side is associated with the Liver and Gallbladder. There are two aspects of Liver function which contribute to the tendency of the qualities of the middle positions to overflow, especially to the distal positions. The first is the Liver's expansive function to continuously spread the qi throughout the body. The second is its function of storing blood. When heat from excess in the Liver increases due to the Liver's effort to overcome qi stagnation, the Liver blood is heated and expands, and the pulse will thereupon overflow (become Hollow Full-Overflowing.) Therefore, heat in the Liver blood contributes to the propensity of the middle positions to occupy a proportionally greater space than the other two positions.

For these same reasons, the qualities of the middle positions tend to flood the other positions; when you place the index fingers flat on the distal positions, you are actually reading the qualities encroaching from the middle. Therefore, in order to get an accurate reading of the upper burner, the index finger must be *rolled* distally toward the thenar eminence and scaphoid bone where the qualities are accessed with the radial side of the index finger, rather than the flat pad. Here the qualities are generally more restricted in the space they occupy. For this reason, special consideration is given to the anatomy, physiology, and method of access. (See the discussion of the left and right distal positions below.)

Dr. Shen demonstrated this to me from our earliest contacts to our last. It is his position that without rolling the finger, the information accessed at the conventional distal position is actually relevant to the Liver and Spleen-Stomach rather than the Heart and Lung. (For a more detailed discussion of rolling the fingers, see Chapters 2 and 4).

PROXIMAL POSITIONS TEND TO BE DEEPER

The proximal positions are frequently experienced as being slightly deeper than the middle positions. Some sources consider this to be normal. Wang Ping states that "It should sound deep and strong like a stone thrown."[1] Except to say that the Kidneys are the 'root,' the reasons for this are not satisfactorily explained anywhere in the literature with which I am familiar.

My explanation is somewhat more pedestrian, but I believe more compatible with the dynamics of Chinese physiology and pathology. Since Kidney qi, which is represented at this position, is the foundation of all of the body functions, it is constantly being used to support our use and abuse of all other functions. The Deep quality is a sign of the depletion of qi, which, for the reasons just cited, would explain why the proximal positions are usually Deeper, at least in older people. However, over the course of my three decades of study and practice, it is clear that the impulses at these positions are becoming Deeper and more Feeble at an increasingly younger age. The proximal position is discussed at greater length below.

QUALITIES

Qualities that range from the most common to the least common are listed below for each position. One exception is the Bean (Spinning) quality, which I have found only three times, once each at the right distal, right middle, and left proximal positions. Because of the infrequency of its occurrence, a discussion of this quality is omitted here (see Chapter 10).

Complementary Positions

The Tight and Wiry qualities in the complementary positions reflect over-activity, irritability, inflammation, and pain. Changes in Intensity, Changes in Qualities, the Empty qualities, other Reduced qualities (Feeble-Absent and Deep), as well as the Unstable and Nonhomogeneous qualities, signify impaired function. Flooding Excess is a sign of acute heat from excess with infection, and Robust Pounding of heat from excess. The Leather-like Hollow quality is always a sign of sudden hemorrhage, but Yielding Hollow is often a sign of excess hydrochloric acid and ulceration, especially in the Stomach-Pylorus Extension and even Intestine positions. The Muffled quality is a sign of molecular chaos, including at the Neuro-psychological position, where it has been recently associated with cerebral palsy and with LSD abuse.

The Thin quality in the complementary positions is interpreted as a Restricted quality, and the Bean (Spinning) quality has the same meaning as in the principal positions. The Inflated quality is usually associated with trapped qi and heat, often of a gaseous nature, in the Special Lung (emphysema), Gallbladder, and Intestine positions. This is attributable to stagnation, or inability to move (the Lung and Diaphragm positions), or to the gases produced by bacteria (Gallbladder position). I have never found the Hollow Full-Overflowing quality in the complementary positions, except at the Neuro-psychological position (rarely). The Choppy quality is a sign of blood stagnation. I have never found the Flat quality in a complementary position.

Left Distal Position

Again, there is considerably more information and detail provided about this position than any of the other principal positions (see Chapter 15). The reason for this is that Dr. Shen had much more to say about the pulse at the left distal position and about the Heart, which is represented at this position, than about any other organ system. The Heart is, after all, the 'emperor.' Unless otherwise stated, what is described below are qualities associated with energy patterns and not with parenchymal damage to the heart. However, some parenchymal damage is a likely outcome if the pattern is not corrected.

In order to avoid the sensory overlap of the medial into the distal aspects of the pulse, the distal positions are not accessed in the distal-proximal axis along the radial artery, as are the proximal and medial positions. Rather, they are accessed horizontally, along a radial-ulnar, medial-lateral axis just under the scaphoid bone, to which position one has rolled the radial edge of the index finger. Here we are not accessing the radial artery, but rather the fluid dynamics of its sudden breakdown into many smaller arteries, which sets up a wave informing us about the physiological integrity of the Heart and Lungs.

LOCATION

To locate the left distal position, the right index finger and entire arm of the examiner must be rolled distally toward and slightly under the left scaphoid bone, where the qualities are accessed with the radial side of the index finger rather than the flat pad. Again, the position is then accessed by rolling the side of the index finger in a medial-lateral direction rather than the proximal-distal direction which we use for the middle and proximal positions. Once in the position, it is important to lighten up slightly to avoid obliterating the impulse.

DEPTH

The three separate depths are not easily accessed in the distal positions due to the diminished space accorded these positions on the wrist. Superficial and Deep are easily recognized, as are those qualities such as Hollow Full-Overflowing which exceed the qi depth, the Inflated quality which seems to expand it, and, less readily, the Empty quality which shows itself only at the superficial aspect and is absent from the deeper aspects.

QUALITIES FOUND AT LEFT DISTAL POSITION

Due to the importance of the Heart, we are including some examples of the qualities commonly found at this position. However, for a more complete and comprehensive discussion the reader is referred to the individual sections which focus on each quality, including rhythm and rate. For a complete discussion of some of the conditions alluded to in this section, such as Heart yin deficiency and Heart qi agitation, refer below to the section entitled "Heart conditions according to Dr. Shen," or to the glossary at the back of the book.

Common qualities

Cotton

This is a sign of superficial qi stagnation due to the causes listed below (Chapter 9).

Resignation pulse ('sad pulse')

This is the most common etiology of the Cotton quality. While Dr. Shen calls it the 'sad pulse,' I have found that it is accompanied by a feeling of powerlessness and a deep sense of despair about changing one's life in a more fulfilling direction. I therefore call it the resignation pulse. When found only at this position, the condition is in its earliest stage and is of recent origin. More frequently, it is found simultaneously at all positions.

Trauma

Another possibility is physical trauma to the left side of the chest. Check the history.

Tense

Heat from excess and qi stagnation in the Heart usually accompanies this pulse quality. Insomnia with difficulty in falling asleep could be a symptom. Robust Pounding often accompanies heat from excess.

Tight in Pericardium position and moderately Rapid

Heat from excess and qi stagnation usually accompanies the Tight quality configuration, again often accompanied by difficulty in falling asleep. The Tight quality in the Pericardium position feels like a pencil point in the middle of the left distal position.

Tight over entire position and slightly Rapid

This is a sign of Heart yin deficiency. Symptoms could include some agitation and a sleep disorder marked by restless sleep and frequent waking during the night.

Thin

This is a sign of Heart blood deficiency. Symptoms could involve waking after four or five hours of sleep and difficulty returning to sleep, dizziness, becoming easily fatigued on exertion, and diminishment of memory and concentration.

Feeble-Absent

Heart qi and yang deficiency and/or (more rarely) advanced essential hypertension (with a Feeble-Absent quality at the left proximal position and high diastolic) are associated with this quality at this position. The distinction is made in the eyes, on the tongue, and with other symptoms.

Feeble with Increase in Rate on Exertion (>8 beats/minute)

Combined Heart qi and Heart blood deficiency is generally associated with this pulse pattern.

Superficial, Smooth, and Transitory Vibration

This is a mild sign of Heart qi agitation marked by transient worry or mild emotional shock.

Less common qualities

Yielding Tense Inflated and slightly Rapid

Qi, or heat from excess, is trapped in the Heart and cannot escape. This is often due to prolonged delivery at birth with the head inside; unresolved grief (more often the Inflation is bilateral with the right distal position); less often to violent unexpressed anger while physically active; and, in rare instances, to one extraordinary episode of excessive lifting primarily with the left side, or trauma to the left side of the chest. Dr. Shen refers to the Yielding Inflated quality and its associated condition as Heart Full.

An Inflated pulse associated with anger, lifting, and trauma is not a serious sign, since these causes imply that the individual's general energy is strong, and probably good enough to open the Heart naturally, or that they will respond to therapy if it is treated within a reasonable time.

If the etiology is prolonged delivery with the head inside, the Inflated quality can be a sign of qi dilation of the Heart, and is usually associated with breech presentation. With this early cause I find the condition more serious symptomatically, with graver consequences in terms of ultimate Heart qi deficiency, and more difficult to treat. This individual is very easily angered, feels tired throughout life, and is more susceptible to hypertension and hemoptysis. The whole body feels uncomfortable and it is hard to lie on the left side (see Inflated quality, Chapter 9).

Flat Wave

This is a pattern of Heart qi stagnation, usually associated with efforts to repress emotional pain early in life, for example, owing to the loss of a parent or parent surrogate. The Flat Wave is a sign that the qi of the Heart was deficient or immature at the time of the incident, as in childhood. This sign is interpreted to mean that qi is unable to enter the Heart. Such people tend to be spiteful. A sudden personal rejection by a loved one in adulthood can also bring about this quality, although it tends to be transient, lasting only until the emotional wound is healed.

The Flat Wave is also found in early stages or in mild cases of Heart blood stagnation when the heart muscles are tense, the coronary arteries are in spasm but not yet blocked, there is transient angina, and difficulty inhaling. In Dr. Shen's terms, the Heart is 'suffocating.' Ultimately, if uncorrected, this will lead to the occlusion of the coronary arteries (heart attack). Even one episode of lifting far beyond one's capacity can produce a Flat quality at the left distal position. However, more often the quality is found in both distal positions with this etiology.

Slippery

The Slippery quality at the left distal position is a sign of the 'misting of the orifices.' Less severe emotional disturbances falling into the category of neurosis accompany dampness 'misting the orifices.' Severe emotional disturbances or epilepsy are associated with phlegm disturbing and confusing the Heart orifices, while stroke is associated with the obstruction of the Heart orifices (see discussion of Slippery quality in Chapter 11). The Slippery quality is appearing more frequently at this position.

Phlegm in the Pericardium or Heart is a consequence of the inability of the Lungs, Spleen, Triple Burner, and Kidneys to move and metabolize dampness, combined in some instances of mania with Liver heat or fire rising to the Heart (phlegm fire).

Slippery with Normal rate

This is associated with phlegm-fire disturbing the orifices of the Heart, with depression and epilepsy.

Slippery and Rapid

Phlegm-fire disturbing the orifices of the Heart

Without a high fever this sign is usually accompanied by an agitated depression or manic type of mental disorder.

Slippery and very Rapid

Especially when accompanied by a very Tight Hollow Full-Overflowing quality, this is a sign of impending stroke.

Change in Intensity or Amplitude and Qualities

Extreme deficiency of Heart qi and yang, with probable separation of yin and yang within the Heart ('Heart disease'), is indicated when these qualities are found more frequently.

Rough Vibration, constant at left distal position at all depths or deep

This configuration is a sign of serious Heart qi and yang deficiency ('Heart disease') associated with parenchymal damage. It is found more frequently now than in the recent past.

Deep Thin Feeble-Absent and very Slow

According to Dr. Shen, this pulse is associated with severe Heart qi deficiency ('Heart large') which has existed for a very long period of time and caused deterioration of peripheral circulation.

Very Tense Hollow Full-Overflowing

This is a sign of hypertension. The quality is usually found simultaneously at the left middle position.

Muffled

At the left distal position this is usually a sign of the Heart type of depression, which is characterized by a lack of joy. It has also been reported with a thickening of the Pericardium (usually with an accompanying arrhythmia) or occlusion of the coronary arteries. This quality is encountered much more frequently now than in the recent past.

Uncommon qualities

Empty

Extreme deficiency of Heart qi and yang with possible separation of yin and yang within the Heart is indicated by this quality.

Wiry

This quality is found at the left distal position with long-term cocaine abuse, with chronic mania, and with the final stages of Grave's disease. The yin of the Heart is extremely deficient. More rarely, the Wiry quality is found here with severe angina.

Rare qualities (usually associated with extreme illness)

Choppy

This quality is rarely found at this position. It is a very serious sign of blood stagnation in the coronary arteries.

Leather-like Hollow

Bleeding from the heart is either imminent (with Rapid rate) or recent (with Slow rate).

Unstable

This is a serious sign of extreme physical deterioration of the heart, such as infarction.

Deep Thin Feeble with Normal rate, slightly Rapid or Slow

This combination of qualities is found with advanced Heart blood stagnation. In Dr. Shen's terms, the Heart is 'suffocating,' and it is this pattern which comes closest to severe coronary artery disease.

Deep Thin Tight with rate >100 beats/minute

Trapped qi and later severe qi deficiency in the Heart due to Heart shock, breech birth, chest trauma, prolonged grief and sudden anger, with fatigue, difficulty exhaling and lying on left side that can lead to enlarged Heart. Often there is a predisposing constitutional Heart qi deficiency.

Yielding Hollow Full-Overflowing with rate >100 beats/minute

This is another combination of qualities associated with severe Heart qi deficiency, which Dr. Shen says is related to suppressed emotion over a long period of time. I have not observed this combination.

Robust Pounding Tight and slightly Inflated with Rapid rate

The greater the Pounding at this position, the more dangerous the condition. This is a sign of severe heat from excess in the Heart found with Grave's disease, acute mania, cocaine addiction, and pericarditis. If accompanied by irregularity in the rhythm (Interrupted and Intermittent) the situation is critical.

Very Tense Inflated

Recently a few cases have been observed when this quality is associated with 'misting of the Heart orifice,' both with a disturbed and confused Heart orifice, and with severe cocaine and amphetamine abuse. However, this is usually a sign of trapped blood in other positions, which must be considered here as well (tamponade).

Bean (Spinning)

This quality has been found at the left distal position with profound emotional shock accompanied by great terror.

COMPLEMENTARY POSITIONS ASSOCIATED WITH LEFT DISTAL POSITION

The reader is referred to Chapter 2, Fig. 2-1 for my version of these positions, and to Fig. 2-2 for Dr. Shen's depiction of them.

Pericardium position

The Pericardium position occupies the center of the left distal position and is accessed by rolling the radial side of one's right index finger from medial to lateral and back again in that position. It has a quality separate from the rest of the position only with the following pathologies.

COMMON QUALITY

Tight

The Tight quality feels as if a pencil point is sticking one's finger in the center of the left distal position. It is a sign of qi stagnation and heat from excess in the Pericardium, and is an early indication of potential heat from excess in the Heart. It has also been found with transient ischemia in the Heart (angina) where the Tight quality is a sign of pain. (By contrast, at most other positions the Tight quality indicates heat from deficiency.)

UNCOMMON QUALITIES

Slippery

The Pericardium surrounds and protects the Heart. Phlegm in the Pericardium has an oppressive and suffocating effect on the Heart and is usually accompanied by neuro-psychological symptoms such as mania, depression, or epilepsy.

Myocarditis

If accompanied by a high fever, this quality can be a sign of myocarditis. The left distal position is Pounding and Tense.

Inflated

While the Inflated quality at the Pericardium position is difficult to distinguish from the Inflated quality over the entire left distal position, it is viewed by Dr. Shen as a specific sign of phlegm misting the orifices of the Heart. The Inflated quality over the entire left distal position rarely affords the same interpretation. (See above under less common conditions at the left distal position.)

Neuro-psychological position

Location

This position is found just above both distal positions on the trapezium bone, in and around a slight depression in the bone. Since the position is not mentioned in the literature or developed to any extent by Dr. Shen, its interpretations below are especially open to further investigation.

Qualities

The qualities set out below are those that are most commonly found. However, increasingly, I am finding Change in Intensity, Slippery, Choppy, Muffled, Robust Pounding, and Tight qualities at the Neuro-psychological position, sometimes accompanying the better understood Vibration and Doughy qualities. Although we have some sign posts, the meaning of these previously unobserved qualities requires considerable research. My inclination is to interpret them as having more serious implications than would either of the qualities standing alone. In one part of the country where I examined seven people, all had a Slippery quality at the Neuro-psychological position. Before and since I have observed only a few with a frequently Slippery quality. Another practitioner has found the Slippery quality here in drug addicts and those suffering from multiple sclerosis.

QUALITIES

Smooth Vibration

Sensation

A very smooth, subtle, and superficial Vibration is the most frequent quality found at this position. Often it is ephemeral and tends to come and go at irregular intervals, requiring one to linger at the position for a short time.

Interpretation

Smooth Vibration at this position is associated with Heart qi agitation, anxiety, and sometimes extreme fear. It is Dr. Shen's contention that the Vibration quality at this position is always related to Heart function. I see this in terms of the traditional relationship between the Heart and mind which says that the Heart controls the mind. He expresses this in terms of Heart qi agitation ('Heart nervous') affecting the 'nervous system,' or of the 'nervous system' affecting the Heart qi.

Rough Vibration

Sensation

A Rough Vibration pulse has the sense of a coarse buzzing under one's fingers.

Interpretation

While speculative due to the early stages of investigation, the impression of Rough Vibration at the Neuro-psychological positions is similar to its interpretation at other individual positions, namely, that there is more damage to the essence (marrow) than to the mind, and more to the tissues than to chemical neurotransmitters. For example, the even rougher Choppy quality has been associated with head trauma, probably involving some degree of blood stagnation. In the context of traditional Chinese medical concepts and terminology, with Rough Vibration we seem to be talking more about the less profoundly damaging condition of qi stagnation, possibly also from trauma, even from birth. Severe, intractable headache somewhat related to the changing status in the strength and circulation of qi would be an associated symptom. However, I have seen it with multiple sclerosis and in a patient with a history of electroshock therapy, and with current deep fear and terror.

Doughy

Sensation

This is the most common quality found in the Neuro-psychological position. It is an ill-defined, undifferentiated impulse that does not correspond in sensation to any of the other qualities described in this book. I would best offer to describe it as an amorphous glob of clay, whose shape is never the same and whose volume varies from very faint to moderately robust.

Interpretation

Most often I have observed the Doughy quality at the Neuro-psychological position with central nervous system disabilities such as multiple sclerosis, and only rarely in people with a history of electroshock therapy, and in cases of intractable headache. At this stage in our investigation it is associated with yang-essence deficiency because it has been frequently observed in very yang-deficient patients with multiple sclerosis. A highly tentative thesis is that the substance of the central nervous system is yin-essence, and that the more active, rapidly moving qi (electrical, circulating in the myelin sheath where the lesions of multiple sclerosis are) is yang-essence.

Choppy

The Choppy quality here has been increasingly associated with multiple past head traumas and chronic intractable headache, probably involving manifold micro loci of intracranial blood stagnation.

Muffled

The Muffled quality at this position has been tentatively associated with the very heavy use of LSD, and more recently with cerebral palsy.

Other qualities

These interpretations are highly tentative. The Robust Pounding Tight pulse seems to be associated with the pain of a current headache. Change in Intensity has been tentatively identified with dizziness. A very Tight quality, which is also rarely found in this position, was present in a person with a glioblastoma.

Mitral Valve complementary position

Location

I have never succeeded in consistently identifying all of the four valves which Dr. Shen mentions in the locations he has assigned to them in Fig. 2-2 above. According to Dr. Shen, the four valves are differentiated by Slipperiness or Vibration from his three Large Vessel positions, which occupy approximately the same area of the left distal position, but which are identified by the Inflated or Full-Overflowing qualities.

The Mitral Valve position described below is one that I discovered over time primarily by checking the quality in this area with objective biomedical data, such as echo cardiogram, and secondarily by relating the quality to symptoms such as panic associated in biomedicine with mitral valve prolapse. Auscultation of the heart has not proven supportive. I offer these observations to the Chinese medical community as experimental data to be tested over time.

The Mitral Valve position I use is located on or around the muscle-tendon (abductor pollicis brevis) passing over the styloid process to the scaphoid bone. While both the

Symptoms

Vibration and Slippery qualities found here are usually accessed very superficially, the Slippery quality has been located more deeply on several occasions.

Anxiety and panic are the only symptoms of the mitral valve prolapse syndrome described in Western medicine. In terms of Chinese medicine it is a more serious sign, primarily of Heart qi deficiency and some blood deficiency (which Dr. Shen generally and specifically treated with Korean ginseng and human placenta). Along with anxiety, Chinese medicine recognizes such additional symptoms as becoming easily fatigued and palpitations on exertion. It is viewed as a sign along the progression to more serious Heart-related conditions.

QUALITIES

Vibration

This is a sign of a mildly incompetent mitral valve and mild Heart qi deficiency.

Slippery

This is a more serious sign of a defective and very incompetent prolapsed valve, and more severe Heart qi deficiency with greater signs of anxiety, panic, and fatigue.

Large Vessel complementary position

Location

I have been able to consistently locate only one of the three Large Vessels to which Dr. Shen alludes in Fig. 2-2, and have felt only two of the qualities discussed below: the Inflated (five times), and the Full-Overflowing (once). Each time I have felt the Inflated quality at this position there have been confirmed aneurysms of the aorta. Others have reported this finding many times. One observer postulated that while the Inflated quality is a sign of an aneurysm in the aorta, a more pin-pointed sensation should be associated with aneurysms of small vessels such as in the brain.

The Large Vessel position is accessed by rolling the index finger medially and distally toward the ulna. At the intersection of the tendon of the flexor carpi radialis and the scaphoid bone is a 'hole' or 'cave-like place' that is palpated by the radial distal edge of the index finger. This 'hole' normally lacks any pulse quality.

QUALITIES

Tense Inflated

Here this combination represents an aneurysm in the vital Large Vessels, especially the aorta. This has been confirmed many times by others.

Hollow Full-Overflowing (rare)

This is associated with true hypertension, with the expansion of veins and arteries due to heat in the blood and not enough fluid in the vessels. According to Dr. Shen, this quality is found here first only when there exists, or is susceptibility to, hypertension, and when the Heart itself is relatively strong.

Robust Pounding, Tight, and slightly Inflated (very rare)

Atherosclerosis

Although outside my own experience, Dr. Shen noted that with atherosclerosis in the Large Vessels this combination of qualities can be felt by rolling the fingers to the Large Vessel position. To best judge this assertion one would need a large sampling of individuals with this diagnosis. The Tense Ropy quality and Rough Vibration and Slipperiness at the blood depth have proven to be effective signs of arterio-artheroschlerosis.

Lifting

Also outside my own experience, Dr. Shen stated that excessive lifting can cause stagnation in the vessels. With this etiology the quality is Tighter and pain can be an accompanying symptom.

Heart Enlarged position

Location and sensation

The Heart Enlarged position is located superficially in the area between the left distal and left middle positions, otherwise known as the left Diaphragm position. The presence of a Heart Enlarged condition is discernible when the distal aspect of the left Diaphragm position is either more Inflated and/or Rougher than the proximal aspect.

Interpretation

A positive finding here indicates that the Heart is enlarged, at least energetically, which will create discomfort in the chest, especially when lying on the left side. The greater the Inflation or Roughness, the more likely the enlargement may be morphological as well as energetic. This finding should be followed by a chest x-ray as well as a referral to a cardiologist.

COMBINATIONS OF QUALITIES AT LEFT DISTAL AND OTHER POSITIONS

Obviously, there are an almost infinite number of combinations of qualities which can occur between the positions. The following are only the most common or important ones.

Left distal and right distal positions

The reader is referred to Chapter 14, and to Table 14-1 (Uniform qualities bilaterally at the same position) for a list of these combinations.

Left distal and left middle positions

SIMILAR QUALITIES

Tense

Although more often associated with a Tense pulse in the left middle position, unexpressed smoldering anger over a long period of time can produce a Tense quality simultaneously in both positions. This represents an early stage in the process by which Liver fire moves to the Heart.

Cotton

This is the 'sad pulse' which usually accompanies a feeling of hopelessness, of about two to three years' duration, and is a form of superficial qi stagnation.

Slippery

This combination occurs with phlegm-fire in the Heart related to Liver fire and Gallbladder damp-heat. If, however, the Slipperiness appears over the entire left side, especially at the organ depth, the more likely etiology is a chronic infection of the yin organs, especially originating in the Liver.

Tense Hollow Full-Overflowing

Hypertension due to heat in the blood with an elevated diastolic pressure is associated with this combination. Robust Pounding often accompanies this pulse.

DISSIMILAR QUALITIES

Left distal Feeble-Absent and left middle very Tense Inflated or Hollow Full-Overflowing

An individual presenting with this combination can become easily and explosively angered. The Heart controls the mind. A weakened Heart is no longer able to control the explosive anger with rational thinking. Hypertension with a high diastolic pressure is also associated with this combination.

HEART-GALLBLADDER QI DEFICIENCY

The left distal position is Deep Slippery Thin, the Gallbladder position is Tense Slippery, and the tongue has a thin white coating. Symptoms are dizziness, blurred vision, timidity, palpitations, sighing, excessive dreams, easily startled, and a quick temper. (See discussion in Chapter 15 under the left middle position.)

Left distal and right middle positions

SIMILAR QUALITIES

Thin Feeble Interrupted and Slow

This combination is found with severe Heart qi and blood deficiency, and Spleen qi deficiency, with palpitations, dyspnea on exertion, depression, spontaneous sweating, watery stools, and anorexia. The tongue body is pale and swollen with a white coating and teethmarks.

Slippery

This indicates phlegm accumulating in the Heart due to Spleen dampness. The tongue body is wet, pale, and swollen with a white coating and teethmarks.

Left distal and left proximal positions

KIDNEY-HEART DISHARMONY

These two positions involve Kidney-Heart disharmony, one of the most important pathological patterns in Chinese medicine (see Chapter 15). Dr. Shen observed that the Heart is "on top" and the Kidney "on the end." If the top and the end are balanced, the entire body is balanced.

Both the Heart and the Kidney control the mind and the brain. If the water of the Kidney cannot control the fire of the Heart, the mind will become restless. If the fire of the Heart cannot warm the water (yin-essence) of the Kidney, it is unable to rise and nourish the brain; normal patterns will thereupon become disrupted. The Triple Burner mediates this relationship and should always be considered in management. The symptoms of this disharmony, or spirit disturbance, are palpitations, insomnia, irritability, fatigue, depression, being easily startled, and anxiety.

The literature of Chinese herbal medicine usually regards Kidney-Heart disharmony as Kidney-Heart yin deficiency. Both positions are Tight with a slightly Rapid rate. However, according to Dr. Shen, and strongly supported in my own experience, Kidney-Heart disharmony occurs as often (or more so) when both the left distal and left proximal positions are both Feeble-Absent. One source of confusion is that, while a Rapid rate occurs more often with yin deficiency, one can have a Rapid rate with either yin or yang deficiency. With yang deficiency the rate can become very Rapid with stress, and, according to Dr. Shen, with an enlarged heart, one form of Heart qi deficiency ('Heart full'). The symptoms are insomnia, anxiety, palpitations, and fatigue. Kidney-Heart disharmony, wherein both positions are Feeble-Absent, is probably more likely of constitutional origin; where both positions are Tight it is more likely related to overworking of the mind and emotional stress.

In my own experience, which is consistent with Dr. Shen's observations, the Kidney-Heart disharmony can also appear with other combinations of qualities on the left distal and proximal positions. One position could have a Feeble-Absent quality and the other a Tight quality, as described below.

Both the Feeble-Absent and Tight qualities are signs of deficiency. This is more obvious with the Feeble-Absent quality, but it is important to reiterate that, despite the hard sensation of the Tight quality, it is just as much a sign of deficiency as the Feeble-Absent quality. (The Feeble-Absent quality is a sign of qi and yang deficiency, while the Tight quality is a sign of yin deficiency.)

COMMON COMBINATIONS OF QUALITIES AT THE LEFT DISTAL AND PROXIMAL POSITIONS

Feeble-Absent in both positions

Except in the elderly, if both the left distal and left proximal positions are Feeble-Absent, the etiology is usually constitutional or congenital. It is, according to Dr. Shen, the principal combination associated with Kidney-Heart disharmony and spirit disturbance.

Tight in both positions

If both positions are Tight it indicates that there is a spirit disturbance with Heart and Kidney yin deficiency due more to constant worry and anxiety during life than to constitutional predisposition. This is the pattern more often alluded to in the literature.

LESS COMMON COMBINATIONS WITH KIDNEY-HEART DISHARMONY

Left distal Feeble-Absent and left proximal Tight

This is another combination I have observed with Kidney-Heart disharmony which can be due to constitutional Heart qi deficiency, or to physical and mental overwork and anxiety, or (most often) to both. Found at an early age, the constitution is the likely etiology. Found later in adulthood, one would look to insults to the Heart such as shock or overwork that have occurred during adulthood. If the left distal position is Feeble while the left proximal position is Tight, we know that the process has existed long enough for the Heart to move from a yin-deficient Heart qi agitation to a qi-and-blood-deficient pattern.

With this combination people will easily wake up at the smallest sound or disturbance because, as Dr. Shen would say, "the Heart is sensitive." The Feeble-Absent quality at the left distal position conforms to Heart qi deficiency. (The Tight quality at that position is an expression of Heart yin deficiency.) Both Heart qi and yin deficiency are expressed by similar sleep disturbances.

Left distal Tight and left proximal Feeble-Absent

This is the least frequent combination I have found in cases of Kidney-Heart disharmony. In all but the elderly or profoundly ill, the Feeble-Absent quality at the left proximal position suggests a constitutional or congenital disorder. I find that a Feeble-Absent left proximal position is more a sign of Kidney qi and yang deficiency than of Kidney yin, whose deficiency is marked more by Tightness at the left proximal position. However, when this position is Feeble-Absent I have found some deficiency of Kidney yin and essence as well as qi and yang.

Tightness in the left distal position suggests that there is simultaneously Heart yin deficiency, which is usually associated with excessive worry, anxiety, or a mild emotional shock. The implication is that the Kidney is unable to support the Heart in withstanding the stresses which are placed upon it. This would suggest a management program in which both the Heart yin and Kidney yin and yang are supported simultaneously.

Left distal and right proximal positions

If both positions are Tight the possible explanation is that there is Bladder heat due to heat from excess in the Heart. The Small Intestine is responsible for removing excessive heat from the Heart, which it tries to eliminate from the body. Due to their greater yang relationship in the six stages, the heat can move from the Small Intestine to the Bladder.

Left distal and all other positions

Left distal and proximal positions Feeble-Absent, remainder Normal

This combination indicates that there is a constitutional factor in the Heart disharmony because of the Feeble-Absent quality in the left proximal (Kidney) position. The constitutional nature of the condition means that it is not entirely correctable, and that the individual will always be vulnerable and have to take care. However, the fact that the remainder of the pulse is Normal indicates that the digestive system is still functioning well, improving the prognosis.

If the person does not take care, for example, by engaging in excessive physical work beyond his energy, the Heart will gradually become seriously deficient, affecting the function of the entire body including the immune system. The entire pulse will gradually become Empty, indicating a 'qi wild' condition, which places the organism in danger of a serious illness such as cancer.

Left distal and proximal Feeble-Absent, and left middle Tense (Short Excess)

LIVER QI STAGNATION

With this condition the problem is not necessarily deficiency of the Heart and Kidney that causes the disharmony, but stagnation in the middle burner, which prevents communication between the upper and lower burners (a Short Excess pulse). It is usually accompanied by anxiety and insomnia. With Liver qi stagnation one also sees passive-aggressive behavior interspersed with explosive anger and digestive disturbances.

A striking example of this involved a well-known entertainer who was concerned by his increasing girth. His pulse showed this picture, and treatment was focused on the extra-channel girdle vessel *(dai mai)*. The pulse became more balanced after treatment, but on his way to catch the train home, his girth had so diminished that his pants fell down on the street!

YIN ORGAN SYSTEMS DEFICIENT

If the left distal and proximal positions are Feeble, the left middle position is Tense, and the right side is Deep or Feeble, the excess in the Liver may be more apparent than real. The true etiology here is that all yin organ systems are deficient with an excess in the Liver, such as qi stagnation due to repressed emotion and the resulting accumulation of heat in the Liver blood.

HEART AND KIDNEY QI DEFICIENCY

The Liver excess may be an illusion, which can be tested by treating for Liver qi stagnation and heat from excess. If, after a suitable period of treatment, the Liver retains a Normal quality and the right side is relatively Robust, the problem is then strictly one involving Kidney and Heart qi deficiency. If, however, the left middle position also becomes Feeble, this suggests a deficient 'organ system' and a relatively healthy, or compensating, 'digestive system.'

Left distal Feeble-Absent and remainder Slippery at blood depth

HEART QI DEFICIENT

Heart qi affects blood flow. If the Heart qi is deficient it cannot push the blood, which becomes stagnant and creates turbulence; this can be expressed as Slipperiness over the entire pulse at the blood depth. The pulse will be moderately Slow (60-65 beats per minute).

CIRCULATION STAGNANT

Stagnation, due for example to a 'blood thick' condition of excess blood lipids, can, in turn, create a Slippery quality at the blood depth over the entire pulse. This stagnation in the peripheral circulation will eventually weaken the Heart (left distal position Feeble-Absent), which will attempt to overcome it.

Left distal position, rate and rhythm

Left distal Tight and Rapid

This is one type of Heart qi agitation ('Heart nervous'), which is usually due to unresolved emotional shock.

Left distal Tight and Slow

The Slow rate is a sign of Heart qi deficiency. One would expect this to be accompanied by one of the pulse qualities associated with Heart qi deficiency at the left distal position, such as the Feeble-Absent quality. The presence of both Heart yin deficiency (left distal position Tight) and qi deficiency (Slow rate) is possible, especially if the left proximal position (Kidney) is also Tight. The harder qualities tend to obliterate the reduced qualities. If, however, there were angina, the left distal position could be Tight from pain. Likewise, if there were a Tight quality over the entire pulse for whatever reason, including a longstanding 'nervous system tense' condition, one would find the Tight quality at the left distal position as well. This combination of qualities would seemingly be complicated if the Slow rate is artificially induced by exercise. In fact, however, Chinese medicine would still regard this as a sign of deficiency.

Left distal Feeble-Absent and Slow

Both of these qualities are congruent with qi deficiency. Together they indicate that the qi deficiency is greater than if only one or the other were present.

Left distal Feeble-Absent and Rapid

With this combination we have deficient Heart qi observed during a period of emotional or physical strain. The increase in rate represents the inability of the qi-deficient Heart to stabilize under stress.

Left distal with a Change in Rate at Rest

OCCASIONAL CHANGE IN RATE AT REST

This is a sign of Heart qi agitation ('Heart nervous'), which is discussed more fully below. It is important to reiterate that over time, a condition of Heart qi agitation can lead to Heart blood or qi deficiency ('Heart weak' or 'Heart large,' respectively), and that both can lead to Heart yang deficiency ('Heart disease'). Early intervention is important.

CONSTANT CHANGE IN RATE AT REST

When the rate change at rest is constant, the condition is one of mild Heart qi deficiency.

Left distal Increase in Rate on Exertion >8-12 beats/minute

HEART BLOOD DEFICIENT ('HEART WEAK')

This is a situation in which deficiency of Heart blood is the principal problem, with slight deficiency of Heart qi. The greater the increase in rate, the greater the deficiency. If the left distal position is Feeble-Absent, the rate Normal or a little Slow, and the change in rate with even slight exertion large, there is a more equal combination of Heart qi and blood deficiency.

Left distal and proximal Thin Feeble, entire pulse Interrupted or Intermittent

This combination is found in cases of Heart and Kidney yang deficiency with palpitations, cardiac asthma, edema of face, eyelids and limbs, cold limbs, scant urine, and spontaneous sweating, especially on the forehead. The tongue body is wet, swollen, and pale with a white coating. The face is ashen white.

Left distal Tight with Hesitant Wave

The Hesitant Wave is associated with observed mental states and mild Heart yin deficiency. The Tight left distal position is a somewhat stronger sign of Heart yin deficiency.

Heart Conditions According to Dr. Shen

The following are conditions described by Dr. Shen which involve Heart function and qualities at the left distal position, by which they are partially distinguished. While I have retained his terminology in parenthesis, I have developed an idiom closer to the language of traditional Chinese medicine. For 'Heart nervous,' 'Heart vibration,' and 'Heart tight,' I have introduced a new term to identify variations in severity: Heart qi agitation. This reflects exactly what Dr. Shen meant to describe with different degrees of agitation.

Several points bear repeating. One is that all shock, emotional or physical, affects the Heart. A second is that with these conditions, one usually finds some Kidney-Heart disharmony. The third is that often, though not always, there is a progression from one condition to another. For example, and in particular, a prolonged condition of mild Heart qi agitation ('Heart tight') can lead to severe Heart qi agitation ('Heart nervous'), and a condition of either prolonged 'Heart nervous' or 'Heart tight' can lead to the other more serious conditions. This is what makes early intervention so important.

MILD HEART QI AGITATION: HEART VIBRATION

Vibration over the entire pulse or at individual positions is defined by whether it is transient or consistent, superficial or deep, and rough or smooth. Transient, superficial, and smooth qualities at the left distal position, or even over the entire pulse, indicates a relatively innocuous process involving passing worries or a tendency to worry which I define as mild Heart qi agitation (very mild Heart yin deficiency). This sometimes begins with a very mild emotional shock, and often there is a background of very mild Heart qi deficiency.

Consistent Smooth Vibration over the entire pulse is a sign that one is highly susceptible to worry, and will find something to worry about even if there is no reason to. Consistent Vibration which is rougher and deeper over the entire pulse is a sign of shock, guilt, or fear, and at individual positions indicates parenchymal damage (severe Heart qi-yang deficiency).

Heart Tight

Pulse qualities

This is moderate Heart qi agitation due to heat from excess or deficiency. With heat from excess, the left distal position will feel Tight at the Pericardium position, as if a strong, sharp point is sticking the middle of the finger with each beat. If the heat becomes overwhelming, the entire position can feel Tense and a little Robust Pounding, and the rate is between 90 to 100 beats per minute.

With heat from deficiency, Tightness is felt over the entire left distal position. If the condition has existed for a short period of time, the pulse is usually relatively Rapid, between 84 to 90 beats per minute. Over a much longer period of time the pulse rate will be Slower, as this condition weakens Heart qi and affects overall circulation. (There may also be some coincidental transient, superficial Vibration at the left distal position from time to time, reflecting episodes of worry.)

Etiology

Heat from excess is usually associated with Liver, Gallbladder, or Stomach fire and a loss of thermostatic control by the Triple Burner. Moderate Heart qi agitation or yin deficiency ('Heart tight') can also be heat from yin deficiency due to overwork of the Heart in attempting to overcome stagnation of circulation from a small emotional shock, or to balancing the heat from excess in the Liver, from worry, Grave's disease, or the manic phase of bipolar disease, and stimulating substances such as cocaine or Herba Ephedra (*ma huang*). Check on general symptoms and other signs to differentiate whether the heat is from excess or deficiency.

Symptoms

Moderate Heart qi agitation or yin deficiency due to heat from excess or yin deficiency is marked by symptoms of constant worry, tension, and restlessness which is more acute with excess, and more chronic with yin deficiency. People complain of a 'racing mind' associated with heat from excess, and of restless sleep with heat from deficiency. With heat from excess the restlessness during the day can reach manic proportions. Occasionally there will be some discomfort in the left side of the chest over a relatively large area. This discomfort is an early form of mild angina, which is due to heat from excess or stagnant qi rising to the Pericardium from the Liver, Gallbladder, or Stomach and causing a mild spasm of the coronary arteries. There may also be some shortness of breath during episodes of anxiety.

Signs

As long as the process is confined to the Heart, the tongue will be normal, except for redness at the tip later in the process, which represents heat from deficiency. The eyes will be normal. Another sign is the depth of facial color. There will be an increasing redness, compared to the color of the hands, especially between the eyebrows and the lower forehead in the area of the acupuncture point M-HN-3 *(yin tang)*. The latter is also a sign that the person is easily angered.

Hesitant Wave ('push pulse')

Sensation

This quality occurs over the entire pulse as the Hesitant Wave, which was described in Chapter 6 (Fig. 6-1). The pulse wave has lost its normal sine wave form, whereby the flow to and from the wave peak becomes sharp and abrupt instead of being a gradual rise and fall. The term Hesitant is used because some people experience this quality as faltering or balking, yet not missing a beat.

Etiology

The Hesitant quality is a form of the 'push pulse' in which individuals push themselves mentally, in contrast to the 'push pulse' associated with the Flooding Deficient quality in which individuals push themselves more physically. Since mental 'pushing' seems to antecede the physical exhaustion, it is my impression that with similar etiologies, and a vulnerable Heart, the Hesitant quality precedes the Flooding Deficient quality.

Interpretation and symptoms

In traditional medical terms the Hesitant quality seems closest to mild to moderate Heart yin deficiency. The left distal position would be Tight-Tense.

I have found that this quality occurs in individuals with a tendency to think incessantly about one subject. Most characteristic of this quality is a monomaniacal obsessive preoccupation with some aspect of life, usually work, sometimes health, in which the person's mind never ceases to rest, even when asleep. Originally, I found this pulse in stockbrokers who never stop thinking about money, and later in high-level political appointees who have no civil service safety net and are extraordinarily exploited by their political masters.

This is to be distinguished from a general tendency to worry about almost anything, real or imagined, which is expressed over the entire pulse by a superficial Smooth Vibration at all depths. In the early stages, except for the symptom of worry or difficulty in falling asleep, there are no other related signs or symptoms. Later, affected individuals seek help because of a strong sense of malaise and a feeling that they cannot keep up the pace they have set for themselves. Individuals with this pulse quality often collapse suddenly, physically or emotionally.

Vibration at Neuro-psychological positions

Smooth Vibration at the Neuro-psychological positions accompanies most other signs of Heart qi agitation.

SEVERE HEART QI AGITATION: HEART NERVOUS

This condition, and its related quality, is one in which the yin of the Heart is deficient and the qi is consequently agitated, erratic, and mildly deficient.

Pulse qualities

There are two types of Heart Nervous pulse qualities. Less serious is the one due to prolonged worry and a 'Heart tight' condition described above, in which the pulse rate will tend to be somewhat Rapid, between 80 to 84 beats per minute. With this type people report feeling nervous. With the second, more serious type due to emotional shock, there is occasional Change in Rate at Rest, with no missed beats. There is a propensity to panic with a large Change in Rate at Rest (see Chapter 6).

Etiology

Often there is a constitutional predisposition. The cause may be worry and 'Heart tight' over a long period of time, moderate to strong emotional shock, or physical trauma, often at birth and sometimes in utero. Over time Heart blood deficiency ('Heart weak') can contribute to the 'Heart nervous' pattern, in which case the left distal position is generally Thin Tight, and the rate on exertion increases by more than 10 beats/minute.

Symptoms

The person will complain of being easily fatigued, especially in the morning when awakening. Sleep is restless, marked by frequent awakenings, so that one is in and out of a state of sleep throughout the night. Palpitations can occur occasionally. People will report feeling frequent and disturbing mood swings, changes of mind about people and their own chosen course of life, and as if they are on a "roller coaster" and mildly out of control. There will also be increased irritability of a relatively mild nature.

Signs

The tongue is usually unremarkable. It can have a thin vertical line, if there is a constitutional predisposition, or a deeper vertical line if the cause is related to life events, such as a 'Heart tight' condition over a long period of time. In chronic conditions there can also be some redness at the end. The eyes are usually normal.

Conversely, Heart qi agitation ('Heart nervous') over a long period of time leads to Heart blood deficiency ('Heart weak'), in which case there is a relatively large increase in rate on exertion, the left distal position is Thin, and the left proximal position is Tight.

HEART BLOOD DEFICIENCY: HEART WEAK

The condition of Heart blood deficiency and its related pulse quality (Heart Weak) is one in which the blood of the Heart is deficient with some consequent Heart qi deficiency, both rendering a deficit in Heart function.

Pulse qualities

The pulse shows a large Change in Rate on Exertion of more than 20 beats/minute if the Heart is very blood deficient, and a lesser change (12-19) if the Heart is slightly blood deficient. The rate may be a little Rapid, Normal, or Slow, depending upon the chronicity of the condition: the longer the condition has endured, the Slower the rate. The left distal position is often very Thin when the blood deficiency is more severe, with Reduced Substance if the Heart qi is deficient. The tongue has a peach color.

Etiology

While constitutional Heart deficiency is sometimes a predisposing factor, Heart blood deficiency is most often due to prolonged Heart qi agitation. With continued Heart qi agitation as the cause, the pulse is generally more Tight and the vessels under the eyes are normal. However, Heart blood deficiency can be due to one, or any combination of, the following factors: Kidney essence deficiency, Spleen qi deficiency, and gradual blood loss over time causing blood deficiency. With generalized blood deficiency as the cause, the entire pulse is Thin and a little Feeble, and the vessels inside the lower eyelid are pale.

Symptoms

The patient may experience palpitations throughout the day, especially with activity, because there is not enough blood in the Heart. There is also a general feeling of weakness, depression, poor concentration, and forgetfulness. The sleep pattern is one in which the individual will sleep steadily for a few hours and then awaken, sometimes unable to return to sleep. There is fatigue in the morning. A long-term 'Heart weak' pattern can lead to serious Heart qi and yang deficiency ('Heart disease'), such as congestive heart failure.

HEART QI STAGNATION: HEART CLOSED

Etiology and pulse qualities

Heart qi stagnation and its related pulse quality (Heart Closed) is a condition in which the Flat quality at the left distal position signifies that qi and blood are slightly stagnant in the Pericardium, and cannot freely enter the Heart. The reason is that circulation of qi, and to a lesser extent blood, in the Heart has been blocked from entering the Heart by a shock. This ultimately leads to Heart qi deficiency and diminished peripheral blood circulation. While with Heart qi agitation ('Heart nervous') the shock affected the nervous innervation of the Heart, with Heart qi stagnation ('Heart closed') the substance (parenchyma) of the Heart is slightly affected by diminished circulation, though much less so than with 'Heart small' and 'Heart full.'

The shock is most often an emotional one in childhood while the body's qi is still immature, and usually involves the loss of someone very close, such as a parent.

However, it can occur later in life due to a major emotional shock, such as sudden bad news or the sudden breakup of a romance in which the person withdraws their 'heart' feelings. Other causes can be Heart qi agitation over a long period of time, or even a physical shock to the chest. The Flat Wave associated with Heart qi stagnation usually occurs in a person whose qi is already deficient or undeveloped.

Symptoms

These people seem to be constantly in some kind of emotional difficulty. Their nature tends to be vengeful and spiteful. The spirit of the eyes can seem somewhat withdrawn or angry. Some chest pain can be experienced in connection with the closing of circulation. The pain will feel either like oppression or shooting pain, which is less serious, or needle-like pain in one spot, which tends to be somewhat more serious. One sometimes finds an irritation at the back of the head in the general area of the acupuncture point GV-16 *(feng fu)*.

HEART BLOOD STAGNATION: HEART SMALL

Etiology and pulse qualities

The condition closest to this disorder and its related pulse quality (Heart Small) in Western medicine would be coronary artery occlusion. There is a mild and temporary form, and a serious and enduring form.

With the mild and temporary form the pattern is usually the result of a sudden shock during which the heart contracts, constricting the arteries of the heart. The constriction of these vessels deprives the Heart of qi and blood, leading to transient blood stagnation in the coronary arteries and capillaries, and an insufficient supply of oxygen to the coronary muscle. The cardiac muscles are tense, the coronary arteries are in spasm, and breathing in is difficult. In Dr. Shen's terms, the Heart is "suffocating." The left distal position can be extremely Flat.

With the more serious form the pulse becomes very Deep, Thin, and Feeble. The rate is Normal, slightly Rapid, or slightly Slow. Less often, a Choppy quality has been observed here in the presence of this condition. The condition will be permanent unless it is treated, and is equated by Dr. Shen to what he calls 'true heart disease,' by which means coronary artery disease.

The etiology of the more serious 'Heart small' condition is a profound shock at birth when there is prolonged labor and the head has already reached the outside of the birth canal, but is being held back by something like the cord around the neck of the infant.

Prolonged fear and unexpressed anger may also lead to this condition, although these emotions may also be the consequence, since one finds in people with the 'Heart small' condition a lifelong, unexpressed, and unexplained fear, and some anger and tension. Night terrors and being easily startled are common complaints. There is shortness of breath, in which it is easy to expel air and difficult to take it in. There may be chest pain, usually of a needle-like or stabbing quality in one spot, in the left shoulder, and/or down the left arm. Other symptoms are palpitations and cold extremities.

Other signs

The tongue shows a deep blue color; the face is red or dusky with blue around the chin and mouth if the cause is constitutional or congenital. The lips are purple. Fingers can show clubbing (swelling of the distal phalanges), and the fingernails show purple under the nails. A short wide thumb is found with a constitutional etiology, especially if a propensity to this condition is found in close relatives for several generations. The inside of the lower eyelids can show some confluence of blood vessels, and there may be some redness in the area of the acupuncture points GV-1 *(chang qiang)* and GV-16 *(feng fu)*.

TRAPPED QI IN THE HEART: HEART FULL

Trapped qi in the Heart and its related quality (Heart Full) is a condition in which the qi is unable to get out of the Heart. In contrast to the 'Heart closed' condition (Flat quality), this tends to occur more often in robust people.

Pulse qualities

Trapped qi in the Heart manifests on the pulse as an Inflated quality at the left distal position. When the condition is less serious the left distal position can be a little Yielding Inflated and slightly Pounding, and the rate Normal or a little Rapid. According to Dr. Shen, when the condition is more serious the left distal position is Deep, Thin, and Tight rather than Inflated, and the entire pulse rate is Rapid. The latter pulse configuration is outside of my own experience with this disorder.

Etiology

The etiology in which there is a prolonged birth with the head inside, such as a breech delivery, is more serious because it begins at such an early age; prolonged grief is another associated condition, usually also involving the right distal position. It can also occur due to sudden, very profound repressed anger at a time when a person is extremely active; trauma to the left side of the chest; or after lifting beyond one's energy. Uncorrected, trapped qi in the Heart can progress to either an enlarged heart ('Heart large') or hypertension, or both.

Symptoms

The patient will feel tired their entire life, have little energy, and be rather depressed. Frequently, these people are very quick to anger. These symptoms are similar to, but will be more severe than, those associated with Heart blood deficiency ('Heart weak'). The patient's entire body can be uncomfortable. They will have more difficulty breathing out and less difficulty breathing in, and experience discomfort when lying down on the left side. When the condition is more advanced they can, at times, cough up blood. The Lungs become secondarily stagnant due to cardio-pulmonary insufficiency from diminished Heart function.

Signs

The tongue is red and a little swollen on the end, and on either side of the vertical line, and the eyes show some confluence of blood vessels inside the lower eyelid. The face is usually very red, with some greenish color around the mouth if the cause is congenital, and around the chin if there is a constitutional factor.

MILD, MODERATE, AND SEVERE HEART QI DEFICIENCY: HEART LARGE

The differentiation of these three types of Heart qi deficiency depends upon different pulse pictures and on an increasing severity of similar symptoms.

Whereas mild and moderate Heart qi deficiency will not manifest in biomedical morphological terms, severe Heart qi deficiency ('Heart large'), although largely a measure of energetic cardiomyopathy and cardiomegaly, is the equivalent of an enlarged heart in biomedical terms, as evidenced by imaging studies.

Pulse types and qualities

There are roughly eight pulse types at the left distal position related to Heart qi deficiency ('Heart large'). The occurrence of Heart qi deficiency in the young and middle-aged usually involves a predisposing constitutional deficit of Heart qi. These eight signs often overlap and are only roughly listed in order of increasing pathology. Here, qi and yang deficiency are in a close continuum.

The first of these pulse types, in which the left distal position has Reduced Substance or is slightly Feeble with a Slow rate, indicates mild to moderate Heart qi deficiency. The Mitral Valve position may show Smooth Vibration.

The second pulse type shows a Change in Rate at Rest that occurs consistently, signifying mild to moderate Heart qi deficiency. The larger the change, the greater the Heart qi deficiency. According to Dr. Shen, despite the mildness of the condition, this can have a constitutional etiology.

The third pulse type indicates significant Heart qi-yang deficiency. This manifests as a Change in Intensity and Qualities, indicating a separation of Heart yin and yang and pronounced functional instability. Rough Vibration at the left distal position indicates parenchymal damage, which is possibly another type of Heart qi-yang deficiency and dysfunction. The Mitral Valve position may be Slippery.

With the fourth type of severe Heart qi deficiency there is a positive Heart Enlarged position. The area between the left distal and left middle positions is very Inflated or Rougher as one rolls the finger from distal to proximal, compared with rolling from proximal to distal ('Heart Large').

The fifth type is a Deep, Thin, and Tight quality with the rate exceeding 100 beats per minute, especially under stress. This is a pattern of severe Heart qi deficiency ('Heart large') and is associated by Dr. Shen with Heart shock, breech birth, chest trauma, prolonged grief, and profound sudden anger. This combination may also occur with an Interrupted or Intermittent quality and a positive Heart Enlarged position.

The sixth pulse type is a Tense Hollow Full-Overflowing quality with a rate exceeding 100 beats per minute. This combination is also associated with severe Heart qi deficiency ('Heart large') and is often attended by hypertension, related by Dr. Shen to long-suppressed emotions.

The seventh type, which also indicates severe Heart qi-yang deficiency, is an irregular rhythm, either an Interrupted quality in which the rate cannot be accurately measured, or an Intermittent quality where the regular missed beat is more often than once every 20 beats. With the Interrupted quality, the more consistent and frequent the interruptions, the greater the difficulty in reading the rate. With the Intermittent quality, the more frequently the beat is missed, the more serious the sign.

The eighth type involves a Change in Rate on Exertion less than eight beats per minute; this is another sign of Heart qi deficiency. The less the rate rises, the greater the deficiency. When it does not rise at all or diminishes on exertion we have a strong sign of Heart yang deficiency.

Etiology

The causes of Heart qi deficiency are constitutional, habitual overwork and/or exercise, extreme emotional repression over a very long period of time, any of the earlier mentioned Heart conditions (especially Trapped qi in the Heart ['Heart full'], long-term Heart blood stagnation with coronary occlusion ['Heart small'], and rheumatic heart disease). Also, more common before the advent of child labor laws, is excessive physical child labor at an early age, together with malnutrition. With the latter etiology there is usually a Hollow Interrupted or Intermittent rhythm (see Chapter 6). Repressed profound anger, which occurs especially while active, will often exacerbate any of the other factors.

Symptoms

Symptoms include extreme shortness of breath, especially on exertion, difficulty breathing if lying flat on the back or on the left side, chronic chest discomfort, as well as becoming easily and extensively fatigued. Hypertension is often present.

Other signs

The tongue is swollen, wet, generally pale, and red on the end with a vertical line (central crease) along which, on either side, the tongue is especially swollen. The eyes have a confluence of blood vessels inside the lower lids, which are simultaneously pale. The nails are round and there is clubbing. The face appears drained of color.

HEART YANG DEFICIENCY: 'HEART DISEASE'

In biomedical terms, what Dr. Shen calls 'Heart disease' overlaps with heart failure, and in Chinese medicine often corresponds to Heart yang deficiency. This is the end of the process of gradual depletion of Heart qi, which has been described in the conditions above.

Pulse qualities

Commonly, the entire pulse is very Rapid, Arrhythmic, either Interrupted or Intermittent, and sometimes Hollow with the most serious forms of Heart yang deficiency. The left distal position is Deep to Absent or Empty, shows Change in Intensity and Qualities, constant Deep Rough Vibration, or an Unstable quality (very serious, see Chapter 13), and possibly Slippery. Both proximal positions are almost always Feeble-Absent. The rate decreases on exertion and the Heart Enlarged position is present.

Etiology

Among the causes are constitutional predisposition, congenital defects, work beyond one's energy as a child and pre-adolescent, rheumatic fever, extreme abuse of drugs, alcohol, and nicotine, prolonged chronic disease, and severe emotional shock to the Heart and circulation early in life. Repressed anger can always be a contributing factor. All of the etiologies listed above lead gradually to an extreme weakening of Heart qi and yang, until the Heart can no longer control the circulation.

Symptoms

The symptoms are the same as those for severe Heart qi deficiency and trapped qi in the Heart, with the addition of greater chest pain, greater fatigue and shortness of breath on exertion, excessive spontaneous cold or beady perspiration during the day with minimal exertion, coldness in the body and especially the limbs, dependent pitting edema, and a greater need to sleep in a sitting position.

Other symptoms are poor concentration and forgetfulness, palpitations with even mild exertion, numbness of the upper limbs, and a suffocating sensation in the chest. If the etiology is constitutional or congenital, the individual is anxious and vulnerable their entire life.

Signs

The tongue has a deep vertical line (central crease), is swollen, very wet, pale with a dark hue, and possibly with some residual redness at the tip. The swelling is often most pronounced on either side of the vertical line. The eyes have a loss of confluence and there is paleness inside the lower eyelids. The nails are blue and round, and the ends of the fingers show clubbing. The face is without color, especially the forehead, except for a greenish color on the chin or around the mouth if the cause is, respectively, constitutional or congenital. The lips may be purple.

SUMMARY OF CONSTITUTIONAL, CONGENITAL, AND LIFE-RELATED CONDITIONS ACCORDING TO DR. SHEN

Constitutional (inherited)

Both the left distal (Heart) and left proximal positions (Kidneys) are Feeble, or, less often, just the left distal position is Feeble and left proximal is unremarkable, with a shallow vertical line in the center of the tongue from the root to the end. If there is a Change in Rate at Rest due to constitutional factors, the change will be large and consistent.

Congenital

HEAD INSIDE

If the head remains inside the birth canal longer than normal, usually associated with a breech birth, the Heart becomes 'large' (to use Dr. Shen's term) because the baby cannot breathe. This is associated with the Inflated quality at the distal positions, especially the left distal.

HEAD OUTSIDE

If the birth process is stopped after the baby's head is outside the mother, usually due to the cord wrapped around the baby's neck, the Heart becomes 'small' because of the shock ("scared"); according to Dr. Shen, fear makes the veins (blood vessels) small. He considers this to be one type of 'Heart disease.'

Life-related

Heart conditions are said to be the result of abuse during life if the left distal position is Feeble and the left proximal position is very Tight, or if the entire pulse reflects Reduced Substance or is Feeble. If there is a Change in Rate at Rest due to abusive lifestyle, the change will be small and inconsistent.

HEART AND 'NERVOUS SYSTEM' AFFECT EACH OTHER

According to Dr. Shen, the Heart and 'nervous system' have a special relationship in that the Heart controls the mind, and the condition of the 'nervous system' is integrally associated with the mind. If the condition is associated with the Heart alone, the left distal position will be Tight. If the condition begins in the 'nervous system,' the entire pulse will be Tense-Tight.

Heart qi-yang deficiency

If the 'nervous system' is intact the physical symptoms of Heart qi-yang deficiency are lassitude, palpitations, shortness of breath, precordial stiffness, edema, and spontaneous sweating which increases on exertion. If the 'nervous system' is weak, the individual will also tend to be quiet, withdrawn, passive, depressed, forgetful with poor concentration, and is easily frightened. The cause may be a long illness, a constitutional weakness, or very advanced old age.

If we have a 'nervous system tense' person with Heart qi-yang deficiency, they will be one of those I saw frequently as an intern who, despite enormous disability, could never stay still and rest, which was essential to their recovery. If they had a business before coming to the hospital, they had to be on the phone conducting business, even though their life depended on surrendering to their illness. After a short while I could unerringly predict which ones would survive and which would succumb, based on their ability to lay back and be cared for.

Heart yin deficiency

Heart yin deficiency increases tension in the 'nervous system.' Yin deficient conditions of the Heart generally coincide with blood deficiency.

The symptoms associated with Heart yin and blood deficiency and their causes are well known. The result is the drying out of the nerves of the heart, which leads to Heart qi agitation and an instability of the mind. This instability in turn leads to life situations which increase daily tension and dry out the nerves, especially those of the autonomic nervous system, creating a variety of pseudo-neurological symptoms such as headache, vertigo, and parasthesia. Gradually, the Kidney yang (adrenal) and yin (steroids) are depleted, leading to parenchymal disease in the vulnerable areas of the body.

On the other hand, a 'nervous system tense' individual will, over many years, owing to the overactive, rapidly moving qi of the body and organs, drain the yin of the most vulnerable organ. All things being equal, the yin of the Liver will be depleted first, which is unable to feed the yin of the Heart, and later both will deplete the Kidneys, which store the yin. The result is a racing mind that has difficulty finding rest in the context of agitated Heart qi.

HEART AND CIRCULATION

The relationship between the effect of the Heart on circulation, and circulation on the Heart, is complex. Over a long period of time the pictures tend to merge. By circulation we refer to the peripheral circulation of both qi and blood outside of the Heart, in the channels and blood vessels. Dr. Shen has referred to this as the 'circulatory system,' a level of energy that is heavier, deeper, and more slow-moving than that associated with the 'nervous system.'

Circulation affects the Heart

When the circulation affects the Heart due to trauma, both physical and mental, the pulse at first will be Tight and Rapid. The shock causes the vessels to contract in response, perhaps partially to control the bleeding. There will be a Change in Intensity over the entire pulse only after the Heart qi is depleted in its effort to overcome the closed circulation.

EMOTIONAL TRAUMA

We know that sudden emotional shock at any time in life drains Heart yin. At this point the face is red, especially at *yin tang*, and the hands are more pale.

If the trauma is emotional the left distal position, especially the Pericardium position, will be Tight, the entire position possibly Slippery, and the Diaphragm position may be Inflated. If the physical condition is good, the left distal position may be Inflated, and Flat if the physical condition is poor. There will be Rough Vibration over the entire pulse if the shock is great, especially if there is an element of fear and guilt. In the beginning, the rate is Rapid. If the shock occurs at birth or early in life and/or is great, the Change in Rate at Rest will be consistent and great. By contrast, if the shock is small and/or occurs later in life, the Change in Rate at Rest will be small and inconsistent.

However, over a long period of time the rate will decrease to very Slow, around 50 to 60 beats per minute, there will be Change in Intensity over the entire pulse, and the left distal position will become Feeble.

PHYSICAL TRAUMA

Again, the vessels contract for the reason cited above. The pulse becomes very Tight and Rapid, depending on the severity. In the affected area the pulse will be Tight and Inflated in a relatively robust individual, and Tight and Flat in an individual with reduced qi. There will be no Rough Vibration over the entire pulse unless there is a simultaneous emotional shock, which is not uncommon. The left distal position will be unremarkable unless the trauma is to the chest. There will be no Change in Rate at Rest.

Over a long period of time the rate will decrease to very Slow, about 50 to 60 beats per minute, the left distal position will be unremarkable, and the entire pulse will show no Change in Intensity unless there are other factors affecting the Heart.

HYPOTHERMIA

The pulse is Firm or Hidden and very Slow, altogether too deep to show a Change in Intensity.

Heart affects the circulation

This is usually a manifestation of deficient Heart qi being unable to move the circulation. It generally reflects a constitutional deficit, disease (rheumatic), overwork, overexercise, a generally poor physical condition (Spleen qi not producing blood), or a long-term mental and emotional drain (worry, obsession).

The entire pulse will eventually show Change in Intensity and Rough Vibration. The rate will be Slow, in the low 60s, except with aerobic exercise, when it will be lower. The left distal position will show varying degrees of deficiency or separation of yin and yang, from Feeble-Absent to Change in Qualities. Eventually the left distal position will be Slippery and have Rough Vibration and greater Change in Intensity than the rest of the pulse.

If the cause is constitutional, the proximal positions will be feeble, and if the cause is chronic debility, the entire pulse may be Reduced, but less so than the left distal position. If there is an obsessional factor the wave will be Hesitant, and if long-term worry is involved the Vibration will be Smooth at first, then moving to Rough. Since the overworking of the mind is the issue here, the proximal positions, especially the left, will be Tight changing back and forth to Feeble (Change in Qualities), expressing both the life stress and constitutional etiologies respectively.

Right Distal, Special Lung, and Pleura positions

We will concern ourselves here with the right distal, Special Lung, and Pleura positions, whose locations are described below. Each tells us, alone and in combination, about the functional integrity of the Lungs, and, together with the left distal position, the energy of the chest and upper burner. Dr. Shen considers the function of the Lungs to be part of what he calls the 'digestive system,' since he speaks of the Lungs as 'digesting' phlegm.

RIGHT DISTAL POSITION

In order to avoid the sensory overlap of the medial into the distal aspects of the pulse, the distal positions are not accessed in the distal-proximal axis along the radial artery, as are the proximal and medial positions. Rather, they are accessed horizontally, along a radial-ulnar, medial-lateral axis just under the scaphoid bone, to which position one has rolled the radial edge of the index finger. Here we are not accessing the radial artery, but rather the fluid dynamics of its sudden breakdown into many smaller arteries, which sets up a wave informing us about the physiological integrity of the Heart and Lungs.

Location To locate the right distal position, the left index finger and entire left arm of the examiner must be rolled distally toward and slightly under the right scaphoid bone, where the qualities are accessed with the radial side of the index finger rather than the flat pad. After slightly lessening pressure, the position is then accessed by rolling the radial side of the index finger in a medial-lateral direction, rather than the proximal-distal direction which we use for the middle and proximal positions.

Depths The three separate depths are not easily accessed at the distal position due to the diminished space accorded this position. Superficial and deep are easily recognized, as are those qualities, such as Full-Overflowing, which exceed the qi depth, or the Inflated, which seems to expand it, and the Empty, which shows itself only at the superficial aspect and is missing at the deeper aspects.

Function

The right distal position represents the current function of the Lungs, and can be used to locate the different lobes of the material lung. However, in my experience the location of the lobes is found more readily and accurately using the Special Lung position, as illustrated in Fig. 2-3 (see Chapter 2).

Etiology

Among the problems which most often affect the Lungs are congenital trauma (prematurity and prolonged labor); working the Lungs beyond their capacity (as with speaking and singing); incorrect breathing and meditation techniques; unresolved external pathogenic factors; smoking and other toxic inhalants; excessive and inappropriate use of medications; lifting; Kidney qi deficiency (and, to a lesser extent, Spleen and Heart deficiency); poor eating habits; unresolved grief; and stagnant Liver qi attacking the Lungs.

One may have Lung disharmony, such as asthma, from disharmonies of the Heart, Liver, or Kidneys, and less often the Spleen or Stomach, especially if the Lungs are vulnerable.

Qualities found at right distal position

The following are qualities that I have found at the right distal position: Inflated, Deep, Flat, Muffled, Feeble-Absent, Floating, Empty, Thin, Slippery, Reduced Substance, Taut, Tense, Tight, Wiry, Vibration, Pounding, Change in Intensity and Qualities. (See the specific sections discussing these qualities for additional information.)

Floating

According to Dr. Shen, this was an extremely common quality at this position before the era of antibiotics, and is a sign of an early attack by an external pathogenic factor such as wind-cold or wind-heat. If the tongue has a thin white coating, the illness is very recent; if the coating is no longer thin and white, the illness has existed for a longer time.

Floating Tense and a slightly Slow rate is a sign of wind-cold. Floating Yielding and a slightly Rapid rate is a sign of wind-heat.

Tense

This is a sign of Lung qi stagnation and an overworking Lung with heat from excess, usually due to an unresolved cold external pathogenic factor. It can be found with excess-type asthma. The Special Lung position is often Slippery at this stage.

Tight

Conditions which dry out the Lungs, such as inhalant irritants (tobacco, nasal sprays), frequent invasions of wind-heat, high fevers, general yin deficiency, and dry climates and tuberculosis will eventually cause yin deficiency and a Tight quality at the right distal (and Special Lung) position.

Stagnant qi of the Liver which attacks a vulnerable Lung will, over time, create the kind of stagnation which drains Lung yin. This in turn will lead to a Tight quality at the right distal position. Yin-deficient asthma may be one outcome of this process.

The Tight quality at this position can also be found with stagnation due to chest trauma with pain. In asthmatics it is a sign of bronchial spasm. I have found this quality in those with a history of premature birth, who spent weeks or months in an incubator. The pulse was Tight-Wiry.

Wiry

This is rare sign of more advanced yin deficiency, with yin-deficient asthma or tuberculosis, and sometimes with a history of premature birth and time spent in an incubator. Severe pain due to chest trauma and excessive use of tobacco and bronchial spasm are important etiologies. This sign should alert the practitioner to investigate an early neoplastic process. With chronic cocaine abuse the Wiry quality will always appear simultaneously at the left distal position.

Yielding Inflated

A Yielding Inflated quality at the right distal position alone is associated with 'trapped qi' due to repressed emotion (probably grief), overworking Lungs (singing, talking), poor breathing techniques, and lifting.

Tense Inflated

A Tense Inflated quality is a sign of 'trapped qi and heat' in the Lungs accumulating over a long period of time. This is found in adult smokers who had inhalant allergies, asthma, and frequent upper respiratory infections as children and were treated repeatedly with antibiotics and other medications. The infections were resolved but the invading cold remained to create stagnation. The heat can come over time from the effort of the Lungs to open the 'trap' and release the qi. Those people for whom the stagnation is not overcome will accumulate heat and qi, and will remain susceptible to future upper respiratory and Lung illness.

The Tense Inflated quality is also specifically associated with emphysema as a manifestation of the later stages of the above pathogenesis.

Flat

The Flat quality in the right distal position is a sign that qi cannot enter the Lungs. It is a form of stagnation which will appear primarily in a deficient or physiologically immature person or yin organ, with the same etiologies that might engender an Inflated quality in a less deficient person.

Emotional repression

If the Flat quality, for this reason, is felt at the right distal position, it is almost always felt simultaneously with the same quality at the left distal position. This occurs with a usually forgotten disappointment or severe emotional loss early in life in which the feelings are automatically repressed at the time by closing off the flow of Heart qi and the qi of the Lungs.

Prolonged birth with head outside the birth canal

This quality can appear in children, and subsequently in adulthood, where at birth the cord is entangled around the baby's neck. If the Flat quality is felt at the right distal position for this reason, it is almost always felt simultaneously with the same quality at the left distal position.

Trauma and lifting

The Flat quality can occur with trauma to the chest in individuals who were qi deficient at the time of the trauma. More often with this etiology, however, the Flat quality is found simultaneously in both distal positions. It can be found in deficient individuals who lift even once far beyond their energy.

Tumor

I have found the Flat quality in the right distal position in individuals with early Lung tumors.

Reduced Substance

This quality is described in Chapter 8, and here is a sign of mild Lung qi deficiency.

Feeble-Absent

This quality is found with moderate to severe Lung qi deficiency associated with deficient Kidney qi, or with overwork of the Lungs due to excessive talking or singing beyond one's energy, or poor breathing techniques (as with the improper practice of meditation, yoga, qi gong) over a long period of time.

Another common cause of Lung qi deficiency, and the Feeble-Absent quality at the right distal position, is the gradual enervation of Lung qi due to the effort required to overcome Lung qi stagnation. One scenario involves the invasion of a cold external pathogenic factor which the Lung qi is not strong enough to expel, and which creates stagnation in the Lungs. This is especially true if the person continues to overwork and drain both the overall energy and specifically the Lung qi. With this deficiency, and with changes in weather and the seasons, the fluids which the Lungs normally disperse and cause to descend through the body are trapped in the upper burner. They exit through the most convenient opening to the outside, the nose, with concomitant allergies and asthma with difficulty exhaling.

Vibration

Vibration at the right distal position is usually a sign of Lung qi deficiency and functional impairment of the Lungs. The degree depends on the Roughness and Smoothness of the Vibration and the depth at which it is found. The Rougher and Deeper the Vibration, the more serious the condition and impairment.

When a Smooth Vibration and Tense quality appear suddenly at the right distal position, one should consider a recent mild trauma to the chest, or lifting beyond one's energy, which has created stagnation in the Lungs. There is temporary poor Lung function with a feeling of chest oppression and inability to expand the chest.

Deep

This is a sign of moderately deficient Lung qi, for all the reasons described above for this condition.

Empty, Change in Intensity and Qualities

These qualities are all signs of the separation of Lung yin and yang, and of extreme Lung qi deficiency and chaotic impaired Lung function. It must be given immediate and serious diagnostic and therapeutic attention due to the danger of tumor formation. A Yielding Empty quality, especially when also found at the left distal position, can also be a sign of unresolved guilt (see also Special Lung position).

Thin

The interpretation of the Thin quality is, at the moment, somewhat ambiguous. Clinically, the Thin quality at the right distal position is a sign of mild to moderately deficient qi rather than blood; it is somewhat less deficient than with the Feeble-Absent quality. Blood deficiency is the usual interpretation of the Thin quality at other positions or over the entire pulse. In the literature I have reviewed there is no mention of Lung blood deficiency. As I am impressed by the obvious fact that lungs do bleed (hemoptysis), I cautiously question the absence in the literature of references to Lung blood.

Slippery

This is a sign of damp-phlegm stagnation in the Lungs. Slipperiness readily occurs with Lung qi deficiency due to its failure to disperse and move the fluids downward. This is compounded if the Heart cannot maintain blood circulation in the Lungs (edema); if the Kidneys cannot assist in the Lungs' downward-moving action, especially in young children with immature Lung qi; if the Spleen qi is deficient in its digestive function and does not adequately 'digest' the fluids in food; if Liver qi stagnates and attacks the Lungs, interfering with their dispersing and downward-moving action; and if the Triple Burner and Internal Duct fail to control food and water metabolism.

Muffled

This is a sign of chaotic qi and extreme stagnation of all substances, and is consistent with the existence of a malignant tumor in the lungs or chest.

Robust Pounding

Robust Pounding is a sign of heat from excess in the Lungs, often associated with allergies.

Common conditions associated with right distal and Special Lung positions

COMMON COLD

Floating Tense and Slow with wind-cold and Floating Yielding and Reduced with wind-heat, with a Taut Floating quality at the Special Lung position.

INFLUENZA

Floating Tense-Tight at the right distal, spreading to most other positions, with a Tense Floating quality at the Special Lung position.

BRONCHITIS

Floating Tight, mild Pounding, mild Slippery, and Smooth Vibration, with a mildly Rapid rate. Depending on the pulmonary history, the Special Lung position is essentially the same.

PNEUMONIA

Tense-Tight, Robust Pounding, Flooding Excess, Slippery and Smooth-Rough Vibration, with a very Rapid rate. Depending on the pulmonary history, the Special Lung position is essentially the same.

ACUTE ASTHMA

Tense-Tight, Pounding, Yielding Inflated, very Slippery, Floating and Rough Vibration. Depending on the pulmonary history, the Special Lung position is essentially the same.

CHRONIC ASTHMA

Qi deficiency

Right distal position is Feeble, Slippery, Rough Vibration, and a Slow rate, with Change in Qualities and Intensity. The Special Lung position is Tight, Wiry, and Slippery, Rough Vibration, and Change in Intensity.

Yin deficiency

Tight-Wiry, Slippery, Rough Vibration, Change in Intensity, and a slightly Rapid rate. The Special Lung position is Wiry, Slippery, Rough Vibration, and Change in Intensity.

EMPHYSEMA

Tense, very Inflated, very Slippery, and Rough Vibration, with a Slow or Normal rate.

TUMOR

Both the right distal and Special Lung positions are Muffled to Dead or Nonhomogeneous, and the Special Lung position may also be Restricted.

OBSTRUCTIVE DISORDER, INCLUDING SMOKER'S OR MINER'S LUNG

The right distal and Special Lung positions are Thin, Tight-Wiry, very Slippery with very Rough Vibration and Change in Intensity. In advanced cases the Muffled quality can begin to appear at both positions, especially the right distal, and the Restricted quality at the Special Lung position (see Chapter 10).

Combinations at the right distal and other positions

RIGHT AND LEFT DISTAL POSITIONS

Refer to Chapter 14 and Table 14-1 for these combinations. One indication specifically mentioned by Dr. Shen is tuberculosis, when both of these positions are Deep and Feeble and the Special Lung position is Floating and Slippery.

RIGHT DISTAL AND LEFT MIDDLE POSITIONS

Right distal Feeble-Absent, left middle Tense to Tight

This combination can occur with asthma due to qi-deficient Lungs being attacked by rising stagnant Liver qi.

RIGHT DISTAL AND RIGHT MIDDLE POSITIONS

Floating Tense and Slow

This combination could be a sign of wind-cold which has moved into both the upper and middle burners, affecting respiration and digestion.

Floating Yielding Rapid

This would suggest that external wind-heat has moved into both the upper and middle burners, affecting respiration and digestion.

Tense

This quality implies qi stagnation and heat from excess in the Lungs and Stomach.

Slippery

This is a sign of phlegm excess due perhaps to Spleen dampness, possibly in combination with Lung qi deficiency. If the right distal position is Feeble, the likelihood is that the Lung qi has been deficient for a long time, and that the Lungs are susceptible to accumulation of dampness.

Feeble-Absent

Generally, the Feeble-Absent qualities are found here when eating habits are irregular over a long period of time. This combination is more commonly found over the entire right side, rather than in just the distal and middle positions. The meaning is the same since the 'digestive system' in Dr. Shen's scheme involves the Lungs, Spleen-Stomach, and Kidneys. The Lungs, according to him, 'digest' mucus, the Spleen 'digests' food, and the Kidneys 'digest' water. At times some other processes, such as a damp-heat in the Bladder (urinary infection), might alter the uniform picture, introducing a more Tense to Tight and possibly Slippery quality in the right proximal position.

Tight

Tightness occurs here when a person eats too rapidly over a long period of time. This quality is also often found over the entire right side with the same significance, for the reasons explained in the previous item involving the extent of the 'digestive system' as conceived by Dr. Shen.[2]

RIGHT DISTAL AND LEFT PROXIMAL POSITIONS

Feeble-Absent

This combination is found in asthmatic and allergic children whose Kidney qi is deficient, and thus unable to assist the Lung qi in bringing the qi from the atmosphere into the body. With this combined Lung and Kidney qi deficiency there is difficulty in both inhaling (Kidneys) and exhaling (Lungs).

Tight

This is a sign of Lung and Kidney yin deficiency. Lung yin deficiency due, for example, to heavy smoking can consume Kidney yin as the Kidneys seek to maintain fluid homeostasis in the Lungs.

RIGHT DISTAL AND RIGHT PROXIMAL POSITIONS

Feeble-Absent

This combination can be found at these positions in asthmatic and allergic children whose Kidney qi is deficient and thus unable to assist the Lung qi in bringing the qi from the atmosphere into the body. It may also be found when there is stagnation in the middle burner blocking the movement of qi between the upper and lower burners.

SPECIAL LUNG POSITION

The Special Lung position informs us primarily of the past medical history of the Lungs. While theoretically it should not be palpable in a normal person, I have found that in my practice its absence is a sign of serious pathology. (Others have not found its absence to be significant.) It must always be considered in relationship to the qualities at the right distal position.

Location

This position is found at the superficial palmar branch of the radial artery, which occurs as an extension of the radial artery medially and upward toward the trapezium, which is part of the lower row of the carpus. I usually begin my examination of the Special Lung position by using the flat pad of my index finger to search lightly for this unpredictable small branch of the radial artery; it can be found medial to the radial artery somewhere between the acupuncture points LU-9 *(tai yuan)* and PC-7 *(da ling)*. Because it is anomalous, it varies considerably from person to person, and from side to side in the same person. The left Special Lung position tells us about the right Lung, and the right Special Lung position about the left Lung. The most frequent qualities found at this position are Floating, Tense, Tight, Thin, Slippery, Feeble, Change in Intensity, and Vibration. Less common are the Inflated, Pounding, Wiry, Restricted, and Muffled qualities.

Palpation

The Special Lung position has an unpredictable number of depths which do not conform to the classic three depths of qi, blood, and organ that are found at the principal positions. I have found that by increasing and decreasing finger pressure, or rolling medially or laterally, one can discern different qualities. For example, you may find the Slippery quality more superficially and the Vibration quality more deeply at one pulse, and just the opposite at another pulse. Or you may find one quality more medial and another more lateral in one person, and just the opposite in another. It is therefore advisable to explore the entire area as well as all depths with the flat pad of your index finger in order to get the most complete picture.

Special Lung position qualities and the right distal position

The presence of the qualities Floating, Change in Intensity, Tight, Tense, Slippery, Thin, Rough Vibration, Wiry, Restricted, and Muffled, in one combination or another, at the Special Lung position always indicates Lung qi stagnation and vulnerability associated with injury to Lung function in the past, even early in life. If the right distal position has no similar signs of current activity, or even if it is just Feeble-Absent, there is probably no current Lung disharmony. (The one exception, according to Dr. Shen, is tuberculosis, which is outside of my experience.)

The presence of the above qualities at the Special Lung position indicates great susceptibility to disease. For example, a Normal right distal position with a Tight-Wiry Slippery quality at the Special Lung position with Vibration might mean a scar from an old tuberculosis. In the final analysis, the condition of the Lungs is drawn from the combined information accessed at both the Special Lung and right distal positions.

There is a considerable amount of material recorded from Dr. Shen on the relationship between the qualities at the right distal and Special Lung positions. Recently, he seemed to have taken a step back from the original detail about this position to a much simpler diagnostic formula. His stance concerning the presence of qualities at the Special Lung position suggests either simply a constitutional Lung qi deficiency, a Lung illness which probably recurred frequently very early in life (infections), or a serious Lung illness that occurred in the past just once, such as tuberculosis. I have chosen to omit the more complex material since I cannot personally confirm much of it. What I can confirm appears under the common conditions discussed a few pages previously.[3]

Morphology

The Special Lung position informs us of the energetic and morphological status of the opposite Lung, including the medial, lateral, upper, and lower aspects, which can be accessed by rolling one's finger in the appropriate direction, as illustrated in Chapter 4.

Specific qualities

Recall that, theoretically, there are no qualities when the Special Lung position is Normal. However, the presence of a Taut quality would be considered as close to Normal as one could expect in this imperfect world, and as I have already said, the absence of the Special Lung position in my experience has attended the most serious pathology.

I also wish to preface this discussion with the observation that smoke or toxic inhalants from any source (tobacco, industrial, moxibustion) will ultimately call forth all of the following qualities, especially the combination of Tight-Wiry, Slippery, and Rough Vibration at the Special Lung position, and Tight-Wiry with Vibration at the right distal position.

Floating

The Floating quality at the Special Lung position is a sign of an an acute external pathogenic factor: Tense Floating and Slow with wind-cold, and Yielding Floating and Rapid with wind-heat. The same qualities are also found at the right distal position.

Slippery

The Slippery quality at the Special Lung position is a sign of stagnation of dampness, usually preceded by qi stagnation related either to an unresolved pathogenic factor or Lung qi deficiency, and sometimes associated Kidney, Spleen, or (more rarely) Heart qi deficiency. Anything that interferes with the dispersing and downward-moving actions of the Lungs, and the water metabolism function of the Triple Burner system, will lead to stagnation of dampness and the appearance of the Slippery quality at the Special Lung position. This includes trauma, lifting, infection, and deficiency for any reason, including overuse of the lungs.

Slipperiness appears more often at the Special Lung position than at any other position on the pulse, except perhaps the Gallbladder position. Slipperiness at the Special Lung position represents an old process, possibly beginning early in life, to which the body has adapted, while Slipperiness at the right distal position speaks more of a current, ongoing process of stagnation of dampness in the Lungs. Together, the two would indicate that the situation is more serious, for we have signs of both a currently active (right distal position) and chronically quiescent, already damaged, and vulnerable Lung (Special Lung position).

Tight or Wiry

A Tight or Wiry quality at the Special Lung position is either a sign of Lung yin deficiency, spasm of the bronchi, or even pain (especially Wiry). The Wiry quality is a sign that, whatever the cause, the pathological process is more advanced than with the Tight quality. The differentiation must be made through other signs and symptoms. Tightness, Slipperiness, and Vibration are often encountered together as a sign of chronicity due to early Lung disharmony, usually childhood asthma, where the Tight quality is also a sign of bronchial spasm, or exposure to Lung irritants such as tobacco.

Rough Vibration

This is a sign that the Lungs have been a repeated site of disease, that Lung qi is very deficient, that Lung alveolar function is impaired, and that the Lungs are presently highly vulnerable to more serious illness.

Empty

The sudden appearance of a Yielding Empty pulse at the Special Lung position usually suggests a recent and profound personal loss, such as the death of someone close. One must be careful to distinguish the Empty from the Floating quality. The Floating quality is more superficial and often presents other qualities on pressure, whereas the Empty quality is less superficial but reveals no other qualities on pressure.

Yielding Inflated

A Yielding Inflated quality at this position is a sign of 'trapped qi' in the Lungs often associated with Lung qi deficiency due to overuse (singing, talking) and misuse (incorrect breathing or meditation) of breathing. Especially when found simultaneously at both distal positions, a congenital etiology (cord around the neck) must be considered.

Tense-Tight Inflated at right distal and Special Lung positions

Unresolved external pathogenic factors

If the pulse is more Tense, this combination may reflect 'trapped' heat. As previously explained, this could be due to repeated, unresolved upper respiratory infections, usually in childhood, in which large amounts of antibiotics and other medications were used that eliminated the infection but left the cold in the Lungs. This creates qi stagnation, which the Lung qi attempts to overcome by using yang qi, or the metabolic heat of the body. When this is unsuccessful, the yang qi accumulates and is perceived as trapped heat from excess, associated with a Tense Inflated pulse quality. At this stage we may have excess-type allergies and asthma.

The effort to balance the heat from excess will at first gradually deplete the yin and lead to yin deficiency (heat from deficiency), reflected in a Tight Inflated pulse, and then eventually deplete the Lung qi, manifested in a Tight Inflated pulse with Rough Vibration at the Special Lung position, but Feeble at the right distal position.

Again, with this deficiency, and with changes in the weather and seasons, the fluids which the Lungs normally disperse and move downward are instead trapped in the upper burner; they emerge through the most convenient opening to the outside—the nose—with concomitant inhalant allergies, sinusitis, and asthma.

Emphysema

The Tense Inflated quality at these positions is a sign of 'trapped' qi and heat in the Lungs, often of emphysema, which is the end product of the aforementioned causes of the Inflated quality.

Restricted

The Restricted quality is found only at the Special Lung position and is a sign of any chronic Lung disease with reduced alveolar capacity, often due to a neoplastic process, including metastatic cancer. Examples from my experience include reduced Lung function in a young man who was born prematurely at 25 weeks, and a 24-year-old woman with ideopathic pulmonary fibrosis.

Muffled

The Muffled quality at the Special Lung position is, in my experience, associated with an already advanced neoplastic process.

PLEURA POSITION

Location

The Pleura position is located superficially in the area between the right distal and right middle positions, otherwise known as the right Diaphragm position. The presence of a pleural pathology is discernible when the distal aspect of the right Diaphragm position is either more Inflated or Rougher than the proximal aspect. More rarely, a deeper Tight quality has been found at this position with a history of pleurisy in the distant past.

Interpretation

According to Dr. Shen, this is a sign of qi stagnation between the Lungs and the chest musculature which can be equated with the biomedical condition of pleurisy. If there is activity at the right distal position—Tight-Tense, Pounding, Slippery, and Rapid—the pleurisy could be active; otherwise it would be a sign of previous pleurisy.

Left Middle Position

This position represents the Liver on the pulse. More than any other yin organ, the Liver is the first line of defense against stress and the one which shows, through its pulse, the vicissitudes of our pressured lives at the dawn of the twenty-first century. These stresses are emotional, chemical, and physical. By physical stress we mean overwork beyond one's energy over a long period of time, and insufficient sleep and rest. According to Dr. Shen, and confirmed by my own experience, Liver qi and blood provide the body's 'second wind' and allow us to recover our spent energy. Chemical stress includes medications, environmental toxins, and the abuse of recreational drugs, including alcohol. Emotional stress affecting the Liver is usually associated with repressed anger and frustration.

In addition to the principal left middle position there are distal, ulnar, and radial aspects of the position (discussed below) which are accessed when there is a Change in Quality while rolling the finger in these directions. Normally they are not present, and are observed only when there is engorgement of the Liver. Efrem Korngold[4] has noted and demonstrated that some people seem to have a second artery medial and parallel to the radial artery on the level of the left middle position, which he finds associated with brain tumor. This finding has now been confirmed many times and seems to be associated most closely with 'near death' experiences in a variety of circumstances.

COMMON QUALITIES AT LEFT MIDDLE POSITION

Taut; Tense; Tight; Wiry; Thin

These are the most common qualities found at this position, all related to repressed emotions (usually anger and frustration), which causes constrained Liver qi. These qualities represent, respectively, a progression from qi stagnation (Taut) to heat from excess (Tense), and finally to stages of yin deficiency (Tight, Wiry) and blood deficiency (Thin). The Wiry quality should also be an alert signal for either abdominal pain, early hypertension, or diabetes, especially if the proximal positions are also Wiry.

Blood Unclear; Blood Heat; Blood Thick; Tense Hollow Full-Overflowing

These are all signs of toxicity in the blood and in the Liver, which stores the blood, with increasing amounts of heat from excess. The reader is referred to Chapter 13 for a more complete discussion of these qualities.

Slippery

Mild Slipperiness at the qi depth in this position, with a Slow rate, signifies only slight Liver qi deficiency. With a more Rapid rate it could indicate elevated blood sugar. At the blood depth, Slipperiness is usually associated with the turbulence in the blood caused by toxic conditions in the Liver and blood. At the organ depth, Slipperiness is found with Liver infection and, more rarely, with concurrent Gallbladder infection. According to Dr. Shen, the Slippery quality at all depths at the left middle position is a sign of general qi deficiency. I am unable to confirm this in my own experience, but I do find Slipperiness at all depths at the left middle position to be a strong sign of infection, including parasites, subclinical chronic hepatitis, or chronic mononucleosis.

Spreading

The Spreading quality at this position is a sign of Liver qi deficiency and early Liver blood deficiency.

Reduced Substance

This quality, defined in Chapter 8, is here a sign of mild Liver qi deficiency. It is found with increasing frequency.

Yielding Partially Hollow

At the left middle position this is a sign of mild blood deficiency. Usually the Hollowness at the blood depth is partial, with separation on pressure, rather than a total absence of sensation.

Tense Inflated

This quality is associated here with a recent episode of great but repressed anger.

Empty

The Empty quality is a sign that the yin and yang of the Liver have separated. This is an indication of chaos in the Liver with progressive Liver qi and yang deficiency, the separation of Liver yin and yang, and increasing vulnerability to lymphomas and tumors.

In our times the Empty quality is found at this position after the chronic use of cooling drugs such as marijuana, with chronic subclinical lingering hepatitis and mononucleosis, and with chronic parasites. Less often it can be found when one has worked beyond one's energy over a long period of time. (Dr. Shen also mentioned "sadness," which is outside of my experience with this quality.)

LESS COMMON QUALITIES AT LEFT MIDDLE POSITION

Change in Qualities and Intensity

These are also signs that the yin and yang have separated in the Liver, leaving that organ highly vulnerable to the chaotic forms of Liver disease, such as cancer.

Diffuse

The Diffuse quality described in Chapter 8 is found at this position more frequently than at any other, and is a sign of moderate Liver qi deficiency, often in combination with Liver blood and sometimes yin deficiency.

Vibration and Choppy

Smooth Vibration at this position is a sign of moderate Liver qi deficiency. A mild or moderate Rough Vibration is a sign of parenchymal damage and perhaps Liver qi deficiency. In this position a Choppy quality, which indicates blood stagnation in the Liver, can be confused with a very Rough Vibration. With blood stagnation and the Choppy quality in the Liver position, one usually finds the Liver Engorged position as a confirming sign.

Muffled and Dead

These qualities are described in Chapter 8. Each time that I have felt the Muffled quality it has been associated with a malignant neoplastic process, and each time I have felt the Dead quality at the left middle position it has indicated an advanced or terminal cancer of the liver or bile ducts.

Flooding Excess and Robust Pounding

At the left middle position, Flooding Excess, a sign of internal heat from excess, usually accompanied by Robust Pounding and a Rapid rate, is a sign of a fulminating liver infection such as hepatitis or mononucleosis.

Floating Tight

A Floating Tight quality at the left middle position has been found with internal Liver wind. This may be accompanied by wind in the channels and is a precursor sign to serious vascular accidents such as stroke.

Leather-like Hollow

If the rate is Rapid, this quality is a sign of impending hemorrhage from the Liver; if the rate is Slow, it represents a recent hemorrhage. The Hollowness is absolute rather than separating at the blood depth, and hospital emergency room evaluation is immediately required.

COMMON COMBINATIONS AT THE LEFT MIDDLE AND OTHER POSITIONS

Left middle and left distal

Refer to the left distal positions in this chapter.

Left middle and right distal

Refer to the right distal positions in this chapter.

Left middle and right middle

Refer to Table 14-1 "Uniform qualities bilaterally at same position" in Chapter 14 for these combinations.

Left middle and left proximal

Deep Wiry

This combination is found with early hypertension or diabetes.

Tense Hollow Full-Overflowing

This combination is found in advanced hypertension or advanced diabetes.

Left middle with left distal and proximal

When the left middle position is Taut to Tense and Inflated, with both left distal and proximal positions being Feeble-Absent, and the right side is Normal, this indicates a Kidney/Heart disharmony. It can also be found with a stagnant middle burner, although this pattern is more commonly found bilaterally.

Left middle and right proximal

A Tense left middle position with a Tight right proximal position can indicate difficulty with urination due to the Liver qi attacking downward to the Bladder, causing urethral spasm with hesitancy. This would occur when there is considerable Liver qi stagnation and weak Bladder or Kidney qi. Constrained Liver qi will attack the most vulnerable organ.

GALLBLADDER POSITION

This position is found at approximately the first interphalangeal joint by laying the right middle finger medially and proximally along and on top of the radial artery, between the left middle and proximal positions. The principal qualities here are Tense, Tight, Wiry, Slippery, Inflated, Pounding, Choppy, Change in Intensity, and Muffled. The Tense and Tight qualities are almost always found in combination with the Slippery quality.

Tense Slippery

This is the most common combination to be found at this position and is a sign of damp-heat in the Gallbladder, usually without any symptoms of Gallbladder dysfunction.

Tight Slippery

This is the second most common combination at this position and is a sign of stone formation and greater inflammation, probably with some digestive symptoms such as discomfort after meals, gas, and bloating. It is in the later stages of the inflammatory process when there is acute infection that one will find Robust Pounding.

Inflated

This occurs with trapped heat in the Gallbladder, a sign of progression in the infectious process, and of increased pressure within the Gallbladder due to trapped qi and heat.

Muffled; Wiry; Change in Intensity; Choppy

I have found these qualities at the Gallbladder position when the gallbladder itself has many stones, severe infection, and especially if it is close to, or is already, necrotic. The Muffled quality is most often associated with tumor formation. In one case that I recall, it was also found at the left middle position with cancer of the bile ducts. The Wiry quality usually attends severe pain as well as necrosis.

Gallbladder-Heart deficiency

The left distal position is Thin and Deep and the Gallbladder position is Tense and Slippery. Symptoms include timidity, dizziness, blurred vision, palpitations, sighing, excessive dreams, easily frightened, and a quick temper. (See Chapter 15.)

LIVER ENGORGEMENT POSITIONS

When Liver blood is moderately stagnant beyond just heat in the blood, these positions will be present. The morphological liver itself is not necessarily physically enlarged.

Distal Engorgement

The Distal Engorgement position is located in the area between the left distal and left middle positions, otherwise known as the left Diaphragm position. The presence of Distal Engorgement of the Liver is discernible when the proximal aspect of the left Diaphragm position is either more Inflated or Rougher than the distal aspect.

Ulnar Engorgement

Finding the radial artery with the middle finger on the left middle position, one rolls the finger very superficially in the ulnar direction searching for another distinctly different impulse coming to the area between the extreme tip of the finger and the nail, from between the flexor carpal radialis tendon and the radial artery. The quality is almost always Inflated. There should be no pulse at this position, but if a distinct Inflated quality is present, one can say that there is Ulnar Engorgement of the Liver.

Radial Engorgement

Rolling the finger from the radial artery at the left middle position in the radial direction, one looks for another separate impulse from the main artery, almost along the radial bone. If present, it is usually rather Thin and a little hard, though sometimes Vibrating. There should be no pulse at this position, but if it is found, one can say that there is Radial Engorgement of the Liver.

LIVER QI 'ATTACKS'

Liver qi is the moving qi of the body, the 'free wanderer.' When Liver qi stagnates (pulse Tense, or rarely, Inflated) it will eventually escape from the Liver, although not through regular channels. Instead, it will tend to 'attack' the most vulnerable organ. Best known is when it attacks the Spleen-Stomach. However, the Lungs, Intestines, and Bladder, and less often the Heart (palpitations at rest), are also well known destinations of this random, unpredictable qi.

Right Middle Position

YANG ORGAN (STOMACH) OCCUPIES PRINCIPAL POSITION

The question is raised as to why, in Dr. Shen's scheme, the only yang organ to occupy a principal position is the Stomach, while all the others occupy complementary positions.

The answer is, simply, experience.

My own experience varies slightly from that of Dr. Shen's in that I find that qualities over the entire right middle position, such as Tense and Tight, which suggest stagnation and heat, are more closely related to the Stomach function, while those representing deficiency, such as Feeble-Absent and Empty, are signs of Spleen qi deficiency. If we have only one or the other, the entire right middle position will be dominated by that quality. Tense-Tight, Pounding, and even Inflated qualities indicate Stomach qi stagnation and heat, while Deep, Feeble-Absent, or Empty qualities indicate Spleen qi deficiency.

If both Stomach heat and Spleen qi deficiency exist simultaneously, there will be a Tense-Tight Pounding and Inflated quality at the more radial Stomach position, and an Inflated quality discernible when one rolls the finger medially to the Spleen position; or even more often, a Change in Qualities between Tense-Tight, Pounding, and Inflated on the one hand, and either Feeble, Reduced Substance, or Empty on the other.

The Stomach position is evaluated in conjunction with the Intestine positions. Heat from excess and abdominal pain often involve the Stomach and one or both of the Intestines similarly and simultaneously.

STOMACH DISORDERS AND THE RIGHT MIDDLE POSITION

'Sour Stomach'

The pulse quality is often Tense, Hollow, and/or Slippery, and slightly Inflated. The Slippery quality is found at the qi depth if the hyperacidity is less severe, and the Hollow quality is also found if it is more severe. If the Slippery quality is found at the organ depth and is a little Tight there is infection, probably also in the pylorus and in the Small Intestine. The tongue may be slightly red with random cracks in the middle area.

Actually, the right middle position is rarely Slippery. During my visit to clinics in China, and acupuncture schools in the United States, I have found that practitioners and teachers alike confuse the Cotton quality and Separating qualities with the Slippery quality. The consequence of Spleen qi deficiency is a damp condition which is more often seen in the Gallbladder, Lung, and Heart positions than in the Spleen position itself. The body's reaction to Stomach heat is to bring fluid to the middle burner, and this damp-heat is reflected primarily in the Gallbladder position as a Tense Slippery quality.

Dr. Shen used the term 'sour' with regard to Stomach conditions. In biomedical terms, he means excess hydrochloric acid, and in Chinese medical terms, stagnant qi. That accumulation is equivalent to excess hydrochloric acid. He associated this phenomenon with the Liver attacking the Stomach-Spleen, or with qi stagnation following physical labor during or soon after eating, and with sitting in one position for long periods of time.

Stomach, pyloric, and duodenal ulcers

The quality associated with stomach, pyloric, or duodenal ulcers is always Slippery and Hollow, and is usually Tight. More often the Stomach-Pylorus Extension position will reflect these qualities. However, there can be a Stomach ulcer with either heat from excess or from Stomach-Spleen qi deficiency. With the former, the pulse is Slippery Hollow Tight-Wiry, and with the latter, Slippery Deep Feeble.

If the ulcer is not serious, the quality is more Tight and Slippery, and the tongue has a patchy coating with many cracks in the middle. If the ulcer is serious and a slow bleeder, the pulse quality tends to be first Partially Hollow, and later Leather-like Hollow and a little Robust Pounding, as well as Slippery. The Rapid Leather-like Hollow quality is a sign of impending bleeding. The Leather-like Hollow and Slow quality is a sign of recent bleeding. With this condition the Hollow quality is absolute, with no sensation at all at the blood depth, rather than just separating on pressure.

More rarely, a Choppy quality can be encountered at this position with a bleeding ulcer. The tongue is moderately to severely red, with cracks in the middle and sides and no coating.

Stomach fire

Full-blown Stomach fire is usually attended by a Robust Pounding, Tense to Tight Flooding Excess quality. Symptoms are subcostal pain intensified by eating, heartburn, great thirst for cold beverages, constant hunger and heavy food consumption, bad breath, chapped lips, constipation, sour regurgitation, and gingivitis. This approaches a yang brightness disorder. The tongue is red with a thick, yellow, dry coating.

Work habits, emotional disturbances, eating habits, and digestion

Irregular eating, emotional disturbances, and mental or physical work engaged in during and soon after meals, have an important effect on digestion. The associated pulse qualities will depend on the individual's overall physical condition, the length of the habit and the age it started, and the amount of work in which one engages, or the degree of emotional stress. If work or emotional stress occurs during meals it tends to affect the esophagus. Emotional stress or work performed immediately after meals will usually affect the Stomach, then the duodenum after about an hour, and the Intestines after that. The symptoms are typically abdominal pain, bloating, and gas, affecting the esophagus least and the Stomach the most.

Reduced Substance

This quality is discussed in Chapter 8. At this position it is a sign of Spleen qi deficiency.

Flat; Inflated; Deep; Feeble-Absent; Empty

Resuming physical labor immediately after eating, lifting after eating, sitting in a bent position for long periods of time, trauma, anorexia and bulimia, and thinking excessively while eating are some of the events which will deplete Stomach-Spleen qi.

The Flat quality is usually associated with the early stages of this etiology in a more deficient physical condition, and an Inflated quality in a more robust condition. Both are signs of 'trapped' qi and heat in the Stomach. With the Flat quality the qi is trapped outside and cannot get into the Stomach-Spleen. With the Inflated quality the qi is trapped inside.

When the habit is of long duration, or especially excessive, or if there is severe deficiency of the 'digestive system' or of the individual generally, the pulse will be Feeble-Absent or Empty due to the depletion of Stomach-Spleen qi in its efforts to overcome the stagnation.

Tense-Tight

Eating too quickly due to constant emotional tension and pressure, either externally or internally driven, will give rise to the Tense-Tight quality at this position, indicating qi stagnation and heat from excess and deficiency. With heat from excess, there may also be Pounding. Over time the Slippery and Hollow qualities associated with ulcer formation will often accompany the Tense-Tight quality.

COMBINATIONS OF THE RIGHT MIDDLE AND OTHER POSITIONS

Right middle and left middle

Refer to Table 14-1 "Uniform qualities bilaterally at same position" in Chapter 14.

Right middle and left distal

Refer to the left distal position.

Right middle and right distal

Refer to the right distal position.

Right middle and left proximal

Deep; Feeble-Absent; Empty

These qualities at the left proximal position will often be accompanied by the same qualities at the right proximal position. Usually this indicates that constitutional Kidney qi or yang deficiency has led over time to Spleen qi or yang deficiency. The degree of deficiency will also depend on eating habits. However, as with the current epidemic of anorexia/bulimia, the Spleen yang deficiency may occur first and be found in very young people, depending on the individual's original constitution.

Tight

The Tight quality at these two positions simultaneously indicates that Kidney yin deficiency is associated with yin deficiency of the Stomach, the end result of heat from excess due to the ill effects of poor long-term eating habits, either too fast, too much, or both.

Right middle and right proximal (or distal)

Feeble-Absent

The appearance of this quality at these two (or three) positions simultaneously is a sign of irregular eating habits and a deficient 'digestive system,' as well as simultaneous Kidney qi-yang and Spleen qi-yang deficiency, described above.

Tight

This quality is a sign of eating too rapidly.

Right middle position and over entire left side

When the entire left side is Feeble-Absent and the right middle position is Robust, the implication is that, even though the 'organ system'[5] is depleted, the 'digestive system' is strong enough to sustain the person because nutrition is good and the nutritive qi and stored qi can be renewed.

When the entire right side is Reduced and the left side is Robust, this is a sign that, despite a deficient 'digestive system,' which is probably due to poor eating habits, the individual began life with a strong constitution.

COMPLEMENTARY POSITIONS OF RIGHT MIDDLE POSITION

Esophagus position

QI STAGNATION

Location — The presence of esophageal qi stagnation is discernible when the proximal aspect of the right Diaphragm position is either more Inflated, Rougher, or Tighter than the distal aspect. A Slippery quality instead of the Rough quality is a sign of esophageal food stagnation. If the body is deficient, the Yielding aspect of the Inflated quality will be greater, which is a sign of a loss of tone in the walls of the esophagus.

Interpretation — This condition is often due to habitual obsessive thinking or repeated emotional stress while eating, although one major episode of emotional shock while eating could give rise to the same condition. It is sometimes confused with angina and heart attack. Heavy lifting while eating, or bulimia, are other possible etiologies.

REBELLIOUS STOMACH QI

Qi stagnation in the esophagus sometimes occurs with rebellious Stomach qi with signs of burping, nausea, and especially vomiting. This condition overlaps with food stagnation and regurgitation.

FOOD STAGNATION AND REGURGITATION

At times, when the Inflated quality at the Diaphragm position can be felt coming equally from both directions, one can also encounter simultaneously another quality, usually a Tight and/or Slippery Roughness, as one rolls the finger distally from the right middle position. This means that, in addition to the presence of diaphragmatic qi stagnation, we have greater spasm and food stagnation in the esophagus. Qi stagnation in the esophagus will, over time, lead to food stagnation.

This pulse picture is compatible with regurgitation, which also occurs with Spleen qi deficiency (without vomiting) and Liver qi stagnation (with vomiting). This is an increasingly serious medical issue with the increase in the occurrence of Barrett's syndrome and adenocarcinoma of the esophagus. Finding this pulse can lead to early diagnosis and treatment.

Spleen Position

The Spleen complementary position is accessed by rolling one's finger very superficially and medially toward the ulna, over the right middle position. An Inflated quality at this position at the extreme tip of the middle finger is a sign of Spleen qi deficiency. On rare occasions I have found a Tight quality here in the presence of a Stomach ulcer, usually in combination with other qualities at the main position and/or at the Stomach-Pylorus Extension position.

It is my impression that in the progression of Spleen qi deficiency, the presence of a pulse at the Spleen complementary position suggests a milder degree of deficiency than when the Deep, Feeble-Absent, Empty, and Change in Qualities and Intensity are found over the entire position. The presence of a pulse at the Spleen position might even suggest a vulnerability—rather than an active deficiency—due to underlying Kidney qi or yang deficiency.

Stomach-Pylorus Extension position

If, as one rolls the middle finger medially, laying the distal interphalangeal joint proximally along and on top of the radial artery, beyond the most proximal part of the right middle position, there is a Change in Quality to that of Yielding Inflated, this probably indicates a stomach prolapse. The prolapse may not be discernible by x-ray or ultrasound, but the individual will have abdominal discomfort several hours after eating, insomnia after the evening meal, and will be tired in the morning. The cause is usually Spleen qi deficiency with the specific loss of the Spleen qi's lifting function.

Occasionally, with inflammation or ulcer of the lower stomach, pylorus, and duodenum, the pulse at this position will be Tight-Wiry Biting Slippery and even Hollow, as well as possibly Inflated and Choppy. A Leather-like Hollow quality at this position is a danger sign of hemorrhage, usually from a bleeding ulcer.

Peritoneal Cavity (Pancreas) position

The simultaneous presence of both the Spleen and Ulnar Engorgement positions should alert one to the presence of pathology in the pancreas, such as pancreatitis or a pancreatic tumor, and/or in the peritoneum, such as peritonitis, tumor, or ascites. A less auspicious pulse sign associated with these conditions is the presence of very similar qualities at the left and right middle positions.

Duodenum

If there are qualities indicating pathology in the Stomach-Pylorus Extension position, and the same qualities appear at the Small Intestine position, we probably have a similar pathology in the duodenum.

Proximal Positions

GENERAL INFORMATION

Depth and root

Root refers to the Kidney position. Because the Kidneys are associated with the foundational basal energy of the body, if their pulse has some strength, the body has root. This implies a greater resistance to disease, or, if a disease has occurred, that the prognosis will be better.[6] According to another source, "Root means there is strength in the deep position. This has two interpretations, the first says that there is some pulse in the deep position; or it can mean the third position is there, basically meaning that the Kidney has energy."[7]

Townsend and DeDonna explain it this way:

> [I]f the Root is in good condition, the Deep level pulse at the Chi position should be clean and reasonably forceful, with a feeling of intrinsic strength and slight elasticity. Now press the pulse more deeply still until it nearly vanishes. The pulse

should disappear slowly as pressure is increased, with a hint of pulse still present even at very deep pressure. If the pulse cuts off sharply on deepening pressure or weakens and fades very significantly, this indicates a weakness of the Root.[8]

On the other hand, the proximal positions are frequently described as being slightly deeper than the middle positions. Wang Ping[9] states that "It should sound deep and strong like a stone thrown." The reasons for this are not explained anywhere in the literature with which I am familiar. The fact that the Kidney is the root energy at the 'end' or bottom of the body does not seem to be a sufficient explanation, since, as I have noted elsewhere, this position, representing the foundation of all the body's qi, gets deeper with age and with abuse.

This certainly explains why the proximal positions are deeper in older people. However, a most disturbing development during the three decades that I have studied and practiced Chinese medicine is the loss of the root at younger and younger ages. I can only attribute this to the stress and pace of modern life, to pollution, fast food, sex at an early age, excessive exercise, and perhaps to the artificial birthing techniques of the past forty years. While people seem to be growing larger and stronger on the outside, they also seem to be growing weaker on the inside.

There is still another aspect to the deeper proximal positions. The Kidneys are traditionally associated with the polarities of fear and courage. Kidney qi deficiency promulgates fear, and fear affects the Kidneys because, of all the emotions, fear descends and is more likely to affect the major organ of the lower burner, the Kidneys. In its effort to cope with fear through courage, Kidney yang (the adrenal medulla) is drained.

Physiology

Kidney energy is as complex as the human central nervous system, and there are an almost infinite variety of Kidney functions, each reflecting its own aspect of that nervous system. Summing it up as Kidney yin, yang, essence, and qi is a massive oversimplification. That is why one can be missing one small aspect and still have the rest intact. How can a person born with such obvious Kidney essence deficiency as, for example, spina bifida have a powerful will, good teeth and bones, an intact endocrine system, good fertility and sexual function, and be a genius?

Kidney yin controls the pituitary, and Kidney yang controls the thyroid and basic metabolic heat. Both are involved with the adrenal gland, the medulla with Kidney yang and the cortex with Kidney yin. Any abnormal quality in this position is diagnostic of an endocrine disorder. It is also my impression that the propensity toward depression is rooted in Kidney qi, especially 'endogenous depression.'

While Kidney essence is generally associated with Kidney yin, I have found that deficiency of either Kidney yin or Kidney yang can be associated with Kidney essence deficiency. Kidney essence is, after all, the stored essence and qi of the entire organism, both from before birth and after, and is the lifelong source of yin and yang. Rather than just yin and yang, there is yin essence and yang essence; and since Kidney qi is a combination of yin and yang, we must also have Kidney qi essence. The essence is everywhere in Kidney physiology and pathology.

Origin of disharmony

This position tells us a great deal about the origin of a disorder, since the Feeble-Absent quality (Empty, Change in Intensity or Qualities) in all but the aged is usually associated with a constitutional etiology, and a Tight quality with postpartum etiology, often due to overwork of the mind and 'nervous system.' This is important in terms of how one advises the patient about self-care.

Especially if the left proximal position is Feeble-Absent (in other than the elderly), the etiology is clearly constitutional, and the individual should understand that he or she does not have the innate strength to do certain things that others can do easily, without becoming ill. I have found this to be one of the most emotionally releasing pieces of information for people who have lived a lifetime burdened by guilt and a sense of inferiority that they were not performing as they were expected to by parents and peers. They are relieved to be released from the guilt and to be able to cease performing disabling activities that enervate them and lead to symptoms and disease.

If the etiology is related to a later stage of development, one can seek for the lifestyle change that would create less stress. Changes in addictive and ego-based lifestyle patterns, such as excessive sex or work, are then the focus of treatment. In such cases, there is usually more resistance to change.

LEFT AND RIGHT PROXIMAL POSITIONS

In some of the classical literature, the left proximal position is associated with Kidney yin and the right proximal position with Kidney yang and qi. However, it is my clinical impression that deficiencies of both Kidney yin and yang can be found at either or both proximal positions, with the former accompanied by a Tight and the latter by a Feeble-Absent quality. Li Shi-Zhen concurs: "Even though the ancients say that the left chi pulse belongs to the kidney and the right chi belongs to the ming men [gate of vitality], actually the weakness or strength of the yang yuan [source] qi can be felt at both pulses."[10]

In the early stages of yin deficiency a Tight quality will appear first at the left proximal position, and as the yin deficiency grows, then also at the right proximal position. It has been my experience that if qi-yang deficiency is developing, the qualities which characterize this condition (Feeble-Absent, Empty, Change in Intensity or Qualities) will appear equally at both proximal positions.

In the early stages of a simultaneous Kidney yin and yang-qi deficiency, the yin deficiency will manifest as a Tight quality at the left proximal position, and the yang deficiency as a Feeble-Absent quality (Empty, Change in Intensity or Qualities) at the right proximal position. In the presence of both deficiencies simultaneously, the harder yin-deficient quality, Tight, might overshadow the more Yielding Reduced qualities, such as Feeble-Absent, and both proximal positions would feel Tight, especially if the yin deficiency is clearly greater than the yang-qi deficiency.

Even more often in the presence of dual conditions of Kidney qi-yang and Kidney yin deficiency I have found a Change in Qualities at one or both proximal positions, such as Tight and Absent, with constant change from one to the other.

On the other hand, but more rarely, the Feeble-Absent quality will dominate if the yang-qi deficiency is significantly greater than the yin deficiency. In chronic conditions, with either sign of deficiency manifesting, the likelihood is that both yin and yang are deficient. For example, Dr. Shen noted that systemic lupus erythematosus is a condition reflecting severe Kidney yin and qi-yang deficiency in which external cold has invaded the Kidneys, which is the most vulnerable organ when the cold invades the body. (He regarded this as a form of chronic fatigue syndrome.) Here the pulse picture is in a state of flux depending upon the stage of the disease.

If acute (or exacerbated chronic) colitis, pelvic inflammatory disease, or prostatitis should occur, the qualities in the proximal positions will take on an entirely different character—Flooding Excess, Robust Pounding, Slippery, Tight-Wiry, and Rapid—reflecting these processes, rather than the innate condition of the Kidneys. Once the acute condition passes, however, the qualities reflecting the true condition of the Kidneys will return.

Qualities commonly found at left proximal position

Tense

Invasion of external heat

A Tense quality, unless found uniformly over the entire pulse, with slight Pounding bilaterally in the proximal positions, and even in the Pelvis/Lower Body position, can be a sign of invading external heat in people who frequently walk barefoot on hot sand or rocks, or sit for long periods in scant clothing such as bathing suits. It can also be an early sign of internal heat associated with subacute pelvic area or intestinal tract infection.

Taut

'Buddha's pulse'

Long-term sexual abstinence found with monks and nuns will be noted on the pulse as a very Taut quality only in the proximal positions. This was demonstrated to me by Dr. Shen. The appearance of this quality was formerly a test in Buddhist monasteries to determine the degree of adherence to the vow of abstinence.

Tight-Wiry

Yin-essence deficiency

In this position the presence of these qualities is usually a sign of yin-essence deficiency. As mentioned above, this is associated with a disharmony which has developed after birth as a result of overwork, usually of the 'nervous system,' driving the yin organs until they become yin-deficient, dry, and function poorly. There is a feedback mechanism at work here in as much as the drying out of the body with increasing yin deficiency seems, in turn, to make the 'nervous system' more irritable.

Kidney yin-essence is the foundation of the yin of the entire body. A Tight or Wiry quality here does not bode well for the function of such other vital organs as the Heart, Liver, Stomach, and Lungs. In this position, these qualities—especially Wiry—are also associated with the early stages of hypertension and diabetes.

On the other hand, any drying process in another organ, such as the Lungs from smoking, the Stomach from eating too rapidly, the Liver from excessive use of alcohol, or the Heart from emotional stress and shock, will drain Kidney yin, since this organ stores and supplies yin to the entire body.

Pain

A Thin, Tight, and (especially) Wiry quality, sometimes Slippery at the left proximal position, with a Rapid rate, can attend a painful kidney stone. The Wiry quality often appears simultaneously with the Choppy quality in the Pelvis/Lower Body position (and more rarely, the proximal positions), indicating pain associated with blood stagnation in the lower burner and menstrual pain.

Yin deficiency turns to yang deficiency

Ultimately, yin deficiency will turn to yang deficiency when the yin can no longer nourish the yang. The increased diastolic blood pressure associated with Kidney pathology can be explained (as we have elsewhere) through the vulcanizing effect of heat from deficiency on the blood vessel walls, and the necessity of the Heart to work harder to move blood through an inelastic, narrowing circulatory system.

Cold stagnation in the lower burner

Although relatively rare, the invasion of cold from excess through the legs to the lower burner due to exposure to cold water, ice, and snow can manifest as a Tight quality in both the left and right proximal positions.

Reduced Substance

This quality is defined in Chapter 8, and here is a sign of mild Kidney qi deficiency.

Deep

The Deep quality at this position is a sign of moderate Kidney qi deficiency evolving to Kidney yang deficiency.

Feeble-Absent

Constitution, excessive sex, and heavy physical labor

While this quality is associated with severe constitutional Kidney qi deficiency at this position, it can become a sign of Kidney qi-yang and essence deficiency due to excessive sex and heavy physical labor, where the Kidneys are already vulnerable for other reasons, including constitutional. Dr. Shen associates this quality with long-term or even lifelong sadness, or what I call 'endogenous depression.' As already mentioned, it is my impression that the propensity toward all types of depression is rooted in deficiency of Kidney qi-yang and essence.

Qualities less commonly found at left proximal position

Flooding Excess; Robust Pounding; Slippery; Tight-Wiry

As mentioned above, if an acute (or exacerbation of chronic) colitis, pelvic inflammatory disease, or prostatitis should occur, the qualities in the proximal positions will be Flooding Excess, Robust Pounding, Slippery, and Tight-Wiry, with a Rapid rate. These qualities reflect these disease processes, rather than the innate condition of the Kidneys. Once the acute condition passes, the qualities that reflect the true condition of the Kidneys will return.

Empty

Rarely encountered at this position, this is a sign of the separation of Kidney yin and yang and of chaotic Kidney function. (Dr. Shen also mentioned 'nervous tension,' which is outside of my experience if found alone at this position. Instead, I have found a 'nervous system weak' condition when Kidney yin and yang separate.)

Change in Qualities and Intensity

These are increasingly common signs of the separation of Kidney yin and yang and of chaotic Kidney function attending a more serious inability to sustain the function of other organs. It is probably equivalent to a severely compromised immune system. Again, these qualities would attend a 'nervous system weak' condition.

Left proximal combined with other positions

LEFT PROXIMAL AND LEFT DISTAL

Refer to the left distal position.

LEFT PROXIMAL AND LEFT MIDDLE

Refer to the left middle position.

LEFT PROXIMAL AND RIGHT DISTAL

Refer to the right distal position.

LEFT PROXIMAL AND RIGHT MIDDLE

Refer to the right middle position.

LEFT PROXIMAL AND RIGHT PROXIMAL POSITIONS

Refer to Table 14-1 "Uniform qualities bilaterally at same position" in Chapter 14. See also the discussion above regarding the left and right proximal positions.

Large Intestine, prostate, and uterus

While the Large Intestine occupies the distal portion of this position, qualities on the left proximal position can also reflect conditions in the Large Intestine, for example, when the disease becomes acute and fulminating, or when there is a flare-up of a chronic disease, such as colitis. Likewise, fulminating prostatitis or pelvic inflammatory disease, normally confined to the left Pelvis/Lower Body area, can dominate the position. Usually the symptoms will help differentiate the cause.

RIGHT PROXIMAL POSITION

Refer to the discussion above regarding the left and right proximal positions.

Bladder position

While the right proximal position is usually associated with Kidney qi-yang, according to Dr. Shen, the position also reflects Bladder function. I have found that Bladder function becomes an issue at this position only when it is very Tight-Wiry, or when there are signs of a more acute process (Flooding Excess, Pounding, Slippery, Tight-Wiry, and a Rapid rate), in which case I will consider disharmony not only in the Bladder, but also in the Large and Small Intestines, prostate, and genital organs. The Small Intestine occupies the distal portion of this position and, under certain circumstances, fulminating afflictions of this organ can manifest over the entire proximal position. It is sometimes difficult to distinguish the two based only on the pulse. Other signs and symptoms may be necessary to make the differentiation.

Qualities commonly found at right proximal position

Tense

The Tense quality, if not a reflection of tension over the entire pulse, could at this position be an early sign of some developing, subacute heat from excess which might unfold to involve an acute inflammatory condition of the Bladder, Small Intestine, or pelvic area and organs. Tension may also be associated with external heat due to walking on hot surfaces.

Flooding Excess; Robust Pounding; Slippery; Rapid

With these qualities we have an acute fulminating inflammatory process involving damp-heat and either the Bladder, Small Intestine, or pelvic area or organs.

Tight-Wiry

Yin-essence deficiency

I have found that as a condition of heat from yin deficiency develops, if severe, it will manifest at the right proximal position simultaneously with, although following, Tightness at the left proximal position.

Pain and acute or fulminating inflammatory condition in lower burner

Tightness with Slipperiness and Robust Pounding can also indicate an acute inflammatory condition. Tightness, and especially Wiriness, at this position is often an indicator of pain in the lower burner, either musculoskeletal or in the urogenital system. The more Wiry the quality, the greater the pain.

Cold stagnation in the lower burner

Although relatively rare, the invasion of cold from excess through the legs or buttocks to the lower burner, due to exposure to cold water, ice, or snow, can manifest as a Tight quality and pain in the right and left proximal positions.

Reduced Substance

This quality is described in Chapter 8, and at this position is a sign of mild Kidney qi deficiency.

Deep

Here the Deep quality signifies moderate Kidney qi deficiency.

Feeble-Absent

Here the Feeble-Absent quality is a sign of severe qi deficiency.

Right proximal combined with other positions

RIGHT AND LEFT PROXIMAL

Refer to Table 14-1 "Uniform qualities bilaterally at same position" in Chapter 14, and to the discussion earlier in this chapter regarding the left proximal position.

RIGHT PROXIMAL AND LEFT DISTAL

Refer to the left distal position.

RIGHT PROXIMAL AND RIGHT DISTAL

Refer to the right distal position.

RIGHT PROXIMAL AND LEFT MIDDLE

Refer to the left middle position.

RIGHT PROXIMAL AND RIGHT MIDDLE AND DISTAL (ENTIRE RIGHT SIDE)

Feeble-Absent

This is a sign that the 'digestive system' is weakened by irregular eating habits.

Tight

This is a sign that the 'digestive system' is overworked from eating too rapidly.

Small Intestine, prostate, and uterus

While the Small Intestine occupies only the distal portion of the right proximal position, qualities on the right proximal position can also be signs of conditions in the Small Intestine, as when the disease in the Small Intestine becomes acute and fulminating, or when there is a flare-up of a chronic disease, such as regional enteritis. Likewise, a fulminating prostatitis or pelvic inflammatory disease, which is normally confined to the right Pelvis/Lower Body area, can dominate the position. Usually the other symptoms will help to differentiate the cause.

Large and Small Intestine Complementary Position

LOCATION

Using the medial edge of the fingertip, the ring finger is rolled distally over the proximal positions to find the Intestine position. Often the proximal positions are also Tense and Tight. To distinguish the presence of the Intestine position, one's attention is drawn to the quality of the tenseness to note a subtle change, since a Tense or Tight quality can feel more focused and Robust at the Intestine position than at a proximal position.

QUALITIES COMMONLY FOUND AT LARGE AND SMALL INTESTINE POSITIONS

These positions are always evaluated in the context of findings on the Stomach, Spleen, and middle burner complementary positions. Signs of heat from excess in the Stomach frequently are found in connection with similar signs in the Intestine positions. The relationship between some of these qualities and their associated functions is still uncertain, as indicated below.

With mild disharmony and a relatively short-term disease process, the qualities listed below are limited to the Intestine positions, as indicated by Dr. Shen. With more acute fulminating illness and flare-ups of more chronic illness, the entire left and/or right proximal positions may show these or other qualities.

Tense

The Tense quality alone is not found with any measurable degree of disharmony, although the quality is usually a sign of some qi stagnation and heat from excess. Expected, but not always found, is some tendency toward a slowing of peristalsis and constipation. Often there are no symptoms associated with this quality.

Tight

The Tight quality is found frequently with symptoms of irritation, irritability, and inflammation of the bowel. In other positions the Tight quality is a sign of yin deficiency with, as in the case of the Heart, accompanying signs of agitation. However, in Chinese medicine yin deficiency in the bowel is associated with small hard stools (constipation), while in our system of pulse diagnosis, the Tight quality in the Intestine position is associated with more frequent and loose stools.

We need to investigate a possible distinction between the two Intestines, whether the Tight quality in the Small Intestine is a sign of irritability and/or inflammation (e.g., Crohn's disease), but in the Large Intestine a sign of dryness (constipation).

Biting

The Tight quality is often accompanied by the Biting quality when there is attending abdominal cramping, discomfort, or pain.

Slippery

The Slippery quality is found here with a damp condition and symptoms of mucus in the stool and very loose stools.

Rough Vibration

Vibration at this position is a sign of significant parenchymal dysfunction of the Intestines and warrants biomedical investigation for a wide variety of often silent pathologies, including polyps and cancer, as well as less silent conditions such as diverticulitis, colitis, and symptomatic tumors.

Choppy

The Choppy quality is usually a sign of blood stagnation. Choppiness at this position is an uncertain sign. However, since it seems to indicate an even more significant dysfunction of the Intestines than does Rough Vibration, it warrants biomedical investigation for a wide variety of silent and active pathologies, including polyps and cancer, where blood stagnation may be a sign of more advanced pathology. While the blood stagnation suggested by this quality is consistent with findings of hemorrhoids, I do not have enough data to support this association, and in fact find a greater correlation between the hemorrhoids and Choppiness in the Pelvis/Lower Body positions.

Change in Intensity

Change in Intensity is another sign of chaos and significant dysfunction in the Intestines, and warrants biomedical investigation.

Robust Pounding

The Robust Pounding quality is usually found in the presence of significant inflammation of the Intestines, as with early fulminating regional enteritis or colitis.

Inflated

The Inflated quality is a sign of trapped qi or heat in the Intestines, which manifests as trapped gas and usually abdominal discomfort.

Muffled

The Muffled quality is always associated with the presence of tumors, although I have found it in the Large Intestine position with some degree of fecal impaction and loss of peristaltic activity.

PELVIS/LOWER BODY POSITION

Location

The left Pelvis/Lower Body position is palpated by laying the right ring finger along the artery medial and proximal to the left proximal position; the area of the finger that is actually used is closer to the distal interphalangeal joint. The right Pelvis/Lower Body position is palpated in the same manner, except that the practitioner uses the left ring finger.

Interpretation and conditions

This position informs us very generally about chronic conditions in the pelvis, lower back, knees, and legs, and less often about chronic fulmination conditions such as pelvic inflammatory disease, tubal pregnancy, and inflamed ovarian cyst. Primarily, it tells us about qi and blood stagnation, and stagnation of dampness in the lower part of the body and legs. This would include dysmenorrhea, endometriosis, leukorrhea, fibroids, ovarian cysts, pelvic inflammatory disease, ovarian, cervical and uterine carcinoma, prostatitis, prostatic hypertrophy, and prostatic cancer. Much more often, signs of acute pelvic inflammatory disease, such as Flooding Excess, are found at the proximal positions.

Given the current state of our knowledge, these conditions are not easily distinguished one from the other on the pulse based on the qualities listed below. We must use other forms of diagnosis to further inform our decisions, and make the appropriate referrals to medical doctors, especially gynecologists, for more complete exploration.

However, the presence of the Choppy, Change in Intensity, and especially Muffled qualities are strong indications of a serious disease process in patients with no pelvic symptoms, whose lives could be saved by prompt referral to a medical doctor and a combination of conventional and other necessary therapies. Many women find themselves with silent advanced ovarian cancer which could have been prevented by the early diagnosis afforded by a sophisticated system of pulse diagnosis. This is also true, to a lesser extent, of generally slower-growing prostate cancer in men.

Qualities

The qualities found are Tense, Tight, Wiry, Slippery, Muffled, Choppy, Robust Pounding, and Change in Intensity. The qualities in this area are not specific as to side. The Slippery quality is a sign of damp stagnation and often infection (PID, candida), and with the Choppy quality, prostatic hypertrophy in men; the Tense quality of qi stagnation and heat from excess; the Tight-Wiry quality of an inflammatory process with pain; the Robust Pounding quality of heat from excess; the Choppy quality of blood stagnation; and the Change in Intensity quality of significant parenchymal dysfunction and physiological chaos in the area. The Muffled quality is the one most often associated with tumors and carcinoma.

TRIPLE BURNER POSITION

There is no specific position for the Triple Burner system in our model of pulse diagnosis. According to Dr. Shen, its function is found in all three burners, and there is no single position for it.

I consider the Triple Burner to be a messenger or servant of the Gate of Vitality for the distribution of yuan qi—source qi or 'original breaths'—the manager and harmonizer of the water and heat functions of the body, and of the functions of the Internal Duct.[11] On a spiritual/mental level, it is the harmonizer of all relationships and acts in synchrony with the corpus collusum of the brain in balancing thoughts and emotions between the right and left brains.[12]

I assess the function of the Triple Burner by examining the relationship between the principal positions and the burners. If the qualities are generally more or less uniform, I consider the Triple Burner to be functioning well. If, on the other hand, the qualities vary considerably from position to position or burner to burner, the functioning of the Triple Burner is greatly stressed. I have found this chaos especially in cases of autoimmune disease and severe chronic fatigue syndrome. Students report associations to the right proximal position, which makes this a reasonable area for exploration. For example, one five element practitioner, treating a patient who she believed to have a Triple Burner causative factor, was unable to make any progress until she found extreme activity in the Gallbladder and right proximal positions. At this point she resolved the pulse and clinical picture by using the exit-entry points for Gallbladder and Triple Burner.

GATE OF VITALITY *(MING MEN)* POSITION

The understanding in much of the literature is of Kidney yin as the left Kidney, and Kidney yang as the right, with the Gate of Vitality associated with Kidney yang on the right side. However, on the pulse I find that the right and left sides, though not consistently corresponding to yin on the left or yang on the right, do express Kidney yin and yang physiology and pathology. And of all the arguments in the literature, that in the *Classic of Difficulties (Nan jing)*, which places the Gate of Vitality between the left and right Kidneys, is the one which is most congenial to me, primarily because I have found that treating the Governing channel in the lower burner is more relevant to spiritual/emotional issues than treating the Kidney *shu* points. Li Shi-Zhen[13] supports this view. Writing in the 16th century, he observed: "According to recent findings, ming men is located between the two kidneys."

For this reason I have begun to explore the areas between the two Kidneys on the pulse by rolling my finger toward the ulna from both left and right proximal positions, looking for the bilateral Inflation similar to that which I find at the Spleen and Liver Ulnar Engorgement positions in the presence of a pancreatic disorder.

I believe that the Gate of Vitality is the source *(yuan)* which at birth resides in the womb and issues forth the Kidney duality associated primarily with the Governing and Conception vessels, and especially the Penetrating vessel *(chong mai),* which is associated with the Kidney channel points K-21~27. These are most effective in treating spiritual/emotional issues and are closely related to the Heart-Pericardium. I was heartened to find this approach reinforced in a discussion of the subject by Larre and Rochat de la Valle.[14]

Other Complementary Positions

DIAPHRAGM POSITION

There are left and right Diaphragm positions which can occur simultaneously, but they are independent positions, so that one can occur without the other. Etiologies may coincide or be separate, as indicated below.

Location bilaterally

The left and right Diaphragm positions are considered present when the Inflated quality is accessed in both directions, by rolling the finger both proximally from the distal position and distally from the middle position. If it is felt to be coming primarily from only one or the other position, it has an additional meaning, as explained under each of the principal positions (Heart Enlarged, Pleura, distal Liver Engorgement, and Esophagus).

PHYSIOLOGY AND PATHOLOGY

Dr. Shen conceived of this position as existing "between the muscle and the skin." He felt that with time and without resolution, the pathology which resides there goes deeper, ultimately to Liver qi or esophageal qi and food stagnation. A mild Inflated quality is considered normal.

LITERATURE

In apparent agreement with Dr. Shen, Larre et al. make the following observations about the significance of the diaphragm:

> Wei [protective] energy plays a role in the functioning of the diaphragm, at the level of the mesenteric formation of the thorax and the belly, and it has a connection with the organs. The texts say that 'the wei energy warms the diaphragm.' The diaphragm and the ensemble of mesenchymatous tissues in the thorax and belly form something like a great mesenchymal curtain in those areas. The text cited should be read in the sense of an optimum metabolic activity allowing the defense processes to play to their maximum capacity, especially the lymphatic defenses that are an inherent aspect of wei energy.... The Chinese concept of the diaphragm is like a sac of membranes 'which undulates like a curtain' uniting with the folds of the peritoneum and with the membranes of the thorax (pleura and the pericardium).... [T]he diaphragm is... also an intermediary between the thorax and the abdomen. Wei energy, therefore, has an important role in the

mesenteric defenses of the pleura and pericardium as well as of the peritoneum. These great mesenchymal curtains of the torso are tied to the three heaters.... Wei energy participates in the defense against attacks on these deep viscera.[14, 15]

Interpretation

SEPARATION

When the Inflated quality increases bilaterally, or only on the left side, in the Diaphragm position, it is usually associated with an acrimonious separation in which the tender feelings formerly felt for the lost person are repressed, and the angry feelings accentuated, in order to make the break without too much pain. Suppression of the diaphragm and breathing are somehow involved. From any single precipitating event, the Inflated quality tends to diminish over time. By five years it is much less noticeable, and is usually gone after seven to ten years.

LIFTING

If the Inflated quality increases only on the right side, the cause is probably repeated episodes of very heavy lifting beyond one's energy.

RAGE

According to Dr. Shen, the appearance of a very Inflated quality with just one episode of great unexpressed, repressed rage can occur in the Diaphragm position rather than in the left distal or middle position, especially when the Liver and Heart qi is strong. Otherwise the quality would appear at the latter two positions. Repeated episodes of rage will also inflate the Diaphragm.

HIATAL HERNIA

I have come to associate hiatal hernia with significant qi stagnation (Inflated quality) in the Diaphragm position. In the majority of people I have treated with this diagnosis, their symptoms have responded well to the treatment for relieving qi stagnation in the diaphragm. Surgery, of course, complicates the clinical recovery.

This biomedical term is ambiguous in clinical practice as a wastebasket for a wide variety of otherwise unexplainable gastrointestinal symptoms, even without clear x-ray evidence for it. It is hard to say how many surgical interventions to repair the hernia are based on hard evidence or have positive outcomes, but certainly in my practice no one benefited from the surgery—or they would not have consulted me.

MUSCULOSKELETAL POSITIONS

I have noted that the Contemporary Chinese Pulse Diagnosis system emphasizes the organs. However, by rolling the fingers to the radial side of the area between the burners, one can detect musculoskeletal disorders. I have tended to ignore these positions while practicing and teaching since the practitioner is usually well aware of these patients' pain and discomfort, which they are only too eager to communicate. It has been my inclination to save our talents as pulse diagnosticians for the less obvious disorders.

The pulse is usually very Tight-Wiry when there is musculoskeletal pathology. The Tight-Wiry quality in these positions is also a sign of pain. Above and radial to the distal positions we can access the neck. Radial to the area between the distal and middle positions we can access the shoulder-arm area. Radial to the area between the middle and proximal positions we can access the hip, and radial to the area between the proximal and Pelvis/Lower Body positions, the knees.

CHAPTER 13

The Three Depths and Common Qualities Found Uniformly over the Entire Pulse

CONTENTS

Introductory Remarks, 457
    Classification and organization, 457
        Fig. 13-1: The three depths, 458
        The three-depth and two-depth models, 458
            Interpretation of the three depths, 459
        Fig. 13-2: The eight depths, 459
        The eight-depth model, 459
        Projection of the organ system on the radial pulse, 460
        Relationship between the harder and more pliable qualities, 460
        Yin qi and yang qi at the organ depth, 460
            Pliable and fluid qualities, 461
            Harder qualities, 461
    Etiology of disharmonies, 461
        Qi stagnation and pulse types, 462
            Physiology of qi stagnation and the pulse types, 462
        Qi deficiency and the pulse types, 463
Qualities Found Simultaneously at All Positions and the Three Depths, 463
    The Normal pulse, 464
    Stability and activity (rhythm and rate), 464
        Rhythm, 465
        Rate, 465
        Circulation, 465
            Qi and blood circulation affecting each other, 466
                Qi affecting blood circulation, 466

Circulation affecting qi and blood, 467
Change in Intensity over the entire pulse and circulation, 468
Blood circulation and the Heart, 468
Qi circulation and the Liver, 468
Stability, 468
Change in Quality, 469
Change in Intensity, 469
Empty Interrupted or Yielding Hollow Interrupted, 469
Yielding Hollow Full Overflowing, 469
Qualities at Each of the Three Depths and Above the Qi Depth, 469
Depths and consciousness, 470
Above the qi depth, 470
Excess above the qi depth, 470
Qi stagnation, 470
Yielding (pliable) sensations above the qi depth, 470
Cotton ('sad pulse'), 470
Floating, 471
Floating Yielding and slightly Rapid, 471
Yielding Hollow Full-Overflowing, 472
Hard sensations above the qi depth, 472
Tense Hollow Full-Overflowing, 472
Flooding Excess, 472
Floating Tense and slightly Slow, 472
Floating Tight, 472
Floating Slippery, 472
Qi depth, 472
Qi stagnation, 473
Taut, 473
Tense, 473
Tense qualities appearing uniformly over the entire pulse, 474
Tense Long, 474
Tense Robust Pounding, 474
Etiology of Tense qualities over the entire pulse, 474
Emotional repression and metabolic disorders, 474
Febrile disorder, 474
Acute anxiety, 474
'Nervous system tense', 474
Stimulants and medications, 474
Robust Pounding and Bounding with Rapid rate, 474
Tense Robust Pounding Suppressed, 474
Robust Pounding at organ depth, 475
Bean (Spinning), 475
Trapped qi, 475
Inflated, 475
Fluid stagnation, 475
Slippery, 475
Agitation at qi depth, 475
Qi deficiency, 476
Yielding (pliable), 476
Diminished Feeble or Absent at qi depth, 476
Yielding Reduced Pounding, 476

    Flooding Deficient, 477
   Yin deficiency, 477
    Tight and Thin at qi depth, 477
Blood depth, 477
Fig. 13-3: Progression of Heat and Toxicity in the Blood, 478
  Blood excess, 478
   Blood stagnation, 478
    Slowed and impaired blood circulation in the tissues and body cavities, 478
     Choppy, 478
     Very Tense Inflated, 479
    Impaired blood circulation in the blood vessels, 479
     Blood Unclear (turbid blood), 479
      Fig. 13-4: Blood Unclear quality, 480
     Blood Heat, 480
      Fig. 13-5: Blood Heat quality, 481
     Blood Thick (exuberant blood), 481
      Fig. 13-6: Blood Thick quality, 482
     Tense Hollow Full-Overflowing, 482
     Slippery, 482
      Fig. 13-7: Tense Hollow Full-Overflowing quality, 483
     Rough Vibration, 483
     Ropy, 483
      Tense Ropy, 483
      Yielding Ropy, 484
  Blood deficiency, 484
   Thin, 484
   Spreading (on pressure), 484
   Absence of the blood and qi depths: Deep, 484
   Yielding partially Hollow, 484
  Instability of blood (blood out of control), 484
   Leather-like Hollow, 484
   Very Tense or Tight Hollow Full-Overflowing, 485
Organ depth, 485
  Stagnation at the organ depth, 486
   Qi stagnation from excess, 486
    Taut-Tense, 486
    Hidden Excess, 486
   Phlegm, food, qi, and/or blood stagnation, 487
   Qi stagnation from deficiency, 487
    Trapped qi, 487
    Flat, 487
   Blood stagnation, 487
    Choppy, 487
   Dampness (stagnation of fluids), 487
    Damp-heat, 487
    Damp-cold, 488
  Heat from excess at the organ depth, 488
   Unconstrained heat, 488
    Flooding Excess, 488
  Deficiency at the organ depth, 488
   Blood deficiency, 488

Thin Yielding, 488
  Thin Tight, 489
Yin and essence depletion, 489
  Tight, 489
  Wiry, 489
Qi and yang deficiency, 490
  Yin and yang in contact, 490
    Short Yielding, 490
    Deep, 490
    Deep Reduced Substance, 490
    Deep Separating, 490
    Feeble-Absent, 490
    Hidden Deficient, 491
  Separation of yin and yang (yin and yang out of contact), 491
    Empty, 491
    Leather, 492
    Empty Thread-like (soggy), 492
    Scattered, 492
    Minute, 493
    Yielding Hollow Full-Overflowing, 493
    Empty Interrupted-Intermittent, Yielding Hollow Interrupted-Intermittent, 493

Conclusion, 493

CHAPTER 13

The Three Depths and Common Qualities Found Uniformly over the Entire Pulse

A significant part of the first day's practicum of my course in pulse diagnosis is devoted to the identification of the various depths, which are accessed by the most subtle movement of the wrist. This exercise is constantly reinforced in succeeding seminars. Unless this technique is mastered, the information coming through the fingers concerning another person's well-being is unreliable within the model of Chinese medicine to which this book subscribes.[1] The sensations and interpretations of each quality that comprise the substance of this book are applicable only if these depths are correctly accessed.

Physiologically, the principal three depths — qi, blood, and organ (Fig. 13-1) — represent the condition of the qi, blood, and the yin and essence of the organs. Qi is the lightest and rises; it is felt at the most superficial or qi depth. Blood is somewhat heavier and is found at the middle depth. Yin is the heaviest and is thus detected at the innermost yin organ depth. The pulse typically feels the thinnest and lightest at the qi depth, becoming increasingly heavier as the fingers press down through the blood depth, and then feeling widest and heaviest with increased resistance at the organ depth. Any other progression in either direction is a sign of abnormality.

Introductory Remarks

CLASSIFICATION AND ORGANIZATION

For teaching purposes, arbitrary decisions are made in this chapter with regard to classification of pulse qualities. Many qualities, such as Slipperiness, can be accessed simultaneously at more than one depth. Therefore, in discussing the pulses, repetition of some of the qualities is unavoidable. Moreover, many of the qualities are more fully described elsewhere in the text (see pulse index).

Qi stagnation and the progression of qi deficiency can often involve both the qi depth and the organ depth, and the progression of yin deficiency can be felt at all depths. Blood deficiency can be associated, for example, with either yin deficiency or qi deficiency, more often one or the other. These facts should be kept in mind while studying the following material in which artificial distinctions are made for the sake of instructional clarity.

Furthermore, in this chapter we are departing from our primary classification of qualities according to sensation and are organizing the material by *interpretation*. At this juncture, we are less interested in identification of a quality and more concerned with emphasizing the *significance* of the quality when found over large segments of the pulse.

Finally, the presentation of the qualities in this chapter is extremely abbreviated. For a full discussion of each, readers are directed to the specific sections of the book that deal with the individual pulse qualities.

Fig. 13-1 The three depths

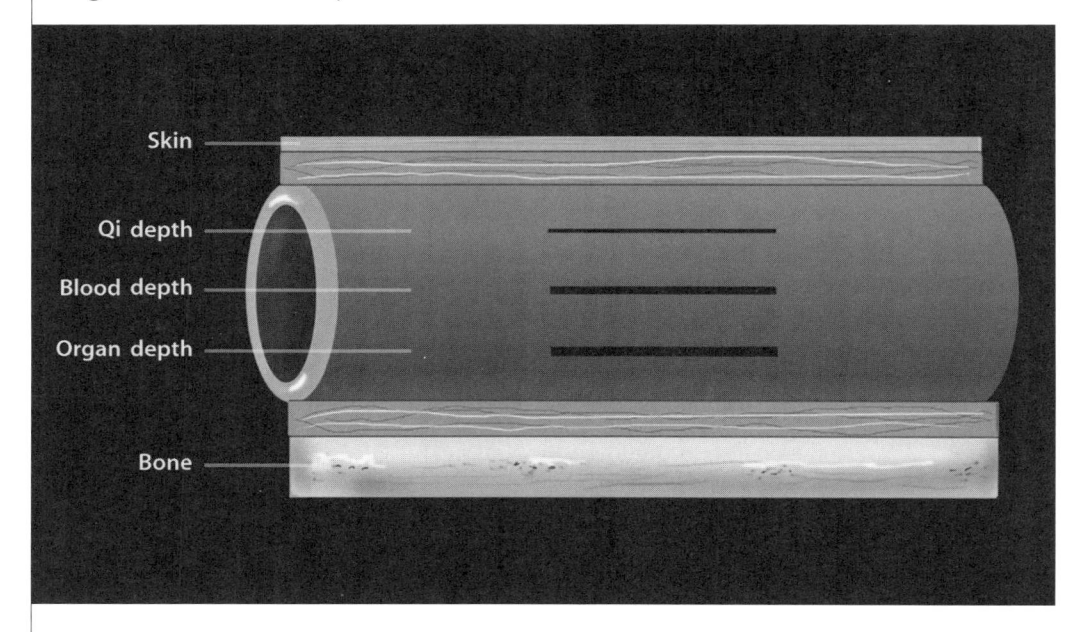

THE THREE-DEPTH AND TWO-DEPTH MODELS

The method of reading the pulse at three depths, which is followed by Dr. Shen and by practitioners in China, yields information that is unavailable through the two-depth system, which simply differentiates between superficial yang and deep yin organs. The diagrams in the Li Shi-Zhen,[2] Kaptchuk,[3] and Cheung and Belluomini[4] source materials all resemble Fig. 13-1 and reflect the widespread use of the three-depth model.

Kaptchuk describes palpation of the three depths as follows:

> The pulse is palpated at three levels of pressure: superficial, middle, and deep. At the first, or superficial, level, the skin is lightly touched. At the second, or middle, level, a moderate amount of pressure is applied. At the third, or deep, level, the physician presses quite hard.... Twenty-eight basic pulses can be felt at three levels in three positions and on two wrists.[5]

Matsumoto and Birch provide further elaboration:

> The nine diagnoses are the floating, middle, and deep depths of the three positions.... There are five relative depths to the pulse corresponding to the Five Elements. The *Nan Ching* differentiates these depths by 'beans of pressure.' The beans of pressure are degrees of pressure applied by the fingers which describe the relative depth.[6]

They go on to describe how these depths are arrived at, and to some extent, what they imply.

Interpretation of the three depths

Palpation of the superficial depth over the entire pulse (all three positions on both wrists) measures the protective and nutritive qi, and the activity of the nervous system, in the body as a whole. It also reflects these same aspects of an individual organ when felt at a single position. In addition, it is generally accepted that the middle depth reflects the blood of the organism, or of a particular organ. The deepest depth provides signs of yin (or parenchyma) of the yin organs. In fact, each of the depths reflects qi, blood, and yin to some extent, however, one of these aspects will predominate at any one depth, as indicated. Especially at the organ depth, the most skilled pulse reader can distinguish with his or her fingers among the most superficial qi, the middle blood, and the deepest yin aspect of this depth.[7]

The idea of the three depths can be traced to antiquity. According to Hua Shou in his commentary to the *Classic of Difficulties (Nan jing)*:

> Heart [with the] lung are both at the surface, that [the movement in the vessels associated with the] kidneys and [with the] liver are both in the depth, and the spleen represents the central region.[8]

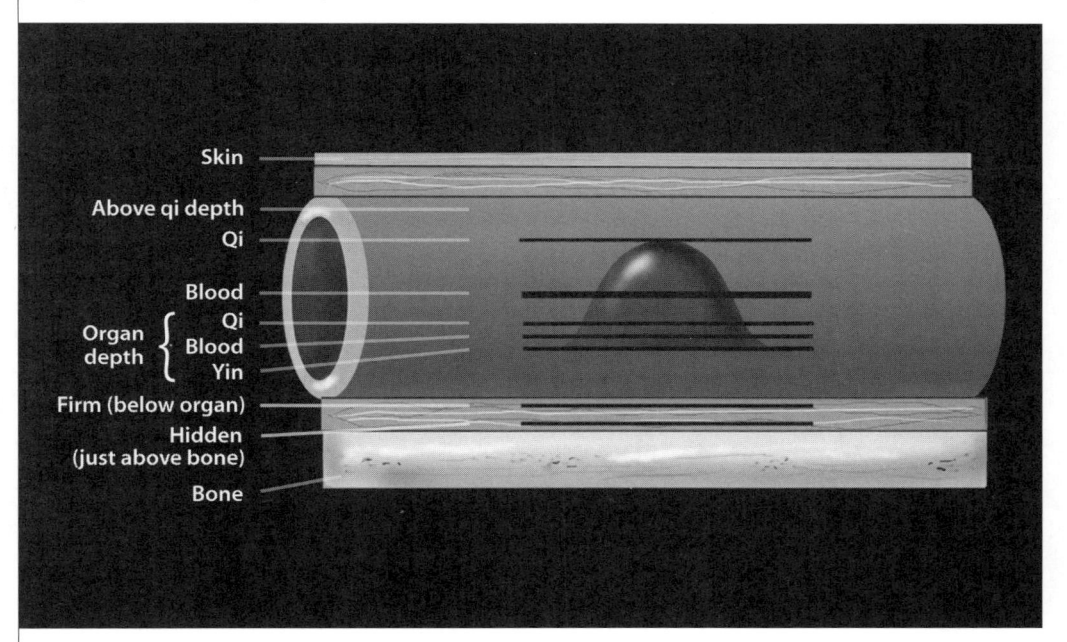

Fig. 13-2 The eight depths

THE EIGHT-DEPTH MODEL

Although the classical literature describes either two or three depths, in fact there are more. In our system there are eight depths, or vertical levels (see Fig. 13-2): above the qi depth, the qi depth, the blood depth, and three levels within the organ depth which correspond to the qi, blood, and yin (parenchyma) of the yin organ itself, and the Firm and Hidden depths below the organ depth. The qi and blood depths of any yin organ represent the organ's contribution to the total qi and blood of the organism. The three levels within the organ depth represent its own internal function. However, teaching and learning the basic three depths is hard enough without introducing a discipline which may discourage even the most hardy.

PROJECTION OF THE ORGAN SYSTEM ON THE RADIAL PULSE

The representation of the physiology of qi, blood, yin, and essence on the pulse is not an exact reflection of the actual physiological state of the organism at that moment. There is a lag between the two, often of a significant period of time. The pulse presents a pathological picture that always appears somewhat worse than the reality. This lag holds true until the pulses associated with impending death appear, when the pulse signs and the reality are finally unified.

A set of correlations has been recognized between what is palpated and what is really occurring physiologically, which we call the pulse qualities. Since these qualities are several steps *ahead* of the physiology of the organism in terms of the process of disease, the pulse serves as an instrument for prediction and prevention. The diagnostic challenge is to correctly match the sign with the fact.

It is important to realize that even with, for example, a Feeble-Absent or Empty pulse, the patient, though possibly unwell, is still functioning and therefore has a considerable reservoir of stored true qi. An Absent quality is a relative measure of yin organ deficiency and does not imply that it is entirely nonfunctional. The yin organs are still there, performing their tasks, at least well enough to sustain life. However, according to Dr. Shen, the implication of the Absent quality is that the patient will be ill within a year, and of the Empty quality that the patient will be ill within six months, if the condition is not resolved. (I find the time lag to be longer by about one to three years.) The development of most chronic diseases is a process, usually a slow one. The pulse is therefore a predictor and the foundation of a preventive medicine.

RELATIONSHIP BETWEEN THE HARDER AND MORE PLIABLE QUALITIES

In considering uniform qualities over large segments of the pulse as well as at individual positions, it should be kept in mind that the harder qualities can override the more pliable (softer) qualities when two disorders exist simultaneously and affect the same position or positions. For instance, if a disorder begins as Kidney yang deficiency, both right and left proximal positions may be Feeble-Absent. If a Kidney yin pattern develops along the way, the quality can change to Tight, masking the Kidney yang condition. However, under these circumstances, especially at the left proximal position, the pulse changes from Tight to Feeble-Absent as the finger is held at that position. Ultimately, in the most advanced chronic state, the Feeble-Absent quality will again be dominant in that position.

It is important to remember that the disorder associated with the pulse quality that is displaced still exists. When pulse signs of stagnation and heat from excess (Tense quality) change to signs of yin deficiency and heat from deficiency (Tight quality), the pattern of stagnation and heat from excess continues to exist, although it may not now be the dominant clinical consideration, which, for the sake of the organism's survival, has shifted to relieving the yin deficiency.

YIN QI AND YANG QI AT THE ORGAN DEPTH

The yin organs contain qi and blood as well as substantial yin. While it is theoretically possible, with great skill, to distinguish among qi, blood, and material yin at the organ depth, it is a difficult undertaking. The lighter, ephemeral yang qi within the yin organ tends naturally to "wander." The organ's yin seems to serve as a gravitational centripetal force, holding the expansive, centrifugally-directed yang qi in functional communication with the yin organs. When the heavier yin of the yin organs is reduced beyond a critical point and cannot hold onto, maintain contact with, and nourish the yang qi, the latter rises to the qi depth and produces the Empty pulse qualities. When the yang is too deficient to push the yin, the result is the same. With either process, the outcome is a state in which the 'qi is wild.' The expression 'wild' in relation to qi indicates the most severe state of depletion of the true qi, the qi of the entire organism. There is a hierarchy of these 'wild' states which is touched on in this chapter and explained more fully in Chapters 6 and 9.

Pliable and fluid qualities

The pliable or yielding qualities which separate and give way to pressure represent deficiency, usually of qi. Diminished or absent qi at the qi depth speaks for itself. The Spreading quality indicates advancing qi and some blood deficiency, and the Reduced Substance and Diffuse qualities are other, slightly greater, signs of qi deficiency. The Yielding Partially Hollow quality is a sign of blood deficiency, in some instances gradual hemorrhage, and in others a separation of yin and yang if the pulse is also Interrupted-Intermittent. The Deep and Feeble-Absent qualities indicate a more advanced qi deficiency.

The Empty qualities are signs of the separation of yin and yang in various degrees, and for different reasons. Leather, Empty and String-like, Scattered, and Minute pulses signify the extremes of separation between yin and yang. All are 'qi wild' pulses.

The only fluid pulse is the Slippery quality, which slides under the finger in one direction. It is confused with pulses which separate under pressure such as the Spreading, Empty, and Hollow qualities. These three qualities can be distinguished from the Slippery quality because, upon separating, the pulse feels as if it is moving in two directions, each away from the finger. By contrast, the Slippery pulse slides in only one direction.

Harder qualities

Some pulses are experienced as non-fluid and resistant to pressure, and are relatively harder to the touch. In fact, the ambiguous term 'hard' has been used indiscriminately without consideration for the nuances that I describe below, and more fully in Chapter 11. The hardness or pliability of the pulse is greatly influenced by both the amount of excess heat and the amount and availability of fluids or yin in the body, a topic that we will expand upon later.

These pulses are experienced and conceptualized in the following sequence: Floating Tense, Flooding Excess Wave, Tense Full-Overflowing, Taut, Tense, Tight, Wiry, and Ropy. The first quality represents qi stagnation at the surface. The second is a sign of deep internal heat, and the third of heat in the blood. The Taut and Tense qualities are signs of internal qi stagnation with developing heat from excess. The Tight and Wiry qualities involve some qi stagnation, some heat from excess, but primarily developing heat from deficiency (discussed below under organ-depth deficiencies). The Ropy quality is the end stage, with heat from both excess and deficiency in the blood, causing hardening of the arteries (discussed below under blood-depth qualities).

ETIOLOGY OF DISHARMONIES

Disharmony arises from two sources. The first is stagnation of substances, attributable to internal conflict, emotional resignation, inability to eliminate external pathogenic factors, trauma (physical or emotional), and deficiency.

The second is deficiency of substances, which can arise from constitutional or congenital defects, energy drains at any age due to illness, recreational drugs that are harmful to physiology (marijuana to the liver, cocaine to the heart), medications that are harmful to physiology (chemotherapy to the bone marrow—the list is endless), overwork of the body or mind, overexercise, and irregularities in living habits such as insufficient sleep and sudden cessation or onset of exercise and physical labor, and from stagnation. Hemorrhage, vomiting, sweating, and diarrhea in the extreme are other obvious drains.

Another important source of deficiency involves poor nourishment of substances, such as results from inadequate Spleen-Stomach qi, poor nutrition, irregular eating habits, eating too rapidly or while under emotional stress, sitting in a bent position or returning to work too soon after eating over a long period of time.

While this is not the appropriate venue for an in-depth discussion of most of these etiologies, we will list here the pulse qualities associated with qi stagnation, some of which do not appear in the literature but are more relevant to our times. We will also explore qi stagnation associated with internal conflict because the physiology of this etiology is also not available in the English-language literature.

Qi stagnation and pulse types

Based on Dr. Shen's ideas, I have developed a concept of qi stagnation in terms of pulse types which includes the Taut-Tense qualities, the Inflated, Flat, Cotton, Muffled, Dead, Short, Bean (Spinning), Firm, and Hidden Excess qualities, a few of which are explored in this chapter. Stagnation may be associated with excess or deficiency. All of the above distinctions are clinically relevant in terms of diagnosis, prognosis, and treatment, and are discussed more fully in Chapters 8 through 11.

Dr. Shen classifies as 'stagnant' a pulse with a diminished wave form. I use the term Flat instead, because it describes the sensation that is being considered, and because Dr. Shen has delineated several other types of stagnant conditions in addition to that associated with the Flat quality.

The condition most commonly associated with the term stagnation is reflected in the Taut and Tense pulse qualities. With these qualities there are two opposing and usually strong forces within an area or organ: the 'irresistible force' engaging the 'immovable object.' The classic example is Liver qi stagnation in which the qi wants to move and spread, but is opposed and restrained, usually by repressive emotional forces such as repressed anger and frustration.

The Inflated quality is a sign of qi or heat trapped in an area or organ in which the qi is initially robust. The Flat stagnant quality is one in which qi is unable to enter an area or organ in which the qi is deficient. The Flat and Inflated qualities can have similar etiologies, but in very different body conditions. An a priori condition of the Flat quality is reduced qi, and the a priori condition of the Inflated quality is robust qi.

The Cotton quality is a sign of profound emotional resignation, or a major physical trauma, in which the free flow of qi at the surface of the body is suppressed throughout the body, especially at the protective and qi levels of circulation. Dr. Shen calls it the 'sad pulse.' The Muffled and Dead qualities are related to potential, imminent, or present tumor formation. The Firm, Hidden-Excess, and Short-Excess qualities are associated with severe internal cold. The Short quality can also reflect qi, blood, or food stagnation between yin organs. The Bean (Spinning) quality is found with severe fright and intense pain.

PHYSIOLOGY OF QI STAGNATION AND THE PULSE TYPES

Qi is the lightest 'energy' of the body. It tends to be expansive and its form is elastic. As this energy starts to stagnate, the normal elasticity of the pulse becomes increasingly

Taut. The body's attempt to overcome this stagnation is real work. Webster defines internal work as that "resulting from the introduction of heat among the molecules of a body, as in a change in condition or an increase in temperature."[9] This strong heat, together with the stagnation that has engendered it, is reflected in the pulse by the development of a Tense quality, which has lost some of the elasticity of the Taut quality.

As the organism begins to fail in its effort to overcome the stagnation, one of two scenarios, or a combination of the two, unfolds. (The development of yin and qi deficiency described below need not necessarily begin with stagnation; it can also arise from overwork of the mind and body respectively.)

One direction is related to yin, which is fluid, and which provides the pulse with the quality of softness. One measure of the integrity of yin in the body is, therefore, the degree of hardness or softness of the pulse. Increasing hardness is noted with the loss of yin, and is accompanied by the concomitant development of heat from deficiency. (The latter is found especially when the work that one does beyond one's energy involves emotional stress and tension in the nervous system.) Another direction involves stages of increasing qi deficiency, particularly when the etiology is physical work beyond the individual's qi. Since qi is expansive and gives the feeling of an elastic resilience to pressure when it is healthy, its depletion results in less resistance to pressure, a sense of yielding, and a diminishment in form.

Where both physical and mental overwork are involved simultaneously, yin and qi deficiency often develop together, but to different degrees, depending on many factors including physical conditioning and the nature of the life experience.

Qi deficiency and the pulse types

These include Yielding or Diminished, Feeble, or Absent at the qi depth, Spreading, Diffuse, Reduced Substance, Flooding Deficient Wave, Deep, Feeble, Absent, and all of the Empty pulses (Leather, Empty and Thread-like, Scattered, Minute), Yielding Hollow Full-Overflowing, Yielding Hollow-Interrupted, and Yielding Hollow Intermittent, Change in Qualities and Intensity, and Rough Vibration (parenchymal damage).

Qualities Found Simultaneously at All Positions and the Three Depths

At the same time that we explore the three depths, we identify those qualities that can be found at *all positions* simultaneously. All of the qualities discussed in this chapter, except Bean (Spinning), Choppy, Inflated, and Short, meet this criteria.

With the exception of the Blood Unclear, Blood Heat, and Blood Thick qualities, as well as the Empty type of qualities, most of the other qualities listed below may appear at all depths. However, due to space considerations, each quality is described in this chapter at only the single depth which is most appropriate to that quality. For example, the Inflated quality is described under the rubric of the qi depth because, although it encompasses all three depths, it is first felt at the highest depth (usually the qi depth) to which it is capable of rising.

These qualities include the following:

Normal	Deep
Cotton	Feeble-Absent
Floating	Yielding Hollow Full-Overflowing
Taut	Vibration

- Tense
- Tight
- Wiry
- Inflated
- Slippery
- Hollow Full-Overflowing Wave
- Ropy
- Flooding-Excess Wave
- Pounding (Robust or Reduced)
- Hesitant Wave
- Suppressed Wave
- Thin
- Wide
- Qi Depth Diminished, Reduced Substance, Feeble-Absent
- Spreading
- Flooding Deficient Wave
- Diffuse
- Reduced Substance
- Blood Unclear
- Blood Heat
- Blood Thick
- Ropy
- Hollow
- Empty
- Scattered
- Leather
- Minute
- Change in Intensity
- Change in Amplitude
- Change in Qualities
- Intermittent
- Interrupted
- Yielding Hollow Interrupted-Intermittent
- Change in Rate at Rest
- Change in Rate on Exertion
- Muffled

Each of these qualities is discussed at greater length in Chapters 6 through 11.

THE NORMAL PULSE

The following characteristics of the Normal pulse serve as a baseline for health. (Each of these attributes is separately discussed in Chapter 5.)

- Regular, consistent rhythm
- Rate is consistent with age
- Amplitude and qualities are stable and consistent over time
- Moderate spirit (amplitude) and substance (intensity), with spirit and substance dependent on body build
- Long and continuous without turbulence
- Compressible, resilient, and elastic (substance and intensity)
- The depths—superficial, middle, and deep—are balanced, with the greatest strength in the root at the deepest or organ depth, and becoming lighter as pressure is released toward the qi depth (the perception of an impulse above the qi depth signifies pathology)
- Balanced between positions, with the middle position occupying the most space, followed by the proximal and distal positions
- Entire pulse is normally deeper in a heavy person and more superficial in a thin person, thus requiring appropriate adjustments in finger pressure
- Normal sine wave form

STABILITY AND ACTIVITY (RHYTHM AND RATE)

We continue our discussion of qualities that involve the entire pulse by re-examining the rhythm (regularity) and rate of the pulse. This is to emphasize a theme that I consider basic, and to which we return frequently. Alterations from normal rhythm (regularity) and rate are primarily signs of disharmony of the Heart. The Heart is the 'emperor,' and though there are exceptions to this rule, it is safest to proceed as if this is the first order of business in any diagnostic and treatment scheme. Until these two qualities, rhythm and rate, are brought into some kind of order and balance, all your efforts in dealing with other signs and symptoms, in making an accurate diagnosis, and in instituting an effective treatment regimen, will be futile. Other parameters of diagnosis are unreliable in the presence of a significantly altered rhythm and rate, and cannot be properly assessed until these have been resolved. Furthermore, clinical experience has shown that the Heart and circulation play a large role in problems never before attributed to them, as discussed at the end of Chapter 3.

Rhythm

Rhythm is the most significant measure of Heart and circulatory function. An unstable emperor causes chaos in the empire and anarchy among ministers and subjects. Unless this issue is attended to first, all other efforts may be in vain. As we have already seen in Chapter 7, irregular rhythm is considered in terms of whether it occurs at rest or on exertion, whether the rate can be accessed, whether the changes in rate are small or large, and finally, whether the irregularity occurs constantly or occasionally. It should also be mentioned that some pulse combinations of the 'qi wild' condition include irregularity (Yielding Hollow Interrupted-Intermittent), but by themselves are only a sign that the Heart and circulation are out of control.

Rate

A uniformly Rapid pulse is classically interpreted to represent a hot disorder and hyperactivity, and a uniformly Slow pulse is usually indicative of a cold disorder and hypoactivity. The pulse increases with acute external pathogenic heat, less so with generalized yin deficiency; it decreases with acute external pathogenic cold and with chronic qi and yang deficiency.

It bears repeating that clinically, alteration from a Normal rate is often a sign of significantly more far-reaching processes than those listed above. Unless you can confirm otherwise, a change in rate from Normal is usually the result of either a shock to the Heart (in utero, at birth, or during life) or some alteration in the circulation of blood and qi due to factors outside of, but ultimately affecting, the Heart. Thus, where a change in rate occurs, focus on the Heart (see Chapter 7).

Circulation

Closely related to the discussion of rhythm and rate is Dr. Shen's concept of the 'circulatory system.' Early in Dr. Shen's career, he began seeing patients who were thought to have problems with this system. They complained of being easily tired, having cold hands and feet, migrating joint pain that worsened when they were not active and improved when they were. They also suffered pain and swelling in the joints that was either passing or more persistent. Their entire bodies were chronically uncomfortable, and they were prone to anger, especially when the pulse was Inflated. Generally, there were no findings that were consistent with conventional Chinese or biomedical diagnosis, and over time, Dr. Shen came to recognize that these symptoms reflected problems in what he called the 'circulatory system.'

Dr. Shen differentiated three conditions involving the 'circulatory system,' which I will hereafter simply refer to as 'circulation.' They include circulation of qi and blood together, circulation of blood alone, and circulation of qi alone. In all three cases, either qi depletion affects the circulation, or insults to the circulation affect the qi. The results, in terms of symptoms, are similar, except that the former tends to develop more slowly and to appear and disappear with the strength of the person's qi, while the latter is more persistent and more acute. The circulation of qi or blood alone is related to Changes in

Intensity over the entire pulse. Changes in Intensity can be divided into two categories, one in which the instability in intensity is always present—a sign of a blood circulation disorder—and the other, when it is inconsistent—a sign of a qi circulation disorder.

When the 'circulatory system' is chronically affected, the pulse is usually Slow, the degree to which varies with the type of circulation that is involved (blood or qi). When the Heart affects the circulation, the pulse tends to be more Feeble; when the circulation affects the Heart, the pulse tends to be more Tight; and when the condition is due to the sudden stoppage of work and exercise, the pulse is Yielding Hollow Full-Overflowing and Rapid. The latter pulse quality is a sign of more serious disharmony.

QI AND BLOOD CIRCULATION AFFECTING EACH OTHER

See the discussion of the Heart and circulatory system in Chapter 12.

Qi affecting blood circulation

When qi affects blood circulation, the primary issue is qi deficiency.

Adult etiology

The principal cause is a deficiency of qi which arises over a long period of time during adulthood and is attributable to overwork, overexercise, protracted emotional stress, or to a long-term, serious illness. The pulse is Slow and can be Spreading or Deep. The tongue is pale.

Childhood etiology ('qi wild')

The second and more serious syndrome exists when young children are subject to the same conditions at a very early age. This occurred more commonly in the past when children worked in factories and mines, and were doing heavy farm labor by the age of six or seven. An immature organism is highly vulnerable to work beyond its qi. Roughly speaking, if the problem begins before the age of five it can be Yielding Hollow and Interrupted/Intermittent. If it begins between the ages of five and ten the quality is more likely to be only Interrupted/Intermittent, and Yielding Hollow Full-Overflowing and Slow if the onset is between the ages of ten and fifteen. The tongue will be extremely pale, and all of the symptoms described above and below will be exaggerated. The qi is very 'wild,' and the probability of a shortened life is great.

If the same circumstances occurred between the ages of fifteen and twenty, the pulse is more likely to be Empty, which is a less grave sign of 'qi wild' than either the Yielding Hollow Interrupted-Intermittent quality or the Empty Interrupted-Intermittent quality. Variations of the Empty pulse are the Leather, Empty and Thread-like (soggy), Scattered, and Minute qualities. The Hollow and Empty Arrhythmic qualities are signs of both 'qi wild' and chaotic Heart qi, which is far more serious than either alone. (The Empty and Hollow qualities are frequently confused. The Hollow pulse is felt at the qi and organ depths, but not in the middle, whereas the Empty pulse is felt only at the qi depth or superficially.)

The pulse and symptom pictures characterized above as more serious are ones in which the qi is 'wild.' These are described more completely in Chapter 6 in the discussion of stability, and in the chapters describing the individual 'qi wild' qualities. The Interrupted Yielding Hollow quality is technically one of these, but only in terms of the Hollow aspect. However, the Interrupted quality is also a sign of severe instability affecting the entire organism, although more particularly the Heart function.

'Qi wild' is, again, a condition in which the yin has lost control of the yang, which is then ungovernable. Another way of describing it is a state in which the material (yin) aspects of the body have lost control of the lighter yang (qi) functional energies, or in which the yang is so deficient that it cannot push the yin, which in turn is unable to nourish and hold onto the yang. This creates a severe imbalance between the inside and the outside, between yin and yang. The yang thereupon floats to the surface and wanders aimlessly through the organism, causing functional physiological chaos. Pulse qualities associated with 'qi wild' include the Empty, Scattered, Leather, Minute, and Change in Qualities (see Chapters 5, 6 and 9).

Circulation affecting qi and blood

When circulation is the primary etiology, stagnation is the issue, and the source is either a severe accident, extraordinary exertion, sudden emotional shock, sudden cessation of heavy exertion and exercise, or a profound weather or climatic event. Pain and ensuing fatigue are the most common complaints. With qi stagnation the pain migrates, and is milder and less persistent than with blood stagnation, which tends to be fixed, severe, and persistent. The pulse tends to be more Tight, except when the cause is the sudden cessation of excessive work or exercise, which leads to the Yielding Hollow Full-Overflowing and Rapid qualities, a more serious pulse.

Shock and trauma

Chinese medicine holds that any shock or trauma causes some degree of diminished circulation. The more severe the trauma, or the weaker the person at the time of the trauma, the greater the effect on circulation. More qi is then required to move the circulation through the areas where it has been blocked or constricted as a result of the trauma. A vicious cycle then develops between the circulation and qi, with intermediate stages of heat from excess and later deficiency: as more qi is consumed in pushing the circulation, the circulation, which is dependent upon the qi, diminishes; and as the circulation diminishes, less qi is delivered to the areas involved. Whereas the effect may not be immediately noticeable, if the circulation is not corrected, the long-term effect either locally in a less severe shock, or generally in a more severe one, can be debilitating. Many unexplained and seemingly mysterious disorders may be traced to trauma occurring as long as decades before, even at birth. I have seen this in individuals with degenerative neurological diseases as well as with neoplasms.

With severe trauma, it is blood circulation that is primarily affected. The pulse is Tight and Rapid initially, then later Slow and very Tight, and the middle or blood depth tends to be Thin. The Thin quality under these circumstances at the blood depth is a false sign of blood deficiency. The issue here is the delivery of blood and not the amount. A Choppy quality can appear at the positions or areas affected after a considerable time. The tongue has a purplish hue with possibly small, purple spots or blisters on the same side as the trauma. On the mucosa inside of the lower eyelid, on the same side of the trauma, a horizontal red blood vessel is superimposed over the usual vertical blood vessels that appear there. Persistent pain and swelling in the most traumatized area is often the chief complaint.

Sudden cessation of excessive exercise

The circulation of qi is affected when a person who has exercised intensively suddenly stops. Consistent exercise causes blood volume to increase and blood vessels to expand. With precipitous cessation of exercise, the blood volume decreases faster than the blood vessels contract, creating a break in contact between yin (blood) and yang. Sudden lifting far beyond one's ability, as in emergencies when people lift heavy objects to free themselves or others from being crushed, can have the same effect. The associated pulse qualities are Yielding Hollow Full-Overflowing and Rapid uniformly over the entire pulse. This is one form of the 'qi wild' state.

Impaired circulation affects Heart function, which, according to Chinese medicine, controls the mind. Thus, the symptoms of this pattern are fatigue and a tendency to become easily exhausted, emotional lability, feeling 'spaced out,' poor concentration, irritability, restlessness, and a sense of being out of control, both physically and mentally. Anxiety and panic is profound, and is increased by feelings of depersonalization, in which parts of a person's body no longer feel connected, especially when the individual is lying down; there is a sensation as if the limbs are floating away. The scenario is similar to and much more turbulent than that associated with the Empty quality over the entire pulse.

Weather and climate

Examples of extreme weather conditions are inadequate clothing and protection in situations such as mountain climbing in the snow (hypothermia), or crossing a desert in high heat (heat exhaustion or hyperthermia). While showing some long-term similarities to the effects of an accident or emotional shock, hypo- and hyperthermia also have characteristic clinical syndromes and acute pulses, such as the Hidden Excess with hypothermia, and very Tense Hollow Full-Overflowing and very Rapid with hyperthermia until shock occurs, when the pulse will become either Feeble or Yielding Hollow Full-Overflowing and Slow.

CHANGE IN INTENSITY OVER THE ENTIRE PULSE AND CIRCULATION

See Chapter 6.

Blood circulation and the Heart

Changes in Intensity over the entire pulse consistently over days and weeks reflects problems with blood circulation, which can be due to the circulation affecting the Heart, or the Heart affecting the circulation.

Circulation affects the Heart

The etiology can be a shock to the circulation from trauma, sudden and powerful emotion, abrupt overexercise or work beyond one's energy, sudden cessation of heavy labor or exercise, heavy labor especially before puberty, or overexposure to extreme weather, such as occurs with hypo- and hyperthermia. Eventually the circulatory deficit affects the Heart, which controls the circulation.

At this later stage, apart from the Change in Intensity over the entire pulse, the pulse tends to be uniform in quality; the left distal position is either a little Inflated and Tense, if the trauma happened to a strong person, or somewhat Flat, if it occurred to a less robust individual. The rate is very Slow, around 50 beats per minute.

Heart affects the circulation

When the Heart qi is weak, circulation is affected secondarily. Usually the entire pulse is more Feeble, the left distal position is more Feeble-Absent than the rest of the pulse, and the rate is in the sixties.

Qi circulation and the Liver

When a Change in Intensity is inconsistent and only occurs occasionally, the cause is usually stress affecting the Liver. According to Dr. Shen, the stress in men is due to overwork, and that in women to emotion—although these concepts are probably no longer valid in these times of increasing gender equality. Qi is more ephemeral and dependent on diurnal qi levels, which rise and fall for many reasons, and is especially dependent on the emotional stresses on the Liver, which also tend to fluctuate. When qi is reduced or stress elevated, the Change in Intensity is more obvious. Since it is one of the functions of the Liver to move the kinetic qi through the body, the circulation of qi and these occasional Changes in Intensity are tied to the vicissitudes of this yin organ system.

Stability

The following are 'qi wild' qualities associated with all three depths (see Chapters 5, 6, and 9).

Change in Quality

Qualities that are changing in one position are a sign of the separation of yin and yang and of extreme dysfunction in the organ which that position represents. Qualities that are changing in many positions indicate a severe 'qi wild' condition, signifying a serious imbalance in which the patient is at great risk. I have also often observed this quality in seriously mentally ill patients on heavy medication.

Change in Intensity

The intensity of the pulse wave is an expression of the substance and resilience of the body. In any one position, a Change in Intensity is a sign of a separation of yin and yang, of physiological instability of the organ which that position represents. (Constant Change in Intensity over the entire pulse is a sign of Heart qi-yang deficiency.)

Empty Interrupted or Yielding Hollow Interrupted

These pulses represent a most severe form of 'qi wild' disorder in that the instability is already in the yin organs, complicated by severe Heart qi deficiency. The imminence or presence of severe disease is great.

Yielding Hollow Full-Overflowing

This form of 'qi wild' involves a dilatation of blood vessels and contraction of blood volume. The symptoms are depersonalization, anxiety, and fatigue, and the prognosis for severe illness within six months is moderately great if the condition remains unresolved.

Qualities at Each of the Three Depths and Above the Qi Depth

As previously noted, in our system there are eight depths. The first is above the qi depth between the skin and the qi depth; the qi depth; the blood depth; the organ depth, which can be subdivided into three parts; between the organ depth and the bone (Firm quality); and just above the bone (Hidden quality). Whereas the qi and blood depths involve the contribution of a particular yin organ to the total organism's qi and blood, the organ depth is again subdivided into qi, blood, and organ depths, informing us respectively of the state of the qi, the blood, and the parenchyma of that organ. The full use of these subdivisions of the organ depth is being explored.

The exact position of the three depths is very subtle, and is poorly conveyed in words. While it is best learned through demonstration, Fig. 13-1 will be our best visual guide. Locating the exact position of the depths relies on the precise movement of the wrist and fingers. The distance between the depths is only about a tenth of a millimeter, and is accessed by very small increases or decreases in pressure by the wrists, and therefore the fingers, of the practitioner on the patient's pulse. The distance from the skin to the qi depth is about one-third greater than the distance between the qi and blood depth, and the blood and organ depth. The qi depth is just below the surface at a precise point, and the organ depth is well above the bone at another precise point. The blood depth is half way between the qi and organ depths. (For the moment, we are ignoring the three divisions of the organ depth.) The Firm quality is found about halfway between the organ depth and the bone, and the Hidden quality is found just above the bone.

In other words, the location of these depths depends on an exact position of the wrists, and not where one first happens to encounter the vessel. For example, by learning to calibrate and standardize our wrist movements we can locate the position of the depth when it present, or even when it is absent. The entire system described in this book depends on mastering this tool, one which we carry automatically wherever we go, and which opens us to all the complexities which make the pulse such a valuable diagnostic device.

DEPTHS AND CONSCIOUSNESS

Psychologically, the deeper a quality is felt, the further we get from awareness and the closer we approach the subconscious, the unconscious, and finally parenchymal tissue damage. For example, the Cotton quality as a sign of despair and resignation is only suppressed and easily brought to consciousness. The Suppressed wave at the qi depth can involve feelings which are only slightly deeper in the consciousness. The Flat quality, which has a flattened wave usually found at the organ depth, is a sign of a very deep repressed hurt, like the loss of a parent at an early age with which a child cannot deal on an emotional level, and is always unconscious. Later in life with a similar loss we might get an Inflated quality which is like a balloon, and which comes to the surface and is of course quite conscious. Smooth Vibration represents a move from a passing worry at the qi depth to a propensity to worry at the organ depth. At the same time, the organ depth represents the place where energy passes into mass, and where our more serious diseases reside.

ABOVE THE QI DEPTH

See Chapter 9.

Excess above the qi depth

QI STAGNATION

Yielding (Pliable) sensations above the qi depth

Cotton ('sad pulse')

The Cotton quality over the entire pulse represents superficial qi stagnation. It is palpated as an amorphous presence above the qi depth, and feels as if the fingers are passing through a substance lacking in form, or as if the skin or connective tissue is thicker and blocking access to the pulse. Over time, with increasing qi deficiency and a Deeper pulse, the Cotton quality can occupy the qi and blood depths. The cause is either emotional suppression or trauma, or a combination of both; Dr. Shen calls it the 'sad pulse.' The long-term physical consequences of an unresolved Cotton quality can be any chronic disease associated with prolonged qi stagnation, including arthritis or cancer, endocrine disorders such as adrenal insufficiency or hypothyroidism, and disorders of the reproductive system.

Etiology

EMOTIONAL SUPPRESSION

The stagnation of qi that leads to the Cotton quality is often related to a life situation which requires the conscious suppression of emotions, often with a profound, unresolved resignation and sadness of one to ten years' duration. Individuals so affected are globally oppressed across the physical and emotional spectrum, and often their lives are on hold due to the unsettled nature of their feelings. Just beneath consciousness they are aware of a sluggishness of function for a long time, both mentally and physically. This is a situation in which individuals are aware of the circumstances that are causing them to divert the evolution of their being from its natural course—the latter in terms expressed by Joseph Campbell's counsel: "Follow your bliss." Thus, it is common for such people to feel helpless to change a life situation which they know is not good for them, such as an unhappy marriage which they cannot leave, even when it is clear that the commitment to make it work is hopeless.

While many can mask their true feelings, often a sense of helplessness, hopelessness, and resignation are associated with this pulse. In the extreme, the picture is one of a quiet despair, and of grieving for a lost self. The tendency is to blame others for their dilemma rather than to take responsibility for change. When this pulse quality is presented in these terms, such individuals are usually more ready to verbalize their physical and mental complaints than are those with other qualities representing emotional problems.

TRAUMA

Another cause of the Cotton quality is severe trauma that has affected qi more than blood circulation, and which has not been resolved either by the organism's own capacity to open the circulation or by therapy.

Floating

The Floating quality is also accessed superficially with less pressure than is normally required to perceive the qi depth. This pulse is a sign that the qi level of function is involved in a pathological process in which the qi of the body, that is, the protective and nutritive qi, is rising to meet an outside challenge, e.g., from external wind, cold, or heat. Whereas this is a normal condition when it lasts a short time, it can interfere with the normal flow of qi if the invading cold or heat lasts long enough to create stagnation. However, the Floating quality can also be a sign of internal wind, in which case it is also Tight, as well other internal conditions described below.

It should be noted that pulses which float above the qi depth can also signify expansion due to heat in the yin organs (Flooding-Excess quality) or heat in the blood (Tense-Full-Overflowing). However, these have a distinct wave pattern (described n Chapter 9) which the Floating quality does not have. The Floating quality can be confused with the Inflated quality, but, although expansive in nature, it is never felt above the qi depth. The Floating quality can also be confused with another series of pulses that are felt only at the surface qi depth and are vacant below. These include the Empty, Leather, Empty and Thread-like, and Scattered qualities, pulses that signify the separation of yin and yang, such that the yin has lost control of the yang, which has floated to the surface of the pulse, but not above the qi depth.

Floating Yielding and slightly Rapid

A Floating Yielding quality that is usually slightly Rapid is a sign of a wind-heat condition, and indicates that the organism is attempting to defend itself against the external pathogenic factor and to expel the wind-heat.

Yielding Hollow Full-Overflowing

The Yielding Hollow Full-Overflowing quality (see Chapters 6, 8, and 9) has the normal sine curve, appears to be coming from the blood depth, and rises above the qi depth. The Yielding Hollow Full-Overflowing pulse has the same surge above the qi depth as the Tense Hollow Full-Overflowing quality, "like the roaring waves of the sea," except that it separates even more easily under pressure than does that quality. It is a sign that yin and yang have separated in the 'circulatory system,' and is one indicator of a 'qi wild' condition.

Hard sensations above the qi depth

Tense Hollow Full-Overflowing

The Hollow Full-Overflowing quality (see Chapter 9) has the normal sine curve and rises above the qi depth. The Tense Hollow Full-Overflowing pulse feels strong, forceful, swollen, blown-up, rising powerfully from the blood depth, both wide and expansive, as well as floating. The expansiveness felt on the middle blood depth moves vigorously, superficial to and past the qi depth, where the finger feels as if it is being pushed away from the wrist. It is a sign of extreme heat in the blood.

Flooding Excess

The Flooding Excess pulse (see Chapter 9) begins by feeling like a Full-Overflowing Pounding pulse but recedes rapidly as it reaches its apogee, lacking the last part of the curve of the normal wave. It has a stronger base at the organ depth than the Full-Overflowing quality, and is also never Yielding or Hollow. It is a sign of heat in the organs, usually of an infectious nature, such as hepatitis.

Floating Tense and slightly Slow

This pulse reflects an excessive condition of increased activity of the superficial quicker energies (i.e., protective qi) for defense against an acute attack of wind-cold.

Floating Tight

This quality is a sign of internal wind, usually associated with Liver heat from either excess or deficiency, and Liver blood deficiency. With this quality there should be concern for wind in the channels and stroke.

Floating Slippery

This combination can be encountered with a wind-damp condition such as hives.

QI DEPTH

The qi depth is the most superficial of the three depths and is felt closest to the skin. The exact position of this depth can be demonstrated, but not located by language. At this depth both the overall status of the moving or functional qi of the body (i.e., protective and nutritive qi) and the status of the 'nervous system' are being assessed. This holds true over the entire pulse, and for the qi depth in any individual position. However, the qi depth of the individual position informs us of the contribution to the qi of the whole body made by the organ which that position represents. As long as we have a qi depth, the relative condition of the true qi is probably good since, as the true qi depletes, the qi and blood depths tend to disappear.

One pathological direction involves stages of increasing qi deficiency, particularly when the etiology is physical work beyond one's qi. Since qi is expansive and gives the feeling of an elastic resilience to pressure when it is healthy, its depletion results in less resistance to pressure, a sense of yielding, and a diminishment in form. The more pliable qualities, such as Yielding, Diminished, Spreading, and Feeble, present a general assessment of the functions of the protective qi and, to a certain extent, the nutritive qi of the body, usually associated with physical overwork.

The harder qualities, such as Tense and Tight, reflect heat from excess and deficiency, respectively, associated with degrees of stagnation of the moving aspect of the qi, which is equated with the 'nervous system.' These qualities are often felt at all depths simultaneously with the same general meaning.

Where both physical and mental overwork are involved simultaneously, yin and qi deficiency often develop together, but to different degrees, depending on many factors including the true qi and the nature of the life experience.

Qi stagnation

The progression along the continuum that extends from the Taut through the Wiry qualities reflects the restorative manipulation of mental and emotional energies known as repression (see Chapter 11 for a discussion of these qualities). This conflict is mostly outside of awareness, and the manifestations are more at the level of irritability, and an agitated depression with sudden outbursts of rage and anger. Repression also leads to physical illness that tends to develop more insidiously and appear suddenly, such as cancer (especially in women), hypertension, and coronary heart disease (especially in men). As the qi stagnation grows, work is required to move the qi and break through the impasse. The progression from Taut to Wiry is one of increasing heat from excess, and then heat from deficiency due to increasing yin and finally essence deficiency, as further described in Chapter 11. Until the sudden manifestation of disease, individuals so affected rarely complain and tend to consider themselves invulnerable and stronger than others.

Taut

The Taut quality is a pulse that has lost some resilience; it is less compressible and is slightly more resistant to pressure. It represents the first stage of resistance to the free flow of qi through the channels. Usually the cause is repression of emotion, however any excessive or prolonged stress on the Liver, whether physical, chemical, or emotional, will interfere with the free flow of qi. This is reflected in an increasing Tenseness in the pulse beginning at the qi depth, and felt initially and most clearly at the left middle position.

Tense

Ordinarily, excessive internal heat is the result of work by, or excessive activity of, the normal heat of the body in a healthy organism attempting to overcome stagnation. The Tense pulse reflects a situation in which the stagnation and excessive heat are almost equally represented, while the Taut pulse is primarily a reflection of qi stagnation. This differentiation is important in selecting the correct treatment.

TENSE QUALITIES APPEARING UNIFORMLY OVER THE ENTIRE PULSE

Tense Long

The Tense and Long combination indicates the early development of heat from excess, usually as a result of qi stagnation due primarily to the repression of strong emotions.

Tense Robust Pounding

A Tense and Robust Pounding combination represents the next step in the progression of heat from excess. While theoretically this can signify movement of heat inward from the qi to the blood and organ depths, in my experience, it is more often a movement outward from the yin organs to the blood and to the qi depth, as the organism tries to rid itself of the excessive heat.

ETIOLOGY OF TENSE QUALITIES OVER THE ENTIRE PULSE

Emotional repression and metabolic disorders

The most common cause of a Tense Robust Pounding pulse is emotional repression, although the metabolic disorders that lead to heat in the blood and the Blood Thick pulse (see below under blood depth) are significant contributors, often concomitantly.

Febrile disorder

A febrile illness is also accompanied by a uniform increase in rate and force. The rate is more rapid with a febrile disorder, and there are more heat signs on the tongue and in the eyes.

Acute anxiety

Uniform Tense and Robust Pounding qualities, sometimes with a very Rapid rate, may accompany an acute anxiety or panic attack, although the tongue and eyes are usually normal.

'Nervous system tense'

A uniformly Tense pulse may also indicate a state of vigilance, which Dr. Shen calls the 'nervous system tense' condition. Often the 'nervous system'[10] is constantly overworking, even since birth, which may be genetically determined.

When the etiology is constitutional or congenital, the rate is Normal or a little Slow, and the eyes and tongue are normal. The rate does not change at rest or greatly on exertion, as with those qualities created by Heart shock such as Heart qi agitation, Heart yin (Heart Tight), and Heart blood deficiency (Heart Weak) (see Chapter 12). When the etiology is attributable to life experience, the rate will be slightly Rapid and the eyes and tongue will be redder (see Chapter 7 for more detail).

Stimulants and medications

Robust Pounding and Bounding with Rapid rate

Stimulants such as coffee that give rise to this pulse may also cause a slight increase in the force and rate, which are felt as Pounding and Bounding. Many medications such as ephedrine have the same effect. Until the stimulant is completely metabolized and excreted the pulse signs are without diagnostic value.

Tense Robust Pounding Suppressed

When the pulse is uniformly Tense, and the pulse wave is subtly Suppressed at the qi depth, the etiology may be synthesized chemicals, usually prescription, though sometimes recreational. Often the pulse reading is superfluous until the substances are completely metabolized and excreted.

Robust Pounding at organ depth

The presence of chemical substances in the body can sometimes be indicated by the presence of a Robust Pounding at the organ depth, and little or no Pounding at the blood and qi depth or above.

Bean (Spinning)

This pulse occupies only one position, or, more commonly in my experience, between and overlapping two positions. While the sensation is inconsistent and sometimes feels like a splinter, it is often Tight or Wiry, Slippery, and Rapid. The depth of this quality is not consistent, but it feels superficial. I have found it in individuals who have experienced severe pain or fright. I have also found it several times with terror, severe intractable pain, and in one case of acute intestinal obstruction (see Chapter 10).

Trapped qi

Inflated

This pattern is reflected in the Inflated quality and indicates that qi is trapped in and unable to move out of an organ or area of the body, such as the chest. It feels like a balloon that fills all three depths. There are three types of Inflated qualities involving trapped qi: Inflated Yielding, Mildly Tense Inflated, and Moderately Tense Inflated. (A fourth Inflated quality, Very Tense Inflated, is a sign of trapped blood.) These are alluded to again below in the discussion of the organ depth, and in more detail in Chapter 8.

This condition is often due to shock to the circulation from a trauma. Sometimes a sudden and great unexpressed anger can cause this quality, especially in the left distal and left middle positions. It is palpated at the left distal position in an individual whose head remained inside the birth canal for a long period, as with a breech presentation. The Inflated Yielding quality is a less serious sign than the Flat quality, which has a similar etiology, because the former quality, in contrast to the Flat, indicates that the qi in the area of the trauma was strong before the shock.

Fluid stagnation

Slippery

This is a pulse which moves quickly under one's finger in one direction. At the qi depth, Tense Slipperiness over the entire pulse with a Normal or slightly Rapid rate is a sign of excess sugar in the blood. With a Yielding and Slow rate, Slipperiness is a sign of qi deficiency. Rarely, wind-dampness in the channels (hives) can be temporarily accompanied by Slipperiness at the qi depth, usually above the qi depth.

Agitation at qi depth

This is characterized by a Smooth Vibration and is usually a sign of transient worry, anxiety, and lack of sleep. This pattern is discussed more completely in Chapter 11.

Qi deficiency

The successive stages of qi deficiency result either from an unsuccessful attempt by local and general energies to overcome the stagnation described above, or when the etiology is physical work or exercise beyond one's qi, including working long hours, lack of sleep, chronic physical illness, and old age. There is a progression of pulse qualities in the evolution of qi, blood, and finally organ deficiency just as there is for yin deficiency (see Chapter 8). With regard to qi deficiency, the qi depth first feels Yielding and Pliable, and then Diminished Feeble and Absent. This is followed by the Spreading quality, marked by separation on pressure at the blood depth. (Further qi depletion is manifested in the Flooding Deficient Wave, the Diffuse and Reduced Substance, Deep, Feeble, and Absent qualities, which are discussed again under organ depth below.) With increasing deficiency of qi and yin, the yin and yang separate and the yang rises aimlessly to the surface, producing the Empty quality. The Empty quality, and such related qualities as Leather, Soggy, Minute, and Scattered, are, as already mentioned, signs of 'qi wild,' and are felt primarily at the qi depth (see Chapter 9).

Listed below are the qualities that reflect the progressive depletion of qi in the organism as a whole, as manifested over the entire pulse at the qi and blood depths. Qi deficiency at individual positions of the pulse indicates a specific depletion of qi in a particular yin organ system, rather than a generalized devitalization.

Yielding (pliable)

The initial stage in the progression of qi deficiency is a gradual increase in the pliability of the qi depth on pressure. This quality results from mild work or exercise beyond a person's qi, or appears during the recovery phase of a moderately severe illness.

Diminished Feeble or Absent at qi depth

When there is a Diminished Feeble or Absent quality at the qi depth, the protective qi and some of the nutritive qi has been compromised. From a biomedical perspective, the individual has a vulnerable immune system. From the perspective of Chinese medicine, the individual is more susceptible to attack from external pathogenic factors, which include any form of external stress, chemical or physical. It is my impression that the nervous system becomes equally vulnerable to internal stress when the qi depth is weakened.

A Diminished Feeble or Absent quality at the qi depth is usually a sign of qi deficiency from overwork—an ubiquitous finding in a society that does nothing but work beyond its qi. When this pulse appears only occasionally in an individual, it may only signify a lack of sleep. But insufficient sleep is in fact a form of working beyond one's energy, since the person is probably engaging in a qi-depleting endeavor when not sleeping. Even when a person lies awake worrying, he or she is overworking, in this instance with the mind, which actually consumes more glucose per unit of work than does the physical body.

Yielding Reduced Pounding

A weaker and stressed organism that is overworking to maintain homeostasis may exhibit this pulse. An organism that is approaching exhaustion manifests a Reduced Pounding pulse, which, on pressure, lacks force. This is a sign of a desperate attempt to maintain function while suffering from severe qi and yang deficiency.

Flooding Deficient

Dr. Shen calls this the 'push pulse' for individuals who push themselves beyond their qi. This pulse, which lacks the force of the Flooding Excess pulse, rises just up to, but not beyond, the surface at the qi depth, and suddenly recedes precipitously.

Yin deficiency

Another substance deficiency which appears at the qi depth is yin deficiency. Yin is fluid and provides the pulse with the quality of softness. One measure of the integrity of yin in the body is, therefore, the degree of hardness or softness of the pulse. At the qi depth of an individual position, the integrity of the yin is a measure of the contribution to the total yin of the body made by the organ represented by that position. Increasing hardness is noted with the loss of yin, and is accompanied by the concomitant development of heat from deficiency. (The latter is found especially when the work that one does beyond one's energy involves emotional stress and tension in the nervous system.) While the qualities associated with yin deficiency are found at the qi depth, the Tight and Wiry qualities are discussed later under the organ depth where the meanings are essentially the same, except suggesting more serious disharmony.

These qualities are signs of early heat from yin deficiency, which occurs over time as the body expends yin to balance the excess heat used to overcome qi stagnation. When found at the qi depth, these qualities are manifestations of overworking of the 'nervous system.' This is usually the result of using the mind beyond one's energy.

Tight and Thin at qi depth

These qualities are a sign of early heat from yin deficiency, which occurs over time as the body expends yin to balance the heat used to overcome qi stagnation. When found at the qi depth, these qualities manifest an overworking 'nervous system.' This is usually the result of using the mind beyond one's energy.

BLOOD DEPTH

The blood depth over the entire pulse informs us of the general state of the blood for the entire organism. In any one position, the blood depth is a measure of the contribution to the total blood of the organism made by the organ represented by that position. The blood depth is accessed with greater finger pressure than the qi depth. Again, the exact position of this depth can be demonstrated, but not accurately located with mere language. As previously mentioned, the blood depth should feel wider and offer more resistance than the qi depth, but less resistance than the organ depth. Under normal circumstances, the organ depth should be more substantial than either the blood or the qi depth. The blood depth is sometimes indistinct as a separate entity unless there is pathology. Initially, the blood depth should be searched with all six fingers simultaneously. When some of the positions are too Feeble to offer anything at the blood depth, the search should be limited to positions where it is potentially available. However, the position which is Feeble should be separately investigated.

Should the blood depth feel less resistant than the qi depth as finger pressure is increased, and the organ depth is present, we are dealing with the Hollow quality. This quality is best accessed descending from the superficial to the deeper aspects of the pulse. As explained later, Hollowness is a quality, depending upon other attending qualities (Leather-like), that signifies potentially serious and dangerous pathology with grave consequences—including sudden heavy bleeding—and should be considered a possible emergency. This quality is discussed in Chapter 9.

Should the pulse seem to increase in size or become Slippery as finger pressure is released from the organ to the blood depth, heat, toxicity, or stasis in the blood is being revealed. In my experience, it is almost impossible to sense this quality when going in the other direction, from the superficial to the deeper aspects of the pulse.

With some qualities, such as the Hollow pulse, only one position or organ may be reflected at the blood depth. I have found isolated Slipperiness at the blood depth at the left and right middle and left proximal positions. Specifically, in terms of the left middle position, what is found there in the blood depth has widespread effects on the blood generally, even if it is not immediately detectable elsewhere, by virtue of the fact that the Liver stores the blood.

Three forms of disharmony can be found at the blood depth: excess (stagnation), deficiency, and instability.

Fig. 13-3 Progression of heat and toxicity in the blood

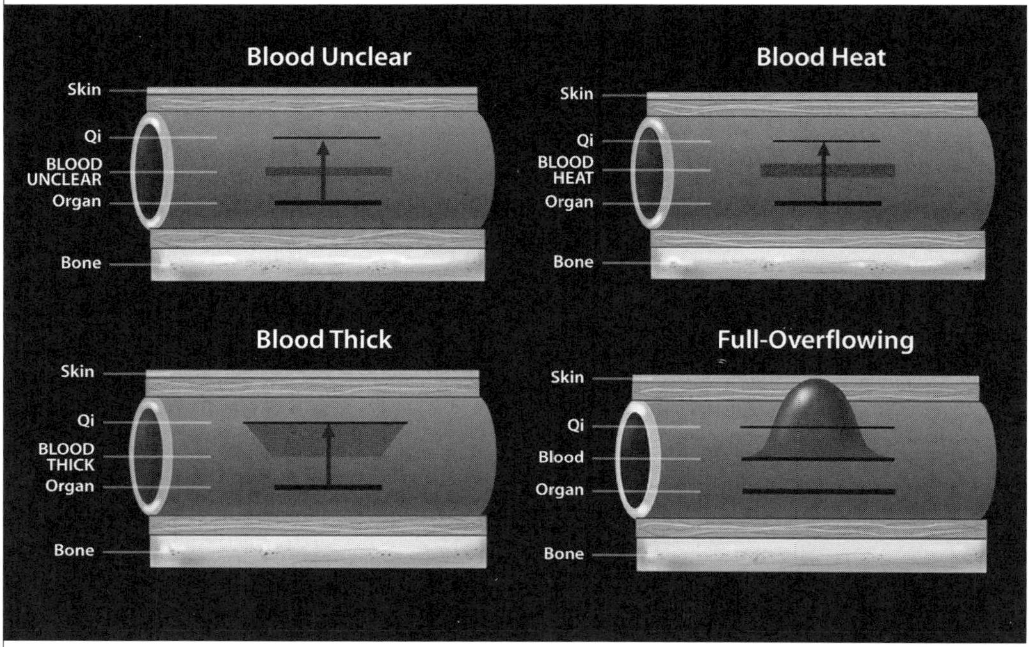

Blood excess

BLOOD STAGNATION

Seven pulse qualities reflecting different forms of stagnation that are mostly discernible at the blood depth are presented here.

Slowed and impaired blood circulation in the tissues and body cavities

Choppy

The Choppy quality is a sign of slowed and impaired circulation of blood in the tissues, rarely found at the blood depth. Usually the individual positions are involved with this pulse: the proximal and Pelvis/Lower Body position with menstrual problems; the left middle with 'dried blood' in the Liver; the right middle with stomach and duodenal ulcers; and the left distal position with coronary artery disease. This quality is rarely felt at all the positions simultaneously; it is most often found at the organ depth.

Very Tense Inflated

This is a rare occurrence that is caused by gradual bleeding into an area or organ, such as with a subdural hematoma in the brain. The associated pulse is the very Tense-Inflated quality.

Impaired blood circulation in the blood vessels

The following qualities—Blood Unclear, Blood Heat, Blood Thick, and Tense Hollow Full-Overflowing—are all accessed by slowly releasing pressure from the organ depth, and then to the qi depth and above. Instead of the orderly diminishment of substance as one moves from deep to superficial, we encounter the opposite trend, and the substance increases. The degree to which it increases, and the depth to which it increases as one releases finger pressure, determines the quality.

However, in searching for the presence of these qualities, an organ depth must be present so that one can determine if there is an increase as one releases finger pressure from the organ to the blood and qi depths. If no organ depth exists, as with the Empty quality, one is unable to evaluate the presence of these qualities. If this is true for the entire pulse, one can only infer its presence if the blood depth is Slippery. If the pulse is Empty at individual positions where one is examining for these qualities (usually the left middle position, as it is the Liver that stores the blood), one can search for a position that is not Empty, particularly the proximal position.

Frequently, the pulse is in a state of transition with Change in Qualities from, for example, Tense at the organ depth to Empty. If one palpates the pulse at the time when it is Tense, one is then in a position to evaluate the presence of the Blood Unclear/Heat/Thick qualities.

The right middle positions are less useful for this purpose, requiring more discernment. One must often distinguish there between the commonly found Inflated quality, which increases like a balloon from the organ to the qi depth, and the Blood Unclear/Heat/Thick qualities, which similarly increase in substance as one goes from the organ to the qi depth. The difference is that, with the Blood Unclear/Heat/Thick qualities, the substance of the pulse feels more dense as one releases finger pressure than with the Inflated quality, which is less defined at each depth, and is compressible like a balloon.

Blood Unclear (turbid blood)

Dr. Shen calls Blood Unclear the condition (and associated pulse quality) in which there is a barely perceptible increase in the size of the blood depth, rather than a decrease, as one's finger is raised from the organ depth toward the qi depth (see Fig. 13-4). Often the pulse is also slightly Slippery. As one releases one's finger from the blood to the qi depth, the size again diminishes.

This sign of toxicity in the blood is usually accompanied by a slightly red tongue that may have a yellow, moist coating. The eyes appear normal (without heat signs), and the symptoms often include fatigue and skin-related problems, such as eczema and psoriasis. Dr. Shen likens this condition to a glass of water that has dirt suspended in it: the quality of the blood is not good.

The most common cause of this quality is exposure to environmental toxins. I first encountered it with artists using highly toxic solvents, often in poorly ventilated rooms, and with the use of acetylene torches in art and industry (e.g., welders). Several practitioners have reported inoculations to be another etiology.

Yet another related origin is Liver stagnation or deficiency that prevents this organ from detoxifying adequately. In addition to storing the blood itself, the Liver also stores the blood toxins that it cannot metabolize. These toxins contaminate the blood and ultimately the entire organism which it nourishes. Skin symptoms are one obvious attempt to discharge that toxicity.

Still another cause of this pattern is Spleen qi deficiency, which prevents the organ from properly building the blood due to poor absorption and digestion of food, especially protein. The protein is only partially digested into small chain polypetides the size of viruses, instead of being completely digested down to amino acids. The small chain polypetides are absorbed and the body reacts to them as if they were viruses by inappropriately mobilizing the immune system. Eventually, auto-immune diseases develop.[11] The Slippery quality at the blood depth is most often associated with Spleen-Gallbladder damp-heat.

Dr. Shen also discussed a form of rheumatoid arthritis which he has found to be caused by toxicity in the blood due to environmental chemicals. Along with the Blood Unclear quality, the entire pulse is Tight, and slightly Slippery at the blood depth, indicating that circulation and the blood are not good. The blood vessels on the mucosa inside the lower eyelids vary in width and color: some are thicker and more brown than others, which are thinner and more red. The greater the toxicity, the greater the variation, and the deeper the brown color.

Fig. 13-4 Blood Unclear quality

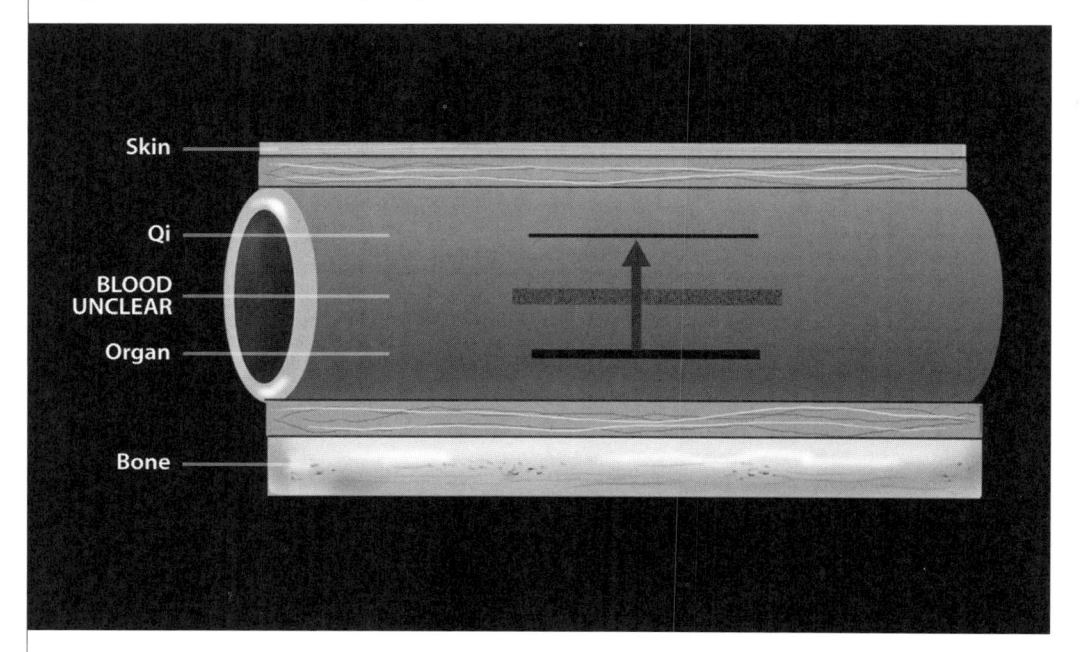

Blood Heat

The next condition and its associated pulse quality, called Blood Heat by Dr. Shen, is one in which the thickness of the blood depth is more readily palpable (Fig. 13-5). As one raises one's finger from the organ depth, the pulse expands even more in the blood depth than with Blood Unclear. Again, as one continues to release pressure to the qi depth, the pulse diminishes. This is a sign of excess Blood heat. Often the blood depth is also Slippery. According to Dr. Shen, Blood Heat without Slipperiness is due to an overworking 'nervous system,' while Blood Heat with Slipperiness is due to metabolism of lipids and digestion.

The tongue is red, and the eyes are congested, both on the mucosa of the lower eyelid and in the sclera. Symptoms are sore throat, canker sores, prickles on the tongue, bleeding gums, flushed face, excitability, pressure headaches, dark urine, and hard and dry bowel movements. Dr. Shen likens this pattern to a glass with hot water, in contrast to the one with dirt, his metaphor for Blood Unclear.

Two patterns can give rise to this pulse. The first is heat from excess associated with foods such as spices, wine, shellfish, coffee, chocolate, and others identified by the Chinese as creating heat. The organs that are usually affected are the Liver, Stomach, Heart, and Lungs. The second pattern is one of heat from deficiency, which is usually due to a nervous system that is extremely tense, and which therefore, from the Chinese perspective, is a system that has been working beyond its 'energy.' Kidney yin depletion usually ensues.

Fig. 13-5 Blood Heat quality

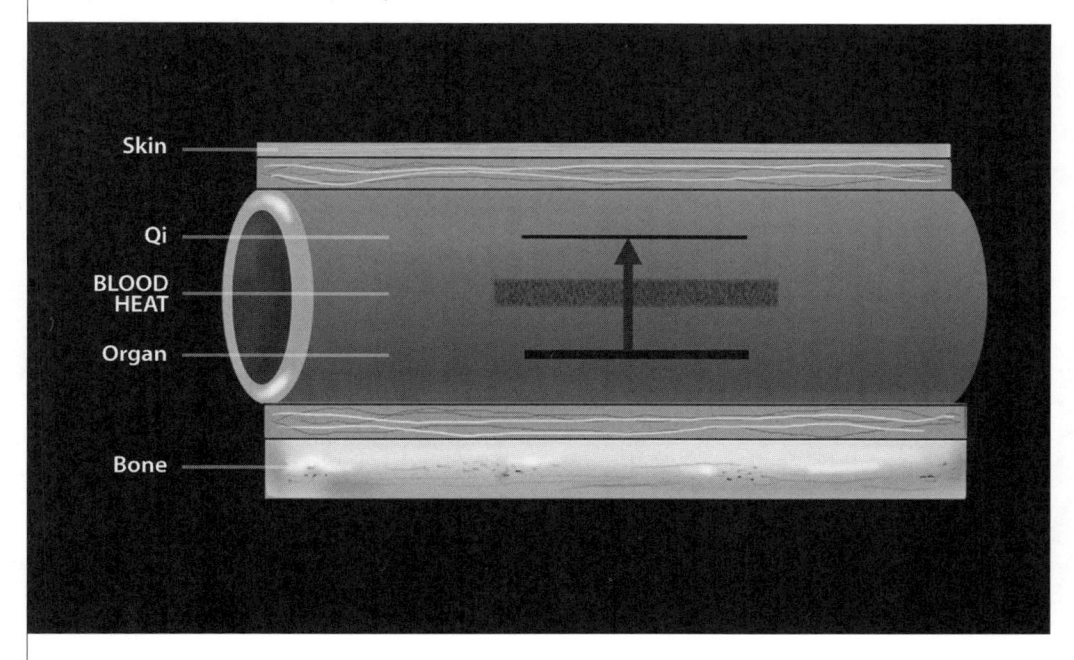

Blood Thick (exuberant blood)

With this pattern and associated pulse quality, the blood depth has become extremely Wide, with Robust Pounding, and Slippery. It is accessed as we did the Blood Heat and Blood Unclear qualities. However, with the condition associated with Blood Thick, the pulse continues to widen, even to the qi depth. Later, it often develops into a Tense Hollow Full-Overflowing quality (wave)—a sign of the later stage of the Blood Thick process in which heat from the blood has overflowed into and above the qi depth, and thereupon becomes a very prominent aspect of the pulse. (See Fig. 13-6.)

The condition associated with Blood Thick is also referred to as exuberant blood. It is accompanied by a scarlet tongue and eyes in which the sclera and vessels on the mucosa of the lower eyelid are very red. According to Dr. Shen, an early sign of this condition can be persistent acne after adolescence. The late signs are usually of a cardiovascular nature, such as hypertension.

Blood Thick has several etiologies and courses. One develops from heat in the blood, and is a damp-heat disorder involving heat from the Liver and dampness from the Spleen and Gallbladder. The causes of Spleen damp-heat are primarily excessive dietary intake of fat and sugar, leading to elevated serum levels of glucose, cholesterol, and triglycerides. The pulse shows more Slipperiness, especially when dampness predominates, and less of the very Tense Hollow Full-Overflowing quality, which is characteristic of advancing hypertension due to other causes described below. This process gradually interferes with Heart function due to increasing resistance in both the peripheral as well as coronary circulation, leading (for this reason) to even higher blood pressure, especially diastolic.

Fig. 13-6 Blood Thick quality

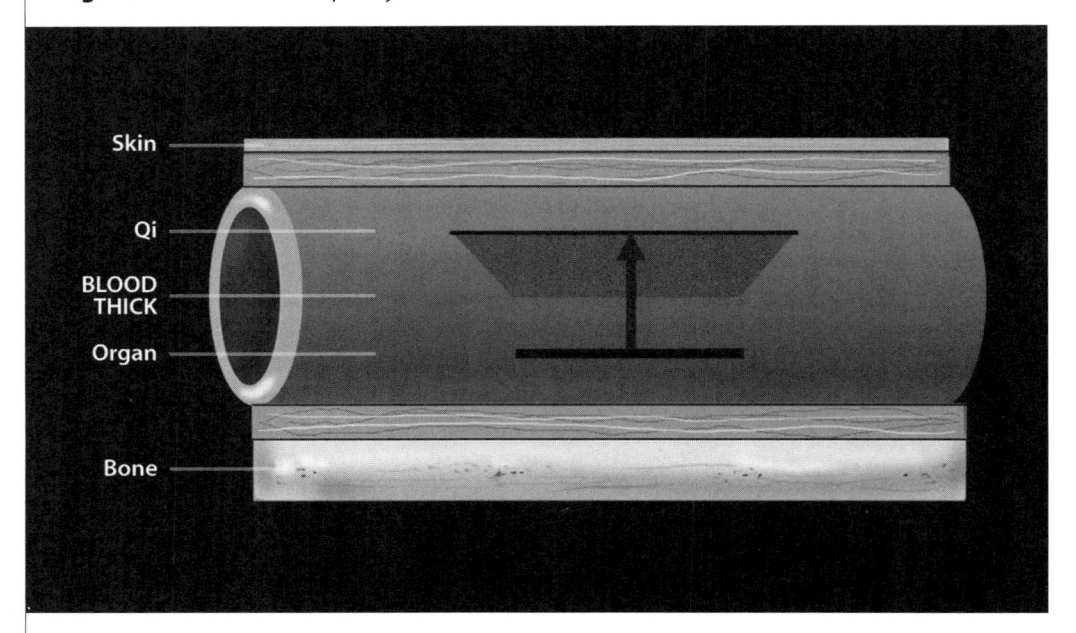

Another contributing factor is a tense nervous system, which causes Liver qi congestion, interfering with the proper digestion and absorption of fats in the alimentary system (Liver attacking Spleen and Stomach), as well as with efficient metabolism of these substances by the Liver. There is a concomitant increase in Liver fire, and later Liver and Kidney yin deficiency, along with the development of the Blood Thick condition. Both processes eventually lead to a Ropy pulse, a sign of arteriosclerosis and atherosclerosis.

Tense Hollow Full-Overflowing

The Tense Hollow Full-Overflowing quality (Fig. 3-7) feels swollen, rising wide and expansive above the qi depth in a sine curve wave, with a Robust Pounding and often slightly Rapid beat. Its expansiveness is felt strongly in the middle blood depth, moving upward vigorously to and past the qi depth, where the finger feels as if it is being pushed away. It does not have the consistently solid sustaining force of the Inflated quality, as it gives way with pressure because of its Hollow aspect.

Tense Hollow Full-Overflowing as a uniform quality over the entire pulse is an extension of the Tense Pounding and Blood Thick pulse. It is a sign of severe heat from excess, which the body is attempting to eliminate from the blood. Since the heat can no longer be contained in the blood, it invades the qi. Over the entire pulse, the sign is one of serious hypertension and imminent stroke, and even death (see Chapter 9).

Slippery

Slipperiness at the blood depth is found whenever there is some alteration in the normal strength or direction of the flow of blood or fluids, which creates turbulence. This can be due to either increased resistance or decreased propulsion. Most of the patterns described in this section are the result of increased resistance to circulation due to an excess such as heat in the blood associated with excessive blood lipids, which increases blood viscosity.

Fig. 13-7 Tense Hollow Full-Overflowing quality

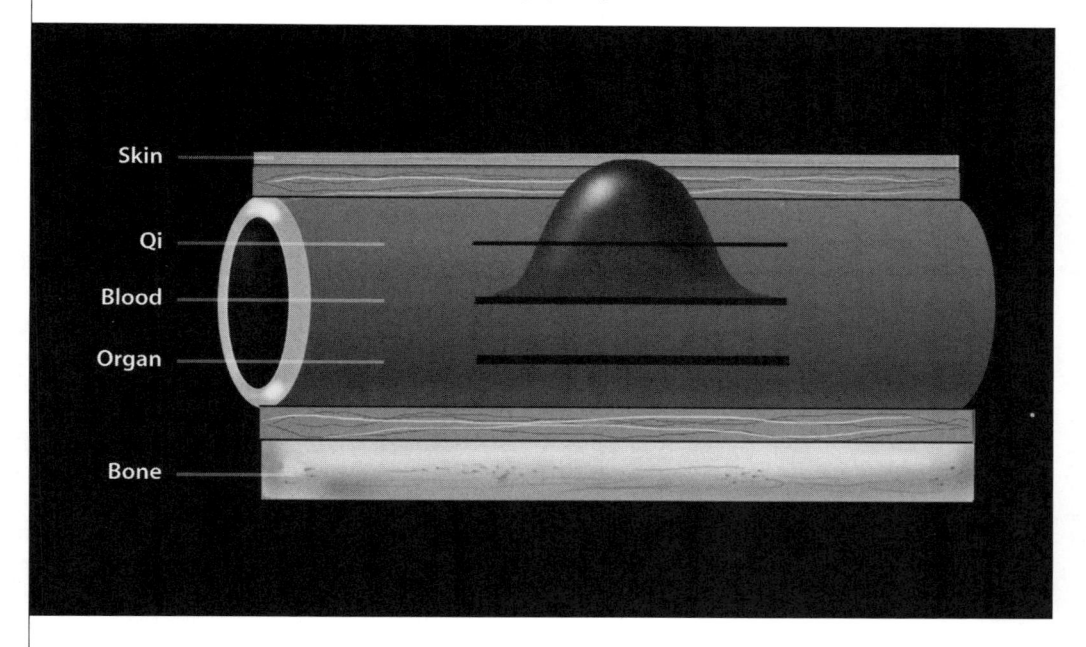

Slipperiness can be found at the qi depth, the blood depth (most commonly), and the organ depth, all three depths together, or in any combination. Slipperiness has slightly different interpretations depending on its location (see Chapter 11).

I have found the Blood Unclear, Blood Heat, and Blood Thick qualities together with Slipperiness occasionally with blood dyscrasias, such as in sicle cell anemia.

Rough Vibration

Rough Vibration confined to the blood depth is a sign that heat in the blood is not only affecting the blood, but is also drying out and damaging the walls of the vessels. This is an early stage of arteriosclerosis.

Ropy

See Chapter 11.

Tense Ropy

The Tense Ropy quality is associated with heat from both excess and deficiency that has 'vulcanized' the walls of the blood vessels over a long period. The heat has caused a loss of elasticity of the smooth muscle fibers. This deterioration has encouraged the development of arteriosclerotic plaques on the vessel walls. Thus, the Ropy quality occurring uniformly over the pulse is associated with the arteriosclerotic process.

Yielding Ropy

The Yielding Ropy quality is due to a separation of yin and yang in the vessels related to exercising beyond one's energy for a very long period of time. The separation deprives the vessel walls of yin nourishment, and the result is a process of drying and consequent fragility, which also leads to the arteriosclerotic process without the heat phase (see Chapter 11).

Blood deficiency

Thin

Thinness at the blood depth is associated with blood stagnation and is a rare form of blood deficiency due to decreased delivery rather than deficiency.

Spreading (on pressure)

With an Absent qi depth and increasing depletion of the nutritive qi, particularly from working beyond one's 'energy' without sufficient rest for extended periods, separating of the blood depth on moderate pressure of a still substantial pulse at the organ depth is manifested. The pulse, although giving way, is still ample and not Empty in the deeper positions. I have found this pulse frequently in medical students and residents, and in physicians who overwork and have little chance to recover through rest. I have also felt it frequently in young women who have had multiple pregnancies, abortions, and miscarriages in whom the quality represents both blood and qi deficiency.

Absence of the blood and qi depths: Deep

According to Dr. Shen, the Absence of the blood and qi depths over the entire pulse is an indication of both blood and qi deficiency. The blood deficiency is more than with a Thin pulse at the blood depth, but less than when all three depths are Thin.

Yielding partially Hollow

When the qi and organ depths are present and the blood depth separates on pressure but is not entirely Absent, the indication is of slight blood deficiency, and the associated quality is Hollow. The blood deficiency is less than when both the qi and blood depths are Absent, and much less than with a Thin quality.

Instability of blood (blood out of control)

The following qualities are both Hollow. In terms of perception, the Hollow quality by definition implies that there is no sensation between the qi and organ depths. This is true, in fact, only of the Leather-like Hollow quality. With all other Hollow qualities the sensation seems to yield and separate between the qi and organ depths, but not disappear entirely.

Leather-like Hollow

This quality (see Chapter 9) over the entire pulse is usually a sign of notable and even massive hemorrhage such as might occur with a bleeding ulcer, sudden massive menorrhagia, ruptured aneurism, trauma, or sudden lifting beyond one's qi. When the pulse is Rapid the bleeding is imminent or in progress, and when the pulse is Slow, the bleeding has already passed. This situation is life-threatening due to shock, which frequently accompanies sudden hemorrhaging, and calls for emergency intervention. With a Leather-like Hollow pulse the lack of control over the blood occurs suddenly, in contrast to the Yielding Partially Hollow quality, which is a sign of the loss of qi with more gradual bleeding. The sensation of Leather-like Hollow is one in which nothing is felt at the blood depth, in contrast to the other Hollow qualities whereby the blood depth is usually only partially Hollow, separating at the blood depth, with intact qi and organ depths.

Dr. Shen believed that with a Leather-like Hollow quality the bleeding is always from a yin organ, and bleeding without a Leather-like Hollow quality indicates that the loss of blood is from other than a yin organ. (Gradual menorrhagia from the uterus is an example of bleeding from other than a yin organ.) More often the pulse quality appears in one position when one organ, yin or otherwise, can no longer control its blood, for example, the stomach with a bleeding ulcer. This quality is always serious whenever it is encountered and calls for emergency measures.

Very Tense or Tight Hollow Full-Overflowing

The uniform appearance over the entire pulse of a very Tense or Tight Hollow Full-Overflowing quality can indicate either hypertension or true insulin dependent diabetes. With this quality the potential for cerebral bleeding, or stroke, is always great; it is another form of 'blood out of control.'

ORGAN DEPTH

The deepest aspect of the pulse is well above the bone and reflects the integrity of the yin organs. Again, the exact position of this depth can be demonstrated but not located precisely with language. These organs are the basic functional units which, working together, create the fluid, blood, and qi, and govern all of the functions that we call life. Large sections of the Intestines, the Stomach, the Bladder, and certainly the Gallbladder may be removed with impunity without regard for life and death. This is not so for the yin organs which, for the most part, cannot be removed without a more immediate threat to life.

Parts of the Lungs and Liver, and sometimes all of the organ identified biomedically as the Spleen, have been removed without life-threatening consequences. It is unclear whether the biomedical and Chinese concepts of the Spleen coincide in any way. The digestive functions ascribed to the Chinese model of the Spleen seem to partially concur with the biomedical physiology of the pancreas, and it is known that removal of the pancreas is inconsistent with life.

Therefore, any alteration at the organ depth of the pulse is clinically very significant. As mentioned above in the discussion of the qi depth, the absence of the organ depth together with the absence of the other two depths is called an Absent pulse, and is a sign of diminished resistance to illness. Its absence with the *presence* of a pulse at the qi depth, known as the Empty quality, is a sign of current serious disharmony and is a form of 'qi wild.' Dr. Shen believed that when the condition remains unresolved, the Absent quality means illness within approximately one year, and the Empty 'qi wild' quality means illness within six months. (My own experience varies from his. With the Absent quality, the time lapse to significant illness can be up to three years, and up to one-and-one-half years with the Empty quality.)

As previously mentioned, through a careful sense of touch, within the organ depth can be found a qi, blood, and more material yin layer, which I equate with the biomedical concept of parenchyma. Here we are passing from the 'energy' to the mass side of the equation. It is worth repeating that qi, blood, and yin deficiency at the qi and blood depths are on a physiological continuum with the more profound organ deficiencies.

When the nervous innervation of an organ is under stress, the qi or surface layer of the organ depth may be extremely Tight. Tension and Tightness in the qi depth is often associated with nervous tension and supports the tenability of Dr. Shen's idea that the qi and the 'nervous system' have common characteristics and functions. I have found this most discernible on the entire left side at the organ depth in individuals whose lifelong tension has moved internally from the musculoskeletal area, affecting the nervous innervation of all the yin organs. Dr. Shen characterized this as the 'nervous system' affecting the 'organ system' (see Chapter 14).

Regarding the relationship between the yin and yang organs, from my perspective the yang organs are there energetically to serve the yin organs by providing contact with the exterior to preserve homeostasis. They act as conduits to remove excess from the yin organs and excrete it from the body. One example is the action of the Small Intestine in removing the excess heat from the Heart.

The yang organs also function as indirect sources of nourishment for their paired yin organs. When the Heart, for instance, is too vulnerable to treat directly, Small Intestine points can be substituted. Additionally, the yang organs assist the mental functions of yin organs; thus, for example, the Small Intestine supports the Heart in its mental function of sorting the important from the irrelevant. In fact, according to Triple Burner theory of the Internal Duct, the yang organs serve to separate the pure from the impure along the entire energetic cycle.

The following are abbreviated descriptions of pulse qualities found in the organ depth. More detail about each of the qualities is found in other chapters.

Stagnation at the organ depth

QI STAGNATION FROM EXCESS

Taut-Tense

The Taut-Tense pulse is an early sign of qi stagnation. The Tense pulse is a sign of qi stagnation, and simultaneously an early indication of mostly heat from excess. This quality is usually associated with emotional stress of a moderate nature, or for a short period of time. While this pulse is more apparent at the qi depth, where it is first encountered, it is usually found simultaneously at all three depths and is strongest at the organ depth.

Hidden Excess

This quality (see Chapter 9) is accessed only by the deepest pressure "to the level of the bone,"[12] and is generally a sign of the most serious disharmony and chronic illness. However, though it is deeper than the organ depth, I place it here because it is described by Li Shi-Zhen as stagnant internal yin cold, or "cold obstructing the channels,"[13] when the pulse is simultaneously Robust. While Li states that with this etiology the condition is easily relieved through sweating, I have found this not to be the case, and find the Hidden quality only with life-threatening hypothermia.

In the context of Dr. Shen's three-depth system, a Hidden quality that is 'behind the bone' is outside the parameters of the Chinese pulse and does not give us any useful information. Dr. Shen did, however, describe a Hidden Deficiency quality, discussed later in this chapter, which in a private communication he identified as my Deep quality, whose characteristics are inconsistent with being 'behind the bone.' Dr. Shen, in discussing the Hidden Deficiency quality, also observed that "If a relatively healthy individual should have the hidden pulse, then it is a congenital lacking."[14] Furthermore, he emphasized the vulnerability of such persons should their lifestyle drain their qi.

PHLEGM, FOOD, QI, AND/OR BLOOD STAGNATION

This pattern is manifested in a Short Excess quality and is attributable to interference in the circulation between organs owing to stagnation of phlegm, food, qi, and blood (see Chapter 10).

QI STAGNATION FROM DEFICIENCY

Trapped qi

Flat

In terms of sensation, this is a Deep pulse with a notably diminished wave. It is a sign of stagnation when qi cannot reach an area of the body due to a shock to the circulation in this area caused by physical or emotional trauma. This quality also suggests that the qi here was deficient prior to the shock. Clinically, I associate it with a neoplastic process that develops over a long period of time. Li Shi-Zhen describes "accumulation diseases" and "lumps, tumors, or hernia" with the Firm (Confined, Prison) quality,[15] one that is similar in sensation to the Flat quality, but very different in interpretation except when there are tumors.

BLOOD STAGNATION

Choppy

Blood stagnation at the organ depth is generally manifested in the Choppy quality. The sensation of the Choppy quality is coarse, uneven, like rolling one's finger across a washboard. In some positions the Choppy quality is confused with Vibration, which generally has a tingling or buzzing, moving sensation (see Chapter 11).

DAMPNESS (STAGNATION OF FLUIDS)

Slipperiness is the quality that is most often associated with stagnation of fluids, a damp disorder. Slipperiness can be found at the qi depth, the blood depth (most commonly), the organ depth, as well as all three depths together or any combination of the same. The significance of Slipperiness varies slightly depending on its location (see Chapter 11).

Damp-heat

Slipperiness found only at the organ depth with a Rapid rate is a sign of damp-heat in the yin organs, or the biomedical equivalent of chronic bacterial, viral, or parasitic infection. Slipperiness found at all depths with a very Rapid rate indicates a more fulminating kind of infection. In pregnancy the Slippery quality is often found over the entire pulse with a slightly Rapid rate.

Damp-cold

The Slippery and Slow pulse at the organ depth is also a sign of chronic infection associated with systemic yeast and fungus infestations. A Slippery and Slow pulse at all depths has been observed in chronic blood dyscrasias such as leukemia, with iatrogenic dampness, or with the use of water-retaining medications such as the corticosteroids (prednisone), estrogen, and progesterone. With Heart qi deficiency, the Slipperiness is a reflection of turbulence in the circulation because of a diminished circulatory force.

Heat from excess at the organ depth

UNCONSTRAINED HEAT

Flooding Excess

There are two kinds of Flooding pulse. The one that I call a Flooding Excess quality is related in the literature to yin organ excess, or less often, to heat from deficiency. In my own and Dr. Shen's experience, there is a Flooding Deficiency quality that is a sign of yin organ qi deficiency, and is described below with the deficient organ qualities.

In this chapter we are not concerned with sensation except to distinguish one quality from another with which it could easily be confused (see Chapter 8). Thus, the Flooding Excess pulse is "like the ocean waves hitting the beach; it comes with force but recedes calmly."[16] This pulse has a strong base at the organ depth, and rises above the qi depth—somewhat like the Hollow Full-Overflowing pulse described above—and then recedes suddenly and precipitously, unlike the Hollow Full-Overflowing pulse, which recedes gradually. On the other hand, the Flooding Excess pulse is not Hollow and does not give way to pressure as easily as the Full-Overflowing quality, suggesting that the rising heat comes from the yin organs rather than the blood.

The Flooding Excess quality is a sign of acute fulminating internal infection identified with the *yang ming* stage of the six stages of disease.

Deficiency at the organ depth

BLOOD DEFICIENCY

A generally Thin pulse usually indicates severe blood deficiency. This quality is associated with a general condition of dryness, especially of the skin, hair, and nails, as well as with other problems, and is described more completely under the quality Thin in Chapter 10. This pattern of blood deficiency is sometimes confused with the biomedical condition of anemia, a distinction also discussed more fully in Chapter 10.

There are two types of Thin pulse: Thin Yielding, which indicates both blood and qi deficiency, and Thin Tight, which is characteristic of blood and yin deficiency. The progression of increasing deficiency leads to the 'wild' and 'reckless' disorders discussed below.

Thin Yielding

This quality reflects blood and qi deficiency, and is often due to Spleen qi deficiency, which results from inadequate digestion, absorption, storage, and metabolism of nutrients. Malnutrition is sadly still a factor in the etiology of this disorder. In women it is often due to hemorrhage associated with menstruation, abortion, miscarriage, and multiple childbirth. The menorrhagia can have several etiologies, including the Liver failing to store the blood, the Spleen failing to govern the blood, and deficiency of Kidney qi failing to support the lower burner, as well as blood stagnation associated with blood deficiency. Another important factor here is the generally neglected but extremely central role of Kidney yin essence in the development and maintenance of the bone marrow, and therefore the hemopoetic system and production of red blood cells. Biomedicine has identified a hemopoetic factor in the Kidneys. Working for long hours with insufficient sleep is another etiology, often accompanied by a peach color on the side of the tongue. The vessels on the inside of the lower eyelids will be pale.

Thin Tight

This quality is usually associated with overwork of the 'nervous system' due to emotional stress over a long period of time, and is a sign of blood and yin deficiency.

YIN AND ESSENCE DEPLETION

Yin and essence depletion is expressed by increasing hardness of the pulse, beginning with the already mentioned Taut-Tense quality, and moving through Tight to Wiry, which is the quality most deficient in yin and essence.

Tight

Tension turns to Tightness as heat from excess evolves into a yin deficient condition, because the yin of the body exhausts itself trying to balance the heat. The first part of this condition can be described as a vigorous disease, and the second is clearly one of yin deficiency and heat from deficiency. The body and/or mind has worked beyond its energy and has therefore depleted the yin fluids. The rate is usually Normal, or perhaps slightly Rapid. This is most commonly encountered as a more advanced stage in the continuum of the situation described above, denoted by Dr. Shen as 'nervous system tense.' Yin deficiency may be envisioned as the 'nervous system' overworking for a period of years, just as qi deficiency is associated with the physical body overworking for a long period of time.

Intense pain throughout the body is another cause of the uniformly Tight pulse. Often the Tightness has an additional, slightly Biting quality. When the pain is acute, the pulse is slightly Rapid, and when it is chronic, the pulse is Slower and the complexion is often dark.

In a drawn out febrile illness with a high fever the pulse may be uniformly Tight, Rapid, Bounding, and Robust Pounding. Tightness in certain portions, such as the Small and Large Intestine positions, can also be a sign of a hyperactive and possibly inflammatory condition of the organs associated with that position.

Wiry

The Wiry pulse is the next stage in the progression of increasing yin deficiency and is the principal sign of the depletion of essence, the energetic substance associated with the development and maintenance of the 'nervous system.' It appears for all of the same reasons that yin deficiency exists in the first place. It represents one step beyond the Tight pulse in the depletion of body fluids, and is especially associated with overworking of the 'nervous system' and exhaustion of Kidney yin. The Wiry quality, more than the Tight quality, can also be associated with pain. Early diabetes/hypertension are considerations.

QI AND YANG DEFICIENCY

One way of viewing deficiency is to distinguish between that which occurs when yin and yang are still in contact, and the more severe form in which yin and yang are separated. The following qualities are associated with the state where yin and yang are still in contact. These can occur over the entire pulse or in just one position. Those qualities that represent the separation of yin and yang over the entire pulse are referred to as 'qi wild' qualities. And those that occur in only one position are signs of extreme dysfunction of the organ represented by that position. The qualities are presented in a sequence of increasing deficiency.

Yin and yang in contact

Short Yielding

This pulse can be felt at any depth as being discontinuous from the distal to the proximal position. When it is 'Short Weak'[17] it is a sign of severe deficiency and reduced qi and blood circulation among the organs (see Chapter 10).

Deep

This pulse can be accessed only at the organ depth and reflects a chronic internal disharmony that is more serious and more difficult to heal. It should be noted that the pulse of an obese person is normally deeper than that of a thinner individual. As previously mentioned, Dr. Shen believes that a person with this pulse is vulnerable, and if not ill, will be symptomatic within a few years if the condition remains unresolved.

There is some question about a Deep pulse that is a constitutional quality, without the usual significance of an advancing disharmony.[18] Dr. Shen, in discussing the Hidden quality, has made similar remarks. I have also had patients with a Deep pulse who are seemingly in good health, although some of them were born prematurely (see Chapter 9).

Deep Reduced Substance

Here the pulse maintains its form but seems to lose its resilience and buoyancy. This is a sign of additional qi and blood deficiency of the yin organ(s).

Deep Separating

Separation at the organ depth, one that is Yielding and gives way to finger pressure moving to the sides, represents an increasing depletion of qi and blood in the organ due to overwork without sufficient rest.

Feeble-Absent

The qualities Feeble and Absent (see Chapter 8) are discussed together because their significance is almost indistinguishable. The Feeble quality is a sign of a process on the same disease continuum that is slightly less serious than the Absent quality. As the pulse separates and gives way more and more easily to pressure, the deficiency increases in severity until one can only find little (Feeble) or no evidence (Absent) of the pulse at any depth. While this phenomenon is more frequently found at individual positions, it can occur over the entire pulse or on one or the other side, and may also occur bilaterally at the same position.

When the entire pulse is Feeble-Absent there is deficiency of the true qi, that is, the qi, yin, and blood of the yin organs of the entire organism. At this point it is a sign of weakened resistance and vulnerability, rather than present disease. Dr. Shen observed that with this quality, illness can be expected within one year since it represents a chronic process such as a prolonged illness or a lifetime of going beyond one's energy in a variety of ways. It is found in people with impaired immune systems and with chronic fatigue syndrome, as well as in women who have given birth to and raised children beyond their ability, although here blood deficiency is likely to be equally pronounced.

Another condition in which this quality is found uniformly over the entire pulse is that described by Dr. Shen as 'nervous system weak.'[19] Again, this is a constitutional disorder in which the pulse goes through a series of stages, eventually ending in a generally Feeble-Absent pulse. This pulse is often found in a person who has a lifelong history of neurasthenia, one whose symptoms are always changing, and who is highly vulnerable, unstable, and easily disturbed or stressed, and subject to constantly fluctuating allergies. The pulse does not represent illness so much as physical and mental instability and vulnerability to stress.

While the Feeble-Absent quality represents a pathological process that must be taken seriously, it is important to note that a chaotic pulse picture that has many different qualities at the various positions and depths may, in some instances, reflect a degree of anarchy indicative of more serious pathology than a completely Absent pulse.

Hidden Deficient

When classified with the deficient organ energies, this pulse quality represents extreme exhaustion of the yang. This quality is mentioned here in deference to its appearance in Dr. Shen's book. He never mentioned or demonstrated it during our eight years together, and always indicated that impulses which felt deeper than the organ depth could not be classified with the other qualities in his pulse system. Dr. Shen confirms in a personal communication that his Hidden quality and my Deep quality are the same.

Separation of yin and yang (yin and yang out of contact)

While the following qualities are not felt at the organ depth, they are signs of pathology in the yin organs which are represented on the pulse at the organ depth. (To reiterate, the organization of this chapter, unlike most of the other chapters, is based on interpretation rather than on sensation.) In fact, in all but two—the Hollow qualities—all of the others have an Absent organ depth.

Separation of yin and yang at one position is a sign of extreme dysfunction of the organ represented by that position. When this quality is found over the entire pulse, it is sign of a 'qi wild' disorder of the entire body, signifying that the qi of the entire organism is in chaos (it may even be considered a pre-cancerous or pre-psychotic sign). Dr. Shen believed that the Empty Interrupted and Hollow Interrupted combinations (see Chapters 6 and 9) are the most serious.

Empty

A serious scenario in the continuum of organ deficiency is a condition reflected by the Empty quality (see Chapters 6 and 9), in which a sensation is palpable at the qi depth, but not at the blood and organ depths. (The Empty quality is classified with the qi depth pulses under the general category of depth, since our classification system is based on sensation. Here, in our discussion of organ-depth qualities, it is classified by interpretation.) This is a condition in which the material aspects of the body—the yin—have lost control of the lighter yang (qi) energies. There is a loss of functional interaction between the yin and yang in which either the yin cannot nourish the yang, or the yang cannot move the yin. The yang then floats to the surface of the body and scatters aimlessly, that is, with a diminished ordered function ordinarily imposed upon it through contact with the organized yin matrix, thus creating a chaotic physiology. This leaves a severe imbalance between the inside and the outside, between yin and yang, known as 'qi wild.' Even without symptoms, when this quality appears over the entire pulse, according to Dr. Shen, significant illness can be anticipated within six months if the condition is not resolved. I have found the timeline to be closer to one-and-a-half years.

The causes of a consistently Empty quality over the entire pulse are usually due to a combination of an impoverished environment, including inadequate nutrition, shelter, and clothing; overwork, and excessive sex, especially between the ages of fifteen to twenty years; and/or constitutional deficiency. Another increasingly common cause is excessive exercise at a young age beyond one's energy, which leads to profound qi depletion, and in many cases severe anxiety and difficulty with attention and concentration. Other increasingly common causes are drug abuse, especially marijuana, and liver infections such as mononucleosis and hepatitis. While the Yielding Empty quality is more common at the left middle position with these etiologies, in the later stages of the process the entire pulse can be Yielding Empty. When the Emptiness over the entire pulse is not consistent, the cause is ordinarily severe emotional stress.

There are five types of Empty pulse. The one we are discussing in this section can be palpated at the qi depth only, and is uniformly Empty and of normal hardness. It is an indication of increasing qi deficiency generally, and particularly in the yin organ system. This form of the Empty pulse is more Yielding than the harder sensation associated with the Leather quality; it is less Yielding than the more pliable sensations of the Empty Thread-like (Soggy or Soft) quality, the Scattered, and the Minute qualities. The latter is found only at the blood depth.

Leather

The Leather quality (see Chapters 6 and 9) is similar in form to the Empty pulse, except that it is much harder at the surface and represents a more severe deficiency of essence, yin, or blood. The 'qi wild' condition is a more advanced disorder than that associated with the Empty pulse.

Empty Thread-like (soggy)

The Empty Thread-like (soggy or soft) quality (see Chapters 6 and 9) is "like a thread floating on water"[20] at the qi depth, which disappears on pressure, and is otherwise like the Empty quality. It is a sign of extreme deficiency of blood, essence, and yang.

Scattered

Of even greater severity (and concern) is the next step in the progression of deficiency, which is represented by the Scattered quality (see Chapters 6 and 9). This quality is felt only discontinuously at the surface and signifies a further disintegration in the continuity of qi within both yin and yang, and of the blood circulation. In this instance, the damage usually occurs before the age of fifteen. This pulse is a more extreme form of the Empty quality associated with 'qi wild.' It is found in AIDS patients, where it is referred to as "ceiling dripping." The prognosis is poor.

Minute

This quality (see Chapters 6 and 9) is Thin and Yielding and is found discontinuously only in the blood depth; it shows little resistance to pressure, and resembles in sensation the Scattered pulse. This is sign of extensive qi and yang deficiency in a seriously ill person. I see it as a stage in the development of a 'qi wild' disorder beyond the Empty pulse, in which there is not enough yang left to rise to the surface.

Yielding Hollow Full-Overflowing

The Empty and the Hollow qualities are frequently confused. The Hollow pulse is felt in the qi and organ depths, but much less in the middle blood depth, whereas the Empty pulse is felt only superficially, in the qi depth. Both the Yielding Hollow Full-Overflowing and the Empty pulses are signs of 'qi wild.' The Yielding Hollow Full-Overflowing and Slow pulse reflects physiological damage beginning sometime between the ages of ten and fifteen. This form of 'qi wild' is considered less serious than the two types involving the Interrupted quality, the etiology of which usually occurs before the age of ten.

The Yielding Hollow Full-Overflowing and Rapid pulse can occur later in life under the following conditions. With excessive exercise the blood vessels dilate, and the Heart pumps with greater vigor. Should such exercise suddenly be discontinued, the blood vessels remain dilated while the blood volume dramatically decreases. This division between the two leaves a gap which is experienced on the pulse as a Hollow quality. The yin has even less control of the yang. More rarely, an episode in which a person is called to suddenly lift a weight far beyond his or her capacity can also cause a Yielding Hollow quality. For a more complete discussion of the Yielding Hollow quality, see Chapter 9.

Empty Interrupted-Intermittent, Yielding Hollow Interrupted-Intermittent

This is a severe form of 'qi wild' in that the instability is already in the yin organs, combined with chaotic qi in the Heart. The presence or imminence of serious, even terminal, disease is great.

Conclusion

It is worth repeating my earlier suggestion: The larger picture of the pulse should be looked at before exploring the more specific. We must first resolve the disharmonies in rate, rhythm, and stability, in the general depletion of the true qi in its various forms as described in this chapter, in the disorders that involve the entire blood and circulation, or in the general separation of yin from yang, before attempting to cope with the individual deficiencies and excesses in particular organ systems. Otherwise, little of lasting value will be accomplished, since the issues that affect the entire pulse (or large segments of it) are the ones of greatest significance to physiology and survival. Furthermore, the unresolved qualities involving large aspects of the pulse render the qualities on the lesser aspects unreliable indicators of disease patterns.

CHAPTER 14

Uniform Qualities on Other Large Segments of the Pulse

CONTENTS

Uniform Qualities on Left or Right Side, 501
    Husband-wife imbalance, 501
    Shen's view, 502
        'Systems' model synopsis, 502
            Balance, 503
            Movement, 503
            'Systems' affecting each other, 503
                Effects of 'nervous system' on other systems, 503
                Effects of 'circulatory system' on other systems, 504
                Effects of 'organ system' on other systems, 504
    Left side: 'organ system', 505
        Robust quality, 505
            Qi stagnation with a Cotton quality, 505
            Pain, 505
            Diabetes, 505
            Hypertension and cerebrovascular accident (stroke), 505
            Toxicity, 505
            Liver wind, 506
        Reduced quality, 506
            'Organ system' deficient, 506
    Right side: 'digestive system', 506
        Physiology, 506
        Robust quality, 507
            Eating too quickly, 507
            Hypertension and cerebrovascular accident (stroke), 507
            Damp-heat in the 'digestive system', 507

    Reduced quality, 508
        Eating irregularly, 508
        Damp-cold in the 'digestive system', 508
    Robust or Reduced quality, 508
        Physical labor immediately after eating, 508
Either side, 508
    Slippery quality, 508
    Very Tense or Tight Hollow Full-Overflowing, 508
    Change in Intensity and qualities from side to side, 508
Uniform Qualities Bilaterally at Same Position, 509
    Overview, 509
        Lower burner: proximal positions, 509
        Middle burner: middle positions, 509
        Upper burner: distal positions, 510
    Floating, 510
        Distal positions, 510
            Floating Tense and Slow, 510
            Floating Tense with Normal or slightly Rapid rate, 510
            Floating Yielding and Rapid, 510
            Floating Yielding and Slow, 510
        Middle positions, 511
        Proximal positions, 511
    Cotton, 511
        Distal positions, 511
        Middle positions, 511
        Proximal positions, 511
    Hollow Full-Overflowing, 511
        Distal positions, 511
        Middle positions, 511
        Proximal positions, 512
    Flooding Excess, 512
        Distal positions, 512
        Middle positions, 512
        Proximal positions, 512
    Inflated, 512
        Distal positions, 512
            Trapped qi, 512
                Yielding Inflated, 512
                    Using the voice incorrectly, 512
                    Unexpressed grief, 512
            Trapped qi and heat, 513
                Tense Inflated, 513
                    Lifting, 513
                    Trauma to upper burner in a strong person, 513
                    Sudden intense, unexpressed anger, 513
                Moderately Tense Inflated, 513
                    Liver attacking upwards, 513
                    Mediastinal or breast tumors, 513
                    Invading cold transforms into heat, 513
                    Emphysema, 513
                Mildly Tense Inflated, 513

                        Breech presentation and prolonged delivery, 513
                Middle positions, 514
                    Trapped qi, 514
                        Yielding Inflated, 514
                            Spleen qi deficiency, 514
                            Ruminating while eating, 514
                    Trapped heat, 514
                        Tense Inflated, 514
                            Liver and Stomach qi stagnation, 514
                            Lifting after eating, 514
                            Trauma, 514
                        Very Tight Inflated, 514
                            Stomach heat, 514
                            Pancreatitis, 514
                            Peritonitis, 514
                Proximal positions, 514
        Flat, 514
            Distal positions, 515
                Sudden emotional trauma, 515
                Umbilical cord around infant's neck at delivery, 515
                Physical trauma, lifting, and chest surgery, 515
                Improper breathing, 515
                Mediastinal or breast tumor, 515
            Middle positions, 515
                Sitting bent over, 515
                Trauma or abdominal surgery, 516
                Lifting, 516
            Proximal positions, 516
                Prolonged standing or walking on hard surfaces, 516
        Tense, 516
            Distal positions, 516
                Moderate or less recent trauma to the chest, 517
                Unresolved internalized cold, 517
                Using the lungs beyond one's energy, 517
                Lifting, 517
            Middle positions, 517
                Trauma and abdominal surgery, 517
                Emotional stress, 517
                Food stagnation and/or cold from excess in the Stomach, 517
                Bending, 517
                Physical labor immediately after eating, 517
            Proximal positions, 517
                Sexual abstinence, 518
                Early stage of infection (heat from excess) in the lower burner, 518
                Trauma and pelvic surgery, 518
                Overexposure to heat, 518
        Tight-Wiry, 518
            Distal positions, 518
                Trauma, 518
                Hypertension and headache, 518
                Severe pain, 519

    Yin deficiency of the Heart and Lungs, 519
    Cardiac asthma and chronic lung asthma, 519
    Emotional stress, 519
    Febrile disease, 519
    Cocaine addiction, 519
  Special Lung position bilaterally, 519
  Middle positions, 519
    Nervous tension, 519
    Infection, 520
    Diabetes and/or hypertension, 520
    Pain, 520
      'Running piglet illness', 520
      Trauma, 520
      Lifting, 520
      Sitting in bent position, 520
      Infection, 520
  Proximal positions, 520
    Kidney yin deficiency, heat from deficiency, and essence deficiency, 520
    Diabetes and and/or hypertension, 520
    Infection, 520
    Pain, 520
      Kidney stones, 521
      Trauma, 521
      Hernia, 521
      Intestinal qi stagnation, 521
      Overexposure to cold, 521
      Blood stagnation, 521
Slippery, 521
  Distal positions, 521
    Lung damp-heat with asthma, 521
    Phlegm-fire disturbing the Heart, 521
    Phlegm confusing the orifices of the Heart, 522
  Bilaterally at Special Lung position, 522
  Middle positions, 522
    Spleen qi deficiency and/or Liver-Gallbladder damp-heat, 522
    Stagnant food, 522
    Stomach or duodenal ulcer, 522
  Proximal positions, 522
    Kidney stones and lower burner infection, 522
Thin, 523
  Distal positions, 523
    Heart and Lung blood deficiency, 523
    Heart and Lung qi and blood deficiency, 523
    Heart yang deficiency with cardiopulmonary insufficiency, 523
    Heart and Lung yin and blood deficiency, 523
    Lung yin deficiency-type chronic asthma affecting Heart blood circulation, 523
    Heart blood deficiency with Heart and Lung phlegm, 524
  Middle positions, 524
    Spleen qi deficiency with Heart and Liver blood deficiency, 524
  Proximal positions, 524
    Kidney qi deficiency, 524

            Kidney yin and essence deficiency, 524
            Deficient-type qi stagnation in the lower burner, 524
Feeble-Absent Deep, 524
    Distal positions, 525
        Early emotional shock, 525
        Physical trauma, 525
        Overwork of the Lungs, 525
        Tuberculosis, 525
    Middle positions, 525
        Spleen and Stomach qi deficiency, 525
        Sitting bent over, 526
        Rumination while eating, 526
        Eating habits, 526
        Anorexia and bulimia, 526
        Parasites, 526
        Liver 'attacks' Stomach-Spleen, 526
    Proximal positions, 526
        Constitutional Kidney deficiency, 527
        Excessive sex, 527
        Menorrhagia and chronic colitis, 527
Empty, 527
    Distal positions, 527
        Overwork of the Lungs, 527
        Physical trauma, 527
        Recent sudden grief, 528
        Emotional trauma, 528
    Middle positions, 528
        Impoverishment, 528
        Sitting bent over, 528
        Rumination, 528
        Resuming work too soon after eating, 528
        Trauma and abdominal surgery, 528
        Liver attacks Spleen, 528
        Anorexia and/or bulimia, 529
        Diet, 529
        Drug abuse, 529
        Parasites, 529
    Proximal positions, 529
        Constitution, excessive sex, chronic colitis, prolonged excessive menorrhagia, 529
Hollow, 529
    Distal positions, 529
        Trauma to the chest with hemorrhage (Leather-like Hollow), 529
        Lifting beyond one's energy (Yielding Hollow Full-Overflowing), 530
    Middle positions, 530
        Abdominal hemorrhage (Leather-like Hollow), 530
        Heavy physical labor after meals (Yielding Hollow Full-Overflowing and Slow), 530
        Advanced diabetes or hypertension (Very Tight Hollow Full-Overflowing), 530
    Proximal positions, 530
        Chronic uterine bleeding and intestinal dysfunction (Yielding Hollow Full-
            Overflowing and Slow), 530
        Imminent hemorrhage in the lower burner (Leather-like Hollow and Rapid), 530

Recent hemorrhage in the lower burner (Leather-like Hollow and Slow), 530
Advanced diabetes or hypertension (Very Tight Hollow Full-Overflowing with Rapid rate), 531

Vibration, 531
    Neuro-psychological position, 531
    Distal positions, 531
    Middle positions, 531
    Proximal positions, 531

Stagnation between the burners, 531
    Between upper and middle positions: diaphragm positions, 532
        Emotional trauma associated with separation, 532
        Lifting beyond one's energy, 532
        Single episode of suppressed and very strong anger, when Heart and Liver are strong, 532
        Hypertension, 532
    Between positions: musculoskeletal disorders, 532

Change in Qualities and Intensity bilaterally, 535
    Distal positions, 535
    Middle positions, 535
    Proximal positions, 535

Table 14-1: Similar qualities bilaterally at same position, 535

CHAPTER 14

Uniform Qualities on Other Large Segments of the Pulse

Uniform Qualities on Left or Right Side

In this section are listed the most common disorders associated with each of the individual pulse qualities when they are found uniformly over one or the other side of the wrist.

HUSBAND-WIFE IMBALANCE

There are several interpretations in the literature concerning the relationship of the right and left sides of the pulse. One view is that a husband-wife (i.e., right and left pulse) imbalance is a sign of eternal difficulties with interpersonal relationships, especially with intimate partners, a phenomenon that I can corroborate clinically through work with many patients. Another view is that a husband-wife imbalance is a reflection of being unbalanced physically, mentally, or both. I once encountered a forty-five-year-old woman with neck and back pain since childhood. She also complained of feeling unbalanced and "discombobulated" down her left side her entire life. The moment the left and right side pulses were balanced after treatment, she broke down in tears and began to talk about her relationship with her husband. Following this, she had no further symptoms.

According to Van Buren,[1] the laws of nature operate to continuously maintain balance. Yang conforms to the right side of the body and yin to the left side. However, in the service of balance, polarized cosmic energy enters a woman's body with the yang distributed to the right side and the yin to the left; in a man, yang is distributed to the left side and yin to the right. Although not explicitly stated, the inference is that in women the right pulse—and in men, the left pulse—should be more Robust. Van Buren believes that in order to maintain balance, in women, yin points are needled on the right side and yang points on the left, and in men, yin points on the left and yang points on the right. Throughout most of my career I have endeavored to follow this rule.

My information concerning Worsley's practice with regard to husband-wife balance and imbalance has been obtained from his students over the course of three decades.

From 1971 through approximately 1981, Worsley taught that in women, the right pulse should feel more Robust than the left, and in men, the left should feel more Robust than the right. Any deviation indicated disharmony. Then in the 1980s, the message changed. The view now seems to be that the left pulse should always be more Robust than the right, the reason being that the yin organs on the right side are more concerned with nurture, and those on the left more with function. Since function is more active than nurture, the functional pulse should normally have a more Robust quality. In fact, any deviation is considered extremely serious, and I have been informed that in Worsley's view, without correction, an individual with a husband-wife imbalance in which the right pulse is more Robust than the left could be expected to live only six months. Some students of Worsley's who also consider this imbalance to be serious take a less cataclysmic view: they speak of grave consequences within three to fifteen years. More importantly, they view (as do I) the husband-wife imbalance as a sign of constant difficulties with interpersonal relationships, especially with the opposite gender.

Li Shi-Zhen's view[2] of the imbalance in left and right pulses is set forth in the following passage:

> Both men and women have a slight yin-yang imbalance which is reflected as a slight difference between the right and left pulses. The left is yang and the right is yin. Men have more yang qi. So, provided their qi is well regulated, their left hand pulse is stronger. Women have more yin blood. In women, provided their qi is well regulated, their right hand pulse is stronger.

It should be mentioned that Worsley's original thesis[3] regarding the relationship between the right and left pulses in men and women seems to reflect Li Shi-Zhen's view.

Amber[4] also lists certain conditions in which there are disparities between the left and right pulses:

> Aneurysm of the arch of the aorta; cervical rib; embolism of the brachial artery; atheroma of the brachial or subclavian artery; aneurism of the subclavian, axillary, brachial, and innominate arteries; mediastinal tumor; fracture of the arm; cicatrices of the arm; tumor or enlarged gland of axilla; pneumothorax; pleural effusion.

SHEN'S VIEW

Dr. Shen's views about the right- and left-side pulses are an integral part of his 'systems' theory in which the right side represents the 'digestive system' and the left side the 'organ system.'[5] When the right pulse is more Robust than the left, the inference is that the 'digestive system' is overworking to compensate for a deficient yin 'organ system.' When the left pulse is stronger than the right, the inference is that the 'digestive system' is more deficient than the 'organ system,' either from poor nutrition or eating habits in a young person, or through resuming work too soon after eating in an older person. Dr. Shen appeared to view the integrity of the 'digestive system' as a predictor of whether a person can or cannot recover from an illness. In other words, while the preference would be for equality between the sides, if the 'organ system' is impaired and the left pulse is Reduced, the preference is for the right-side 'digestive system' to be more Robust than the left side. This is in direct contrast to Worsley's view of the husband-wife imbalance, in which the left side should normally be more Robust for both men and women.

'Systems' model synopsis

Remember that a 'system' problem does not yet involve organ pathology but is only a sign which explains otherwise unexplainable symptoms, such as migrating joint pain, which occurs with circulatory disharmony. The systems are prognostic signs of a pathologic process which will end in disease if not interrupted.

BALANCE

Balance between the left and right pulses is dependent on the proper functioning of the 'digestive system' and 'organ system.' Balance between the upper and lower portions of the body is dependent on the ability of the 'circulatory system' to maintain a steady and smooth flow of qi and blood through the three burners.

MOVEMENT

When the movement of qi and blood is inadequate, the problem is with the 'circulatory system' and the pulse is Slow. When the movement of qi is too quick, the problem is with the 'nervous system' and the pulse is too Rapid.

SYSTEMS AFFECTING EACH OTHER

The sequence that follows—initiated in the 'nervous system'—is the one that occurs when all the systems are approximately equal in strength. Otherwise, the system that is affected first is the weakest, and there is no further progression through this sequence.

If the 'nervous system' is not treated effectively, it first affects the 'circulatory system.' If the 'nervous system' and 'circulatory system' are not treated effectively, it will affect the 'digestive system.' If the 'nervous system,' 'circulatory system,' and 'digestive system' are not treated, it will affect the 'organ system.' Finally, if one of the yin organs in the 'organ system' is especially vulnerable, serious disease ensues.

The system whose symptoms first appear is the root source. For example, one deciding factor between the 'nervous system' and 'digestive system' is whether the tension preceded the digestive disorder or vice versa. If the tension came first, the root source is the 'nervous system,' but if the digestive disorder came first, the root source is the 'digestive system.'

While disorders of the four systems can result from life experiences, those experiences most commonly affect the 'circulatory' and 'digestive' systems. The 'organ' and 'nervous' systems are more often influenced by constitutional factors than are the other two systems. The 'digestive system' (the earth) nourishes the others.

Effects of 'nervous system' on other systems

The effects described below are related to a 'nervous system tense' disorder. The cause may be constitutional or based on life experience. With the former, the person is tense only under stress; with the latter, the person is always tense (see Chapter 7).

With respect to life experience, due to the increasing demands of the modern industrial and technological revolutions that we become hyperactive supermen and women, it is the 'nervous system' that is most often the primary culprit that adversely affects all of the other systems. And, over the centuries, as a species adaptational adjustment, life experience becomes constitutional.

On the 'organ system'

Over the entire left pulse there is one very Thin, Tight line on the surface of whatever depth is first accessed, usually moderately deep, especially in the left middle and proximal positions. This is a situation in which the 'nervous system' is affecting the 'organ system' over a period of time, causing the nervous innervation of the yin organs to overwork and thus gradually develop heat from deficiency. The qi of the yin organs is being accelerated. Such symptoms as agitation, irritability, excitability, and fatigue ensue from this drying of the yin in the yin organs, and in particular of their nervous innervation. This is a vicious circle in which nervous tension depletes the yin, the absence of which makes the superficial qi less controlled and more aimless, which in turn makes the nerves more irritable. The symptoms of fatigue are essentially the same as when the 'organ system' affects the 'nervous system,' except that when 'organ system' deficiency is primary, the fatigue arrives earlier, and is more prominent than the tension which characterizes the 'nervous system.' When the 'organ system' is the etiology, the pulse, especially on the left side, is Slow, Deep, and Feeble-Absent, and the person is more depressed than agitated.

On the 'digestive system'

Habitually eating too quickly due to a tense 'nervous system' can cause the entire right side to be Tight at the surface of whichever depth is first accessed. Irregular eating caused by a tense 'nervous system' can lead to the right side being Feeble. The left side is probably Long, Robust, and Tight in either circumstance, unless the 'organ system' is deficient. Historically, tension will precede a digestive disorder.

On the 'circulatory system'

The rate is Normal, the qi depth is Tight, the middle depth separates on pressure (partially Hollow), and the organ depth is Tense or Tight. Dr. Shen stated that the pulse is also superficial, which I cannot corroborate.

Effects of 'circulatory system' on other systems

On the 'nervous system'

A deficient 'circulatory system' will make the 'nervous system' more vulnerable to emotional stress. Diminished circulation impairs the Heart, which controls the mind, and in turn further diminishes circulation to the brain (marrow) and to the peripheral nerves. The pulse is generally Slow and Tense-Tight.

On the 'digestive system'

A deficient 'circulatory system' along with poor eating habits can affect the 'digestive system' by reducing circulation to the splanchnic plexus, causing digestive problems. The right side is Feeble and the entire pulse (both wrists) is Slow.

On the 'organ system'

Deficiency of the 'digestive system' due to an impaired 'circulatory system' eventually affects the 'organ system,' although a very Slow pulse rate over a long period of time—which indicates poor circulation in the organs—can weaken the 'organ system' directly. In that case, the pulse is Slow and the left side is Feeble.

Effects of 'organ system' on other systems

On the 'nervous system'

Deficiency of the 'organ system' can lead to poor nutrition in the 'nervous system.' When there is stress on Kidney qi (due to constitutional factors and/or excessive work—mental or physical—or sex), or a 'nervous system tense' or weak condition, the 'nervous system' is adversely affected by a deficient 'organ system.' The left side is Deeper and more Feeble, the right side slightly Tense-Tight, and the entire pulse is perhaps slightly Slower than normal. The symptoms include severe fatigue, emotional tension, lassitude, depression, labile emotions, and anxiety. The fatigue is essentially the same as that associated with the 'nervous system' affecting the 'organ system,' except that when 'organ system' deficiency is primary, the onset of fatigue is earlier and is more prominent than the tension which characterizes the 'nervous system.'

On the 'circulatory system'

Deficiency of the 'organ system' leads to a deficiency of true qi. To compensate, the circulatory system must work harder to nourish the organism. Especially if accompanied by overexercise, this can deplete the 'circulatory system.' The pulse is exceptionally Slow and Feeble. In addition to extreme fatigue, other symptoms include cold hands and feet, migrating joint pain, and quick temper.

On the 'digestive system'

If the 'organ system' is unable to sustain metabolic function, the functioning of the 'digestive system' will likewise diminish. One must check to see whether the first symptoms were associated with 'organ system' deficiency—fatigue and weakness—or with 'digestive system' deficiency, where erratic digestive symptoms in which appetite and bowel function fluctuate precede the fatigue. The entire pulse is Feeble-Absent or Empty. If the 'organ system' is the cause of a generally deficient condition, the left side is Deeper and more Feeble. If the 'digestive system' is the cause, the right side is Deeper and more Feeble.

Left side: 'organ system'

As mentioned above, Dr. Shen identifies the left side of the pulse with the 'organ system,' which includes the most essential yin organs. On the left pulse there are two frequently found pathological situations in which there is a uniformity to the pulse. In the first, the pulse tends to be more Robust, and in the second, more Reduced. When the left side 'organ system' is very Reduced, the cause is generally constitutional, except in the aged and among those with chronic debilitating illness.

ROBUST QUALITY

Qi stagnation with a Cotton quality

This is a sign of qi stagnation on the left side which can be due to a trauma to that side, or it can be a sign of resignation (the 'sad pulse') that has existed for a short time (less than five years). As the condition worsens or persists, the Cotton quality spreads to the right side.

Pain

The pulse is uniformly Tight to Wiry, and possibly slightly Rapid if there is pain. The exact location of the pain corresponds to the position that is Tightest. The cause is usually a recent trauma. Facial color is dark.

Diabetes

The left side is moderately Wiry in the early stages, and very Tight Hollow Full-Overflowing and possibly Slippery at the blood depth in the later stages. These qualities are more prominent in the middle and proximal positions, especially the proximal.

Speculatively, the Slippery quality, especially at the blood depth, seems to represent interference with the free-flow of the blood, a form of turbulence caused by elevated sugar levels, elevated lipids, plaque, or other impurities (ketone bodies) in the blood.

Hypertension and cerebrovascular accident (stroke)

In the early stages the pulse is Wiry, especially in the left distal and middle positions. Later the pulse is Rapid and very Tight Hollow Full-Overflowing on the left side, especially in the distal and middle positions. Slipperiness, especially at the blood depth, can be found here also, particularly if there is simultaneous dampness in the Spleen and Gallbladder. Again, the Slippery quality seems to represent interference with the free-flow of the blood, a form of turbulence caused perhaps by excessive dampness and phlegm (lipids, in biomedical terms). When the pulse is very Tight, there is a high risk of a paralytic stroke of the entire left side of the body. If the rate is Rapid, stroke on the side with this quality is imminent. After the stroke the pulse will be Feeble and Slow.

Toxicity

The conditions and associated pulse qualities Blood Unclear, Blood Heat, and Blood Thick described in Chapter 13 are relevant in this case, although the qualities usually appear over the entire pulse. Slipperiness over the entire left side at the blood depth is a sign of blood toxicity in the Liver. On the other hand, when found only at the organ depth, it is usually associated with infection (parasites or low grade hepatitis), especially in the liver. A Yielding Slipperiness at the qi depth on the left side is a sign of Liver qi deficiency when the rate is Slow, and of elevated sugar levels in the blood when the rate is Normal or Rapid and the pulse is Tense.

Liver wind

A moderate Liver wind condition may be indicated by a Tight Floating quality on the left side, especially at the left middle position.

REDUCED QUALITY

'Organ system' deficient

The pulse is Slow, the entire left side is Deep and Feeble-Absent, Empty or Slow Yielding-Hollow Full-Overflowing with increasing fatigue. The tongue tends to be pale, swollen, and wet. The vertical blood vessels on the mucosa of the lower eyelids also tend to be pale. General weakness prevails although there may be no concurrent evidence of disease.

The causes may be a constitutional 'nervous system weak' condition (see Chapter 15); a prolonged recovery from a serious illness that has weakened the yin organs; an ongoing, chronic, draining illness such as paraplegia; or a degenerative disease such as multiple sclerosis. When the condition arises after twenty years of age, the quality is more Feeble-Absent; between fifteen and twenty years, it is more likely to be Empty; and between ten to fifteen years, Yielding Hollow Full-Overflowing and Slow. When there is a slightly greater Reduction in the distal and proximal positions than in the middle positions, if accompanied by depression, the cause is probably constitutional with a genetically deficient Kidney qi and Kidney-Heart disharmony. The etiology can also be traced to emotional trauma and severe illness very early in life. When the Reduction is more equally distributed, the disharmony can be attributed to life experience, specifically either excessive sex, overwork, or overexercise at an early age.

Right side: 'digestive system'

PHYSIOLOGY

Dr. Shen identifies the right-side pulse with the 'digestive system.' He arrived at this correlation after many encounters with a syndrome in which the appetite fluctuated between an increased and a diminished desire for food, bowel movements tended to be irregular (sometimes constipated, sometimes loose), and the patient complained of general discomfort in the abdomen, but nothing specific or acute. In these patients, Dr. Shen found a consistent uniformity over the right pulse which led him to postulate the 'digestive system,' one of the four 'systems' that he identified.

In my opinion, Dr. Shen's picture of the 'digestive system' falls within the domain of the Triple Burner.[6] Dr. Shen views all of the organs represented on the right wrist as being involved in digestion: the Lungs 'digest' mucus, the Spleen and Stomach digest food and move dampness or fluids, and the Kidney-Bladder system 'digests' water. Dr. Shen's concept of the 'digestive system' as a discrete unit is one in which pathology occurs when these different aspects fall out of balance with each other. The scenario in which the Liver attacks the Spleen/Stomach can also be present here.

It should be recalled that in traditional Chinese medicine the Triple Burner controls the separation of the pure from the impure and the entire process of water distribution among the three burners and each of the relevant organs, including the Spleen, Lungs, and Kidneys, as well as controlling water absorption from the Small and Large Intestines.

Several patterns, attributed largely to personal habits, can affect the 'digestive system.' Some of these are related to a tense 'nervous system.' Among these are eating too quickly, eating irregularly, resuming work immediately after eating, and excessive thinking or rumination while eating. Others include lifting or sitting for extended periods of time after eating. The resulting patterns may be reflected in the following pulse qualities on the right side.

ROBUST QUALITY

Eating too quickly

My experience with patients who eat too quickly is that their pulses are often generally Tense. Eating too quickly is usually part of a generally unrelaxed approach to life, sometimes constitutionally determined 'nervous system tense,' and sometimes based on life experience, in which case the pulse is also slightly Rapid. These are people who are driven, who generally overwork, and who have very little left for the more pleasurable pursuits in life.

The pulse over the entire right side tends to be very Tight, especially in the right middle Stomach position. This Tightness, in my experience, is frequently just above the depth at which the pulse is accessed; below this, it may be Reduced. This may be accompanied by a uniform Tense quality on the left side, which is present at all depths but primarily at the left middle position, reflecting a tense 'nervous system.' This can be regarded as signaling the Liver attacking the Spleen/Stomach, although it must be remembered that systems, not organs, are involved: an overworked 'nervous system' is affecting the nervous innervation of the digestive functions associated with the Triple Burner system.

The heat from excess in the Stomach from this hyperactivity consumes the gastric secretions and contributes to poor digestion, partially due to the Stomach's consequent inability to moisten and soften food. At this stage of the pattern the individual is often hungry immediately after eating. The Stomach may then develop a condition of heat from yin deficiency. The dryness creates a need for fluids in the Stomach, which feels empty. This increases the hunger, apparently for food that consists mostly of water. There is also a feeling of fullness such that, although there is hunger, only small amounts can be eaten. Individuals so affected often consume snack after snack, filling up, but still experiencing hunger. This condition is exacerbated by eating dry foods.

Hypertension and cerebrovascular accident (stroke)

A very Tight Hollow Full-Overflowing quality on the right pulse is a precursor to a paralytic cerebrovascular accident (stroke) on the right side of the body. If the rate is Rapid, stroke on the side that this quality is found is imminent. If the rate is Slow and the pulse is Feeble, the stroke may have already happened.

Damp-heat in the 'digestive system'

Though rare, a Slippery and Tense combination over the entire right pulse can also indicate 'digestive system' damp-heat and infection developing in the culture medium that dampness creates. In this case the eyes are injected. Slipperiness at the qi depth over the entire right side is a sign of elevated sugar levels in the tissues, and Slipperiness at the blood depth is a sign of elevated sugar and lipids in the blood, which causes turbulence.

REDUCED QUALITY

Eating irregularly

A Reduced pulse over the entire right side that reflects a 'digestive system' pathology can be felt on individuals who ignore their internal needs in the interest of external ones. They eat irregularly, when it suits their ego-oriented schedule, rather than the schedule of their 'digestive system.' They eat when the 'digestive system' is not ready, and do not eat when it is. The result is an impaired digestion that leads to an accumulation of dampness, since food consists primarily of water (food stagnation); the dampness eventually injures the Spleen, causing a qi-deficient damp Spleen.

Damp-cold in the 'digestive system'

Slipperiness, again rarely, and Feebleness over the entire right side may indicate a severe damp-cold disorder in the 'digestive system.' This is indicative of a failure of fluid metabolism and regulation in the Spleen, Lungs, and Kidneys. With this pattern the eyes are normal.

ROBUST OR REDUCED QUALITY

Physical labor immediately after eating

Another habit that can affect the 'digestive system' appears in individuals who resume physical labor too soon after eating. Over a very long period of time, an Empty or Yielding Hollow Full-Overflowing and Slow pulse develops over the entire right side. This pulse is a sign of extreme deficiency and indicates that the qi in the 'digestive system' is 'wild.' Spleen dampness with damp-cold in the Lungs, Bladder, and Intestines is possible. This is often preceded by qualities at the middle position (bilaterally) such as Inflation, Flat, Feeble-Absent, and Empty, depending on the physical condition, other aspects of lifestyle, and the duration of the habit.

Either side

SLIPPERY QUALITY

A Slippery quality on one side at the organ or at all depths indicates infection if the pulse is slightly Rapid. Slipperiness at the qi depth indicates elevated blood sugar if the pulse is Normal or Rapid, and qi deficiency if it is Slow.

VERY TENSE OR TIGHT HOLLOW FULL-OVERFLOWING

Found over either the entire right or left side, this pulse indicates hypertension and what Dr. Shen calls 'vein tight.' More often, however, it is found on the left side only. The Tenseness involves heat from excess, and the Tightness indicates heat from deficiency. If the rate is Rapid, stroke on the side where this quality is found is imminent. After the stroke the pulse will be Slow and Feeble.

CHANGE IN INTENSITY AND QUALITIES FROM SIDE TO SIDE

Patients in whom the intensity is stronger first on one side and then the other have great current difficulty with interpersonal relationships, which are dominating their lives at the time. Other causes are a sudden excessive expenditure of energy beyond one's available true qi. An example is firefighters battling a forest fire for days or weeks on end with little rest (less exertion in a physically weaker person would yield the same result). Dr. Shen has used the expressions 'qi wild,' 'circulation of qi and blood not balanced,' and 'relation to organs not good' to describe this phenomenon. He has indicated that when there are Changes in Qualities first on one side and then the other, it is a weak 'nervous system' disorder similar to a 'qi wild' state, and is much more serious. This is one of the pulses that is reminiscent of the husband-wife imbalance debate. The significance of a Change in Qualities from side to side requires further investigation.

Uniform Qualities Bilaterally at Same Position

In contrast to the presence of a quality in just one position on one wrist, the presence of a quality bilaterally at the same position is regarded as being more a sign of pathology in an *area* of the body rather than in a specific yin or yang organ (see Table 14-1 at the end of this chapter). However, both types of pathology can of course occur at the same time. For example, trauma or heavy lifting can affect the entire chest, while sparing or damaging either the Lungs and/or the Heart.

The appearance of a quality bilaterally at a particular burner is usually a more serious sign than when it appears on only one side.

Each bilateral position, hereafter referred to alternatively as a burner, is discussed in terms of the following commonly-found qualities. Many of the etiologies of these multiple qualities are similar. The variables that determine the differences in pulse qualities are the strength of the person when the etiology began, and the amount of time that has passed since the event, or the duration of the detrimental activity.

OVERVIEW

One can also scan the burners for similarities and differences. The greater the similarity of qualities in the same burner and over the pulse as a whole, the greater the inherent stability of physiology, even if the entire pulse is Feeble-Absent. The presence of pathology in the complementary positions associated with a burner informs us that the disease process in that burner is more advanced and serious than otherwise.

Lower burner: proximal positions

I evaluate the proximal positions to get a sense of the root, the ground on which this person must stand (the Kidneys). If it is reduced in qi at a young age (Deep, Feeble), even up to the age of forty-five depending on degree, I suspect that the constitutional qi is deficient and that recovery will be more difficult. If the person is older, I assume that some of this deficiency is a more gradual draining due to overwork, overexercise, or some other form of abuse (drugs, sex), and that there may be more basic qi with which to work (Reduced Substance).

If the deficiency is primarily that of yin, with harder qualities such as Tight, I realize that this person has probably been overworking their mind and central nervous system. At times, one of these deficiencies is so much more characteristic of the person that it alone will appear. This is especially true if yin is being depleted, since the harder qualities overshadow the more pliable ones (qi deficiency).

More often, in keeping with the realities of life, there are signs of both deficiencies, which informs us that both processes are occurring simultaneously. One proximal position may be Tight and the other Feeble, or the qualities may constantly change from one to the other during the examination.

Middle burner: middle positions

The integrity of the middle burner tells us about how centered this person is in life, and of course about the relationship between the moving and recovering qi (Liver) and the nurturing qi (Spleen-Stomach). It tells us how easily this person can handle stress and toxicity, mental and physical, the organism's capacity for recovery on a day to day basis (Liver), and how well it can replenish itself over time (Spleen).

Upper burner: distal positions

The integrity of the upper burner tells us how well we can reach out to the world, with awareness of our creative being, with the strength to communicate and protect our being, and to maintain mental and emotional stability despite the 'slings and arrows of outrageous fortune' with which we are constantly bombarded. For example, it will tell us how well we can handle shock or recover from grief.

Floating

The Floating quality (Chapter 9) is often a sign of an external pathogenic factor. It indicates increased activity of the superficial, quicker energies (e.g., protective qi) of the organism for defense to help the body rid itself of pathogenic wind, cold, and heat. I have also included conditions with bilateral signs, especially in the middle and proximal positions, which are not related to external pathogenic factors. Thus, along with the Floating quality attributed—mistakenly, in my view—in the literature to these conditions, I present what I consider to be the more accurate quality, based on sensation and interpretation.

Distal positions

These Floating qualities are usually encountered at the right distal positions. Found bilaterally, the condition is more serious.

Floating Tense and Slow

This is a sign of a current wind-cold external pathogenic factor with symptoms of a wind-cold upper respiratory infection. The tongue is wet with a thin white coating.

Floating Tense with Normal or slightly Rapid rate

This can be a sign of a recent, unresolved external pathogenic factor. The indication is that cold has entered the deeper channels, the chest, or the Lungs, creating qi stagnation. In attempting to overcome the stagnation, the body brings heat to the area, which eventually accumulates if the stagnation is not resolved. This quality is more likely to be found in a stronger person whose body is capable of mobilizing the heat. The tongue coating is thin and light yellow.

Floating Yielding and Rapid

This is a sign of external wind-heat with symptoms of a wind-heat upper respiratory infection. The tongue is dry and red with a thin yellow coating.

Floating Yielding and Slow

This combination is probably attributable to a recent cold pathogenic factor in a weak person, which has not been properly cleared from this burner.

Middle positions

Although it is outside of my own experience, the Floating quality is rarely found bilaterally just in the middle positions, although Li Shi-Zhen did observe that "Deficiency and weakness of Spleen qi, affecting the middle heater, or an excess of Liver qi, will show as a floating pulse on the guan [middle] position."[7]

Proximal positions

Although it is outside of my own experience, the Floating quality is rarely found bilaterally in the proximal positions. Again, however, Li Shi-Zhen describes "difficulty in passing urine or stools" associated with this pulse.[8]

Cotton

If found bilaterally at one of the three burners, the Cotton quality (Chapter 9) is an indication of qi stagnation in that area. Whatever the etiology, the Cotton quality found bilaterally only indicates a process which is not yet extensive in its pathological consequences.

Distal positions

The Cotton quality bilaterally at the distal positions is usually due to a recent emotional trauma involving some sense of loss and helplessness rather than anger. A minor local trauma to the chest could also result in a Cotton quality bilaterally in the distal positions.

Middle positions

The Cotton quality at these positions bilaterally involves some digestive discomfort due either to eating while upset or ruminating (Cotton and Tight), eating and talking too much, sitting continuously over a long period of time, resuming work too soon after eating (Cotton and Feeble), or minor trauma to the abdomen.

Proximal positions

The Cotton quality alone in the proximal positions bilaterally is rare and is more often due to mild Kidney qi deficiency, although an injury to the lower part of the body could also bring the same result.

Hollow Full-Overflowing

The Hollow Full-Overflowing quality is a sign of heat in the blood. The Hollow quality is perceived as an absence or as separating on pressure.

Distal positions

I have observed this quality once in a person with severe headache due to hypertension. The middle and lower burner pulses were Feeble or Absent.

Middle positions

A Hollow Full-Overflowing quality bilaterally in the middle position is a sign of impending or current hypertension. Frequently the pulse is also Slippery at the blood depth. Most likely there is a Spleen dampness component to this type of hypertension, although the Slippery quality at the blood depth is more a sign of turbulence in the blood than of Spleen dampness, which would be more convincingly confirmed by a greasy tongue. Diabetes must also be considered as a possibility with this combination of qualities at the middle position bilaterally.

Proximal positions

Hypertension and diabetes must also be considered here.

Flooding Excess

The Flooding Excess quality (Chapter 8) is associated with heat from excess in the yin organs.

Distal positions

This quality may accompany acute fulminating myo-pericarditis or acute bacterial pneumonia.

Middle positions

Here, the quality is associated with acute infection in the area, such as the peritoneum (peritonitis) or appendix (appendicitis), or in a yin organ, such as with hepatitis, cholecystitis, or pancreatitis.

Proximal positions

The possibility of acute fulminating prostatitis, nephritis, bladder and urinary tract or pelvic inflammatory disease (PID) should be considered when a Flooding Excess quality at this position is accompanied by pain and urinary difficulty. Less often, this pulse may appear with an acute, overwhelming ulcerative colitis or regional ileitis with the accompanying symptoms.

Inflated

The Inflated quality (Chapter 8) indicates a situation in which qi is trapped inside of an organ or a particular area and is unable to move out, or heat is trapped in one area or organ and cannot be dissipated. With trapped qi, the quality is more Yielding; with trapped heat, more Tense. The Inflated quality is usually found in a person with a strong constitution at the time the qi was trapped.

Distal positions

TRAPPED QI

Yielding Inflated

Using the voice incorrectly

A Yielding Inflated quality can occur in strong individuals who misuse their voices when they sing or talk, or when they meditate with erroneous breathing techniques. In such cases, the pulse is Inflated and Yielding.

Unexpressed grief

Unexpressed and unresolved grief can give rise to a Yielding Inflated quality bilaterally in the distal positions, usually in an adult with good energy in the chest area at the time of the emotional episode.

TRAPPED QI AND HEAT

Stagnation related to trapped qi brings heat from excess to an organ or area as part of the body's effort to overcome the stagnation caused by the impaired circulation. At some point, this will manifest as trapped heat in the form of a Tense Inflated quality. Over time, all of the etiologies listed above under trapped qi can lead to trapped heat.

Tense Inflated

Lifting

Moderate amounts of trapped qi, and later heat, can occur with one major episode of lifting beyond one's energy. Repeated episodes are more often reflected in stagnation between burners at the Diaphragm area. The pulse is Tense Inflated.

Trauma to upper burner in a strong person

Trauma, including surgery, is a shock to which the body reacts by restricting circulation in the area of the shock. In a strong individual with trauma to the chest, this sudden restriction of circulation causes the excess qi (and later heat) to be trapped in the chest. The pulse is Tense Inflated.

Sudden intense, unexpressed anger

Extreme Inflation can be a sign of a sudden and intense, unexpressed anger which occurs while a person is in motion, such as while exercising or engaged in physical labor. The pulse in this case is very Inflated and moderately Tense.

Moderately Tense Inflated

Liver attacking upwards

Liver qi is the moving qi of the body, the 'free wanderer.' When Liver qi stagnates it will eventually escape from the Liver, although not through regular channels, and will tend to 'attack' the most vulnerable organ. Best known is when it attacks the Spleen-Stomach. However, the Lungs, Intestines, and Bladder are also well-known destinations for this random, unpredictable qi.

Mediastinal or breast tumors

A moderately Tense quality in the upper burner can be a sign of a mediastinal or breast tumor.

Invading cold transforms into heat

Internal retention of heat following repeated upper respiratory infections can sometimes produce this quality bilaterally. For example, the infection has been eliminated by antibiotics but the cold remains, causing obstruction. In the process of trying to overcome the stagnation, the cold eventually transforms into heat. More often this pattern is reflected only on the right distal and Special Lung positions.

Emphysema

With severe emphysema there is extreme trapped qi and possibly heat, and the pulse is very Inflated and Tense, and sometimes Slippery.

Mildly Tense Inflated

Breech presentation and prolonged delivery

Persons who were delivered by breech presentation causing the head to be retained for an excessively long period in the birth canal may present this quality bilaterally in the upper burner; often with this etiology, however, the quality is found only in the left distal position. The pulse is Inflated and mildly Tense.

Middle positions

TRAPPED QI

Yielding Inflated

Spleen qi deficiency

Spleen qi deficiency with consequent qi stagnation may gradually lead to abdominal distention with accumulated gas and a Yielding Inflated pulse. While this quality can occur bilaterally with this etiology, it usually appears at the right middle position alone.

Ruminating while eating

This quality occurs in strong individuals who ruminate excessively and obsessively while eating.

TRAPPED HEAT

Tense Inflated

Liver and Stomach qi stagnation

Liver qi stagnation causing Spleen and Stomach qi stagnation interferes with the movement of qi in the gastrointestinal system and causes abdominal distention, gas, and an Inflated elastic pulse bilaterally; the symptoms are more acute than would be the case from just Spleen qi deficiency alone. Both sides may reflect this quality, as each is highly susceptible to qi disharmonies in the other. If the Liver is the source of the stagnant qi, it is usually attributable to repressed emotion, especially anger and frustration. Stomach qi stagnation can often be traced to resuming work too soon and/or overworking after meals. With Liver qi stagnation, the pulse also tends to be more Tense to Tight at the left middle positions than with Stomach qi stagnation.

Lifting after eating

In strong individuals, frequent lifting of heavy objects or overworking too soon after eating can cause the pulse in the middle burner to be Inflated bilaterally. This pulse is firmer and less elastic than that associated with Spleen qi deficiency.

Trauma

Trauma to the abdomen in a strong person may give rise to this quality bilaterally in the middle positions.

Very Tight Inflated

Stomach heat, pancreatitis, peritonitis

This can occur with Stomach heat pancreatitis or peritonitis.

Proximal positions (see Table 14-1)

An Inflated pulse in the lower burner is rare, although this quality can appear with intestinal obstruction leading to excessive gas in the Small and Large Intestines due to the obstruction or slowed peristalsis. In such cases, the pulse is Inflated and Slow.

Flat

The Flat quality (Chapter 8) is a sign of qi stagnation and deficiency in which qi is unable to reach into the involved area or organ. This pulse occurs with some of the same etiologies associated with the Inflated quality, but is more likely to appear if the individual is already weak at the outset of the process. All of the following patterns are predicated on the qi being deficient at or around the time of the events described.

Distal positions

Over a long period of time, the qi in the upper burner can become very deficient and lead to such serious conditions as a neoplasm in the mediastinum. For this reason, a Flat pulse at these positions is a much more serious sign than, say, an Inflated pulse. It represents the stoppage of circulation of qi and blood such that little of either can enter the area.

SUDDEN EMOTIONAL TRAUMA

The Flat pulse is found when a severe and sudden disappointment has occurred, such as the loss of a parent early in life, especially before the energetic systems have reached full strength and mature stability. A young person's inexperience with grief, hurt, anger, and other emotions forces them to repress the outward expression or even inner awareness of such needs as crying, screaming, or shouting. These children often control their emotions by holding the breath, which creates stagnation of qi in the chest, Lungs, Heart, and diaphragm. In adults, this pulse is frequently found in those who had such experiences when they were very young, and which in many cases they have long since forgotten. Unfortunately, the energy systems remember, and the effect of this stagnation on the circulation of qi and blood can have long-term and widespread pathological ramifications. These include unexplained depression and profound fear, arthritic conditions, difficulty in healing, and ultimately even neoplasms. With this etiology the pulse is slightly more Rapid than with those listed below.

UMBILICAL CORD AROUND INFANT'S NECK AT DELIVERY

The Flat quality can occur in the distal position bilaterally in persons whose umbilical cords were wrapped around their necks during delivery.

PHYSICAL TRAUMA, LIFTING, AND CHEST SURGERY

An accident such as a blow to the chest in a weak person, or lifting beyond one's energy, can create a Flat quality bilaterally in the upper burner positions.

IMPROPER BREATHING

Less often than the Inflated quality, the Flat quality can occur when individuals who are deficient and use their voices and lungs a great deal breathe improperly, such as singers or those who use improper meditative breathing techniques. Whereas individuals who develop an Inflated quality for this reason began with relatively good Lung qi, those who develop the Flat quality began with significantly deficient Lung qi.

MEDIASTINAL OR BREAST TUMOR

The Flat quality can occur with either of these conditions in a deficient individual.

Middle positions

The Flat pulse bilaterally in this position signifies that qi is unable to enter the area. Sometimes this is eventually accompanied by secondary swelling in the area of the diaphragm due to an accumulation of qi which cannot descend. Occasionally, this is diagnosed as a diaphragmatic hernia.

SITTING BENT OVER

Those whose work involves leaning forward in a sitting position for extended periods, and who are qi-deficient in this area before initiating these positions, can develop a Flat pulse in the middle positions. Slow-developing Stomach and Intestinal disorders are frequently found in this group of people. It is recommended that they break up their routine by standing and moving about frequently.

TRAUMA OR ABDOMINAL SURGERY

The Flat quality can also be palpated in a person who has experienced a trauma and whose general energy, or energy in this area of the body, was not strong before the trauma. Usually the patient complains of pain in the area soon after the trauma, which makes it easy to trace. This pain is caused by qi going to the diaphragm where it becomes stuck and accumulates because it cannot move downward.

LIFTING

Frequent lifting beyond one's energy in a deficient person using the abdominal muscles, especially just after eating, may produce a Flat quality in these positions over a period of time. Abdominal pain may appear soon after the episode, although usually its onset is more gradual.

Proximal positions

PROLONGED STANDING OR WALKING ON HARD SURFACES

Though rarely encountered nowadays, in deficient individuals, a Flat quality bilaterally at the proximal positions may be due to standing in one place or walking for long periods on hard surfaces. Soldiers standing motionless on guard duty, and policemen who regulate traffic, are two examples. This phenomenon was also common for the policeman ('flat foot'), who used to walk the beat before the use of squad cars. The resulting pattern is often intestinal qi stagnation leading to constipation, fecal impaction, and hemorrhoids. If impaction takes place over a period of time, there may be watery fecal matter, which is leakage around the impaction. This can also occur in the prostate leading to prostatic hypertrophy and its associated urinary complications.

Another consequence of prolonged standing or walking on hard surfaces is blood stagnation. Menstrual blood stagnation, varicose veins, or hemorrhoids can also develop. The Flat quality is rare under these circumstances, or in a strong person. Choppiness is more common.

Tense

The Tense quality (Chapter 11) is a sign of qi stagnation and heat from excess. This stagnation represents an internal conflict in which two opposing forces create a stalemate. Constrained Liver qi due to emotional repression is a classic example. The Tense quality is less hard and more resilient than the Tight pulse. Tenseness is usually associated with a person who is relatively strong and has experienced the types of precipitating events listed below as recently as a few months to at most a few years prior to the appearance of the pulse.

Distal positions

A Tense pulse at this position can indicate stagnation of qi and heat from excess in a strong person due to the following causes.

MODERATE OR LESS RECENT TRAUMA TO THE CHEST

A Tense quality may be associated with this etiology.

UNRESOLVED, INTERNALIZED COLD

External pathogenic cold that has been internalized relatively recently can cause stagnation and heat from excess, leading to asthma.

USING THE LUNGS BEYOND ONE'S ENERGY

Excessive talking or singing by a strong person over a short period of time can lead to a Tense quality.

LIFTING

A very Tense quality can be found bilaterally in the distal positions after a single extraordinary episode of lifting beyond one's ability.

Middle positions

The Tense pulse at this position is attributable to the following causes.

TRAUMA AND ABDOMINAL SURGERY

Trauma to the abdomen can cause moderate abdominal pain due to qi stagnation.

EMOTIONAL STRESS

Emotional stress affects the Liver, which then attacks the Stomach-Spleen.

FOOD STAGNATION AND/OR COLD FROM EXCESS IN THE STOMACH

Stagnation due to food accumulation or cold from excess (e.g., iced beverages) can result in heat from excess. The Tense quality signifies that the process has existed for a moderate amount of time. Referring to the 'full' pulse—which is the quality in the literature that is closest to Tense in this system—Li Shi-Zhen[9] observed, "Stagnant heat in the spleen and stomach—excess perverse heat in the middle heater—causing symptoms of stuffiness and distention in the abdomen, will reflect in a full pulse at the guan [middle] position."

BENDING

Prolonged periods of bending by strong individuals, or for a few months by deficient individuals, can be signaled by a Tense pulse at the middle position.

PHYSICAL LABOR IMMEDIATELY AFTER EATING

Stagnation caused by resuming work too quickly after meals, without leaving time for reasonable digestion, gives rise to qi stagnation and heat from excess, evidenced in the Tense quality.

Proximal positions

A Tense quality at only this position is the result of qi stagnation associated with the following events.

SEXUAL ABSTINENCE

A very Tense quality bilaterally only in the proximal positions can be a sign of sexual abstinence, or 'Buddha's pulse.'

EARLY STAGE OF INFECTION (HEAT FROM EXCESS) IN THE LOWER BURNER

In this case, the rate is slightly more Rapid than with the other events associated with a Tense quality in the proximal position.

TRAUMA AND PELVIC SURGERY

Tenseness can arise because of a less recent or moderate pelvic trauma, or following pelvic surgery that has left scar tissue.

OVEREXPOSURE TO HEAT

People who walk barefoot or sit on hot sand or rocks will often have pain and/or a rash in the lower part of the body, and a Tense pulse bilaterally in the proximal positions.

Tight-Wiry

In our times, the Tight quality (Chapter 11) most often represents heat from deficiency due to a reduction in the fluids or yin of the body. The Wiry quality is the extreme manifestation of deficient yin and deficient essence. This is usually attributable to the same causes that lead to the Tense quality over a longer period of time, such as stagnation and overwork, and is often related to a tense 'nervous system' over a long period of time.

Pain is another cause of the Tight quality, which presents a special sharper, Biting quality with pain that is absent when the Tight quality is associated with other causes. In some positions, such as the Small and Large Intestines, the Tight quality can also represent hyperactivity, irritability, and inflammation. Infection (fire toxin) is another condition that is sometimes associated with a Tight pulse, especially in the Stomach, Gallbladder, Large and Small Intestine.

With the following etiologies, a more severe disorder will be indicated by a quality that is between Tight and the thinner and harder Wiry pulse. This is especially true of intense pain, such as with an acute kidney stone, but can also be found with very severe hypertension, diabetes, or asthma.

Distal positions

TRAUMA

Trauma with pain in a relatively strong person, occurring neither very recently nor in the too distant past, can lead to a Tight-Wiry quality in the distal positions.

HYPERTENSION AND HEADACHE

If the two distal positions are Tight-Wiry and the other positions are Feeble-Absent, hypertension can be the cause, especially when the tongue and the mucosa inside the lower eyelids are red. If neither is red, severe headache from rising qi is probably a principal cause. With hypertension, the Tight-Wiry quality will also be found in the middle positions, especially on the left side.

SEVERE PAIN

If the conjunctiva, inside of the lower eyelids, and the tongue are not red, pain from severe headache without rising heat is probably a main symptom. Brain tumor should always be considered in such cases, and the Neuro-psychological positions explored for other signs of tumor, such as the Muffled quality.

YIN DEFICIENCY OF THE HEART AND LUNGS

The Tight quality found bilaterally at the distal position is often associated with a yin-deficient type of asthma with a very dry cough and/or inhalant allergies marked by dryness. I have found this in an extreme form with people who were born prematurely and spent a considerable part of the first few weeks or months of their lives in an incubator.

CARDIAC ASTHMA AND CHRONIC LUNG ASTHMA

If the rate is paradoxically Rapid, this is usually indicative of asthma that is related to cardiac function (cardiac asthma). Other signs and symptoms of cardiac insufficiency (Heart qi and/or yang deficiency) should be looked for to confirm the diagnosis. With very severe, chronic lung asthma and the use of pharmaceutical medications, the quality may be closer to Wiry.

EMOTIONAL STRESS

Depletion of yin in the upper part of the body due to excessive emotional stress, particularly prolonged excitement (mania) and anxiety, can lead to a Wiry pulse in these positions. If the pulse is slightly Rapid or lacking stability (an arrhythmia), a history of emotional shock, either recently or a long time in the past, may be the cause. (Overworking of the nervous system depletes the yin and essence.)

FEBRILE DISEASE

A Tight-Wiry quality in the upper burner can also result from chronic febrile disease in the Pericardium or Lungs, which consumes Kidney yin (as in tuberculosis) and thus cannot supply yin to the Heart and Lungs.

COCAINE ADDICTION

A very Tight-Wiry and Rapid quality bilaterally in the upper burner positions has been found in people who frequently use cocaine over several years.

Special Lung position bilaterally

Tightness at this position is a sign of lingering stagnation and heat from deficiency in the Lungs, usually of long duration, such as chronic asthma or allergies and the heavy use of drying medications or exposure to lung irritants such as nicotine. If the regular Lung position (right distal) is abnormal, it may indicate a current as well as chronic illness, with progressive stagnation and increasing heat from deficiency.

Middle positions

NERVOUS TENSION

Heat from deficiency and dryness of the organs due to nervous tension, usually associated with Liver qi stagnation and the Liver attacking the Stomach-Spleen over a long period of time, can lead to Tightness in the middle positions.

INFECTION

A Tight, Slippery, and Rapid pulse at the organ depth, with accompanying fever, are signs of an infection in the area or in one or more of the organs, for which one must search further. Pancreatitis, peritonitis, and appendicitis are important considerations, often accompanied by pain.

DIABETES AND/OR HYPERTENSION

A very Tight pulse in the middle burner positions, extending to the lower burner, may indicate an early stage of diabetes or hypertension.

PAIN

Pain associated with the following precipitating factors may lead to a Tight-to-Wiry pulse in an individual who was relatively strong before the onset of pain. The more intense the pain, the closer to Wiry the pulse. The same disorders in a person affected by deficiency give rise over time to a Flat or Feeble-Absent pulse.

- Eating too rapidly and/or emotional upset while eating
- Ulcer or tumor
- Trauma which results in qi and blood stagnation (with a Choppy quality)
- Constant lifting too soon after eating can cause stagnation
- Sitting in a bent position for long periods over many years can lead to qi stagnation
- Infection (e.g., appendicitis)
- Intermittent pain from navel to throat, associated in my experience with Kidney yang deficiency, is known as 'running piglet illness.'[10]

Proximal positions

KIDNEY YIN DEFICIENCY, HEAT FROM DEFICIENCY, AND ESSENCE DEFICIENCY

With Kidney yin deficiency there is more often a Tight quality only at the left proximal position, but it often occurs bilaterally. Kidney yin deficiency is the most common cause of the Tight quality at the proximal positions. Essence deficiency is associated with the Wiry quality.

DIABETES AND/OR HYPERTENSION

Early diabetes or hypertension are considerations when this quality is found bilaterally at the proximal positions. As the Tightness moves toward Wiriness, and later toward a very Tight Hollow Full-Overflowing quality, the illness will become more severe and the diagnosis more certain, especially when the latter quality is also found at the left middle position.

INFECTION

Tightness at these positions, along with a Rapid rate, can indicate an inflammatory condition, even infection, in or near such organs as the Kidneys, Bladder, Intestines, or prostate. This usually involves a mild acute flare-up of a chronic infection such as ulcerative colitis or enteritis, prostate inflammation, or pelvic inflammatory disease.

PAIN

With pain, the pulse will often be closer to Wiry.

Kidney stones

A Tight-Wiry pulse bilaterally, often accompanied by Slipperiness, can indicate severe stagnation associated with kidney stones. This type of pulse may also be associated with severe stagnation in the Bladder.

Trauma

Pain from unresolved past trauma, including surgery, may eventually lead to this quality.

Hernia

Pain associated with hernia can cause a Tight-Wiry quality at these positions as well.

Intestinal qi stagnation

If the rate is Slow, there may be severe pain associated with a digestive problem, such as qi stagnation and gas in the Large and/or Small Intestine. At the same time, the Tight quality here has a sharp, Biting sensation in the Large and/or Small Intestine position.

Overexposure to cold

Pain in the feet and lower legs, with a Tight pulse bilaterally in the lower burner position, can occur in people whose feet have been overexposed to cold. With frostbite, the pulse is Hidden and Wiry in these positions.

Blood stagnation

Blood stagnation in the lower burner caused by trauma, poor Heart and circulatory function, Liver qi stagnation, or heat in the blood can be accompanied by a Tight-Wiry quality, often Choppy, in the proximal positions and the Pelvis/Lower Body positions.

Slippery

Except during pregnancy, Dr. Shen considered the presence of the Slippery quality (Chapter 11) to always indicate a pattern of disharmony and impaired function. Generally, the interpretation of Slipperiness depends on the depth. At the blood depth I associate this pulse with turbulence in blood flow due to any cause that increases viscosity—such as dampness and heat causing phlegm, elevated lipids and sugars, or infection—or due to blood flowing in the wrong direction, as with a faulty heart valve. Ultimately, turbulence in the blood due to any cause, for example 'blood heat' or 'blood thick,' overworks and weakens the Heart. Where the Slippery quality occurs bilaterally at only one burner, depth is not a relevant consideration.

Distal position

LUNG DAMP-HEAT WITH ASTHMA

A Slippery quality that is Tense and slightly Rapid at both distal positions simultaneously can be a sign of asthma due to damp-heat in the Lungs.

PHLEGM-FIRE DISTURBING THE HEART

Phlegm-fire disturbing the Heart is sometimes accompanied by a Rapid pulse that is Slippery and Tense in both distal positions, although it is usually greater at the left distal position. In this disorder the orifices of the Heart are obstructed or disturbed, leading to neurosis, mental illness such as schizophrenia, or to a neurological condition such as epilepsy. The pattern is one of stagnant qi, phlegm, and heat in the chest, usually from longstanding Liver qi stagnation or food stagnation in the middle burner. This pulse can also be found in pre- and post-stroke patients, whose patterns stem from phlegm as well as from fire and wind.

PHLEGM CONFUSING THE ORIFICES OF THE HEART

A Slippery, Tense, and Slow quality can be a sign of phlegm alone veiling the orifices of the Heart; depression is usually the primary symptom. Although Spleen dampness is often present, neither fire nor Liver qi stagnation is involved.[11]

Bilaterally at Special Lung position

Slipperiness at these positions alone indicates the presence of dampness and phlegm in the Lungs from earlier pathology.

Middle positions

SPLEEN QI DEFICIENCY AND/OR LIVER-GALLBLADDER DAMP-HEAT

Though rare, Slipperiness at this position bilaterally indicates severe Spleen qi deficiency and dampness with a Slow rate. A Rapid rate reflects damp-heat in the Liver-Gallbladder system, with signs of Liver-Gallbladder and/or pancreatic and peritoneal infection.

STAGNANT FOOD

Stagnant food is a possible but less likely cause of bilateral Slipperiness at both middle positions. With stagnant food, Slipperiness is often found at the Esophagus position.

STOMACH OR DUODENAL ULCER

A Slippery quality, often accompanied by a Tight, Hollow, and Rapid pulse (usually in the Stomach-Pylorus Extension position), is found in cases of ulcers in the stomach and duodenum.[12]

Proximal positions

KIDNEY STONES AND LOWER BURNER INFECTION

Slipperiness bilaterally at this position, usually accompanied by a Wiry or Flooding Excess and Robust Pounding pulse, is associated with kidney stones or infection or fulminating inflammation in the intestines, such as ulcerative colitis, regional enteritis, or pelvic inflammatory disease. Differentiation is made by symptoms: if accompanied by severe flank pain, for example, the condition is usually a kidney stone. In rare instances, diabetes can give rise to Slipperiness, but the Slipperiness observed in such cases is always found at the blood depth and is usually accompanied by a Hollow Full-Overflowing quality. While the blood depth separates on pressure, a sensation of a sliding movement in one direction occurs simultaneously[13] when releasing pressure from the organ depth.

Thin

The Thin quality (Chapter 10) is indicative of blood deficiency, especially when it is found across the entire pulse. Blood deficiency is almost always accompanied by either yin or qi deficiency. If the pulse is Thin and Tight, the condition is blood and yin deficiency. If it is Thin and Yielding, there is a deficiency of blood and qi.

Distal positions

The following conditions and pulse signs all involve cardio-pulmonary disharmony or disease.

HEART AND LUNG BLOOD DEFICIENCY

Blood deficiency in the Heart and Lungs is accompanied by a pale and/or peach-colored tongue and paleness of the mucosa of the lower eyelids. Other symptoms include fatigue, impaired concentration and memory, palpitations, anxiety, insomnia, excessive dreaming, and dizziness. The Thinner the pulse, the greater the blood deficiency. The Thinness is found on the right side—designated as the Lung position—because of the insufficiency of blood traveling from the Heart through the pulmonary circulation and back again. The rate can also increase excessively on exertion with Heart blood deficiency ('Heart weak').

HEART AND LUNG QI AND BLOOD DEFICIENCY

A Thin, Deep, and Feeble quality bilaterally at the distal position often points to qi and blood deficiency. Symptoms include shortness of breath on exertion, excessive perspiration, fatigue, an oppressive sensation in the chest, and a pale and somewhat flabby or slightly swollen tongue. Li Shi-Zhen noted that a Thin quality in the distal position may be due to qi deficiency resulting from severe vomiting.[14] With qi deficiency, the rate may increase only slightly, stay the same, or decrease on exertion.

HEART YANG DEFICIENCY WITH CARDIOPULMONARY INSUFFICIENCY

A Slow and Arrhythmic pulse that is Thin bilaterally at the distal position is a sign of Heart yang deficiency and cold from deficiency. The symptoms include shortness of breath, excessive spontaneous perspiration, fatigue, an oppressive sensation in the chest, chills, and coldness throughout the body. This can cause cardiac asthma due to the inability of the Heart to move qi and blood through the Lungs.

HEART AND LUNG YIN AND BLOOD DEFICIENCY

A Thin, Tight, and Rapid pulse with facial pallor, confluence of vessels on the mucosa inside the lower eyelids, and a peach-colored and red-tipped tongue may indicate deficiency of the yin and blood of the Heart and Lungs. If there is more blood deficiency than yin deficiency, the pulse rate will be closer to Normal or slightly Slow. If there is a greater degree of yin deficiency and more heat from deficiency, the pulse will tend to be slightly Rapid and perhaps Tighter.

LUNG YIN DEFICIENCY-TYPE CHRONIC ASTHMA AFFECTING HEART BLOOD CIRCULATION

Severe Lung yin deficiency-type chronic asthma that affects the circulation of the Heart blood will present a Thin, Wiry quality bilaterally at the distal position. The tongue is thin, with a thin white to slightly yellow coating; the tongue body is pale, but with a slight bright red shining through the coating; often there is a slight swelling at the front of the tongue, with a depression behind the swelling. The Heart controls the vessels. It is more difficult for the Heart to push blood through dry, contracted Lungs than through Lungs in which the tissue is normal.

HEART BLOOD DEFICIENCY WITH HEART AND LUNG PHLEGM

A combination of Thin and Slippery qualities usually indicates Heart blood deficiency with an accumulation of damp-phlegm in both the Heart and Lungs. If the phlegm is more in the Heart the symptoms are emotional and/or neurological; if the phlegm affects the Lungs more, the symptoms are associated with asthma.

Middle positions

SPLEEN QI DEFICIENCY WITH HEART AND LIVER BLOOD DEFICIENCY

Over a long period of time, Spleen qi deficiency can give rise to deficiency of blood in the Liver as well as the Heart, with a Thin and Feeble quality bilaterally in the distal as well as the middle positions. Kaptchuk[15] and Li Shi-Zhen[16] both associate Spleen and Stomach qi deficiency with a Thin pulse at this position.

Proximal positions

KIDNEY QI DEFICIENCY

With this pattern the pulse is usually Feeble and Slow, but in cases of extreme deficiency it can also be Thin. This may be attributable to severe constitutional Kidney qi deficiency, very poor nutrition as a young child, extremely long-term debilitating illness, or to old age.

KIDNEY YIN AND ESSENCE DEFICIENCY

Thin, Deep, Tight-Wiry, and slightly Rapid bilaterally at the proximal position can be a sign of Kidney yin and essence deficiency from excessive sex or masturbation in the young, and overworking of the nervous system (marrow) in older people.

DEFICIENT-TYPE QI STAGNATION IN THE LOWER BURNER

Dr. Shen has noted the Thin, Deep, Feeble, and Slow qualities bilaterally in these positions due to deficient-type stagnant qi in the lower abdomen. Such a pattern can be caused by chronically sluggish bowels owing to a long-term improper diet of, for example, refined foods lacking in fiber, or to excessive lower abdominal exercises such as sit-ups.

Feeble-Absent Deep

A Feeble-Absent quality bilaterally usually indicates longstanding organ qi and blood deficiency. True qi and blood are already deficient and the disease process has long since become chronic. This is usually both a Deep and Reduced pulse. (See Chapters 8 and 9.)

The origin of this condition often begins much earlier with qi stagnation. The body's attempt to overcome stagnation over a long period depletes the qi. Overwork or overexercise beyond one's capacity for many years may also be attended by a Feeble-Absent quality. Constitutional deficiency and prolonged or chronic deteriorating illness (e.g., multiple sclerosis) are other common etiologies.

The Feeble-Absent quality is a sign of vulnerability. Often a person with this quality has no current symptomatology. According to Dr. Shen, a Feeble-Absent pulse left unattended portends illness within one year.

Distal positions

Bilaterally, this quality at the distal position may indicate qi deficiency of the Heart, Lungs, and chest.

EARLY EMOTIONAL SHOCK

This pattern, found in older people, may be attributable to severe emotional shock in childhood that impaired the circulation of qi into this area, resulting in the burying of disappointment, sadness, hurt, loss, or trauma which the young child was ill-equipped to deal with emotionally. In adulthood these events have been largely forgotten, and the individual is unaware of the associated emotions. Posture is often marked by the shoulders being bent forward such that the chest appears sunken, a physical phenomenon due to unconscious sadness. This further stagnates the qi in that area, which in turn exacerbates the sadness and qi deficiency, the result of a mind-body feedback mechanism involving inefficient air and qi exchange.

Initially the pulse is usually Inflated or Flat, becoming Feeble-Absent over time as the energy in the area is exhausted trying to break through the stifled circulation.

PHYSICAL TRAUMA

Trauma to the chest of an individual who is already weak, or trauma which occurred in the distant past and was untreated, can manifest with this pulse in the distal position. Again, the energy in the area is exhausted by trying to break through the stifled circulation.

OVERWORK OF THE LUNGS

This quality can be palpated bilaterally at this position in deficient individuals, such as teachers or singers, who use the qi of the Lungs and chest beyond capacity over a long period of time.

TUBERCULOSIS

According to Dr. Shen, but outside my own experience, a Feeble quality in both distal positions combined with a Floating and Slippery quality at the Special Lung position is a sign of tuberculosis.

Middle positions

At an earlier stage when diminished circulation of qi is the more central process, Inflation or Flatness precedes the Feeble-Absent Deep quality. The latter derives from an unsuccessful attempt by local and general energies to overcome the obstructed circulation in the area. Gastrointestinal difficulties, depending partly on other variables such as constitution, are the usual consequence. These conditions range from gas, distention, pain, and reflux to gastritis, ulcer, and cancer over a period of time.

SPLEEN AND STOMACH QI DEFICIENCY

Deficiency of Spleen and Stomach qi resulting from either poor nutrition or irregular eating habits in childhood, adolescence, or mid-life may be reflected in these positions by the Feeble-Absent Deep quality. Ultimately, the Liver-Gallbladder is affected, probably due to dampness as a consequence of the Spleen qi deficiency.

SITTING BENT OVER

Another cause of this quality is sitting in a bent-over position for long periods of time over many years. As previously noted, office workers and drivers are often affected. Some people who suffer depression also tend to sit bent over, holding their head with their hands. This posture is especially damaging during mealtime.

RUMINATING WHILE EATING

According to Dr. Shen, ruminating while eating depletes the Spleen-Stomach qi. One must choose between a ruminating mind or stomach.

EATING HABITS

A Feeble-Absent Deep and Slow pulse can be found in an individual who, over a long period of time, resumes work too soon after meals. With more recent onset, the pulse is Feeble-Absent at the qi depth, or Spreading at the blood depth, and the rate is close to Normal. Individuals on a diet of foods that are difficult to digest (such as brown rice) or who drink too much water are prone to severe digestive problems over time, as manifested by this pulse quality. This represents depletion of Spleen qi.

ANOREXIA AND BULIMIA

Either of these conditions, as well as extreme dieting, can lead to a Feeble-Absent pulse in the middle positions.

PARASITES

Parasitic infection in deficient individuals will, over a moderate period of time, lead to a Feeble-Absent quality at the middle positions, reflecting qi deficiency in the middle burner.

LIVER 'ATTACKS' STOMACH-SPLEEN

While initially the qualities encountered with this condition are Tense, Tight, and Inflated, over a long period of time and in a very deficient person the middle burner will become Feeble-Absent.

Proximal positions

Deficiency in the lower burner is a phenomenon that I have encountered more frequently in recent years in younger and younger people, suggesting that even before or at the very beginning of life there are serious insults to the genetic make-up of the organism. This may well be due to the proliferation of environmental toxins and overuse of antibiotics, as well as to individual toxicities associated with drugs, alcohol, or nutritional deficits to which the essence is exposed as the individual develops toward child-bearing age, and to which women are subject during pregnancy. This is further complicated by the use of traumatic delivery techniques during the past sixty years, including the use of drug induction, forceps, and unnecessary caesarean sections, often performed for the convenience of the obstetrician. Recent reports in the media even implicate the loss of the ozone layer as a cause of immune deficiency disorders.

CONSTITUTIONAL KIDNEY DEFICIENCY

Except in the elderly, a Feeble-Absent Deep quality in this position is usually a reflection of constitutionally deficient Kidney qi, essence, or yang. Since the Kidneys are the foundation of original and stored qi and essence for the entire organism, the Kidney qi-deficient individual is vulnerable to many defects. These can include menstrual difficulties, hernia and low back problems, heart and respiratory disorders such as childhood asthma, as well as digestive problems, since Kidney yang and qi support Spleen qi and yang.

A range of mental and emotional problems are also related to constitutionally deficient Kidney qi and essence. These include endogenous depression and schizophrenia, as well as severe neurological deficits including retardation. Kidney essence is responsible for the development and maintenance of the central nervous system. Deficiency of Kidney yin and yang are also associated with endocrine problems, especially in women.

EXCESSIVE SEX

Another cause of deficiency in the lower burner is excessive sexual activity over an extended period in a healthy person, or an inappropriate amount of sex by one whose energy was compromised to start with.

MENORRHAGIA AND CHRONIC COLITIS

Likewise, any drain on qi, yin, blood, and essence through conditions such as excessive menstruation, chronic colitis, or diarrhea over a long period can manifest as a Feeble-Absent quality at these positions, since the Kidney qi controls the lower burner and is intimately affected by lower burner pathologies.

Empty

Wherever it is found—simultaneously at all three burners, at any single position, or bilaterally at any position—the Empty quality (Chapter 9) is a sign of the separation of yin and yang and of potentially serious illness in the associated area or organ system(s). It is a 'qi wild' sign if found over the entire pulse, and even without symptoms, illness can be anticipated within six months if the condition remains untreated. The etiology usually begins between the ages of fifteen and twenty before the organism has fully matured, and occurs among those who are already deficient.

Distal positions

The Empty quality is rare in the distal position, although the following causes may give rise to this quality.

OVERWORK OF THE LUNGS

Extreme work beyond one's energy involving the upper burner—such as singing, talking, or playing a wind instrument—can, over a very long period, result in a Yielding Empty quality at the distal position bilaterally, especially if the Lungs are already weak.

PHYSICAL TRAUMA

Unresolved circulatory stagnation due to trauma to the chest area in a very deficient person over a very long time in the past may be expressed as an Empty quality simultaneously in these positions. Earlier stages will manifest as Inflated, Flat, and Feeble-Absent qualities.

RECENT SUDDEN GRIEF

The Yielding Empty quality can appear bilaterally in the distal positions with very recent grief, such as the loss of a loved one. More often I have found this quality in the Special Lung positions.

EMOTIONAL TRAUMA

In very deficient individuals, emotional trauma, especially during childhood, can, over a very long period of time, lead to this quality in late adulthood. (See the Feeble-Absent quality above for a fuller discussion.)

Middle positions

The Yielding Empty quality found bilaterally at this position is usually a sign of extreme Spleen qi deficiency and exhaustion of pancreatic enzyme function.

IMPOVERISHMENT

Impoverishment due to inadequate nutrition, especially in childhood and adolescence, though in extreme circumstances even mid-life, can, over a long period of time, lead to a Yielding Empty quality at the middle positions bilaterally.

SITTING BENT OVER

As with the Feeble-Absent quality in the upper and middle burners, an Empty quality in the middle position can also be due to sitting bent over for very long periods of time, especially in an initially deficient person. Gastrointestinal difficulties are the usual consequence.

RUMINATION

Emptiness in the middle positions can occur, usually in a very deficient person, after years of ruminating excessively while eating. With many individuals the onset of this habit is in adolescence. The mechanism of this pattern is severe Spleen qi deficiency which has secondarily caused Liver energies to overwork in an effort to move the qi in the digestive system.

RESUMING WORK TOO SOON AFTER EATING

A longtime habit, by a very deficient individual, of resuming work too soon after eating can lead to a Yielding Empty and Slow quality at the middle position.

TRAUMA AND ABDOMINAL SURGERY

In a very weak individual, trauma in this area or protracted, unresolved circulatory shock can give rise to this quality at the middle positions.

LIVER ATTACKS SPLEEN

Both middle positions are Empty when, in a very deficient person, the Liver attacks the Spleen over a long period of time. On the surface, the Liver pulse is usually slightly Tight and the Spleen-Stomach position more Yielding Empty. Digestive symptoms such as belching, distention, and hypochondriac pain are typically present.

ANOREXIA AND/OR BULIMIA

I have observed a Yielding Empty quality bilaterally at the middle positions in persons suffering advanced anorexia or bulimia, although with bulimia the quality is Tighter, and with anorexia more Yielding Empty.

DIET

Individuals on a diet of foods that are difficult to digest (such as brown rice), who drink too much water over a long period of time, or whose weight-loss diets are extreme, are prone to severe digestive problems, as reflected in this quality over time. It represents exhaustion of Spleen qi and pancreatic enzyme function.

DRUG ABUSE

A common cause of the Yielding Empty quality in the middle burner position is the use of marijuana and LSD, especially in childhood and adolescence. I say "use" rather than "abuse" because most people who are damaged in this fashion rationalize the abuse as "use."

PARASITES

A very long-term parasitic condition in the bowel, in a very deficient person, can lead to separation of yin and yang in the middle burner and a Yielding Empty quality bilaterally.

Proximal positions

An Empty quality at these positions is rare, although the following factors can give rise to the quality.

CONSTITUTION, EXCESSIVE SEX, CHRONIC COLITIS, PROLONGED EXCESSIVE MENORRHAGIA

Constitutional deficiency, continual sexual activity beyond one's energy, chronic colitis, excessive prolonged menorrhagia, and with the lesser and absolute yin stages of the four stages of disease.

Hollow

With a Yielding Hollow Full-Overflowing quality the qi is more 'wild,' or the separation of yin and yang greater, than with an Empty quality. In all of the following etiologies, the Yielding Hollow Full-Overflowing and Slow quality represents extreme deficiency, meaning that the process has taken place over a long period, the events are very severe, and the individual is massively deficient overall. (See Chapter 9 for a discussion of the Hollow quality.)

A Leather-like Hollow pulse is always a sign of bleeding, and is indicative of a life-and-death situation that must be attended to immediately. When the pulse is Rapid, the bleeding is imminent; when Slow, the bleeding is recent.

A Tense or very Tight Hollow Full-Overflowing quality is found with heat in the blood from either excess or deficiency, and with hypertension and diabetes.

Distal positions

TRAUMA TO THE CHEST WITH HEMORRHAGE (LEATHER-LIKE HOLLOW)

A Leather-like Hollow quality bilaterally in the distal position is a sign of trauma to the chest with internal bleeding.

LIFTING BEYOND ONE'S ENERGY (YIELDING HOLLOW FULL-OVERFLOWING)

A Yielding Hollow Full-Overflowing quality can result from one remarkable episode of lifting beyond one's energy. Repeated heavy lifting usually causes this quality in just the Diaphragm position, especially on the right side.

Middle positions

ABDOMINAL HEMORRHAGE (LEATHER-LIKE HOLLOW)

The Leather-like Hollow quality bilaterally at the middle position can reflect bleeding in the abdominal area.

HEAVY PHYSICAL LABOR AFTER MEALS (YIELDING HOLLOW FULL-OVERFLOWING AND SLOW)

The Yielding Hollow Full-Overflowing and Slow quality occurs bilaterally in a very deficient person at the middle position, in one who either performs heavy physical labor immediately after eating, or who sits for long periods of time and is chronically angry. If accompanied by hyperacidity ('sour stomach'), the pulse, especially in the Stomach-Pylorus Extension position, may also be Slippery, and with an ulcer, might change to Tight Hollow and Slippery.

ADVANCED DIABETES OR HYPERTENSION (VERY TIGHT HOLLOW FULL-OVERFLOWING)

A very Tight Hollow Full-Overflowing pulse bilaterally at the middle position can sometimes be a sign of advanced diabetes and/or hypertension. This quality is found at the left side with these conditions, especially in the middle and proximal positions, and less often on the right side.

Proximal positions

CHRONIC UTERINE BLEEDING AND INTESTINAL DYSFUNCTION (YIELDING HOLLOW FULL-OVERFLOWING AND SLOW)

A Yielding Hollow Full-Overflowing and Slow quality at both proximal positions with a Normal rate may be due to moderate and chronic uterine bleeding. (Intestinal dysfunction due to heavy physical work immediately after eating, with alternating constipation and diarrhea, is also associated by Dr. Shen with this quality at the proximal position, which I cannot corroborate.)

IMMINENT HEMORRHAGE IN THE LOWER BURNER (LEATHER-LIKE HOLLOW AND RAPID)

A Leather-like Hollow quality bilaterally at the proximal position with a Rapid rate may be a sign of imminent bleeding from the Kidneys, Intestines, Bladder, ovaries, or uterus.

RECENT HEMORRHAGE IN THE LOWER BURNER (LEATHER-LIKE HOLLOW AND SLOW)

A Leather-like Hollow quality bilaterally in the proximal position with a Slow rate indicates that bleeding has already occurred in the Kidneys, Intestines, Bladder, ovaries, or uterus.

ADVANCED DIABETES OR HYPERTENSION (VERY TIGHT HOLLOW FULL-OVER-FLOWING WITH RAPID RATE)

A Very Tight-Hollow Full-Overflowing quality with a Rapid rate bilaterally at this position signifies advanced diabetes or hypertension.

Vibration

Rough Vibration (Chapter 11) at any single position or bilaterally is a sign of severe parenchymal dysfunction or disease. Dr. Shen has used the expression "organ dead" to refer to this pulse.

Neuro-psychological position

Smooth Vibration at this position is associated with Heart qi agitation and extreme anxiety. Dr. Shen contended that Vibration at this position is always related to Heart function. I view this at least in terms of the traditional relationship between the Heart and mind (the Heart controls the mind). Sometimes this position has Rough Vibration, indicating possible organic brain disease, which may be neurologically subtle or gross and involve central nervous system essence deficiency.

Distal positions

When the Vibration is very Smooth, comes and goes, and is superficial, this can mean that the individual is worried about a current problem. When the quality is slightly Rougher, slightly Deeper, and more consistent, then the individual has a propensity to obsessive worry. When the Vibration is found at all depths, or just at the deep position, and is Rougher, the indication is a parenchymal disease process that is serious, such as a tumor, and affecting the mediastinal area and/or the Heart and Lungs (cardio-pulmonary disease). It can, however, also occur with very severe trauma to the chest.

Middle positions

The appearance of Deep Rough Vibration bilaterally at this position usually indicates serious physical deterioration in the digestive system (including the Liver-Gallbladder) which requires immediate biomedical investigation and possibly intervention. It can also reflect severe trauma to the abdomen.

Proximal positions

Here, the Deep Rough Vibration is again a sign of a serious disorder, such as a malignant tumor, in the pelvis or any of the organs in the area, including the entire urogenital system and the lower bowel. It may also reflect severe trauma to the lower burner, pelvis, and lower back.

STAGNATION BETWEEN THE BURNERS

The following qualities (and associated etiologies) appear bilaterally between the burners.

Between upper and middle positions: Diaphragm positions

EMOTIONAL TRAUMA ASSOCIATED WITH SEPARATION

A Tense Inflated quality bilaterally between the distal and middle positions is related to recent emotional trauma, usually a breach in a relationship that had strong attachments, such as a divorce, and represents an attempt to control feelings by inhibiting the breath. While the separation can be attended by strong hostility and resentment, the pulse quality is, I believe, caused more by a need to suppress the inevitable love that had to exist for the relationship to start. Furthermore, the relationship is difficult to end while the individual continues to have tender feelings. When the pulse is less Inflated and more Yielding, the separation is less recent or less important, usually the former. The Inflation diminishes over time, and in my experience can often last even as a small Inflation for up to ten years after the event.

HIATAL HERNIA

I have come to associate hiatal hernia with significant qi stagnation (Inflated quality) in the Diaphragm position. In the majority of people that I have treated with this diagnosis, their symptoms have responded well to the treatment for relieving qi stagnation in the diaphragm. Surgery, of course, complicates the clinical recovery.

This biomedical term is ambiguous in clinical practice and is a wastebasket for a wide variety of otherwise unexplainable gastrointestinal symptoms, even without clear x-ray evidence. It is hard to say how many surgical interventions to repair the hernia are based on hard evidence or have positive outcomes, but certainly in my practice no one benefited from the surgery, or they would not have consulted me.

LIFTING BEYOND ONE'S ENERGY

Another cause of the Inflated quality bilaterally between the distal and middle positions may be repeated episodes of lifting, by a healthy person, with the upper part of the body, which was beyond his or her energy. In my experience, Inflation due to lifting is usually greater on the right side; after a period of time, the quality can be found on both sides.

SINGLE EPISODE OF SUPPRESSED AND VERY STRONG ANGER, WHEN HEART AND LIVER ARE STRONG

When the Heart and Liver qi are strong and not vulnerable, an enormous and violent feeling of anger that cannot be expressed may lead to a Tense and very Inflated pulse bilaterally in the Diaphragm positions. Repeated episodes of rage will also inflate the Diaphragm.

HYPERTENSION

A Tense-Tight Hollow Full-Overflowing quality bilaterally at the Diaphragm positions may be a sign of hypertension in a person with strong Heart and Liver qi.

Between positions: musculoskeletal disorders

By rolling the fingers to the radial side of the area between the burners, one can detect musculoskeletal disorders. The pulse is usually very Tight-Wiry when there is musculoskeletal pathology. The Tight quality in these positions is also a sign of pain. Above and radial to the distal positions we access the neck. Radial to the area between the distal and middle positions we access the shoulder girdle. Radial to the area between the middle and proximal positions we access the hip, and radial to the area between the proximal and Pelvis/Lower Body positions we access the knees.

CHANGE IN QUALITIES AND INTENSITY BILATERALLY

Distal positions

This finding is ordinarily associated with separation of yin and yang and very deficient qi in the upper burner, or both the Lungs and Heart. It is accompanied by such symptoms as severe asthma and allergies. Several times in my experience it has coincided with breast tumors. However, I have had patients presenting with these symptoms with a history of bipolar disease, and others—usually professional singers—who have used their voices far beyond the qi available in the upper burner. In one instance, I found this in a well-known teacher of yoga breathing technique, which would imply that the technique was faulty. Together with excessive smoking, the voice and breathing etiologies can lead to a malignant neoplasm.

Middle positions

This is a sign of chaos (separation of yin and yang) in the middle burner, which can lead to malignant tumor formation in the abdomen, such as stomach or pancreatic cancer.

Proximal positions

This is a sign of chaos (separation of yin and yang) in the lower burner, which can lead to malignant tumor formation in the pelvis, such as cancer of the uterus, ovaries, or even Intestines, as well as the Kidneys and Bladder.

Table 14-1 Similar qualities bilaterally at same position

Quality	Distal Position	Middle Position	Proximal Position
Floating Floating Yielding and Rapid	Current wind-heat	Rare	Rare
Floating Yielding and Slow	Unresolved external pathogenic factor in deficient person	Rare	Rare
Floating Tense and Slow	Current wind-cold		
Floating Tense with Normal or Rapid rate	Unresolved cold from excess causes internal stagnation and heat in strong person		
Cotton	Recent emotional trauma Minor accident to chest	Emotional stress while eating Ruminating while eating Sitting in one position continuously Resuming work too soon after eating Minor trauma to abdomen	Mild Kidney qi deficiency Minor trauma to lower body

Table 14-1, cont. Similar qualities bilaterally at same position

Quality	Distal Position	Middle Position	Proximal Position
Hollow Full-Overflowing	Headache w/ hypertension	Hypertension and/or diabetes	Hypertension and/or diabetes
Flooding Excess Heat from excess in organ	Acute fulminating myo-pericarditis Acute bacterial pneumonia	Acute infection Peritonitis Hepatitis Cholecystitis Pancreatitis	Fulminating PID, prostatitis, nephritis, urinary tract infection, colitis

Inflated
 	
Trapped qi or heat in organ or area in person strong at the time the qi is trapped
 	
Trapped blood
	1. Yielding
	  • talking, breathing or singing incorrectly
	  • unresolved grief
	2. Mildly Tense
	  • breech birth
	3. Moderately Tense
	  • Liver qi attacking upward
	  • breast pathology
	  • trapped heat (invading cold turns to heat)
	  • emphysema
	4. Tense
	  • sudden extreme anger and active
	  • one major episode of lifting beyond one's energy
	  • trauma or surgery to upper burner
	5. Very Tense
	  • extravasated blood in chest
		1. Trapped qi
		  Yielding
		  • Spleen qi deficiency with distention
		  • ruminating during meals
		2. Trapped heat
		  Tense
		  • frequent lifting of heavy objects after eating
		  • Liver-GB attacks Spleen-Stomach
		  • trauma-surgery
		  Very Tight
		  • trapped heat
		  • pancreatitis or peritonitis
		  • Stomach fire
		3. Very Tense
		  • extravasated blood in peritoneum
			1. Rare: excessive gas in Intestines from obstruction:
			  • Inflated but Slow
			  • Bean [spinning] with total obstruction
			2. Rarer: acute episode in chronic PID, prostatitis or colitis:
			  • mild Tight-Wiry and Rapid
			  • usually severe Flooding Excess
			3. Very Tense
			  • extravasated blood in peritoneum

Flat Qi cannot get into an organ or area in a person deficient at the time of the causative event	1. Severe disappointment when very young; event outside of awareness 2. Physical trauma to the chest when energy not strong 3. Improper breathing, misuse of voice 4. Cord around neck at birth 5. Mediastinal or breast tumor 6. One episode of excessive lifting by a weak person	1. Sitting position leaning forward for a long time (e.g., typists) 2. Abdominal trauma or surgery 3. Lifting frequently too soon after eating	Rare: standing in one place or walking for a long time on hard surfaces

Table 14-1, cont. Similar qualities bilaterally at same position

Quality	Distal Position	Middle Position	Proximal Position
Tense Qi stagnation and heat from excess, usually in strong person	1. Moderate or less recent chest trauma 2. Unresolved cold with internal heat from excess: asthma 3. Excessive use of voice by strong person for a relatively short time 4. Lifting: single extraordinary episode beyond one's energy (very Tense)	1. Emotional stress with Liver 'attacking' Spleen 2. Trauma and surgery w/ pain 3. Qi & food stagnation or excess cold with slight pain 4. Repeated prolonged bending 5. Physical work during or right after eating	Pain from: 1. Trauma or surgery to lower burner or pelvis 2. Overexposure to heat in lower burner, especially feet 3. 'Buddha's pulse' (sexual abstinence over a long period of time) 4. Early stage of inflammatory condition in lower burner (more Rapid)
Tight-Wiry Heat from deficiency and diminishing yin-essence due to overwork, especially of 'nervous system' Pain Hyperactivity and infection	1. Cardiac asthma and chronic lung asthma (Rapid rate, Wiry with medication) 2. Hypertension and/or headache 3. Trauma with pain 4. Special Lung position: long-term heat from deficiency 5. Cocaine abuse (Wiry) 6. Excessive emotional stress & yin depletion in upper burner, esp. shock & mania 7. Febrile disease in upper burner consumes Kidney yin, which fails to nourish Heart & Lung yin 8. Severe pain in upper burner: local tumor	Heat from deficiency: 1. Nervous tension w/ Liver qi Stagnation, Liver qi attacking Stomach 2. Hypertension or diabetes 3. Infection in area or organ, pancreatitis (Slippery) 4. Pain due to: • eating (long time) • lifting too soon after eating • sitting in bent position • eating rapidly • tension while eating 5. Trauma 6. Tumor 7. Inflammation; ulcer 8. 'Running piglet disease' (rare)	1. Kidney yin deficiency & heat from deficiency 2. Infection in area or organs (e.g., colitis), especially with Rapid rate 3. Pain due to: • blood stagnation: Choppy at Pelvis/Lower Body position • qi stagnation in intestines • kidney stones • trauma • hernia • overexposure to cold (feet) 4. Very early diabetes or hypertension
Slippery	1. Asthma w/ damp-heat in Lungs and chest: Slippery & Rapid 2. Phlegm or phlegm-fire in Heart obstructing Heart orifices: Slippery Tense and slightly Rapid 3. Phlegm-cold disturbing orifices of Heart: Slippery Tense and Slow 4. Special Lung Position: phlegm in Lungs	1. Spleen qi deficiency: Slow rate 2. Spleen & Liver-GB damp-heat: Rapid (w/ infection of local organs: liver, gallbladder, pancreas, appendix, peritoneum) 3. Ulcer: Tight Hollow and Rapid, esp. Stomach-Pylorus Ext. position 4. Stagnant food: Slippery at Esophagus position	1. Kidney stone w/ severe pain: Wiry & Rapid 2. Infection w/ colitis, enteritis, PID, prostatitis

Table 14-1, cont. Similar qualities bilaterally at same position

Quality	Distal Position	Middle Position	Proximal Position
Thin Blood deficiency	1. Blood deficiency in Heart and Lungs 2. Qi and blood deficiency (Deep Thin Feeble) 3. Heart yang deficient (Thin Slow Arrhythmic); cardiac asthma 4. Heart & Lung yin and blood deficient w/ asthma (Thin Tight, and slightly Rapid) 5. Severe Lung yin deficiency asthma w/ obstruction of blood circulation in Lungs and Heart (Thin Wiry) 6. Heart blood deficiency & Heart, Lung phlegm (Thin Slippery)	Prolonged Stomach-Spleen qi deficiency w/ Heart & Liver blood deficiency	1. Kidney qi deficiency due to constitution or poor nutrition: Thin Deep Feeble and Slow 2. Stagnant qi & sluggish bowel due to chronic poor diet & improper exercise: Thin Deep and Slow 3. Kidney yin & essence deficiency: Thin, Deep, Tight-Wiry, and slightly Rapid
Feeble-Absent Long-term qi deficiency in a very deficient person	1. Found later in life in those with large emotional shock in early childhood out of awareness (e.g., loss of parent) with stagnant qi due to suppressed breath from unconscious sadness 2. Physical trauma in distant past 3. Long-term overwork of Lungs such as excessive singing or talking 4. Tuberculosis: Floating Slippery at Special Lung position (Dr. Shen)	1. Spleen qi deficiency from poor nutrition or irregular eating habits in childhood affecting Liver 2. Sitting in bent position for long time, possibly from sadness, especially during mealtime 3. Resuming work too soon after eating (long-term) 4. Mild anorexia, bulimia or extreme diet 5. Rumination while eating 6. Parasites 7. Liver attacks Spleen long-term	1. Constitutionally deficient Kidney qi, essence, yang affecting many systems 2. Long-term excessive sexual activity 3. Menorrhagia or chronic active or quiescent colitis
Empty Separation of yin & yang; advanced qi deficiency found with long-term conditions (in a very deficient person)	1. Extreme overwork of Lungs & Heart 2. Physical trauma to chest in distant past 3. Emotional trauma as child: Feeble-Absent 4. Grief for recent loss of loved one, especially Special Lung position	1. Impoverishment in childhood 2. Sitting in bent position (e.g., secretary, sadness) 3. Rumination while eating 4. Working too soon after meal 5. Trauma to abdomen 6. Liver 'attacks' Spleen 7. Severe anorexia-bulimia (or very destructive dieting) 8. Chronic parasites 9. Pancreatic enzyme function fails 10. Drug abuse	1. Serious yin & yang deficiency in greater & lesser yin stages of six stages 2. Constitutionally deficient Kidney qi affecting many systems 3. Long-term excessive sexual activity in weak person 4. Menorrhagia 5. Chronic sub-clinical colitis

Table 14-1, cont. Similar qualities bilaterally at same position

Quality	Distal Position	Middle Position	Proximal Position

Hollow
 	
1. Leather-like Hollow
  a. Rapid: imminent bleeding
  b. Slow: bleeding in recent past
2. Yielding Hollow Full-Overflowing: separation of yin & yang
3. Tight Hollow Full-Overflowing: heat in blood
	1. Trauma to chest with possible bleeding: Leather-like Hollow
	2. Lifting well beyond one's energy (once): Yielding Hollow Full-Overflowing
		1. Bleeding in abdominal area: Leather-like Hollow
		2. Heavy physical labor after eating: Yielding Hollow Full-Overflowing
		3. Hyperacidity in Stomach: Tight Hollow; with ulcer: Slippery Tight
		4. Hypertension, diabetes: very Tight Hollow Full-Overflowing
			1. Leather-like Hollow: acute sudden bleeding in pelvis
			2. Yielding Hollow Full-Overflowing:
			  a. Slow: menorrhagia
			  b. very diminished intestinal function from heavy work after eating
			3. Hypertension, diabetes: very Tight Hollow Full-Overflowing

Vibration
 	
Smooth superficial: worry
 	
Rougher & deeper: serious pathology
	1. Smooth & Superficial:
	  a. Distal position: worry & anxiety
	  b. Neuro-psychological Position: Heart qi agitation & anxiety
	2. Rougher or Deeper:
	  a. Distal position:
	    • 'Heart disease'
	    • mediastinal disease (tumor)
	    • very severe trauma (rare)
	  b. Neuro-psychological position
	    • central nervous system (essence) damage
		1. Serious physical illness in abdominal area
		2. Severe trauma to the abdomen
			1. Serious physical illness in Kidney or pelvic area, including tumor
			2. Severe trauma to pelvis/lower body area

Table 14-1, cont.   Similar qualities bilaterally at same position

1. Stagnation between burners bilaterally
    A. Inflated between upper and middle burners (Diaphragm position)
        1. Separation and suppression of tender feelings with anger
            a. Tense Inflated is more recent
            b. Yielding and less Inflated is less recent
        2. Repeated episodes of lifting beyond one's energy using upper part of body
        3. Hypertension when Liver and Heart are strong
        4. Strong, sudden, unexpressed anger when Heart and Liver are both strong
    B. Musculoskeletal
        Radial side of area between burners
            Above distal position: neck
            Between distal and middle positions: shoulder girdle
            Between middle and proximal positions: hip
            Between proximal and Pelvis/Lower Body positions: knees

2. Change in Qualities and Intensity bilaterally
    A. Distal positions
        1. Separation of yin and yang of Heart and Lungs: severe asthma or allergies
        2. Breast tumor
        3. Bipolar disease
        4. Extreme abuse of voice or improper meditation breathing techniques
        5. Mediastinal and lung tumors usually associated with excessive tobacco abuse
    B. Middle positions
        Neoplasms of stomach or pancreas
    C. Proximal positions
        Neoplasms of uterus, ovaries, intestines, bladder, kidneys

3. Change in Intensity from side to side
    A. Current severe interpersonal dislocation
    B. Recent work beyond one's energy

CHAPTER 15

Qualities as Signs of Psychological Disharmony

CONTENTS

The Heart and the Nervous System, 546
The Central Role of the Heart in Human Psychology, 547
    Awareness, psychology, and the Heart, 547
    The pulse: a summary, 547
        Mild to moderate psychological disorders, 548
        Severe psychological disorders, 548
        Very severe psychological disorders, 548
            'Qi wild': disrupted circulation, separation of yin and yang in the entire organism, 548
            Separation of yin and yang in the Heart, 548
            Pathogenic influences, 549
Emotional States, 549
    Depression, grief, melancholia, anguish, and sadness, 549
        Grief, anguish, and melancholia, 549
            Distinctions, 549
            Recent grief and anguish, 549
            Long-term unexpressed repressed grief, 549
            Melancholia, 550
            Grief associated with a past loss later in life, 550
        Depression, 550
            The existential condition, 550
            Pathophysiology, 550
            Endogenous depression, 551

Psychopathology, 551
Kidney essence, 552
Other forms of depression described in *Dragon Rises, Red Bird Flies*, 553
    Primary anaclytic depression (profound despair), 553
    Cyclothymic depression, 553
    Agitated depression, 553
    Hysterical and reactive depression (uncertain pulse qualities), 553
    Dysphoric depression (lack of joy), 554
        Lack of joy without fatigue, 554
            Flat, 554
                Early loss and disappointment, 554
                Sudden bad news and rejected love, 554
                Delivery with umbilical cord around neck, 554
            Inflated bilaterally at distal positions, 555
                Early loss and disappointment, 555
                Sudden bad news and rejected love, 555
            Muffled at left distal position or over entire pulse, 555
        Lack of joy with fatigue (including post-menopausal depression), 555
            Heart blood deficiency, 555
            Heart qi deficiency, 555
    Post-menopausal syndrome, 556
    Secondary anaclytic depression (despair) and narcissistic depression, 556
    Intra-individual failure, loneliness in middle and old age, 556
        Muffled at left distal position, empty at left middle position, 556
        Cotton over entire pulse, 556
        Heart blood stagnation ('Heart small') at the left distal position, 556
    Post chemical intoxication, post hepatitis, and post mononucleosis depression, 556
    Depression associated with the 'qi wild' condition, 556
    Bipolar and acute Grave's disease, 557
        Manic phase, 557
        Depressive phase, 557
Anxiety (apprehension, worry, fright, phobia, panic, shock) and fear (terror, panic), 557
    Differentiation of anxiety and fear, 557
    Anxiety, phobia, and fright, 558
    Anxiety and panic, 558
    Anxiety (phobia, panic, and fright), 558
        General symptoms, 558
        Conditions and qualities pathognomonic of anxiety, 558
            Heart qi agitation, 558
                Smooth Vibration, 558
                Rapid, 559
                Occasional Change in Rate at Rest, 559
            Heat from excess in Heart, 559
                Pericardium Tight or left distal position Tense with Robust Pounding, 559
            Heart yin deficiency, 560
                Tight at left distal position (Heart Tight), 560
            Heart blood deficiency ('Heart weak'), 560
                Left distal position Thin and/or Increase in Rate on Exertion >8–12 Beats/Min, 561

     Thin over entire pulse, 561
    Heart qi deficiency, 561
     Feeble-Absent at left distal position, 561
     Constant Change in Intensity over entire pulse, 561
     Yielding Hollow Full-Overflowing, 561
     Slow, 561
     Change in Qualities and Intensity at left distal position, 562
     Vibration and Slippery at Mitral Valve positions, 562
     Arrhythmic qualities, 562
    Heart-Gallbladder deficiency (timidity), 562
   Worry, 563
    Vibration, 563
     Smooth Vibration (mild Heart qi agitation), 564
      Progression of Smooth Vibration at the qi depth, 564
      Entire pulse at all depths, 564
      Vibration at the Neuro-psychological positions, 564
     Tightness at Pericardium Position and Tense at left distal position, 564
     Occasional Change in Rate at Rest, 564
   Fear, 564
    Types of fear, 564
    Fear and Heart blood stagnation ('Heart small'), 565
    Profound guilt and fear, 565
     Consistent Rough Vibration over entire pulse at all depths, 565
      Differentiation of etiology of Rough Vibration (Heart qi deficiency), 566
       from guilt and fear, 566
      Guilt and terror for perpetrators of transgressions against others, 566
      Guilt and terror in the victims of transgressions, 566
   Terror (without guilt), 567
    Bean (Spinning), 567
    'Qi wild' qualities, 567
    Rough Vibration at the Neuro-psychological positions, 567
   Horror, 567
  Roller-coaster feeling, 567
   Physiology, 567
   Psychopathology, 567
   Pulse, 568
  Post-traumatic stress syndrome, 568
   Acute, 568
   Chronic, 568
  Vengefulness and spite, 568
  Paranoid personality, 568
  Psychosis, schizophrenia, and dissociated mental states involving boundaries, 569
   Symptoms and pathogenesis, 569
   Stagnant etiology of psychotic disorders, 569
    Qi stagnation, 569
    Food stagnation, 570
    Phlegm-fire (phlegm disturbs the Heart), 570
    Phlegm-cold (phlegm confuses the Heart), 571
  Bipolar disease, 571
   Psycho-energetic pathology, 571
   Pulse, 572

Deficient etiologies of psychotic states, 572
    'Qi wild', 572
        Introduction, 572
        Etiology, 572
        'Qi wild' qualities, 573
        Symptoms, 573
Tension, 573
    Liver qi stagnation and tension, 573
        Taut or Tense at left middle position, 573
        Inconstant Change in Intensity over entire pulse, 573
    'Nervous system tense', 574
        Tense to Tight over entire pulse, 574
        Etiology, 574
            Constitution, 574
            Daily stress, 575
    'Nervous system' affects 'organ system', 576
Neurasthenia or 'nervous system weak', 576
    Etiology, 576
        Constitution, 576
            Early in childhood, 577
            Later in adulthood, 577
        Life experience, 577
            Very mild, 577
            Moderate, 577
            Severe, 577
Anger, 577
    Sudden anger: trapped qi in the Heart, or 'Heart full', 577
    Propensity to anger: trapped qi in the Heart, or 'Heart full', 578
    Gradually developing anger, repression, and passive-aggressive behavior, 578
        Strong individual, 578
            Short time, 578
            Moderate time, 578
            Long time, 578
        Deficient individual, 578
    Separation and divorce, 578
    Inflated at Diaphragm position, 578
    Explosiveness and impotent rage, 579
        Psychogenesis, 579
        Pulse, 579
Indecision, 580
    Liver-related, 580
    Gallbladder-related, 580
    Heart-related, 580
Resignation, 580
    Cotton, 580
Obsessive thinking (reflection), 580
    Hesitant quality and obsessive thinking, 581
    Spleen-Stomach and obsessive thinking, 581
        Physiology, 581
        Pathogenesis and symptoms, 581
        Spleen-Stomach and obsessive thinking, 581

Withdrawal and the Deep quality, 582
Denial and the Empty quality, 582
Physical pain, 583
Addictions, 583
    Alcoholism, 584
    Marijuana, 584
    Hallucinogens, 584
    Cocaine, 584
Central nervous system disorders, 584
Emotional disharmonies related to left-right imbalance, 584
    Changes in Intensity shifting back and forth between sides, 585
    Left side, 585
        Resignation for a moderate period, 585
        'Organ system' deficient, 585
    Right side, 586
        Eating too rapidly: 'nervous system' affecting the 'digestive system', 586
        Eating irregularly, 587
        Physical labor immediately after eating, 587
        Emotion, timing, and gastro-intestinal dysfunction, 587
Qualities associated with Kidney-Heart disharmony, 587
    Physiology and symptoms, 587
    Common combinations, 588
        Feeble-Absent at left distal and proximal positions, Normal at left middle position with a Slow or Rapid rate, 588
        Feeble-Absent at left distal and proximal positions, Tense Inflated at left middle position, 588
        Tight at left distal and proximal positions, and slightly Rapid, 588
    Less common combinations, 588
        Feeble-Absent at left distal and Tight at left proximal positions, 588
        Tight at left distal position, Feeble-Absent at left proximal position, 588
Heart patterns affecting sleep, 589
    Introduction, 589
    Summary, 589
    Common patterns, 589
        Heart heat from excess ('Heart fire'), 589
        Heart yin deficiency and Heart qi agitation, 589
        Heart blood deficiency ('Heart weak'), 589
    Less common patterns, 590
        Kidney-Heart disharmony and sleep, 590
Recently acknowledged emotional and mental conditions, 590
The Three Burners, 590
    Lower burner (proximal positions), 590
    Middle burner (middle positions), 591
    Upper burner (distal positions), 591
Summary of Pulse Qualities Associated with Psychological Disharmony, 591
▪ Table 15-1: Pulse qualities and associated psychological states, 592

CHAPTER 15

Qualities as Signs of Psychological Disharmony

According to Amber, "The Sanskrit rule observes, 'The learned physician should read the happiness and misery of the body by feeling the pulse at the root of the thumb which stands as the witness of the soul'."[1] Referring to the Dao,

> The Emperor said, "I desire to hear about their way!" Ch'i Po replied: "In order to make all acupuncture thorough and effective one must first cure the spirit. Then after one has established [the pulse] of the five viscera and determined the nine subdivisions, one can apply the needle."[2]

This chapter addresses those pulse qualities which are signs of emotional, mental, and spiritual problems that I have individually observed over the years. Apart from their obvious diagnostic value, I have found that by referring to the pulse as an indicator of problems about which people ordinarily do not speak freely, patients have responded by opening their hearts and minds with little or no reluctance. This instantaneous unveiling, in the context of saying "Your pulse tells me" rather than "It is my impression," is in sharp contrast to the experience that my psychiatric colleagues and I have had within the context of various psychotherapies, which has given rise to the vast literature on the subject of 'resistance.' Having practiced both disciplines, I can attest to the remarkable value of pulse diagnosis as a rapid and consonant avenue into the vital emotional issues in people's lives.

On the other hand, the human condition is so complex with so many unknowns, including unidentified strengths and resources, that making predictions with regard to the mind and emotions is problematic. With any of the pulse qualities described here, there can be unpredictable emotional disturbances. Those mentioned are the ones most often encountered, although the presence of the quality is by no means an absolute guarantor of certain consequences, nor does the presence of a mental or emotional disorder guarantee the appearance of a specific quality.

This chapter is organized around 'emotional states' for easy reference. Therefore, one would refer to anxiety, depression, or anger for associated pulse qualities, which are then described in detail elsewhere in the book. Issues involving pulse positions, specific qualities, and the vicissitudes of the various organs are placed within this context. At times some of the pulse states apply to more than one emotion or mental condition. Arbitrary decisions have been made based on the dominant alignments of pulse and condition. And although each quality is discussed within the parameters of psychological issues, each of them is also a sign of a physical condition, usually of equal severity. There is frequent reference to my book *Dragon Rises, Red Bird Flies*. It does not include a detailed discussion of psychological states, only enough to correlate with associated pulse combinations, which is the purpose and goal of this chapter.

Emotional states will present different associated pulse pictures depending upon whether the individual is deficient or robust, and whether the etiology is before or at birth, or at a later age, and with the acute or chronic stage. Where possible, these distinctions have been made.

Some of the information in this chapter is necessarily repetitive of earlier material due to the reference nature of the book. The best expression of an issue is repeated here more conveniently than searching for it elsewhere in the volume.

The Heart and the Nervous System

What Dr. Shen refers to as the 'nervous system' is the superficial and most rapidly moving qi (protective qi), corresponding to the qi flowing in the channels. It is the first layer of qi affected by pernicious influences, including all of the abusive habits we bring to bear on ourselves. These abusive behaviors may involve eating habits, work, exercise, sleep, study, drugs, sex, relationships, and emotions. They can arise from within, for example, in the form of phlegm-cold or heat. If the 'nervous system' is vulnerable, these behaviors will create significant psychological problems. If it is strong, they will only cause physical disorders, especially if another 'system' or organ is at risk.

If the 'nervous system' is weak, the function of the entire organism will be disturbed. After all, this qi is directly engendered and nourished by Kidney essence, which is the foundation of the entire physiology. With a defective 'nervous system,' even the smallest stress will affect the most vulnerable organ, and the smallest organ dysfunction will lead to a psychological problem.

On the other hand, the Heart governs the mind. In Chinese medicine this is a different order of function relating more to the spirit *(shén)*, which comes from heaven rather than the earth. The 'nervous system' develops slowly from below, from Kidney essence, while the mind (spirit) comes from above and through the Heart down to the *ming men* or 'gate of vitality.' These must, of course, be balanced; they depend on each other for emotional as well as physical stability. In my opinion, the Triple Burner functions to monitor and maintain this balance.

We have said that Kidney essence, both yin and yang, are the foundation of the 'nervous system.' A robust 'nervous system,' when stressed either by life or genetics, is associated with excessive tension. This infers a strong foundation. A deficient 'nervous system' is associated more with collapse and a strong propensity to severe depressive states, often marked by diminished psychomotor activity and profound exhaustion. This infers a weak foundation. We have also said that Heart qi, blood, and yin are the foundation of the mind. A robust Heart and mind, when stressed, will tend to be expressed as agitation, which serves an adaptive function by alerting the mind to action. However, in its extreme form, agitation becomes anxiety, panic, and neurosis. A mildly deficient Heart and mind will be expressed in mild and transient depressions. In extreme Heart deficiency we find the life-instigated milder psychotic states, especially with the accumulation of phlegm. With the more severe psychotic states involving the breakdown of boundaries between the inner and outer worlds, self and others, we find the overlap between Kidney essence and Heart qi-blood deficiency, between genetics and life experience, between nature and nurture.

If either the 'nervous system' (Kidney essence) or the mind/spirit (Heart) is depleted, stress will easily cause psychological problems. If both are strong, the organism may bend under pressure, but psychologically stay intact. And staying intact psychologically is the most important issue in life, because when one's mind and nerves are stable, one can solve any problem. Furthermore, in our society, the lifetime repercussions of a mental breakdown are extraordinarily more far-reaching than those of a physical illness.

The important message to learn from these observations is that one should not be misled by specific emotional states such as anger, depression, or mania into treating these states without first or simultaneously addressing the larger issue of the 'nervous system' and the Heart. The tendency to say that one should treat the Liver if a person is angry, or the Spleen if a person is obsessive, is missing the underlying and larger issue of what makes the person vulnerable to emotional and psychological problems in the first place. A stagnant Liver will not give rise to anger if the Heart and 'nervous system' are intact. (Moreover, anger, or any emotion for that matter, will affect the organ which is most defective.) Any program of psychological treatment must rest on the balance between the Heart and 'nervous system,' and the Triple Burner as the intermediary, or it will fail.

The Central Role of the Heart in Human Psychology

This chapter is not a treatise on 'mind, body, and spirit' and deliberately avoids the concepts of spirit *(shén)*, ethereal soul *(hún)*, corporeal soul *(pò)*, intention or intelligence *(yì)*, and purpose or will *(zhì)*, each of which deserves special consideration in a different context. Here we are concerned primarily with pulse diagnosis and identifiable emotional conditions. However, in considering the following emotional states, we cannot overlook, and must begin by pointing to the dominance of, the force of the spirit of the Heart in the development and function of all the other energetic forces related to the mind, spirit, and soul (see also Chapter 12).

AWARENESS, PSYCHOLOGY, AND THE HEART

In Chapter 2 of my book *Dragon Rises, Red Bird Flies* I wrote that "Perhaps the most important consequence of the introduction of acupuncture into my practice was the flowering of awareness in my patients and my own appreciation of its significance to growth and development."[3] Awareness is the centerpiece of Zen Buddhism and is almost synonymous with the concept and experience of enlightenment.

Almost all psychological disorders can be understood as a function of awareness, either in quantity, quality (perception and distortion), or form. In fact, the Greek word for insanity is alienation, which is a loss of awareness of the inner or outer world, and of the difference between them.

The principal problems which attend human relationships fall mostly into the realm of awareness and communication. Fire energies are all about awareness and communication. Heart yang and Pericardium yang, Triple Burner and Small Intestine energies, as discussed in *Dragon Rises, Red Bird Flies,* are all involved in the appropriate and effective expression of thoughts and feelings. And where the clarity of communication is involved, all of the distortions attending maladaptive discourse are rooted in awareness; they are thus also ineluctably rooted in the integrity of the Heart and fire phase. Hence, all human problems, from marital and family conflicts to the most serious neurosis and psychosis, are to some extent the manifestations of defects in fire energy performance.

THE PULSE: A SUMMARY

The emotional, mental, and spiritual states associated with the following pulse qualities are a direct consequence of the physiological principle which states that the Heart controls the mind and the mind affects the Heart. All of these qualities are signs of disturbed Heart function and, consequently, chaotic or diminished spirit.

Mild to moderate psychological disorders

Heart qi agitation, Heart yin deficiency, and mild qi and blood deficiency of the Heart are associated with the less serious, emotionally-troubled states. These include anxiety neurosis, transient depressions, worry and the tendency to worry, irritability, difficulty with memory and concentration, recurrent inter-individual conflicts, and some sleep disturbances.

Among the associated pulse qualities are a Rapid rate, a Tight quality at the Pericardium position, and Tight and occasionally Slippery left distal position, Smooth Vibration over the entire pulse at all depths, and occasional small Changes in Rate at Rest, occasional Slipperiness, and Smooth Vibration at the Neuro-psychological positions. The 'nervous system tense' condition often affects the Heart and circulation, giving rise to a Rapid rate, a Tight quality at the Pericardium position, and, at a later stage, Tightness at the left distal position. Heart qi agitation in the various forms discussed in Chapter 12 makes the 'nervous system' more tense.

Severe psychological disorders

More serious, fixed mental and emotional problems are found with the Hesitant quality (a wave abnormality discussed in Chapter 6 with the pseudo-arrhythmias, with which it is often confused, and which is associated with obsessions), Rough Vibration over the entire pulse (Heart-related shock, terror, and guilt), the Bean (Spinning) quality, especially at the left distal position (terror), and mild to moderate Slipperiness at the left distal position (phlegm veiling the orifices). With regard to phlegm veiling the orifices, I have come through experience to include in my treatment of all emotional disorders measures to remove dampness from the Heart, even without clear evidence of a Slippery quality at the left distal position.

Very severe psychological disorders

'QI WILD': DISRUPTED CIRCULATION, SEPARATION OF YIN AND YANG IN THE ENTIRE ORGANISM

The Yielding Hollow Full-Overflowing quality (severe anxiety and panic) is a 'qi wild' disorder involving the separation of yin and yang, and chaos in the circulation, and consequently of the Heart qi and blood. With this condition the Yielding Hollow Full-Overflowing quality overwhelms the pulse picture, obviating more specific qualities at the left distal position. Also in the realm of the separation of yin and yang is constant Change in Qualities over the entire pulse. The Intermittent and Interrupted qualities are signs of severe Heart dysfunction, and may also be identified with mental and emotional disturbance.

SEPARATION OF YIN AND YANG IN THE HEART

Instability of the mind reflects the condition of the Heart, which is also suggested by the following signs of chaos at the left distal position: the Unstable quality, Change in Qualities or Intensity, and Rough Vibration at all depths. All of these qualities are evidence that Heart function is erratic; they are associated with a wide variety of severe mental and emotional disturbances including overwhelming, debilitating anxiety and psychosis. The Slippery quality almost always accompanies these pulses under these circumstances.

PATHOGENIC INFLUENCES

The most serious problems are associated with pathogenic influences, such as phlegm and fire, which affect the mind through their effect on the Heart with symptoms of severe depression, mania, and schizophrenia. All involve the presence of an intense Slippery quality at the left distal position. The Tense-Tight Hollow Full-Overflowing and the Ropy qualities are signs of atherosclerosis and hypertension, and are often the result of life-long tension leading to the ultimate psychological insult: stroke and death.

Emotional States

Emotion will most adversely affect the most vulnerable organ system and does not usually follow the correspondences according to the five phase system, with the following caveat: although another weaker organ may be more affected, grief will also secondarily usually touch the Lungs, worry will also affect the Heart, and reflection (rumination) will also usually have some effect on the Spleen.

The emotional states discussed below create pathological patterns of disharmony only when repressed or suppressed. The time frames mentioned are approximations and depend on many variables including body condition and the presence in an individual's life of positive mitigating experience.

DEPRESSION, GRIEF, MELANCHOLIA, ANGUISH, AND SADNESS

Depression is a term which encompasses all of these states and more, and exists whenever there is an inhibiting or muffling of the life force, for a day or over a lifetime.

Grief, anguish, and melancholia

DISTINCTIONS

Freud differentiates between grief and melancholia. Grief is appropriate mourning that is self-limited, while melancholia is grief that has gone both temporally and in degree beyond what is appropriate. Melancholia is one form of depression. As I noted in *Dragon Rises, Red Bird Flies*:

> Repressed grief, which we will arbitrarily call sadness for the sake of discussion, is a most important source of deep-seated and lifelong personality problems. With anguish, one knows and remembers, and with sadness one forgets. With disappointment we have an individual who could not speak, but who may have eventually cried; with true sadness we have a child who may have spoken but could not feel or cry. With the latter, on the energy level, we have stagnation deep inside the Lung and Heart where the feeling and crying is hidden and blocked. The Lung and Heart pulses are deep and the wave either Flat or Feeble.[4]

RECENT GRIEF AND ANGUISH

After a lecture a young Chinese woman asked me to demonstrate to her the Special Lung positions: they were Empty with no abnormal qualities at the right distal position. I asked her if she was grieving after a recent and profound individual loss. She explained that her mother had died two weeks before.

LONG-TERM UNEXPRESSED REPRESSED GRIEF

Dr. Shen noted that sadness which comes early in life, and is held deep inside with no sound, affects the Lungs. In my experience I have found that it more often affects the entire upper burner.

The left and right distal positions are usually Flat, and possibly Feeble, much later in life. Dr. Shen reported an association, which I have not observed, between the combination of Empty right distal position and Inflated Special Lung position on the one hand, and repressed grief from very early in life "with no sound" on the other. I have rarely found an Empty right distal position, and never with this history, except at an advanced age.

MELANCHOLIA

An Inflated quality bilaterally in the distal positions can mean melancholia or grief that is inappropriately prolonged. Dr. Shen noted that sadness or grief expressed with a whimpering sound (groan), which is often heard in melancholia, affects primarily the Kidneys. Kidney qi deficiency at the proximal positions, such as with a Feeble-Absent quality, could be a cause for the lack of life-force required to move on, past a loss.

GRIEF ASSOCIATED WITH A PAST LOSS LATER IN LIFE

My own experience finds either a Flat quality (deficient individual) or a Yielding Inflated quality (robust individual) at the distal positions. According to Dr. Shen, but outside my own experience, sadness later in life due to the failure of inter-individual relationships or loss of a close individual is attended by an Empty left middle position, and affects the Liver more than the Lungs.

Depression

I cannot emphasize enough that vulnerability to all depressions, with the possible exception of the primary anaclytic, is rooted in a deficiency of Kidney essence, especially Kidney qi-yang essence. This is closely associated with the 'nervous system' and underlies all of the following discussion of depression.

THE EXISTENTIAL CONDITION

Depression is a statement that "If I cannot be myself (within reason), I will be nothing."[5]

> Under some circumstances, for example, if assertion might bring destruction from more powerful forces, the retreat (into depression) may be the safest and most expedient tactic.
>
> Life, on the other hand, has another agenda. It is perforce a growth process which, despite periodic strategic retreats, is basically expansive. Depressions, therefore, tend to be short lived. Prolonged retreats such as depression cannot resist the forward thrust of these drives, and it is the pain that ensues from this struggle that becomes unbearable and leads to suicide, the final retreat on, and from, earth. It is a monumental paradox that in depression the stronger the life-drive, the greater the chance of an individual taking his own life.[6]

PATHOPHYSIOLOGY

The propensity toward depression is rooted in Kidney qi-yang and Kidney essence deficiency. Kidney energy is as complex as the human central nervous system and there are an almost infinite variety of Kidney functions, each connected to its own aspect of that nervous system. Summing it up as Kidney yin, yang, essence, and qi is a massive oversimplification. That is why one can be missing one small aspect of the Kidney realm and keep the rest intact. I would consider that *yuan* qi (original qi) comes into living beings as essence. Qi, yin, and yang are differentiated aspects of essence and should, therefore, be alluded to as qi-essence, yin-essence, and yang-essence, to clarify and emphasize the relationship, and to point the way for further investigation.

> The origin of the depressive individuality lies in the failure of genetics or very early intra-uterine life to provide these energies adequately. This adversity is the root of all habitual depressions and the source of the spiritual poverty (Kidney qi) which we call 'endogenous' depression.
>
> More specifically, the loss of 'will' and 'drive' associated with Kidney yang (the fire of *ming men*) deficiency is an intrinsic deficit associated with all sustained, profound, or recurrent depressions. Kidney 'fire' is the functional heat energy that 'drives' the entire physical plant to provide the force behind the 'will to live.' Without this 'will,' the inclination is to collapse well before retreat is expedient.
>
> Kidney yin provides the substance, the basic grounding material, upon which we must all depend when we go down, and the fundamental stored essence *(jing)* that is the principal reserve with which to bounce back after defeat. It can make strategic retreats (in conjunction with Liver yin) in situations where advance would lead to major defeat and subsequent grounds for depression. Kidney yin endows the spiritually evolved individual with the capacity for the Divine Love needed to 'forgive us our trespasses' when we falter. Kidney qi endows us with the ability to live in the present, to confront issues now, to live with our feet on the ground even when we are dreaming, all qualities which stand us well in the face of defeat and the inclination to withdraw into depression.[7]

The nervous system is developed and sustained by Kidney essence.

ENDOGENOUS DEPRESSION

Psychopathology

Genetic or intra-uterine

As alluded to above, 'endogenous depression' is the most profoundly enduring expression of the genetic, or intra-uterine, failure of Kidney essence and yang to sustain the spiritual requirements for the desire and willingness to see life through fully and let fate rule, to carry us beyond despair.

The depressions which have been identified as 'endogenous' often do not reveal a particular precipitating event. One is left to speculate whether the etiology is entirely internal: in biomedical terms, some innate disharmony in neurotransmitters, or in Chinese terms, a subtle energy drain of the Kidney yin, essence, and yang, which brings the energies below a critical level necessary to sustain the will 'to be.'

There also seems to be an inability to sustain will and drive, especially in the face of real, or more often, imagined, failure or adversity. Getting up off the floor after being knocked down is difficult. However, even when considered successful by others, these people often feel like failures, convinced that they are fooling people into believing they are competent when they know they are not. Their sense of worthlessness is profound.

Post-partum

The debate which has persisted since at least my earliest exposure to psychology has been between the advocates of Nature and those of Nurture as the etiology of emotional and mental illness. My training at Bellevue Hospital with Loretta Bender (of the Bender-Gestalt Test), and later with Stella Chess, was strongly oriented to the Nature side of the argument. The seven years I spent at the William A. White Psychoanalyic and Psychatric Institute heavily exposed me to the Nurture argument. After eight years as medical director of a child guidance center I realized that both arguments were correct. Part of my attraction to Chinese medicine is that it embraces both, while focusing on the energetic disharmony.

The energetic psychopathology involves Kidney-essence, whether the cause be Nature or Nurture. However, during my twenty years as a child psychiatrist when the overwhelming weight of opinion was with Nurture, I was deeply impressed by the preponderance of intra-uterine and birth insults to disturbed children and adolescents. In *Dragon Rises, Red Bird Flies* I referred to research by Lee Salk, M.D., et al., at Cornell

University Medical College and Payne-Whitney Psychiatric Clinic reported in an article in the journal *Lancet* entitled "Relationship of Maternal and Perinatal Conditions to Eventual Adolescent Suicide." About this article I wrote:

> Salk... along with several colleagues, claims to have found a link between respiratory distress for more than one hour at birth and the increased incidence of adolescent suicide. Other factors also related were the absence of prenatal care before the twentieth week of pregnancy and chronic disease in the mother during pregnancy. All of this would make absolute sense in the Chinese system inasmuch as the Lungs are directly associated with the emotion of sadness.[8]

Furthermore, as indicated by research published in *Crying Baby, Sleepless Nights*, evidence for Nature has continued to mount:

> For most babies the ill effects of oxygen deprivation or drugs are measured in weeks or months, but for other babies the results may be more long lasting. A British study has found that 48 percent of preschool children who have sleeping disorders such as waking up over and over had suffered from anoxia or complications at birth. Anoxia at birth has also been implicated in hyperactivity in school-age boys. A survey of the drug intake of over fifty-thousand pregnant mothers has found that those who took drugs such as Compazine, a potent antinausea medication, had twenty percent greater chance of their babies becoming hyperactive and impulsive at school age.
>
> It may well be that for some babies crying and sleeplessness, colic, is a prolonged physical reaction to events that have happened before they are even brought home from the hospital.[9]

Kidney essence

The essence of both the Kidney yin and yang build, nourish, and protect the central nervous system. Again, yin-essence is the substance, yang-essence is the drive, and, together with the qi of the Triple Burner, essence is the regulator.

Pulse Both Kidney qi-yang-essence and Kidney yin-essence deficiency can appear simultaneously so that one proximal position might be Tight-Wiry and the other Feeble-Absent, or in one or both proximal positions there may be a Change in Qualities back and forth from Tight-Wiry to Feeble-Absent.

KIDNEY QI AND YANG-ESSENCE DEFICIENCY (SEE CHAPTER 12)

The left and right proximal pulses may be Feeble-Absent, have Reduced Substance, and be Diffuse, Empty, and show a Change in Intensity or Qualities. These are signs of Kidney qi-yang-essence deficiency. Kidney yang-essence is the fire aspect of Kidney 'breaths' or energies, and is responsible for the drive and will which carries us beyond despair.

The depression associated with Kidney yang-essence deficiency is marked by considerable fatigue, lassitude, psychomotor retardation, and pain since the potential (yin-essence substance) is there but the drive to use it is lacking. This pain can lead to suicide. This is the more common cause of 'endogenous depression.'

KIDNEY YIN-ESSENCE DEFICIENCY

A Wiry quality at the left or right proximal position is a sign of Kidney yin-essence deficiency. Kidney essence is responsible for the substance and maintenance of the central nervous system. The clinical picture involves more agitation. Here we have the drive but not the substance, which ultimately leads to failure. Here again, the associated pain can lead to suicide. This is the less common cause of 'endogenous depression.'

OTHER FORMS OF DEPRESSION DESCRIBED IN *DRAGON RISES, RED BIRD FLIES*

The forms of depression discussed in Chapter 15 of *Dragon Rises, Red Bird Flies* are briefly reviewed below. Some have not been sufficiently tested for typical pulse qualities to present with any degree of certainty. The Slippery quality with a Slow rate (major dysphoric) and Muffled quality at the left distal position (minor dysphoric) are frequently associated with depression, as well as other mental-emotional states.

Primary anaclytic[10] depression (profound despair)

This is found in infancy before the pulse can be accurately assessed except for rate and rhythm. The Interrupted or Intermittent qualities are associated with this condition. Apart from a 'broken heart,' the extreme cachexia in infancy with anaclytic depression leads to Yielding Hollow Interrupted and Intermittent pulse qualities. Much more observation is required.

Cyclothymic depression

The pulse quality associated with this form of depression is the large occasional Change in Rate at Rest with the overall rate of Normal or Slow. With this pulse quality people are subject to frequent mood swings.

Agitated depression

Mild heat from excess in the Heart and Liver

The left middle position is Tense and Robust Pounding due to suppressed emotion (anger or frustration); this leads to mild Liver fire which moves to the Heart and creates a mild Heart fire (left distal pulse Tense and Robust Pounding, with a Rapid rate). The body attempts to compensate for this heat by bringing yin (damp) to bear, which eventually creates a phlegm condition in the Heart due to the congealing effect of the heat. At this point we have a Slippery quality and phlegm-fire reflected at the left distal position, associated with a broad range of emotional disturbances including agitated depression and manic behavior.

At both earlier and later stages of chronic suppressed anger affecting the movement of Liver qi (stagnation), the clinical picture is also agitated depression with less explosive behavior in which the anger is often expressed by passive-aggressive behavior. We see this most obviously in children and adolescents still subject to parental authority, although with some the suppressed feelings are 'acted out' in externally-directed destructive behavior. When acting out occurs, the tense quality at the left middle position is probably less prominent. Of course, we see a great deal of this impotent rage in adults, as discussed in *Dragon Rises, Red Bird Flies*.[11]

Heat from deficiency in the Heart

Another scenario for an agitated depression is a Tight left distal position and Feeble-Absent proximal position. Both the Heart and the Kidneys control the mind and the brain. If the water of the Kidneys cannot control the fire of the Heart, the mind will become restless. (On the other hand, if the water of the Kidneys is excessive, it will diminish the fire and cause depression, marked by a lack of joy.)

Hysterical and reactive depression

Returning to *Dragon Rises, Red Bird Flies*:[12]

> The 'hysterical' depression is partially a manipulative threat to create guilt and make us all unhappy 'if I do not get my own way.' It is characterized by strongly seductive overtones and is most obvious in women who have not succeeded in winning a fulfilling love relationship with the parent of the opposite sex. These are people who often wear their 'hearts on their sleeves,' and who succeed in repeatedly 'losing in love.'

The Pericardium position is Tight and probably a little Slippery. There is a small occasional Change in Rate at Rest. During the depressive phase, depending upon the individual's energy, the entire left distal position is temporarily Flat (reduced energy) or Inflated (robust energy) for a short time. With the Flat quality the individual is disposed toward jealousy and vengeance. Dr. Shen referred to the Flat quality in the left distal position as 'Heart closed,' and I call it Heart qi stagnation. With the Inflated quality the tendency is to be quick to anger. The Inflated quality at the left distal (or more rarely, Pericardium) position has also been observed in individuals who have symptoms of 'disturbed' Heart orifices, which could be a sign of the depression that occurs with this condition. During the euphoric phase there could be some Smooth Vibration.

I once treated a 45-year-old divorced mother whose pulse was Flat at both the left and right distal positions. She had been rejected by lovers, which had occurred several times since her divorce. She reported that to protect herself emotionally, she could extend or withdraw the energy through her arms (Heart channel) at will, outward toward or away from the world. I was able to perceive this happening at the left distal position, which changed from Normal to a Flat quality as she withdrew. When she was again 'in love,' the Flat quality at the left distal position disappeared.

Dysphoric depression (lack of joy)

Lack of joy without fatigue

Flat

An ongoing Flat quality bilaterally at the distal positions signifies Heart qi stagnation ('Heart closed') and early blood stagnation ('Heart small') (see Chapters 8 and 12). With Heart qi stagnation it is associated with spite and vengefulness. With Heart blood stagnation, it is associated with fear.

Early loss and disappointment

The Flat quality found bilaterally at the upper burner or left distal position with dysphoria is associated with a repressed, very early loss or disappointment, such as a child's loss of a parent, when organ qi was immature and weaker. These events are frequently forgotten in adulthood except upon persistent questioning. (The Flat quality at these positions could also be due to an early physical shock to the chest.)

Sudden bad news and rejected love

This a depression or dampening of joy associated with chronic disappointment in love. This causes a withdrawal of 'heart' feelings in individuals suffering from deficiency, some of whom are jilted and rejected frequently, and who tend to pick unsuitable partners. These individuals differ from the hysterical and reactive depressive in that they are unhappy even when they are in a relationship, anticipating the worst, which may be self-fulfilling; moreover, the Flat quality is always there. Ongoing vengeance and spitefulness are associated emotions.

Delivery with umbilical cord around neck

This etiology occurs at birth and has more serious physical consequences, including Heart blood stagnation ('Heart small') as well as Heart qi stagnation ('Heart closed'). Unless corrected this sign can last a lifetime, and the clinical consequences of this stagnation can remain and evolve into severe pathology in the upper burner, including constant emotional problems, vengeful or spiteful tendencies, fearfulness, and shooting chest pain—oppressive, which is less serious, and needle-like, which is more serious. With this etiology the facial color is green-blue around the mouth.

Inflated bilaterally at distal positions

The Inflated quality at the left distal or bilaterally at both distal positions is associated with a single episode of great unexpressed anger. Once the Inflated quality appears at the left distal position ('Heart full'), the person is prone to quick anger their entire life (see Chapters 8 and 12).

Early loss and disappointment

The Inflated quality can occur when there is unexpressed and unresolved grief due to a deep-seated individual loss at a time when the organ qi is more mature and stronger. Again, the Inflated quality at the left distal position has also been observed in people with symptoms of veiled Heart orifices, which could be a sign of the depression that occurs with this disorder.

Sudden bad news and rejected love

This is a depression or dampening of joy associated with chronic disappointment in love, causing a withdrawal of 'heart' feelings in robust individuals, some of whom have been jilted and rejected frequently, and who tend to pick unsuitable partners. Again, such individuals differ from the hysterical and reactive depressive in that they are not happy even when they are in a relationship, anticipating the worst, which may be self-fulfilling; also, the Inflated quality is always there. With the Inflated quality, the tendency is to be quick to anger.

Muffled at left distal position or over entire pulse

I have found a minor dysphoric lack of joy to be associated with a low level Muffled quality, especially at the left distal position, but also more rarely over the entire pulse.

Lack of joy with fatigue (including post-menopausal depression)

HEART BLOOD DEFICIENCY

The pulse is Thin or shows Change in Rate on Exertion (see Chapter 12), increasing more than 8-12 beats per minute. The sleep pattern is one of waking up and being unable to return to sleep after five hours of solid sleep. The depression involves more withdrawal.

The classic scenario for this pattern is found in cases of Heart blood and Spleen qi deficiency with palpitations, dyspnea on exertion, depression, spontaneous sweating, and anorexia. Any combination of qualities at the left distal and right middle positions—such as Thin, Feeble, Empty, Change in Qualities or Intensity, with a Slow rate—would be a sign that the digestive and transformative aspects of Spleen qi are incapable of producing and supplying sufficient blood to the Heart.

HEART QI DEFICIENCY

With Heart qi deficiency the depressions are more profound, with greater psychomotor retardation. At the left distal position the pulse will include one or more of the following characteristics: Feeble-Absent, Change in Qualities or Intensity, and Rough Vibration. There could be Slipperiness, or to a lesser extent Vibration, at the Mitral Valve position. With severe Heart qi deficiency the rate rises slightly, stays the same, or decreases with exertion, and the left distal position could be Empty. The sleep pattern is one of being up and down all night. If the fire of the Heart cannot warm the water (essence) of the Kidneys, it will be unable to rise and nourish the brain, and normal patterns will be disrupted.

Post-menopausal syndrome

This syndrome results from the profound loss of qi and blood during pregnancy and childbirth, aggravated by further loss with Cesarean deliveries and toxic medications, breast feeding, and lack of sleep. Very common in the West, this form of depression is almost unknown in Asia. There the care of a woman after childbirth involves complete rest for at least a month, with total care of the new baby and household assumed by a surrogate mother. Furthermore, supplementing the mother's qi and blood with herbs has always been routine.

Secondary anaclytic depression (despair) and narcissistic depression

The pulse for these conditions has not been substantiated.

Intra-individual failure, loneliness in middle and old age

This would include grieving for oneself, involutional depression, despair, and depression of the soul and spirit.

Muffled at left distal position, Empty at left middle position

These types of depression, associated with midlife crisis, all involve a failure to individuate in one or another way. The qualities most often associated with these conditions are Muffled at the left distal position and primarily Empty at the left middle position.

Cotton over entire pulse

While a thick Cotton quality above the qi depth over the entire pulse is more often associated with suppressed emotion and resignation, by late middle age the stagnation of the life force over such a long period can manifest in depression.

Heart blood stagnation ('Heart small') at the left distal position

Heart blood stagnation ('Heart small') appears at a later stage of an unresolved midlife crisis with either a Flat quality or, according to Dr. Shen (but not substantiated in my own experience), a Deep, Thin, Feeble pulse with a Normal, slightly Rapid, or Slow rate. In my own experience, I find at the left distal position a Deep quality with a very Rough Vibration (possibly Choppy), and sometimes the pulse is Interrupted or Intermittent at a later stage. Lifelong fear and coronary artery disease are associated symptoms.

Post-chemical intoxication, post-hepatitis, and post-mononucleosis depression

The pulse associated with these conditions is Empty at the left middle position. This form of depression is experienced as a psychomotor paralysis arising from an inability to turn plans and decisions into action. I have found the Empty quality at the left middle position in individuals who have used a great deal of marijuana or have a history of severe hepatitis or mononucleosis. With hepatitis and mononucleosis, a Slippery quality may attend the presence of a chronic low grade infection. In such cases the qualities change from Empty back and forth to Slippery at the organ depth.

Depression associated with the 'qi wild' condition

Yielding Hollow Full-Overflowing or Yielding Ropy qualities reflect a separation of yin and yang ('qi wild') due to either exercising vigorously for a long time and then stopping suddenly (Rapid rate), or exercising beyond one's energy for a very long time (Slow rate).

Severe anxiety, panic, and depersonalization is the earliest clinical manifestation of this disorder, and depression will follow the initial agitation and instability.

Bipolar and acute Grave's disease

Manic phase

Here we find Tight, Robust Pounding, and Slippery qualities at the left distal position and a Tight quality at the left proximal position associated with phlegm-fire disturbing the Heart orifices. The left middle position would be Flooding Excess with Robust Pounding due to suppressed emotion (anger) that leads to severe Liver fire, which rises to the Heart and causes Heart fire. However, depression is sometimes associated with these qualities here just before the 'burned out' phase begins. If the water of the Kidneys is relatively excessive, it will diminish the fire, which it is already trying to control. The Triple Burner mediates this relationship and should always be considered in management.

Depressive phase

Qualities of Heart qi deficiency (Feeble-Absent, Change in Qualities or Intensity, Rough Vibration) and Slipperiness appear at the left distal position. The left middle position is Empty, the left proximal position Tight and Deep, and the right proximal position Feeble-Absent. This is known as Heart phlegm confusing the Heart orifices.

ANXIETY (APPREHENSION, WORRY, FRIGHT, PHOBIA, PANIC, SHOCK) AND FEAR (TERROR, HORROR)

The distinction which I am making here between anxiety and fear is a progressive departure from my discussion of anxiety and fear in *Dragon Rises, Red Bird Flies*.

Differentiation of anxiety and fear

Both of these emotions are intrinsic to life and survival. Anxiety reawakens associated dangers from the past. Fear in humans is inherent to the mystery of our existence, of the great unknown, and all of the lesser unknowns.

Fear, in Western psychology, is distinguished from anxiety as a condition when there is a real rather than imagined source of dread. With anxiety there is usually a history of past trauma, re-evoked as a warning sign of danger by experiences in later life. Often, with free-floating anxiety, the connection is obscure.

In Chinese medicine the issue is more complicated. Anxiety or apprehension rises and more often stimulates the Heart and circulation, while fear descends and affects the Kidneys. Anxiety is associated with an agitation of the 'nervous system' while fear is more often associated with a dampening of that system. Fear is associated with cold, anxiety with heat. Fear is associated with heaviness, anxiety with quickness. Fear has a slowly developing dread, and anxiety a rapidly developing apprehension.

Existential atavistic fear is always with us, and whether or not we are controlled by it depends to a large extent on the integrity of Kidney yang-essence—the courage, fire, and will—and of Kidney qi—the faith and hope. When Kidney yang-qi-essence is deficient, hatred of and discrimination against the 'other' is the coping mechanism. Kidney yin and essence nourish the central nervous system and control the endocrine system through the pituitary gland; in a sense, therefore, they are masters of it all.

Anxiety, by contrast, has more to do with shock, fright, something imminent rather than something profound slowly taking hold. The free-floating anxieties are physiologically induced primarily as a result of shock to the Heart, which is initially experienced as fright. The instability in the Heart makes for instability in the mind, which affects the 'nervous system.'

Discussion of fright will be subsumed under Heart shock, and phobia considered as an isolated form of anxiety, with a susceptibility to phobia due to an underlying instability of the Heart.

Anxiety, phobia, and fright

Phobia is regarded as an isolated form of anxiety, with a susceptibility to phobia due to underlying instability of Heart qi. The principal pulse sign of phobia is Slippery at the Mitral Valve position, known in biomedicine as mitral valve prolapse. Phobic anxiety is a warning system of danger from either without or within, which is associated with the known rather than the unknown. For example, although we may not know why we are afraid of crowds, we do know that it is crowds that frighten us, a fright possibly engendered by some past experience and triggered by a familiar association.

Anxiety and panic

In terms of response to medication, psychiatry makes a distinction between anxiety and panic. There are also distinctions made in Western psychology among phobia, emotional shock, terror, and horror. In Chinese medicine these distinctions are less clear.

The patient with anxiety has an ongoing, low-level discomfort with occasional exacerbations. The pulse picture is, therefore, more enduring than the individual with panic, which is a sudden, shortlived experience associated with a particular situation such as fear of flying. To take the pulse just at that moment is a nearly impossible task without extensive preparation. In the following discussion we will consider panic as an accelerated anxiety.

GENERAL SYMPTOMS

Anxiety is attended by irregular breathing, palpitations, changes in perspiration, salivation, and trembling. Although this subject is controversial, the symptoms are generally thought to fall into two categories of autonomic responses, sympathetic (fight) or parasympathetic (flight). Larre et al. quote Lavier saying that "the master-heart [Pericardium] plays an essential role in the physiology of the sympathetic nervous system, the three heater [Triple Burner] playing an analogous role for the parasympathetic nervous system."[13]

According to Dr. Shen, whose observations I can corroborate, palpitations that occur at rest are related to Liver patterns, and those that occur during activity are Heart related.

CONDITIONS AND QUALITIES PATHOGNOMONIC OF ANXIETY

Heart qi agitation

Physical shock to the Heart at birth or during a heart operation, emotional shock to the Heart, and prolonged worry will all cause Heart qi agitation (see Chapter 12). A 'nervous system tense' condition will also accelerate the qi of a Heart that is already vulnerable, gradually depleting the yin of the Heart and creating a more severe form of Heart qi agitation. Some of the pulse pictures associated with Heart qi agitation are listed below.

Depending upon when the shock occurred and its severity, one finds a green hue around the chin, mouth, between the eyes and temples, or over the entire face.

Smooth Vibration

Smooth Vibration (see Chapters 11 and 12), especially when confined to the left distal position and at the qi depth, is the mildest form of Heart qi agitation. It is a sign of worry.

Rapid

Heart shock and Heart qi agitation is most often accompanied by a Rapid pulse rate. This condition is associated with emotional symptoms of anxiety, irritability, and worry. (It is important to remember that the pulse can sometimes be very Rapid with Heart qi deficiency, especially upon exertion, due to the instability of an organ with deficient qi. In our times, heat from either excess or deficiency is far less important as a cause of a Rapid rate.) If emotional shock has existed a short time the rate is between 84-90 beats/minute, although for short periods it can rise to as much as 140. Over a longer time the pulse is slower because the Rapid rate weakens the Heart and circulation. It is also slower when a small emotional shock, chronic anxiety, or worry is the etiology.

Occasional Change in Rate at Rest

Etiology — This is another, more serious sign of Heart qi agitation ('Heart nervous') (see Chapters 6 and 12). One day the pulse rate Changes at Rest and the next day it does not. With this quality the individual tends to become nervous, increasingly so as the Change in Rate is larger and more constant. Mood swings are common and the individual finds herself unrooted and constantly changing what she wants and where she is going in life. In the past the term 'grasshopper mind' was applied to people with this disorder. (Coincidentally, the eyebrows often touch in those with this quality. This is a sign in people with a constitutional propensity to self-doubt and therefore the inability to make up their mind.)

Symptoms — When shock is the etiology the individual is more easily scared; always worried, nervous, insecure; there are moderate to severe palpitations upon light exertion which are relatively persistent; readily and frequently awakens through the night due to very light sleep, then readily returns to sleep; tired in the morning; infants are up and down all night if shock occurs from around birth to the first few months; greater fatigue upon moderate exertion than with a mild agitated qi disharmony, although fatigue is less of a concern than anxiety to people with this condition.

Pulse — There is occasional Change in Rate at Rest. With worry as the etiology the rate is generally more stable, changing less often than when the etiology is shock, where the rate change is larger, constantly accelerating and slowing. The entire pulse can be a little Tight and Rapid, especially the left distal position in the central Pericardium area if the body condition is good. If the body is weak, the left distal position can be more Feeble and less Rapid.

Heat from excess in Heart

Pericardium Tight or left distal position Tense with Robust Pounding

Tightness at the Pericardium position in the middle of the left distal position, where one feels a sharp sensation like a pencil point hitting the middle of one's finger, is a sign of heat from excess in the Heart. With overwhelming heat, the entire left distal position is Tense with Robust Pounding. The heat will cause the 'nervous system' to accelerate, increasing general tension.

The accumulation of heat from excess in the Pericardium is attributable either to heat in the Liver or Stomach moving to the Heart, or to the Heart overworking to overcome the stagnation from a small shock, or to chronic worry.

Mild angina symptoms are usually due to heat from the Liver, Stomach, Triple Burner, Small Intestine, and Pericardium passing through internal channels connecting the Heart and Stomach, causing spasm of the coronary arteries. Other symptoms include shortness of breath during episodes of anxiety, flushing with feelings of heat in the face, and sometimes irritability and being easily angered.

Heart yin deficiency

Tight at left distal position (Heart Tight)

This is a sign of Heart yin deficiency (see Chapters 11 and 12).

Symptoms — Irritability, nervousness, and agitation with moderate to intense stress; fatigue after strenuous exertion; mild sporadic palpitations upon heavy exertion, which does not persist; light sleep and easily awakened, but also returning easily to sleep, therefore tending to be up and down all night; frequently a little tired in the morning; mild roller-coaster feeling and some difficulty in focusing thoughts and actions.

Etiology — Emotional shock primarily affects the Heart, creating a significant Heart yin deficiency. The effect on the Heart depends upon the prior status of Heart qi and blood, the size and duration of the shock, and the time that has elapsed since the shock.

Another principal cause is prolonged tension. If all of the yin organ systems are equally strong, this tension affects the Liver first. Liver qi stagnation creates heat which moves to the Heart where the yin of the Heart attempts to balance the heat. This depletes the Heart yin, which gives rise to Heart qi agitation. When the nerves innervating any organ become dry, they are more easily irritated and excited. Where the Heart is concerned, this manifests as agitation; where the Liver is concerned, it manifests as irritability. This drying out process depletes Kidney yin-essence and the 'nervous system' thereby becomes more irritable.

Prolonged worry is one way of overworking the Heart qi, causing agitation. Rapid movement of the Heart qi (nerves) creates heat, eventually depleting the Heart yin.

Heart blood deficiency ('Heart weak')

Condition and symptoms — This is primarily a condition of Heart blood deficiency ('Heart weak'), and to a lesser extent of Heart qi deficiency, both of which render Heart function unstable. Sleep is steady for a few hours, with early morning waking and difficulty returning to sleep, and with excessive dreaming. Apart from anxiety and some depression, other symptoms include impaired memory, concentration, and attention; frequently tired in the morning; easily startled; a roller coaster feeling and lack of focus; and unsettling palpitations upon mild to moderate exertion due to insufficient blood circulating to the Heart. Physically, there is minimal numbness and coldness in the extremities due to diminished circulation, and fatigue to the point of exhaustion even without significant exertion, partially due to inadequate sleep.

Etiology — Heart blood deficiency can be due to one or any combination of the following: Kidney essence deficiency; Spleen qi deficiency; chronic disease; excessive gradual blood loss over time; Heart qi agitation ('Heart nervous' and 'Heart tight') over an extended period of time. Constitutional Heart deficiency could be a predisposing factor. Again, prolonged and uncorrected Heart blood deficiency ('Heart weak') can eventually lead to serious Heart disease, such as congestive heart failure.

Thin at left distal position and/or Increase in Rate on Exertion >8–12 beats/min

If the blood deficiency is localized to the Heart, the left distal position will be Thin and/or there will be an Increase in Rate on Exertion more than 8–12 beats/minute. With a persistent 'Heart nervous' disorder as the cause, the pulse is more Thin and Tight.

Thin over entire pulse

With general blood deficiency as the cause, circulation is reduced and Heart blood is inadequate, leading to the above listed symptoms. Here, the entire pulse is Thin and a little Feeble, or Thin and Tight.

Heart qi deficiency

Feeble-Absent at left distal position

Next to a consistent Change in Rate at Rest, this is a sign of the mildest form of Heart qi deficiency with attendant emotional fragility and susceptibility to anxiety.

Constant Change in Intensity over entire pulse

This is a more serious sign of Heart qi deficiency accompanied by a disturbance of the Heart spirit, wherein one easily becomes anxious and emotionally unstable. Other symptoms of this Heart circulatory disorder are cold hands and feet, and migrating pains. The Heart is the 'emperor,' and illness in this organ will eventually affect the entire organism.

Yielding Hollow Full-Overflowing

Anxiety is traditionally associated with a Rapid rate, which is true for the more acute states. However, chronic low-grade anxiety can be found with qi deficient and 'qi wild' states, and may have a Slow rate, depending on etiology. (See Chapters 6, 8, and 9.)

Rapid pulses are related to a shock to the circulation, such as the sudden cessation of heavy, prolonged exercise. The abrupt reduction in blood volume without a concomitant reduction in blood vessel volume seems to predispose to depersonalization and dissociation most heavily. Prolonged exercise and work beyond one's energy are associated with a Yielding Hollow Full-Overflowing and Slow pulse.

Both etiologies of the Yielding Hollow Full-Overflowing pulse are accompanied by the most severe emotional and mental symptoms such as profound anxiety, depersonalization, dissociative experiences, and, especially when the exercise is suddenly stopped, a tendency to explosive anger. These symptoms develop more slowly when the etiology is prolonged exercise and work beyond one's energy.

Slow

Slow pulse rates associated with heavy exercise such as running are not regarded in Chinese medicine as beneficial to Heart function. The Slow rate is a sign of either Heart qi deficiency or a shock to the circulatory system. Experience has shown that the addiction to aerobic exercise begins with a sluggish circulation due to Heart qi deficiency, accompanied by lethargy and depression. Running temporarily increases circulation, transiently assuaging the lethargy and depression but further depleting Heart qi, resulting in even more profound listlessness and a need to run longer and farther to achieve the same euphoria to which the individual has become habituated.

Change in Qualities and Intensity at left distal position

These are serious signs of severe Heart qi deficiency indicating that the Heart yin and yang have separated, seriously interfering with Heart function and leading to emotional instability and fragility. (See Chapters 6, 12, and 13.)

Vibration and Slippery at Mitral Valve positions

The mitral valve prolapse syndrome in biomedicine, with which the Slippery quality at this position is associated, often has as its only symptoms phobia, anxiety, and panic. In Chinese medical terms it is a sign of Heart qi and blood deficiency.

Vibration is a less serious sign here, indicating a mild valvular insufficiency; the tendency to anxiety and panic is less than with the Slippery quality. The Slippery quality is a sign of more severe mitral valve prolapse, suggesting a congenital gross pathological defect or rheumatic fever with considerable panic and anxiety.

Arrhythmic qualities

These qualities represent severe Heart qi deficiency and separation of yin and yang. With highly Arrhythmic qualities the physical disability often overshadows the emotional. However, an individual with Intermittent or Interrupted qualities is more prone to anxiety and more emotionally fragile due to the relationship between the stability of the Heart and the stability of the mind. Again, the Heart is the 'emperor' whose well-being is reflected in the well-being of all physiology ('subjects' and 'officials'), spiritually, mentally, and physically. Chaotic Heart qi is not conducive to a quiet mind.

Heart-Gallbladder deficiency (timidity)

Physiology

The description of this syndrome in traditional Chinese medicine offers little explanation, in my experience, of the physiological relationship between the Heart and Gallbladder. However, the divergent channel of the Gallbladder passes through the Heart, and the divergent channel of the Heart uses GB-22 *(yuan ye)* as a connecting point with the Small Intestine.[14] The other obvious relationship between the Heart and Gallbladder is the Chinese clock. According to the 'law of midday-midnight' there is a special relationship between organ energies which are in ascendency twelve hours apart. The Gallbladder occupies this period of maximal flow of qi between 11 P.M. and 1 A.M., while the Heart occupies it between 11 A.M. and 1 P.M.

In *Acupuncture: The Ancient Art of Chinese Healing and How It Works Scientifically*, Felix Mann points out the relationship between the Heart and Gallbladder in Western medicine. Within the realm of Chinese medicine,

> If an organ is stimulated by a moderate stimulus only the organ itself is stimulated. If the same organ is strongly stimulated, the organ with which it is connected by the law 'midday-midnight' is stimulated in the opposite sense.[15]

I liberally interpret this to mean, in terms of traditional Chinese medicine, that stagnation (excess) in the Gallbladder would sedate the Heart qi. Chronic excess in the

Gallbladder would suppress Heart qi sufficiently to produce the mental-emotional components mentioned here. It is of interest in this regard that the herbal compound associated with a Heart-Gallbladder disharmony is Warm the Gallbladder Decoction *(wen dan tang)*, also known as Bamboo and Hoelen Combination. In this formula, Fructus Zizyphi Jujubae *(da zao)* tonifies the Heart, Rhizoma Pinelliae Ternatae *(ban xia)* and Sclerotium Poriae Cocos *(fu ling)* dispel dampness from the Heart and Gallbladder, Fructus Citri seu Ponciri immaturus *(zhi shi)*, Pericarpium Citri Reticulatae *(chen pi)*, and Rhizoma Zingiberis Officinalis Recens *(sheng jiang)* move stagnant qi from the Gallbladder, and Caulis Bambusae in Taeniis *(zhu ru)* and Rhizoma Coptidis *(huang lian)* clear Gallbladder heat. The formula, I believe, bears out the above association of Heart and Gallbladder through the 'law of midday-midnight' and 'Heart-Gallbladder timidity.'

Psychopathology — Symptoms include dizziness, blurred vision, timidity, palpitations, sighing, excessive dreams, easily startled, and a quick temper.

Pulse — The left distal position is Deep and Thin, the right middle Feeble, the Stomach-Pylorus Extension position Slippery-Hollow, and the Gallbladder position Tense and Slippery. The tongue has a white, thin coating. (Spleen qi deficiency and Spleen damp-heat and Gallbladder damp-heat are almost always found together clinically.)

Worry

Physiology — Worry is inordinate thinking, tinged with fear. Worry involves the process of rehearsing, mentioned by Freud, and is a talisman whose message is, "As long as I worry, I am safe."

Pathogenesis — Worry accelerates an organ's work while, at the same time, divesting it of energy, deharmonizing the smooth nervous innervation of that organ, and leading to a degree of chaos, rather than smoothness of operation. The principal effect of anxiety is upon the Heart, whose metabolism is accelerated. The principal effect of thinking is upon the Spleen-Stomach, whose physiology is at first accelerated, and later diminished, from working beyond its energy.

Dr. Shen observed that worry first affects the most vulnerable yin or yang organ. All organs being roughly equal in strength, sudden, short-term worry tends to affect the Heart first while ongoing, long-term worry will impugn the Liver, and through the Liver will eventually affect other organs such as the Spleen and Stomach.

However, I find the distinction between worry and thinking, in particular, too arbitrary. Excessive use of the mind as, for example, by students and academics, is certainly going to affect the Spleen more than the Heart, other things being equal. However, worry is a form of unproductive thinking, especially when it becomes chronic, and is bound to affect Spleen qi as well as the Heart.

Vibration

Superficial Smooth Vibration at the left distal position is the earliest and principal sign of worry, which can extend to other parts of the left side, and eventually to the right side, if the worry persists over time.

Vibration is a quality whose interpretation varies depending on the degree of its smoothness, consistency, position, depth, and response to treatment, as well as the time it has existed. We will not attempt to discuss each variable separately in this context (see Chapter 11 for elaboration). As with all qualities, its interpretation also depends diagnostically on other signs and symptoms, and on the history.

Generally, the causes of Vibration on the pulse are worry, Heart qi and blood deficiency ('Heart disease'), shock, terror, and guilt. Over time these will affect the 'nervous system.'

Smooth Vibration (mild Heart qi agitation)

PROGRESSION OF SMOOTH VIBRATION AT THE QI DEPTH

Sudden worry, such as bad news or concern over the next day's events (e.g., a test or job interview), is one important cause of Smooth Vibration at the left distal position. In its earliest phase the Vibration will occur first at the left distal position superficially as very Smooth and superficial. If the worry continues for a considerable period of time, and the effect on the Heart is not corrected, the quality will spread. Smooth Vibration at the qi depth will continue first down the left side to the left middle and left proximal positions. If the worry is not alleviated, over time the Smooth Vibration will continue progressing to the right distal position, and finally down the right side to the right proximal position.

ENTIRE PULSE AT ALL DEPTHS

When Smooth Vibration is found at all depths over the entire pulse we have a sign of an individual who is by nature a worrier, and who will find something to worry about even when there is nothing.

VIBRATION AT THE NEURO-PSYCHOLOGICAL POSITIONS

Smooth Vibration at these positions is associated with all of the symptoms of Heart qi agitation, especially anxiety, which may have been preceded by prolonged worry.

Tightness at Pericardium position and Tense at left distal position

Longer-term signs of worry on the pulse are Tight at the Pericardium position, and Tense or Tight over the entire left distal position.

Occasional Change in Rate at Rest

Profound worry over a long period of time will cause an occasional Change in Rate at Rest ('Heart nervous'), described just above, and later a Change in Rate on Exertion of over 8–12 beats per minute ('Heart weak').

Fear

TYPES OF FEAR

The ontogenetic separations from one stage of development to another concern themselves always and inevitably with the 'unknown,' which is the area of existence signaled by fear. I therefore define fear as that emotion which is signaled by the more fundamental unknowns of our existence, such as birth and death and all the great transitions in between.

Kidney yang is associated with the adrenal medulla, which secretes epinephrine, the arousal mechanism in adaptation. It also controls the thyroid, which maintains the metabolic heat of the body. A deficiency of Kidney yang is associated with a loss of courage and lack of will, with endogenous depression, and with deep internal cold.

Fear is our natural atavistic state from the dawning of the consciousness. We cannot avoid living with the ultimate unknowns. We do not know who we are, where we are or why, and what will happen to us. Only courage, faith, and hope have been the antidotes which allow us to live. Fear, therefore, is involved with a loss of courage, a loss of internal fire to face life, an endless challenge to deal with the unknown, and fear is the natural reaction before courage responds. Kidney energies are always involved with the courage to live with the essential challenges of life, which, in their most significant moments, involve change and the journeys into the unknown.

I refer to this classification of fear as the phylogenetic model because it is built around the ineluctable, intrinsic 'evolution of the self.' Each phase of this evolution is a culturally ritualized rite of passage. In this framework, fear is understood as a threat to 'becoming,' as explained by Gordon Allport in his book *Becoming*.[16] There are many threats to becoming discussed in some detail in *Dragon Rises, Red Bird Flies* under the aegis of the water, wood, fire, earth, and metal phases. These rites of passage are transitions which always involve the unknown in the process of separation from the known. This involves the issue of the transformation of bonds and boundaries.

While all energies are involved everywhere along the line of development and individuation, in all transitions and transformations, the energies which are always most ineluctable to the process are water, which provides courage (controlled fear), and metal, which drives toward change.

The water phase, and the courage to undergo the rites of passage, or what Joseph Campbell called the "hero's journey," is the most essential energetic issue where the primordial 'fear of the unknown' dominates an individual's life. This phase is highly vulnerable to insult, either constitutional, intra-uterine, or congenital, which injures the Kidney qi and compromises an individual's capacity to deal with the unknown and make the passages to full realization. Bonding with the earth (Mother Nature) and with God (Sun and fire-Father) involves love and faith, which are the only counteragents to fear.

In summary, with regard to bonds and the five phases, metal involves accepting and letting go; earth involves the substance and quality of the bond; wood determines the direction of the bonding; water its power and potential; and fire its passion.

Some of the the various stages of 'fear of separation,' which are included in *Dragon Rises, Red Bird Flies*, are mitosis, birth, infancy, and early childhood, assertion, Oedipal conflicts, surrogate parents bonding, peer bonding, and 'chumship.'

FEAR AND HEART BLOOD STAGNATION ('HEART SMALL')

Heart qi stagnation ('Heart closed'), with a very Flat left distal position, progresses to Heart blood stagnation ('Heart small'). The Flat quality at this position becomes either Deep, Thin, and Feeble, or Deep with a very Rough Vibration (possibly Choppy) at the left distal position. The rhythm is sometimes Arrhythmic at a later stage, and the rate is slightly Rapid or Normal. There is lifelong unexpressed and unexplained fear and tension, and coronary artery heart disease.

Heart blood stagnation ('Heart small') is associated with excessive heat in the Heart and circulation (blood vessels) over a long period, often due to a diet rich in saturated fats and to emotional tension. Sudden, profound, and early shock, such as prolonged labor with the umbilical cord around the neck, is another predisposing factor.

PROFOUND GUILT AND FEAR

Consistent Rough Vibration over entire pulse at all depths

Etiology

A consistent Rough Vibration over the entire pulse at all depths can also be due to profound guilt and fear, and is found in individuals who have committed a major violent crime, or experienced terror for another reason. Profound shock to the Heart often accompanies these extraordinary experiences.

Differentiation of etiology of Rough Vibration, Heart qi deficiency from shock, guilt, and fear

According to Dr. Shen, this extreme guilt and fear manifests as Vibration only if the Heart is qi or yang deficient. He said that guilt and fear without Heart dysfunction would show only with a very Tight and Rapid quality over the entire pulse. In my own limited clinical experience with these states of guilt/terror, consistent Rough Vibration, pervasive over the entire pulse at all depths, is more often associated with a profound sense of guilt and/or terror than with just severe Heart disease.

Vibration due to shock, guilt, or fear is differentiated from Heart disease by the pulse, facial color, and eyes. With fear the entire face has a green color. With guilt the facial color is normal but the spirit in the eyes is dull and the individual cannot look you directly in the eye. One would expect to find none of these characteristics with Heart qi deficiency. Instead, with Heart qi deficiency one might find a Slow pulse, constant Changes in Intensity over the entire pulse, *and* a Feeble-Absent quality at the left distal position, as well as loss of facial color (pallor).

Guilt and terror for perpetrators of transgressions against others

A distinction must be made between the Rough Vibration which appears in individuals whose terror concerns transgressions against others, and those where the Vibration appears in the victim of those transgressions.

The former is related, as far as I know, to some real, and not imagined, antisocial act, with guilt and fear concerning a major transgression of societal rules and laws up to and including murder. Such people, Dr. Shen said, cannot look you directly in the eye, which he relies upon as a vital diagnostic sign of guilt. (I *have* found people who, despite having this guilt and fear, are able to look others directly in the eye.)

The guilt and fear do not seem to be out of immediate and current concern with being caught and punished for their crimes. One of my patients, with Rough Vibration over the entire pulse, had murdered someone in North Africa some thirty years prior to his examination, and was in no danger of being prosecuted for his crime.

While the possibility that a major crime had been committed should be considered when a consistent Rough Vibration is found over most or all of the positions and depths, I believe that guilt and worry based on *imagined* rather than real acts is another possibility that must be explored. My own experience here is too circumscribed to form a firm opinion. However, based on my limited clinical exposure, it is my strong hunch that the pervasive presence of these qualities is more likely to reflect a real rather than imagined act.

Guilt and terror in the victims of transgressions

Recent experience indicates that consistent Rough Vibration over the entire pulse should be investigated as a shock to the Heart in connection with rape, childhood sexual abuse, and multiple personality syndrome (see below). With this etiology the Rough Vibration often appears in a setting of a 'qi wild' disorder (Change in Qualities, Yielding Hollow Full-Overflowing, Empty) or where the Heart shows instability manifested in Changes in Rate at Rest ('Heart nervous'), or more seriously Interrupted-Intermittent, and more rarely with a Bean (Spinning) quality. Smooth Vibration is also often present at the Neuro-psychological positions.

Terror (without guilt)

Terror is associated with extreme Kidney deficiency where the fear of the unknown is extreme. In addition to the qualities already described at the proximal positions which are associated with fear, the following qualities suggest more extreme fear.

Bean (Spinning)

The Bean (Spinning) quality combined with moderately Rough Vibration over the entire pulse, Vibration at the Neuro-psychological positions, and Slipperiness or Vibration at the Mitral Valve positions, is a class of qualities which I have found in individuals who are in a state of terror.

'Qi wild' qualities

Another group that may also be experiencing terror are those individuals exhibiting the 'qi wild' qualities. These include the Empty, Yielding Hollow Full-Overflowing, Interrupted-Intermittent Yielding Hollow, Change in Rate at Rest, and Change in Qualities. The Interrupted-Intermittent Yielding Hollow pulse represents the greatest instability.

Rough Vibration at the Neuro-psychological positions

This has been observed in people experiencing profound fear and terror.

Horror

Horror attends situations which are not personal threats, but which are emotionally upsetting to watch or hear about. An example is watching tragedies occurring to others, such as pictures of the Holocaust. The pulse rate increases, and the pulse may feel as if it is Bounding (Racing). There is general Robust Pounding and possibly a Change in Rate at Rest. Rage (or outrage) and its attendant qualities sometimes occurs under these circumstances. (See discussion of anger below.)

ROLLER-COASTER FEELING

Physiology

The Heart controls the mind. When Heart qi become unstable, the mind also loses its equilibrium.

Psychopathology

Loss of balance by the Heart causes instability in the mind, which tends to race and speed up mental processes. As mentioned above, an individual loses control over his thoughts, which tend to skip too quickly from one subject to the next, the proverbial 'grasshopper mind.' One day they want to do one thing with their lives and the next day something different. This leads to confusion and to a breakdown in the orderly conduct of life. The syndromes of Heart qi agitation and Heart blood deficiency are usually involved (see above and Chapter 12).

Pulse

With Heart qi agitation, the less serious of the etiologies, there is an occasional Change in Rate at Rest with no skipped beats, and the rate is measurable. The change increases with the amount of Heart qi agitation.

With Heart blood deficiency there is a Change in Rate on Exertion of more than 8-12 beats/minute. The greater the blood deficiency, the greater the increase, and the greater the emotional instability. The roller coaster feeling can also occur with the Interrupted and Intermittent qualities.

POST-TRAUMATIC STRESS SYNDROME

Acute

The typical finding includes Heart shock with a Rapid Bounding (Racing) rate, Change in Rate at Rest, and a Tight Pounding quality at the left distal position.

Chronic

In certain situations the Empty quality is a marker for the anarchy of severe ongoing post-traumatic stress syndrome. An example of this was a woman I met whose pulses were all Empty. I then took the pulses of her teenage son, which were also completely Empty. I was alarmed at the implications of extensive qi deficiency and therefore treated the woman and her son for deficiency, but nothing changed.

I learned quickly that here again I was dealing with an Empty quality which had nothing to do with its classical interpretation. It was, instead, a sign of a person who had a severe trauma (husband left suddenly and without warning) and had lost her center, and was literally floating aimlessly, with accompanying extreme anxiety and somatic manifestations. Upon resolution of the stress, the Empty quality disappeared within days (son) to weeks (mother).

VENGEFULNESS AND SPITE

Heart qi stagnation ('Heart closed') is described above, and in Chapter 12, in connection with the Flat quality at the left distal position.

PARANOID PERSONALITY

While there is no specific pulse picture to share due to the tendency of paranoid people to avoid contact with the helping professions, it is my sense that, in terms of their personality configuration, they would present the uniformly Tense quality over the entire pulse of the 'nervous system tense' condition.

The paranoid personality is a particular method of coping with fear that is highly organized and involves an otherwise intact organism. A system of intense vigilance is developed, similar to the 'nervous system tense' person, except that here it is difficult for the person to distinguish between what is genuinely dangerous from what is benign. All stimuli from the outside are regarded as threats, so that rather than belonging to a community of threatened people who act and sort as a group, the paranoid personality will at most allow only one other person in, what is known as a *folie a deux*, or 'us against the world': "Of all the world I trust only thou and I, and I am not so sure of thou."

The issue of fear and lack of trust and faith would lead one to anticipate that the pulse picture would be one of Kidney qi-yang deficiency, with Deep and Feeble-Absent qualities at the proximal positions from an early age. The pulse configuration is closer to a 'nervous system weak' picture in which the paranoid personality shows no obvious signs. They are more often very hardy individuals who can live long lives.

Based on rather extensive experience with paranoid personalities during my years as a psychiatrist, I would place them in the category of people who have a strong 'nervous system' but who have not made the first transition from self to other. This is probably more to do with psychological insults during the transition from the wood dominated to the fire dominated stages of development. This involves the transition from the negative relationship ("no") to the positive ("yes") relationship in which the child becomes attached to the parent of the opposite sex. The child, and subsequently adult, does not develop Heart connections, and all of their fire energy is focused into a heightened awareness. In psychiatry it has long been known that the eyes of paranoid people are especially and uniquely intense: the intact Liver qi which controls the eyes enhances the fire's keen and exaggerated awareness. Experienced psychotherapists know to avoid eye contact with paranoid patients.

In another sense, both the substance, Kidney yin, and the drive, Kidney yang, are sufficient. However, the drive is stopped. Metal energies cannot make the transition from wood to fire, and the accumulated substance is used less as a supply depot for the organism than it is to build defensive fortifications.

The paranoid schizophrenic is far less organized because of the inherent inability to build and maintain the paranoid's strong boundaries, which creates extraordinary disorientation with regard to reality, and consequently profound terror. The pulse picture is similar to that associated with the 'nervous system weak' condition and represents a more fundamental insult involving the deficient Kidney essence, both yin and yang.

Paranoia is essentially a defensive mechanism which is sustained until the essence is depleted and the fortification threatened, at which point the paranoid personality and the paranoid schizophrenic may strike out aggressively. However, this is not their first choice.

PSYCHOSIS, SCHIZOPHRENIA, AND DISSOCIATED MENTAL STATES INVOLVING BOUNDARIES

In biomedicine the term schizophrenia is a "waste basket" diagnosis for disorders involving boundaries between the inside and outside that vary in etiology from purely genetic and congenital damage to the central nervous system, to unbearable and unresolvable life conditions from which there is no escape except into an ultimately terror-filled inner chaos. Most are a combination of the genetic, congenital, and life experience etiologies, in varying degrees along a continuum of mild to severe inner anarchy. We shall consider two conditions in Chinese medicine which are associated with schizophrenia, the stagnant and the deficient.

Symptoms and pathogenesis

Severe anxiety, terror, hallucinations, delusions, paranoia, depersonalization, and dissociation are some of the symptoms of the inner chaos associated with a defect in boundary delineations between the internal and external environments.

Stagnant etiology of psychotic disorders

QI STAGNATION

This condition of qi stagnation in relation to psychosis was known to Dr. Shen, but is outside of my own experience.

> Qi stagnation in the middle burner (Stomach) occurs most often when the qi in the Liver becomes stagnant. While this may be the result of chemical stress (e.g., alcohol) or trauma, it is most often the result of suppressed feelings, especially unexpressed anger. Liver qi stagnation causes stagnation in the entire middle burner and is eventually accompanied by some heat, which may be likened to the heat of friction caused by two strong opposing forces. The qi is unable to move down to the lower burner (Intestines) and may either stay in the middle, causing physical discomfort, or, if the Heart is vulnerable, will rise with the heat and move to the Heart; because the Heart controls the mind, mental symptoms will then occur.
>
> These symptoms include mental confusion that occurs periodically, clearing and clouding on and off throughout the day. There may even be days when the individual is entirely well, interspersed with days when these symptoms appear. Qi problems generally tend to come and go, depending on whether the qi is stronger or weaker at any one time. And since qi is relatively unsubstantial and ephemeral, its strength, and therefore its stagnation, responds to influences much more readily than blood or water stagnation. This process can be likened to a fire in a house in which the windows are closed. The smoke is unable to escape and will tend to rise with the heat to the attic.[17]

In psychotic disorders associated with qi stagnation, the pulse will be Tense or Tight in both middle positions, changing in the degree of Tension depending on the amount of stress the individual is experiencing. The left distal position will be discontinuously Tense, again, depending on the level of stress.

FOOD STAGNATION

This condition of food stagnation in relation to psychosis was known to Dr. Shen, but is outside of my own experience.

> This occurs most often as the result of a severe emotional shock while eating, or just after, sharply curtailing digestion. The stagnation is of both food and qi and occurs actually in the esophageal area and is an upper qiao [burner] chest distress problem.... The symptoms are the same as those mentioned under qi stagnation except that the periods of confusion are more frequent, last longer, and are more severe.[18]

The Esophageal position is Slippery and the right middle position is particularly Tense and Inflated. The left middle position is also Tense and the left distal position Tense or Tight.

PHLEGM-FIRE (PHLEGM DISTURBS THE HEART)

This condition in relation to psychosis is well known to me.

Pathogenesis

We have already discussed phlegm-fire under the aegis of anxiety, depression, and palpitation. Phlegm-fire congestion is the result of stagnant dampness from poor digestion (Spleen qi deficiency or poor habits, and Gallbladder damp-heat), which accumulates into mucus, combined with excessive heat from Liver qi stagnation. Since food is eighty percent water, a weak Spleen (and/or Triple Burner), or excessive fluids or food that is difficult to digest can leave the digestive tract with more dampness (water) than it can handle. Chinese medicine teaches that this dampness (water) normally ascends to the Lung with Spleen energy to be 'digested' or, more accurately, 'misted.' If, in addition to poor digestion, the Lungs are weak and cannot digest this dampness that is normally dispersed through sweat or moved downward to the Kidneys, the dampness accumulates into mucus. Long-standing heat from Liver qi stagnation transforms into fire and combines with the mucus to become the more viscous substance referred to as phlegm-fire, which goes to the Heart where it disturbs the orifices. Especially if the nervous system is already compromised, there will be mental confusion that is continuous and unabating.

These are the severe, long-term psychoses that in Chinese medicine are on a continuum with epilepsy, which is thought to represent an even greater aggregate of phlegm-fire in the Heart orifices. These mental illnesses are usually marked by greater agitation.

Treatment — Therapeutic intervention, especially with herbs removing phlegm from the Heart orifices, was very effective in treating the most as well as the less severe cases of mental-emotional disorders.

Pulse — The left distal position is Tense-Tight and Slippery, the left middle position Tense with Robust Pounding, the right middle position Feeble or Empty, and the right distal position is probably Feeble and Slippery.

PHLEGM-COLD (PHLEGM CONFUSES THE HEART)

Pathogenesis — This condition is essentially the same as phlegm-fire without the heat from the Liver. It involves only dampness rising to the Heart. The psychological symptoms are of a more quiescent nature, such as depression.

Pulse — The left distal position is Feeble and Slippery, the right middle position Feeble or Empty, and the right distal position is probably Feeble.

BIPOLAR DISEASE

Psycho-energetic pathology

Within the framework of the concepts expressed in *Dragon Rises, Red Bird Flies,* the bipolar disorder is a manifestation of the interference with the development of creative expression associated with the fire element ("yes") by the inhibition of the psychomotor wood element ("no"). Stagnation of the qi of wood and fire creates heat from excess in its effort to overcome the stagnation. Eventually, the water (Kidney yin) is unable to control the fire (mind) which, during the *manic phase*, burns out of control and thereby depletes the wood, water, and finally the fire, which is now deprived of fuel. We then enter the *depressed phase* until the wood is replenished, at which point the conflagration begins again. In people with strong wood, the manic phase may be longer and more pronounced than the depressive phase, and they may report anxiety during the non-manic phase, rather than depression.

Bipolar episodes may be precipitated by stress in another vulnerable energy sphere, such as abandonment on the Spleen energies or separation on the Metal energies.

I believe that bipolar disease is often a constitutional defect of the Triple Burner's thermostatic control of the wood-fire cycle. However, the Triple Burner, as the harmonizer of relationships, is itself injured by the conflicts which led to the interference and inhibition of wood and fire described above. It has been pushed beyond its capacity to maintain control of the thermostat, through its governance of water metabolism, and is therefore an integral part of the solution. Supporting the Triple Burner's ability to regulate the consumption of wood by fire may help avoid this psychological and physiological catastrophe.

Pulse

During the manic phase the left middle and distal positions are Tense with Robust Pounding, possibly Flooding Excess with Change in Intensity, and the rate is very Rapid. During the depressed phase the left proximal position is Tight, the left middle has Reduced Substance or may even be Empty, and the left distal is Feeble-Absent. The disorder in the Triple Burner is manifested by less similarity in qualities at the different positions, which tend to be wildly different.

Deficient etiologies of psychotic states

'QI WILD'

Not all 'qi wild' qualities are necessarily associated with psychosis, although all lend themselves to mental instability. The Yielding Hollow Full-Overflowing quality is the one most often found with severe depersonalization and terror.

The reader is referred to Chapter 6 for a detailed discussion of 'qi wild,' and to Chapter 12 for a discussion of many of the qualities mentioned below.

Introduction

'Qi wild' is a condition characterized by chaos representing the most serious disorganization and disruption of overall physiology. Mental illness is one form of that chaos. It is a statement that the yin and yang of the entire organism have separated and lost functional contact.

What has become particularly frightening is the frequency of the most serious forms of 'qi wild' pulses, such as Change in Qualities and Arrhythmic rhythm, in the young, especially among those on medication.

It is also interesting that over the years I have found an increase in 'qi wild' disorders among my patients, as I travel around the country doing seminars, and especially in those places which have a reputation for anarchy. The inferences are unclear, although one wonders what is taking place on this planet that can be responsible for the apparent escalation of such widespread dispersal of our energies. It also raises the possibility that in certain places on earth the *feng shui* is more chaotic than in others. In my experience, the greatest instability is found in earthquake-prone San Francisco and Berkeley.

Etiology

Most of the pulse qualities described below will have their etiology prior to the age of twenty. The more severe the condition, the earlier the etiology. An individual with an Empty pulse probably worked or exercised beyond their energy between the ages of fifteen and twenty, while an individual with a Yielding Hollow Full-Overflowing pulse is more likely to have had a problem between the ages of ten and fifteen.

On the other hand, the etiology associated with an Arrhythmic rhythm, and a Yielding Hollow Interrupted pulse, for example, is either constitutional or occurs between birth and age ten. Heavy labor for a long period of time beyond one's energy, or frequent pregnancies and deliveries without rest and recovery, can (more rarely) also produce these qualities after the age of twenty.

The primary etiologies are severe early deprivation of food and shelter in utero, during infancy and in early childhood (from conception to age five), overwork in early childhood (e.g., child labor in Indian quarries), prolonged heavy exercise beyond a child's energy, sudden cessation of such exercise (common among high school athletes after starting college), serious long-term illness, a sudden extraordinary episode of lifting (heroic life rescues), protracted menorrhagia especially in adolescent girls, and substance abuse.

'Qi wild' qualities

The following qualities meet the criteria of 'qi wild' provided they appear over the entire pulse at all or almost all positions. They include the Empty, Leather, Empty and Thread-like, Scattered, Minute, Yielding Hollow Full-Overflowing, Yielding Ropy, Change in Qualities, and the Yielding Hollow Interrupted and Yielding Hollow Intermittent qualities. Again, these are all discussed in Chapters 6 and 9.

The terminal scenarios of delirium and coma when the pulse rate is Slow with high fever, or Rapid with a low temperature, occur with serious, often life-threatening, disease and are among the most profound 'qi wild' disorders.

Symptoms

Although they vary with the form of 'qi wild,' the following is a summary of symptoms associated with this state which can occur in both men and women. (For more specific symptoms, refer to the qualities listed above.)

There will be complaints of emotional fragility, labile emotions, severe anxiety, quick temper, a confused sensorium with feelings of being "spaced out" and losing one's mind, lives marked by anarchy and of being out of control. Sometimes, especially when such individuals lie down, they feel as if their bodies and arms are floating away, or are unreal (depersonalization). Often they become profoundly terrified by this experience. In addition, they are easily fatigued, and suffer extreme tiredness and migrating pains. The mental and emotional symptoms are particularly severe if the 'nervous system' is already 'tense' or especially 'weak.'

The result is physiological chaos which disrupts the orderly circulation of yang to the channels and the yin organs, impairing their ability to function. This chaos is especially disruptive to the 'nervous system,' which depends on the organized, coherent integrity of the lighter, fast-moving qi energies, which is lost with the 'qi wild' disorder.

People with a 'qi wild' disorder are often seen by psychiatrists and are diagnosed with anxiety neurosis, panic attacks, and psychosis. This disorder, which is totally misunderstood in Western medicine, will lead to lifelong emotional problems that are compounded by the treatments offered in the form of drugs and shock therapy.

TENSION

Liver qi stagnation and tension

Taut or Tense at left middle position

The Taut and Tense qualities at the left middle position are the most common signs of Liver qi stagnation due to the repression of an internal conflict. It is as if the irresistible force has met the immovable object. Tension is the felt experience.

Inconstant Change in Intensity over entire pulse

When the Change in Intensity is occasional, the cause is usually stress affecting the Liver. According to Dr. Shen, the stress in men is due to overwork and that in women to emotion. (These concepts probably no longer hold in a unisex world.) The inconstancy of the finding points to a problem in qi circulation. Qi is more ephemeral and dependent on diurnal energy levels, which rise and fall for many reasons, and on stresses on the Liver, which also tend to fluctuate.

When energy is reduced or stress elevated, the Change in Intensity is more obvious. Since it is one of the functions of the Liver to move the kinetic qi through the body, the circulation of qi and these Changes in Intensity are tied to the vicissitudes of the yin organ system.

'Nervous system tense'[19]

Tense to Tight over entire pulse

When Tension is found uniformly over the entire pulse I refer to it as the 'vigilance' pulse, having found it to be constitutional among members of oppressed minority ethnic groups whose survival through the centuries has required extraordinary vigilance. A similar quality can be found today in almost anyone living in a large city, or living constantly with the need to be vigilant. Therefore, a differential diagnosis is required between a constitutional 'nervous system tense' and that which is associated with ongoing chronic stress. With the constitutional etiology the pulse tends to be Slower than with the etiology associated with chronic stress.

Making the distinction is important since one can ask an individual whose tension is due to life experiences to alter their lifestyle as part of the treatment. By contrast, telling the individual who is constitutionally 'nervous system tense' that they will feel less tense if they alter their environment will be an exercise in frustration for the individual, and possibly counterproductive to their accepting other helpful treatment.

One test of a constitutional etiology is made when the patient's distress decreases after a few treatments, but the pulse stays the same. However, the principal distinction is made through facial diagnosis and color. According to Dr. Shen, when the etiology is constitutional the eyebrows are extraordinarily thick such that one cannot see the roots of the individual hairs, and the color around the chin and mouth is blue-green. When the etiology is based on life experiences, the roots of the hairs in the eyebrows are easily distinguishable and there is no blue around the chin or mouth. While I have often observed these relationships, there have been many instances when the constitutional 'nervous system tense' condition was found in the absence of these signs.

ETIOLOGY

Constitution

In the United States I have found this pulse most often among Jews and Israelis, who, along with the gypsies, are the only people who have not had a "home" for the past two thousand years. Examining the pulses of other displaced peoples would be an interesting test, although the time spans may be shorter.

The former German Jews should know that vigilance is not something that a minority gives up in this world without risk. In a sense it seems to document the process of the survival of the fittest, and the fittest were those most vigilant to external danger.

I consider this pulse quality to be equivalent to a state of readiness, and regard it as a reflection of a survival mechanism in which people are in a state of alert for danger and are therefore more likely to survive. I know, for example, from studying medieval history that the Jews benefitted from living together closely in ghettos from which they organized a spy system in the country in which they lived to warn of impending attacks. When they left the ghettos and were "assimilated," they developed a false sense of security and were paradoxically in greater danger. Nazi Germany is the inescapable prototype of this thesis. It is for this reason that I refer to it as the 'vigilance' quality, a necessary evil for survival for those few who have it.

As with everything in life, too much of a good thing is not good. Beyond a certain level of the 'nervous system tense' condition, this strong personality becomes impulsive. The best diagnostic signs are the eyebrows and, to a lesser extent, the pulse itself, which is described below.

Over the course of a lifetime this tension takes its toll on the 'nervous system,' and ultimately on other vulnerable systems. While I consider the Tense quality to be a sign of vigorous essence, in the long run eternal vigilance will deplete the essence, and profound fear and paranoia, increasing in intensity, will be its inevitable companions.

Symptoms

The principal symptom is an ongoing tension which is unrelated to any particular externally-generated life stress. Accompanying symptoms will depend on the vulnerability of other organ systems, affected by the heat from excess, and especially from deficiency, which can be a consequence of this condition over a long period of time.

Signs

The pulse rate is Normal to slightly Slow, and the pulse is otherwise mildly Robust Pounding, and uniformly Tense. This uniformity is enduring even when other problems, such as overwork or trauma, complicate the clinical picture. Some changes can be anticipated, especially in the proximal positions, if the intervening events are prolonged and severe. As mentioned just above, if the circulatory system is vulnerable, some form of heat in the blood is possible with a Blood Heat and Hollow Full-Overflowing and ultimately Tense Ropy quality. Especially at an early age, the likelihood of the impulsive behavior described above being involved with the exaggerated 'nervous system tense' condition manifests on the pulse as a greater Tightness and more Rapid rate.

The tongue and eyes will be normal. The eyebrows may be thicker than normal, increasing in thickness with the increasing degree of inherited tension in the nervous system, and a commensurate tendency toward impulsive behavior. The individual hairs are not easily distinguishable, especially in the impulsive person. There are often vertical lines between the eyes, two if the problem is profound, and one if it is less serious. If the line has a bright color, the condition is less severe than if it is dull. The color of the face is generally darker, and the color around the chin and mouth is blue-green.

Daily stress

Hypervigilance over a long period of time can give rise to mild heat from excess. The concept is that the vigilance causes the qi to move too fast, generating external heat. Paradoxically, vigilance also requires great control over one's spontaneity, which involves suppression of emotion primarily in the channels of the Liver where it is recognized as stagnation. The body mobilizes internal metabolic heat to overcome the stagnation. If the circulatory system is vulnerable, the heat can easily affect the blood vessels and the blood.

The difference between the constitutional etiology and that rooted in life experiences is that in the latter case the tongue and eyes will show more signs of heat, and a more Rapid rate, and will not exhibit the facial signs listed above that are pathognomonic of the constitutional etiology.

Symptoms

Tension associated with living under conditions which promote stress, and only with stress; mild flushing; intolerance of heat; mild headache; dryness of eyes; thirst which is easily quenched; tendency to constipation; difficulty getting to sleep; readily perspires; eczema.

Signs

The pulse is Tense and essentially the same as with the constitutional etiology, except possibly a little more Rapid, because here the 'nervous system' is affecting the Heart. If the condition is mild and in the early stages, the Tension can feel stronger at the qi depth. When the tense situation has existed a moderate length of time, the Tense quality will be felt more at the blood depth. When it has existed a very long time, the Tension will be strongest at the organ depth. The blood depth can be slightly expanded over time into a 'blood heat' and 'blood thick' disorder with these qualities.

In contrast to the constitutional origin of this quality, when it is based on daily stress the pulse will become less Tense with treatment that relieves the patient's distress. The eyebrows are normal in thickness and there are no lines between the eyes. Facial color is normal.

'Nervous system' affects 'organ system'

Etiology

This is a situation in which the 'nervous system' is affecting the 'organ system' over a period of time (i.e., the qi innervation of the yin organs causes them to work too rapidly), causing heat from excess, and later the gradual progression to heat from deficiency. Signs of tension precede the signs of fatigue. (See Chapter 14.)

Symptoms

Symptoms of agitation, irritability, and being easily excitable ensue from this drying of the yin of the yin organs, and, in particular, their innervation. This is a vicious cycle in which nervous tension depletes yin, the absence (dryness) of which makes the nerves more irritable. With this condition, considerable fatigue accompanies the agitation and irritability because the vital yin organs cannot fully contribute to the true qi. The face has vertical lines between the eyes. The skin is thin and transparent and the face and body are pale with a bluish color, especially around the chin and mouth. The deeper the blue color, the more serious the condition. The tongue is normal unless complicated by another problem.

Pulse

The entire pulse is only slightly Deep, and there is one very Thin Tight line on the surface of the organ depth, on the left side. The pulse may also be a little Rapid.

NEURASTHENIA OR 'NERVOUS SYSTEM WEAK'

Etiology

CONSTITUTION

This is constitutional Kidney yin, yang, and qi essence deficiency associated with constitutional vulnerability to stress. It is often found in people who were extremely shy and sensitive as children, easily picked on and intimidated. An entire array of mental and emotional problems are related to constitutionally deficient Kidney yin, yang, and qi essence. These include endogenous depression and schizophrenia, as well as severe neurological deficits including retardation. Kidney essence is responsible for the development and maintenance of the central nervous system. Deficiency of Kidney yin and yang are associated with endocrine problems, especially in women.

Symptoms

The symptoms are always changing. For example, there are constantly changing allergies. The individual is vulnerable, easily disturbed, and unstable emotionally from childhood, at which time they appear sickly and unable to physically compete with children their own age. When the yang is more deficient, there is more lassitude; when the yin is more deficient, there is more agitation; and when the qi (and Triple Burner) regulator is more deficient, there is greater instability.

The face has vertical lines between the eyes. The skin is thin and transparent and the face and body are pale with a bluish color, especially around the chin and mouth. The deeper the blue color, the more serious the condition. The tongue is normal unless complicated by another problem.

Pulse in left margin.

'Nervous system weak,' which is characterized by these qualities, is roughly the same pattern as neurasthenia with lifelong, continuously changing symptoms and fatigue.[20] These individuals are never quite able to function, care for themselves, or lead independent lives.

Early in childhood

In the beginning the entire pulse is a little Floating because, as Dr. Shen noted, "the nervous system *(tai yang)* is on top, the fastest moving qi." By this, I believe he means superficial at the qi depth. The rate varies from 88 to 120 beats/minute. There is superficial Smooth Vibration and the proximal positions are Feeble. I have not personally encountered this stage.

Later in adulthood

Gradually the 'organ system' is affected and the pulse is Deep with Reduced Substance and Thin, finally Feeble-Absent, with a Tight line above the organ depth. If it affects the 'circulatory system' the rate is Slow. I also find Change in Intensity and Qualities at the proximal positions, which is a sign of yin and yang separating.

LIFE EXPERIENCE

Very mild

Qualities of Yielding or Absent at the qi depth and Spreading at the blood depth are signs of mild qi and some blood depletion, usually due to working beyond one's energy. The depletion of qi and blood makes the individual's 'nervous system' more vulnerable to emotional as well as physical stress.

Moderate

Qualities of Deep or Feeble-Absent over the entire pulse, or with a Normal or Slow rate, are due to work beyond one's energy over a long time, or to prolonged and serious illness. The qi and blood deficiency is severe and the individual is even more vulnerable to stress, to which he reacts with collapse or depression.

Severe

The Empty quality is a 'qi wild' pulse, a sign of psychological and physiological chaos with greater mental disorganization as a reaction to stress.

ANGER

Sudden anger: trapped qi in the Heart, or 'Heart full'

The qualities associated with sudden, great, unexpressed anger tend to manifest mostly on the left distal and left middle positions with a very Inflated quality. With this etiology, the Diaphragm position will show this quality when the Heart and Liver qi are particularly strong. The more recent the sudden anger, the more pronounced the Inflated quality.

    Sudden and great, unexpressed anger which occurs when one is active causes the left distal position to be very Inflated (trapped qi in the Heart, or 'Heart full'). If it occurs when one is quiet it will cause the left middle position to have a very Inflated quality, and if it occurs while eating it will be signaled by a very Inflated quality in the right middle positions.

Propensity to anger: trapped qi in the Heart, or 'Heart full'

Prolonged delivery with the head inside, as with a breech presentation, can cause mild qi dilation of the Heart, which presents at the left distal position as a Yielding Inflated quality. This is a sign of trapped qi in the Heart. The consequences are being quick to anger, lifelong fatigue and bodily discomfort, with difficulty lying on one's left side.

Gradually developing anger, repression, and passive-aggressive behavior

The qualities associated with gradually developing anger are Taut, Tense, and Tight, and tend to manifest in the left middle position, less often in the left distal position, and rarely in the Diaphragm position. They have already been mentioned in connection with agitated depression and irritability.

These qualities are associated with repressed conflict and emotion, especially anger. The Taut and Tense qualities are more connected to a gradually developing anger or frustration, and are a sign of internal conflict between two opposing emotions, such as anger at one's boss and fear of expressing it out of concern for losing one's job.

Repressed emotion, especially chronic anger, requires a variety of adaptive maneuvers to express the anger without direct confrontation. Humor is one avenue, passive-aggressive undermining behavior is another, and 'acting out' is probably the least adaptive. All are associated with these qualities in the left middle position.

STRONG INDIVIDUAL

Short time

The Taut quality represents qi stagnation due to repressed anger for up to a few (five) years.

Moderate time

The Tense quality (qi stagnation and heat from excess) is associated with low-level anger for a relatively moderate period of time, up to ten or twenty years. Taut-to-Tense and Inflated qualities bilaterally in the middle positions are associated with repressed anger and Liver qi stagnation causing Stomach qi rebellion.

Long time

The Tight quality (yin deficiency) is associated with low-level anger beyond approximately twenty years.

DEFICIENT INDIVIDUAL

The Tense with Reduced Substance or Tight and Diffuse qualities are most often associated with prolonged repressed anger in a deficient individual. The pulse is Deep and the Tension is found primarily at the organ depth.

Separation and divorce

Inflated at Diaphragm position

The Inflated quality found at the Diaphragm position is usually associated with an acrimonious separation in which the tender feelings formerly felt for the lost individual are repressed, and the angry feelings accentuated, in order to make the break without too much pain. Suppression of the diaphragm and breathing are somehow involved.

This is found more often on the left side, although it can appear bilaterally. The degree of Inflation depends on two factors. First is the length of time between the episode and the examination of the pulse, with the Inflation decreasing over time. Second is the importance of the separation to the individual: the Inflation increases in proportion to the importance of the relationship. For this reason, Inflation diminishes over the years, but, in my experience, will usually last even as a small Inflation for up to ten years.

At a recent conference where I was demonstrating pulse diagnosis a woman presented with a very prominently Inflated left Diaphragm position. She and others asked me what it meant and I said that one of the possibilities was a recent separation or divorce. She began to cry almost uncontrollably, and whispered that she was in the midst of a very difficult and painful divorce.

If it is found only on the left side, the cause is probably as mentioned here. If it is found only on the right, the cause is probably repeated episodes of very heavy lifting beyond one's energy. This quality is sometimes found at the Diaphragm position bilaterally, or only on the left side, with a sudden, great, unexpressed anger for reasons other than separation, when the Liver and Heart qi are strong.

Explosiveness and impotent rage

The individual flies into violent rages with the least provocation.

PSYCHOGENESIS

The factors involving explosive rage are the degree of impotence that the person feels prior to the outburst, and the stability of the mind and the nervous system. With regard to the stability of the mind we are concerned with Heart qi agitation, trapped qi in the Heart, and with phlegm in the Heart. With regard to the nervous system we are concerned with the basic integrity of Kidney essence and with Liver qi stagnation transforming into Liver fire and wind. As with bipolar disease, I find the consistency of the thermostatic and homeostatic functions of the Triple Burner to be an essential factor in maintaining emotional balance.

PULSE

Concerning the Kidneys, there are central nervous system defects which lend themselves to impulsive violent rages about which I have no direct knowledge of the pulse, but which I assume are a form of Kidney yang-essence deficiency in which the thermostatic function of the Triple Burner in the hind brain is damaged or undeveloped. Where the water cannot control the fire and nourish the Liver yin (fire turning to wind), we would also find a Kidney yin-essence deficiency. With Kidney yang-essence deficiency the proximal positions would be Feeble and the Neuro-psychological positions possibly Doughy; with Kidney yin-essence deficiency, the proximal positions would be Tight.

With regard to the Triple Burner, one will find widely disparate qualities from one position to another. Heart dysfunction will manifest as inconsistent Change in Rate at Rest, and Tense Inflated Robust Pounding Slippery at the left distal position.

Liver involvement will manifest as Tense Inflated Robust Pounding qualities at the left middle position, and possibly a Floating Tight quality above the left middle position, the left side, or over the entire pulse.

An impaired 'circulatory system' with a very Slow pulse rate, and a 'circulatory system' experiencing a separation of yin and yang with the Yielding Hollow Full-Overflowing (Slow or Rapid) qualities, are both attended by uncontrollable anger. People with trapped qi in the Heart ('Heart full') are prone to anger and explosive rage throughout their lives, presumably when some of the trapped qi suddenly escapes.

INDECISION

Liver-related

The Empty quality is associated with extensive decisions and plans that are made but not executed. The cause of this quality in our times is usually substance abuse, especially the abuse of marijuana. Overwork, chronic hepatitis, mononucleosis, and parasites can also be accompanied by an Empty quality at this position.

Gallbladder-related

According to Larre et al., the Gallbladder is one of the singular organs and "is given a particular value because it works with that special energy having rapport with the nervous system and the cerebral system: jing (essences)."[21] This relates to its important function as decision maker. A passage in Chapter 13 of the *Su Wen* declares that "the eleven other organs take for themselves the decision made by the gallbladder."[22] Larre goes on to say that "biliary function is not uniquely limited to the receptacle of the gallbladder but concerns the entire 'hepatic gland'" and "in the large organic functional ensemble, the gallbladder is dominant" over the liver.[23]

In my experience, agonizing over profound life decisions over time can cause serious Gallbladder pathology, including necrosis, with Tight Robust Pounding, Choppy, Wiry, and even Muffled or Change in Intensity qualities at the Gallbladder position. At the same time, Gallbladder pathology due to other causes such as chronic heat from excess in the Liver will also make decisions more problematic. Frequently, when the problem is constitutional, the eyebrows cross over and touch.

Heart-related

With those who cannot make decisions because they are constantly doubting themselves, and therefore can never make up their minds, the problem of decision making is related more to instability of the Heart than to the Gallbladder, where the problem is one of stagnation and not moving forward.[24]

The rate here occasionally Changes at Rest ('Heart nervous'). When this constant doubting is constitutionally determined, the eyebrows will touch. Other members of the family will have the same facial diagnostic sign.

RESIGNATION

Cotton

This is a sign of a 'sad pulse' according to Dr. Shen. I have found that it conveys the experience of oppression out of a sense of hopelessness and helplessness to change specific onerous conditions of life. Thoreau expressed this in his observation that "the mass of men lead lives of quiet desperation."[25] I have found that people with a thick, heavy Cotton quality over the entire pulse tend to blame others rather than take responsibility to extricate themselves from the burdensome condition of their own lives.

This pulse is a sign of superficial qi stagnation, and, if uncorrected over a long period of time, is prognostic of tumors, especially cancer.

OBSESSIVE THINKING (REFLECTION)

Obsessive thinking is one form of an excessive use of the mind.

Hesitant quality and obsessive thinking

With this individual there is a monomaniacal preoccupation with some aspect of life, usually work, though often health, in which the individual's mind never ceases to rest even when asleep. I have found this pulse in individuals working for the stock market who never stop thinking about money, and in high level government political appointees who have no civil service safety net, and who are extraordinarily exploited by their political masters. I have also recently found it in mature acupuncturists who are attempting to balance school, other work, and family. These people tend to collapse suddenly (nervous and physical breakdowns). The Hesitant quality is a sign of mild Heart yin deficiency.

Spleen-Stomach and obsessive thinking

PHYSIOLOGY

The brain is nourished by rising Spleen qi and Heart blood. Sharpness of thought, concentration, and attention is a function of Heart blood. 'Spaciness,' on the other hand, depends on the integrity of rising Spleen qi. This is roughly equivalent to the Western concept of glucose, which is the only nutrient which crosses the blood-brain barrier, and therefore the only energy source for the central nervous system. The use of the mind in the form of thinking consumes more glucose than any other activity. Obsessive thinking is a form of excess that depletes the Spleen qi. The clouding of consciousness is partly due to the accumulation of fluids owing to deficiency of the Spleen qi, which inhibits the rising of clear Spleen qi to the brain. Also, these fluids frequently accumulate in the Heart and 'mist' the orifices, which further interferes with clear consciousness.

PATHOGENESIS AND SYMPTOMS

> Since the mind consumes more energy than any other process in the organism, excessive thinking has the effect of depriving organs of the quantity and quality of energy necessary to their optimum productivity.... [A]ll organs must sacrifice their energy to the mind, which has first call on it. Those organs that are most vulnerable will suffer the most apparent dysfunction and will produce the most immediate and severe symptomatology. However, since thinking requires an energy that is entirely reliant upon a supply of glucose, there is a greater likelihood of it having an effect upon the 'digestive system' (Spleen-Pancreas, Stomach, and Liver) than on any other system, however vulnerable it may be.... This would tend to preclude thinking during mealtime, the time when thinking has its greatest effect upon the 'digestive system.'[26]

During mealtime the ruminating mind has to compete with the ruminating stomach. Symptoms include those which affect the mind—sharpness of thinking, concentration, and attention—leading to complaints of feeling 'spaced out' or 'spacy.' Digestive complaints are wide ranging from mild burping, gas, distention, flatulence, and mild abdominal discomfort to severe discomfort and the extremes of regurgitation, nausea and vomiting, diarrhea or constipation, food allergies, and anorexia.

SPLEEN-STOMACH AND OBSESSIVE THINKING

The entire right side will exhibit abnormal qualities, especially the right middle position. These will vary depending on the type and severity of the symptoms. In the earlier stages when the 'digestive system' is overworking, the quality will probably be Tight. Later, a Cotton and Feeble Empty quality will indicate greater deficiency. The expected Slippery quality appears at the left distal and Gallbladder positions.

The left distal position could also be Thin and Tight, since Spleen qi deficiency eventually produces Heart blood deficiency. In this case, the rate will increase disproportionately to the amount of exertion.

WITHDRAWAL AND THE DEEP QUALITY

Early in my career as a practitioner of Chinese medicine I observed that people who coped with life and stress through withdrawal would often present a Deep quality over the entire pulse, even though the rest of their signs and symptoms would suggest a more Robust quality. This would usually occur on the first visit and in the first encounter with the pulse. However, the Deep quality, as a sign of emotional withdrawal, usually cannot be sustained and will ordinarily last for only a relatively short time, after which the pulse will reveal its entire message. In my experience, this would continue during the first few minutes of the pulse examination until, during subsequent visits, the individual felt safe and comfortable with me, at which time the Deep quality was no longer in evidence at the beginning of the pulse-taking procedure.

With a few people this withdrawal of qi was more persistent. One patient, who I met within the first year of my practice, was a middle-aged woman whose entire pulse was uniformly Deep and which did not revert quickly, as described above. Ordinarily one would interpret this as a sign of significantly deficient qi. I sensed a notable emotional component, which made me entertain the possibility that some aspect of the depth of her pulse represented an even more profound retreat than that which I found when the Deep pulse lasted only a short time. At the time, I interpreted the physiologic effect as an imbalance between her protective and nutritive energies.

Her presenting complaint was immobility and pain in the neck. Her other chief complaint was anorexia nervosa. The question was whether she was qi deficient due partly to the damage to her digestion and assimilation, or whether all of her qi was locked inwardly due to her general retreat from life, rendering her protective or true qi unavailable.

The test was to see how easily one could raise the qi with acupuncture. The treatment would reveal the diagnosis. If it rose quickly the diagnosis would be 'retreat'; if it did not rise quickly the diagnosis would lean toward severe qi deficiency, although a combination was probable. The initial task, to 'raise the yang,' was made using a combination of S-12 *(que pen)*, S-36 *(zu san li)*, and GV-14 *(da zhui)*, all reunion ('meeting') points of yang energy.

Her pulse almost immediately became less Deep, more balanced, and calm, with good quality. Within a short time she revealed some of her profound life difficulties, involving a broken marriage and an emotionally disturbed child. Her anorexia disappeared and her emotions and life in general began to stabilize. The rapid response to this 'test' revealed that the larger part of this Deep pulse was related to emotional withdrawal and less to qi deficiency.

DENIAL AND THE EMPTY QUALITY

During this early period in my practice I observed another transient quality in people who seemed to meet the world as always cheerful and effervescent, even when they were in profound difficulty, thereby keeping others from knowing their vulnerability. The Empty pulse quality, in which all the qi seems to be at the surface, represented this method of coping with stress; it would also last only briefly before giving way to the true pulse picture.

An example of this occurred when I worked with a young woman in her mid-twenties who came because of insomnia and because she could not open her heart to a man out of fear of "losing my freedom." She was unmarried and unattached and functioned as an extension of a large family clan that ran an extremely successful business. She had become a key part of that business as the 'front' which met the public, always with a cheerful smile and glad handshake, while she suffered inwardly. She was hardly "free."

Her pulse was Empty, which from all other evidence was a sign of putting all of her energy on the surface rather than a sign of a separation of yin and yang ('qi wild') and severe qi deficiency. The left side was more excessive than the right, which Dr. Worsley would (at that time) interpret, in a woman, as a sign of a husband-wife imbalance.

I suspected this pulse of being partially an expression of denial (the happy 'front') and partially an expression of a rigid, tough outer shell. She was not going to surrender to her tender feelings, partially out of fear of being hurt, and partially from fear of separating from her family.

The test in this instance was to see if the issue was one of balance or deficiency. To accomplish this I would first attempt to balance the yin and yang by increasing the yin (her tender feelings) and softening the yang (her tough outer shell) so as to stabilize the husband-wife imbalance (inter-individual relationships) and to move the heat from excess out of the Heart. Moving the fire to the water and building water (courage) and wood yin, and balancing within the fire phase using the fire point of the Triple Burner (harmonious relations), accomplished this and also reversed the husband-wife imbalance.

Within six sessions, which was the total length of treatment, her pulse was balanced in all respects. Her insomnia disappeared almost immediately and her rigidity (the tough shell) began to soften. She met a man with whom she fell in love and subsequently married, and began to communicate her tender feelings for the first time. While I cannot say that they lived happily ever after, at least she entered into the stream of life and lived in the real world.

This therapeutic 'test' revealed that her pulse picture was an expression of imbalance between her tender heart feelings and the need to defend herself. The Empty quality was for her a sign of a culturally-induced need to always present a pleasant front, to deny all, or at least never communicate, any unpleasant feeling.

PHYSICAL PAIN

When an individual is experiencing pain, the pulse is uniformly Tight to Wiry, and possibly a little Rapid. For the exact location one would search for the position which is most Tight, including the musculoskeletal positions. The cause is usually a recent trauma. The facial color is dark. (See Chapter 12 for a discussion of the musculoskeletal positions.)

Physical pain is an important emotional issue on many levels, including the irritability which accompanies it from day to day, and the depression which ultimately sets in if it is not resolved. While most people will voice their complaint, the pulse, tongue, and eyes can sometimes be useful when dealing with those who deny their feelings, including (especially) chronic pain. The Cotton quality can develop in people with chronic pain who are given the familiar biomedical balm, "just learn to live with it." A Muffled quality at the left distal position, or even over the entire pulse, would be a commensurate sign of the depression.

ADDICTIONS

There is no simple pulse picture related to the propensity to addiction. As I have previously stated, the essence qi associated with the functioning of the central nervous system is so infinitely more complex than anything I have read in the Chinese medical literature that it seems impossible to pinpoint all the different central nervous system defects on the pulse. What follows is only a statement of the results rather than the cause.

It is my impression that most people susceptible to addictive chemicals have an aversion to pain and a condition of the central nervous system somewhere in the continuum of 'nervous system weak' with regard to the fragility of their essence. The left side would be Deep and Feeble with a Tight quality at the surface.

People who crave stimulants are similar to those who are not content unless they are constantly taking risks. With those who I have known, they are often severely detached from feeling, especially Heart feeling, which is perhaps why so many like heart stimulants such as cocaine and amphetamines. The left distal position would probably be Flat before the onset of the effects of the drugs.

Alcoholism

The left middle position is Tight to Wiry due to the drying out of liver parenchyma from alcohol abuse.

Marijuana

The left middle position is Empty.

Hallucinogens

With hallucinogens the left middle position is Empty and the Neuro-psychological position is Muffled.

Cocaine

The left distal position is Tense with Robust Pounding, and Slippery with Rough Vibration until the burnt-out stage when this position exhibits all the qualities of deficiency, from yin-deficient Tight-Wiry (which I encountered most frequently) at first to qi-deficient Feeble-Absent much later. The pulse rate is Rapid in the Tense and Wiry stages, and Slow when the pulse is Feeble-Absent.

CENTRAL NERVOUS SYSTEM DISORDERS

The Doughy quality at the Neuro-psychological positions, while not specifically a sign of emotional or mental disharmony, is frequently a sign of pathology in the central nervous system which inevitably has emotional-mental sequelae and is often confused with neurosis or psychosis. This quality at this position requires much further investigation. As stated above, the Muffled quality at this position is associated with excessive use of hallucinogens. Change in Intensity has been associated with dizziness, and the Choppy quality at the Neuro-psychological positions has been associated with trauma.

EMOTIONAL DISHARMONIES RELATED TO LEFT-RIGHT IMBALANCE

The husband-wife concept (see Chapter 14) involves several inconsistencies in the literature concerning the relationship of the right and left sides of the pulse. My own experience supports what Worsley taught during the 1970s, that for a woman, the right side of the pulse should be stronger than the left side, and vice versa for a man. This is in agreement with Li Shi-Zhen who observed, "Men have more yang qi. So, provided their qi is well regulated, their left hand pulse is stronger. Women have more yin blood. So, provided their qi is well regulated, their right hand pulse is stronger."[27] Van Buren essentially says the same (see Chapter 14). However, during the 1980s Worsley shifted his position, stating that the left side should be stronger in both men and women.

Worsley and Van Buren generally share the view that a husband-wife imbalance is a sign of eternal difficulties with inter-individual relationships, especially with the opposite sex, which I can corroborate clinically with many patients. Associated with a husband-wife imbalance is a sense of being unbalanced physically, mentally, or both. A 45-year-old woman came complaining of back and neck pain since childhood. She also complained of having felt unbalanced and "discombobulated" down her left side all her life. The left side pulse was much stronger than the right side. The moment that the pulses of her right side became stronger than her left side, she broke down and began to cry and talk about her relationship with her husband. After this she no longer felt "discombobulated" and had no further symptoms during the ensuing fifteen years of our acquaintance.

Changes in Intensity shifting back and forth between sides

There are two clinical scenarios associated with this pulse picture. One, which I find most commonly, is a currently ongoing, severe inter-individual conflict. The other, much less common scenario is the sudden onset of overwork or overexercise very far beyond one's energy, in the recent past.

LEFT SIDE

Resignation for a moderate period

The Cotton quality on the left side is a sign of qi stagnation on that side, which can be due to a trauma to that side, or can be a sign of the 'sad pulse' (resignation) which has existed for less than approximately five years. As the condition worsens or lasts longer, the Cotton quality spreads to the right side.

'Organ system' deficient

Remember that a 'system' problem does not yet involve organ pathology, but is only a sign explaining otherwise inexplicable symptoms, such as fatigue in this case. The symptoms are prognostic signs of a pathological process which, if not interrupted, will lead to disease.

Pulse — The pulse is Slow, the entire left side is Deep Thin and Feeble-Absent or Empty, with an increasing degree of deficiency. The tongue tends to be pale, and the vertical vessels under the lower eyelid also tend to be pale.

Etiology — The causes may be constitutional, a prolonged recovery from a serious illness which has weakened the yin organs, an ongoing chronic draining illness such as paraplegia, or a degenerating disease such as multiple sclerosis.

When there is a slightly greater reduction in the left distal and proximal positions than in the other positions, and when accompanied by depression, the cause is probably constitutional, in which case there is genetically deficient Kidney qi and a Kidney-Heart disharmony. When the reduction is more equally distributed, the disharmony is attributable to abusive life experiences, in which case there was either excessive sex, excessive work, or excessive exercise at an early age.

Symptoms — The individual feels emotionally vulnerable, depressed, generally weak, although there is often no concurrent evidence of disease.

'Organ system' and 'nervous system' affect each other

Pathogenesis and symptoms

When the 'organ system' is deficient there will be diminished nutrition to the 'nervous system,' which will ultimately be adversely affected if that system has any vulnerability. The symptoms are lassitude and depression, as well as fatigue. When the 'nervous system' affects the 'organ system,' the qi (nerves) to the yin organs become overworked, drier, tighter and hyper-irritable.

When the 'organ system' affects the 'nervous system,' there is more passivity, lassitude and depression, emotional tension, irritability, labile emotions and quick anger, anxiety, and greater fatigue. When the 'organ system' deficiency is primary the fatigue comes earlier, and when the 'nervous system' is primary the emotional disharmonies appear first.

Pulse

When the 'nervous system' is affecting the 'organ system,' the entire left side of the pulse ('organ system') is Deep Thin and Feeble-Absent or Empty, with a Thin Tight quality at the surface of the entire pulse. The pulse is more Rapid (less Slow) than when the 'organ system' affects the 'nervous system,' where the pulse on the left side is Deeper and more Feeble.

RIGHT SIDE

Apart from eating foods too difficult to digest, there are three etiologic scenarios: a tendency to eat too rapidly, working immediately after eating, and a tendency to eat irregularly. All three of these habits affecting the 'digestive system' reflect the condition of a mechanistic industrial society in which man has rewritten the laws of the universe, as if the natural, physiological requirements of the human body can be ignored and overridden by the requirements of production and output. All involve disharmonious mental and emotional states. (See 'digestive system,' Chapter 14.)

Eating too quickly: 'nervous system' affecting the 'digestive system'

My experience with patients who eat too fast is that they are generally those whose pulses are Tense and who live in the fast track in all areas of life. The rapid eating is usually part of a generally unrelaxed approach to life, sometimes constitutionally determined ('nervous system tense'), and sometimes due to life experiences, in which case the pulse is also a little Rapid. These are people who are driven, who generally overwork, and who have very little time to give to the more pleasurable pursuits in life, one of which is eating leisurely.

At first the pulse over the entire right side tends to be very Tight, especially in the right middle Stomach position. Over a longer period of time the pulse is Deep, and the Tightness, in my experience, is frequently found just above the organ depth. The organ depth itself may be reduced. This may be accompanied by a uniform Tenseness on the left side, which is present at all depths, and primarily at the left middle position, reflecting a tense 'nervous system.' This sometimes represents the Liver attacking the Spleen-Stomach.

The heat from excess in the Stomach associated with this hyperactivity consumes the gastric secretions and contributes to poor digestion, partially due to the Stomach's consequent inability to moisten and soften the food. At this point the individual is hungry immediately after eating.

Later the Stomach will become yin deficient. The dryness creates a need for fluids in the Stomach, which feels empty. This increases the hunger, apparently for food which is eighty percent water. This is accompanied by a feeling of fullness; thus, although there is hunger, often only small amounts can be eaten. People with this pattern quickly consume snack after snack, getting full yet remaining hungry. This condition is exacerbated by eating dry foods.

Eating irregularly

Another situation is one in which the pulse over the entire right side is Feeble-Absent or Empty. This is found in people who ignore their internal needs in the interest of external ones. They eat irregularly when it suits their ego-oriented schedule, and not the schedule of their alimentary rhythms. They eat when the digestive system is not ready, and do not eat when it is. This impairs digestion, which eventually hurts the Spleen by causing qi deficiency and accumulation of dampness.

Physical labor immediately after eating

Individuals who habitually engage in physical labor as soon as they finish eating will eventually develop an Empty pulse over the entire right side. This pulse is a sign of extreme deficiency, and that the qi in the digestive system is chaotic. Spleen dampness with damp-cold in the Heart, Lungs, and Bladder, as well as the Intestines, is possible. This is often preceded by such qualities bilaterally at the middle position as Inflated, Flat, and Feeble-Absent, depending on the physical condition, other aspects of lifestyle, and the length of time one has had this habit.

This, again, is a sign either that one is driving oneself, or that one is being driven by the industrial social system. In either case, one is out of touch with one's feelings and being (the inner 'wise observer'). Moreover, this insensitivity to everything but work will affect one's entire life, including relationships and health. Today this scenario is being extended by the information age to a larger percentage of the population than ever before, when, instead of engaging in physical labor after eating, the stagnation which leads to depletion and the Empty quality in the middle burner on the right side is associated with sitting in front of a computer.

Emotion, timing, and gastro-intestinal dysfunction

If there is an emotional disturbance before eating it will affect the esophagus and the associated pain is moderate. If the disturbance occurs while eating the Stomach will be affected and the pain is severe. If the upsetting event occurs after the meal it will affect the Intestines and the pain is mild.

QUALITIES ASSOCIATED WITH KIDNEY-HEART DISHARMONY

Physiology and symptoms

The left distal and proximal positions reflect Kidney-Heart disharmony, one of the most important psycho-pathological patterns in Chinese medicine (see Chapter 11). Dr. Shen said that the Heart is "on top" and the Kidneys "on the end." If the "top" and the "end" are balanced, the entire body is balanced.

As previously mentioned, both the Heart and the Kidneys control the mind and the brain. If the water of the Kidneys cannot control the fire of the Heart, the mind will become restless. If the fire of the Heart cannot warm the water (essence) of the Kidneys, it will be unable to rise and nourish the brain, and normal patterns will be disrupted. If the water of the Kidneys is excessive, it will diminish the fire. It is the latter condition which is the cause of one type of depression. The Triple Burner mediates this relationship and should always be considered in management.

The symptoms of this disharmony, or spirit disturbance, are palpitations, insomnia, irritability, fatigue, depression, being easily startled, and anxiety. Manic depression or bipolar disease is another manifestation.

Common combinations

All of the following qualities are signs of deficiency. With the Feeble-Absent qualities this is more obvious. It is important to reiterate that the Tight quality is just as much a sign of deficiency as the Feeble-Absent quality: the Feeble-Absent quality is a sign of qi and yang deficiency, while the Tight quality a sign of yin deficiency.

Feeble-Absent at left distal and proximal positions, Normal at left middle position with a Slow or Rapid rate

It has already been mentioned that, except in the elderly, if only the left distal and left proximal positions are Feeble-Absent the etiology is usually constitutional or congenital. (If the entire pulse is Feeble-Absent the etiology is based on other factors.) In contrast to most teaching, but supported by experience, this is, according to Dr. Shen, the principal combination associated with Kidney-Heart disharmony.

Feeble-Absent at left distal and proximal positions, Tense Inflated at left middle position

Here the cause is not necessarily deficiency of the Heart and Kidneys, but qi stagnation in the middle burner, which prevents communication between the upper and lower burners. It is usually accompanied by anxiety and insomnia. With Liver qi stagnation one generally also sees passive-aggressive behavior interspersed with explosive anger.

Tight at left distal and proximal positions, and slightly Rapid

If both positions are Tight it indicates that there is a disturbance of the spirit with Heart and Kidney yin deficiency, which is more likely due to emotional shock, prolonged worry, and anxiety than to constitutional predisposition. With yin-deficient qualities there is greater agitation than with the qi-deficient qualities.

Less common combinations

Feeble-Absent at left distal and Tight at left proximal positions

This is another combination that I have observed with a Kidney-Heart disharmony which can be attributed to constitutional Heart qi deficiency in the young, and other factors in life with adults. Most likely, both positions were originally Feeble-Absent with a constitutional etiology. With overworking of the mind and nervous system, yin is depleted and the dominant Kidney problem changes from qi to yin deficiency with a Tight quality at the proximal position.

Tight at left distal position, Feeble-Absent at left proximal position

This is the rarest combination I have found with Kidney-Heart disharmony. It can occur with shock to the Heart when there is Kidney qi deficiency, and during the manic stage of bipolar disease.

HEART PATTERNS AFFECTING SLEEP

Introduction

Qualities found at the left distal position, and at the Heart complementary positions, are often signs of sleep disorders, since most sleep patterns involve Heart function. In Chinese medicine the Heart controls the mind, and all Heart conditions affect sleep.

Insomnia—the absence of rest—gradually enervates the Heart qi, eventually rendering the afflicted individual with deficient true qi and a wide variety of emotional disorders, including irritability and depression. In the literature these disturbances are mostly associated with blood and yin deficiency. Even the sleep disorder associated with the Gallbladder is related to Liver blood supporting the 'ethereal soul.' Here we are introducing some other Heart patterns described by Dr. Shen that are not, to my knowledge, mentioned elsewhere. The reader is referred to the appropriate sections of the book for a discussion of the pulse patterns associated with each of the following conditions.

Summary

According to Dr. Shen, Heart qi and yin deficiency are associated with a pattern in which it is easy to get fall asleep, but just as easy to awaken. Such individuals are up and down all night, though the yin-deficient person is more emotionally agitated. Heart blood deficiency and blood stagnation are associated more with the pattern of falling asleep for several hours, waking, and not easily returning to sleep. Those with Heart heat from excess (Heart fire) and Heart stagnant qi have a hard time falling asleep in the first place. (For the specific qualities, refer to the Heart pattern involved, such as severe Heart qi agitation.)

Common patterns

HEART HEAT FROM EXCESS ('HEART FIRE')

With the excess-type heat associated with Heart qi agitation, brought on by worry or Liver fire, it is hard to fall asleep. The mind is racing, worried, and the individual is restless and uptight. If one does get to sleep, one also tends to wake easily and be up and down all night. When one awakes, one is thinking obsessively about a real problem.

HEART YIN DEFICIENCY AND HEART QI AGITATION

With the Heart yin-deficient Heart qi agitation (Heart Nervous, Heart Tight, and Hesitant Wave qualities), the Heart qi is excited and/or erratic. The individual is very sensitive to sound, restless, up and down all night, irritable, nervous, and of course tired. An individual with a Change in Rate at Rest ('Heart nervous') type of Heart qi agitation may also have difficulty falling asleep if she is overworked, or has been under great stress the previous day.

HEART BLOOD DEFICIENCY ('HEART WEAK')

Heart blood deficiency is characterized by a pattern of mild difficulty in falling asleep, and then waking after four or five hours, sometimes unable to return to sleep. Often there is nothing on the mind when one awakes, unless one also has some Heart heat from excess or deficiency. There is a propensity to mild depression, but they feel less tired in the morning than those with Heart yin and qi deficiency, or either Heart qi or blood stagnation.

Heart blood deficiency is often involved directly due to Heart qi agitation or Heart shock over several years. It can also occur indirectly, through Spleen qi deficiency causing Heart blood deficiency, a Liver which cannot store the blood, chronic hemorrhage, or Kidney essence disturbance which affects the haemopoetic function of bone marrow.

Less common patterns

People with stagnant Heart qi ('Heart closed') cannot sleep at all some nights, and are preoccupied with real or imagined hurts and thoughts of vengeance. Those with stagnant Heart blood ('Heart small') wake up exhausted, even after sleeping through the night, but often awaken after four or five hours of sleep and remain awake, experiencing considerable fear, especially in the early hours of the morning after they awake.

People with trapped qi/heat in the Heart ('Heart full'), Heart qi deficiency ('Heart large'), and Heart yang deficiency ('Heart disease') find that their body is uncomfortable because they cannot lie flat, and wake up to find a more comfortable position. They too awake tired in the morning, even when they have slept through the night. Those with Heart qi and yang deficiency are very depressed in the early morning after they awake.

KIDNEY-HEART DISHARMONY AND SLEEP

Physiology We can also consider sleep patterns in terms of Kidney-Heart disharmony. Both the Heart and the Kidneys control the mind and the brain, which was previously discussed.

Pulse With regard to the pulse and one type of Kidney-Heart disharmony, Dr. Shen made the following observations. If both the left distal and proximal positions are Tight, the individual will easily wake at the smallest sound or disturbance because, in his words, "the Heart is sensitive." Here we have the form of Kidney-Heart disharmony of the yin-deficient type.

We previously mentioned that both Heart qi and yin deficiency are expressed by similar sleep disturbances. Therefore, if both the left distal and proximal positions are Feeble-Absent, we will have a similar sleep disturbance, although for very different reasons, and with far less agitation and more depression. With qi deficiency, as well as trapped qi, the individual is physically very uncomfortable in the reclining position, and accordingly finds it difficult to sleep for long periods of time. However, they are less emotionally restless than with Heart-Kidney yin deficiency (the Tight quality).

RECENTLY ACKNOWLEDGED EMOTIONAL AND MENTAL CONDITIONS

With the few documented cases of both multiple personality and sexual abuse which I have treated, I have found one or more of the following qualities: very Rapid rate and Rough Vibration over the entire pulse; Vibration at the Neuro-psychological position; Vibration and Slipperiness at the Mitral Valve position; an Unstable quality at the left distal position; a Bean (Spinning) quality anywhere, but especially at the distal positions; a significant Change in Rate at Rest; and, in one case, an Interrupted quality.

The Three Burners

LOWER BURNER (PROXIMAL POSITIONS)

I evaluate the proximal positions to get a sense of the root, the ground on which this person must stand (the Kidneys). If it is reduced in qi at a young age (Deep, Feeble), even up to the age of forty-five depending on degree, I suspect that the constitutional qi is deficient and that recovery will be more difficult. If the person is older, I assume that some of this deficiency is a more gradual draining due to overwork, overexercise, or some other form of abuse (drugs, sex), and that there may be more basic qi with which to work (Reduced Substance quality).

If the deficiency is primarily of yin, with harder qualities such as Tight, I realize that this person has probably been overworking their mind and central nervous system. At times one of these deficiencies is so much more characteristic of the person that it appears by itself. This is especially true if yin is being depleted, since the harder qualities overshadow the more pliable ones (qi deficiency).

More often, in keeping with the realities of life, there are signs of both types of deficiency, which informs me that both processes are occurring simultaneously. One proximal position may be Tight and the other Feeble, or the qualities might constantly change from one to the other during the examination.

MIDDLE BURNER (MIDDLE POSITIONS)

The integrity of the middle burner qi reflects how centered this person is in life, and of course about the relationship between the moving and recovering qi (Liver) and the nurturing qi (Spleen-Stomach). It tells us how easily this person can handle stress and toxicity, mental and physical, and the organism's capacity for recovery on a day-to-day basis (Liver), and how well it can replenish itself over time (Spleen).

UPPER BURNER (DISTAL POSITIONS)

The integrity of the upper burner qi tells us how well we can reach out to the world and take it in, with awareness of our creative being, with the strength to communicate and protect our being and to maintain mental and emotional stability. It will, for example, tell us how well we can handle shock or recover from grief.

Summary of Pulse Qualities Associated with Psychological Disharmony

The following associations between specific qualities and psychological states should be used, with the patient's cooperation, only as a starting point for exploration, rather than as conclusive evidence of disharmony.

The following list is offered here as a tentative association of pulse qualities and emotional-mental states (psychological disharmonies); it is a work in progress. Those qualities marked with an asterisk are those with which I have the least experience or confidence in presenting, but I nonetheless do so in the hope of stimulating thought and response.

Table 15-1 Pulse qualities and associated psychological states

Pulse qualities	Associated psychological states
Occasional Change in Rate at Rest	Racing, constantly shifting and agitated ('grasshopper') mind, mood, and behavior
Interrupted-Intermittent	Fear; shifting moods
Hesitant	Obsessive
RATE ON EXERTION	
Increase in Rate >20 beats/minute	Memory and attention span diminished; focus wanders mildly to moderately
Increase in Rate <8 beats/minute, stays same, or decreases	Concentration impaired after short time; severe mental lethargy
Occasional Change in Intensity (entire pulse)	Tension; occasional external stress responding with internal conflict
Constant Change in Intensity (entire pulse)	Concentration impaired after moderate period of time; moderate mental lethargy
EMPTY QUALITIES	
Empty (mild to moderate)	Losing center; feelings unbalanced; cannot find place in life; feeling lost; post-traumatic syndrome
Empty Thread-like (moderate to severe)	Losing center; feelings unbalanced; cannot find place in life; feeling lost
Leather (moderate to severe)	Memory and attention span severely diminished; focus wanders in extreme; agitated; losing center; feelings unbalanced; cannot find place in life; feeling lost
Minute and Scattered (very severe)	Losing center; feelings unbalanced; cannot find place in life; feeling lost
Yielding Hollow Full-Overflowing and Slow	Gradually developing anxiety, panic, labile emotions and quick to anger, depersonalization, delusions
Yielding Hollow Full-Overflowing and Rapid	Rapidly developing anxiety, panic, labile emotions and quick to anger, depersonalization, delusions
Sides vary greatly in substance (husband-wife imbalance)	Severe intra- and interpersonal conflict and anguish
Muffled (slight)	Depression, lack of joy
*Empty Interrupted-Intermittent & Yielding Hollow Interrupted-Intermittent	Possible immature/stunted emotional development
Very high fever and very low rate, or very low fever and very high rate	Delirium, coma

Qualities as Signs of Psychological Disharmony

Pulse qualities	Associated psychological states
EMPTY; CHANGE IN QUALITIES, INTENSITY, OR AMPLITUDE; CHANGE IN ONE POSITION (ALL INDICATE SEPARATION OF YIN AND YANG)	
Left distal position (Heart)	Mental instability, confusion
Right distal position (Lungs)	Intractable grief; difficulty making transitions, taking in the new and letting go of past due to lack of strength to change and evolve
Left middle position (Liver)	Tendency to live in mild delusional state with grandiose plans that are never executed; easily frustrated; emotional lability (especially anger)
Right middle position (Spleen)	Tendency to ruminate aimlessly and unproductively
Proximal positions (Kidneys)	Tendency to profound, recurrent, unexplained (endogenous) depression
UNSTABLE	Profound unexpressed fear
Change in Intensity shifting from side to side	Current significant interpersonal conflict
RATE	
Rapid (Bounding)	Tendency toward anxiety
Slow	Tendency toward depression
MISCELLANEOUS	
Hollow Full-Overflowing	Repressed hot labile emotions; hot temper expressed rarely or unpredictably
Flooding Excess with Robust Pounding	Sudden, explosive (but enduring) outward rage
Inflated	Controlled anger
Flat (left distal)	Vengeance; slow, hidden rage
Suppressed Wave at qi depth and Suppressed Pounding	Emotions muted
Qi depth Yielding, Feeble-Absent, Spreading (at blood depth), Flooding Deficient, Diffuse, Reduced Substance, Reduced Pounding, Deep, Feeble, Absent	Tendency toward depression increases with increasing qi deficiency
Deep	Tendency toward withdrawal, especially under stress
Partially Hollow at blood depth	Mildly diminished memory and attention span; focus wanders
*Leather-like Hollow	Emotions eating away at person inside (gastric-duodenal ulcer)
*Floating	Relates in a superficial and extroverted way as a coping mechanism, especially under stress
Cotton ('sad')	Feeling stuck
*Blood Unclear	Thoughts and emotions imprecise and vague
Blood Heat, Blood Thick	Repressed hot emotions
*Tense Ropy	Emotionally obdurate and rigid, especially under pressure
*Yielding Ropy	Rigid, but yielding under pressure

Pulse qualities	Associated psychological states
THIN	
Thin Tight	Diminished memory and attention span, focus wanders moderately to severely, agitated
Thin Yielding	Diminished memory and attention span, focus wanders moderately to severely, tendency toward depression, cannot protect self
*Restricted (Special Lung position)	Difficulty making transitions, taking in the new, and letting go of past due to rigidity
Long	Stable but slightly tense
*Short (Brief)	Personality is compartmentalized, not integrated, and each part out of touch with others; in its extreme form, a Dr. Jeckyl and Mr. Hyde or multiple personality
Bean (Spinning)	Sudden terror; recent profound shock; horror
SLIPPERY	Mentation clouded and unclear <u>Upper burner</u> Slow—depression Rapid—manic, driven, creativity out of control and burns self out
Taut	Slightly tense, vigilant
Tense	Driven; hypervigilant; repressed internal conflict
Tight-Wiry	High strung; agitated; becoming hardened against the world but supersensitive. There is an extreme deficiency of Kidney yin-essence which in turn dries out the Pericardium. This makes it difficult to access or release Heart feelings, which manifests as the inability to accept or give love and tenderness.
*Wiry	In diabetes, of which the Wiry quality in the lower and sometimes middle burner is an early sign, where the body has lost control of sugar metabolism, the sweet taste, perhaps metaphorically, is of love. In pain but cannot accept love and tenderness from others [essence (love)]; sweetness is leaving body ['sugar me'].
Choppy	Fixed, obstinate, unmoving
VIBRATION	
Smooth	Worry and tendency to worry
Rough	Guilt, fear, past shock

CHAPTER 16
Prognosis and Prevention

CONTENTS

The long-range view, 599
Time lag, 599
Logic, medical models, and the pulse as communicator, 600
Estimated times of arrival of symptoms, 600
Seriousness, 600
    Literature, 600
    Consistency, 601
    Children, 601
Denial, 601
The pre-eminence of the cardiovascular system in the disease process, 601
Qualities, 602
    Any time, 602
    Distant future, 602
        Cotton, 602
        Flat, 603
            Bilaterally in upper burner, 603
            Right distal position, 603
        Yielding Inflated, 603
        Yielding or diminished qi depth, 603
        Taut, 603
        Tight, 604
        Arrhythmia: Constant Change in Rate at Rest, 604
        Slow, 604
        Rapid, 604
    Semi-distant future, 604

Spreading over entire pulse, 604
Flooding Deficient Diffuse and Reduced Substance, 605
Empty at left middle position, 605
Thin-Tight, 605
Thin Yielding, 605
Flat, 605
    Left distal position (Heart), 605
        Stagnant qi, 605
        Stagnant blood, 606
    Right Distal Position (Lungs), 606
Doughy, 606
Blood Unclear, 606
Blood Heat, 606
Blood Thick, 606
Tense Hollow Full-Overflowing, 607
Smooth Vibration at Mitral Valve position, 607
Slippery at qi depth over entire pulse, 607
Slippery at blood depth, 607
Arrhythmias: Interrupted or Intermittent, 607
Rough Vibration at blood depth, 607
Inflated, 607
Tense, 608
Tense Slippery at Gallbladder position, 608
Wiry, 608
Yielding Ropy, 608
Occasional Change in Intensity over entire pulse, 609
Constant Change in Intensity, 609
Excessive Increase in Rate on mild Exertion >8–12 beats/minute, 609
Rhythm, 609
Choppy at Neuro-psychological position, 609
Muffled at Neuro-psychological position, 610
  Systems, 610
Immediate future, 610
  Less serious prognosticators, 610
      Occasional Change in Rate at Rest, 610
      Hesitant, 610
      Muffled, 610
        Left distal position, 610
        Neuro-psychological position, 610
      Smooth Vibration, 611
        Left distal progressing to entire pulse, 611
        Neuro-psychological position, 611
      Choppy, 611
      Floating Tense and Slow, 611
      Floating Yielding and Rapid, 611
      Inflated at distal aspect of right Diaphragm position, 611
  More serious prognosticators, 611
      Floating Tight, 611
      Wiry, 612

Slippery qualities, 612
    Slippery at Mitral Valve position, 612
    Slippery Tight at Gallbladder position, 612
    Slippery at left distal position, 612
    Slippery at organ depth, 612
Muffled qualities, 612
    Muffled at Gallbladder position, 612
    Muffled at left distal position, 613
Rough Vibration qualities, 613
    Rough Vibration at Neuro-psychological position, 613
    Rough Vibration over entire pulse, 613
    Rough Vibration at individual positions, 613
Flooding Excess, 613
Deep, 613
Feeble-Absent qualities, 613
    Feeble-Absent over entire pulse, 613
    Feeble-Absent at individual positions, 614
Inflated qualities, 614
    Inflated at Large Vessel positions, 614
    Inflated at distal aspect of left Diaphragm position, 614
Empty qualities, 615
    Empty over entire pulse, 615
    Empty at individual positions, 615
    Empty Thread-like; Leather; Minute; Scattered; Hollow Yielding
      Full-Overflowing and Slow, 615
Leather-like Hollow, 615
      Rapid, 615
      Slow, 615
Very Tense Tight, or Wiry Full-Overflowing Hollow and Rapid, 615
      Left middle and proximal positions, 615
      Left distal and left middle positions or entire pulse, 616
      Either side, 616
Tense Ropy, 616
Tense Hollow Full-Overflowing at Large Vessel positions, 616
Increase in Rate on Exertion <8 beats/minute, 616
Change in Qualities, 616
      Entire pulse, 616
      Individual positions, 616
Yielding Hollow Full-Overflowing and Rapid, 616
Choppy qualities, 617
    Choppy at Pelvis/Lower Body positions, 617
    Choppy at left middle position, 617
    Choppy at left distal position, 617
    Choppy at Gallbladder positions, 617
Bean (Spinning), 617
Unstable, 617
Interrupted or Intermittent, 617
Intermittent or Interrupted Yielding Hollow, 618
Dead, 618

Positions, 618
> Left middle position, 618
>> **Slippery at organ depth**, 618
>> **Floating Tight**, 618
> Liver Engorgement positions, 619
> Right middle position and Stomach-Pylorus Extension position, 619
> Esophagus position, 619

Paradox, 619
Signs of a Positive Prognosis, 619

CHAPTER 16

Prognosis and Prevention

With the role of the pulse in prevention as our central theme, I will review some of the pulse qualities which are useful prognosticators. However, I wish to make clear that while the thrust of this chapter is on the pulse as prognosticator, the information from the pulse is useful in many other ways. It will reveal acute diseases with qualities such as Flooding Excess and Floating. Changes in the pulse give us a picture of therapeutic progress. And perhaps most importantly to the practitioner, on a day to day basis the pulse can direct us to the often not-so-obvious source of the patient's current symptoms. While this book is concerned with all of these aspects, this chapter is focused primarily on the pulse as a tool for prevention. Based on what has come before, there is necessarily some repetition here.

The following observations are based on clinical experience. Without therapeutic intervention or change in lifestyle the outcomes are predictable, although, due to the mysteries of our complex being, not inevitable.

All of the qualities described here have been felt by me with some frequency in the absence of other symptoms that are often associated with their occurrence. I therefore consider them to be of some prognostic significance. While they can foretell future infirmities, once the projection comes true, these qualities may continue to be present alongside the illness which they have foreseen. Thus, they are often both diagnostic and prognostic depending on the presence or absence of other symptoms.[1]

THE LONG-RANGE VIEW

A pulse reading is essentially a 'printout' reflecting the course of deterioration in the health of an individual person, the relative triumph of catabolism over anabolism in each organ over time. Whether or not accompanied by symptoms, the reading is the truth. This is often unsettling to practitioners, to have such a profound and revealing picture of the inner person who, on the surface, may have only minor complaints.

TIME LAG

The representation of the physiology of qi, blood, yin, and essence on the pulse is not an exact replica of the actual physiological state of the organism. There is a lag between the two, often of a significant period of time. The pulse presents a pathological picture that always appears somewhat worse than the symptomatic reality of the organism. This lag holds true until the pulses associated with impending death appear, when the pulse signs and the reality become a unity.

A set of correlations has been recognized between what has been palpated and what concretely occurs in physiology. These correlations are what we call the qualities. The signs accessed from the pulse are several steps ahead of the symptomatology of the organism in terms of the process of disease. The pulse is therefore an instrument for prediction and prevention. The diagnostic challenge is to correctly match the sign with the fact.

It is important to realize that, even with a Feeble-Absent or Empty quality, the patient, although possibly unwell, is still functioning, and has, therefore, a considerable reservoir of stored true qi. The Absent quality merely describes the sensation on the pulse. It is a measure of moderately severe qi deficiency and does not imply that the qi is entirely absent. The yin organs are still there performing their tasks at least well enough to sustain life. However, according to Dr. Shen, the implication of the Absent quality is that the person will be ill within a year, and of the Empty quality that the person will be ill within six months. Hence, the pulse is, perhaps most importantly, a prognosticator and the foundation of a preventive medicine.

LOGIC, MEDICAL MODELS, AND THE PULSE AS COMMUNICATOR

Furthermore, although the pulse is a precise instrument transmitting signals about the organism of which it is a part, it is not to be gainfully contemplated as a digitally logical expression of energic physiology. Over the years each model of Chinese medicine (eight principles, five phases) has attempted to fit the pulse into its parameters, with, in my opinion, limited results.

The pulse is a message center transmitting many signals simultaneously, which are deciphered only by experiment based on trial and error and trial and success. For example, paradoxically, during the same pulse taking, as one increases finger pressure from the qi through the blood to the organ depth, one can find a Hollow quality at the blood depth; but, as one releases pressure from the organ to the qi depth, the blood depth could fill out, become wide, and give us a Blood Heat or Blood Unclear quality. No paradigm of Chinese medicine applied rigidly can accommodate this paradox. A model is only a guide which must be tested over and over against the often unpredictable, and frequently contradictory, messages transmitted to our fingers from the pulse.

ESTIMATED TIMES OF ARRIVAL OF SYMPTOMS

The time periods we are giving—such as six months until disease is in evidence, with an Empty quality—have a wide tolerance. They are relative measures. Six months can mean three months to two years depending upon variables which no one can predict, and are too numerous to catalogue with each quality. In general, constitution, vulnerability, life habits, treatment, fortune, and fate are the principal considerations. (There is a saying that "Man can cure disease but cannot cure fate.") However, the time frame does give us a sense of the relative seriousness of the condition and the urgency of intervention.

SERIOUSNESS

Literature

Li Shi-Zhen qualifies the seriousness of pulse signs as follows:

However, when analyzing the seasonal and disease pulses, the most important factor is the state of the stomach qi. When the pulse contains stomach qi it has shen [spirit], and pulse with shen is regular, not too fast and not too slow. For instance, a weak and minute pulse with regularity indicates shen (stomach qi). This means that although the symptoms are very severe they can still be treated.[2]

The reader is referred to Chapter 5 for a discussion of Stomach qi.

Consistency

Here, seriousness is considered with each individual quality. However, all of the qualities discussed in this context are considered only as they appear consistently on the pulse from day to day and week to week. This consistency is in itself a sign of seriousness. The interpretation of the same qualities occurring inconsistently is different, and usually less consequential in terms of pathogenesis.

Some of the signs we read on the pulse, often the ones that are inconsistent, can disappear if the organism is strong enough to resolve the pathological process even without outside intervention. However, strong organisms have a handicap in that while they have the capacity to heal themselves more easily than a weak organism, they are often capable of coping with, and tend to ignore, warning signs of disharmony which a weaker organism cannot. The weaker organism, therefore, will be more likely to take steps sooner to interrupt a pathological process.

Children

On review of my records I now consider children's pulses somewhat differently than those of adults. While the interpretation of specific qualities may be the same, chaos in the pulse may reflect a child's immaturity and state of constant change, rather than being a sign of serious disease. However, each case must be taken individually since I have in my records cases in which this chaos was pathognomonic of serious disease.

DENIAL

Some of the qualities indicate current pathology which the patient may presently deny. Especially for people who are reluctant to reveal their psychological states, these pulse qualities provide objective readings of their emotional state. We can predict that the denial will break down under the pressure of reality, often sooner than later. However, informing people that their condition is indicated by an objective reading of their pulse, rather than as a personal impression, usually bypasses the resistance to interpretation encountered in psychotherapeutic practices, and hastens the rapid dissolution of the denial.

THE PRE-EMINENCE OF THE CARDIOVASCULAR SYSTEM IN THE DISEASE PROCESS

As previously observed, it has been my experience over the past three decades that the two systems which seem to bear the brunt of both constitutional deficits and self-abuse are the Heart and the Kidneys. Unexpectedly but irrefutably, the cardiovascular system is the one which shows signs of depletion of qi, yin, and blood at an earlier age and far exceeding that of any other system, including the Kidneys. Because the Kidneys are associated with storage of the essence upon which all other systems draw when under stress, we have come to expect that the Kidneys would be the first organ system to show signs of depletion. However, this is not borne out by the pulse, which shows that the Heart— the 'emperor'—is the critical system.

I have also observed that, perhaps because of this lofty status recognized and endowed by the ancients, a large number of disorders, as diverse as gynecological, neurological, headaches, and arthritis, as well as chronic fatigue syndrome, but including any pathology, are due primarily to deficits in Heart (cardiovascular) function. This diagnostic discovery has assisted a great many patients to recover from conditions previously resistant to treatment. By adding small amounts of herbs for the Heart and circulation to other formulas, some students report greater success in treating sinusitis, migraines, arthritis, neurologic manifestations, diabetes, and depression.

Qualities

There are qualities which tell us about the very distant future, the semi-distant future, the more immediate future, and about any time. The ultimate outcome of a disease process is, of course, complicated, so that these must be viewed as warning signs which are not etched in stone. While this is not the venue for an in-depth discussion of each quality (see specific chapters), I hope that the following will convey a flavor of the pulse as prognosticator and pillar of a preventive medicine.

ANY TIME

In some positions a quality can be a sign of danger at any time. A good example is the Inflated quality at the Large Vessel position, which is a reliable sign of an aneurism. While we have included this under the aegis of the Inflated quality in the section 'immediate future,' an aneurism can rupture at any time and must therefore be considered with the 'distant' and 'semi-distant' prognostic categories. While experience to date would have us associate this sign with aneurisms of the aorta, we must consider the possibility of this quality appearing at this position for aneurisms in smaller vessels, including the cerebral circulation. This could become a valuable diagnostic tool in combination with modern brain visualization techniques.

DISTANT FUTURE

By the distant future we are thinking roughly in terms of twenty to thirty years. Most disharmonies are progressive if not corrected either by the organism, by change in lifestyle, or by therapeutic intervention. For example, the long-term effect of all of the less serious Heart disharmonies—a Tight quality at the left distal position ('Heart tight'), occasional Change in Rate at Rest ('Heart nervous'), the Hesitant quality discussed below—is depletion of Heart qi and yin, and eventual Heart disease.

Cotton

The Cotton quality (see Chapter 9) conveys a spongy, amorphous, formless resistance from the surface through the qi depth. This quality tells us that there is general stagnation of the qi which, uncorrected over a very long time, will lead to those diseases, especially cancer, which are associated with the general extended slowing of the circulation of qi. The cancer will occur in those areas of the body which are vulnerable for other reasons.

Sluggishness, a sense of oppression, resignation, and a tendency to blame external forces for their dilemma can be earlier symptoms. Hopelessness and depression may occur later before the serious physical consequences are manifest. Depression has often been associated with cancer.

Flat

BILATERALLY IN UPPER BURNER

Pathogenesis and prognosis

When this loss of the pulse wave is felt bilaterally, qi cannot get into an area or organ where the qi is already deficient, coincident with the etiological event. The area affected in this case is the chest.

In the upper burner, this form of stagnation affects the efficiency of the circulation of blood and qi in the chest. Mediastinal and breast tumors are associated with this sign when it is present for a long time.

Furthermore, the Heart and Lungs have to work harder to overcome the resistance in the stagnant chest circulation. Circulatory difficulties are therefore predictable, including slow healing there, and ultimately elsewhere.

Etiology

The Flat quality (see Chapter 8) in the upper burner is usually due to an attempt to repress emotional pain, often early in life, associated with the loss of a parent or parent surrogate. The Flat wave is a sign that the qi of the Heart was deficient or immature at the time of the incident. A sudden personal rejection by loved ones in adulthood can bring about this quality, although it tends to be transient, lasting only until the emotional wound is healed, and appears most often only at the left distal position. Another common cause is the cord tied around the neck at birth during delivery. Trauma and heavy lifting are less common causes.

RIGHT DISTAL POSITION

A Flat quality here is a sign of stagnation in Lungs with weak qi, and can augur a neoplasm if present over a long period of time.

Yielding Inflated

The Yielding Inflated quality (see Chapter 8) is a sign that qi is trapped in an organ or area of the body and cannot get out. This stagnation will eventually lead to heat trapped in the organ (Tense Inflated quality) and poor function (qi deficiency).

For example, in the left distal position this quality is often associated with a breech delivery resulting in trapped Heart qi ('Heart full'). Predictable symptoms are fatigue, depression, discomfort in the entire body, especially when lying on the right side, quick temper throughout one's life, and hypertension. Without correction, the heart could become enlarged.

Yielding or Diminished qi depth

This indicates early deficiency of true qi. While this makes them more vulnerable to mild ephemeral illnesses, if uncorrected, the distant future holds all of the possibilities of chronic fatigue syndrome and other chronic diseases. (See Chapter 8 and 13.)

Taut

Entire pulse

The Taut quality (see Chapter 11) found over the entire pulse is a sign of an early or mild 'nervous system tense' condition.

Individual position This is a very early sign of qi stagnation which will, if not corrected, eventually lead to dysfunction of the organ in the position where it is found. For example, on the right middle position, it foretells a slowing of peristalsis with food stagnation, gas, and distention.

Tight

A common long-term effect of the heat from deficiency associated with the Tight quality over the entire pulse is hypertension (see Chapter 11). In any single position the associated yin deficiency will lead to a drying out and increased excitability of that organ. For example, the Tight quality at the left distal position is associated with agitated Heart qi and symptoms of irritability and insomnia.

Found simultaneously in the left middle and proximal positions, one must consider future glucose tolerance problems such as diabetes, and possibly hypertension. Found simultaneously at the left middle and distal positions the Tight quality is again an early sign of possible future hypertension.

Arrhythmia: Constant Change in Rate at Rest

This is an early sign of potential Heart qi deficiency ('Heart disease') which will manifest early with anxiety and emotional vulnerability, and much later with being easily fatigued, shortness of breath, dependent edema, spontaneous sweating, coldness, and chest pain. (See Chapter 6.)

Slow

A rate under 55 beats/minute, depending on age, is a sign of deficient circulation and vulnerability to disease, especially chronic fatigue syndrome, fibromyalgia, migrating arthritis, volatile anger, and circulatory diseases. While a Slow rate is associated with a healthy heart in biomedicine, it is my impression that exactly the opposite is true (see Chapter 7). The average life span of athletes is far less than that of the general population. (See discussion of the distal positions in Chapter 12.)

Rapid

A persistently Rapid rate, for any reason, including Heart shock, will gradually cause an exhaustion of Heart qi. Symptoms include varying degrees of fatigue, even after long sleep. If uncorrected it can lead eventually to Heart disease.

SEMI-DISTANT FUTURE

By the semi-distant future we are thinking roughly in terms of five to twenty years.

Spreading over entire pulse

This quality (see Chapters 8 and 13) is a sign of a mild to moderate progression in the diminishment of qi with some blood deficiency due to overwork, which is a step toward chronic fatigue syndrome or some other chronic disease in the semi-distant future. The possibility of illness has been accelerated in areas which are already vulnerable. Heart attacks in young adults, especially physicians, athletes, and driving young businessmen, are related outcomes.

Flooding Deficient Diffuse and Reduced Substance

This pulse is a sign of moderate qi, blood, and essence deficiency in an individual who is pushing himself far beyond his energy, with physical overwork in the form of long hours, and little rest and relaxation, even sleep (see Chapter 8). Dr. Shen calls the Flooding Deficient quality the 'push pulse.' The wave rises normally almost to the qi depth and then suddenly falls off. Without a change in the drain of the qi, chronic fatigue or other chronic disease is predictable.

In those who have particular vulnerabilities, the possibility of physical and emotional collapse, including heart attacks, fulminating blood dyscrasias, and neurological diseases, is a more immediate concern.

Empty at left middle position

This is often a sign of the use of marijuana or hallucinogens, or of chronic hepatitis/mononucleosis, with gradually developing symptoms of lassitude, indecision, and inability to carry out plans and visions. The danger of primary liver cancer and lymphomas with an Empty quality at the left middle position is increasing in frequency.

Thin-Tight

Blood and yin deficiency with circulatory and deficient-type heat symptoms will be encountered in the not too distant future with this pulse (see Chapters 10 and 11). Symptoms may eventually include dryness, irregular menstruation, vision problems, palpitations, vertigo, parasthesias, afternoon fevers, night sweats, and symptoms of Liver wind, including hypertension and adult onset diabetes. If found only at the qi depth over the entire pulse, it is a more advanced sign of a 'nervous system tense' condition, which will eventually contribute to a blood heat disorder and then to hypertension.

Thin Yielding

This combination (see Chapters 10 and 13) portends symptoms of blood deficiency listed just above, and symptoms of qi deficiency including being easily fatigued, shortness of breath, diarrhea or constipation, prolonged scanty menstruation, and urinary frequency.

Flat

LEFT DISTAL POSITION (HEART)

Stagnant qi

In the left distal position this quality (see Chapter 8) is often associated with stagnant Heart qi ('Heart closed,' see Chapter 12) in which the individual has withdrawn their

Heart energy from the channels in response to some emotional trauma, frequently in the distant (and long forgotten) past, or to a cord tied around their neck at birth. Constant interpersonal problems, including a tendency to spitefulness and vengeance, is often the result.

Stagnant blood

Another condition which can begin with a Flat quality in the left distal position is stagnant Heart blood ('Heart small'), associated with prolonged labor with the head outside of the mother and the cord around the neck. Often found in childhood, symptoms of life-long unexplained fear, tension, shortness of breath especially on inhalation, and chest pain will occur sooner or later.

RIGHT DISTAL POSITION (LUNGS)

When pathology is found at this position, respiratory and kidney problems, such as asthma, chronic bronchitis and nephritis, which are often recalcitrant to therapeutic intervention, will ensue from the inability of the Lungs to grasp the qi.

Doughy

I have found this quality only at the Neuro-psychological position where it is accessed with the sensation of play-dough or soft clay. It has no clearly differentiated shape. (See Chapter 11.)

To date this quality is associated with central nervous system defects and could be a precursor to such diseases as multiple sclerosis. Headaches with a history of cerebral trauma is another possible etiology. We need further data for this and all other qualities at this position to delineate it as a sign of other central nervous system disorders such as tumors, or even psychosis.

Blood Unclear

This sign is identified with skin diseases such as eczema and psoriasis, which can affect any part of the body, being easily fatigued and severe malaise, arthritis, and headaches. It is a sign of toxicity in the blood and stress on the Liver (liver), and hepatic complications may be anticipated.

Blood Heat

Symptoms of sore throat, canker sores, tongue sores, bleeding gums, excitability, pressure headaches, hard dry stools, and dark scanty urine as well as some skin diseases are to be expected as early outcomes of this sign. It is also a sign of future hypertension and stroke.

Blood Thick

In adolescence one will imminently encounter severe acne. Severe hypertension and possible stroke later in adulthood is a strong possibility.

Tense Hollow Full-Overflowing

When the pulse is Tense Full-Overflowing there is heat in the blood which the body is having difficulty eliminating, putting a burden on the Heart, Liver, and Kidneys. There is the likelihood of eventual hypertension and stroke.

Smooth Vibration at Mitral Valve position

Vibration indicates that the valve is insufficient and is a mild sign of Heart qi deficiency, which should be corrected before it progresses to mitral valve prolapse, with a Slippery quality, which is a more serious portent of heart disease.

Slippery at qi depth over entire pulse

If the pulse is slightly Rapid, this can be a sign of excessive sugar in the blood and an early sign of diabetes. (See Chapter 11.) If the pulse is Slow it is a sign of general qi deficiency and mild immune system deficiency.

Slippery at blood depth

This a sign of turbulence in the blood often found with the Blood Heat and Blood Thick qualities (see Chapter 11). The turbulence is an indication that the conditions for the laying down of plaque already exist and that arterio-atherosclerosis is well on its way. Damp-heat in the Spleen-Gallbladder is frequently involved.

Arrhythmia: Interrupted or Intermittent

When the Interrupted quality does not interfere with the ability to read the rate but has more than five irregularly missed beats per minute, or the Intermittent quality misses a beat less often than every 15 beats but more often than every 30 beats, we can predict that the onset of symptomatic Heart disease will occur within the next five to ten years.

Rough Vibration at blood depth

This is a sign (see Chapter 11) usually found with the Slippery quality at the blood depth indicating that not only is the circulation of blood affected by blood heat, but the vessels are also damaged, which further presages the development of arterio-atherosclerosis.

Inflated

An Inflated quality (see Chapter 8) at the right distal position or bilaterally at the distal positions can be a sign of developing emphysema.

Tense

Entire pulse

When the Tense quality (see Chapter 11) is found in almost all of the positions the condition is 'nervous system tense.' The long-term effect of this constant overworking of the nervous system is a gradual wearing down and loss of the functional ability of a vulnerable organ through the hyperactivity of the nerves associated with that organ. This leads to blood heat and Hollow Full-Overflowing hypertensive disorders.

Individual position

This will be a slightly greater sign of qi stagnation with some excess-type heat, which will lead to the same outcome as described above with the Taut quality, except sooner. For example, if found at the left middle position, in the semi-distant future one will find symptoms of headache, irritability, quick to anger, cold hands and feet, difficulty recovering one's energy, distention and pain in the sides, suffocating sensation in the chest, sighing, and depression, all signs of Liver qi stagnation and heat from excess. Eventually, inability to overcome the stagnation will lead first to Liver yin and blood deficiency, and finally to Liver qi deficiency with extreme fatigue, especially around 4 P.M., and an inability to recover one's energy.

Tense Slippery at Gallbladder position

This combination here (see Chapter 12) is a sign of cholecystitis and cholelithiasis in progress at a relatively early stage.

Wiry

The Wiry quality (see Chapter 11) is a sign of either deficient yin-essence or of pain.

Entire pulse

A Wiry quality over the entire pulse can be a sign of developing hypertension or diabetes, or severe pain. With pain, prognostication is not an issue, but it is important to know the connection so that one considers diabetes or hypertension. The differential is made after the pain is resolved, when the Wiry quality should disappear if pain is the cause.

Individual position

A Wiry quality in the left proximal position, and often the left middle position or bilaterally in the proximal positions, is evidence of deficient essence and future adult onset diabetes or hypertension. The condition is not as far advanced as when the Wiry quality appears over the entire pulse.

A Wiry quality at the left distal and/or left middle position is a sign of cocaine abuse, Grave's disease, or advanced manic-depressive illness.

Yielding Ropy

I have found a Yielding Ropy quality (see Chapter 11) in individuals who have exercised far beyond their energy over a long period of time. With overactivity the qi and blood are depleted. This is reflected in less blood flowing through the vessels. The vessel wall shrinks more slowly than did the quantity of blood, and there is thus a separation of the yin (blood) from the yang (wall of the vessel). Therefore, the vessel wall is less well-nourished than before, and, having less yin, becomes harder. The hardness makes for the Ropy quality, and it is Yielding because of the depletion of the circulating blood and qi.

This causes a hardening of arteries for reasons other than heat. I have had one patient exhibit this quality prior to the symptoms and diagnosis of Parkinson's disease, raising the question of the role of the circulatory system in this disease and other neurological diseases. However, this patient had also been exposed to solvents during her career as an artist.

Occasional Change in Intensity over entire pulse

If the change is occasional over the entire pulse the associated condition is Liver qi stagnation. Within a moderate period of time, all of the concomitant symptoms of quickness to anger and irritability, flank and breast pain, PMS, dysmenorrhea, and depression will become manifest.

Constant Change in Intensity

Entire pulse

If the change is constant, either a deficiency of Heart qi is affecting circulation, or insults to circulation, such as trauma, are affecting the Heart. Initial problems with circulation, including migrating joint pain and cold hands and feet, can be anticipated. Intermediate signs include disturbance in mental activities, insomnia, palpitations, emotional vulnerability, and fatigue (especially in the morning). Eventually, heart disease is possible.

Individual position

Here the change indicates a separation of yin and yang and a deterioration in function of the yin organ associated with the position at which it is found.

In the left middle position, for example, problems with the recovery of energy and healing, menstrual difficulties, impaired planning and decision-making will eventually manifest. Uncorrected, Liver cancer and lymphomas are possible, as well as one form of chronic fatigue syndrome.

Excessive Increase in Rate on mild Exertion >8–12 beats/minute

This is sign of Heart blood deficiency ('Heart weak') with eventual palpitations, insomnia, weakness, fatigue, loss of memory and concentration, and numbness, which, over a moderate period of time, will lead to Heart yang deficiency. (See Chapters 6, 12, and 15.)

Rhythm

An Intermittent quality whose beats miss more than once every thirty seconds, or an Interrupted quality that occurs more than once a minute, portend heart disease in the semi-distant future. (See Chapter 6.)

Choppy at Neuro-psychological position

The Choppy quality at this position is a sign of previous head trauma (usually multiple) which has not been resolved in terms of cerebral blood stagnation and cerebral circulation. Conditions ranging from intractable headache to tumors are possible.

Muffled at Neuro-psychological position

The Muffled quality here is associated with excessive use of hallucinogens, and foretells an eventual deterioration in mental activity, including concentration, clarity, and purpose.

Systems

Dr. Shen's systems—'nervous,' 'circulatory,' 'digestive,' and 'organ'—were previously discussed in Chapters 7, 14, and 15. Here it is only necessary to mention that Dr. Shen described these systems because a large number of his patients experienced symptoms of, respectively, nervous tension, migrating joint problems, alternating digestive disorders, and fatigue, with no evidence of organ disease either by Chinese or biomedical diagnosis. These systems are a relatively benign step in a process that begins at conception and ends at death, and which tells us that if we do not treat these systems, greater disharmony is not far away. The systems are therefore prognosticators of serious pathology.

IMMEDIATE FUTURE

Less serious prognosticators

Occasional Change in Rate at Rest

This is a predictable sign (see Chapter 6) of impending emotional instability with a 'grasshopper' changing mind and roller coaster feeling, fear, borderline psychological states, palpitations, insomnia, and fatigue.

Hesitant

This quality (see Chapter 6) is a sign of a person who has a tendency to be obsessed with one theme, such as money, health, or religion. This is a form of what Dr. Shen calls the 'push pulse,' in which the 'push' is primarily mental, rather than the physical 'push' one finds with the Flooding Deficient quality.

The long-term effect on Heart qi and blood is unpredictable, except that this quality is associated with massive and often fatal heart attacks in young professionals. Mild Heart yin deficiency symptoms of hyperactivity, irritability, insomnia, and palpitations should be expected.

Muffled

LEFT DISTAL POSITION

This is a sign of impending depression. (See Chapters 8 and 12.)

NEURO-PSYCHOLOGICAL POSITION

This is a sign of excessive use of hallucinogens and increasing loss of mental clarity and purpose, and possible developing central nervous system pathology.

Smooth Vibration

LEFT DISTAL PROGRESSING TO ENTIRE PULSE

Qi depth — This is a sign of worry, which, as it progresses to the entire pulse, is more and more likely to be associated with insomnia and anxiety.

All depths — Individuals with this sign are predictably those who will find something to worry about even when there is nothing to worry about. They are always rehearsing for disaster.

NEURO-PSYCHOLOGICAL POSITION

Smooth Vibration is a sign of Heart qi agitation. Like Smooth Vibration at the left distal position, it is usually soon accompanied by worry, anxiety, and insomnia. (See Chapter 12.)

Choppy

Indicating blood stagnation wherever it is found, the incidence of the following disorders can be anticipated soon after the appearance of this quality: fixed pain, especially menstrual or joint, intermittent menstrual bleeding with purple clots, spider veins, purpura, ropy stools, flushing up with migraine headache (qi and blood separate, and the qi rises), bleeding gums, and rectal bleeding with hemorrhoids. (See below for the more serious consequences associated with the Choppy quality.)

Floating Tense and Slow

When the pulse is Floating, Tense, and Slow the likelihood is an imminent upper respiratory infection with cold symptoms.

Floating Yielding and Rapid

When the pulse is Floating, Yielding, and Rapid the likelihood is an imminent upper respiratory infection with heat symptoms.

Inflated at distal aspect of right Diaphragm position

When the distal aspect of the Diaphragm is greatly Inflated or Rougher compared to the proximal part, we can anticipate pathology of the pleura. (See Chapter 16.)

More serious prognosticators

Floating Tight

A Floating Tight quality, especially at the left middle position or left side, is associated with Liver wind, a rising yang condition attended by headache, flushing, and by stroke in the longer run.

Wiry

A Wiry quality (see Chapter 11) at an individual position can coincidentally involve pain in one part of the body. For example, at the proximal positions a Wiry quality can be a sign of pain due to a Kidney stone or to blood stagnation in the pelvis/lower body where a Choppy quality is usually also present. If the Wiry quality continues after the pain goes away, or is present in a patient without pain, one must prognostically look ahead to other causes, including the early stages of diabetes or hypertension.

SLIPPERY QUALITIES

Slippery at Mitral Valve position

Slipperiness at this position (see Chapter 12) is a sign of mitral valve prolapse, that blood is regurgitating into the ventricle. Panic disorder, anxiety, and palpitations are predictable. Since this a moderate sign of Heart qi deficiency, one can predict heart disease if the condition is uncorrected.

Slippery Tight at Gallbladder position

With the Tight quality (see Chapter 12), this is a sign of more advanced cholecystitis and cholelithiasis when, in my opinion, a severe gallbladder attack could occur at any time.

Slippery at left distal position

This quality (see Chapter 11) is a sign that the Heart orifices are blocked by phlegm-heat or phlegm-cold. In either case, one can expect severe emotional problems or epilepsy, and, with other signs of yang rising, even stroke.

Slippery at organ depth

This is usually a sign of infection and is found most often at the left middle position or entire left side at the organ or all depths, where one must consider parasites or chronic hepatitis. Liver cancer is the long-term consideration; episodic fatigue and irritability is found in the short term.

MUFFLED QUALITIES

In my experience this quality (see Chapter 8) is associated with the late stages in the process of tumor formation, malignancy, and severe auto-immune disease such as lupus. I have found that malignancy is usually accompanied by the Muffled or Dead quality when cellular chromosomal damage is well along. This finding is so consistent that when I find it, I fear for the person and suggest an active search for a tumor. This is easier to do when the Muffled quality is in a particular area, such as the Pelvis/Lower Body, where a gynecological exam, ultrasound, and pap smear are such reliable diagnostic tools. The Lungs (right distal and Special Lung positions), Stomach, Prolapse, and Intestine positions are other places that are easy to localize malignancy with the Muffled quality. Earlier stages are indicated by the Choppy and Slippery qualities, and, in the Lungs, a very Rough Vibration.

Recently, I saw a woman who complained of fatigue who had been diagnosed and hospitalized with diverticulosis a few weeks earlier, but whose entire pulse was Muffled. I recommended ultrasound of her liver because it seemed slightly enlarged. She was then diagnosed with metastatic liver disease and given three months to live. She died about five weeks later.

Muffled at Gallbladder position

Here the progression of cholecystitis and cholelithiasis has reached the stage of imminent necrosis of the gallbladder with the danger of peritonitis. Tumors of the gallbladder bile duct and the liver bile duct have followed the finding of the Muffled quality at this position.

Muffled at left distal position

A mild Muffled quality here is a sign of the dampening of the spirit and the emergence of a depression marked by a lack of joy.

ROUGH VIBRATION QUALITIES

Rough Vibration at Neuro-psychological position

Rough Vibration (see Chapter 12) at this position is associated with extreme fear, even terror, and Heart shock, and is a sign of severely agitated Heart qi.

Rough Vibration over entire pulse

Rough Vibration over the entire pulse (see Chapter 11) is a prognosticator of severe Heart qi deficiency provided there are other signs of Heart dysfunction, for example, the Interrupted quality, or Change in Intensity over the entire pulse or at the left distal position. If there are no other signs of Heart dysfunction, extreme fear, shock, and guilt may be involved.

Rough Vibration at individual positions

Rough Vibration is a sign of severe qi deficiency in the organ represented by the position, a marker of parenchymal damage and a very serious collapse of function (a 'broken' organ, according to Dr. Shen). For example, Deep Rough Vibration at the left distal position can anticipate failing Heart function within the near future, and a shutting down of Kidney function and anuria if found in the left proximal position.

Flooding Excess

With this quality (see Chapter 8) there is heat in an organ with the possibility of imminent deep infection such as a hidden appendicitis, peritonitis, and septicemia.

Deep

The Deep quality (see Chapter 9), if not already accompanied by illness, is a sign that there will be illness within one to three years, unless the person learns to conserve his or her qi and accept therapeutic intervention. The illness will involve the organ associated with the position in which it is found, or, if found over the entire pulse, the position with the most Feeble-Absent quality.

FEEBLE-ABSENT QUALITIES

Feeble-Absent over entire pulse

The individual with this quality (see Chapter 8) over the entire pulse will be ill within one to three years without intervention. It is another prognosticator of a near future pervasive chronic fatigue syndrome, or other chronic disease.

Feeble-Absent at individual positions

Found in one position it foretells a functional breakdown of the associated yin organ within one year. For example, if it is found at the left middle position, one would expect to find fatigue, especially after work or later in the day, with difficulty recovering or getting one's second wind, and musculoskeletal problems including being easily injured and slow to recover.

One would also anticipate menstrual problems with delayed or missing periods, sensitivity to light and other eye problems, and digestive difficulties such as stagnant gas and distention. A Feeble-Absent quality in this position is also associated with lassitude, and with depression due to a lack of what Porkert calls 'active' moving energy.

I have found the Feeble-Absent, and especially Empty, qualities in the left middle position to be increasing along with the proliferation of drug use, especially marijuana, with environmental toxins, and with what seems to be an epidemic of mononucleosis and hepatitis. As mentioned above, the danger of primary liver cancer and lymphomas with a Feeble-Absent quality, and even more so with an Empty quality, in the left middle position, is increasing.

INFLATED QUALITIES

Inflated at Large Vessel positions

With an Inflated quality (see Chapter 8) at the Large Vessel positions one can expect an aneurysm and anticipate rupture. In my experience the aneurysm has always been in the ascending aorta even as far away as the mid-epigastric area. This finding has been confirmed by me many times, and by other practitioners even more often.

Inflated at distal aspect of left Diaphragm position

When the distal aspect of the left Diaphragm position (see Chapter 12) is greatly Inflated or Rougher compared to the proximal part, we can anticipate symptoms of an enlarged heart.

EMPTY QUALITIES

Empty over entire pulse

This quality (see Chapter 9) found consistently over the entire pulse portends a profound loss of contact between yin and yang ('qi wild') with major illness predictable within three months to two years. The sudden appearance of the Empty quality over the entire pulse can occur when a person is under great stress, during which time they bring to the surface all of their available energies in order to cope and maintain their sanity, as in post-traumatic stress syndrome.

Empty at individual positions

In one position this quality foretells major dysfunction of the associated yin organ in which the yin and yang have lost contact. Found consistently at the left middle position, for example, one could anticipate vulnerability to major infection, auto-immune diseases, and neoplasms, both benign and malignant.

Empty Thread-like; Leather; Minute; Scattered; Hollow Yielding Full-Overflowing and Slow

These qualities represent increasing degrees of the 'qi wild' disorder, a profound separation between yin and yang, with major illness likely within six months. The Scattered quality is associated with the terminal stages of AIDS and other illness, and is known as the 'ceiling dripping' pulse.

Leather-like Hollow

Rapid

This quality (see Chapter 13) portends imminent hemorrhage in the organ or area associated with the position in which it is found, and should be treated as a medical emergency.

Slow

This suggests recent past severe hemorrhage in the organ or area associated with the position in which it is found, and warrants emergency investigation and treatment since the hemorrhage could soon recur.

Very Tense Tight, or Wiry Full-Overflowing Hollow and Rapid

Left middle and proximal positions

This combination (see Chapter 13), especially at the left middle and left proximal positions simultaneously, is a sign of severe Liver wind and a prognosticator of early adult onset diabetes or hypertension.

Left distal and left middle positions or entire pulse

If found at the left distal and left middle positions, or over the entire pulse, and the rate is very Rapid, a stroke may be imminent.

Either side

If these qualities are accessed only on one side, there is imminent danger of a stroke on that side.

Tense Ropy

This quality (see Chapter 11) is a sign of a developing arteriosclerosis in the later stage, and is a serious prognostic sign, especially in a younger person.

Tense Hollow Full-Overflowing at Large Vessel positions

This combination (see Chapter 12) is a sign of cardiac hypertension affecting the large vessels. According to Dr. Shen, the Hollow Full-Overflowing quality is found here first when Heart qi is relatively strong. Of course, without immediate therapeutic intervention the Heart will weaken and fail.

Increase in Rate on Exertion <8 beats/minute

If, on exertion, the rate increases less than eight beats per minute, stays the same, or decreases, we have an increasing degree of Heart qi deficiency. If it stays the same or decreases, this is a sign of severe Heart qi-yang deficiency with expectant heart disease, including symptoms of fatigue, spontaneous daytime perspiration, shortness of breath on exertion, weakness, and a suffocating sensation in the chest. (See Chapters 6 and 12.)

Change in Qualities

Entire pulse

This pulse (see Chapter 6) indicates a 'qi wild' disorder with separation of yin and yang, in which case there will be serious illness within six months to two years.

Individual positions

This quality signifies the separation of yin and yang and the deterioration in function of the yin organ associated with the position in which it is found, with illness possible within several months to a year.

Yielding Hollow Full-Overflowing and Rapid

This combination (see Chapters 6 and 8), associated with the sudden cessation of extended and heavy exercise, will be found with near-term rapidly developing severe anxiety, episodes of depersonalization and dissociation, severe fatigue, and migrating joint pains.

CHOPPY QUALITIES

Choppy at Pelvis/Lower Body positions

Found here at its most common position, the Choppy quality (see Chapter 11) involves potential endometriosis, fibroid tumors and ovarian cysts in women, and prostatic enlargement and prostatic tumors in men.

Choppy at left middle position

A rare finding, the Choppy quality at this position is associated with 'dried blood in the Liver' or with blockage of the portal system to the heart, both usually due to a rare asymptomatic cirrhosis. Sudden fatal hemorrhage is possible, especially if the pulse is also Leather-like Hollow.

Choppy at left distal position

Even rarer is the Choppy quality at this position, where it is a sign of severe asymptomatic coronary artery blockage and a high expectation of an early heart attack.

Choppy at Gallbladder positions

The Choppy quality here is a sign of many large gallstones and necrosis of the gallbladder with the threat of peritonitis.

Bean (Spinning)

The Bean (Spinning) quality (see Chapter 10) is found in only the most emergent situations. I have felt it at the right middle position with severe gastric pain related to an ulcer, at the left and right distal position with profound terror, and at the left proximal position with intestinal obstruction. I found it recently at the radial extremity of the left distal position in a 36-year-old type-1 diabetic, who also had an Inflated Large Vessel position and a rate that decreased on exertion. I am concerned about an imminent heart and circulatory collapse. While it is unlikely that the Bean (Spinning) quality will be felt without symptoms, it is mentioned in this context to alert the reader of its seriousness.

Unstable

This sign (see Chapter 6) indicates imminent extremely serious illness in the particular yin organ associated with the position in which it is found. At the left distal position, for example, coronary occlusion or heart failure can be anticipated at any time.

Interrupted or Intermittent

When the Interrupted quality (see Chapter 6) reaches the stage when the rate consistently cannot be accurately read, or the Intermittent quality occurs less than every five beats, this is a sign of serious heart disease and possibly a short life.

Intermittent or Interrupted Yielding Hollow

This is a very serious sign of heart disease and indicates a short life expectancy, combining chaotic Heart function and a serious 'qi wild' condition. (See Chapter 6.)

Dead

The sensation of this quality (see Chapter 8) is that of touching a dead body in which there is no movement. The diagnosis is usually a malignant carcinoma and the prognosis is early death.

Many years ago I examined a woman whose left middle position was Dead. Dr. Shen confirmed my impression. She was referred back to her Park Avenue internist who laughed at her for taking this finding seriously. Reluctantly, he did liver function tests, all of which were negative, and he declared her perfectly well. For this reason she refused herbal and acupuncture treatment, although she returned regularly for a check-up. For two and a half years I insisted that she pursue this finding, with the same result, until on one occasion this same internist became alarmed, and, after much further testing, concluded that she had carcinoma of the bile ducts. She died about a year later, after radium implants failed to halt the disease.

Positions

The following are qualities or combinations thereof found only at special positions.

LEFT MIDDLE POSITION

Slippery at organ depth

This is a sign of an acute exacerbation of a chronic infection such as parasites or hepatitis.

Floating Tight

See Floating Tight in the section 'More serious prognosticators' above.

LIVER ENGORGEMENT POSITIONS

A positive finding in these positions is a sign of a Liver engorged with stagnant blood and qi, causing diminished Liver function with menstrual difficulties and being easily fatigued.

RIGHT MIDDLE POSITION AND STOMACH-PYLORUS EXTENSION POSITION

A Tight Hollow and Slippery combination in both or either of these positions, sometimes accompanied by Inflation at the Stomach Extension position, suggests the onset of gastritis and an ulcer.

ESOPHAGUS POSITION

An Inflated Rough or Slippery quality here is a sign of increasing stagnation in the esophagus, with short-term implications of reflux, and long-term ramifications of Barrett's syndrome and a neoplasm.

Paradox

When the signs and symptoms correspond to each other in terms of their Robust or Reduced aspects, the illness is less serious. But when they vary, whereby one is Reduced while the other is inappropriately Robust, the illness is more serious. In an acute illness the pulse should be Robust and Pounding, and in a chronic disease it should be Reduced.[3] This is discussed more fully in Chapters 3 and 17.

The age, weight, and sex of the patient have already been discussed in connection with this paradox. Other findings which are serious indicators of impending illness include the Ropy quality in a young person, the Reduced qualities in a young person (Deep, Feeble-Absent, and all the Empty qualities), and the chaotic qualities (Interrupted-Intermittent, Change in Qualities or Intensity, Unstable). Likewise, finding one of the hard qualities in a young person (Tight, Rough Vibration, Choppy, Wiry) or the very Robust qualities (Hollow Full-Overflowing, Flooding Excess) would be inappropriate.

When, at any age, the rate stays the same, rises less than eight beats, or decreases, we can expect Heart disease relatively soon. A Thin pulse in a man, or a Wide pulse in a woman, is usually a sign of current or at least certain-to-be illness. Especially in the terminal stage of the six stages, the presence of a very high temperature and a very low pulse rate, or a very low temperature and a very high rate, are signs of extreme physiological disorder ('qi wild') and imminent death.

Signs of a Positive Prognosis

It is unfortunate that our discussion of prognosis is weighted so heavily in the direction of increasing pathology. It is true that the pulse record is a statement of a person's condition at a particular point along the continuum from birth to death, and that our principal concern as physicians is to diagnose and treat the disharmonies revealed by the record. Since we must all eventually die, the picture is usually not a pretty one, inasmuch as the record is telling us how we are dying and how far along we are in the process.

However, the pulse record also tells us about our *strengths*. Strong proximal positions (lower burner) tell us that we have root, ground on which to stand and heal. Strong middle positions (middle burner) tell us that we can restore and cleanse ourselves. Strong distal positions (upper burner) tell us that we can reach out to the world with awareness of our creative being, with the strength to communicate and protect our being, and to maintain mental and emotional stability despite the 'slings and arrows of outrageous fortune' with which we are all constantly bombarded.

Even with signs of Heart disharmony, a Normal rhythm tells us that there is strength to recover. A Normal rate, consistent with the person's age, indicates the ability to maintain cardiovascular stability under stress.

Another important sign is the integrity of the right side of the pulse, especially the right middle position. This informs us that the digestive system and Spleen-Stomach qi (see Chapter 5) are capable of restoring qi and blood when the organism is under stress. And clearly, when overly Robust or Reduced pulses approach the signs that approximate those of the Normal pulse described in Chapter 5, we are on the road to healing.

The Tense quality over the entire pulse tells us that there is enough true (upright) qi, or sufficient metabolic heat, to sustain the organism under adverse circumstances. Normal complementary positions inform us that the pathology found in the associated principal positions is not as serious as it first seemed, and that the chances for restoration are favorable. The presence of a Normal sine wave is another positive sign when the person is ill.

When the qualities in the same burner tend to be more similar than different, we are witnessing less chaos than when the qualities in all the positions are significantly different. When there is little change in qualities and intensity and few Empty-type qualities, we have a more stable organism. Further stability is indicated when the pulse and other signs and symptoms are synchronous and not paradoxical. This is also true for the synchronicity of age, sex, height, and weight with the pulse qualities. The relative absence of qualities that indicates excess or deficiency is another positive sign.[4]

CHAPTER 17

Interpretation

CONTENTS

    The process of disease and prevention, 625
    Pulse as life record, 626
Methodology for Pulse Interpretation, 626
    Data, 626
        Preliminary considerations, 626
            Collecting the data, 626
            Interpreting the data, 626
            Age, gender, and weight, 626
            Degree of presence, 627
            Location, 627
                Seriousness of condition, 627
                Relation of a quality in one position to the same quality over the entire pulse, 627
                A common quality in one position assumes special significance, 627
            Integration of the pulse data, 627
            Integration with other diagnostic parameters, 627
    Procedure, 628
        Beginner: list substances and activity, 628
            Substances (includes broad, closer, and closest focus), 628
                Qi, 628
                Blood, 628
                Yin, 628
                Yang, 628
                Essence, 629
                Wind, 629

Food, 629
Parenchyma, 629
Activity, 629
Heat, 629
Cold, 629
Advanced: quick overview, 629
Scan for qualities suggestive of serious conditions, 629
Stability (activity and change), 629
Primarily qi, 630
Primarily blood and circulation, 630
Other qualities implying potentially serious conditions, 630
Common and less common qualities and prevention, 630
Burners: preliminary examination, 630
Paradoxical qualities, 631
Age, 631
Ropy in a young person, 631
Deep and/or Feeble-Absent; Empty (Leather, Scattered, Minute) in a young person; Interrupted-Intermittent (Hollow or not); and all pulses associated with 'qi wild' and separation of yin and yang, 631
Very Tight quality in a young person, 631
Pounding in a young person, 631
Robust Pounding, 631
Reduced Pounding, 631
Tense Tight Hollow Full-Overflowing in a young person, 631
Increase in Rate on Exertion of >8-12 beats/minute in a young person, 632
Rate stays the same, rises <8 beats/minute, or decreases at any age, 632
Gender, 632
Thin in a man and Wide in a woman, 632
Size (weight and height), 632
Heavy person with very superficial pulse, and thin person with very deep pulse, 632
Temperature, rate, 632
Acute and chronic, 633
List preliminary diagnostic impressions, 633
Systematic approach: all levels of experience, 633
Broad focus: initial impressions, 633
Specific qualities and the broad focus, 633
Rhythm (Chapter 6), 633
Change in Rate at Rest: consistent or not?, 633
Interrupted: can you determine the rate or not?, 634
Intermittent: how frequently are the beats missed?, 634
Rate (Chapter 7), 634
Slow: how slow?, 634
Fast: how fast?, 634
Sides vary in rate?, 634
Rate at end compared with rate at beginning, 634
Rate on exertion: consistent or not? small or large?, 634

With disharmonies of rhythm and rate, 634
Uniform qualities over the entire pulse, 635
Closer focus (depths, sides, wave forms), 635
Depths, 635
Above the qi depth, 635
External etiology, 635
Internal etiology, 635
Qi depth, 635
Blood depth, 635
Organ depth, 635
Sides, 635
Left side, 636
Right side, 636
Intensity shifting from side to side, 637
Qualities shifting from side to side, 637
Wave form, 637
Flooding Deficient Wave, 637
Hesitant Wave, 637
Flooding Excess Wave, 637
Hollow Full-Overflowing Wave, 637
Suppressed Wave and Suppressed Pounding, 638
Areas, 638
Diaphragm, 638
Pelvis/Lower Body, 638
Burners, 638
Existential, 638
Specific: similar qualities bilaterally at burners, 638
Examples, 639
Systems, 639
Psychology, 639
Closest focus, 640
General considerations, 640
Specific considerations, 640
Organs: principal and complementary positions, 640
Relationships between individual positions, 640
Chronic disease, 640
Acute disease, 640
Revisiting broad/closer/closest focus, 641
Interpretation, 641
Summary of findings, 641
Formulation, 641
Current prevailing issues or patterns, 641
Root issues and etiology of disharmonies, 641
Derivative issues ('branches'), 641
Primary derivative issues, 641
Secondary derivative issues, 641
Analysis and synthesis, 641
Management, 642
Lifestyle strategies, 642

Referrals, 642
Acupuncture, herbal, and other healing strategies, 642
Immediate interventions, 642
Intermediate interventions, 642
Long range major interventions, 642
Long range minor interventions, 642
Review patient's history and complaints, 642
Amend previous synthesis, 642
Conclusion, 642
- Table 17-1: Methodology for interpretation, 643
- Appendix: Case Illustrations, 647

CHAPTER 17

Interpretation

The purpose of this chapter is to discuss how, in practice, to interpret the information that is found in pulse examination. Case histories set forth in an appendix to this chapter demonstrate how this may be done in practice. It would be wise for the serious student to analyze these cases for yourself before reading the interpretation.

The presentation in this chapter involves many details which cannot be absorbed quickly; they must be studied in conjunction with the illustrative cases. The actual practice of interpretation is far quicker and easier than the slow, plodding, and often repetitive steps outlined in this book. Skill in diagnosis will be enhanced by taking the examination presented at my web site, *www.dragonrises.com,* and attempting to analyze the case histories from the records prior to reading the solutions given in the book.

After some important preliminary considerations, this chapter is divided into three sections. First, we begin by examining and gathering data with a *broad focus*, or what might be called initial impressions, including the rhythm, rate, uniform qualities, and wave of the pulse. Then we examine, with a *closer focus*, the depths and sides of the pulse. Finally, we take the *closest focus* by examining the individual positions, both principal and complementary. Included in these examinations is a summary assessment of the *stability, substances, activity, areas,* and what Dr. Shen calls *systems* of the body. This is followed by a discussion of the relationship of these data with each other, which is meant to serve as a guide and stimulus to the thought process involved in using the pulse as a diagnostic tool.

No single diagnostic method is designed to act alone. In Chinese medicine all four of the diagnostic methods are meant to be used in concert to arrive at a reasonable assessment of alterations in the patient's physiology. Remember also that the didactic study of pulse diagnosis is insufficient to master the ineluctable step of learning to identify the qualities, which must be accomplished by training the sense of touch.

THE PROCESS OF DISEASE AND PREVENTION

Many disease processes exist simultaneously in the same organism. This may be difficult to understand at first; however, these processes are set in motion before birth, since life from its inception encounters obstacles to normal maturation. The pulse reflects each of these threads of the disease process. It therefore serves not only to illuminate the current symptomatic situation, but also as a valuable tool in prevention, since we can see the direction.

The possibility of prevention is further enhanced by the fact that the pulse picture often precedes the onset of related symptoms. For example, if the quality of the pulse is Absent, the implication is that the person is already ill, while in fact it may be telling us only that the person is highly vulnerable to illness.

PULSE AS LIFE RECORD

Above all, remember this: An accurate pulse record is a precise and faithful catalog of an individual's physiology and pathology at a given moment in life. It is the royal road to early diagnosis and prevention. This is the true reality of who we are along the passage from birth to death, and the basis upon which management is more fruitfully guided than by any other diagnostic parameter or therapeutic pursuit of symptoms.

Along this passage of life the pulse records consistently illustrate that the cardiovascular system shows the earliest and most pervasive signs of constitutional or congenital insult, and seems to absorb the greatest punishment from abusive living. Students are stunned by the consistency of this finding in the young as well as the old. Yet, considering that the Heart is the 'emperor' serving its 'subjects,' one should not be surprised that it is the organ most affected by the exigencies of living. It is therefore not remarkable that the most frequent cause of death is heart disease.

Methodology for Pulse Interpretation

DATA

Preliminary considerations

COLLECTING THE DATA

First we must have data, which we gather from the patient's pulse, regarding the substances (qi, blood, yin, yang, wind, food and essence, both in general, as well as in and between specific organs), stability (changes in rhythm, rate, qualities, and intensity), activity (heat and cold, excess and deficiency), body areas, and systems. The method of taking the pulse is described in Chapter 4.

INTERPRETING THE DATA

The ultimate goal of pulse diagnosis is interpretation in the service of management and treatment. While it will be necessary here to repeat the most common, less common, and rarely encountered qualities in each position without exposition, in this chapter we will primarily discuss the meaning of the qualities in relation to the conditions which they represent. However, based on my teaching experience, where I have found that the interpretation of a quality in relation to a position bears emphasis because it is particularly unfamiliar to students trained in other traditions, or often misunderstood (as with the blood depth), the discussion of the quality is expanded. Therefore, all qualities are not treated equally here, but only as it serves our object to expand interpretation. The reader is referred to recommended chapters for elaboration.

AGE, GENDER, AND WEIGHT

Consider and record the age, gender, and weight of the person in terms of what is appropriate or paradoxical, which you must always keep in mind throughout the exam. While no one piece of data is necessarily more useful than another, I find the age and gender of the patient to be essential factors in arriving at a meaningful diagnosis.

DEGREE OF PRESENCE

The degree of presence of a quality is important to note. Muffled at a five is a far more important sign of physiological chaos than Muffled at a one, which, when found over the entire pulse, may merely represent a sign of depression.

LOCATION

Seriousness of condition

The seriousness of a quality can also depend upon its location. In a woman, a Choppy quality is of much more concern at the left distal position (Heart) than at the Pelvis/Lower Body position where, if found only occasionally, might just be a sign of concurrent menstruation. Whereas a Muffled quality at most positions is often associated with a neoplastic process, when found at the left distal position, it might only be a sign of depression.

Relation of a quality in one position to the same quality over the entire pulse

We must be alert to the possibility that the findings in one position are not just a reflection of something that is characteristic of the entire pulse, or a larger segment of the pulse. Change in Intensity is a common example of a quality found in individual positions. On re-examination of our initial impressions, it may be a quality which occurs generally over the entire pulse, which has a different meaning than if it appeared in only one position. On the other hand, within this general context, there may be one position where the change is especially dramatic, which then requires that we focus on the special condition which is affecting the organ associated with that position.

A common quality in one position assumes special significance

There are instances in which one position alone shows a quality that, while ordinarily not unusual, appears nowhere else on the pulse. For example, a generally Reduced pulse in which the proximal positions are very Taut could be a sign of a deficient person who abstains from sex.

INTEGRATION OF THE PULSE DATA

Integration involves an exploration of relationships among the data, for which the pages below are meant as a guide. We compare the findings from the initial impression, then the findings from the individual positions, and then combine the findings from the initial impressions and the individual positions for a consolidated picture in terms of energetic drains, circulation (stagnation), nourishment, and storage. From this we formulate a diagnosis which identifies the root and current prevailing issues, etiology, and possible prognosis.

INTEGRATION WITH OTHER DIAGNOSTIC PARAMETERS

Finally, we integrate the diagnosis of the pulse with other diagnostic signs, the patient's history, and physical and psychological symptoms. With this information we attempt to refine the root and current prevailing issues that were based on the pulse alone. We must then connect all of this to the patient's life in terms of constitution and life habits in order to recommend a rational management program, as outlined below.

PROCEDURE

There are several ways that one may approach interpretation. Table 17-1 provides the simplest outline.

Beginner: list substances and activity

For the beginner, I suggest that you first list the substances and activity of the body. If this is as far as you can go, you will at least have information which is immediately useful in formulating a treatment plan, especially with herbs, since you will know which substances are excessive and need to be moved or reduced, and which are deficient and need to be supplemented. Many serious mistakes in prescribing can thereby be avoided. For example, supplementing the qi in someone who has stagnant qi, or yang in someone with heat from excess, or removing dampness in someone who is already yin deficient, will exacerbate their disorders.

SUBSTANCES (INCLUDES BROAD, CLOSER, AND CLOSEST FOCUS)

Qi

Excess (stagnation)	EXTERNAL
	Cotton, Floating, or Slippery
	INTERNAL
	Taut, Tense, Tight, Wiry, Muffled, Bean (Spinning), or Short Excess; Inflated or Rough at Esophagus position
Deficiency	Yielding, Diminished, or Absent at qi depth; Spreading, Flooding Deficient, Diffuse, Reduced Substance, Reduced Pounding, Deep, Feeble-Absent, Short Deficient, Yielding Ropy

Blood

Excess (stagnation)	Choppy; Blood Unclear, Blood Heat, or Blood Thick; Hollow Full-Overflowing, Slippery, and Rough Vibration at the blood depth; Tense Ropy, Muffled, Liver Engorgement, Very Tense Inflated
Deficiency	Yielding Partially Hollow, Thin, Leather, Minute, Rate on Exertion <8–12 beats/minute

Yin

Excess (stagnation [damp-phlegm])	Slippery, Muffled
Deficiency	Tight, Wiry, Ropy; Empty Thread-like, Leather, Minute, Tight Ropy

Yang

Excess (stagnation)	Very Taut-Tense in proximal positions ('Buddha's pulse')
Deficiency	Deep, Feeble-Absent, Empty, Yielding Hollow Full-Overflowing, Hidden Deficient, Empty Thread-like, Minute, Scattered, Hollow Interrupted-Intermittent, Change in Qualities

Essence

Excess (stagnation) — Very Taut-Tense in proximal positions ('Buddha's pulse')

Deficiency — Wiry, Leather, Doughy (Neuro-psychological positions)

Wind

External — Floating

Internal — Floating Tight, Tight-Wiry Hollow Full-Overflowing

Food

Food stagnation is most clearly identified by a Slippery quality at the Esophagus position. Any signs of qi stagnation in the gastrointestinal tract, such as Inflated at the right middle position (trapped qi in the Stomach), would imply some concomitant food stagnation.

Parenchyma

Damage to the parenchyma is signalled by the presence of Rough Vibration at individual and complementary positions.

ACTIVITY

Heat

Excess — Tense, Blood Heat and Blood Thick, Hollow Full-Overflowing, Flooding Excess, Tense Ropy, Robust Pounding, Moderately Tense Inflated

Deficiency — Tight, Wiry, Tight Ropy

Cold

Excess —
External: Floating Tense
Internal: Tense or Tight (usually in one position [rare]), Hidden Excess

Deficiency (Qi-yang deficiency) —
External: Yielding or Absent at qi depth, Spreading
Internal: Deep, Feeble-Absent, Empty, Yielding Hollow Full-Overflowing, Hidden Deficient, Empty Thread-like, Minute, Scattered

Advanced: quick overview

SCAN FOR QUALITIES SUGGESTIVE OF SERIOUS CONDITIONS

To get some quick sense of the degree of disability one is encountering, scan the pulse record for qualities which suggest potential or current serious illness.

Stability (activity and change)

In glancing over the individual positions our attention is drawn first to the positions with the greatest activity, and the greatest degree of change, especially for those qualities which are signs of chaos.

Physiological chaos, far more than deficiency or excess (stagnation, heat), is the greatest threat to health and life. Following are some of the qualities that are signs of chaos, all of which indicate either a separation of yin and yang, or 'blood out of control,' and the highest degree of dysfunction. (It is understood that the absolute yin conditions of very high fever and very Slow rate, and the reverse, are the most extreme, almost always found near death.)

Primarily qi

Muffled, Unstable, Change in Intensity and Amplitude at individual positions, Change in Qualities, Empty (including Empty Thread-Like, Leather, Scattered and Minute), Hollow Interrupted-Intermittent, Dead, sides vastly different in strength, burners vary greatly in qualities

Primarily blood and circulation

Leather-like Hollow, and very Tense or Tight Hollow Full-Overflowing, are signs of the instability of the blood ('blood out of control'). Interrupted-Intermittent rhythms, constant Change in Intensity over the entire pulse, Change in Intensity shifting from side to side, and a difference in rate on different sides are signs of the instability of the circulation.

Other qualities implying potentially serious conditions

Wiry, Choppy, Restricted, Bean (Spinning), Ropy, Floating Tight, Nonhomogeneous, little or no Increase or Decrease in Rate on Exertion, Heart Enlarged and Large Vessel positions present, Robust Pounding, abnormal wave form, especially Flooding Excess, Hollow Full-Overflowing and Suppressed

Common and less common qualities and prevention

Apart from chaos or other signs of the functional unraveling of the organism, it is equally important that we distinguish less disturbed organs, and especially the disease process at an earlier stage, by identifying positions with lesser degrees of deficiency and stagnation.

Qualities such as Flooding Deficient Wave (qi), Deep (qi) and Feeble-Absent (qi), or Tight (yin) or Thin (blood), are evidence of just such a stage earlier in the process of disease than chaos. These qualities can be prognostic of impending disease or appear simultaneously with the earlier stages of disease.

Likewise, stagnation in the form of the Flat, Inflated, and Cotton qualities has been associated by Dr. Shen with the formation of cancer over a long period of time. This characteristic of pulse diagnosis provides an opportunity for early intervention and prevention.

BURNERS: PRELIMINARY EXAMINATION

One can also scan the burners (see Chapter 14) for similarities and differences, discussed below under the heading of 'Areas.' The greater the similarity of qualities in the same burner and on the pulse as a whole, the greater the inherent stability of physiology, even if the entire pulse were Feeble-Absent. Similarity of a particular quality bilaterally in one burner, exclusive of the other burners, indicates a problem in the area associated with that burner, or that one of the pair of organs in the burner is significantly affecting the other.

You may also obtain a general impression of the person's existential place in the world. For example, I evaluate the proximal positions to get a sense of the root, the ground on which this person must stand (the Kidneys). The integrity of the middle burner tells us how centered this person is in life, and the upper burner tells us how well she can reach out to the world and take it in.

PARADOXICAL QUALITIES

Age

While any of the qualities mentioned above under 'Stability' and 'Other serious qualities' would be paradoxical in a young person, the following are some of the more common ones.

Ropy in a young person

A Ropy quality, either Yielding or Tense, in a young person is a sign of serious illness. Both, for different reasons, indicate a separation of yin and yang in the vessels with ensuing deterioration of those vessels, the entire circulation, and finally the cardiovascular system.

Deep and/or Feeble-Absent; Empty (Leather, Scattered, Minute) in a young person; Interrupted-Intermittent (Hollow or not); and all qualities associated with 'qi wild' and separation of yin and yang

When confronted by deficiency or chaos of this magnitude in a young person, Dr. Shen would express surprise. The only explanation could be significant constitutional or congenital insult.

Very Tight quality in a young person

Whereas Tightness is normally associated with yin deficiency, it takes many years of worry, rumination, and overworking of the nervous system to exhaust the yin. Especially if the Tight quality is extreme and found over the entire pulse, in a young person one must consider other causes. In my experience this is usually associated with intractable pain, often due to inexplicable arthritis.

Pounding in a young person

ROBUST POUNDING

The quality is a sign of heat from excess which the body is trying unsuccessfully to eliminate. In a young person, apart from an obvious acute illness, the presence of this quality usually denotes a chronic illness, one in which the body is overworking to create the metabolic heat to control or eliminate a pathogenic factor, internal or external. A chronic illness in a young person is usually grave.

REDUCED POUNDING

The scenario described above with regard to Robust Pounding is even more serious when there is Reduced Pounding in a young person. The implication is that this person, even at a young age, is struggling and barely able to create the metabolic heat required to cope with a threatening pathogenic factor.

Tense-Tight Hollow Full-Overflowing in a young person

This quality, rarely found earlier than middle age, is usually a sign of accumulated extreme heat from excess in the blood, most often associated with hypertension. The etiology is usually an overworked nervous system and/or digestive system heat. The source of this quality, which is extraordinary in a young person, would require a different explanation, usually one associated with a major physiological defect. Early onset, insulin dependent diabetes is another possible explanation which should be investigated.

Increase in Rate on Exertion of >8-12 beats/minute in a young person

An increase of more than 8 to 12 beats per minute on exertion is a sign of Heart blood deficiency, which is a slowly developing condition due to overwork, lack of sleep, and poor nutrition. The greater the increase, the greater the deficiency. Unless there is a congenital etiology or a serious systemic blood deficiency associated with a dyscrasia, or serious, ongoing blood loss as with menhorragia in teenage girls, Heart blood deficiency would be almost impossible to find in a young person.

Rate stays the same, rises <8 beats/minute, or decreases at any age

With exertion (swinging one arm vigorously ten times) the pulse rate should normally increase between 8 and 12 beats per minute. When cardiovascular function cannot respond to the need for increased circulation, or the rate does not rise 8 beats per minute, stays the same, or decreases, the indication is Heart qi, and more likely Heart yang, deficiency.

Gender

Thin in a man and Wide in a woman

A Thin quality in a man and a Wide quality in a woman are signs of illness. Conventional Chinese medical wisdom associates women with blood and men with qi. Therefore, one would normally expect that a woman's pulse would be Wide and a man's Thinner, if perhaps more forceful. In practice, however, the opposite seems to occur, for reasons which I cannot explain.

In cultures where blood is not specifically supplemented with herbs or food, women's pulses are Thinner in part because, after menarche, the loss of menstrual blood and the loss of blood in childbirth, which is considerable, is never completely replaced. This blood deficiency is also partially due to the loss of sleep during the first years of each child, and breast feeding without sufficient replacement nourishment. Also, in practice, nervous tension seems, in women, to consume more yin and blood. All of these factors lead to Thin pulses in women. A Wide pulse in women is found with the abnormal creation of heat and dampness in the blood (hyperlipidemia and hypertension) or with blood dyscrasias such as thrombocythemia and polycythemia vera.

In practice, in adult men I find the Thin pulse to be a sign of qi and especially yang deficiency (loss of metabolic heat), as well as blood deficiency, often occurring in autoimmune diseases such as HIV, and often previously undetected.

The expected difference in the width of arteries between men and women is also partially due to the anatomical differences between the sexes. Men are generally larger, as is the size of their vessels, which is necessary due to their greater muscle mass.

Size (weight and height)

Heavy person with very superficial pulse, and thin person with very deep pulse

The depth of the pulse is determined to some extent by the amount of connective tissue between the body surface and the vessels. There is more tissue in obese people, in whom the pulse therefore feels deeper, and less tissue in thin people, in whom the pulse feels more superficial. In contrast to the Cotton quality, which appears as an amorphous spongy sensation between the skin and vessel, increased connective tissue creates a harder sensation.

Temperature, rate

A very high temperature and a very low pulse rate, or a very low temperature and a very high pulse rate, are signs of physiological chaos ('qi wild,' see Chapter 6) of the most serious kind, frequently found in the terminal yin stage of illness.

Acute and chronic

In an acute disease the pulse should be Robust and Pounding, and in a chronic disease the pulse should be Reduced. If the pulse and the disease are corresponding, the prognosis is better than when they are incompatible.[1]

LIST PRELIMINARY DIAGNOSTIC IMPRESSIONS

Include: Robust (Excess), Reduced (Deficient), or Mixed

Systematic approach: all levels of experience

The following is the most thorough method, which I recommend to even the most advanced practitioner, and in practice includes both approaches described above. From the preliminary scan just discussed it moves from a *broad focus,* which are impressions of qualities which appear to characterize the entire pulse and the wave form, to a *closer focus* on the qualities which seem to characterize the various depths and sides, to the *closest focus,* which involves an examination of the individual principal and complementary positions.

BROAD FOCUS: INITIAL IMPRESSIONS

We first consider the qualities that appear simultaneously over the entire pulse when we access both wrists simultaneously. Most important of all are the rhythm and rate, which inform us to a reasonable extent about the status of the Heart and circulation, the 'emperor' on whose well-being rest all of physiology and psychology.

Another aspect of the importance of qualities found over large segments of the pulse, especially the rhythm and rate, is that unless the imbalances represented by these general qualities are resolved therapeutically, the treatment efforts made by attending to the qualities on the principal and complementary positions will usually not hold. It is a question of first things first, and the message delivered by the larger sections of the pulse generally comes first.

Here we sense the width of the pulse, which immediately tells us something about the condition of the blood (Thin or Wide); the hardness of the pulse, which tells us about the yin and heat from deficiency (Tight-Wiry); the tenseness or pliability of the pulse, which tells us about the strength of the qi; and the force of the pulse, which tells us about the strength of the qi and heat from excess (Tense or Reduced Substance, Robust or Reduced Pounding).

However, since these are first perceptions, we then proceed to examine the principal and complementary positions so as to augment and correct the initial impressions. In practice, we can move back and forth between the broad, closer (depths, areas, and sides), and closest (principal and complementary positions) to gain a complete and balanced interpretation.

Specific qualities and the broad focus

Rhythm

The abnormalities in rhythm (Chapters 6 and 12) include the following qualities:

- CHANGE IN RATE AT REST: Consistent or not?
  Inconsistent: Heart qi agitation
  Consistent: Mild Heart qi deficiency

- INTERRUPTED: Can you determine the rate or not?

  With rate: Moderate Heart qi deficiency and severe Heart qi agitation
  Without rate: Severe Heart qi-yang deficiency

- INTERMITTENT: How frequently are the beats missed?

  Infrequent: Mild Heart qi deficiency
  Frequent: Severe Heart qi-yang deficiency

Rate

See Chapter 7.

- SLOW: How slow?

Most frequently associated with qi deficiency, especially of the Heart and circulation, and not, in this day and age, with cold from excess, contrary to what is stated in the literature.

- FAST: How fast?

Most frequently associated with Heart qi agitation and shock. (Clinically, in our times, much less frequently found with heat from excess associated with an acute pathogenic factor, and infrequently with heat from deficiency.)

SIDES VARY IN RATE?

Associated with congenital anomalies or work situations involving extreme chronic physical distortion (see Chapter 7).

RATE AT END COMPARED WITH RATE AT BEGINNING

Large differences suggest either Heart qi deficiency, especially if the rate varies considerably during the exam or on exertion, or Heart qi agitation, if it is Rapid at first and Slower later and at the end of the examination.

RATE ON EXERTION: CONSISTENT OR NOT? SMALL OR LARGE?

Rate increases more than 8-12 beats per minute on exertion: An increase of more than 8 to 12 beats per minute on exertion is a sign of Heart blood deficiency, which is a slowly developing condition due to overwork, lack of sleep, and poor nutrition. The greater the increase, the greater the deficiency.

Rate stays the same, rises less than 8-12 beats, or decreases: With exertion (swinging one arm vigorously ten times) the pulse rate should normally increase between 8 and 12 beats per minute. When cardiovascular function cannot respond to the need for increased circulation, and the rate does not rise 8-12 beats per minute, stays the same, or decreases, the indication is Heart qi, and more likely Heart yang, deficiency.

With disharmonies of rhythm and rate

Check for other qualities that are associated with Heart dysfunction such as a Rough Vibration or Change in Intensity over the entire pulse.

Check the left distal and Heart complementary positions for:

Tense, Tight, Wiry, Inflated, Flat, Deep, Feeble, Absent, Change in Qualities or Intensity, Slippery, Vibration (Rough or Smooth), Unstable

Uniform qualities over the entire pulse

Qualities found most frequently over the entire pulse (Chapter 13) that are signs of lesser disharmony are the Tense, Tight, Thin, Smooth Vibration, mild Robust Pounding, Reduced Substance, Diffuse, inconsistent Change in Rate at Rest, Floating, Cotton, Flooding Deficient Wave, Suppressed and Hesitant Wave.

Qualities found over the entire pulse that reflect the most serious conditions, either existing or imminent, include alterations in rhythm (such as Interrupted and Intermittent), very Rapid and very Slow rates, large or minimal Changes in Rate on Exertion, Muffled, Empty, Scattered, Minute, Hollow, Interrupted-Intermittent, Rough Vibration (superficial or deep), Changes in Intensity, Changes in Qualities, Leather-like Hollow, Choppy, Blood Heat, Blood Unclear, Blood Thick, Ropy, Wiry, Slippery, Flooding Excess Wave, Full-Overflowing Wave, as well as the paradoxical findings listed above.

CLOSER FOCUS (DEPTHS, SIDES, WAVE FORMS)

See the appropriate chapters for a more complete discussion of individual qualities.

Depths

Above the qi depth

- EXTERNAL ETIOLOGY

These are signs of activity at the protective level. They are without a wave and include the Cotton quality from physical trauma, and the Floating qualities (Floating Tense and Slow, Floating Yielding and Rapid).

- INTERNAL ETIOLOGY

Without a wave: Floating Tight, Cotton (emotional resignation)
With a wave: Hollow Full-Overflowing, Flooding Excess

Qi depth

Qualities found at the qi depth (Chapter 13) are Diminished to Absent, Thin Tight, Thin Yielding, Taut, Tense, Tight, Wiry, Robust Pounding, Slippery, Vibration, Empty (all the Empty qualities)

Blood depth

Qualities found at the blood depth (Chapter 13) are Spreading (qi depth Absent), Yielding Partially Hollow (blood depth separating), Leather-like Hollow, Blood Unclear, Blood Heat, Blood Thick, Hollow Full-Overflowing, Slippery, Vibration at the blood depth, Pounding (Robust or Reduced).

Organ depth

Qualities found at the organ depth (Chapter 13) are Taut, Tense, Tight, Thin, Wiry, Slippery, Diffuse, Pounding Robust or Reduced, Feeble-Absent, Vibration (Smooth or Rough), Choppy, Muffled, Dead. The Tense Slippery quality found at this depth, and so frequently missed, is a sign of heat from excess and damp stagnation associated with chronic infection (parasites, hepatitis).

Sides

Uniform qualities found only on one side (Chapter 14) usually involve one of the 'systems,' in Dr. Shen's parlance. Frequently, in the earlier and middle stages of 'system' disharmonies, no one organ is found to be distressed, so that a search for problems in individual positions may be unrevealing.

Again, in my opinion the right side should be slightly stronger than the left in women, and the left side slightly stronger than the right in men. However, major differences in strength between the sides suggest a husband-wife disharmony, which, according to one five element school (with which I agree), is a sign of potential or current serious disease. This is a separation of yin and yang in terms of sides of the body, and is a form of chaos ('qi wild').

Left side

ENTIRE LEFT SIDE DEEP, FEEBLE-ABSENT, OR EMPTY

This is a sign that the 'organ system' is deficient, an overall diminishment of the most vital yin organs: Heart, Liver, and Kidneys.

In the very elderly, a deficient 'organ system' may be due to aging, but in others it is a sign that we are handicapped by constitutional factors, or by early insults (as during pregnancy, delivery, or infancy), by long-term illness, chronic excessive work, early malnutrition (e.g., in the various gulags and concentration camps), or child labor; with the latter there is often an irregular rhythm (Arrhythmic).

A constitutional etiology could be identified if both proximal positions (Kidneys) are extremely qi deficient (Deep, Feeble-Absent, Change in Intensity), especially if the person is relatively young (up to the age of 50). However, today we are finding these signs of Kidney deficiency in increasing numbers of young people, including children. Dr. Shen refers to this condition as 'nervous system weak.'[2]

One might inspect the right side to see if the source of the problem is digestion and nourishment, by examining the principal and complementary right middle positions. If the left side is Reduced and the right side Robust, we know that we can rely upon the 'digestive system' to help us in our efforts to restore function to the 'organ system.' If both sides are Reduced, the process of healing is more difficult.

ENTIRE LEFT SIDE IS THIN TIGHT AT THE SURFACE

This is a sign that the 'nervous system' is affecting the 'organ system.' The symptoms are usually both tension and fatigue. As for which system affected the other, one would first have to inquire as to which symptom came first. If tension is first, it is the 'nervous system' affecting the 'organ system'; if the earliest symptom is fatigue, it is the 'organ system' affecting the 'nervous system.'

Right side

ENTIRE RIGHT SIDE IS DEEP, FEEBLE, EMPTY

If the entire right side is Deep, Feeble, Empty, the indication is of a 'digestive system' deficiency and a potential lack of nourishment from air, food, and stored essence. The causes are usually irregular eating habits such as not eating when hungry or eating when not hungry. Anorexia, bulimia, extreme diets and severe nutritional deprivation as a young child are other etiologies. One would search for the most deficient organ: Lungs, Spleen (middle principal and complementary positions), or Kidneys, although usually in the earlier stages of system disharmonies no single organ is found to be disturbed.

Examine especially those complementary positions associated with the Spleen-Stomach and Intestines including the Esophagus, Spleen, Stomach-Pylorus Extension, Peritoneum, and Duodenum positions.

ENTIRE RIGHT SIDE WITH A THIN TIGHT LINE AT SURFACE

This is a sign of overworking of the nerves of the 'digestive system,' usually due to eating too rapidly; this is frequently due to a 'nervous system tense' condition affecting the 'digestive system.' One would especially check the Liver (left middle position very Tense) for signs of emotional tension affecting the 'digestive system' (Liver attacking the Spleen), although, as just noted, often in the earlier stages of 'system' disharmonies no one organ is found to be disturbed. The question concerning which system is affecting the other can also be determined by asking which came first, the tension or the digestive disorder.

Intensity shifting from side to side

If the Changes in Intensity occur first on one side and then on the other, we must consider especially the presence of a strong current interpersonal conflict, or that recently (during the past few weeks or months) this person engaged in some physical activity that was considerably beyond their capacity.

Qualities shifting from side to side

When the qualities are shifting from side to side we are usually dealing with a 'qi wild' condition of considerable magnitude which I have encountered only rarely in connection with advanced stages of auto-immune disorders such as Lupus Erythematosus and other chronic, usually fatal, diseases.

Wave form

We are concerned about the wave form as part of the larger picture, since deviations from the norm also direct us to more serious or compelling issues.

Flooding Deficient Wave

This is a sign of moderate qi deficiency. Although the source could be general, from working long hours or insomnia, one must examine individual positions for the primary origins of deficiency. One searches for such qualities as Deep, Absent, Empty, and Changes in Quality and Intensity, which are indications of the failure of a yin organ that is draining the entire organism. This is the physical form of what Dr. Shen calls the 'push pulse.'

Hesitant Wave

This quality represents the mental form of the 'push pulse' which I find associated with obsessional states of mind, sometimes of monomaniacal proportions. Often we find this quality in patients who are preoccupied with their health, though the quality itself suggests the tendency to become fixated on a single idea.

Flooding Excess Wave

If the pulse wave is Flooding Excess we must search for the individual positions, or the blood, for the source of an infection. If the rate is Rapid, the cause is current or very recent, and if Slower, the infection is more chronic. Slipperiness and heavy Robust Pounding at the organ depth are often adjunctive indications of infection.

Hollow Full-Overflowing Wave

The cause of this is usually 'Blood heat' or 'Blood thick.' Look for signs of tension and heat (Tense-Tight quality) and turbulence of blood (Slippery at the blood depth, especially at the left middle position), as well as congestion of blood at the Liver Engorgement positions. Also look for signs of dampness (Slippery) and heat (Tension, Pounding) in the Spleen-Stomach (left middle, Spleen, Stomach-Pylorus Extension, Peritoneal, Duodenum, and Gall Bladder positions), and a 'nervous system tense' condition (entire pulse or most positions Tense, or Tense to Tight if the condition has existed for a long time).

Suppressed Wave and Suppressed Pounding

If found over the entire pulse, these are indications of the current use of chemicals, such as medications. One is a wave that is cut off at the top so that it feels as if it has not rounded off against one's finger. Recently I have observed this with suppressed emotions. The other sign of the use of chemicals is Robust Pounding at the organ depth, which drops off precipitously at the blood and qi depths.

Areas

Areas refer to the three burners, each as a unit, rather than to their constituent organs; to the Neuro-psychological positions; to the Special Lung positions; to the diaphragm area as indicated by the Diaphragm positions; and to the pelvic organs and structure as indicated by the Pelvis/Lower Body positions. For example, a similar quality in both the right and left middle positions—Wiry, for example—might indicate pancreatitis rather than a specific disharmony in the Liver and Spleen.

The following qualities are most frequently found bilaterally in these areas.

Diaphragm

Inflated, Rough, Slippery, and less often Tight and Hollow Full-Overflowing. (See Chapter 12.)

Pelvis/Lower Body

Tense, Tight, Slippery, Choppy, Muffled, Change in Intensity. (See Chapter 12.)

Burners

EXISTENTIAL

The reader is referred to the discussion of the three burners at the end of Chapter 15.

Specific: similar qualities bilaterally at burners

Examine the burners to see if there is a quality bilaterally in one burner that is distinctly different from the other burners and positions. (See Chapter 14, Table 14-1.) If there is, that has a special significance involving the entire area of that burner, as well as the organs in that burner. For example, if there is a Cotton quality at both distal positions, the source is recent emotional stress that is causing a superficial stagnation in the entire chest.

Among many other qualities in these positions, one sometimes finds an Inflated or Flat quality at both distal positions, an Empty quality at both middle positions, or a Wiry quality at both proximal positions. Each of these has a special meaning which is different than if they appeared at only one individual position in the same burner. (For further information, see Chapter 14.)

If we find deficiency in the upper and lower burners, we must look at the middle burner for signs of stagnation due either to excess or deficiency. The deficiency in the other burners can be more apparent than real due to the middle blocking connections between the upper and lower; this is known as the Short quality. The Short quality can be due to excess or deficiency. With excess, the middle burner would be Robust, and with deficiency, it would be Reduced. Therefore, despite the signs of deficiency, we would consider treating for stagnation, especially if treatment for deficiency had been tried and was unsuccessful.

Upper burner, bilaterally	Floating, Cotton, Hollow Full-Overflowing, Inflated, Tense, Tight, Wiry, Flat, Slippery, Thin, Feeble-Absent, Vibration, Change in Intensity or Qualities

Middle burner, bilaterally	Floating, Cotton, Hollow Full-Overflowing, Inflated, Tense, Tight, Wiry, Flat, Slippery, Thin, Feeble-Absent, Vibration, Empty, Yielding Partially Hollow, Change in Intensity or Qualities
Lower burner, bilaterally	Tense, Tight, Wiry, Hollow Full-Overflowing, Flooding Excess, Deep, Thin, Feeble-Absent, Change in Intensity or Qualities

Examples

Upper burner	If both distal positions are Flat or Inflated, compare the finding with the person's age. In a person under the age of 40, the causes of the Flat quality are either severe disappointment and loss during childhood, or a nuchal cord. In an older person it suggests a more recent trauma to the chest. If both distal positions are Inflated in a young person, the cause is more likely to be a breech birth; in an older person, sudden extreme but repressed anger, lifting beyond one's energy, and emphysema should be considered.
Middle burner	If both middle positions are Empty, check the age of the person. Of the many possible causes for such a finding, with a younger person the cause is more likely to be early impoverishment (rare but still possible in the West), anorexia or bulimia (especially in women), trauma, lifting after eating (more likely in a man), drug abuse, and parasites. For an older person the more common etiologies are sitting in one position for a long time, persistent worry while eating, and pancreatic disturbance.
Lower burner	If both proximal positions are Wiry, in a younger person this could represent pain due to blood stagnation in the pelvis or lower body, possibly due to trauma, with considerable pain. In an older person one would consider early hypertension, diabetes, or a kidney stone with pain.

Systems

There are four systems identified by Dr. Shen: the 'nervous system,' digestive system,' 'circulatory system,' and 'organ system' (Chapter 13). Dr. Shen developed the systems model to explain the relatively mild and shifting complaints of patients who showed no signs of illness either by Chinese or biomedical diagnostic methods. A search for problems in individual positions is unrevealing.

Two of the systems ('organ' and 'digestive') are mentioned above in our discussion of sides. The 'nervous system' is either tense or weak, the first associated with lifelong or stress-related tension due to hyper-vigilance, and the second, weak, associated with lifelong physical and emotional constitutional vulnerability. The 'circulatory system' is marked by occasional migrating joint pain, quick to anger, and a Slow pulse with no other signs.

Psychology

In this category we include all mental, emotional, and spiritual issues which are discussed in Chapter 15. Briefly, and by way of example, the Cotton quality indicates a state of emotional resignation. Change in Rate at Rest indicates a restless mental and emotional state associated with Heart qi agitation, the Hesitant quality with an obsessive-compulsive condition, or Smooth Vibration associated with either transient worry or a personality marked by worry, depending on the extent of the Smooth Vibration. The existential issues discussed above under the aegis of 'burners,' the awareness implications of the Slippery quality at the left distal position, and the suggestion of depression with a mild Muffled quality at the same position, are other examples.

CLOSEST FOCUS

General considerations

We have discussed these above in the 'quick overview' section.

Specific considerations

This encompasses the interpretation of individual and complementary positions and their relationships. Below are the qualities and conditions associated with the individual principal and complementary positions and their related organs. The presence of pathology in the complementary positions associated with an organ informs me that the disease process in that organ is more advanced and serious than otherwise.

Each organ is considered in terms of the most and least common qualities and the most frequently encountered conditions. (See Chapter 12 for more detail.) A trend has been observed by many that the qualities which are more serious and were once uncommon are now becoming more common, especially those indicating the separation of yin and yang (Change in Qualities) and parenchymal damage (Rough Vibration).

Later, within the context of these individual positions, we consider the relationships between them. We ask ourselves if the Liver is affecting the Spleen (or vice versa), whether stagnation in the Lungs could create deficiency in the Heart, or deficiency in the Heart lead to Lung qi and damp stagnation. Is there evidence of a Kidney-Heart disharmony with the left distal or proximal positions being either especially Tight (yin deficient) or especially Feeble (qi deficient)? Generally, but not exclusively, the source of the problem is the position where there is the greatest chaos or deficiency.

Organs: principal and complementary positions

See Chapter 12.

Relationships between individual positions

See Chapter 12.

Chronic disease

The organs showing the greatest chaos or deficiency (Empty, Feeble) are most likely to be identified with the etiology or root of a chronic disease process. Often in chronic disease, but less reliably, those positions and associated organs with the harder qualities (very Tense, Tight, or Wiry) may reflect the secondary or branch issues. We often find the highest degree of current compelling symptomatology in those organs associated with these branch-related organs. One example is cardiac asthma in which the left distal and Heart-related complementary positions can show signs of considerable deficiency (e.g., Feeble-Absent) while the right distal (Lung) and Special Lung positions are Tense-Tight, Slippery, Inflated, and have Rough Vibration. The obvious symptoms are Lung related, though the root condition is in the Heart.

Acute disease

In acute diseases the organs associated with positions with the most Robust or hard qualities are probably the source (root), and the less Robust or hard qualities are secondary (branch). For example, a recently appearing very Tense-Tight quality at the left middle (Liver) position caused by a current new stress can cause a mildly Tense Inflated quality (stagnation) at the right middle (Spleen-Stomach) position in the syndrome known as Liver attacking Spleen (the controlling cycle of the five phases). In this case, the symptoms would again be in the organ-associated secondary aspect of the process, with more acute indigestion, abdominal pain, and signs of Stomach heat such as penetrating frontal headaches, mouth ulcers, bad breath, nausea, and vomiting.

REVISITING BROAD/CLOSER/CLOSEST FOCUS

Finally, one returns to the broader initial impressions and searches again for connections between those qualities and the findings in the individual positions. As a reminder, for example, a Deep right side and clear signs on the right middle position would indicate that the condition affecting digestion goes beyond the Spleen to include the Kidneys and Lungs. Liver qi stagnation is often rooted in a 'nervous system tense' condition, with Tension over the entire pulse, perhaps exaggerated in the left middle position.

INTERPRETATION

Summary of findings

This is a summary of specific diagnostic categories or conditions culled from the previous diagnostic impressions. For example: qi deficiency, blood stagnation, Lung damp-heat.

Formulation

The formulation is based on the summary.

CURRENT PREVAILING ISSUES OR PATTERNS

As shown in the case histories, these are the diagnostic categories which require more immediate intervention, including emergencies and urgent matters such as imminent hemorrhage, acute diseases, and various forms of intolerable pain, physical and emotional. The latter includes threatened suicide or homicide.

ROOT ISSUES AND ETIOLOGY OF DISHARMONIES

These are the fundamental patterns which underlie the patient's condition and which are often the least obvious without the aid of the pulse.

DERIVATIVE ISSUES ('BRANCHES')

These are the resulting conditions, which are often the most obvious in the form of symptomatology, but misleading in terms of essential pathological process.

Primary derivative issues

These may require some immediate attention in terms of relieving serious symptoms such as pain, vomiting, diarrhea, and severe itching.

Secondary derivative issues

These are the less serious and incapacitating symptoms and conditions for which attention can be delayed.

ANALYSIS AND SYNTHESIS

Here we attempt to present a coherent statement of the patient's overall condition and the factors that led to it. We will relate the current, root, and derivative issues to each other to form a single explanation of this person's physiology, pathology, and being.

Management

The following is based first on the pulse as an exercise, but the final management is deferred until the integration of the pulse with the patient's history, symptoms, and other signs.

LIFESTYLE STRATEGIES

These are recommendations for changes in the patient's lifestyle which have led to their current state of mental, emotional, spiritual, and physical health.

REFERRALS

These are made for diagnostic or treatment purposes that will enhance those already available to the practitioner within their own scope of practice.

ACUPUNCTURE, HERBAL, AND OTHER HEALING STRATEGIES

Immediate interventions

These involve those treatments which place more emphasis on relieving current symptomatology, combined with some treatment aimed at the underlying root condition, as circumstances will allow.

Intermediate interventions

Here the emphasis shifts to the root problems while continuing to relieve debilitating symptoms.

Long-range major interventions

With the major relief of the debilitating derivative problems the treatment strategy moves primarily to the enduring root issues.

Long-range minor interventions

These involve disharmonious conditions which are important to resolve over the long term, but which are not the primary sources of the patient's pathology. The Cotton quality, and the superficial stagnation it reflects, would be an example of a condition probably not primary to the patient's current dilemma, but which, if not resolved, could cause great difficulties such as cancer in the distant future.

Review patient's history and complaints

Relate pulse as explanation and clarification of specific symptoms.

Amend previous synthesis

Here we integrate the patient's history, symptoms, and pulse and alter our management recommendations accordingly.

CONCLUSION

This chapter has been concerned with the method of interpreting the data revealed by palpation of the radial pulse. Teaching this skill with the written word is unavoidably complex and repetitious. This methodology is illustrated in two patient records set forth in an appendix to this chapter. Each case uses a slightly different approach, while holding true to the basic principles of bringing the pulse signs into a coherent picture of the patient's physiology, pathology, history, prognosis, and management.

The process of learning involves a dynamic interplay between the didactic material found in these chapters and direct, practical experience. While some rote learning is required, the acquisition of this skill involves a gradual absorption and integration of experience below direct consciousness, interrupted by epiphanies of great insight and awareness, and by the diligent application of the rational and intuitive tools with which we are all blessed in different quantities and qualities. For the serious student, I would advise analyzing the cases in the appendix before consulting the listed interpretation.

The work is not as difficult in practice as implied by the inescapable attention to detail found in this book. The reward for the dedicated practitioner is a world of exciting and very useful knowledge, and as far beyond our routine diagnostic assessments as the observation of a drop of water was to scientists after the invention of the microscope.

Table 17-1   Methodology for interpretation

I. Quick Overview of the Entire Pulse
   Sex and age in terms of what is appropriate or paradoxical
   Unusual qualities
   Paradoxical findings

II. Broad Focus and Closer Focus
   In-depth evaluation
      A. Observations
         1. Rhythm and rate: outstanding abnormalities
         2. Uniform qualities
         3. Unusual wave form
         4. Above qi, qi, blood, and organ depths
         5. Areas
             Neuro-psychological
             Burners: similar qualities bilaterally at upper, middle, and lower
             Diaphragm
             Pelvis/lower body
         6. Sides
         7. Systems
             'Nervous system'
             'Circulatory system'
             'Digestive system'
             'Organ system'
         8. Stability
             Separation of yin and yang
             'Qi wild'
             Blood out of control (hemorrhage)
      B. Diagnostic impressions

III. Closest Focus

A. Substances
   1. Qi
   2. Yin
   3. Yang
   4. Blood
   5. Dampness
   6. Wind
   7. Food
   8. Essence
   9. Parenchyma

B. Activity
   1. Heat
      Excess
      Deficiency
   2. Cold
      Excess: internal, external
      Deficiency

C. Organs (principal and complementary positions)
   1. Heart-circulation
   2. Lungs
   3. Liver
   4. Spleen-Stomach
   5. Kidneys

D. Diagnostic impressions

IV. Psychology

Mind, emotion, and spirit

V. Interpretation

Initial formations are not set in stone and serve primarily as a starting point for a flexible process that increases with precision in the course of the success and failure of treatment strategies. Consider multiple etiologies.

A. Summary of specific diagnostic categories
B. Formulation
   1. Current prevailing issues
   2. Root issues and etiology of disharmonies
   3. Derivative issues
      a. Primary derivative issues
      b. Secondary derivative issues
   4. Analysis and synthesis of significant patterns and overall diagnostic concept

VI. Management

A. Lifestyle strategies
B. Referrals
C. Acupuncture, herbs, and other healing strategies

For the sake of discussion these strategies are separated into stages that in reality must be flexible and generously blended as the clinical situation unfolds into a clearer diagnostic picture:
1. Immediate interventions

If these interventions succeed, proceed to the next step:
2. Intermediate interventions

If these interventions succeed, proceed to the next step:
3. Long-range minor and major interventions

VII. Client History and Integration with Pulse Interpretation
   A. Client history—age, gender, occupation
      1. Chief complaints
      2. Medical history
         a. Review of systems
         b. Habits
         c. Childhood
         d. Family
   B. Symptoms and the pulse
      1. Analysis of symptoms with pulse diagnosis
      2. Amendments to analysis and synthesis of significant patterns and diagnostic concepts

APPENDIX

Case Illustrations

Introduction

Two case histories are presented in this appendix as exercises in interpretation. They follow the procedures used in actual classes that I teach on the pulse to practitioners of Chinese medicine. The first case is based on a personal consultation. The second case was selected at random from one of my seminars. The 'asking' aspect of Chinese diagnosis is neglected almost as much as the pulse. This neglect is reflected in the difference in detail between the histories of the first case, when I took the history, and the second case, when I did not.

I suggest that you begin by reading and analyzing the pulse record (chart) through the section on management, but not the client history, in accordance with the precepts that are set forth in Chapter 17 and in Fig. 17-1. Then compare your analysis and management recommendations with those presented here, and use the comparison to explore aspects that you may have overlooked. (It is of course possible that you may discover issues that I have missed, in which case a message to my website would be appreciated.)

Next, read the client history and its correlation with the pulse. In the context of my classes, the goal here is to explain the patient's problems based on the findings from the pulse so as to provide the referring practitioner with a fresh perspective on a clinical situation which has thus far resisted their efforts to resolve. Again, compare your findings with mine. Additional case illustrations will be posted from time to time on my website, *www.dragonrises.com*.

Figure 18-1 Case 1: Female, Age 27

P = Present   ---- = Absent   (1 → 5) = Difficulty of access by degree: 1=low, 5=high

Name:	Gender: Female	Age: 27	Date:	Refer:
Weight: 160 Height: 5' 10" Occup: Housewife				

Rhythm: Interrupted (Arrhythmic about 5x/min)

First Impressions of Uniform Qualities

  Entire Pulse: Thin; Tense-Tight; Robust Pounding (2); Rough Vibration at all depths; Change in Intensity (2)

  Sides, Left: -------

     Right: -------

Principal Positions

  Distal Position

   Left (Pericardium):
   Tense: Slippery (4-5)

   Right:
   Tight; Rough Vibration; Slippery

  Middle Position

   Left:
   Reduced Substance ⟷ Thin
   Qi depth: Tight-Tense
   Blood depth: Thick; Slippery; Rough Vibration (2)
   Organ depth: Tense-Tight

   Right:
   Tense; Robust Pounding (4)

  Proximal Position

   Left:
   Tight ⟷ Absent
   Qi depth: Diminished

   Right:
   Qi depth: Diminished
   Tight
   Change in Intensity (2)

 Three Burners
  Same Qualities Bilaterally

   Upper: Slippery

   Middle: -------

   Lower: Tight

 Other:

Rate/Min:	**Begin:**	60
	End:	66
	W/exertion:	72
OTHER RATES DURING EXAM:		

Three Depths

  Above qi depth: Cotton (3-4)
  Qi depth: Tense-Tight
  Blood depth: Thick
  Organ depth: Tense

Wave: Normal → Flooding Deficient

Complementary Positions

  Neuro-psychological
   Left: Smooth Vibration; Doughy

   Right: Smooth Vibration; Doughy

  Heart
   Mitral Valve: Slippery
   Large Vessels: -------
   Enlarged: P

  Lung
   Special Lung position
    Left: Tight; Rough Vibration; Slippery

    Right: Tight; Rough Vibration; Slippery
   Pleura: -------

  Diaphragm, Left: Inflated (1-2)
           Right: Inflated (1-2)

  Liver
   Engorged, Radial: ?
              Ulnar: -------
              Distal: P
   Gallbladder: Tight; Slippery

  Spleen-Stomach
   Esophagus: -------
   Spleen: -------
   Stomach-Pylorus Extension: -------
   Peritoneum-Pancreas: -------
   Duodenum: -------

  Intestines
   Large: Tense; Slippery
   Small: Tight; Biting; Slippery

  Pelvis/Lower Body
   Left: Change in Intensity (5); Muffled
   Right: Change in Intensity (5); Choppy

Case 1 Female, Age 27

Broad Focus

INITIAL IMPRESSION OF LARGE SEGMENTS AND UNIFORM QUALITIES

Rhythm

The rhythm is Interrupted, irregularly skipping beats approximately five times per minute. Ordinarily this would be a sign of moderate Heart qi deficiency, but since we are still able to get the rate we would evaluate this finding by itself as severe Heart qi agitation with mild Heart qi deficiency.

Rate

The initial rate is only 60 beats/minute and 66 at the end. On exertion the rate goes up six points to 72. The Slow rate in a 27-year-old woman is a sign of Heart qi deficiency, and the increase of only six beats on vigorous exertion is borderline for mild Heart qi deficiency.

Uniform qualities over the entire pulse

COMMON QUALITIES

The Tense-Tight combination is a sign of qi stagnation and heat from excess (Tense) and developing heat from deficiency (Tight). If the principal positions bear out the Tense-Tight quality, a 'nervous system tense' condition is possible, with the origin most likely being constitutional since the rate is Slow.

Robust Pounding (2) is a mild sign of heat from excess which the body is unable to eliminate completely through the normal processes.

The Thin quality is a sign of blood deficiency.

LESS COMMON QUALITIES

Rough Vibration over the entire pulse at all depths is a sign of Heart shock and possibly Heart qi deficiency.

Change in Intensity over the entire pulse (2) is another mild sign of Heart qi deficiency.

UNUSUAL QUALITIES

See 'rhythm' above.

PARADOXICAL QUALITIES

'Blood thick' is a form of blood heat and congestion that is rarely found in a young woman.

A rate rising 6 beats/minute on exertion is a paradoxical finding in a 27-year-old woman.

The developing Flooding Deficient wave is a sign of growing true qi deficiency, an unusual though mild sign in a 27-year-old woman.

The Interrupted and Change in Intensity qualities are evidence of considerable instability related almost entirely to the Heart/circulatory system.

Were the quality primarily Tight in a 27-year-old woman, one would consider pain as the cause, perhaps from arthritis.

Closer Focus

Depths

ABOVE THE QI DEPTH

Cotton quality

This is a sign of superficial qi stagnation associated with either a major physical trauma, or more often, a sense of resignation with regard to a less than satisfactory life situation.

QI DEPTH

Tense-Tight quality, as above.

BLOOD DEPTH

Blood Thick is a sign of turbidity in the blood that could be implicated in part in the Slow circulation.

ORGAN DEPTH

Tense quality, as above.

Sides

Nothing significant

Three burners

Nothing significant

SUMMARY OF INITIAL IMPRESSIONS

The principal finding here are the signs of Heart qi deficiency, Heart shock, and Heart qi agitation, including the Interrupted rhythm, Slow rate, Rough Vibration at all depths, and the Change in Intensity, over the entire pulse.

The Tense-Tight quality is a sign of a 'nervous system tense' condition moving at a rather young age from a heat from excess (Robust Pounding) to a heat from deficiency condition (Tense to Tight). Blood deficiency is evidenced by the Thin quality. There is considerable superficial qi stagnation (Cotton), general moderate qi deficiency (Flooding Deficient Wave), and 'blood thick' (Blood Thick quality), which is a sign of turbidity in the blood circulation.

Closest Focus (Individual Positions and Organs)

RAPID OVERVIEW

All of the principal positions were either Tense (qi stagnation and heat from excess), Tight (yin heat from deficiency), or somewhere between these two qualities (Tense-Tight or Tight-Tense), which indicates the presence of both excess and heat from deficiency. The complementary position is not mentioned when the qualities are Normal.

Unusual qualities

The presence of the Heart Enlarged position is probably the most unusual and potentially serious sign. The Muffled quality at the Pelvis/Lower Body position is relatively unusual and is a sign of extreme stagnation of all substances. It is often associated with tumors.

Instability: where there is the most activity and change

The most change can be found in the left proximal (Tight Absent) and left middle positions, which show Reduced Substance becoming very Thin. The Change in Intensity is extreme at the right Neuro-psychological and Pelvis/Lower Body positions, indicating serious physiological disturbance respectively in the central nervous system and organs of the lower burner.

Other more serious qualities

The Choppy quality at the Pelvis/Lower Body position (blood stagnation in the lower burner), and the Doughy quality at the Neuro-psychological positions (disturbance of essence), are potentially serious signs.

The Slippery quality at both distal positions is a sign of phlegm in the chest, Heart, and Lungs. Rough Vibration at the right distal (Lung alveolar damage and qi deficiency) and blood depth of the left middle positions (damage to the intima of the vessels) are serious signs.

Paradoxical findings

All of the above are paradoxical in a 27-year-old woman, especially an enlarged Heart position.

INDIVIDUAL POSITIONS (PRINCIPAL AND COMPLEMENTARY)

Heart/circulation

The Slippery quality at the left distal position is a sign of phlegm blocking the Heart orifices. The presence of the Heart Enlarged position, and the Slippery quality at the Mitral Valve position, are signs of Heart qi deficiency. The Smooth Vibration quality at the Neuro-psychological positions is a sign of Heart qi agitation.

Lungs

The Tight quality at the right distal position and at the Special Lung positions is a sign of Lung yin deficiency. The Slippery quality at both of these positions is a sign of Lung damp stagnation, and the Rough Vibration quality at both positions is a sign of Lung qi deficiency and parenchymal damage.

Liver-Gallbladder

This position has Reduced Substance and is becoming very Thin, which indicates developing Liver qi and blood deficiency. One position is Engorged, indicating some slight blood stagnation in the Liver. The Gallbladder shows signs of damp-heat (Slippery, Tight). In this position the Tight quality is usually a sign of moderate inflammation. The Change in Qualities from Tight-Tense to Reduced Substance to Thin suggests that the Liver yin and yang are in an early stage of separating.

Spleen/Stomach/Intestines

The Robust Pounding quality at this position, and the Biting and Slippery qualities at the Intestine positions, are indications of heat from excess and dampness (irritation or inflammation) in the gastro-intestinal tract. This is in keeping with the finding of inflammation in the Gallbladder.

Kidneys/Bladder

There are signs of Kidney yin (Tight quality) and qi deficiency (Absent quality). The Change in Intensity (2) is the same as that mentioned under 'initial impressions.' The Change in Qualities at the left proximal position, from Tight to Absent, is a sign that Kidney yin and yang are separating.

SUMMARY OF INITIAL IMPRESSIONS OF INDIVIDUAL POSITIONS

We must consider an enlarged Heart with phlegm blocking the Heart orifices and Heart yang deficiency, damp-heat in the Lungs, damp-heat and damage to the intima of the blood vessels, heat from excess and inflammation of the gastro-intestinal system, Kidney-Liver qi deficiency, chaotic Kidney qi, and tumor in the pelvic area.

Substances (includes broad, closer, and closest focus)

Qi

Stagnation

EXTERNAL

The Cotton quality (3-4) is a sign of external qi stagnation, discussed above and below.

INTERNAL

The Tense quality is a sign of internal qi stagnation, which pervades the entire pulse.

Deficiency

The Flooding Deficient wave is a sign of general qi deficiency. The Change in Intensity over the entire pulse, the Slow rate, the Slippery quality at the Mitral Valve position, the Interrupted rhythm, the rise on exertion of the rate of only 6 beats/min., and the presence of the enlarged positions are signs of Heart qi deficiency. Other signs of qi deficiency are found in the Lung (Rough Vibration), Liver (Reduced Substance), and Kidneys (Absent).

Blood

Stagnation

The Choppy quality at the Pelvis/Lower Body position is a sign of blood stagnation in the pelvis, and the presence of the distal Engorged position indicates mild blood stagnation in the Liver. The Blood Thick quality is a sign of blood stagnation in the general circulation and turbulence (Slippery at the blood depth).

Deficiency

The Thin quality mentioned under 'initial impressions' is a sign of blood deficiency.

Yin

Excess (dampness)

The Slippery quality is a sign of damp stagnation in the Heart, Lungs, Gallbladder, and Intestines. The Slippery quality at the Mitral Valve position is a sign of valve prolapse and regurgitation of blood. The Slippery quality at the blood depth is a sign of turbulence in the blood. The Muffled quality suggests stagnation of all substances at a cellular level, and dampness in the pelvis and lower burner.

Deficiency

The Tight quality found especially in the Lungs and the Kidneys is a sign of yin deficiency. Generally, and in several positions, the Tense-Tight qualities appear, indicating a trend toward yin deficiency.

Yang

Excess

None

Deficiency

The presence of the Enlarged Heart position could be a sign of developing Heart yang deficiency. The Interrupted quality, and the increase of less than 8 beats/minute (6 on exertion), could be another indication of the same trend. The Absent quality and Change in Qualities at the left proximal position is an indication of a trend toward Kidney yang deficiency.

Essence

The Doughy quality at the Neuro-psychological positions, and the Change in Qualities at the left proximal position from Tight to Absent, are signs of yang-essence deficiency.

Parenchyma

The Rough Vibration at the right distal and Special Lung positions is a sign of parenchymal damage to the alveoli of the lung.

Activity

Heat

Excess

The Tense quality throughout the pulse, Robust Pounding, and Blood Thick qualities are signs of heat from excess.

Deficiency

The Tight quality found at the right distal, Special Lung, and proximal positions is a sign of heat from yin deficiency.

Combined excess and heat from deficiency

The Tense-Tight and Tight-Tense qualities, found generally and at the left middle position, are signs of simultaneous excess and heat from deficiency.

Cold

Excess

If accompanied by pain, the Tight quality is sometimes a sign of cold from excess, especially in the lower burner (proximal positions). This is a rare finding in the modern world.

Deficient

Cold from deficiency is equivalent to yang deficiency, one piece of evidence for which is the occasionally Absent quality and Change in Qualities at the left proximal position. The presence of the Enlarged Heart position could be a sign of developing Heart yang deficiency. The Interrupted quality, and increase of less than 8 beats per minute (6 on exertion), could be another indication of the same trend.

Areas

BURNERS: SIMILAR QUALITIES BILATERALLY AT SAME BURNER

Upper burner — The Slippery quality bilaterally at both distal positions is a sign of dampness in the chest. Emotionally, this could also indicate some inhibition of the normal impulse to open one's heart and arms to the world.

Middle burner — None

Lower burner — The presence of both the Tight quality and Diminished quality at the qi depth reflects the simultaneous presence of Kidney yin and qi deficiency.

Diaphragm — The bilateral minimal Inflation (1-2) at the Diaphragm position is a sign that there is *no* current ongoing stress associated with separation and the acrimonious suppression of tender feelings associated with it.

Pelvis/Lower Body — The extreme Change in Intensity (5), and the Muffled and Choppy qualities bilaterally, are signs of extreme stagnation of qi and blood and physiological disorganization in the female pelvic organs.

Sides

The left side is slightly more robust than the right, but not sufficiently to make any inferences.

Systems

'Nervous system'

The ubiquitous Tense or Tense-Tight quality at this pulse suggests a 'nervous system tense' condition, probably of constitutional origin because of the Slow pulse rate.

'Circulatory system'

The Slow pulse rate and the Rough Vibration quality at all depths over the entire pulse are signs of impairment of the 'circulatory system,' the latter due probably to shock.

Interpretation

SUMMARY OF SPECIFIC DIAGNOSTIC CATEGORIES

- Heart qi/yang deficiency with Mitral Valve prolapse & enlargement
- Heart qi agitation
- Phlegm obstructing orifices of the Heart, and dampness in the chest
- 'Circulatory system' deficient
- 'Nervous system tense'
- 'Blood thick,' turbulence in the blood, and vessel wall damage
- Blood, qi, and probably damp stagnation in the lower burner (Pelvis/Lower Body position)
- Blood deficiency
- General qi stagnation and deficiency
- Lung yin and qi deficiency and stagnation of dampness
- Liver blood and qi deficiency and blood congestion
- Gallbladder damp-heat
- Moderate inflammation and heat from excess and dampness (irritation and inflammation) in the gastro-intestinal tract
- Kidney yin, essence, and qi/yang deficiency; separation of Kidney yin and yang
- External qi stagnation (moderate)

DIAGNOSTIC FORMULATION

It must be clear at the beginning of this discussion of diagnosis that one's initial formulations are not set in stone. They serve primarily as a starting point for a flexible process that becomes increasingly precise over the course of treatment, which is part of the diagnostic process.

Current prevailing issues

EXCESS DAMP-HEAT IN GALLBLADDER AND GASTRO-INTESTINAL SYSTEM

The Tight and Slippery qualities in the Gallbladder and Intestines, the Biting quality in the Intestines, and the Robust Pounding (4) at the right middle position (Stomach) are signs of heat from excess in the gastro-intestinal system.

BLOOD STAGNATION AND ORGAN DYSFUNCTION IN THE LOWER BURNER

The Muffled and Choppy qualities, and the great Change in Intensity (5) at the Pelvis/Lower Body positions, suggest an active pathological process.

PHLEGM OBSTRUCTING THE ORIFICES OF THE HEART, HEART QI AGITATION

The Slippery quality at the left (and right) distal positions, and the minimal Interrupted quality, are signs that are consistent with current emotional disturbances.

BLOOD THICK, TURBULENCE IN THE BLOOD (SLIPPERY AT BLOOD DEPTH), AND VESSEL WALL DAMAGE (ROUGH VIBRATION AT BLOOD DEPTH)

These findings are probably related to the Heart qi deficiency, to the 'nervous system tense' condition, and to the damp-heat in the Gallbladder, Intestines, and Stomach. They compound the more critical Heart deficiencies and stagnation.

EXTERNAL QI STAGNATION (MODERATE)

The Cotton quality is sufficiently strong to suggest that either this young woman is resigning herself to a lifestyle which is harmful to her health, and/or she has experienced a major trauma.

Root Issues and Etiology of Disharmonies

Heart qi-yang deficiency with Mitral Valve prolapse and enlargement

The Interrupted quality, Change in Intensity, Rough Vibration over the entire pulse, Slow rate, enlarged Heart, failure of the rate to increase more than 8 beats per minute (6 on exertion), and Slippery quality at the Mitral Valve position are all signs of Heart qi-yang deficiency. For this degree of disharmony in a 27-year-old woman, the suggestion is either a constitutional or congenital insult, or rheumatic heart disease. The seriousness of this condition is reflected in the ability to get the rate.

Kidney yin, essence, and qi-yang deficiency

The Change in Qualities at the left proximal position back and forth from Tight to Absent suggests both Kidney qi and yin deficiency. This is a sign that Kidney yin and yang are separating. The Doughy quality at the Neuro-psychological positions is a sign of Kidney yang-essence deficiency. The Change in Intensity has been associated with dizziness and extreme Changes in Intensity, probably indicating more extensive essence efficiency.

'Nervous system tense' condition

The prevailing Tense-Tight quality over the entire pulse is a sign of a 'nervous system tense' condition, probably of constitutional origin because of the Slow pulse.

Derivative issues

PRIMARY DERIVATIVE ISSUES

Lung yin and qi deficiency and damp-heat stagnation

The Tight quality at the right distal and Special Lung positions is a sign of Lung yin deficiency. The Rough Vibration quality at both positions is a sign of Lung qi deficiency and alveolar insufficiency, while the Slippery quality is a sign of Lung damp stagnation.

Liver blood and qi deficiency and blood congestion

The Reduced Substance quality at the left middle position is a sign of early Liver qi deficiency, and the Thin quality which alternates with the Reduced Substance quality is a sign of Liver blood deficiency. The clear presence of one Blood Engorgement position suggests blood congestion, which is usually secondary to Liver qi deficiency and stagnation or heat from excess in the blood. The Change in Qualities from Tight-Tense to Reduced Substance to Thin suggests that Liver yin and yang are separating. In a 27-year-old woman, one would suspect a history of substance abuse, hepatitis, or mononucleosis, although lack of sleep and overwork could contribute to this finding.

SECONDARY DERIVATIVE ISSUES

General qi stagnation and deficiency

Signs of general qi stagnation are the general Tense quality. The Muffled quality at the Pelvis/Lower Body positions is a sign of stagnation at a cellular-molecular level of function. The evidence for qi deficiency can be found in the signs listed above for the Heart, Lung, Liver, and Kidneys of qi deficiency and the Flooding Deficient Wave.

Blood deficiency

Blood deficiency is evidenced by the initial impression of an overall Thin quality, borne out on further examination by the Thin quality at the left middle position.

Analysis and synthesis

The primary vulnerability for this woman is her Heart qi and yang deficiency within a setting of a probable inherited 'nervous system tense' condition and Heart shock (Rough Vibration). The latter has affected Liver qi (stagnation) and contributed to Heart qi agitation. The damp-phlegm condition in the Heart, Lungs, and chest is associated with the Heart and Lung qi deficiency. The bilateral Slippery quality in the upper burner is a signal that her Heart feelings, which normally reach out through one's arms to the world, are somewhat withdrawn.

Damp-heat from excess in the Gallbladder, Stomach, and Intestines, and both the 'nervous system tense' and the Heart qi deficiency, have caused the 'blood thick' condition. The nervous system, 'blood thick,' and Heart/circulation conditions have contributed to the blood stagnation in the lower burner and Liver. The Heart qi agitation, 'nervous system tense,' heat from excess, and 'blood thick' condition have probably contributed to the Kidney yin deficiency. Separately, Liver qi and blood are depleted and Liver yin and yang are separating, suggesting a history of drugs and/or infection, since she is so young.

The early age of this seemingly significant Heart qi deficiency, and the Change in Qualities to Absent at the left proximal position, suggest the early onset of this problem with concomitant Kidney qi deficiency.

MANAGEMENT

Lifestyle strategies

OVERWORK, PREGNANCY, AND BIRTH CONTROL

The significant deficiencies of qi and blood in several organs, especially the Heart, and the degree of blood stagnation in the lower burner, make it imperative that she rest and avoid the stresses of pregnancy and the blood-stagnating side effects of birth control medications.

HABITS

Avoiding alcohol, tobacco, and recreational drugs, eating a low fat, low sugar diet, and avoidance of spices are also imperative in terms of the damp-heat in the blood, the damp-heat in the Gallbladder and Intestines, the heat in the Stomach, and both Lung yin deficiency and Lung damp-heat, as well as the separation of yin and yang in the Liver.

EMOTIONAL STRESS

See 'referrals' below (counseling).

Referrals

GYNECOLOGICAL ASSESSMENT

The considerable stagnation of qi and blood in the lower burner warrants regular gynecological examination.

COUNSELING

The Cotton quality, the 'nervous system tense' condition, and Heart qi agitation all suggest the advisability of psychotherapy.

ULTRASOUND OF GALLBLADDER

The damp-heat from excess in the Gallbladder suggests inflammation and stones, which should be investigated with ultrasound.

Acupuncture, herbs, and other strategies

IMMEDIATE INTERVENTIONS

One should begin with the Heart and circulation in terms of possible early trauma, using Yunnan Bai Yao and Sheng Mai San for a limited period of time. If there are problems digesting the herbs, treating the damp-heat in the Gallbladder and Intestines and the heat in the Stomach might precede all else.

INTERMEDIATE INTERVENTIONS

Assuming the immediate interventions succeed, the following must be considered. The Heart (including phlegm in the Heart and Lungs, and Heart qi agitation) and circulation, the blood stagnation in the lower burner (and Liver), and the 'blood thick' conditions are the basic issues to deal with at this stage. Combining treatment of the Heart, Liver, and Kidney deficiencies (qi, blood, yin, essence) is desirable.

LONG-RANGE INTERVENTIONS

Assuming the immediate and intermediate interventions are successful, the following must be considered.

Long-range major interventions

Continuation of the treatment of the intermediate interventions related to the Heart, Kidneys, circulation, 'blood thick,' blood stagnation, and separation of Liver yin and yang must continue. The 'nervous system tense' condition would receive major attention at this stage, which often resolves the external qi stagnation (Cotton quality), especially if the etiology is emotional, and with the addition of surface-moving herbs (such as siler) and Kidney qi herbs (already included with the Heart formula).

Long-range minor interventions

Treating the general qi and blood deficiency by also supporting the Liver blood and qi and Lung qi and yin, and removing the damp-heat from the Gallbladder and Intestines and heat from the Stomach, will improve digestion and assimilation.

History and Previous Treatment

COMPLAINTS

Tiredness

SYMPTOMS

- 50 percent of time: trouble getting up even after a good sleep
- Could sleep all day but doesn't because then she would not sleep at night
- On 'empty' all of the time for no reason in terms of activities, including sex
- Body is in slow motion, as if carrying a heavy weight
- Hard to concentrate, organize. Feels discombobulated and frazzled
- Cannot finish a project
- Hands have lost strength
- Patience is greatly diminished at these times
- Good times (50%): On good days she is tired only after activity or at end of day, and goes to sleep at 10 P.M.
- Somewhat worse before menstrual period when her husband reports increased irritability.
- Feels that tiredness is due to stress, too much on her mind, so that she wants to "close my eyes, sleep and hide." In the past she dealt with stress through activity, not talk.

HISTORY

- Began three years ago before pregnant with latest child, now two years old.
- Routine physical revealed very low platelets, under 100,000
- Thought IUD led to fatigue and low platelets. IUD removed with no benefit, and then became pregnant.

Adolescence: Rebellious, dropped out of school and partied, which involved heavy drugs (cocaine, marijuana, alcohol, and cigarettes). Once slept five days. Went to live with father who remarried and had new family.

Birth control: Ortho-Nova from age 16-20. Nausea, headaches, weight gain and sluggish; Depro-Prevara at age 22 for one year with same symptoms, some worse, some less. IUD used from age 23-25 and now.

Stress: Pregnant and delivered at age 20 with 60 pound weight gain, restricted activity due to back injury. Left father of child when baby was eight months old due to verbal and physical abuse, followed by vicious custody battle. Shortly after, her father died.

EXPLANATION

Fatigue, especially even after a good night's sleep, is associated with Heart qi deficiency for which there is abundant evidence on the pulse. Difficulty organizing and concentrating, and feeling discombobulated, is a sign of Heart qi and blood deficiency and Heart phlegm, and the decrease in patience is due in part to Heart qi agitation.

The history of birth trauma (see 'pregnancy and birth history' below) reveals prolonged delivery under anesthesia with the cord wrapped around her neck several times. The multiple pregnancies in the presence of significant Heart qi deficiency is extremely draining. The heaviness and "body in slow motion" is related to the damp condition which we see in the Gallbladder, Intestines, and Lungs, and to diminished circulation, partly due to Heart qi deficiency, and partly to the 'blood thick' condition.

The fifty percent of the time when she feels at her worst and is most irritable is when she is premenstrual or under great stress, which I believe to be related to the Liver qi and blood deficiency and blood stagnation, both in the lower burner and the Liver. These symptoms began in the context of a custody battle for her first child.

Kidney essence deficiency, with its effect on the bone marrow (drop in platelets), and Lung qi deficiency, are contributory factors, as is the superficial qi stagnation.

Easily bruises

SYMPTOMS

- Spontaneous and unrelated to trauma
- Sometimes painful and sometimes not
- Platelets normal recently, with less bruising

HISTORY

- Always bruised easily and just assumed that she was clumsy
- Current increase began three years ago when platelets dropped
- Bone marrow biopsy normal, no spider varicose veins, or phlebitis

EXPLANATION

Spontaneous bruising is classically due either to Spleen qi deficiency, for which there is no great evidence on the pulse, or blood stagnation, for which there is much pulse evidence (IUD, birth control pills). My experience closely ties the easy bruising and low platelets to Liver qi and blood deficiency and the separation of Liver yin and yang.

Body aches

SYMPTOMS

- Several joints at once
- Almost constant
- Dull ache in knees, hip, elbows, shoulders, and hands
- With activity the dull ache becomes a deeper soreness, pain
- Stiffness without activity
- Worsens with cold, stress, and fatigue
- Constant with cold
- Relieved by warm bath, which relaxes her

HISTORY

- Hands have always hurt with cold
- Symptoms began one year ago and have become progressively worse.

EXPLANATION

Slow circulation is the foundation for these symptoms (stiffness without activity), which have become fixed because her Kidney qi-yang deficiency has created an internal cold condition which makes her more susceptible to external cold (hands always hurt with cold). This internal cold condition has been with her all her life. The fixed aspect is also enhanced by the damp condition in her Gallbladder, Intestines, and Lungs.

Dizziness

SYMPTOMS

- Like a hot wave which washes over her; head tingles, feels flushed from chest up
- Has to hold on, then fuzzy-headed and unsteady

HISTORY

- Began three months ago
- Three occasions: sitting in kitchen, sitting at dinner table, talking to husband

EXPLANATION

These episodes of a "hot wave washing over me" are consistent with blood stagnation in the lower burner, which enhances a separation of qi and blood since the qi wants to move and the blood cannot. The qi is light and rises rapidly, and is experienced as a wave of heat.

REVIEW OF SYSTEMS

Head

- Frontal headaches, which are persistent and interfere with functioning; pressure and sitting up helps; becoming less intense.
- Frontal headaches are associated with damp-heat in the gastro-intestinal system (Gallbladder and Intestinal damp-heat).

Eyes

- Sensitive to bright light (Liver blood deficiency); difficulty reading, needs glasses

Ears

- Clog easily (Lung and Gallbladder damp-heat stagnation)

Nose and inhalant allergies

- Allergic to cats, animal hair, dust, and feathers (Kidney and Lung qi deficiency)

Mouth

- Canker sores on gums occasionally (damp-heat in the gastro-intestinal system; Gallbladder and Intestinal damp-heat)
- Canker sores on tongue after dental surgery
- Lump inside back of jaw, painful, and lasts for a few days; occurred four times last month ('nervous system tense')

Upper respiratory

- Head cold once or twice a year (not throat) that progresses to the chest and tends to last a long time (Kidney and Lung qi deficiency)

Lungs

- Shortness of breath twice in past few months, once with dizziness, again doing nothing at the time (Heart, Lung qi, and Kidney yang deficiency)

Digestion

- No complaints

Urinary

- Two bladder infections; candida with antibiotics led to painful urination (damp-heat from excess pouring down from impaired digestion; Robust Pounding at right middle position; Gallbladder and Intestinal positions Slippery)

Skin

- Excema in the winter; upper arms (rarely face) is dry, itches, and occasional circular patch; helped by moisturizer. Acne now on face and shoulders; more now than as adolescent (blood stagnation and deficiency, Gallbladder damp-heat, and heat from excess in the Stomach-Intestines)

Trauma

- Accident at age 15, went through the windshield (Cotton quality, Rough Vibration, and diminished circulation)
- Surgery:

Tonsils, age 5
Carpal tunnel, age 14
Back, age 23 (related to car accident)
Wisdom teeth, age 27

Liver

No history of mononucleosis or hepatitis; drug abuse (see below)

Temperature

(All symptoms below due primarily to Kidney qi-yang deficiency and diminished Heart/circulatory qi, and cold hands and feet secondary to Liver qi stagnation and deficiency)

- Deep chill when others are warm
- Hands, fingers, feet, and toes are generally cold
- Especially cold in winter when she feels stiff
- Prefers warm climate
- Never overexposed to the cold

Perspiration

- Sweats easily (normally)

Thirst

- Frequently drinks a great deal, depending on activity (probably due to heat from excess, especially in the Stomach)

Exercise

- Past: gym machine and walking
- Now: crunches 100 several times/week (further depleting her general extreme deficient qi and blood); plays with children and takes walks

Diet

- Eats a lot of dairy, cheese, yogurt, and red meat, because of husband (damp-heat in Gallbladder and Intestines)

Habits

- Currently does not use drugs, cigarettes, or alcohol
- Past: marijuana use several times/week (2-3 joints); sniffed cocaine 4 to 5 times/week; cigarettes from age 14 to 25, from a few to a pack/day; used all forms of alcohol from age 14 to 20, paralyzed briefly from bourbon, gave up alcohol when she became pregnant at age 20. (This explains the separation of Liver yin and yang.)

Obstetrical and Gynecological

MENSTRUAL

- Menarche at age 12, lasted days with no problems
- Cycle: 31-33 days, heavy flow for two days (Kidney qi deficiency), lasts at least one week, deep red first three days, then brownish
- Blood stagnation in Pelvis/Lower Burner from birth control: IUD ages 23-25 and now: cramping increasing, with clots ranging from small to large, and very dark with heavy bleeding. Ortho-Nova from age 16-20: nausea, headaches, weight gain, and sluggish; Depro-Prevara from age 22 for one year with same symptoms, some worse, some less

PREGNANCIES:

Two full term
1. Female, age 6½ years, overdue 3½ weeks; induced; gained 60 pounds, greatly stressed
2. Male, age 2 years, didn't breathe, cord around neck and incubated

INFECTION

Candida one time with antibiotics; no venereal disease

SEXUAL ENERGY

Low (Kidney, Heart, and Liver qi deficiency)

Pregnancy and birth history

- Mother had morning sickness, bronchitis, and tonsillitis
- Medication for morning sickness, no drugs or alcohol
- Birth took 12 hours after water broke, with anesthesia
- Umbilical cord wrapped several times around neck

Childhood

Breast-fed; tonsillitis

Family history

Mother: migrating joint pains, sinusitis, chronic fatigue
Father: alcoholic, died at age 37 from liver failure due to hepatitis
Maternal grandfather: agranulocytosis, brain tumor, died of heart disease at age 77
Maternal grandmother: breast cancer, died at age 44

Biomedical medications and treatments

Surgeries and birth control as listed above

Alternative treatments

None

COMMENTS

The original impression of an early insult to the cardiovascular system is borne out in the history of a cord wrapped around the neck at a prolonged birth performed under anesthesia. The Blood Thick quality and damp-heat in the Gallbladder and Intestines is partially explained by the diet high in milk products, animal protein, and fat, and the Liver qi deficiency by the history of recreational drugs. The Kidney qi-yang deficiency is compatible with the history of feeling a deep chill and cold since childhood and the birth trauma. The blood stagnation in the lower burner is partially explained by the presence of an IUD, a history of birth control medication, and severe trauma, including the accident and low back surgery, as well as the other causes (Heart, Kidney, and Liver qi deficiency, and 'blood thick') listed earlier.

Figure 18-2 Case 2: Female, Age 42

P = Present   ---- = Absent   (1 → 5) = Difficulty of access by degree: 1=low, 5=high

Name:	Gender: Female	Age: 42	Date:	Refer:
Weight: Height: Occup:				

Rhythm: Normal	**Rate/Min: Begin:** 75 **End:** 60 **W/exertion:** 68

First Impressions of Uniform Qualities
 	
Entire Pulse: Tense-Tight; Robust Pounding; Hollow Full-Overflowing [2]; Empty (more on left); Change in Intensity [3]
 	
Sides, Left: More Empty
 	
         Right: Reduced
	OTHER RATES DURING EXAM:
	Three Depths
	   Above qi depth: Cotton [1]
	   Qi depth: Tense-Tight
	   Blood depth: Empty; Thick when pulse Tense & Intensity is high
	   Organ depth: Empty ⟷ Tense
	
	Wave: Hesitant → Hollow Full-Overflowing

Principal Positions
 	
Distal Position
   Left (Pericardium):
   Tense; Change in Intensity [3]
 	
   Right:
   Feeble
 	
Middle Position
   Left:
   Change in Intensity [3]; Change in Qualities:
   Tense-Tight ⟷ Hollow Full-Overflowing ⟷ Empty
 	
   Right:
   Change in Intensity [3]; Change in Qualities:
   Thin, Tight-Wiry ⟷ Empty ⟷ Tense
 	
Proximal Position
   Left:
   Deep; Thin; Tight
 	
   Right:
   Deep; Thin; Feeble
 	
Three Burners
   Upper: -------
 	
   Middle: Tight → Empty
 	
   Lower: Deep; Tight
 	
Other:
	Complementary Positions
	
	Neuro-psychological
	   Left: Smooth Vibration (ephemeral)
	   Right: -------
	
	Heart
	   Mitral Valve: Smooth Vibration (ephemeral)
	   Large Vessels: -------
	   Enlarged: -------
	
	Lung
	   Special Lung position
	      Left: Tense; Robust Pounding
	      Right: Tense; Robust Pounding
	   Pleura: -------
	
	Diaphragm, Left: P [2]
	                 Right: P [2]
	
	Liver
	   Engorged, Radial: P
	                Ulnar: -------
	                Distal: -------
	   Gallbladder: Tense
	
	Spleen-Stomach
	   Esophagus: -------
	   Spleen: Yielding Inflated
	   Stomach-Pylorus Extension: -------
	   Peritoneum-Pancreas: both middle positions Empty
	   Duodenum: -------
	
	Intestines
	   Large: Tight
	   Small: Tense
	
	Pelvis/Lower Body
	   Left: Tense [5]
	   Right: Tense [5]

Case 2 Female, Age 42

Broad Focus

INITIAL IMPRESSION OF LARGE SEGMENTS AND UNIFORM QUALITIES

Rhythm

Hesitant quality indicates Heart yin deficiency and obsessive preoccupation.

Rate

Rate of 75 beats/minute in beginning and 60 at rest at end indicates instability of Heart qi, a sign of Heart qi deficiency.

Change in Rate on exertion from 60 to 68 is Normal.

Uniform qualities over the entire pulse

COMMON QUALITIES

Robust Pounding is a sign of heat from excess which the body is having difficulty eliminating.

The Tense-Tight quality is a sign of qi stagnation and heat from excess (Tense) at the onset of heat from yin deficiency (Tight).

The Hollow Full-Overflowing quality is another sign of heat from excess, this time in the blood, which the body is having difficulty eliminating.

UNUSUAL QUALITIES

The Empty quality is either a sign of a 'qi wild' condition if it is enduring, or severe emotional stress if temporary. (Further examination of the individual positions indicates that the Emptiness is found only at the middle positions.)

PARADOXICAL FINDINGS

Tense, Robust Pounding, and Hollow Full-Overflowing combined with an Empty quality on the left side indicates simultaneous qi stagnation and heat from excess, heat in the blood and a seriously deficient 'organ system,' or ongoing severe emotional stress (Empty on the left side). The Empty quality is most often a sign of the separation of yin and yang. (Further examination of the individual positions indicates that the Emptiness is found only at the middle positions.)

INSTABILITY

Change in Intensity over entire pulse is a sign of Heart qi deficiency if consistent, and Liver qi stagnation if inconsistent.

UNUSUAL WAVE FORM

Hesitant quality (see rhythm and rate above) changing to Hollow Full-Overflowing (heat in the blood). When the intensity was Robust, the wave was Hollow Full-Overflowing, and when the intensity was Diminished, the wave was Hesitant.

Closer Focus

Depths

ABOVE QI DEPTH

Cotton (2) is usually a sign of mild external qi stagnation associated with resignation and suppression of self. Physical trauma is another less likely etiology.

QI DEPTH

Tense-Tight indicates qi stagnation and heat from excess changing to heat from deficiency.

BLOOD DEPTH

Absent

ORGAN DEPTH

Absent. The absence of both the blood and organ depth is the Empty quality.

Sides and systems

The left side is more Tense at qi depth, but also more Empty than the right side. The Empty quality on the left, is a sign of 'organ system' qi deficiency and separation of yin and yang, or ongoing severe emotional stress. (Further examination of the individual positions indicates that the Emptiness is found only at the middle positions.)

SUMMARY OF INITIAL IMPRESSIONS

'Nervous system tense'

'Nervous system tense' (entire pulse Tense-Tight) creates heat in the blood (Hollow Full-Overflowing and Pounding).

Separation of yin and yang or post-traumatic stress

The separation of yin and yang ('qi wild'), especially of the 'organ systems,' or post-traumatic severe emotional stress are possible. The latter is severe emotional stress in which all of one's energy comes to the surface, or separation of yin and yang, especially involving the 'organ system' (Empty quality, especially on the left side). If the Emptiness is consistent, the diagnosis of separation of yin and yang is more likely. If the Emptiness is inconsistent, the diagnosis of current extreme post-traumatic emotional stress is more likely.

The fact that the pulse is also Tense, Hollow Full-Overflowing, with Robust Pounding rather than Yielding suggests that the diagnosis of extreme emotional tension is more likely than separation of yin and yang. However, the presence of the Empty quality on only the left side favors the 'qi wild' diagnosis. (Further examination of the individual positions indicates that the Emptiness is found only in the middle positions, but I have found that first impressions seem to have a validity of their own which must, of course, be tested in the context of the history.)

Heart and circulation

QI DEFICIENCY

The rate decreases during the four-hour examination from 75 to 60, and the circulation is Slow. This is a sign of Heart/circulatory instability leading to Heart qi deficiency.

Change in Intensity is constant

MILD HEART YIN DEFICIENCY WITH OBSESSIVE ACTIVITY

Hesitant quality

'Blood heat' and 'blood thick'

BIOMEDICAL CONDITION

Very early hypertension or diabetes

PULSE

Middle burner Tense and Hollow Full-Overflowing; lower burner Tight

Kidney yin deficiency

BIOMEDICAL CONDITION

Very early diabetes, hypertension; kidney stones and/or pain

PULSE

Lower burner Tight. (On closer examination of the proximal positions, we find the Tight quality only on the left.)

Closest Focus (Individual positions and Organs)

OVERVIEW

Unusual qualities

Wiry quality in right middle position may be a sign of abdominal pain or (much less likely) a very early sign of diabetes.

Instability (where there is the most activity and change)

CHANGE IN QUALITIES AT BOTH MIDDLE POSITIONS

This is a sign of a separation of yin and yang and qi deficiency at the middle burner.

Other more serious qualities

EMPTY AT BOTH MIDDLE POSITIONS

This is another sign of the separation of yin and yang and qi deficiency of the middle burner.

Paradoxical findings

Hollow Full-Overflowing changing to Empty at the left middle position is a combined sign of heat in the blood occurring simultaneously with separation of yin and yang in the Liver and in the middle burner, since the right middle position is also Empty.

INDIVIDUAL POSITIONS (PRINCIPAL AND COMPLEMENTARY)

Left distal, Large Vessel, Enlarged, Neuro-psychological, Mitral Valve (Heart-circulation) positions

HEART QI DEFICIENCY

A rate of 75/minute in the beginning and 60 at the end is a sign of mild Heart qi deficiency. Change in Intensity over the entire pulse, if constant, and especially at the left distal position, and the Smooth Vibration quality at the Mitral Valve position, are also signs of Heart qi deficiency. The Slow circulation (60/minute) further supports this view.

HEART YIN DEFICIENCY

The Hesitant quality indicates mild Heart yin deficiency with obsessive activity.

HEART HEAT FROM EXCESS

There is heat from excess in the Heart, as evidenced by the Tense quality at the left distal position.

HEART QI AGITATION

The ephemeral Smooth Vibration at the Neuro-psychological position suggests mild Heart qi agitation.

Right distal and Special Lung positions (Lungs)

Lung qi deficiency is signified by a Feeble quality at the right distal position, and Lung heat from excess by a Tense Robust Pounding quality at the Special Lung position.

Left middle, Gallbladder, and Liver Engorgement positions (Liver-Gallbladder)

The Change in Intensity and Qualities, and Emptiness, at the left middle position signify a separation of Liver yin and yang, which is probably due to Liver qi deficiency. The simultaneous Emptiness at the right middle position indicates qi deficiency over the entire middle burner, and is also a specific sign of Liver and Spleen qi-yang deficiency. The Tense quality at the left middle position (and Change in Intensity over the entire pulse if inconstant) indicates simultaneous Liver qi stagnation and heat from excess.

The Hollow Full-Overflowing quality at the left middle position suggests 'blood heat' or 'blood thick' in at least the Liver, and a consideration of either very early hypertension or diabetes. The engorgement of the Liver distally further indicates blood congestion in the Liver.

Right middle, Intestines, Esophagus, Spleen, Stomach-Pylorus Extension, Peritoneum (Spleen-Stomach) positions

The Thin Tight-Wiry quality at the right middle position, along with Tightness and Tension in the Intestine positions, suggests irritation/inflammation and pain along the alimentary canal, including gastritis, and, with the Wiry quality, possibly a stomach ulcer. This impression is mitigated by the unremarkable Stomach-Pylorus position.

The Empty quality in the right middle position and the Inflated Spleen position suggest Spleen qi deficiency and separation of Spleen yin and yang. The simultaneous Emptiness at the left middle position indicates qi deficiency and separation of yin and yang of the entire middle burner, as well as a specific sign of Spleen and Liver qi deficiency.

Proximal positions (Kidneys)

With both proximal positions Deep, and Feeble in the right, we have Kidney qi deficiency. The Thin Tight quality on the left is a sign of Kidney yin deficiency.

DIAGNOSTIC IMPRESSIONS FROM INDIVIDUAL POSITIONS

- Gastritis (possible stomach ulcer) and irritability in the intestines
- 'Digestive system' deficiency and separation of yin and yang in the middle burner
- Lung qi deficiency and lung heat from excess
- Heat in the blood
- Heart qi deficiency
- Kidney qi-yang and kidney yin deficiency
- General qi stagnation

The Tense quality in general and at the left distal, left middle and Gallbladder positions, and the very Tense quality at the Pelvis/Lower Body position can also indicate qi stagnation and/or may only be an expression of the general tension of the pulse associated with the 'nervous system tense' condition.

Substances (includes broad, closer, and closest focus)

Qi | ### Stagnation

EXTERNAL

Cotton quality

The slight Cotton quality (2) indicates minimal external qi stagnation associated with a mild emotional state of resignation.

INTERNAL

Tense-Tight quality

The Tense-Tight quality can be a sign of qi stagnation and heat from excess wherever it is found, related to unexpressed internal conflict and/or a 'nervous system tense' condition.

Diaphragm area Inflated (2)

The slight qi stagnation here is associated with the mild repression of tender feelings and the exaggeration of angry ones, usually associated with interpersonal separation.

Blood

Excess

Hollow Full-Overflowing and Robust Pounding suggest a 'blood heat-thick' condition. The distal engorgement suggests mild congestion of blood in the Liver.

Deficiency

The Thin quality at the proximal positions I believe to be more associated with the Tight yin deficiency quality rather than with blood deficiency since the Thin quality appears only in those positions. However, the Thin quality at this and the right distal and Special Lung positions may be more a sign of qi deficiency since, in TCM theory, there is no recognized blood deficiency in the Kidney and Lungs (with which I personally disagree).

Yin

Excess

There is no evidence of yin excess (no Slippery quality) which in itself is unusual in a 42-year-old woman, unless she is taking diuretic medication.

Deficiency

Tightness at the proximal positions, and the Tense-Tight qualities at the middle position, suggest yin deficiency and heat from deficiency.

Yang

Excess

There is no evidence on the pulse of yang excess.

Deficiency

The Deep quality at the proximal position, the Empty quality at the middle burner, and Feeble quality at the right distal position are signs of qi-yang deficiency of the Kidney, Liver, Spleen and Lung respectively. A complaint of coldness would be one deciding factor in determining whether this is a sign of qi or yang deficiency.

Wind

There is no evidence of internal or external wind.

Food

There is no evidence of food stagnation.

Activity

Heat

Excess

Tension at many positions is a sign of heat from excess associated with qi stagnation. The Hollow Full-Overflowing quality is a sign of heat in the blood, and Robust Pounding is a sign of heat from excess.

Deficiency

Tightness at many positions indicates yin deficiency and heat from that deficiency.

Cold

Excess

None. The Tight quality, indicating cold from excess in the lower burner, is a rare finding at the proximal positions, and with this etiology is usually bilateral.

Deficiency

See yang deficiency above.

Areas

Middle burner — The simultaneous Emptiness at the right and left middle positions indicates qi deficiency and separation of yin and yang over the entire middle burner.

Diaphragm — The slight Inflated quality at the Diaphragm position is a sign of minimal trapped qi in the diaphragm area, the implications of which were discussed above.

Pelvis/Lower Body — The very Tense quality at the Pelvis/Lower Body positions is a sign of qi stagnation and mild blockage in the pelvic area.

Systems

'Nervous system' — The almost uniformly Tense quality throughout the pulse is a sign of a 'nervous system tense' condition, the implications of which are explained below under root issues.

'Digestive system' — The qualities on the right side of the pulse, which is identified as the 'digestive system,' are all signs of deficiency (Feeble and Empty), which is explained below under root issues.

Interpretation

SUMMARY OF FINDINGS

- 'Nervous system tense'
- 'Digestive system' deficiency and separation of yin and yang in the middle burner
- Blood Heat, Blood Thick, and blood congestion in the Liver (all signs of blood stagnation)
- Heart qi deficiency
- Heart yin deficiency with obsessive activity and slight Heart qi agitation
- Lung qi deficiency
- Lung heat from excess
- Liver qi stagnation

- Liver yang deficiency
- Spleen qi/yang deficiency
- Gastritis (or stomach ulcer) and irritability in the intestines with abdominal pain
- Kidney yin deficiency
- Kidney qi-yang deficiency
- Qi stagnation at the Pelvis/Lower Body position
- Possible very early signs of diabetes, hypertension
- Possible pancreatic or peritoneal pathology
- Heat from excess
- Mild external qi stagnation
- Trapped qi in diaphragm area
- Qi stagnation and mild heat from excess in the Gallbladder
- Severe emotional stress or separation of yin and yang, especially of the 'organ system'

FORMULATION

Current prevailing issues

GASTRITIS (POSSIBLE STOMACH ULCER) AND IRRITABILITY IN THE INTESTINES

Gastritis and a possible stomach ulcer, and irritation/inflammation and pain along the alimentary canal, are suggested by the Tight-Wiry quality at the right middle position, along with Tightness and Tension at the Intestine positions, and Robust Pounding over the entire pulse.

'BLOOD HEAT,' 'BLOOD THICK,' AND BLOOD CONGESTION IN THE LIVER

Possibly very early hypertension or diabetes, suggested by the Tense Hollow Full-Overflowing qualities at the middle burner positions, and the Tight quality at the left proximal position. However, with early diabetes the proximal positions are usually more Wiry. These are also signs of blood stagnation, especially in the Liver.

HEART QI DEFICIENCY OR LIVER QI STAGNATION

The pulse should be checked at frequent intervals over the period of a week to determine if the Change in Intensity is constant, which would tell us whether it is a sign of Heart qi deficiency or Liver qi stagnation.

SLOW CIRCULATION AND TRAUMA

The Slow circulation should be evaluated in terms of etiology. If it is due partially to trauma, herbs to overcome the effects of trauma should be used immediately.

CURRENT ONGOING LUNG CONDITION

The Pounding at the Special Lung position suggests either heat from excess in the Lungs or a compensatory attempt to function, which, along with the Feeble quality at the right distal position, suggests an ongoing chronic Lung condition (asthma or allergies).

QI STAGNATION AT THE PELVIS/LOWER BODY POSITION

It is difficult to differentiate the Tense quality at this position from that of the pulse in general, and the absence of a Choppy or Slippery quality here reduces our concern. Nevertheless, the degree of Tension is high at this position, warranting consideration of severe qi stagnation and its biomedical consequences.

SEVERE EMOTIONAL STRESS ('ORGAN SYSTEM' DEFICIENCY)

Severe emotional stress, in which all of one's energy comes to the surface, or separation of yin and yang, especially involving the 'organ system,' is indicated by the Empty quality, especially on the left side. If the Emptiness is consistent, the diagnosis of separation of yin and yang is more likely. If the Emptiness is not consistent, the diagnosis of current and extreme emotional stress is more likely.

The initial impression of Emptiness on the left side ('organ system' separation of yin and yang or 'qi wild') was not supported by examination of the individual positions, but I have found that often this first impression is borne out by the history.

ROOT ISSUES

'Nervous system tense' condition

'Nervous system tense' (entire pulse Tense) creates stagnation of qi (especially Liver qi), which eventually leads to 'blood heat' and 'blood thick' conditions. This conviction is supported by the presence of the Hollow Full-Overflowing and Robust Pounding qualities. At the relatively young age of forty-two, the Slow rate and Deep proximal positions suggest a constitutional etiology.

Over time the 'nervous system tense' state will cause overworking and depletion of other systems, in this instance the 'circulatory system' (Slow rate), the 'digestive system' (reduced qualities on the right side), and possibly the 'organ system' (initial impression of Empty quality on the left side). With regard to the 'digestive system,' the irritability in this system could be due to an increase in peristalsis and hydrochloric secretions from the tension promulgated by the 'nervous system tense' condition' affecting the Liver, which is then 'attacking' the Spleen-Stomach-Intestines. It almost always leads to a general, and specifically Kidney-yin, condition.

Spleen qi and 'digestive system' deficiency

The Reduced qualities on the right side, the Empty quality at the right middle and left middle positions, and the Inflated Spleen position suggest deficiency of the 'digestive system' and Spleen qi deficiency.

The potential causes, in a 42-year-old woman, of the Empty quality bilaterally at the middle positions, and of the 'digestive system' deficiency, are many. Her relatively young age suggests Spleen deficiency due to constitutional Kidney qi-yang deficiency. There could also be a substantial contribution from her harmful eating habits: the irregularity, excessive dieting, perhaps reaching the extremes in anorexia and bulimia, and the 'nervous system' affecting the 'digestive system' (Liver attacking the Spleen). Drug abuse is also a major consideration with the Empty qualities in the middle burner, especially the left middle position.

Pancreatic involvement must be considered when we have a similar quality in both middle positions. Other (less likely) etiologies are impoverishment in childhood (usually with an arrhythmia); sitting in a bent-over position at work (e.g., a secretary); excessive rumination while eating; resuming physical labor too soon after eating; and trauma. These etiologies are unlikely because they would not have existed long enough in a 42-year-old to cause an Empty quality in the middle burner.

Kidney qi-yang and yin deficiency

Kidney qi-yang and yin deficiency are evidenced by the Deep and Tight qualities at the proximal positions. The Deep quality here in a 42-year-old woman suggests a constitutional or congenital qi-yang deficit, or it may be attributable to very early insults due to illness or trauma. The yin deficiency is probably the result of overworking the mind (Hesitant wave) and the 'nervous system,' both of which deplete yin, which is supplied by the Kidneys. Were it not for the latter, and the fact that the resultant harder qualities associated with yin deficiency override the reduced qualities in the early and middle portions of a disease process, the left proximal position would be Feeble.

Heart qi and yin deficiency, very slight Heart qi agitation, and mild blood deficiency

There is Heart qi deficiency evidenced by the Slow rate, a reduction from 75 to 60 beats/minute, and another reading of 68, during the four-hour seminar at which the pulse was taken, and a Change in Intensity over the entire pulse (if it is constant).

The Hesitant quality is a sign of mild Heart yin deficiency with overworking of the mind, possibly in the form of obsessive activity. There is also heat from excess in the Heart (Tense quality at the left distal position). The initial higher rate and ephemeral Smooth Vibration at the Neuro-psychological position suggests mild Heart qi agitation. While the Change in Intensity at the left distal position usually suggests the more serious separation of Heart yin and yang, it is less likely to be the case here due to the sense of Change in Intensity of the same degree over the entire pulse.

The Slow circulation could be due to trauma, overexercise, overwork, Heart qi deficiency, or chronic illness. In view of the simultaneous presence of Kidney qi deficiency, the Heart qi deficiency, if it exists, is more likely attributable to an early (even constitutional or congenital) physiological insult, or (much less likely) rheumatic heart disease in childhood, than to trauma to the circulation.

'Qi wild' condition

If the initial impression of Emptiness at the left side (separation of yin and yang of the 'organ system') is valid and lasting over time, and if it is supported by medical history, the 'qi wild' condition, of which it is a sign, could be the most serious of all the pulse findings in terms of morbidity and mortality. This is so because this state is potentially coincident with the most severe diseases, including neoplasms, autoimmune, and degenerative neurological disorders.

DERIVATIVE ISSUES

Liver qi deficiency, qi stagnation, heat from excess, 'blood heat,' or 'blood thick'

The Liver qi deficiency is the result of the same process as that which gave rise to the Spleen qi and 'digestive system' deficiency, although one must also consider a history of recreational or other drug abuse, and hepatitis or mononucleosis, as well as the eating disorders. The absence of a Slippery quality at the organ depth reduces the likelihood of hepatitis/mononucleosis or chronic infection and qi depletion from parasites.

The Liver qi stagnation is probably related to the 'nervous system tense' condition and to internal conflicts, which have affected the qi of the Stomach, Intestines, and Spleen; thus the qi deficiency and separation of yin and yang in the middle burner. The heat from excess is a consequence of the effort by the Liver to overcome the stagnation. The Liver stores the blood and the left middle position will be the first and most evident pulse position to reveal problems in the blood such as toxicity, heat, and increasing denseness ('blood thick'). Mild congestion of blood in the Liver is present, as indicated by the radial engorgement.

Heat from excess in the blood and body

Heat from excess (Tense at most positions, plus the Hollow Full-Overflowing and Robust Pounding qualities) is probably the result, in part, of the 'nervous system tense' condition over a long period of time. It is also partly the result of poor eating habits and incomplete digestion, as indicated by the deficient 'digestive system' and Spleen qi, and the signs of inflammation in the alimentary canal.

Mild external qi stagnation

The very slight Cotton quality suggests a very mild state of resignation with regard to compromises she is making in her current life situation.

Trapped qi in the diaphragm area

This is mild, which suggests some retention of anger and repression of tender feelings associated with a previous separation.

Qi stagnation in the Gallbladder

The absence of Slipperiness with the Tense quality mitigates the possible seriousness of the qi stagnation in the Gallbladder.

Analysis and synthesis

One underlying issue which has led to some of the others is the constitutionally derived 'nervous system tense' condition. This has given rise to heat in the blood (and possibly very early signs of hypertension), to Liver qi stagnation (and blood congestion), to irritability/inflammation of the alimentary canal, and to eating habits which produced the middle burner chaos and deficiency of the 'digestive system.' The Liver qi stagnation and heat in the blood has led to stagnation in the area of the pelvis and lower burner. This could lead to gynecological/menstrual difficulties of a deficient nature.

Another underlying issue involves the Heart-Kidney axis. The Kidney qi-yang deficiency indicates an early defect in development, which is probably related to the deficiencies in the middle burner and 'digestive system,' the Lung qi deficiency, and Heart qi deficiency. The slowing of the circulation will also increase stagnation in dependent areas such as the pelvis and lower body.

The yin-deficient aspects of this axis involve the overworking 'nervous system' and a vicious cycle between Heart and Kidney yin deficiencies, which have contributed to the Hesitant quality and to the obsessive, agitated personality which it represents.

As already indicated, the possible 'qi wild' condition (separation of yin and yang in the 'organ system') is probably the summation of the deficiencies listed above. The 'qi wild' condition ('danger pulse'), if true, is the most serious threat to her life and well-being. At this point, the separation of yin and yang is confined to the middle burner, but with the Feeble right distal position and the Deep proximal position, the circumstances are auspicious for the development of the 'qi wild' condition.

MANAGEMENT

Lifestyle strategies

- Relaxation techniques for 'nervous system tense'
- Explore emotional causes for stagnation in diaphragmatic area (divorce, separation), Hesitant quality (obsessive nature and pushing self mentally), and possible post-traumatic stress (Empty quality on left side).

- Investigate energy drains, including eating habits, that have led to the 'digestive system' deficiency, the separation of yin and yang in the middle burner, and irritability in the alimentary canal (Wiry quality in the left middle position, indicating possible gastritis and/or stomach ulcer with abdominal discomfort). Provide nutritional counseling, and intervene immediately if there is danger of hemorrhage.
- Investigate lifestyle causes of slow circulation (overexercise, overwork, medications).

Referrals

- Do a complete drug history and a history of liver disease to explain the Empty and Change in Qualities at the left middle position.
- Blood chemistry to explore the status of liver, kidney, and lipid function, and glucose tolerance (diabetes), including a complete blood count and thyroid profile, would be useful.
- Rule out hypertension with a complete biomedical physical examination.
- Gynecological examination to explore the stagnation in the lower burner and other menstrual implications of the kidney, spleen, liver, and heart/circulation deficiencies.
- Chest x-ray and tests of lung capacity and function to explain the Feeble left distal position and Robust Pounding at the Special Lung positions.

Acupuncture, herbal, and other healing strategies

IMMEDIATE INTERVENTIONS

Stomach ulcer

If biomedical techniques reveal a stomach ulcer it should be treated immediately to prevent rupture and hemorrhage. Treat gastritis and the irritable alimentary canal first so that she will better tolerate the other herbal treatments that follow.

Hypertension and/or diabetes

While signs of blood stagnation such as heat in the blood, blood congestion in the Liver, and 'blood thick' must be treated as an intermediate and long-range intervention, the presence of current hypertension and/or diabetes brings these interventions into the realm of the immediate.

INTERMEDIATE INTERVENTIONS

Heart yin deficiency and Heart qi agitation

Mitigate the process of obsessive thinking that is affecting the Heart and Kidney and creating agitation, when her recovery depends on inner quiet.

'Nervous system tense'

The relaxation of the nervous system is the single most important intermediate intervention, and should begin with acupuncture from the beginning, and with herbs as soon as the digestion is stabilized.

Heat in the blood, blood congestion in the Liver, and 'blood thick' conditions

Since these signs of blood stagnation can lead to serious consequences (hypertension) they must be treated with some urgency and be ongoing, more in the short term than long, in the service of prevention.

LONG-RANGE MAJOR INTERVENTIONS

Kidney qi-yang and yin deficiency

Kidney qi-yang deficiency is the single most important intervention for the long term and is a primary constitutional issue for this patient, giving rise to and affecting all other pathological processes. Kidney yin should be included in the plan to offset the depletion of yin by her overworking mind, which affects all function, especially the Heart.

'Nervous system tense'

The relaxation of the nervous system is the second most important intervention over the long run, and should continue as long as she lives.

Heart qi deficiency, slow circulation, and Heart yin and blood deficiency

It is important to treat these conditions as part of correcting the Kidney-Heart imbalance, and because the Heart is the 'emperor' whose well-being affects all other 'subjects' (organ function).

'Digestive system' middle burner chaos and irritable alimentary canal

Continued treatment of these disharmonies must be ongoing until they are resolved.

Heat in the blood, blood congestion in the Liver, and 'blood thick' conditions

Since these signs of blood stagnation can lead to serious consequences (e.g., hypertension), they must be treated as an ongoing issue, in the service of prevention.

'Qi wild'

Exploration of the validity of this impression must be ongoing, and if found to be accurate, treated vigorously in terms of reducing this current energetic chaos and healing all the etiologies listed above.

LONG-RANGE MINOR INTERVENTIONS

Liver qi-yang deficiency

This disharmony should already be a focus of the treatment for the middle burner separation of yin and yang and probably accounts for some of the blood stagnation mentioned below. The Empty quality at the left middle position has been associated with lymphomas.

Stagnation of qi and blood in the Liver, and qi in the pelvis and lower body areas

Open the stagnation in the Liver and pelvis and lower body areas, which also makes more qi available for healing.

Lung qi deficiency

This disharmony should likewise already be a focus of the treatment for the 'digestive system' deficiency (Lung, Spleen, and Kidney yang).

Client History

CHIEF COMPLAINTS

Gynecological

Amenorrhea for several months (with normal period after treatment with herbs and acupuncture)
Hot flashes and sweats

Obstetrical

Infertility

Gastro-Intestinal

Abdominal distention

MEDICAL HISTORY

Gynecological

Eight years ago a fluid cyst was found one ovary and two blocked tubes, one of which was cleared.
Irregular periods

Psychosomatic

She has often had intense emotional crises, resulting in sinus infections with chest tightening simulating asthma, the symptoms of which are relieved after the emotional crisis passes.

Relationships

A recent conflict with an authority at school, where she was supported by her fellow students, resulted in her expulsion. For years she fought unsuccessfully to be reinstated, and is finally, after considerable difficulty, trying to put this behind her. This is being helped by a new satisfying relationship.

Oncology and operations

Ten years ago a melanoma was removed from her side.

Family history

Father alcoholic and parents divorced when she was young.

TREATMENTS

Treatment by the referring practitioner focused on Liver qi stagnation, blood and yin deficiency, and heat from deficiency.

SYMPTOMS AND THE PULSE

Amenorrhea for several months

Amenorrhea, which develops suddenly and passes relatively quickly, is most often the result of Liver qi stagnation which we have commented upon above in the section describing current prevailing issues as Liver qi stagnation and qi stagnation in the pelvis and lower burner. The Liver yang deficiency would increase her susceptibility to Liver qi-stagnant amenorrhea.

Symptoms associated with blood stagnation come on more gradually, usually involving more pain, and with Choppiness at the Pelvis/Lower Body position, and less often at the proximal positions, and are resolved more slowly. With heat in the blood and Slow circulation, as well as Liver qi and blood stagnation and Kidney-Spleen qi deficiency, I would anticipate some blood stagnation. This in fact is indicated as already occurring by the history of a fluid cyst on the right ovary and two blocked tubes. Treatment with Chinese medicine has altered the original picture of blood stagnation, which probably included a Choppy quality at the Pelvis/Lower Body positions.

Hot flashes and sweats

If the hot flashes and especially the sweats continue after awakening (they usually occur at night, though this is not specified) they are signs of qi deficiency. If they stop upon awakening they could be signs of heat from deficiency due to yin deficiency. Since she shows signs of both Kidney yin and qi-yang deficiency, we can only go by the percentages, which are heavily in favor of yin heat from deficiency.

Irregular periods

It is not clear whether "irregular periods" refers to skipping periods, variable lengths, or to an on-off pattern during one period. Skipping of periods is more often associated with Liver qi stagnation, and the on-off pattern with blood stagnation. Irregularity that involves periods that are longer and shorter from month to month indicates Kidney yang deficiency (with variable amounts of pale blood), unmentioned in the history.

The pulse at this time indicates that qi stagnation in general, in the pelvis/lower body, and Liver qi stagnation are more pressing issues than is blood stagnation. However, Kidney qi-yang deficiency is indicated by the Deep, Thin, and Feeble qualities in the proximal positions, and 'blood thick,' and mild blood congestion in the Liver are conditions favorable to the development of a blood stagnation process in the lower burner.

Infertility with history of a fluid cyst on one ovary and two blocked tubes

Stagnation of qi is the primary finding at the moment, but as previously mentioned, the probability is that blood stagnation due to slow circulation, 'blood thick,' Heart blood deficiency, Kidney-qi yang deficiency, and Liver qi stagnation, and Liver yang deficiency would contribute to these gynecological disorders. We have clear findings for all of these etiologies. (According the referring practitioner, Chinese medical treatment has diminished the signs of blood stagnation in the pelvis.)

Abdominal distention

The separation of yin and yang in the middle burner, 'digestive system' deficiency, Spleen qi deficiency, and Liver qi stagnation and qi-yang deficiency are all contributing to stagnation and irritation in the alimentary canal with resultant qi stagnation and abdominal bloating. I would anticipate increasing gastro-intestinal difficulties in the near future unless she changes the lifestyle engendering the chaos, irritability, and deficiency in this function, in the absence of therapeutic intervention.

Intense emotional crises

This resulted in sinus infections with chest tightening, almost asthmatic, improving with the passing of the emotional crises. Chest tightening is often a sign of Liver qi attacking upward to the chest and Lungs. The Liver is the yin organ most affected by frustration, tension, and inner emotional conflict. Since the Lungs govern the nose and sinuses, an attack upward by Liver qi on the already qi-deficient Lungs can affect the sinuses, especially in the presence of Lung heat, which we observe at the Special Lung positions (Robust Pounding).

Melanoma

Melanoma is one of the most virulent forms of cancer, which I have found increasingly in young people. Cancer is traditionally thought of as a condition involving stagnation of substances, a conception with which I partially agree. However, I have found it more often in situations in which the yin and yang have separated, either in one organ or area, or as a 'qi wild' condition affecting the entire organism. Despite six years of treatment, this patient continues to show signs of separation of yin and yang in the middle burner. There was also one initial impression of Emptiness over the entire left side, possibly a sign of a 'qi wild' condition in the 'organ system' of the fundamental Heart, Kidney, and Liver organs.

My experience with this form of cancer in young people includes a history of heavy abuse of recreational drugs. The conditions exist now for some other form of chaos—such as cancer, auto-immune disease, or degenerative neurological disease—to occur within the next five to ten years unless therapeutic attention is given to these findings.

AMENDED ANALYSIS AND SYNTHESIS

Our findings of severe stagnation of qi in the pelvis/lower body and of general and Liver qi stagnation, support a history of ovarian cysts and blocked fallopian tubes which contributed to her irregular periods and occasional amenorrhea and infertility. Qi problems have an ephemeral aspect due to the susceptibility of qi to stress.

A history of qi deficiency (of the 'digestive system,' Lungs, Heart, Spleen, Liver, and Kidneys) associated with the separation of yin and yang, especially in the middle burner and 'organ system,' is obviously related to her infertility and other menstrual difficulties. More importantly, this deficiency, especially of the Liver and Kidney qi-yang, is associated in my experience with cancer (melanoma).

The constitutional 'nervous system tense' condition made her vulnerable to her intense emotional crises. The effects on her sinuses and lungs (asthma) were discussed above with regards to Lung qi deficiency, heat from excess in the digestive system, and

Gallbladder and Liver qi attacking upward. Of course, this hypervigilant state was augmented by early family trauma (alcoholic father, parents' early divorce). The 'nervous system tense' condition has affected the Heart, resulting in a tendency toward obsessive preoccupation (Hesitant quality), interpersonal conflict (enduring struggle with authority), and interpersonal failures (unmarried at age forty-two). Another sign of the ongoing and ephemeral effects of emotional stress is the initial impression of an Empty quality on the left side.

Without therapeutic intervention, a recurrence of severe chronic disease (degenerative neurological, autoimmune, or neoplasms) and digestive disorders is on the horizon.

Epilogue

Soulié De Morant stated the case concisely when he wrote:

> The knowledge of pulses is absolutely indispensable for the practice of true acupuncture, which is based on treating the root condition. Using only memorized formulae and treating only visible problems does not constitute true acupuncture.[1]

One of my missions in life is to reawaken an awareness of the importance of pulse diagnosis, which was recognized since antiquity and in all cultures as necessary to gaining a profound knowledge of a person. Yet it is also necessary for traditions to evolve and remain relevant to the times in which they are practiced.

Knowledge of Chinese pulse diagnosis has steadily diminished in recent times. In part, the problem has been that it relies on ideas that are expressed in an archaic language that is often incomprehensible to a practitioner of the twenty-first century. Moreover, the ideas themselves are based on texts and traditional lore that were passed down from an agrarian civilization whose daily life was so different from our own that the information is often no longer relevant in the modern clinic. To that extent, Chinese medicine has increasingly lost its ability to predict and thereby prevent illness.

During the modern era, the industrial, information, nuclear and `space' revolutions have made new demands on every aspect of our physiology, particularly our nervous and immune systems, demands which are historically sudden and cataclysmic. This has happened to a creature, homo sapien, who has otherwise evolved in a remarkably stable and slowly-changing cultural environment for at least the last ten thousand years. While the human organism has remained more or less constant, the stresses to which it is subject have changed radically in recent times.

The only thing that never changes is change itself. Pulse diagnosis must be brought up to date to reflect our current situation. The human organism has a limited reservoir of

---

1. George Soulié de Morant, *Chinese Acupuncture,* trans. Lawrence Grinnell et al. (Brookline, MA: Paradigm Publications, 1994) 56

symbols with which to express its internal anguish. We call these symptoms. The causes of each symptom are legion, and a patient can rarely tell you that they have an ulcer or a tumor, to say nothing of its cause. This limitation is the genesis of the art and science of diagnosis.

The pulse qualities themselves, likewise, limited in the variety of sensations, have not changed. What has changed in many cases are the causes for these qualities, our ability to distinguish them from one another, and the language we use to communicate them. Many of the images, metaphors, and interpretations of the past no longer resonate with modern man.

Even the best of traditions must evolve to remain relevant. And while the contents of this book mark a significant departure from the past, its goal is to return Chinese medicine to its diagnostic roots. It draws upon the written classics, but even more from the clan-based, oral tradition with its emphasis on learning from actual practice. It is based on the work of a teacher from the Ding (Ting) clan, Dr. John H.F. Shen, and the work of his student. The goal is to bring pulse diagnosis into the twenty-first century in terms of sensation, expressed in modern, easily identified terminology, and interpretation, which is in accord with the enormous changes in all aspects of our existence since ancient times.

Students in my classes tell me that their otherwise competent teachers discourage them from pursuing the study of pulse diagnosis because "it is really not that important." For those who do not know pulse diagnosis, it cannot be very important. Furthermore, the time and patience necessary to master Chinese pulse diagnosis are not synchronous with a culture such as ours, which encourages short-term vision and short-term investment in all positive human attributes. Yet, within the traditional Chinese diagnostic system of asking, looking, listening, and touching, pulse diagnosis is the most informative and profound diagnostic modality concerned with the physical, emotional, and mental status of an individual.

The Normal pulse is the most sensitive indicator of the state of our health. Of all diagnostic modalities, it provides the most reliable basis of a preventive medicine by giving us the most precise picture of every subtle and complex deviation from this standard. In addition, the pulse provides information about the root cause of any deviation, allowing our patients the opportunity to change their lives and their habits, or adapt to constitutional deficits, in the direction of health. And the more precise the diagnosis, the more precisely we can design a therapeutic regime for the patient. The pulse record is an instant picture of the current status of a person's voyage from birth to death. It permits us to diagnose and treat people as individuals, rather than diseases.

When practiced with dedication, quiet patience, and consistency, becoming attuned to pulse qualities is an ongoing meditation, a training ground for the development of awareness and mindfulness. Finally, pulse diagnosis is an opportunity for practitioners to obtain the ultimate satisfaction of being one with their patients, one with themselves, one with the diagnostic process, and perhaps with the universal forces which are expressed through the pulse.

Dr. Shen once asked the question, "Why did God put eyes in front of our head instead of behind?" The answer, he said, is that "We were meant to always look ahead, not behind." In a similar vein, Martin Prechtel, who lived and studied in Guatemala for many years with a Mayan shaman, recorded these words from his teacher:

> If God gives us life and we continue as we have, some day when I'm a pile of ashes and the smell of smoke in your memory is all you have left of these days, then you will see situations and sicknesses never seen before. I've no idea what they may be; I have no way of recognizing them with our very old ways and traditional

roots. But you're the new one who's going to have to find special medicines to deal with them, instead of just using the old things because they're old. You must find new ways to do old things, and new medicines with old roots to cure the bad times made by new things.[2]

---

2. Martin Prechtel, *Secrets of the Talking Jaguar: Unmasking the Mysterious World of the Living Maya* (New York: Penguin-Putnam, 1998)

Endnotes

Chapter 1

1. According to *The Stories of Rabbi Nachman of Breslov* (Brooklyn: Breslov Research Institute, 1983), the art of using pulse diagnosis is discussed in the following sections of the Kabbalah: Tikkuney Zohar 69, 109a; Shgar Ruach Ha Kodesh 14; Likutey Moharan 56:9; Likutney Halakhoth, Tefillah 4:22. Among other passages are the following:

   > Laying on of hand confers wisdom. Thus, Moses laid his hand on Joshua to give him wisdom. The Torah says, 'Joshua, son of Nun, was full of the spirit of wisdom because Moses had laid his hands upon . . . him' (Deuteronomy 34:9). Joshua thus became a man 'who has wind-spirit in him' (Numbers 27:18). This meant that he knew how to determine each person's wind-spirit, which is manifested in that person's pulse (*Likutey Halakhoth, Tolaim* 4:2). (Nachman, 416).

   > There are ten types of pulse. . . . These ten types of pulse beats correspond to the ten Hebrew vowel points. The pulse beat is related to the shape of the vowel point." (Nachman, 420) "Human life depends on the pulse. The ten pulse types parallel the types of song (see *Likutey Moharan Tinyana* 24). Therefore, healing requires knowing the pulses, and then knowing what *song* to use as a remedy (*Likutey Halakhoth, P'ru U'R'vu* 3:1). (Nachman, 417)

   It is clear that the pulse was considered a singularly significant resource for accessing the human spirit and physiology in the Jewish and other ancient traditions.

   R.B. Amber asserts "The Easterner uses the pulse as a very significant and direct diagnostic tool for the whole man: physical, emotional, and spiritual. Every other procedure is ancillary to it." *The Pulse in Occident and Orient* (New York: Santa Barbara Press, 1966) 100.

   The Tibetan physician Yeshi Donden had this to say about his training: "But it was mastery of the second trunk, pulse diagnosis, that was the hallmark of a leading physician." Yeshi Donden, *Healing from the Source: The Science and Lore of Tibetan Medicine* (Ithaca, NY: Snow Lion Publications, 2000) 144.

   Since undertaking the writing of this book I have also encountered Korean pulse diagnosis through the writings of Peter Eckman and Jiang Jing. From these sources I have come to appreciate this model as a remarkably precise and richly endowed diagnostic tradition that is also worthy of study. See Peter Eckman, "Korean Acupuncture" *Traditional Acupuncture Society Journal* 1990;7:1, and Jiang Jing "A Brief Survey of the Korean Dong Han System of Pulse Diagnosis" *Oriental Medicine* 1993;2(1):8.

2. One such original and interesting approach to pulse diagnosis was developed by Townsend and DeDonna during eighteen years of practice, described in their book *Pulses and Impulses* (Northamptonshire: Thorsons Publishing Group, 1990).

3. Wang Shu-He, *The Pulse Classic,* trans. Yang Shou-Zhong (Boulder, CO: Blue Poppy Press) 4.

4. Li Shi–Zhen, *Pulse Diagnosis*, trans. Hoe Ku Huynh (Brookline, MA: Paradigm Publications, 1981) 70; Ted Kaptchuk, *The Web That Has No Weaver* (New York: Congdon and Weed, 1983) 309; Wu Shui-Wan, *The Chinese Pulse Diagnosis* (San Francisco: Writers Guild of America, 1973) 20; Deng Tietao, *Practical Diagnosis in Traditional Chinese Medicine*, trans. Marnae Ergil (Edinburgh: Churchill Livingstone, 1999) 119–21.

5. Lu Yubin, *Pulse Diagnosis* (Jinan: Shandong Science and Technology Press, 1996) 70–71.

6. Leon Hammer, "Tradition and Revision" *Oriental Medicine* 2001;8(3&4):27.

7. Manfred Porkert calls this pulse 'tense.' *The Essentials of Chinese Diagnostics* (Zurich: Chinese Medicine Publications, 1983) 216.

8. Li, 80.

9. Examples of this abound in books on pulse diagnosis. One example can be found in *Practical Diagnosis in Traditional Chinese Medicine* (Edinburgh: Churchill Livingstone, 1999) by the contemporary Chinese physician Deng Tietao. In his review of the Hidden pulse (108–9), there is extensive discussion of cholera-related symptoms, a disease that few of us in the West are likely to ever see in our clinics. Yet there is no mention that this pulse is an extreme rarity in our times, and that if we were to see it at all, it would most likely be associated with cold from excess due to extreme hypothermia.

10. Deng, 88.

11. For example, Deng Tietao (95), referring to the Empty quality, says that it is "tangled like the thread of a spider web or a pulse that is continuous like flowing liqueur." And elsewhere (106) he observes that "the descriptions of a drumskin pulse provided by the ancients were not all the same."

12. Some characteristic examples from Ilza Veith's translation of *The Yellow Emperor's Classic of Internal Medicine* (Berkeley: University of California Press, 1966) include the following (209):

> Wang Ping explains: The five pulses should correctly appear in the following ways: The pulse of the liver should sound like the strings of a musical instrument; the pulse of the heart should sound like the blows of a hammer (continuous); the pulse of the spleen should be intermittent and irregular; the pulse of the lungs should be (soft) like hair (and feathers); the pulse of the kidneys should sound like a stone.

And in another of many similar descriptions, Wang Ping says the following (174):

> When man is ill the pulse of the kidneys flows like the sound that is made by touching the stretched fibers of beans and its strength is increased; and then one can speak of sick kidneys.

13. Wu, 34.

14. Amber, 2.

15. Leon Hammer, *Dragon Rises, Red Bird Flies* (Barrytown, NY: Station Hill Press, 1990) Chapter 14. See also the glossary at the back of the present volume.

16. Veith, 151–52, 195, 215–16, 221. "The Sanskrit rule observes, 'The learned physician should read the happiness and misery of the body by feeling the root of the thumb which stands as the witness of the soul'." Amber, 6.

17. Amber, 103.

18. Attributed to Xu Da-Chun in Paul Unschuld, *Forgotten Traditions of Chinese Medicine* (Brookline, MA: Paradigm Publications, 1990) 321. Xu observes:

> Those experts who discussed the [movement in the] vessels through the ages have all contradicted one another, and they differed in what they considered right and wrong. They all cling to their specific doctrine, and their advantages and errors balance each

> other. All this results from their ignorance of the essential meanings of changing relationships [among movements in the vessels, pathoconditions, and illnesses], and the more detailed [their discourses become], the further away [they move from perfection]....
> If one clings, though, to the [movement in the] vessels in order to [gain the information needed to] treat an illness, one will never reach a state of security.

While I agree that some of the claims of Xu's contemporaries carried a significant degree of mystification, on closer examination of his criticisms, it is my opinion that his own knowledge of the pulse may also have left something to be desired.

19. Amber (10) notes that "Solomon, a recognized authority on the pulse, observed that in the absence of instruments and other aids for diagnosis, the ancient healer had to rely on the pulse for the interpretation of disease."

20. Ibid., v–vi.

21. Veith, 151.

22. Personal communication from Miles Roberts, 1993.

23. Amber, 2, 132.

24. Ibid., 107.

25. "In traditional Chinese medicine, examination of the patient's pulse is the keystone in the diagnostic procedure." Anton Jayasuria, *Textbook of Acupuncture Science* (Dehiwala, Sri Lanka: Chandrakanthi Industrial Press, 1981) 515.

Chapter 2

1. Wang Shu-He, *The Pulse Classic,* trans. Yang Shou-Zhong (Boulder, CO: Blue Poppy Press, 1997).

2. As cited in Ted Kaptchuk, *The Web That Has No Weaver* (New York: Congdon & Weed, 1983) 300.

3. Joseph Needham and Lu Gwei-Djen, *Celestial Lancets* (Cambridge: Cambridge University Press, 1980) 141, 148-49. The following opinion—which I share—appeared in course materials of the former North American College of Acupuncture (Vancouver) under the title "Chinese Philosophy and Principles of Diagnosis" (1972). It suggests that Wang Shu-He developed his system of pulse diagnosis based on a theoretical misinterpretation of what he felt:

    > In the Wang Shu-Hu method, the assigning of a Fou organ to the superficial pulse and Tsang organ to a deep pulse was based on a theory as to the positions that they received on the wrist. The Li Shi-Chen method on the other hand, has evolved through practical experience and the anatomical positions of the Three Burning Spaces [Triple Burner]. As has been mentioned before, the pulses were originally meant to reveal the condition of the five Yin organs or viscera. A Tsang which suffers from a lack of Yin or an abundance of Yang will show a floating pulse. If Yang is damaged however, the pulse will be sunken (Yin). When considering the husband/wife relationship of the Tsangs/Fous (which matches a Yin Tsang with a Yang Fou) it can be seen how Wang Shu-Hu decided that the superficial pulses belong to the Fous and the deep pulses to the Tsangs.

    According to this perspective, Wang Shu-He, within his five-phase model, misinterpreted yin deficiency with yang rising (Floating or Empty pulse), or yang deficiency with yin sinking (Deep pulse), as representing a disharmony between the yin and yang pair of a phase. In the left middle position he would have interpreted an Empty quality to signify excess of the Gallbladder and deficiency of the Liver, while the opposite would have been true for a Deep quality at that position.

4. Jiang Jing, "A Brief Survey of the Korean Dong Han System of Pulse Diagnosis" *Oriental Medicine* 1993;2(1):14, 62.

5. Paul Unschuld, trans., *Nan-Ching* (Berkeley: University of California Press, 1986) 248.

6. Ibid., 250–51.

7. John Shen, *Chinese Medicine* (New York: Educational Solutions, 1980).

8. Ilza Veith, *The Yellow Emperor's Classic of Internal Medicine* (Berkeley: University of California Press, 1966)

9. Li Shi-Zhen, *Pulse Diagnosis*, trans. Hoe Ku Huynh (Brookline, MA: Paradigm Publications, 1981)

10. The confusion about pulse positions is apparently also found in the Ayurvedic tradition:

    The reader is reminded that in Ayurvedic medicine, too, there is a controversy about the position of the pulse; the important thing to remember is that it is not the position but its movement that is the key to the pulse, and on that there is no disagreement among Ayurvedists.

    R.B. Amber, *The Pulse in Occident and Orient: Its Philosophy and Practice in India, China, Iran, and the West* (New York: Santa Barbara Press, 1966) 110.

11. Unschuld, *Nan-Ching*, 155.

12. Jiang Jing (18) notes that "The lower level of the Mingmen should copy or balance the lower level of the kidney pulse, which represents the ovaries." This seems to correspond to the Pelvis/Lower Body position in our system. He also mentions the position between the distal and middle positions, which we call the Diaphragm position: "The pulses in between the CHUN [distal] and KWAN [middle] locations are representative of the yang energy...." Of the position between the middle and proximal positions, he adds (25), "The pulses between KWAN [middle] and CHI [proximal] locations are representative of yin energy." The positions seem to be the same, although the interpretations are apparently different.

13. Shen, 43, 45.

14. Manfred Porkert does include a limited reference to rolling the finger into auxiliary positions. *The Essentials of Chinese Diagnostics* (Zurich: Chinese Medicine Publications, 1983) 236.

15. Van Buren received this information from Lavier, who got it from Soulié de Morant.

16. Unschuld, *Nan-Ching*, 258.

17. Wang, 23.

18. Deng Tietao, *Practical Diagnosis in Traditional Chinese Medicine*, trans. Marnae Ergil (Edinburgh: Churchill Livingstone, 1999) 90.

19. George Soulié de Morant, *Chinese Acupuncture*, trans. Lawrence Grinnell et al., (Brookline, MA: Paradigm Publications, 1994) 61–63.

20. Giovanni Maciocia, personal communication.

21. John Shen, personal communication.

22. Ibid.

Chapter 3

1. Deng Tietao, *Practical Diagnosis in Traditional Chinese Medicine*, trans. Marnae Ergil (Edinburgh: Churchill Livingstone, 1999) 85.

2. R.B. Amber, *The Pulse in Occident and Orient: Its Philosophy and Practice in India, China, Iran, and the West* (New York: Santa Barbara Press, 1966) 97, 107, 114–15.

3. Amber (2) sums up this dilemma:

    The Westerner is inclined to write off Chinese and Ayurvedic medicine as a mass of superstitious ignorance which should be scuttled or excised from the cultural matrix of healing as though it were a vermiform appendix—no longer serving a purpose. The Oriental physician regards Western medicine as an offshoot of its own system, and a bad one at that, without any theory and with a reliance on gadgets and instruments to cover up its lack of competence in diagnosis and prevention of disease. To the indigenous physician, Western medicine is wrong both in theory and practice: In theory because it is based on morbid anatomy, the science of death, and the laboratory instead of on the science of living. Man does not live in a laboratory or in a vacuum, but in the world of society which molds his mental and physical state either in health or in disease.

[T]he Occident does not have a theory of medicine; therefore the result, to use the cybernetic vernacular, is "garbage–in and garbage–out."

4. Deng, 90–91.

5. Jiang Jing, "A Brief Survey of the Korean Dong Han System of Pulse Diagnosis" *Oriental Medicine* 1993;2(1):19, 21.

6. Ibid., 21–22.

7. This section is based on Leon Hammer, "The Paradox of the Unity and Duality of the Kidneys According to Chinese Medicine" *American Journal of Acupuncture* 1999;27(3&4): 179.

8. Giovanni Maciocia, *The Foundations of Chinese Medicine* (London: Churchill Livingstone, 1989) 40.

9. What are some of the abuses of this basic energy that can account for the ever-increasing Kidney deficiencies across the spectrum, including Kidney essence and yang deficiency, and ultimately the separation of Kidney yin and yang ('qi wild')? What accounts for the regrettable increase in the frequency of pulses that are deficient in Kidney energies, especially in the very young? While this is not the focus of our inquiry here, we are justified in speculating that industrial and post-industrial stresses in the form of pollution, incredible pace, depleted foods, and unnatural conception, pregnancy, delivery, and early childhood practices are some of the places to begin the search.

10. Leon Hammer, "The Unified Field Theory of Chronic Disease with Regard to the Separation of Yin and Yang and 'The Qi is Wild'" *Oriental Medicine* 1998;6(2&3):15.

Chapter 4

1. Deng Tietao's recommendation of an average of three minutes does not provide the practitioner of this exquisite art-science the time it requires and deserves. *Practical Diagnosis in Traditional Chinese Medicine*, trans. Marnae Ergil (Edinburgh: Churchill Livingstone, 1999) 89.

2. Anton Jayasuria, *Textbook of Acupuncture Science* (Dehiwala, Sri Lanka: Chandrakanthi Industrial Press, 1981) 526.

3. R.B. Amber, *The Pulse in Occident and Orient: Its Philosophy and Practice in India, China, Iran, and the West* (New York: Santa Barbara Press, 1966) 111–32.

4. Jayasuria, 529.

5. "Jet lag is another consideration in terms of the Chinese clock and biorhythms. Likewise, night workers can show a reversal of these rhythms. Individuals under stress associated with combat, political campaigns, and those in isolation can also show bizarre variations of the pulses." Ibid., 526.

6. Amber, 160–61. Elsewhere (106) he elaborates:

The best time of the day for taking the pulse was considered the early morning from three to nine o'clock, local mean time, when the physician himself was cool and collected .... It is at this time that the meridians are calm and the conjunctive vessels are empty and no energy is transmitted between the coupled meridians. It is at this moment only that the circulation of the blood and energy channels are calm and that a correct diagnosis can be made. The pulse reveals whether the five Tsang are in excess or deficient and whether the six bowels are strong or weak....

Since the doctor is called upon at any hour of the day or night, he must remember and use the horary cycle or the tides of energy, all discernible by the pulse. The pulse of the stomach, for example, if taken at three o'clock in the afternoon may indicate an exaggerated condition .... [T]he hour of zenith, which is the time for the maximum flow of energy, is 0800 [eight in the morning] for the stomach.

7. According to Amber (128):

   The position of the patient influences the frequency of the beat on an average of eight per minute between the standing and recumbent positions. It beats ten or twelve times faster when one is standing than it does when one is sitting, and beats faster when one is sitting than when one is lying down. As a general rule, the better the posture, the lower the pulse.

8. While Korean and Chinese pulse diagnosis are quite different, Jiang Jing seems to agree with the concept of accessing all positions simultaneously: "When applying pressure make sure that all three fingers exert the same amount of force at all times. The method of releasing a finger or two while reading a pulse is generally very wrong, unless the reader is looking into rather complex chakra or genetic circumstances." Jiang Jing, "A Brief Survey of the Korean Dong Han System of Pulse Diagnosis" *Oriental Medicine* 1993;2(1):15.

9. Deng, 90.

10. Amber, 106.

11. The finding of Heart Enlarged at this position, or for that matter a positive finding in almost any position, is often concurrent with a biomedically-defined 'organic' problem. When such qualities are found on the pulse they are assessed in terms of the total pulse picture, in conjunction with other signs and symptoms. However, I always recommend that a thorough physical examination, with all appropriate testing, be performed to determine which of these findings are energetic and which are 'organic.'

Chapter 5

1. Ted Kaptchuk, *The Web That Has No Weaver* (New York: Congdon and Weed, 1983) 167.

2. Li Shi–Zhen, *Pulse Diagnosis*, trans. Hoe Ku Huynh (Brookline, MA: Paradigm Publications, 1981) 81.

3. C.S. Cheung and Jenny Belluomini, "An Overview of Pulse Types Used In Traditional Chinese Medical Diagnosis" *Journal of the American College of Traditional Chinese Medicine* 1982;1:31.

4. Felix Mann, *Acupuncture: The Ancient Art of Chinese Healing and How It Works Scientifically* (New York: Vintage Books, 1971) 169.

5. Various sources categorize the Normal pulse differently from what has been described here. For example, Li Shi-Zhen (81) refers to the Leisurely quality as the Normal pulse. It is, he says,

   slightly faster than a slow pulse, with exactly four beats per respiration. It is like a thread on a loom which has not been tightened, it ambles beneath the fingers and is normal in every respect. It is elegant and relaxed like a weeping willow branch, swaying in a gentle spring breeze.

   Basically, according to Li (24), this quality indicates "an abundance of shen qi" and that "the stomach qi is still functioning and that the kidney qi is abundant." It is "an indication of health." However, if the Leisurely quality is combined with other qualities, it is a sign of pathology.

6. Manfred Porkert, *The Essentials of Chinese Diagnostics* (Zurich: Chinese Medicine Publications, 1983) 245.

7. Paul Unschuld, trans., *Nan-Ching* (Berkeley: University of California Press, 1986) 245.

8. Ilza Veith, trans., *The Yellow Emperor's Classic of Internal Medicine* (Berkeley: University of

California Press, 1966) 209.

9. Leon Hammer, "The Unified Field Theory of Chronic Disease with Regard to the Separation of Yin and Yang and 'The Qi is Wild'" *Oriental Medicine* 1998;6(2&3):15.

10. Porkert, 243.

11. Dan Bensky, "Editors' Introduction to Chinese Medicine" *Acupuncture: A Comprehensive Text*, trans. and ed. John O'Connor and Dan Bensky (Chicago: Eastland Press, 1981) 28.

12. Deng Tietao, *Practical Diagnosis in Traditional Chinese Medicine*, trans. Marnae Ergil (Edinburgh: Churchill Livingstone, 1999) 93.

13. Richard Van Buren, personal communication, 1973.

14. Graham Townsend and Ysha DeDonna, *Pulses and Impulses* (Northamptonshire: Thorsons Publishing Group, 1990) 73.

15. Ralph Alan Dale, "The Demystification of Chinese Pulse Diagnosis" *American Journal of Acupuncture* 1993;21(1):65.

16. Mann, 169.

17. Bensky, 28.

18. Porkert, 244.

19. Richard Van Buren, personal communication, 1973.

20. Townsend and DeDonna, 73. They assess the spirit at "the Middle level pulse." They observe, "When examining factors related to the Heart, it is the FORCE of the pulse that interests us …. If the Heart, and therefore the Shen [spirit], is in good condition, the pulse will possess an easy strength, with slight elasticity and shortness, and no misbeats."

21. Deng, 94.

22. Porkert, 244.

23. Deng, 94.

24. Richard Van Buren, personal communication, 1973.

25. Townsend and DeDonna, 73.

26. R.B. Amber, *The Pulse in Occident and Orient: Its Philosophy and Practice in India, China, Iran, and the West* (New York: Santa Barbara Press, 1966) 127. Deng (92) concurs.

27. Richard Van Buren, personal communications, 1971–73.

28. Townsend and DeDonna, 70, 71, 74.

29. Porkert, 246.

30. Ibid., 245.

31. John Shen, *Chinese Medicine* (New York: Educational Solutions, 1980) 60.

32. Richard Van Buren, personal communication, 1973.

33. Describing the pulses of pregnancy, Amber (173) quotes from the *Classic of the Pulse:*

> When the pulse of the left wrist … is hurried without slowing down, she will give birth to a boy. When the pulse of the right shows these characteristics … a girl may be expected. If the Tsun pulse is delicate and concealed, the Kuan pulse slippery and the Ch'ih pulse accelerated, there is pregnancy.

See also Li, 50.

34. "Deep, firmer than the firm pulse and has a strong beat." (Li, 14) He continues: "The pulse becomes full at all three levels when perverse qi and upright qi are fighting each other" and deep "when internal heat blocks the spread of qi." (Li, 108) This is technically correct but hardly justifies classifying the Inflated quality with deep, which clinical experience shows is actually uncommon. He then says, "When a pulse is felt both deeply and superficially and has big, long, wiry, strong beats, it is called a full pulse." (Li, 73) Other assertions by Li that are outside of my experience, such as comments about the Slippery and

Tight pulses, I have found are not always Rapid, the Choppy pulse is certainly not always Slow, and the classification of Arrhythmic pulses under the Slow category does not seem to be accurate or useful.

Chapter 6

1. R.B. Amber, *The Pulse in Occident and Orient: Its Philosophy and Practice in India, China, Iran, and the West* (New York: Santa Barbara Press, 1966) 115.

2. Leon Hammer, *Dragon Rises, Red Bird Flies* (Barrytown, NY: Station Hill, 1990) 346.

3. Ibid., 347.

4. This occurs especially in individuals whose eyebrows are continuous from one side to the other; such eyebrows are a sign of a constitutional propensity to constantly change one's mind. Both Dr. Shen and I confirmed this correlation time and again in our practices.

5. John Shen, *Chinese Medicine* (New York: Educational Solutions, 1980) 64.

6. C.S. Cheung and Jenny Belluomini, "An Overview of Pulse Types Used In Traditional Chinese Medical Diagnosis" *Journal of the American College of Traditional Chinese Medicine* 1982;1:34.

7. Ted Kaptchuk, *The Web That Has No Weaver* (New York: Congdon & Weed, 1983) 165.

8. Ibid., 312.

9. Ibid., 165.

10. Li Shi-Zhen associates this pulse with "failure and weakness of the zang qi with deficiency of yuan yang ... deficiency and damage of the lower yuan qi with abdominal pain ... weakness and deficiency of the stomach and spleen [which] causes diarrhea ... weakness of the central yang qi [which] causes vomiting and diarrhea ... after three months of pregnancy it indicates deficiency of yuan qi." *Pulse Diagnosis*, trans. Hoe Ku Huynh (Brookline, MA: Paradigm Publications, 1981) 101. He speaks vaguely and inconclusively when he observes that "the intermittent pulse, which cannot recover its lost beat, stops at regular intervals and it pauses for a little longer than one beat." He also notes (25):

    The intermittent pulse occurs when the yuan qi is failing. If there are symptoms of chronic diarrhea with blood and pus in the stools, caused by severe damage to the yuan qi, or chronic yang deficiency palpitations caused by a cold injury, or extremely severe morning sickness and vomiting [caused by qi stasis] after three months of pregnancy, the pulse is intermittent. This occurs because the channel qi cannot communicate with the mai qi.

    Manfred Porkert adds another etiology: "the consequences of either intense emotions or of mechanical lesions and wounds." *The Essentials of Chinese Diagnostics* (Zurich: Chinese Medicine Publications, 1983) 223. Both are outside of my own experience and are conceivable as short-term reactions to overwhelming physical and emotional trauma leading to shock.

11. The following is a discussion of the Hurried (Hasty Interrupted-Running Rapid) and the Knotted (Adherent) qualities in the literature. These two qualities are both subsumed under the heading of Interrupted in Dr. Shen's system, as he does not distinguish between an irregularly irregular pulse that is Rapid (Hurried) or Slow (Knotted). This discussion is therefore included only for the sake of completeness, since, as explained earlier, I consider these other categories to be no longer relevant in the clinic.

    The Hurried and Knotted qualities express conditions in which the circulation of all or some of the essential substances of the body are diminished, either because of a loss of yin substance due to heat from excess, or a surfeit of yin substance due to cold from excess or deficiency. The diminished circulation ultimately stresses the Heart and causes irregularities in Heart rhythm.

    HURRIED

Li Shi-Zhen (17) classifies this quality with the rapid pulses and calls it 'hasty.' Porkert (222) refers to it as 'agitated,' and Cheung and Belluomini (33) as 'accelerated.'

This is a Rapid pulse that consistently skips beats on an irregular basis. Li Shi-Zhen (98) describes it as "a person who stumbles while walking briskly; the flow is interrupted." He also says the hasty pulse is one that "feels rapid but loses a beat at irregular intervals."

This quality primarily occurs over the entire pulse. When a single position has this quality, it indicates a profound instability in the function of that organ system, which is described below under the category of Unstable.

Kaptchuk (165, 312) considers it to be a "sign of Heat agitating the Qi and Blood." Li Shi-Zhen (98) believes that it "results from fire stasis, qi accumulating in the three heater. Therefore the yin fluid (blood) can be easily damaged. The circulation of qi and blood is obstructed." Accumulations of "thick phlegm, thin phlegm and food" may also be involved. Li (99) continues to say that with loss of consciousness, coma, and delirium, "perverse fire has penetrated the Zang," and that if there are ulcers and abscesses, the heat "has penetrated the muscles and caused accumulation of blood and qi and disintegration." Elsewhere (25) he notes that "the hasty pulse occurs whenever excessive yang heat damages the yin, for example, in lung carbuncles with symptoms such as tidal fever, coughing, spitting of sticky, bad smelling mucus, or chest pain, and also in yang poisoning with purple skin spots, sore throat and possibly vomiting of blood."

Porkert (222) believes that

> If an agitated pulse is strong and large, it may indicate an excess of active energies; if it is weak and small, we may conclude, on the contrary, that structive energies are present in excessive middle position or intensity; or we may infer *inanities algoris* ('cold induced by a depletion of active energy').

This may mean that if the qi cannot move the fluids and blood, they can accumulate and become stagnant.

Felix Mann calls this a 'fast' pulse, which he attributes to "a serious over-abundance of Yang Ch'i, and Yin Ch'i diminished to the point of exhaustion." *Acupuncture: The Ancient Art of Chinese Healing and How It Works Scientifically* (New York: Vintage Books, 1971) 171.

COMBINATIONS OF THE HURRIED QUALITY

Kaptchuk (312) lists the following combinations of the Hurried quality, with his interpretations:

- Hurried, Flooding, and Full: "Pernicious Influence Obstructing Meridian"
- Hurried and Weak: "Deficiency approaching separation of Yin and Yang"
- Hurried and Floating: "Yang Brightness Heat or full Heat and 'Heat Evil' stuck in the meridians."

12. The knotted quality is a Slow pulse that skips beats irregularly. Li Shi-Zhen (99) describes it as "a pulse which feels leisurely, but loses a beat at irregular intervals." Porkert (223) calls this pulse 'adherent.' The knotted quality is felt mainly over the entire pulse. When a single position presents this quality, there is a profound instability in the function of that yin organ system, which is described later in our text under the category of unstable.

    There are a number of interpretations of this pulse, all of which involve stagnation due to cold from either excess or deficiency. The latter includes deficiency of qi, blood, essence, or yang, either individually or in combination. This pulse occurs where the natural current of the body's operation has been interfered with, causing accretion, coagulation, and impediment.

13. Ted Kaptchuk (313) describes combinations with which I have had no experience. He indicates that the Intermittent, Thin, and Sinking combination is associated with deficiency and diarrhea; the Intermittent, Minute, and Thin combination with dry fluids; and the Intermittent and Moderate combination with exhaustion of Spleen qi.

14. Leon Hammer, "The Unified Field Theory of Chronic Disease with Regard to the Separation of Yin and Yang and 'The Qi is Wild'" *Oriental Medicine* 1998;6(2&3):15.

15. Hammer, *Dragon Rises,* 311–22.

16. The *Inner Classic* addresses the 'qi wild' condition in the following reference. Says Qi Bo:

Those who act contrary to the laws of the four seasons and live in excess have insufficient secretions and dissipate in their duties. When they go beyond the mark in the fulfillment of their duties or when they perform their duties incompletely, their secretions are small. When their performance of their duties is incomplete, they live in excess and this causes dissipation. And since under these conditions yin and yang *do not correspond* to each other, a disease results which is known to influence the center [bar] pulse. [italics mine]

Ilza Veith, trans., *The Yellow Emperor's Classic of Internal Medicine* (Berkeley: University of California Press, 1966) 161.

Here, it is the phrase "yin and yang do not correspond to each other" to which we are referring, and the thoughts that precede this phrase are an apt summary of the etiology.

Porkert (215) refers to the 'qi wild' condition at least twice. The first is in his discussion of the Flooding quality, which he associates with "profuse Heat." He also describes this as a sign of deficiency and "grave danger" if this quality persists during convalescence following a serious illness, which he fears is a period of "dissociation of active and structive energies." This corresponds to what Dr. Shen describes as the 'qi wild' dissociation of yin and yang.

Porkert's second reference (223) is in his discussion of the Racing pulse. This is "an extremely excited and accelerated pulse attaining seven to eight beats per respiration in the adult." He continues, "After a collapse of the Yin, the Yang, having lost its foundation, is mobilized in the extreme: a symptom of the imminent collapse of the Qi primum." He explains further (224) that the Kidney essence is exhausted such that the "Yang active energies disperse uncontrolled. At the same time, it is a symptom that this Yang, this active energy has already been greatly depleted or is about to be depleted", and that if it is accompanied by a high fever or terminal tuberculosis, "it must be considered a very serious symptom."

Jiang Jing speaks of "wild movement" as follows: "If the liver pulse is feeding the kidney with a 'wild' movement and the kidney is wildly feeding the Sanjiao [Triple Burner] strongly, then very likely a menstrual period is arriving." He also notes, "So the only way to accurately tell if a woman is pregnant is to distinguish whether the liver is feeding the kidney mildly or wildly." "A Brief Survey of the Korean Dong Han System of Pulse Diagnosis" *Oriental Medicine* 1993;2(1):25.

Li Shi-Zhen (59–60) discusses the separation of yin and yang in the section of his book called "Exhausted Pulses of Yin and Yang." In the following passages, he does not make it clear whether he is talking about pulse qualities which involve the entire organism, or just one organ: "If the pulse beats only at the chi position and is unable to reach the guan position" and "If the pulse beats only at the cun position and is unable to reach the guan position." With respect to both pulses, he continues, "In these two diseases the 'yin and yang separate.'" Other pulse qualities similarly implicated in this separation are "deep, hidden and intermittent" in which the "entire body is in danger of breaking down;" and "floating and scattered, but has no root—it cannot be felt under heavy pressure," which is a sign that "the entire body is already suffering from severe damage." (88)

Not included here are the scenarios when the pulse rate is Slow with high fever, or Rapid with a low temperature. These occur with serious, often life-threatening disease and are among the most profound 'qi wild' conditions, often occurring terminally.

17. Li, 88.
18. Russell Jaffe, in a personal communication, claimed that if on inhalation the pulse increases in intensity and/or amplitude, the direction of transition is positive, and if the pulse decreases in strength, the direction is negative.
19. In the early 1990s I began to do seminars in Berkeley, California. There I found for the first time the ubiquity of these 'qi wild' qualities in a way that I had never encountered elsewhere during the nearly twenty years that I had used this system. It was not so prevalent elsewhere in California, although more so than in the Eastern United States, Europe, China, Japan, or Australia.
20. Amber (114) has commented on the amplitude in terms of biomedical physiology.
21. I have not come across a descriptive quality for this phenomenon in any of the literature.

The closest is the description of Tung by Amber (164): "a tremulous pulse, quick and jerky; its pulsation covering a space no longer than a pea." It is interesting that this description is extraordinarily similar to my own, particularly considering that I wrote my description of the Unstable quality before reading Amber. A personal communication from five element practitioners informs me that in their tradition, the Unstable quality is associated with an Akabane disharmony, an imbalance within a phase (element) between one side of the body and the other. Thus, this quality seems to have been subsumed unofficially under the categories of Hurried and Knotted, which only confuses the clear interpretation of all three. But because the Unstable pulse is relatively common and sufficiently significant, it deserves its own place in the spectrum of qualities.

22. Amber (164) says that the Tung pulse "is indicative of pain caused by internal heat or excessive sweating and hemorrhage."

Chapter 7

1. Deng Tietao, *Practical Diagnosis in Traditional Chinese Medicine*, trans. Marnae Ergil (Edinburgh: Churchill Livingstone, 1999) 84.

2. Deng (112) mentions the heart only once in connection with a rapid rate, and then only as a sequela of diphtheria, rheumatic heart disease, or myocarditis.

3. Li Shi-Zhen describes Rapid pulses at individual positions. *Pulse Diagnosis*, trans. Hoe Ku Huynh (Brookline, MA: Paradigm Publications, 1981) 68. Deng Tietao (112) describes the Rapid pulse with respect to the Lung.

4. John Shen, *Chinese Medicine* (New York: Educational Solutions, 1980) 50, 57.

5. R.B. Amber observes:

    The pulse [rate] is higher in children and as a rule decreases with age.... the [rate] is slower in tall persons and faster in short ones. A glance at the table [below] shows that the pulse rate by itself is meaningless unless it is correlated with age, sex, posture, temperature, altitude, food, kind of beat, chemical, physical and electrical agencies, etc.

    The Pulse in Occident and Orient: Its Philosophy and Practice in India, China, Iran, and the West (New York: Santa Barbara Press, 1966) 130.

6. Li, 17–18.

7. J.R. Worsley, *Acupuncturists' Therapeutic Pocket Book: The Little Black Book* (Columbia, MD: Center for Traditional Acupunture, 1975) D–4.

8. Manfred Porkert, *The Essentials of Chinese Diagnostics* (Zurich: Chinese Medicine Publications, 1983) 211, 223.

9. Li (66, 67) states that the Rapid pulse "results when excessive or yin fluid is damaged. Clinically, there are symptoms of restlessness, mental confusion and delirium." He also associates a Rapid pulse with excessive "yang qi" as with "heart or kidney fire" which can be a "deficient or excessive condition." He attributes a Rapid quality during autumn to "excess internal fire burning the lung yin," which he says is difficult to treat. Elsewhere (22), he notes that a rapid pulse accompanies hot diseases of the yin organs, especially when the pulse is also strong. A Rapid pulse without strength is felt when a small amount of heat in the blood remains, as after pus is discharged from an abscess.

    In addition, Li (66, 67) alludes to a Rapid rate in individual positions and bilaterally at the same burner, which are outside of my experience. Therefore, I have not included it here, but refer readers to the source.

    Ted Kaptchuk says that the Rapid pulse reflects the presence of "Heat accelerating the movement of Blood." "A rapid pulse with strength signifies Excess Heat; a rapid but weak pulse points to Deficient Heat or Empty Fire." The exception is when it accompanies a pattern of cold from deficiency, "in which it is a serious sign of extreme Deficient Yang floating to the outside of the body." *The Web That Has No Weaver* (New York: Congdon and

Weed, 1983) 162, 304.

10. Li, 67.

11. Leon Hammer, *Dragon Rises, Red Bird Flies* (Barrytown, NY: Station Hill, 1990). Chapter 14 discusses the 'nervous system.'

12. Porkert (245) refers to something akin to what we are describing:

> If on a very active individual all six sites uniformly show flooding or uniformly show large pulses—and, after very careful diagnosis, the total absence of any other pathological symptoms—such pulses must be considered to be normal pulses for this individual.

Jiang Jing, in his discussion of pregnancy, notes that "These pulses indicate that there is clear communication between the nervous system, liver and uterus." "A Brief Survey of the Korean Dong Han System of Pulse Diagnosis" *Oriental Medicine* 1993;2(1):24. He is making a clear distinction between the 'nervous system' and the organ systems we usually refer to in Chinese medicine, in a manner similar to that of Dr. Shen.

Jiang Jing (62) also appears to describe the 'nervous system tense' quality that is uniform in all positions and at all depths:

> If a person has a chronic emotional blockage you can usually pick it up on the superficial level of the pulse. Once it progresses to the organic level it will be stored as a deeper stress. In that case, the pulse movement will be sinking down and staying there. The movement of that pulse will not be a typical organic movement, rather it will be a light movement at the deeper level. That kind of movement describes an emotional block that has already settled in the organic level.... When you press deeper, the pulse should be striking the fingertips hard but instead it keeps the same shape and the flexibility of the original pulse, as if it was a miniature copy of that pulse on the lower level. If the emotional pulse is sinking down, it is the time when the stress is not being expressed. Instead, the emotional energy movement is becoming a part of the organic movement.

Under ordinary circumstances the yang energy of the body keeps the yin from leaving through perspiration. The energy of the sun assists the yang of the body in performing this function. Yin energy on the other hand tends to act centrifugally to control the centripetal expansion of yang energy. With yin deficiency, false heat tends to rise to the surface and go out of control. The yin attempts to balance the heat by rising to the surface where the yang accumulates. Because the yang of the body is now out of control it cannot keep the yin from leaving through perspiration, except during the day when the sun provides the necessary yang energy. Thus, there are night sweats.

13. Giovonni Maciocia, *Tongue Diagnosis in Chinese Medicine* (Seattle: Eastland Press, 1987) 138.

14. Li, 18.

15. Shen, 52. Li Shi-Zhen (67) makes the following associations:

- Rapid and Floating: superficial heat
- Rapid and Sinking (Deep): internal heat
- Rapid and Strong: heat from excess
- Rapid and Lacking Strength: heat from deficiency

Kaptchuk (304) makes the following associations:

- Rapid and thin: Deficient Yin (Empty Fire)
- Rapid and floating: likely presence of carbuncle or skin ulcers
- Rapid and slippery: Mucus [phlegm] Fire
- Rapid and hollow: severe loss of blood
- Rapid and wiry: Liver Fire

Wu Shui-Wan indicates that the combination of Rapid and Wiry with intermittent fever reflects a lesser yang symptom, while the same combination by itself is a sign of overpowerful Liver fire. *The Chinese Pulse Diagnosis* (San Francisco: Writers Guild of America, 1973) 43.

16. Shen, 50.

17. Li, 65.
18. Shen, 50. Li Shi-Zhen (65) defines the Slow quality as one that appears when "yang qi is too weak to defeat yin–cold perverse qi, or when deficiency of qi and blood causes a deficient cold condition." He adds that it usually appears in diseases involving the qi of the organs. If the pulse is strong, it indicates the "internal accumulation of excessive pain-inducing cold." If it is lacking in strength, it indicates "deficiency of yang qi causing deficient cold." Slow rates, he notes, can be observed in either the upper, middle, or lower positions, independent of the rate elsewhere in the pulse. I, however, have never heard of or observed such a phenomenon.

    Kaptchuk (303) states that the Slow quality "represents Cold. If this pulse is weak, it signifies insufficient Yang to move the Qi and Blood. If ... strong, it is a sign that Excess Cold is restraining the Qi and Blood," which is often associated with pain. A damp-heat pattern can also be accompanied by a Slow "soft" quality. A Slow quality with "great strength" may signify a "Heat Pernicious Influence getting 'stuck,'" a rare event which can appear in acute heat patterns with abdominal distention or constipation.

19. Li, 79–80.
20. Kaptchuk, 303.
21. Ibid.
22. Li, 65.
23. Dr. Shen's (51) interpretation of the Slow pulse rate with other qualities:

    - Slow, Feeble-Absent, and Thin: internal organs are malfunctioning
    - Slow, Tight, and Full-Overflowing: dilation of the blood vessels, which in the elderly can lead to the hardening of the blood vessels

    Li Shi-Zhen's (65) interpretation:

    - Slow and Floating: superficial perverse cold qi
    - Slow and "Sinking" (Deep): internal perverse cold qi

    Kaptchuk's (303) interpretation:

    - Slow and floating: Exterior Cold
    - Slow and choppy: Deficient Blood
    - Slow and slippery: Phlegm
    - Slow and thin: Deficient Yang
    - Slow and wiry: pain due to Coldness

Chapter 8

1. Though not immediately relevant to this discussion of volume, for those who are interested, R.B. Amber has commented upon volume from a Western perspective. *The Pulse in Occident and Orient: Its Philosophy and Practice in India, China, Iran, and the West* (New York: Santa Barbara Press, 1966) 114.
2. Li Shi-Zhen, *Pulse Diagnosis*, trans. Hoe Ku Huynh (Brookline, MA: Paradigm Publications, 1981) 73.
3. Wu Shui-Wan, *The Chinese Pulse Diagnosis* (San Francisco: Writers Guild of America, 1973) 25.
4. Li, 24, 73.
5. Ted Kaptchuk, *The Web That Has No Weaver* (New York: Congdon and Weed, 1983) 307.
6. Ibid.
7. Leon Hammer, *Dragon Rises, Red Bird Flies* (Barrytown, NY: Station Hill Press, 1990) 313.
8. Amber, 98.

9. Kaptchuk, 163.

10. Hammer, *Dragon Rises,* 344–48.

11. Ibid., Chapter 14.

12. Ibid., 344–48. See also the discussion of the left distal position in Chapter 16 of the present volume.

13. Wu, 26.

14. Kaptchuk, 307.

15. Li (74): "Excessive wind heat in the upper heater causing symptoms such as headache, fever, sore throat, stiffness at the root of the tongue or stuffiness in the chest and diaphragm will reflect in a full pulse at the cun [distal] position."

16. Ibid.: "Stagnant heat in the spleen and stomach—excess perverse heat in the middle heater—causing symptoms of stuffiness and distention in the abdomen, will reflect in a full pulse at the guan [middle] position."

17. Ibid.: "Severe accumulations of excessive heat in the lower heater which cause symptoms such as lumbago, abdominal pain and constipation will reflect in a full pulse at the chi [proximal] position."

18. John Shen, *Chinese Medicine* (New York: Educational Solutions, 1980) 54.

19. Li, 77.

20. Kaptchuk, 315.

21. Li, 12.

22. Ibid., 76.

23. Everyone seems to be in agreement with Li Shi-Zhen (76) that the Flooding pulse "is like the ocean waves hitting the beach, it comes with force but recedes calmly." Kaptchuk (168) says that it "surges with the strength of a big pulse to hit the fingers at all three depths, but it leaves the fingers with less strength, like a receding wave." Manfred Porkert says that "The pulse feels like a tidal wave; it arrives with great power and only recedes slowly and gradually; it is a wide and flooding pulse." *The Essentials of Chinese Diagnostics* (Zurich: Chinese Medicine Publications, 1983) 214. J.R. Worsley reports a pulse which "floats with power. It comes like a flood, but it is weak and long when it goes away." *Acupuncturists' Therapeutic Pocket Book: The Little Black Book* (Columbia, MD: Center for Traditional Acupuncture, 1975) D–8.

24. Li Shi-Zhen (77) considers this pulse to be normal in the summer, and otherwise a sign of fire or heat from excess. This heat may be accompanied by fever during a febrile illness, which gradually depletes yin, or "when blood deficiency produces heart fire blazing upwards." It is my impression that with heat from deficiency, the pulse may show a tendency to recede more quickly.

Kaptchuk's (168) principal assertion is that "heat has injured the Fluids and Yin of the body." Although it can accompany the heat from excess which I normally associate with this quality, it has not been my experience to identify a condition of yin deficiency as the principal pathology associated with the Flooding quality.

According to Kaptchuk (314), with a febrile illness the Flooding pulse is accompanied by symptoms of "thirst, irritability" and "red swollen skin ulceration" and signs of "vomiting of blood." He states that "Heart disharmonies" and "Heat in the Interior being restrained or bottled up by Cold on the Exterior" are other etiologies of this quality. He also describes a Flooding pulse "whose surging forward movement is big but lacks strength and which recedes like a regular flooding pulse. If this pulse is accompanied by such signs as diarrhea, the interpretation is that the bigness signifies deficiency [as does an empty pulse], and the pulse is then considered a sign of deficiency." This is possibly the deficient Flooding 'push pulse' observed by Dr. Shen when a person is literally pushing themself in work or exercise beyond their energy. (This quality is discussed with the reduced volume qualities.)

Porkert (214), who otherwise associates this quality with "profuse heat," also describes it as a sign of deficiency and "grave danger" if the quality "persists for some time" during the convalescence of a seriously ill person. Here he fears the "dissociation of active and structive energies," which is essentially what Dr. Shen describes as 'qi wild.'

Worsley (D–8) calls this the "Large" pulse characterized by constipation, mania, anxiety, headache, thirst, and dry throat.

25. According to Kaptchuk (315), a Flooding and Big pulse is a sign of ascending heat, while a Flooding and Floating pulse signifies exterior heat from yin deficiency. A Flooding and Tight pulse can be felt when heat from excess has persisted for a long time, depleting the fluids and giving rise to heat from yin stasis and deficiency. A Flooding and Sinking pulse indicates "Internal Heat or Cold Restraining Heat," and a Flooding and Slippery pulse indicates "Heat/Mucus."

26. Li, 78.

27. Li Shi-Zhen (77) speaks of "heart fire blazes upward, causing symptoms of dryness in the throat, sore throat and cracked or ulcerated tongue." He also describes Heart problems such as "when blood deficiency produces heart fire blazing upwards."

28. Ibid., 78.

29. Worsley, D–9.

30. Li, 78.

31. Worsley, D–9.

32. Li, 78.

33. Worsley, D–9.

34. Ibid.

35. Ibid.

36. Porkert, 212.

37. Ibid.

38. Ibid.

39. Wu Shui-Wan (45) comments on other combinations of what she calls the 'Full' pulse. This quality is a mixture of what I would classify as Inflated and Tense, the latter because she describes the quality as 'Full' and 'Hard' like the Inflated quality, but 'Long' like the Tense quality. I include the following in discussions of both qualities.

   - FULL AND TIGHT: "The Full Pulse combines with the Tight Pulse. It denotes that there is an accumulation [or congealing] due to the internal chill."
   - FULL AND SLIPPERY: "The Full Pulse combines with the Slippery Pulse. It denotes that there is a coagulating of phlegm fluid. It indicates that the functions of the body are so low that the patient will probably be unconscious, and death is imminent."
   - FULL, RAPID, AND BIG (WIDE): "The Full Pulse combines with the Rapid Pulse and the Big Pulse. It denotes that there is fever in the stomach or intestines."

40. Hammer, *Dragon Rises,* 330.

41. Ibid., 316. See also the glossary in the present volume.

42. Ibid., 330.

43. The Tense Inflated quality was found in this position in one patient with severe cocaine and amphetamine abuse.

44. For example, Deng Tietao notes that "Whether the pulse occurs with force or without force differentiates vacuity [deficiency] and repletion [excess]." *Practical Diagnosis in Traditional Chinese Medicine,* trans. Marnae Ergil (Edinburgh: Churchill Livingstone, 1999) 107.

45. Shen, 55.

46. Wu, 32.

47. Felix Mann, *Acupuncture: The Ancient Art of Chinese Healing and How It Works Scientifically* (New York: Vintage Books, 1971) 169.

48. Giovanni Maciocia, *The Foundations of Chinese Medicine* (London: Churchill Livingstone, 1989) 170.

49. Kaptchuk, 169.

50. Li, 88.

51. Porkert, 219.

52. Kaptchuk, 169, 319.

53. Porkert, 220.

54. Li, 90.

55. Maciocia, 170.

56. Worsley, D–12.

57. Li Shi-Zhen (77–78) refers to a "flooding pulse with deficient symptoms" in connection with deficient Kidney essence. Kaptchuk (314) says "there is a flooding pulse whose surging forward movement is big but lacks strength and which recedes like a regular flooding pulse," adding that "the bigness signifies Deficiency (as does the empty pulse), and the pulse is then considered a sign of Deficiency" if accompanied by such signs as diarrhea. Porkert (215), who otherwise associates this quality with "profuse heat," also describes this as a sign of deficiency and "grave danger" if the quality "persists for some time" during convalescence from a serious illness. Here he fears the "dissociation of active and structive energies," which is essentially what Dr. Shen describes as 'qi wild.'

58. Wu, 35.

59. Kaptchuk, 307.

60. Shen, 55.

61. Ibid., 55–56.

62. Ibid.

63. Mann, 169.

64. Hammer, *Dragon Rises*, 324.

65. Li, 91.

66. I must disagree with Kaptchuk (169) who asserts that this quality "signifies a more extreme Deficient Qi condition" than the Empty quality "because the Qi cannot even raise the pulse." The Empty quality I was taught represents the more extreme condition of qi deficiency in which yang has separated from yin, and qi physiology is in a "wild" and chaotic condition.

    Both Li Shi-Zhen (91) and Kaptchuk (316) elaborate on the kinds of qi deficiency which may predominate. Li states that deficiency of yang qi will lead to a concomitant diminishment of the nourishing and protective qi, with susceptibility to external pathogenic factors and "fear of cold and fever," and spontaneous sweating. Deficiency of essence qi would cause a failure to "nourish the bone marrow" with atrophy of the legs, and to "nourish the tendons or connective tissue" causing atrophy and spasticity. Blood deficiency would cause a failure to "nourish the heart and calm the shen [spirit]," and Spleen qi deficiency would cause prolapses and lassitude. Kaptchuk adds that these deficiencies are seen "primarily in Deficient Kidney patterns along with such symptoms as sore bones, weak back and legs, asthma, tinnitus, or dizziness."

67. Hammer, *Dragon Rises*, 319.

68. Ibid., 344–48. See also the discussion of the left distal position in Chapter 16 of the present volume.

Chapter 9

1. Li Shi–Zhen, *Pulse Diagnosis*, trans. Hoe Ku Huynh (Brookline, MA: Paradigm Publications, 1981) 13, 88.

2. Ted Kaptchuk, *The Web That Has No Weaver* (New York: Congdon and Weed, 1983) 169.

3. Henry David Thoreau. *Walden* (White Plains, NY: Peter Pauper Press, 1966) 12.

4. Kaptchuk (161) classifies the Floating quality under the aegis of depth as "yang" because of its "exteriorness." Other descriptions of the Floating quality are "floating like a log or piece of dry wood on water" (Paul Unschuld, trans., *Nan-Ching* [Berkeley: University of California Press, 1986] 245); "like a piece of dry stick floating on the surface of the water" (C.S. Cheung and Jenny Belluomini, "An Overview of Pulse Types Used In Traditional Chinese Medical Diagnosis" *Journal of the American College of Traditional Chinese Medicine* 1982;1:14); and "like bird's feathers being ruffled by wind" (Li, 61). In addition to these characterizations, Li observes that it is "steady and moves gently like a slight breeze blowing over a feather on the back of a bird."

5. Li, 61.

6. Manfred Porkert, *The Essentials of Chinese Diagnostics* (Zurich: Chinese Medicine Publications, 1983) 210.

7. Deng Tietao, *Practical Diagnosis in Traditional Chinese Medicine*, trans. Marnae Ergil (Edinburgh: Churchill Livingstone, 1999) 97.

8. Li, 71.

9. Cheung and Belluomini, 15.

10. Ibid., 18. The deficient Floating pulse does indeed yield on pressure, but, by definition, it never separates to the extent that it does with the Empty 'qi wild' qualities, and is never absent below the surface. In further support, Wu Shui-Wan states that when slight pressure is exerted, "the pulse will diminish in strength, but it is not so Empty and it is not so soft as touching the cotton." *The Chinese Pulse Diagnosis* (San Francisco: Writers Guild of America, 1973) 14. It should also be noted that, even while defining the Floating pulse as "losing its strength when pressure is increased," Li Shi-Zhen (61–2) differentiates the Floating pulse from most of the 'qi wild' pulses mentioned later in this chapter. His reasoning is that the 'qi wild' pulses are less substantial at the inner depths than is the Floating quality. For example, he notes that "a floating pulse which is without root, coming and going without distinct form, is called a scattered pulse" which separates or is absent beneath the qi depth.

11. Felix Mann, *Acupuncture: The Ancient Art of Chinese Healing and How It Works Scientifically* (New York: Vintage Books, 1971) 169.

12. Giovanni Maciocia, *The Foundations of Chinese Medicine* (London: Churchill Livingstone, 1989) 170

13. Wu, 32.

14. Maciocia (167) adds another deficient Floating quality to the list in the following passage: "In rare cases, the pulse can be Floating in Interior conditions, such as anemia and cancer. In these cases, the pulse is Floating because qi is very deficient and 'floats' to the surface of the body."

15. Kaptchuk, 161, 301.

16. Li, 61.

17. Kaptchuk, 161.

18. Li, 103.

19. Ibid., 61.

20. Ibid.

21. Li Shi-Zhen (20) and Wu Shui-Wan (41) list many combinations of the Floating quality,

but their interpretations of these combinations differ markedly. For example, Li attributes the 'Floating rapid pulse' to "injury due to external wind and heat," while Wu attributes it to "wind, with an abundance of heat (including inflammation) internally." The 'floating slow pulse' for Li indicates "empty qi and injury by wind," and for Wu, "infection due to 'wind' or 'dampness.'"

22. Kaptchuk (301) identifies the following combinations:

    - Floating and Rapid: invasion of external heat
    - Floating and Tight: invasion of external cold
    - Floating and Slippery: wind and phlegm of internal origin, or stagnant food
    - Floating and Long: excess
    - Floating and Short: deficiency, especially of qi
    - Floating, Flooding, and Big: summerheat

23. Li Shi-Zhen (12) classifies the Empty pulse quality as one of the seven floating pulses; by floating, he clearly means superficial. Kaptchuk (306) refers without specific citation to an Empty pulse that is superficial and one that is not, each being a sign of distinctly different conditions. Porkert (220) has no specific reference to the Empty quality, but it is indistinguishable from his own category of the Dispersed pulse, which he describes as being superficial. Wu Shui-Wan (22) notes two types, Soft Empty and Real Empty. *Essentials of Chinese Acupuncture* calls it "Pulse of the Xu Type." Beijing College of Traditional Chinese Medicine, *Essentials of Chinese Acupuncture* (Beijing: Foreign Languages Press, 1980) 58.

24. There is considerable disarray in the classification of the Empty quality. Some of the characteristics have simply been restated through the centuries, without serious and critical clinical investigation. Kaptchuk (163) describes it as "big but without strength" and "weak and soft like a balloon partially filled with water." Kaptchuk, Wu Shui-Wan (22), Cheung and Belluomini (18), R.B. Amber, and J.R. Worsley also characterize the Empty pulse as being slow. R.B. Amber, *The Pulse in Occident and Orient: Its Philosophy and Practice in India, China, Iran, and the West* (New York: Santa Barbara Press, 1966) 164. J.R. Worsley, *Acupuncturists' Therapeutic Pocket Book: The Little Black Book* (Columbia, MD: Center for Traditional Acupuncture, 1975) D–12. Cheung and Belluomini refer to this pulse as deficient, using the same descriptive language as Kaptchuk. Others beside Kaptchuk who allude to it as big are Wu Shui-Wan (23) and Li Shi-Zhen (12). Worsley (D–12) uses the term 'weak' for this quality, and says further: "The pulse is slow without power. It is soft, thin and it sinks. No pulse is felt when the fingers are pressed down." *Essentials of Chinese Acupuncture* (58) describes this pulse as "weak and forceless and disappears on heavy pressure." Porkert (220) indicates that what he calls the 'dispersed' pulse is a "superficial, dispersed or dispersing pulse without root. When the pressure of the palpating finger is gradually reduced, this weak pulse can only be felt after some time and vaguely; if pressure is increased again, it disappears completely." Mann (167) speaks of a pulse that "comes with a floating and soft movement [that] disappears on pressure." Wu Shui-Wan (22) alludes to a 'Soft Empty' pulse, which is consistent with Kaptchuk's description, and a 'Real Empty' pulse that "does not respond to the finger when pressed lightly on the superficial position at the three zones. If a little pressure is exerted to feel the deep position, the doctor can still feel the weak pulse beating."

25. Wu, 22.

26. Cheung and Belluomini, 18.

27. With regard to the Empty pulse and qi deficiency, Li Shi-Zhen (72) observes: "The Empty pulse appears when the upright qi is damaged—after perspiration caused by unconsolidated Wei [protective] qi, after palpitations caused by heart blood deficiency, or after fear or fright caused by heart shen [spirit] deficiency."

    Some sources also allude to blood deficiency as a cause of the Empty quality, as in the following passage from Kaptchuk (306):

    > In general, if the Empty pulse is especially superficial, it is said to signify Deficient blood (that is, to have a Deficient yin aspect); if it is less superficial, then it signifies Deficient qi (that is, it has a Deficient yang aspect). Compared with a thin pulse, an Empty pulse is more indicative of Deficient qi; compared with a frail pulse, it is more indicative of Deficient blood.

    Wu Shui-Wan (22) speaks of two kinds of Empty pulse: "The Soft Empty pulse denotes that the blood is deficient while the Real Empty Pulse indicates that the patient is very weak or weakness due to long illness." Porkert (220), who refers to this as the Dispersed pulse, believes that "the structive part of the qi nativum (the resources of energy acquired at birth and stored in the renal orb) has dispersed, has become diffuse." In addition, Wu, Li, and Kaptchuk all mention this pulse in connection with attack of summerheat.

28. Kaptchuk (306) mentions the following Empty pulse combinations:

    • Empty and very Soft: deficient protective qi, with spontaneous sweating
    • Empty and Rapid: deficient yin
    • Empty and Slow: deficient yang

29. Li, 72. Worsley (D–12) also mentions symptoms of yin and essence deficiency such as "asthenic fever, pollution [spermatorrhea], night sweats, low energy."

30. Li, 72.

31. Kaptchuk (307) notes that the Empty quality in this position is a sign that the "Blood cannot get to the Heart," while Li Shi-Zhen (72) indicates it is due to "heart blood [being] unable to provide nourishment."

32. Kaptchuk (307) says that the Empty pulse in the second position means "Deficient Qi with distended abdomen." Li Shi-Zhen (72) identifies the source of the pulse as "food stagnation and stomach swelling caused by qi deficiency and loss of transforming function."

33. Li Shi-Zhen (72) notes, "When numbness caused by steaming bone heat results from damaged jing [essence] and blood, the pulse becomes empty at both chi positions."

34. Kaptchuk, 307.

35. Ibid.

36. Worsley, D–12.

37. According to Kaptchuk (306):

    The organ most associated with an Empty pulse is the Spleen. This association further contributes to the identification of an Empty pulse with Deficient qi, because the Spleen, in itself, is frequently associated with Deficient qi or with a combination of Deficient qi and Deficient blood patterns, but rarely with Deficient blood patterns alone.

    Worsley (D–12) mentions the symptoms of fatigue, gas pain, shortness of breath, poor appetite, and dyspepsia in connection with the Empty quality at this position.

38. Kaptchuk (307) notes an association between this quality here and symptoms of soreness or atrophy of the low back and knees, while Worsley (D–12) mentions incontinence, impotence, tinnitus or hearing defects, and rheumatism.

39. Kaptchuk, 307.

40. Worsley, D–13.

41. Kaptchuk (169) calls this quality Soggy, and categorizes it as one of the ten less important pulses. Li Shi-Zhen (188) refers to it as the Soft pulse. Cheung and Belluomini (21) use the term synonymously with "Soft–floating." Wu Shui-Wan (32) and Mann (169) refer to the pulse as "Weak–Floating," and Wu says further that it can also be called "Soft." She categorizes this with the "Empty Kind." Although not mentioned by its English name, Amber (164) spells it in the Wade-Giles transliteration as *ju*, which is the same as *ru* in pinyin.

42. Amber (164) describes this quality as "a soft pulse, superficial and fine—like a thread floating on water." The "thread floating on water" is the description that comes closest to my own experience. Kaptchuk (169) describes the Soggy pulse as

    a combination of the Thin, Empty, and Floating pulses. It is extremely soft, is less clear than a Thin pulse and is perceptible only in the superficial position. The slightest pressure makes it disappear. A Soggy pulse feels like a bubble floating on water.

    Li Shi-Zhen (88) and Wu Shui-Wan (32) are consistent with both of the above descriptions. Li (61) adds that this quality "is like a bubble, which bursts when pressure is lightly increased." Under the Floating quality he says that the "floating pulse which is spongy, weak and thin is called a soft pulse." Worsley (D–12) calls this the Soft pulse and notes that it is "insufficient, weak and soft; it is without power like a lump of cotton wool dipped in water." Although he does not allude directly to the Empty quality of this pulse, his expression "without power" can be interpreted to have this meaning.

For beginners, this pulse quality is relatively obscure. The following comparisons of this quality with other similar superficial and deficient pulse qualities may be helpful. They are drawn from Li Shi-Zhen and Wu Shui-Wan. The Empty pulse is "bigger" (Wu, 32), the Minute pulse is "intermittently indistinct" (Li, 89), the "Weak" (Feeble-Absent) pulse is deep (Li, 89), and the Thin pulse "can be clearly felt at a sinking position" (Li, 89).

43. Kaptchuk (317, 169) asserts that this pulse is a sign of extreme deficiency of blood, essence, and to a lesser extent yang. This is due primarily to a loss of fluids and blood after a serious illness, childbirth or miscarriage (including abortion), or after surgery, when the patient has not received rest and nourishing therapy. Li Shi-Zhen (89) attributes the deficiency to "damage to the ying–blood and severe deficiency of yin jing," and "with deficiency in the sea of marrow and deficiency of dan–tian." Even in the absence of disease, the pulse "is said to be without root, due to failure of the kidney and spleen", which should be treated promptly.

Li (89) has also found this pulse with "Spleen deficiency with inability to control dampness." Kaptchuk (317) adds that the Soggy quality can accompany a "damp pattern, because the dampness 'spreads everywhere' and obstructs qi and blood movement.... In this case, the Soggy pulse is likely to have a tight, hindered quality." With this pattern, the dampness is interfering with the free flow of qi and blood, and there may be water stagnation at the surface in the form of non-pitting edema in the connective tissue. Thus, the patient is not as wasted as when the pulse is due to depletion of fluids and blood.

Finally, Worsley (D–12) describes a Soft pulse to which he ascribes "anemia, bleeding, internal wounds caused by damp and moisture," and Wu Shui-Wan (32) always regards this quality as "a sign of danger," independent of the duration of the illness.

44. Below are references to those with direct experience of this quality at individual positions.

Bilateral at the Same Position

DISTAL

The Empty and Thread-like quality at this position is to be found when "the yang qi is weak and the surface cannot be consolidated, nonstop sweating appears." (Li Shi-Zhen, 90)

MIDDLE

At the middle position, Li (90) associates this pulse with deficient Stomach, Spleen, and "central qi."

PROXIMAL

At the proximal position, Li (90) notes that this quality signifies injury to the essence and blood, and deficiency and cold in the lower burner.

Sides

The Empty Thread-like quality does not appear on either side alone.

Individual positions

The following material is drawn from Worsley (D-12). His source is unknown, and although I do not make immediate associations with all of these symptoms from my own experience, they do largely coincide with the general meanings of yin, blood, and essence deficiency previously discussed in the summary descriptions of this pulse.

LEFT DISTAL

Associated symptoms are palpitations, phobia, nightsweats, fatigue, shortness of breath, low energy, and anxiety.

RIGHT DISTAL

Associated symptoms are fever, feeling cold, and weakness.

LEFT MIDDLE

Associated symptoms are quick temper, dizziness, impotence, and aspermic paralysis.

RIGHT MIDDLE

Associated symptoms are poor appetite, stomach pain, vomiting, and diarrhea.

LEFT PROXIMAL

Associated symptoms are spermatorrhea, bleeding, and nightsweats.

RIGHT PROXIMAL

Associated symptoms include diarrhea and frigidity.

45. Worsley D–11.

46. Porkert, 218.

47. Amber, 164.

48. Kaptchuk, 170.

49. Li, 87.

50. Ibid.

51. Kaptchuk, 170

52. Cheung and Belluomini, 29.

53. Porkert (219) agrees with this assessment, stating that this quality reflects "outward strength with inward depletion" which shows that "extremely exhausted resources of structive energies fail to control active energy, a situation corresponding to a vicious circle which pushes active energy to the surface, permitting it to disperse completely." The heightened severity of this condition over that signified by the Empty quality suggests greater deficiency.

    In all of the literature the Leather quality is identified as a sign of deficient yin, essence, or blood. It is said to occur more frequently in women as a result of prolonged uterine bleeding, especially after miscarriage or abortion, or even normal childbirth. This quality is also found in older men as a sign of deficient essence "after emissions cause deficiency and damage of ying qi." (Li Shi-Zhen, 24, 87) This quality can also appear at the end of life when the marrow is consumed and the essence is impaired. Thus, the Leather quality is considered to be one of the eight pulses of death.

    When the pulse is Leathery and Slow, cold stagnation with pain can be present due to interference with the circulation. Mann (169) refers to this when he says of this quality, there is "extreme excess of excess cold." Li (24, 87) also speaks of its association with "cold perverse qi."

    Blood deficiency can also cause diminished circulation and blood stagnation with pain. Li (25) observes, "The leather pulse in women occurs after severe blood loss, when the blood and qi are deficient and there is penetration by perverse cold. In this case, the deficiency and cold fight each other." According to Dr. Shen, when accompanied by the Moderately Tense Hollow quality, bleeding is always from a yin organ, whereas bleeding unaccompanied by this quality signifies loss of blood from other than a yin organ. Menorrhagia from the uterus is an example of bleeding from other than a yin organ.

    Finally, Cheung and Belluomini (29) note that this quality "may indicate systemic arteriosclerosis of the vessel. The pulse strength and amplitude are increased; the blood volume is low and there is insufficient vessel filling." Again, the Tense Ropy quality is called to mind.

54. The following combinations are based on Kaptchuk's (317) interpretation:

    - Leather Slippery and Wide: accompanied by excess perspiration or diarrhea
    - Leather and Moderate without Spirit: "dead" yin, which is not treatable

- Leather and Slow: cold stagnation

55. Li Shi-Zhen (12) classifies this pulse among the Floating pulses. Kaptchuk (172) includes it among the "other pulses" which he considers to be less important refinements of the first eighteen pulses. Porkert (220) calls it the Dispersed pulse.

56. John Shen, *Chinese Medicine* (New York: Educational Solutions, 1980) 57–58. While all sources agree about the discontinuous, diffuse nature of the sensation at the surface, and its increasing lack of substance as pressure is applied, there are differences as to whether it is "big" (Kaptchuk and Li Shi-Zhen) or "small" (Maciocia, Shen, and myself).

    Kaptchuk (319) cites other sources to the effect that this pulse "can have the uneven quality sometimes associated with a choppy pulse." Worsley (D–13) says it "does not appear to meet and is scattered." Maciocia (170) notes that it "feels very small and is relatively superficial. Instead of feeling like a wave, the pulse feels as if it were 'broken' in small dots." Li (92) describes it somewhat differently:

    > A pulse which feels indistinct, big and without strength when slight pressure is applied, but vanishes when pressure is increased, is called a scattered pulse.... It is like dandelion seeds in the wind, it feels diffuse. Sometimes its beats rise with strength and fall without strength, and sometimes vice versa. They are therefore indistinct.

    Porkert (220) describes it as "a superficial, dispersed or dispersing pulse without root. When the pressure of the palpating finger is gradually reduced, this weak pulse can only be felt after some time and vaguely; if pressure is increased again, it disappears completely." Kaptchuk (172) mentions that it "is similar to an empty pulse because it is floating, big and weak. It is larger and much less distinct than the empty pulse, however, and tends to be felt primarily as it recedes."

57. Shen, 57–58. All sources concur that this is an extremely serious sign. Li (92) states that it is an indication that the source qi—or what Porkert (220) calls "qi primum"—has been irrevocably destroyed. The latter says that "the resources of energy acquired at birth and stored in the renal orb have dispersed," indicating "that the energy of all orbs is about to be depleted."

    Li (92) believes that when this quality appears during a chronic illness, Spleen yang, which is dependent upon Kidney yang, has also been severely injured. And when this pulse is found during pregnancy, "it indicates that child delivery is imminent. If it is too early for delivery, miscarriage can result."

    Kaptchuk (173, 319) agrees with Li, adding, "Kidney yang [is] exhausted and along with normal qi is 'floating away'." He continues:

    > Unlike the weak [Feeble-Absent] pulse mentioned earlier, in which matching pulse and pattern meant the condition would be relatively easy to treat, this is extreme weakness, and the pattern is difficult to reharmonize.... This pulse is usually seen in chronic patterns or in patterns of exhaustion.

    Cheung and Belluomini (27) note that "Chi and essence are [at] termination."

58. Kaptchuk, 319.

59. Li Shi-Zhen (93) and Worsley (D–13) have the following observations about the Scattered quality at the individual positions.

    LEFT DISTAL

    Here, the Scattered quality reflects Heart yang deficiency with such symptoms as palpitations and phobias.

    RIGHT DISTAL

    Dysfunctional protective qi can lead to the Scattered quality at this position. Accompanying symptoms may include spontaneous sweating, nightsweats, and deficiency-type asthma.

    LEFT MIDDLE

    Worsley reports that this quality accompanies paralysis. He also mentions insomnia with the Scattered quality at this position.

RIGHT MIDDLE

Li associates this quality with "swelling and edema of the legs or the dorsal surface of the foot...when spleen yang is deficient and water-damp pours downward." Worsley mentions "dyspepsia [and] debility."

LEFT PROXIMAL

According to Li, the Scattered quality at this position indicates "chronic diseases [that] are caused by scattered qi." Worsley mentions "weakness [in the] loins and knees."

RIGHT PROXIMAL

For Li, the indications associated with the right proximal position mirror those on the left. Worsley finds "fatigue [and] tinnitus aurium."

60. Kaptchuk, 168.

61. Cheung and Belluomini, 23.

62. In obvious contradiction, however, Li Shi-Zhen (14) classifies the Minute quality with the Floating pulses. Kaptchuk (168) includes it as one of the "ten other" pulses which he considers refinements of the others, and therefore "less important." Porkert (221) does not mention a single pulse description similar to that described in the literature. Instead, his Exhausted, Evanescent, Frail, Small, and Minute qualities each shares some of the characteristics of the Minute quality that is described in our system here. Porkert, incidentally, classifies the Small quality with the Minute, and then says that "the actual distinction between these two pulses, however, quite often has significance." The "significance" is not explained, however. Worsley (D–9, 10) describes a number of pulse qualities in which there is "no pulse when the fingers are pressed down"; but the closest to the Minute quality seems to be his Small pulse.

63. The Minute pulse is felt only at the middle blood depth according to the diagrams of Kaptchuk (168), Li Shi-Zhen (78), and Cheung and Belluomini (23), and disappears under slight pressure. Li describes it as being "like a fine thread [that] breaks when pressure is applied, and [it] becomes intermittently indistinct fading in and out." Kaptchuk says that it is very Thin but "lacks the clarity of the thin pulse." Worsley (D–9) adds that it "probably [is] not a pulse when the fingers are pressed down." He also indicates that it is "slow," a characteristic not mentioned by any other source. Wu Shui-Wan (26) and Mann (168) describe its quality as "blurred," and Cheung and Belluomini (23) describe its amplitude as "small."

64. Kaptchuk (315) points out that this quality can appear either at the final stage of the depletion of qi and yang, or at the end stage of "Vanquished Yin" and "Vanquished Yang," as an example of the principle that at their extremes, conditions transform into their opposites. The reason for this is the interdependence of yin and yang, such that a severe depletion of one will force the other into almost complete dysfunction. It is at this point that the yin and yang separate and can no longer interact to preserve and enhance life. This condition is signaled by cold symptoms such as extreme weakness, oily perspiration, loose stools, intolerance of cold, shallow respiration, or what Kaptchuk calls "Vanquished Yang."

For this pulse quality Li Shi-Zhen (24, 79) refers to "the five types of fatigue and the six types of extreme fatigue in men." Wu Shui-Wan (27) mentions "that the body has very weak metabolism ... [that] may lead to death." She also states that if this quality appears suddenly in the course of an acute illness, the prognosis is better than if the quality appears when "the patient has been ill for a long time." Cheung and Belluomini (23) include "shock or pre–shock due to decreased blood volume" as the source of this quality.

According to Dr. Shen, who concurs with Li Shi-Zhen, one etiology is excessive menstrual flow at a very early age, which depletes the blood and qi at a vulnerable time in energetic development. Li (24, 79) says that "both blood and qi are Empty." Thus, the patient has less resistance to disease and more difficulty recovering, thereby draining the system continuously throughout life, which may itself be shortened by this vicious cycle of devitalization.

65. The following combinations and their interpretations are taken from Kaptchuk (315):
    - Minute and Soggy: spasms
    - Minute and Soft: spontaneous sweating
    - Minute and Choppy: great loss of blood

66. The following information is from the literature, which I cannot personally corroborate.

    Bilaterally at the same position

    DISTAL POSITION

    Li Shi-Zhen (24, 79) states that this quality can be a sign of Heart qi deficiency causing Lung qi deficiency, and in turn, dyspnea and fright. He states, "The Minute cun pulse indicates that the yang is deficient (the cun position belongs to yang). There is accompanying fear of cold." Kaptchuk (316) mentions that it signifies "asthma and heart palpitations."

    MIDDLE POSITION

    Li (79) and Kaptchuk (316) say that the Minute pulse at this position may signify Spleen qi deficiency with abdominal distention.

    PROXIMAL POSITION

    Indicates severely injured yang with cold symptoms, severely injured yin and essence with extreme dryness characteristic of "triple parching" diabetes (Li, 24, 79). Li (24) writes, "The yin is deficient (the chi position belongs to yin). There is usually accompanying fever."

    Individual positions

    LEFT DISTAL

    Kaptchuk (316) associates the pulse at this position with deficient Heart blood and qi with anxiety and palpitations, and Worsley (D–10) adds fatigue and phobia.

    RIGHT DISTAL

    Kaptchuk (316) links stagnation caused by phlegm and deficiency-type asthma with this position, while Worsley (D–10) mentions "cold [in the] upper chest and head" and "gas-like pain [in the] chest."

    LEFT MIDDLE

    Worsley (D–10) reports "[l]ow in energy; chagrin; cold at limbs; cramp or convulsion." Kaptchuk (316) adds "sensation of pressure in chest; spasms in four limbs."

    RIGHT MIDDLE

    Deficiency-type pain in the abdomen and poor digestion due to severe deficiency of the Stomach and Spleen are associated with the Minute quality at this position. Kaptchuk (316) says the etiology can be "Stomach cold and food not [being] transformed," while Worsley (D–10) indicates that the accompanying symptoms are indigestion, stomach pain, oppressive sensation in the chest, and cold-type pain in the abdomen.

    LEFT PROXIMAL

    The literature is in agreement that this pulse is associated with deficiency-type uterine bleeding and leukorrhea, depleted essence with impotence, spermatorrhea, and weakness of the lower limbs. For example, Worsley (D–10) mentions "frigidity, hematuria, menorrhagia, leukorrhea, and anemia," while Kaptchuk (316) alludes to "injured sperm and uterine bleeding."

    RIGHT PROXIMAL

    In the literature, associated symptoms include early morning diarrhea, cold and pain from deficiency below the umbilicus, and a deep-seated feeling of internal cold due to severe yang deficiency. Kaptchuk (316), for example, attributes "kidney diarrhea, pain in navel region, and extremely Deficient yang" to this pulse, while Worsley (D–10) identifies diarrhea and cold-type pain in the abdomen.

67. Porkert, 232.

68. Li, 83.

69. Wu, 83.

70. Porkert (218) agrees with my picture of the Hollow quality as being completely or partially missing at the blood depth. As he says, "This is a long superficial pulse which readily collapses under the exploring finger and disappears, only to reappear in depth upon increased pressure of palpation." Mann (175) describes "the sensation [as] being shaped like an onion stem; either floating or deep with a hollow area in the middle."

   In their diagrams and written material, neither Li Shi-Zhen (83) nor Kaptchuk (172) says that the pulse has a bottom. This is a clear departure from Porkert, Mann, and my own experience. Cheung and Belluomini (28) refer to this quality as "Leakstalk" and say that it is an "Empty-centered quality," but in their diagram, they show no organ depth. This is somewhat puzzling since Li, Kaptchuk, and Cheung and Belluomini all use the terms "spring onion," "green onion," "onion stem," and "green leakstalk" in describing this quality; these terms imply a hollowness in the center only.

71. Kaptchuk's (319) interpretations of Hollow combinations include the following:

    - Hollow, Empty and Soft: deficient essence, loss of blood
    - Hollow and Rapid: deficient yin
    - Hollow and Knotted: stagnant blood

    Jiang Jing (21) indicates that the Hollow and Stringy quality "means there is an imbalance between qi and blood, and usually extreme deficiency of blood."

72. Wu Shui-Wan (29) captures the essence of this quality when she says, "This pulse shows that the volume of blood is less than the actual volume of the artery. It denotes that there has been a great loss of blood" and reflects either the actual or imminent loss of blood. Li Shi-Zhen (84) refers to "perverse fire" invading either the three yang or the three yin channels, leading to either external or internal bleeding. He also notes that the heavy bleeding can cause external excess and internal deficiency. Kaptchuk (172, 319), in agreement with Porkert, mentions that this quality signifies "Deficient blood, and is often seen after great loss of blood, but not in chronic patterns of Deficient blood." However, all authors fail to make the distinction between the moderately Tense Hollow and the Yielding Hollow (often Full-Overflowing) qualities, and associate the moderately Tense Hollow quality with acute loss of blood and the Yielding Hollow (Full-Overflowing) quality with chronic blood loss.

73. Shen, 57.

74. Worsley, D–9.

75. Worsley (ibid.) associates it with "irregularity of menstruation with heavy bleeding [and] anemia."

76. However, several authors, including Li Shi-Zhen (63), Mann (166), Wu Shui-Wan (16), and Maciocia (167), speak of detecting this quality at the bone, muscle, or tendons. Li (21) has the most to say concerning sensation. He notes enigmatically that

    > it feels like a ball of cotton wool on sand, soft at the surface, but strong and rigid below. It can only be felt when searched for, and is comparable to a stone in water. It is deep and depressed, like water, which sinks by nature.

77. Worsley, D–13.

78. Li Shi-Zhen (21) states that this combination, which he calls "the sinking pulse without strength," is indicative of qi stagnation, and that "the yin jing [essence] is deficient or damaged." Wu Shui-Wan (42) believes that "the deep pulse combines with the weak pulse [denoting] the extreme debility of the internal organs."

79. Kaptchuk (302) indicates that this quality is present when "Pernicious Influence is strong and qi is Deficient; [the patterns is] usually accompanied by pain." Li Shi-Zhen (21) adds "stagnant cold (cold pain)" and Wu Shui-Wan (42) "internal chill" as causes of this quality.

80. As to other sources who mention this combination and its causes, Kaptchuk (302) indicates "Constrained Liver qi," and Li Shi-Zhen (21) "pain caused by phlegm," with which Wu Shui-Wan (42) agrees.

81. Kaptchuk (302) believes that this combination represents "Cold Dampness/Mucus or stag-

nant food." Li Shi-Zhen (21) states that "Diminished digestive ability causes symptoms of accumulation," adding that the "sinking leisurely pulse indicates accumulated thin phlegm." Wu Shui-Wan (42) says that a Deep and Slippery combination "denotes internal obstruction that is caused by phlegm."

82. Li Shi-Zhen (21) mentions "deficiency cold," Kaptchuk (302) "Interior cold," and Wu Shui-Wan (42) "internal chill," as causes of this combination.

83. Li, 21.

84. Kaptchuk (302) mentions "Interior heat" as the cause of this combination, a notion with which both Li Shi-Zhen (21) and Wu Shui-Wan (42) agree.

85. Kaptchuk (302) mentions "Deficient qi/Congealed blood" and Wu Shui-Wan (42) "poor circulation of blood." Other combinations of the Deep quality that I have not encountered, but which are found in the literature, include Deep and Firm, and Deep and Full. Wu Shui-Wan (42) says that this quality "denotes that a dense accumulation has formed internally," while Li Shi-Zhen (64) says that it "indicates chronic cold disease." Only Li (64) mentions the combination of Deep and Full, saying that it "indicates internal heat."

86. Shen, 48.

87. Kaptchuk (303) alludes to "Mucus Obstructing the Chest," and Li Shi-Zhen (64) mentions "water retention or phlegm obstructed between the chest and diaphragm" associated with the Deep quality at this position.

88. Shen, 49.

89. Ibid.

90. Shen, 50.

91. Li, 64.

92. Hammer, 344–48.

93. Worsley (D–3) lists "cardialgia, pain [in] the chest and ribs owing to phlegm," and Kaptchuk (303) mentions "Deficient Heart yang" with a "desire for sleep" as signs of the Deep quality in this position.

94. Kaptchuk (303) identifies deficient Lung qi, cough, shortness of breath, and asthma, with this quality, and Worsley (D–3) asthma and gasping. Dr. Shen (48) describes a "deep and fine pulse at the bean-bone, [which means that] the individual may have had or is about to have tuberculosis."

95. Kaptchuk (303) mentions "Constrained Liver qi [and] pain," and Worsley (D–3) pain in the ribs, in connection with the Deep quality at this position.

96. Worsley (D–3) states that the Deep quality at this position can be due to "gastric troubles or dilation [distention] of the stomach," while Kaptchuk (303) attributes it to "Deficient Spleen qi [and] diarrhea."

97. Personal communication.

98. Worsley (D–2) mentions that the Deep quality in the left proximal position indicates "lumbago and a sensation of coldness in the back, and frequency of urination." Kaptchuk (303) states that this quality means "Deficient Kidney qi, difficulty in urination, lumbago, vertigo, menstrual irregularities."

99. Worsley (D–3) indicates that the Deep quality at the right proximal position signifies sciatica and lumbago, while Kaptchuk (303) repeats the indications for the left proximal position.

100. Porkert, 219.

101. Kaptchuk, 171.

102. Cheung and Belluomini, 29.

103. Mann, 169.

104. Li, 87.

105. The Confined and Prison pulses are defined by Kaptchuk (171) as being "opposite of the leather pulse and is a form of the hidden pulse ... This pulse is basically a subcategory of the hidden pulse with strength."

106. Worsley, D–11.

107. Wu, 31.

108. Wu (ibid.) writes of "an internal chill which causes poor blood circulation and poor functioning of the organs, forming accumulation internally." She and others who refer to cold are not clear on the pathogenesis of the "internal chill" or internal cold. Li Shi-Zhen (88), for example, regards this pulse as a sign of excess, and alludes to an undefined "excessive perverse qi" causing "excessive internal cold with symptoms like cold pain in the heart region and abdomen," in addition to symptoms "like hernia and lumps in the abdomen." The latter could be interpreted as a neoplastic process, but the translation is not clear. He states that this pulse can exist with excess, as above, which is not serious because the pulse is going "with the current" (meaning with the etiology of internal cold from excess), or with diseases of deficiency, in which case the problem is more serious because the pulse is going "against the current."

Kaptchuk (171) believes that the Firm quality is a sign of obstruction due to cold, characterized as yang within yin. Porkert (219) mentions "painful blocks in the abdomen," and indicates that when found in a pattern of deficiency "as part of a general 'exhaustion' diagnosis, there is immediate danger of death."

Whether this quality can be associated with deficiency is unclear. None of the sources seems to refer explicitly to cold from deficiency, such as chronic Spleen or Kidney yang deficiency, although it is suggested. Li (88) and Kaptchuk (318) mention the possible association of this quality with deficiency, including "running piglet disease."

109. Worsley (D–11) is the only source who mentions individual positions and the associated symptoms as follows:
    - Left distal: "thirst, baked tongue, bifid tongue"
    - Right distal: "suffocation, diabetes"
    - Left middle: "abdominal pain"
    - Right middle: "poor appetite, palpitations"
    - Left proximal: "rupture (e.g., of the appendix), tumor"
    - Right proximal: "sore loin and knee, constipation, and dysuria"

110. Shen, 57.

111. The Hidden pulse is classified as the deepest of the Deep or Sinking pulses. Worsley (D–14) calls it the Prostrate pulse, Mann (170) uses the term Buried, Cheung and Belluomini refer to it as both Hidden and Latent, and Porkert (221) as recondite. The Hidden quality is of two types, one known as Hidden Excess and the other as Hidden Deficient. Shen (57) and Maciocia (170) discuss only the Hidden Deficient pulse, while Li (95) and Mann (170) mention only the Hidden Excess type. The other sources mention both types of the Hidden quality.

112. Worsley, D–14.

113. Kaptchuk (318) observes, "If the hidden pulse is without strength, it is usually a sign that yang qi is insufficient to raise the pulse." Wu (37) writes:

> It also denotes that the body is extremely weak with internal chill and at the same time the exterior part of the body catches cold [such that] the Interior and Exterior parts of the body are cold. The 'yang qi' means that the organic function is extremely weak.

114. Although Porkert (222) speaks mostly of the Hidden Excess quality, he concludes that "if the pulses on the sites of both hands show reconditeness, if in addition the pulse in the foramina 'yang impedimentalis' and 'rivulus major' can no longer be felt, this indicates imminent death."

115. According to Kaptchuk (318), the latter situation is found after a cerebrovascular accident due to "a chronic pattern combining Arrogant Liver yang and Deficient Kidney yin" and is a sign of severe collapse. He continues, "when an extreme heat situation displays a hidden rapid pulse, it is a situation in which the pattern and pulse do not match and is therefore serious and difficult to treat."

Li Shi-Zhen (95) observes, "The hidden pulse is usually caused by perverse cold obstructing the jing luo or zang fu," thus "preventing yang qi from surfacing." Stagnant internal yin-cold is accompanied by "cold sensations around the navel or in the abdomen with ice cold limbs." Internal stagnation of cold transformed into heat may block the channels, causing obstruction of blood and qi. He adds that the Hidden pulse may appear with "food accumulation or in intermittent abdominal pain caused by phlegm stasis." He also speaks of "perverse cold generating heat, when internal stasis of perverse qi blocks the jing mai, obstructing the blood and qi."

Li (96) states that the Hidden pulse is a sign that the cause is "external cold blocking the channels," which may be preventing yang energy from reaching the surface, "in which case it disappears as soon as the yang qi clears the cold and produces perspiration."

116. Kaptchuk, 318.

Chapter 10

1. Li Shi-Zhen does not list the terms 'wide' or 'big' among his categories of twenty-seven pulse qualities, but he often does use the word 'big' in his book on the pulse. *Pulse Diagnosis*, trans. Hoe Ku Huynh (Brookline, MA: Paradigm Publications, 1981)

2. For example, Wu Shui Wan says that it is "twice as wide as a normal pulse." That is why I use the term Wide to represent that group of pulses that are wider than normal. *The Chinese Pulse Diagnosis* (San Francisco: Writers Guild of America, 1973) 34.

3. The Wide Excess pulse is referred to as 'large' by Manfred Porkert, *The Essentials of Chinese Diagnostics* (Zurich: Chinese Medicine Publications, 1983) 215, and by C.S. Cheung and Jenny Belluomini, "An Overview of Pulse Types Used In Traditional Chinese Medical Diagnosis" *Journal of the American College of Traditional Chinese Medicine* 1982;1:26. It is not mentioned as a separate quality by Dr. Shen, or by Li Shi-Zhen.

4. Porkert, 215. Li Shi-Zhen (76, 102) specifically mentions it as an alternate term for Flooding, which he says has a "very large base" and which "is rough and big with beats that rise strongly but fade out as they fall." He calls the Flooding pulse 'big' and goes on to say that "Abundant Internal heat causes the arteries to expand. Therefore, excessive heat causes a strong superficial pulse [referring to the 'big' pulse]."

   The dilemma is that "abundant internal heat in the arteries" is associated by many with a Wide quality at the blood depth. For example, in the diagrams of both Ted Kaptchuk, *The Web That Has No Weaver* (New York: Congdon and Weed, 1983) 163, and Cheung and Belluomini (26), the Wide pulse is shown at the blood depth. Therefore, in agreement with these writers and with Porkert, who emphasizes the distinction from the Flooding quality, I see the Wide pulse more closely related to heat in the blood, and consequently to the Full-Overflowing quality as defined in this book, than to the Flooding Excess quality whose heat or fire comes from the organs. However, our discussion will include both.

5. Cheung and Belluomini, 26.

6. Wu Shui-Wan (34) observes, "It is twice as wide as a normal pulse, and felt as full below the fingers, but the pulse beat is not too strong." Porkert (215) agrees that "it does not well up" and adds that it is "longer than the ordinary pulse." Kaptchuk (162) says also that it is "broad in diameter, very distinct, and suggests Excess."

7. Cheung and Belluomini (26) support Dr. Shen and the thesis laid out concerning the relationship of heat and the circulation under the aegis of the Full-Overflowing quality. They note: "This pulse indicates a dilation and thickening of the arterial wall, increased filling of blood and increased stroke volume."

   Porkert (215) mentions "a rampant heteropathy (vigor heteropathiae)" and "a spreading, rapidly increasing heteropathy." Nowhere in the indexes of his book is there a definition of these terms.

   Richard Van Buren (unpublished lecture notes, 1971–74) associates the Big quality with arthritis, which is identified with heat. It signifies a "strong personality"—not disease— "up to the age of forty-two for women and forty-nine for men," and "warmth in the artery." He adds that "If big and long, the patient will live long, with a very quick recovery." Li Shi-Zhen (23) states that "The big pulse indicates that the disease is intensifying." Both Li and Van Buren view this pulse as a testament to the patient's strength and ability to resist disease.

Other examples of the use of the term 'big' by Li Shi-Zhen are instructive. "When extravasated blood coagulates internally, the pulse is usually firm and big, excess symptoms with excess pulses. The prognosis is favorable." (34) He adds that "Triple parching is commonly caused by excessive dry heat. The pulse is usually floating, and big or rapid and big, in which case the prognosis is favorable." (35) With respect to edema, Li states that "When analyzing edema, the disorder is not severe if the related pulse is floating and big. The excess pulses correlate with excess symptoms, the upright qi has not been damaged by the perverse attack, and the treatment is straightforward." (44) Under the heading "Symptoms and Pulses in Edema and Fullness and Swelling," Li notes, "In diagnosing these conditions [Fullness and Swelling] a floating, big pulse indicates that although the perverse qi has not diminished, the upright qi has not been damaged. In this case, treatment is possible." (45)

8. Li, 67. The Tense Full-Overflowing pulse is akin to both the Full pulse ("big and also strong, pounding hard against the fingers" [67]) and the 'big' pulse. Its Full aspects are discussed in Chapter 9. Here we are concentrating on the 'big' or Wide aspect, but some overlap is inevitable in our discussion.

■ Big Slippery Wiry

Li Shi-Zhen (85) refers to this heat from excess as "yang perverse qi," and suggests that it is accompanied by Slipperiness, which I have also noted. Kaptchuk (305), in keeping with this interpretation, mentions "Shao–yang Disharmony" with the "Big and Wiry" combination.

■ Big and Sinking

Kaptchuk (305) attributes this combination to "Interior Heat or Kidney Disharmony."

9. Kaptchuk (306): "Irritability; epilepsy; Wind Heat."

10. Ibid.: "Wind with vertigo; Hernia."

11. Ibid.: "Rebellious Qi; swollen face; cough; asthma."

12. Kaptchuk, ibid., relates this pulse at this position to "Kidney qi obstructed."

13. Ibid.: "Stagnant qi; Excess Stomach qi; distended abdomen." In my experience these conditions are attended by the Inflated quality.

14. Ibid. The Wide Excess category at this position is rare. Kaptchuk refers to "dark urine; constipation."

15. The Moderate Wide quality is described only by Kaptchuk (305), who recognizes the clinical value of this subtle distinction between Wide Excess and Wide Deficient. He uses the terms 'Big strong' and 'Big weak.' Although Wu Shui-Wan (35) mentions the yang brightness symptoms in connection with the Wide Moderate quality, she does not make the sensory distinction made by Kaptchuk.

16. William Philpott and Dwight Kalita, *Brain Allergies: The Psychosomatic Connection* (New Canaan, CT: Keats, 1980) 71–72.

17. A Wide Moderate quality is in between the excess and deficient. Kaptchuk (305) says that it "signifies excess (also heat) in the yangming Meridians (the Stomach and Large Intestine)." These meridians, he continues, "are said to have the most qi and blood and to most easily manifest and/or register excess/heat. If there are no accompanying signs of excess, this pulse may be considered the sign of a strong constitution."

Other combinations from the literature include the following:

■ Big Moderate

Kaptchuk (305) suggests damp-heat with this combination.

■ Big Floating

Deficiency or exterior heat

According to Kaptchuk (305), this is a sign of deficiency or exterior heat. However, Li Shi-Zhen (40) speaks of Floating and Big, indicating that "Upright qi is deficient and perverse qi is very severe. Therefore prognosis is poor."

Stomach excess

This is a sign of Stomach excess, according to Kaptchuk (305).

Big Sinking

This is a sign of interior heat and Kidney disharmony, according to Kaptchuk (305).

Big Wiry

This is a sign of lesser yang disharmony, according to Kaptchuk (305).

18. Kaptchuk (305) notes, "A Big pulse is usually strong, which makes it similar to a Full pulse, or weak, which makes it similar to the Empty pulse." However, he also says that "clinically, it is possible for a Full pulse to be part of a Deficiency pattern if all the other elements of a configuration indicate Deficiency. Such a pulse is illusionary and is thought to be a sign that the prognosis is poor." (307) I believe that Kaptchuk's deficient Full pulse and deficient Big pulse are compatible with the Wide (Big) Yielding Hollow (Deficient) and the Full-Overflowing (Full) qualities described in our text.

19. Kaptchuk (162) notes that "The pulse feels like a fine thread or line that is distinct and clear." Porkert (221) pictures it as "A narrow and short pulse which can be felt clearly, independently of its level." Giovanni Maciocia says that it is "thinner than normal." *The Foundations of Chinese Medicine* (London: Churchill Livingstone, 1989) 169. The word 'soft' is not used in these sources as a defining characteristic. John Shen speaks of one kind of Thin pulse which indicates "that the individual's condition is weak." *Chinese Medicine* (New York: Educational Solutions, 1980) 53.

    For other sources, however, the quality of softness, which implies qi deficiency, is an inherent part of the definition. It is likened by Li Shi-Zhen (15) to a "spider web." Wu Shui-Wan (35) describes the sensation "as thin as a hair or a thin thread," and further defines it as "straight and soft." But she seems to qualify this by adding (36) that there is also a Thin pulse with "strength."

20. Shen, 53.

21. Kaptchuk, 41. He (162) also observes that "the Blood is Deficient and unable to fill the pulse properly. Often the Qi is Deficient." Porkert (221), discussing the 'small' pulse, mentions a deficiency "of the active, of the active and structive, or primarily of the structive energies." Felix Mann asserts that "If found in conjunction with disease due to debility and absence of vitality, the disease is severe." *Acupuncture: The Ancient Art of Chinese Healing and How It Works Scientifically* (New York: Vintage Books, 1971) 170.

    Li Shi-Zhen (94), Wu Shui-Wan (36), Mann (170), and Kaptchuk (304) mention dampness as an etiology, and Li Shi-Zhen (94) discusses the role of the circulation of qi in producing blood deficiency, and a Thin pulse quality. (These are described more fully in connection with the pulse combination Thin and Yielding.)

    Li Shi-Zhen (94) says that the Thin quality can appear in

    > Disharmony and damage of the seven emotions, causing deficiency and fatigue; weakness and deficiency of yang qi and penetration of water damp, causing diseases of the loins and kidneys; and internal injury of jing qi, which prevents yang from consolidating the surface, causing spontaneous perspiration.

    Elsewhere (24) he observes:

    > The third pulse can be divided into the soft and weak pulses.... The thin soft pulse indicates that the yin blood has been damaged. The thin weak pulse indicates failure of the yang qi. When the yang qi fails it cannot nourish the body. Fear of cold easily develops. When the yin is deficient and cannot harmonize the yang, there are hot symptoms.

22. Shen, 53.

23. Ibid.
24. Ibid., 54.
25. Li, 94.
26. Ibid.
27. Kaptchuk, 304.
28. Personal communication.
29. Cheung and Belluomini, 24. The following secondary combinations are based on other sources, which I cannot corroborate.

    ▪ Thin Tense and/or Slippery

    Kaptchuk (304) and Wu Shui-Wan mention the Thin quality "with strength" as a sign of a damp condition, which Kaptchuk says is "associated with dampness Obstructing qi and blood."

    ▪ Thin Choppy

    According to Kaptchuk (304) this is a sign of "extreme Deficient blood" probably causing blood stagnation.

30. Claude Larre and Elisabeth Rochat de la Vallée, *The Lung* (Cambridge: Monkey Press, 1989) 78.
31. Li, 94.
32. Kaptchuk, 305; Li, 94.
33. Li Shi-Zhen (94) observes, "When severe failure of yuan yang causes cold dantian, diarrhea and emissions, or collapsed yin jing causes excessive bleeding, the thin pulse can be felt at the chi position." Kaptchuk (305) adds, quoting Li Shi-Zhen, "'Cinnabar Field' (Original qi) cold; yin collapsed."
34. Kaptchuk, 305.
35. J.R. Worsley mentions "Short of Chi; fatigue." *Acupuncturists' Therapeutic Pocket Book: The Little Black Book* (Columbia, MD: Center for Traditional Acupunture, 1975) D–14. Kaptchuk (305) refers to "Qi exhausted from vomiting."
36. Kaptchuk (305) calls it "Liver Yin exhausted," and Worsley (D–14) "Defects of vision; paralysis."
37. Kaptchuk, 305.
38. Worsley, D–14.
39. Kaptchuk (305) mentions "Kidney Yang Cold and exhausted," and Worsley (D–14) "impotence diarrhoea."
40. A Tight Empty and Thread-like quality at this position is outside of my own experience, but according to Li Shi-Zhen (89), it is due to a damp condition arising from Spleen qi deficiency.
41. **Combinations**

    ▪ Long Hollow Full-Overflowing

    This combination denotes heat from excess in the blood, which can be found with such disorders as hypertension. It can also be a sign of diabetes, especially if found on the left side, and especially if it is more Wiry.

    LONG TENSE

    These qualities may indicate a 'nervous system tense' condition if found over the entire pulse (see Chapter 7 for elaboration).

    ▪ Long Tense with Normal rate

    This is a 'nervous system tense' condition, usually constitutional in origin.

- Long Tense and Rapid

This is another 'nervous system tense' condition, usually associated with tension from daily stress.

LONG SLIPPERY

- Long Slippery and Rapid

This combination is a sign of heat from excess associated with subacute infection, such as hepatitis. (Acute infection would be associated with Flooding Excess.)

- Long Slippery and Slow

This is a sign of a lower grade chronic infection, such as parasites or candida, where there is lingering heat from excess in a deficient person.

- Long Tight

This combination usually indicates stagnation of Liver qi with symptoms of heat from both excess and deficiency.

- Long Tense (Wiry) and Rapid

Kaptchuk (313) states that with this pulse there may be signs of "Lung Heat with coughing of blood," which I have not encountered. Bleeding, in my experience, is usually accompanied by a Leather-like Hollow quality. Kaptchuk reports that this pulse also accompanies "Cold/Excess with pain and asthma."

- Long Floating

This combination signifies a lingering external pathogenic factor, such as a cold or flu, which has been partially internalized with some heat from excess.

- Long Flooding

This combination is a sign of yang brightness syndrome with severe heat symptoms in the Stomach and Large Intestine, as with appendicitis, dysentery, and peritonitis. Kaptchuk (314) mentions "Yang insanity or epilepsy." He also notes the following combinations, which are outside my own experience: Long Soggy, described as indicating "alcohol intoxication or Cold;" Long Sinking Thin, a combination said by Kaptchuk to be a sign of "lumps and tumors;" and Long Slippery, a quality which he associates with "Mucous Heat."

Positions

BILATERALLY AT SAME POSITION

By definition, the Long quality cannot be confined to a single position or burner.

SIDES

When one side is longer than the other, some disease process is indicated.

Left: If the left is Long and the right side is shorter and the rate and other qualities are Normal, this is an indication of a strong 'organ system' and a deficient 'digestive system.' If the rate is Rapid and the pulse is Tight, then we have heat from both excess and deficiency in the yin organs, usually due to an overworking 'nervous system.'

Right: The 'digestive system' has good qi if the right side is Long and the rate and other qualities are Normal. If the left side is shorter, we can say that the 'organ system' is deficient and that the 'digestive system' is supporting it. If the rate is Rapid and the right side is Tight, then we have heat from excess and deficiency in the 'digestive system,' usually due to eating too rapidly.

INDIVIDUAL POSITIONS

By definition, the Long pulse would not be limited to one position at a time.

42. Li Shi-Zhen, 19.

43. Mann (168) says in this regard, "If long, yet clear and round, as though feeling along a thin cane to the tip, it is a sign of health and not disease."

44. Li Shi-Zhen (19) categorizes this pulse with the long and wiry pulses. Elsewhere he associates Wiry with the Tight quality, and in yet another place (23) includes it among the long, short, big, small, flooding, empty, and full qualities and their associated diseases. He does this without any explanation. Porkert (214) classifies the pulse as 'brief.'

45. Kaptchuk, 313.

46. Wu Shui-Wan (25) observes, "The short pulse feels little and short, the middle arising and both ends descending, seeming unable to fill its natural place in the Inch, Bar and Cubit Zones." She also notes that "the pulses in the Inch, Bar and Cubit become short and the spacing between the Inch, Bar and Cubit increases."

    Li Shi-Zhen (75) says that "The short pulse always feels dissatisfying—its beats are strong, but it rises and falls abruptly." In a personal communication, Richard Van Buren described it as being "little and short," and Mann (168) as "having no head and tail."

Chapter 11

1. John Shen, *Chinese Medicine* (New York: Educational Solutions, 1980) 53.

2. Ted Kaptchuk, *The Web That Has No Weaver* (New York: Congdon and Weed, 1983) 164, 308.

3. Li Shi-Zhen classifies it as a subcategory of the Rapid pulse, which in my own experience does not hold true. *Pulse Diagnosis*, trans. Hoe Ku Huynh (Brookline, MA: Paradigm Publications, 1981) 18. Li (69) qualifies this by noting that "In a Slippery pulse the beats do not necessarily increase in number."

4. The classical description of the Slippery quality, described to me by Richard Van Buren, is one which "feels like a pearl in a porcelain basin under your finger." Li Shi-Zhen (68) describes it as "a pulse which feels round and smooth and flows evenly" and "like a greasy ball which slides under the fingers. It always remains even, like a smooth stream of water." Kaptchuk (163) calls it "extremely fluid ... it feels smooth, like a ball bearing covered with viscous fluid" and "[i]t slithers like a snake."

5. William Philpott and Dwight Kalita, *Brain Allergies: The Psychosomatic Connection* (New Canaan, CT: Keats, 1980) 71–72.

6. C.S. Cheung and Jenny Belluomini also associate the Slippery quality with blood. They observe, "The Su Wen describes the Slippery pulse as present in cases of overabundance of yin Chi, so it must follow that blood volume necessarily increases. Other sources describe the Slippery pulse as reflecting Excess blood and Congestion of Chi." "An Overview of Pulse Types Used In Traditional Chinese Medical Diagnosis" *Journal of the American College of Traditional Chinese Medicine* 1982;1:20. Wu Shui-Wan notes that "If a normal person has a slippery pulse, it denotes that his blood is abundant" and "If a patient has a slippery pulse, it generally denotes that he suffers from disease due to phlegm." *The Chinese Pulse Diagnosis* (San Francisco: Writers Guild of America, 1973) 19.

    Li Shi-Zhen (69, 22) states that "The Slippery pulse usually results when there is an abundance of yang qi... when yuan qi fails and is unable to hold the liver and kidney fire, causing heat at the blood level." It is also from "internal abundance of wind-phlegm blocking upward or food stagnation, counterflowing upward, causing vomiting, or remaining below, causing stasis" and from pregnancy. He also notes that "The slippery pulse occurs with internal excesses of perverse qi. These include accumulation or stagnation of phlegm, qi stagnation due to damaged digestion, accumulation of extravasated blood and qi stagnation due to vomiting."

    Kaptchuk (308) also mentions "Damp Heat pouring into the Bladder, and Damp Heat in the Intestines." Giovanni Maciocia observes that "Generally speaking, the slippery pulse is Full by definition, but in some cases it can also be Weak, indicating Phlegm or Dampness with a background of Qi deficiency." *The Foundations of Chinese Medicine*

(London: Churchill Livingstone, 1989) 168.

7. Slipperiness in individual positions is generally associated with excess or accumulation, usually of dampness or food retention, which clinically appears either internally, externally, or both, as phlegm (mucus). Internally-generated dampness is almost always due to a failure of Spleen qi. J.R. Worsley describes its nature as "the yin between the yang." *Acupuncturists' Therapeutic Pocket Book: The Little Black Book* (Columbia, MD: Center for Traditional Acupunture, 1975) D–4.

8. Slippery Deep

    Li Shi-Zhen (22) attributes this combination to "damaged digestive ability."

    Slippery and Rapid

    Wu Shui-Wan (44) speaks of "glandular inflammation and phlegm." This is a phlegm-heat disorder.

    Slippery Wiry

    This is reported by Kaptchuk (308) as "Stagnant Food or Mucus with Constrained Liver qi." The latter is previously referred to as the "plum pit" sensation.

    Slippery Tight

    This combination is described without elaboration by Kaptchuk (308) as "Cold Mucus Obstructing." In my own experience, when found in one position, it is associated with infection.

    Slippery Short

    Wu Shui-Wan (44) says this combination means deficiency of qi, which he defines as "poor function of the organs, with phlegm in the lungs and chest."

    Slippery Big (Wide)

    Wu Shui-Wan (44) says this combination signifies "an over-abundance of internal heat and phlegm-fluid."

    Slippery Floating Scattered

    Wu Shui-Wan (44) says that this combination "is a sign of poor to weak functioning of the internal organs, with phlegm dormant internally. In the case of serious illness, it is a sign of paralysis."

9. Kaptchuk (308) associates this combination with "vomiting; belching with sour taste; stiff tongue; cough," which I have never observed. Quoting Li Shi-Zhen (69), the distal position usually becomes Slippery "when tan [phlegm] yin collects between the chest and diaphragm, preventing heart yang and lung qi from descending and causing vomiting, acid reflux, stiff tongue, coughing, etc." Elsewhere, Li (22) speaks of "vomiting due to counterflow."

10. Li Shi-Zhen (69) observes that "the guan [middle] position usually becomes slippery when liver heat blocks the spleen, causing indigestion." He adds (22) that "The slippery guan pulse indicates accumulation of blood." Kaptchuk (308) mentions "Liver Spleen Heat; Stagnant food."

11. According to Kaptchuk (308), this pulse may signify "'wasting and thirsting' (diabetes), diarrhea, hernia, and urinary problems." According to Li Shi-Zhen (69), "the chi [distal] position usually becomes Slippery when damp heat pours down to the Kidney and Bladder and Large Intestines, causing triple parching, dysentery, hernia, or dysuria."

12. Kaptchuk (308) attributes Slipperiness here to "Heart heat; fitful sleep."

13. Kaptchuk (308) mentions "Mucus with vomiting or nausea," with which Worsley (D–4) concurs.

14. Kaptchuk (308) associates Slipperiness in the left middle position with "Liver fire and Vertigo." Worsley (D–4) adds "heat at the liver; sore eye; headache."

15. Kaptchuk (308) includes "Spleen Heat; Stagnant Food", and Worsley (D–4), "[b]ad breath; vomiting; weak digestion."

16. Richard Van Buren, personal communication.

17. Ibid.

18. Kaptchuk (308) finds this sign with "dark urine" and "difficult urination." Worsley (D–4) mentions "[b]urning stools at rectum; urethralgia; gravel."

19. Kaptchuk (308) speaks of "diarrhea; Fire Ascending," meaning Kidney fire, heat from deficiency moving upward with tinnitus, and a sore, dry throat. Worsley (D–4) mentions "[t]hirst; cold at the umbilicus; gaseous sound inside the belly; dysentery. (Female: hot of blood; obstruction by gas; retention of menses; pregnant if the pulse slips with gentleness)."

20. Beijing College of Traditional Chinese Medicine, *Essentials of Chinese Acupuncture* (Beijing: Foreign Languages Press, 1980) 58.

21. Kaptchuk, 164.

22. Ibid.

23. Manfred Porkert, *The Essentials of Chinese Diagnostics* (Zurich: Chinese Medicine Publications, 1983) 216.

24. Kaptchuk, 164.

25. Porkert, 217.

26. It is interesting that Wu Shui-Wan (30) mentions, in connection with her interpretation of the Wiry quality, that "it [Liver] means the nervous system."

27. Jiang Jing, "A Brief Survey of the Korean Dong Han System of Pulse Diagnosis" *Oriental Medicine* 1993;2(1):21–22.

28. *Essentials of Chinese Acupuncture*, 58.

29. According to the descriptions of sensation in the literature, our Tense quality would correspond to the Tight quality described by Kaptchuk (164, 310), Li Shi-Zhen (79), and Wu Shui-Wan (27). Porkert (216) also uses the term Tense for the same quality. However, their descriptions of the sensation and their interpretations vary considerably from those of Dr. Shen and my own experience.

30. Li Shi-Zhen (80) describes a Tight pulse as being "like a tightly stretched rope and feels twisted" and "vibrates to the left and right." In the hierarchy of increasing loss of flexibility, a Tight pulse feels thinner and harder than a "stretched rope," which I call Tense, and which does not feel "twisted." It should be noted that in extreme cases of life-threatening cold, such as hypothermia, I find that the pulse is Hidden Excess (Tense) near the level of the bone, and does feel as Li described it. The "vibrating left and right" with extreme internal cold is akin to the Rough Vibration quality, which, in my system, is associated with parenchymal damage, or what Dr. Shen calls 'organ dead.' Closely allied would be the Choppy quality associated with blood stagnation, which, at the Hidden position, would represent the congealing of blood in the vessels and impending death.

31. Richard Van Buren, in a personal communication, related that in one position this combination can indicate "a putrescent hot and painful abscess in that area of the body."

32. Shen, personal communication.

33. Wu, 46.

34. R.B. Amber, *The Pulse in Occident and Orient: Its Philosophy and Practice in India, China, Iran, and the West* (New York: Santa Barbara Press, 1966) 113.

35. Kaptchuk, 163, 309.

36. Li, 70.

37. Porkert (213) calls it 'grating,' and Cheung and Belluomini (20) use the term 'difficult' to describe the Choppy quality. It is also sometimes alluded to as a 'rough' pulse by Felix Mann. *Acupuncture: The Ancient Art of Chinese Healing and How It Works Scientifically* (New York: Vintage Books, 1971) 167.

It has been described by Kaptchuk (163), quoting the classics, as "Like taking a knife and scraping a bamboo pole" or "a sick silkworm eating a mulberry leaf," and as "uneven, rough, sometimes irregular in strength and fullness." He also portrays it as "unclear," "not flowing smoothly with irregular amplitude," and "not smooth—the opposite of slippery."

Li Shi-Zhen (16, 70) describes the Choppy pulse as "slow, thin with uneven beats (beats that do not flow evenly)," having "root although it seems to scatter," "rough and jagged," "like an ill silkworm eating a leaf," and "can be felt at the floating and deep levels." I differ with Li Shi-Zhen concerning the Slowness and Thinness of this quality and its appearance at the 'floating' depth, which I have not observed as a defining characteristic of the Choppy quality.

Porkert (213) notes that the pulse "comes and recedes gratingly, chafingly, or scrapingly—as if there were friction." He explains the sensation by saying "If the individually specific structive energy (xue) is reduced, if consequently the fluids are depleted, a grating, rasping pulse results."

Maciocia (169) says it feels as if "it had a jagged edge to it." Wu Shui-Wan (20) characterizes it as "short and not fluent" and therefore "just the opposite of the Slippery Pulse."

38. Wang Shu-He, *The Pulse Classic,* trans. Yang Shou-Zhong (Boulder, CO: Blue Poppy Press, 1997) 4.

39. Lu Yubin, *Pulse Diagnosis* (Jinan: Shandong Science and Technology Press, 1996) 70–71.

40. Kaptchuk, 309.

41. Most sources, including Kaptchuk (309), refer to this quality as a sign of either excess or deficiency. Porkert (213) states that "If this pulse is strong there is repletion, if it is weak, inanitas."

    Excess

    With regard to the Choppy 'strong' quality, Kaptchuk (309) suggests that it is "generally a sign of Congealed Blood Obstructing Movement." The Choppy 'strong' quality is also described by Porkert (213) as "stagnant active energy," by which he means "inveterate, hardened pituita, stases, hematomas, concretions (i.e. structive, hence somatic, material neoplasms), keloids."

    According to Kaptchuk (309), it is more rarely reported as "Dampness Obstructing Movement"—presumably of the flow of qi and blood—"which is the same signification carried by its opposite type of pulse (i.e., slippery)." Li Shi-Zhen (70) adds "cold damp as penetrating to the ying level causing blockage and stagnation of blood circulation (blood bi)," which Mann (167) supports with "qi obstructed with cold and damp symptoms."

    Li Shi-Zhen (70) mentions "severe stomach obstruction," with which Porkert (213) concurs, mentioning that "pituita, affecting the stomach orb in infants, produces a block of digestion." Elsewhere, Li Shi-Zhen (22) notes that "Whenever cold and dampness penetrate the blood, stomach disorders develop with constipation due to yin deficiency."

    Deficiency

    Kaptchuk (309) states that the Choppy quality associated with deficiency is due to "insufficient Blood and Jing [essence] to fill the Blood Vessels," especially when the pulse is also "weak or thin." He also alludes to "illnesses accompanied by great loss of blood or fluids, and with Kidney exhaustion (great Deficiency), especially when related to sexual functions."

    With regard to deficiency, Li Shi-Zhen (70) refers to "when severe sweating damages yin and yang" (which I have not observed) and "deficiency of ying [nourishing qi] and blood with damaged jin ye [fluids]." Elsewhere (22) he speaks of "the jin becomes damaged due to excessive perspiration, or convulsions occur due to deficiency and damage of the ying and wei [protective qi]." Mann (167) also mentions that "Jing [essence] is injured" and he concurs with Wu Shui-Wan (20) who notes that "the patient's blood is deficient or his organic function is very weak (weak vital activity)." Porkert (213) also speaks of "an impaired structive potential (jing) or deficiency of the individually specific structive energies (xue)."

    Cheung and Belluomini (20) describe the clinical significance of both types as "blood Deficiency, blood stasis or ecchymosis, and increased blood viscosity with a slow dilation and constriction of the arterial wall."

Kaptchuk (309) also refers to this quality as one kind of irregular pulse, "the three and five not adjusted," in which "in any one breath beats a different number of times." This sounds similar to what I have described in the discussion of rate and rhythm as either the Unstable quality, which hits the finger irregularly in different places at an individual position, or the Heart Nervous quality, where there is a Change in Rate at Rest over the entire pulse.

42. In this connection, Li Shi-Zhen (71) observes that "A choppy pulse in pregnancy means that the woman has insufficient blood to nourish the fetus." He goes on to say that "A choppy pulse in a non-pregnant woman means the essence and blood are drying up and it would be difficult for her to conceive." Wu Shui-Wan (20) states that "If a person has this pulse, pregnancy will be difficult."

43. Kaptchuk (309) associates "Constrained Liver Qi, Congealed Blood" with the 'choppy and wiry' combination. Other combinations from the literature:

    Choppy Feeble (Frail)

    This combination, which is rare in my experience, is regarded as a sign of "Qi exhausted (great Deficiency)" by Kaptchuk (309), one of several causes of blood stagnation listed earlier. At times, this combination is actually Vibration and not Choppiness.

    Choppy Minute

    According to Kaptchuk (309), this combination suggests "Deficient Blood" and "Deficient Yang." Again, qi deficiency can cause blood stagnation.

    Choppy Thin

    This combination, according to Kaptchuk (309), is a sign of "Dried Fluids (Deficiency)," which I interpret to mean blood and yin deficiency, especially of the Liver in the left middle position. I have experienced Choppy and Thin combined with Tight or Wiry, as mentioned above. Blood deficiency is a major etiology of blood stagnation.

    Choppy Rapid 'Big' 'Firm'

    According to Wu Shui-Wan (44), this combination "denotes that there is real internal heat, including 'inflammation,' and there is an invertebrate accumulation (or congealing, or constipation) internally."

    Choppy Rapid Empty 'Soft'

    Wu Shui-Wan (45) describes this combination as "a sign of 'yin-empty.' It means a deficiency of bodily fluids due to inflammation or fever of an internal organ."

44. **Distal position**

    Kaptchuk (309) reports bilateral Choppiness at this position as indicating "Deficient Heart Qi; chest pain."

45. According to Li Shi-Zhen (71), this pulse indicates "weakness and deficiency of the spleen and stomach" and "qi stagnation on both sides of the rib cage" causing "fullness and swelling," with which Kaptchuk (309) concurs.

46. Li, 71.

47. Li Shi-Zhen (71) notes that the distal position becomes Choppy "when damaged heart blood causes chest pain." Kaptchuk (309) mentions "Heart pain; Heart palpitations."

    Right distal position

    I have not observed Choppiness in this position. Kaptchuk (309) speaks of "Deficient Lung Qi; cough with foamy sputum." This is presumably a 'choppy deficient' quality, which Dr. Shen and I classify as Vibration.

48. Kaptchuk (309) also refers to this as "Deficient Liver blood."

49. Kaptchuk (309) describes a "weak Spleen; inability to eat" associated with his category of a 'choppy deficient' quality, which I classify as Vibration.

50. Kaptchuk (309) notes "lower back is weak and sore," which is his 'choppy deficient' quality, which I classify as Vibration.

51. Kaptchuk lists symptoms of a "weak Life Gate fire; Jing [essence] injured." I associate these with the Vibration quality, rather than the Choppy.

52. Vibration does not exist as a category in the literature. It is my contention, as mentioned earlier in the chapter, that what Kaptchuk and others refer to as a 'choppy deficient' quality is closest to what Dr. Shen and I allude to as Vibration. Kaptchuk (309) notes that "Although primarily a Yin pulse, a choppy pulse can have effects of either Deficiency or Excess." The sensation is similar. But the interpretation coincides only in the sense that we are both describing a quality which is a sign of deficiency. However, the interpretation of the deficiency described here differs from that in the literature.

53. Kaptchuk, 171, 318.

54. Mann, 170.

55. Wu, 37.

56. Li, 96.

57. Ibid., 19.

58. Porkert, 222.

59. Cheung and Belluomini, 30.

60. Worsley, D–15.

61. Li, 96.

62. Li Shi-Zhen (97) describes the fundamental meaning of this pulse when he says that it appears only "when yin and yang qi [are] fighting with each other." What they are fighting about, he says, is

> when pain is caused by excessive cold winning over yang; when fright or palpitations are caused by qi confusion; when spontaneous perspiration is caused by yang not winning over yin; when fever is caused by yin not winning over yang; when diarrhea is caused by disharmony between the spleen and stomach; when dysentery is caused by qi and blood disturbing each other [the transportive and transformative functions of the zang-fu are impeded]; when jing mai contractions are caused by yin-cold perverse qi injuring the channel qi; when failure of jing (in men) or uterine bleeding (in women) is caused by yin deficiencies and yang excesses.

When either aspect wins, one gets this pulse. Elsewhere (25) he notes, "The moving pulse indicates stagnation of yang qi at the level of the blood."

Porkert (222) also sees this as "dissonance, disharmony, a clash between active and structive energies." However, he puts an interesting and I feel appropriate twist on this theme by ascribing this pulse to "the incompatibility of outward stimuli with the constitutional or momentary disposition of an individual." He goes on to say that

> any excessive or, in whatever way, inappropriate medication, in particular the excessive use of tonics or of antiphlogistic drugs, also very often the use of cortisone, induces a mobile pulse, thereby indicating that the individual cannot integrate the therapeutic influence.

Kaptchuk (318) agrees that this pulse is "a result of the chaotic movement of Yin and Yang. When severe pain interrupts the Blood flow, or fright causes the Qi to 'sneak' away, the Qi and Blood lose their mutual nourishing function and generate this unharmonious pulse." He points out that the rapidity of the pulse denotes imbalance more than heat. Wu Shui-Wan (37), however, attributes heat from both excess and deficiency to this pulse without further elaboration, as well as "pain, palpitation and great horror," the latter with which I am in total agreement. Mann (171) also attributes the Moving quality to pain symptoms and notes that it is "also present in disease due to fright."

Cheung and Belluomini (31) limit the pulse to the middle position and add pregnancy and palpitations as conditions where it may be found.

63. The following are drawn from Kaptchuk (318):

- Spinning Bean and Frail (Feeble)

This is associated with "palpitations."

- Spinning Bean and Full (Inflated)

This combination is a sign of "pain obstruction."

- Spinning Bean and Hollow

Here we have a "loss of Jing."

- Spinning Bean and Floating

This appears with an "External Pernicious Influence."

64. Li Shi-Zhen (25) offers the following:
    - Distal position: "The cun pulse occurs during non-stop sweating which is also called movement of yang."
    - Middle position: "The moving guan pulse indicates pain and palpitations, heavy bleeding or blood in the stools."
    - Proximal position: "The moving chi pulse occurs during a constant high fever which is also called movement of yin."

65. Worsley (D–15): "Phobia; night–sweat."

66. Ibid.: "Night–sweat; asthma; cough."

67. Ibid.: "Fever; gas pain."

68. Ibid.: "Repression; dyspepsia; suffocation."

69. Ibid.: "Prostration; asthenic fever."

70. Ibid.: "Menorrhagia; hot urine."

71. See, e.g., Li at 7, 12, 16, 48, 58, 65, 70, 76.

72. Ibid., 88.

73. Ibid., 92.

74. Ibid., 93.

75. Deng Tietao describes these briefly in terms of the "pulse on the back of the wrist *(fan guan mai)*." *Practical Diagnosis in Traditional Chinese Medicine*, trans. Marnae Ergil (Edinburgh: Churchill Livingstone, 1999) 91.

Chapter 12

1. Ilza Veith, trans., *The Yellow Emperor's Classic of Internal Medicine* (Berkeley: University of California Press, 1966) 209.

2. Leon Hammer, *Dragon Rises, Red Bird Flies* (Barrytown, NY: Station Hill Press, 1990) 316.

3. According to James Ramholz, the Special Lung pulse is also found in the Korean Dong Han system of pulse diagnosis. In a personal communication, he described it as follows:

    Frequently, it is a wiry pulse mixed with other movements. We interpret it as energy constricting (when wiry in the internal channels) and usually blocking at S-12 *(que pen)* or GV–14 *(da zhui)* depending on the depth and direction; or, if the movement is horizontal, there is an exchange going with the heart. Usually, when the pulse movement passes the wrist crease at PC–7 *(da ling)*, it means that the energy movement is entering the head (which can be verified by comparing the Sanjiao or other involved pulses).

4. Personal communication, 1996. More recently, Celia Dermont reported similar findings with similar results. Dermont has documented the unifying thread between these findings as the reinterpretation of near-death experiences, including suicide.

5. Hammer, *Dragon Rises*, 317.

6. Manfred Porkert, *The Essentials of Chinese Diagnostics* (Zurich: Chinese Medicine Publications, 1983) 244.

7. Richard Van Buren, personal communication, 1973.

8. Graham Townsend and Ysha DeDonna, *Pulses and Impulses* (Northamptonshire: Thorsons Publishing Group, 1990) 73–74.

9. Veith, 209.

10. Li Shi-Zhen, *Pulse Diagnosis*, trans. Hoe Ku Huynh (Brookline, MA: Paradigm Publications, 1981) 7.

11. Leon Hammer, "The Paradox of the Unity and Duality of the Kidneys According to Chinese Medicine" *American Journal of Acupuncture* 1999;27(3&4):151–79.

12. Hammer, *Dragon Rises*, 221–24.

13. Li, 7.

14. Claude Larre, Jean Schatz, and Elisabeth Rochat de la Vallee, *Survey of Traditional Chinese Medicine* (Paris: Institut Ricci and Columbia, MD: Traditional Acupuncture Foundation, 1986) 128.

15. Ibid., 30.

Chapter 13

1. Anton Jayasuria, *Textbook of Acupuncture Science* (Dehiwala, Sri Lanka: Chandrakanthi Industrial Press, 1981) 517:

   > The distinction between the deep and superficial pulses requires a discriminating sense of touch and the ability to vary in a controlled manner the pressure exerted by the examining finger.... Little wonder then that many Western physicians after a few trials, or no experiment at all, have dismissed Chinese pulse diagnosis as an impracticable art, based on highly subjective impressions, derived wholly from the amount of pressure exerted by the examining finger and therefore not worth bothering about.

2. Li Shi-Zhen, *Pulse Diagnosis*, trans. Hoe Ku Huynh (Brookline, MA: Paradigm Publications, 1981).

3. Ted Kaptchuk, *The Web That Has No Weaver* (New York: Congdon and Weed, 1983) 161–72.

4. C.S. Cheung and Jenny Belluomini, "An Overview of Pulse Types Used In Traditional Chinese Medical Differential Diagnosis" *Journal of the American College of Traditional Chinese Medicine* 1982;1:31.

5. Kaptchuk, 160, 173.

6. Kiiko Matsumoto and Stephen Birch, *Five Elements and Ten Stems* (Brookline, MA: Paradigm Publications, 1983) 115–18.

7. A different interpretation is offered by Ralph Alan Dale, who does not cite any source for his point of view; it seems to represent his own logical projection of the five phase system upon the pulse. He crosses over between the two-depth and three-depth systems. In concurrence with the two-depth system, he associates the superficial depth with the yang organs and the deepest part of the pulse with the yin organs. The middle depth, in his view, is identified with Stomach and Spleen qi, rationalizing that earth is in the center of "one of the earliest ancient Chinese concepts of the Five Phases." He adds that:

   > Earth [Spleen and Stomach] is in the middle position, but that it is functionally part of each of the other four Element–Phases. Therefore, the middle level of palpation not only indicates the Stomach but also the nature of all the Vital Energies of the body.

"The Demystification of Chinese Pulse Diagnosis" *American Journal of Acupuncture* 1993;21(1):63.

Another disparate view is offered by Graham Townsend and Ysha DeDonna, who access both the Stomach qi and the quality of the *shen* (spirit) at the middle depth. They also cite no authority for their information. With regard to the Stomach qi, they note:

> Using all three fingers, take the middle level pulse. Count 50 beats, while feeling carefully for misbeats. If there are misbeats, note the frequency of the misbeat (e.g., roughly every 10 beats, or every 15 beats, etc.) Note whether the pulse is smooth and comes and goes easily, or whether it feels rough, sharp or uneven. Check the middle level pulse at the other wrist and note any differences between the wrists.
>
> It is the smoothness and regularity of the middle level pulse that tells us that the Stomach qi is healthy. Any deviation from this, in terms of lack of smoothness or irregularity, infers some disorder of the Stomach qi. It may, of course, infer other things as well, depending on the specific quality of the pulse.

Pulses and Impulses (Northamptonshire: Thorsons Publishing Group, 1990) 73.

With regard to the quality of the *shen,* they recommend (ibid.):

> Examine the middle level pulse. When examining factors related to the Heart, it is the FORCE of the pulse that interests us. Note, therefore, if the pulse is reasonably forceful, with a quality of underlying strength. If the Heart, and therefore the Shen, is in good condition, the pulse will possess an easy strength, with slight elasticity and softness, and no misbeats.

Jiang Jing, on the other hand, speaks of "superficial, middle and deep levels":

> When we divide the pulse position into three levels, the superficial level expresses the emotional state of a given organ, or an emotional influence exerted upon that organ. Depending on the direction, it can indicate that the syndrome is in a surfacing mode as emotion, or that the emotional stress is affecting the organic function. It can also indicate that the disease activity is in the exterior or energetic level, without damaging the organic structure or causing a foreign mass.... The middle level indicates the current organic level and its functioning. The deep level describes a chronic, settled or adopted situation, one that the patient is no longer even aware of. It refers to an inward direction, implying that a disease is about to be hidden, stored or adopted by the body.... If the pulse wave moves above the superficial level, it indicates a higher expression, at which point the situation is totally emotional. If it goes lower then the deep level, it shows deeper hiding and means that the situation has totally adopted organic characteristics.... In this point of view the superficial level belongs to the surface of the body, the middle belongs to the muscles and joints, and the deep belongs to the core of the body, especially the internal organs.

"A Brief Survey of the Korean Dong Han System of Pulse Diagnosis" *Oriental Medicine* 1993;2(1):10, 13.

8. Paul Unschuld, trans., *Nan-Ching* (Berkeley: University of California Press, 1986) 250.

9. *Websters New Twentieth Century Dictionary* (New York: The World Publishing Co, 1983)

10. Leon Hammer, *Dragon Rises, Red Bird Flies* (Barrytown, NY: Station Hill Press, 1990) 311–82.

11. William Philpott and Dwight Kalita, *Brain Allergies: The Psychosomatic Connection* (New Canaan, CT: Keats, 1980) 71–72.

12. Li Shi-Zhen, 95.

13. Ibid.

14. John Shen, *Chinese Medicine* (New York: Educational Solutions, 1980) 57.

15. Li, 88.

16. Ibid., 76.

17. Ibid., 115.

18. Dr. Jong Hon, personal communication regarding Korean constitutional medicine.

19. Hammer, *Dragon Rises*, 324.

20. R.B. Amber, *The Pulse in Occident and Orient: Its Philosophy and Practice in India, China, Iran, and the West* (New York: Santa Barbara Press, 1966) 164.

Chapter 14

1. Personal communications, 1973, 1995.

2. Li Shi–Zhen, *Pulse Diagnosis*, trans. Hoe Ku Huynh (Brookline, MA: Paradigm Publications, 1981) 4.

3. Jiang Jing offers this view:

   The more common of the two methods compared RENYING on the left radial artery and CHUNKOU on the right radial artery. In this method, the yin and yang energy balance is analyzed through the comparison of left and right sides: right side being yin and left side being yang. Because there are two positions on each hand when Shenmen is included, four types of energy can be distinguished: yang of yang, yin of yang, yang of yin and yin of yin.

   "A Brief Survey of the Korean Dong Han System of Pulse Diagnosis" *Oriental Medicine* 1993;2(1):18.

4. R.B. Amber, *The Pulse in Occident and Orient: Its Philosophy and Practice in India, China, Iran, and the West* (New York: Santa Barbara Press, 1966) 102.

5. Leon Hammer, *Dragon Rises, Red Bird Flies* (Barrytown, NY: Station Hill Press, 1990) 311.

6. Crossing models of Chinese medicine to the Worsley school, it is interesting to note that within their framework of a husband/wife imbalance they bring energy to the right side—which is Reduced in the condition described in the text—by stimulating the horary (TB–6 *[zhi gou]*, P–8 *[lao gong]*), and/or the source point of the Triple Burner (TB–4 *[yang chi]*) and the Pericardium (P–7 *[da lin]*).

7. Li, 62.

8. Ibid.

9. Ibid., 74.

10. Ted Kaptchuk, *The Web That Has No Weaver* (New York: Congdon and Weed, 1983) 311.

11. Kaptchuk (308) indicates that Slipperiness in the distal positions can signify "mucus in the chest; vomiting; belching with sour taste; stiff tongue; cough," although I have never observed any of these symptoms. Li Shi–Zhen (69) states that the distal position usually becomes Slippery "when tan yin [fluids] collect between the chest and diaphragm, preventing heart yang and lung qi from descending and causing vomiting, acid reflux, stiff tongue, coughing, etc."

12. Li Shi–Zhen (69) states that "the middle position usually becomes slippery when liver heat blocks the spleen, causing indigestion." He adds, "The slippery guan [middle] pulse indicates accumulation of blood." Kaptchuk (308) mentions "Liver Spleen Heat [and] Stagnant Food" giving rise to Slipperiness in this position.

13. According to Kaptchuk (308), Slipperiness in this position may be associated with "'wasting and thirsting' [diabetes]; diarrhea; hernia; urinary problems." Li Shi–Zhen (69) indicates that "the chi [distal] position usually becomes slippery when damp heat pours down to the kidney and bladder and large intestines, causing triple parching, dysentery, hernia, or dysuria."

14. Li, 94.

15. Kaptchuk, 305.

16. Li, 94.

Chapter 15

1. R.B. Amber, *The Pulse in Occident and Orient: Its Philosophy and Practice in India, China, Iran, and the West* (New York: Santa Barbara Press, 1966) 6.

2. Ilza Veith, trans., *The Yellow Emperor's Classic of Internal Medicine* (Berkeley: University of California Press, 1966) 215–16.

3. Leon Hammer, *Dragon Rises, Red Bird Flies* (Barrytown, NY: Station Hill Press, 1990) 370.

4. Ibid., 302.

5. Ibid., 300.

6. Ibid.

7. Ibid., 302.

8. Ibid., 330–31.

9. Sandy Jones, *Crying Baby, Sleepless Nights* (New York: Warner Books, 1983) 21.

10. Hammer, 302.

11. Ibid., 163.

12. Ibid., 303–4.

13. Claude Larre, Jean Schatz, and Elisabeth Rochat de la Vallee, *Survey of Traditional Chinese Medicine* (Paris: Institut Ricci and Columbia, MD: Traditional Acupuncture Foundation, 1986) 175.

14. Royston Lowe, *Secondary Vessels of Acupuncture* (Northamptonshire: Thorsons Publishing Group, 1983) 135, 140.

15. Felix Mann, *Acupuncture: The Ancient Art of Chinese Healing and How It Works Scientifically* (New York: Vintage Books, 1971) 105–7.

16. Gordon Allport, *Becoming* (New Haven: Yale University Press, 1955).

17. Hammer, 376–79.

18. Ibid.

19. Ibid., 326.

20. Ibid., 324.

21. Larre, 220.

22. Ibid.

23. Ibid.

24. See Hammer, ibid. at 160, where Liver yang is equated with the Gallbladder.

25. Henry D. Thoreau, *Walden* (White Plains, N.Y.: Peter Pauper Press, 1966) 12.

26. Hammer, 362.

27. Li Shi-Zhen, *Pulse Diagnosis*, trans. Hoe Ku Huynh (Brookline, MA: Paradigm Publications, 1981) 4.

Chapter 16

1. R.B. Amber observed:

    The pulse as a vital diagnostic aid of great prophetic significance was recognized in the Orient, and this lesson has now spread to England, France, Russia and Germany. True, the pulse changes often with every treatment and prescription. But whether the state of health has changed for better or worse can always be determined by the pulse reading.

The Pulse in Occident and Orient: Its Philosophy and Practice in India, China, Iran, and the West (New York: Santa Barbara Press, 1966) 104. "Always" is more than a slight exaggeration, but "almost always" is not far from the mark for a skilled practitioner.

2. Li Shi–Zhen, *Pulse Diagnosis*, trans. Hoe Ku Huynh (Brookline, MA: Paradigm Publications, 1981) 9.

3. Deng Tietao, *Practical Diagnosis in Traditional Chinese Medicine*, trans. Marnae Ergil (Edinburgh: Churchill Livingstone, 1999) 85.

4. Deng, 140. Another sign of prognosis is the effect of the breath on the intensity and amplitude of the pulse. According to Russell Jaffe, if, upon taking a deep breath, both of these aspects increase, the prognosis is good; if they decrease, the prognosis is unfavorable. I cannot confirm this.

Chapter 17

1. Deng Tietao, *Practical Diagnosis in Traditional Chinese Medicine*, trans. Marnae Ergil (Edinburgh: Churchill Livingstone, 1999) 85.

2. Leon Hammer, *Dragon Rises, Red Bird Flies* (Barrytown, NY: Station Hill Press, 1990) 324.

APPENDIX: 1

Pulse Qualities: Sensation & Interpretation

QUALITY	SENSATION	INTERPRETATION
Normal (slowed down)	Consistently regular; rate consistent with age; consistently stable quality, amplitude, and intensity; moderate spirit; resilient, compressible; Long, continuous; no turbulence; balanced among qi, blood, and organ depths, with qi the lightest and organ depth with root and the most dense; balanced among positions; Normal wave	Health

RHYTHM (Entire pulse)
    I. ARRHYTHMIA
        A. AT REST: RATE MEASURABLE, WITHOUT MISSED BEATS
            1. OCCASIONAL CHANGE IN RATE

Small change	Speeds up and slows down moderately Left distal: Tight	Mild Heart qi agitation from mild shock between ages 15-20; scared inside
Large change	Speeds up and slows down greatly; Left distal: Feeble	Moderate Heart qi agitation from early moderate shock, or severe shock between ages 15-20; very scared; large mood swings

            2. CONSTANT CHANGE IN RATE

Small change	Speeds up and slows down moderately Left distal and left proximal: Tight Left distal: Vibration	Severe Heart qi agitation; strong shock; mild Heart qi deficiency; vacillating, always changing mind, restless; fatigue

QUALITY	SENSATION	INTERPRETATION
Large change	Speeds up and slows down greatly Left distal: Absent	Moderate Heart qi and some blood deficiency due to constitution, severe shock between ages 10-15, long-term Heart blood deficiency, and/or severe Heart qi agitation; fatigue

B. AT REST: RATE MEASURABLE, WITH MISSED BEATS

QUALITY	SENSATION	INTERPRETATION
Intermittent	Misses beat regularly	Heart qi, blood, and yang deficiency
Frequent	Misses every 2-20 beats	Severe Heart qi, blood, and yang deficiency
Infrequent	Misses every 21-60 beats	Milder Heart qi, blood, and yang deficiency
Interrupted	Misses beats irregularly: 1. Occasional 2. Constant	 1. Moderate Heart qi agitation and mild Heart qi deficiency 2. Moderate Heart qi deficiency

C. AT REST: RATE NOT MEASURABLE
1. CONSTANT: DUE TO SHOCK, OVERWORK, OVEREXERTION, AGE 5-10 YEARS

QUALITY	SENSATION	INTERPRETATION
Interrupted	Missed beats too irregular to measure rate	Severe Heart qi and yang deficiency; Heart blood stagnation Etiology: 5-10 years
Hollow Interrupted-Intermittent	Missed beats too irregular to measure rate, and Hollow	Most severe Heart qi-yang deficiency Etiology: 5-10 years
Literature: Knotted	Interrupted and Slow	Stagnation of circulation due to cold from excess or deficiency; qi, blood, essence, and yang deficiency
Hurried	Interrupted and Rapid	Fire from excess and/or stagnation of qi, blood, food, and phlegm

2. OCCASIONAL: SAME AS CONSTANTLY INTERRUPTED BUT LESS SEVERE, DUE TO:
i. SHOCK, OVERWORK, OR OVEREXERCISE, AGES 10-15, AND/OR
ii. MODERATE TO SEVERE HEART QI AGITATION

D. ON EXERTION: LARGE INCREASE IN RATE

QUALITY	SENSATION	INTERPRETATION
Constant	1. Rate increases on exertion more than 8-12 beats/ minute 2. Large change >20 beats 3. Small change 8-20 beats	1. Heart blood deficiency (some Heart qi deficiency) 2. Moderate-severe Heart blood deficiency 3. Mild Heart blood deficiency
Occasional	Rate increases on exertion	Same interpretation as constant, but less serious

QUALITY	SENSATION	INTERPRETATION

E. ON EXERTION: SMALL INCREASE (< 8 BEATS/MIN.), SAME, OR DECREASE IN RATE

1. Rate stays same, or slight increase	1. No change or slight increase on exertion	1. Mildly severe Heart qi deficiency
2. Small decrease	2. Decreases 1-5 beats/min.	2. Severe Heart qi deficiency
3. Large decrease	3. Decreases > 5 beats/min.	3. Very severe Heart qi-yang deficiency

II. PSEUDO-ARRHYTHMIAS: QUALITIES MISTAKEN FOR ARRHYTHMIAS

Hesitant Wave	Faltering, balking, without a missed beat; wave is up and down without bell-type curve	Excessive rumination about one thing; obsessive personality; worry, insomnia; mild Heart yin deficiency; ('push pulse'–mental overwork)
Change in Intensity over entire pulse	1. Pulse always increases and decreases in width (substance) 2. Pulse occasionally increases and decreases in width (substance)	1. Always: Heart qi deficiency 2. Occasional: Liver qi stagnation
Change in Amplitude over entire pulse	Pulse increases and decreases in height	Yang force, metabolic heat, and spirit in state of transition
Unstable in one position	Impulse continually shifts under finger at individual position	Severe parenchymal damage; separation of yin and yang

STABILITY

Change in Intensity 1. Entire pulse 2. Individual positions	1a. Constant increase and decrease in width (substance) of pulse at all positions 1b. Occasional change in above attributes 2. Constant increase and decrease in width of pulse at one position	1a. Circulation diminished due to Heart qi deficiency 1b. Liver qi stagnation: stress 2. Separation of yin and yang of organ which position represents
Change in Amplitude 1. Entire pulse 2. Individual positions	1. Constant increase and decrease of height (force) of entire pulse 2. Constant increase and decrease of height (force) of pulse at one position	1. Constant change of 'spirit,' functional heat and yang force 2. Separation of yin and yang of the organ which that position represents
Change in Intensity and/or Amplitude from side to side	Change in intensity or amplitude first on one side, then the othck and forth	Either profound interpersonal conflict or recent extraordinary exertion
Change in Qualities ('qi wild,' separation of yin and yang in entire organism)	1. Qualities constantly changing over entire pulse 2. Qualities changing in one position 3. Qualities changing from side to side	1. 'Qi wild': prolonged work and exercise beyond one's energy from early age 2. Separation of yin and yang: extreme deficiency of yin organ qi and blood 3. 'Qi wild': severe husband-wife imbalance
Hollow Intermittent-Interrupted ('qi wild')	Regular or irregular missed beat, with Yielding Hollow quality	Most extreme 'qi wild' condition, also associated with severe Heart disease
Unstable	At individual position the impulse is erratic, constantly hitting a different part of the finger	Separation of yin and yang in the yin organ corresponding to that position; often associated with cellular chaos and neoplasms

QUALITY INTERPRETATION

RATE

I. RAPID: CIRCULATION ACCELERATED

Bounding, as if pulse running away faster than the actual rate	*See* trauma, emotional shock, fever, pain below

    A. EXTERNAL ETIOLOGY
        1. EXTERNAL PATHOGENIC FACTORS

Slightly Rapid Yielding Floating	Wind-heat
Very Rapid Tense Full-Overflowing or Flooding Excess; Robust Pounding	Heat stroke

        2. PHYSICAL TRAUMA

Very Rapid, Bounding, and Tight or Wiry	Extensive trauma (very recent); severe pain (Wiry = more pain)
Rapid, Bounding, and Tight or Wiry	Extensive trauma (after short time); pain (Wiry = more pain)
Less Rapid, and Tight or Wiry at one position	Local trauma; pain (Wiry = more pain)
Rapid, Inflated, and Tight or Wiry	Physical condition strong at time of trauma (Wiry = more pain)
Rapid, Flat, Tight	Physical condition weaker at time of trauma

        3. SEASONAL FACTOR: RAPID IN AUTUMN
        4. EMOTIONAL TRAUMA (Heart Shock)

1. Very Rapid; entire pulse very Tight, right Vibration	1. Extreme emotional trauma
2. Tight at Pericardium and left distal position, Bounding	2. Extreme anxiety and panic
Slightly Rapid, Pericardium Tight	Mild emotional trauma

    B. EXTERNAL/INTERNAL ETIOLOGY: e.g., shock from birth trauma (external) and emotional reaction (internal)
        1. HEART CONDITIONS (all pulses are Rapid)

(SENSATION AT LEFT DISTAL POSITION)

Tight at Pericardium	Mild heat from excess due to very mild Heart shock with worry, insomnia, and restlessness
Superficial Smooth Vibration	Very mild Heart qi agitation, transient worry

QUALITY	INTERPRETATION
Change in Rate at Rest	Moderate to severe Heart qi agitation due to mild Heart shock with anxiety, fatigue, roller coaster feeling and life
Flat Wave	Heart qi stagnation due to moderate shock with spite, vengeance, chest pain
Very Flat Wave, Rough Vibration at all depths	Heart blood stagnation and severe Heart qi deficiency due to severe unresolved Heart shock with fear, guilt
Deep, Thin, Feeble, and slightly Rapid or Slow	Severe Heart blood stagnation due to old unresolved Heart shock with constant fear, chest pain, difficulty inhaling
Inflated (early) or Deep, Thin, Tight (later)	Trapped qi in Heart due to moderate Heart shock with chronic fatigue, easily angered, difficulty exhaling, body discomfort, difficulty lying on left side

C. INTERNAL ETIOLOGY
1. HEAT FROM EXCESS

QUALITY	INTERPRETATION
Rapid, Tense, Flooding Excess, Robust, Pounding, Bounding, and Slippery at organ or all depths	Heat from excess in organ (high fever)
Slightly Rapid, blood depth moderately expanded and Slippery	Heat in blood from excess or deficiency; turbulence in blood (Slippery)
Rapid, blood depth very expanded and Slippery to Tense-Tight Hollow Full-Overflowing Robust Pounding	Blood circulation severely impaired due to severe damp-heat in blood ('blood thick') from excessive lipids (Slippery) or severe Heart qi deficiency
Moderately Rapid and Tense uniformly over entire pulse	'Nervous system tense' due to daily stress (affects Heart)

2. HEAT FROM DEFICIENCY

QUALITY	INTERPRETATION
Slightly Rapid, Thin, and slightly Tight	'Nervous system tense' due to daily stress over longer time
Floating, slightly Rapid, Tight to Wiry	Internal wind: mild (wind in channels)
Very Tight Hollow Full-Overflowing	Internal wind: severe (stroke)
Slightly Rapid, very Tight to Wiry	Low grade fever in chronic illness (e.g., tuberculosis)

D. OTHER ETIOLOGIES

QUALITY	INTERPRETATION
Leather-like Hollow and Rapid	Imminent hemorrhage

QUALITY	INTERPRETATION
Acute: Biting, Wiry, Bounding and Rapid	Acute pain (Wiry = greater pain)
Chronic: Tight, Biting and less Rapid	Chronic pain
Sudden appearance of Rapid rate	Temporary mobilization of qi to fight acute aggravation of chronic disease (e.g., fulminating colitis with chronic colitis)
	Emotional shock, paradoxically with chronic Heart qi deficiency
Sudden appearance of Rapid rate: Yielding Hollow Full-Overflowing	Sudden cessation of heavy, prolonged exercise and/or work
Very Rapid (> 120/min), Deep, Thin and Feeble, or Deep, Thin, Tight	Lesser yin stage of six stages (paradoxically low temperature)

II. SLOW
    A. CIRCULATION DIMINISHED
        1. HEART-CIRCULATION

Slow, and Tight or Rough Vibration	Unresolved shock, either physical (Tight) or emotional (Rough Vibration) after many years (20-30), with paradoxical yin deficiency
Slow, Yielding Hollow Full-Overflowing	Heavy work or exercise beyond one's energy beginning early in life (5-10 years of age)
Slow, Feeble (especially left distal & proximal)	Heart qi and/or yang deficiency, circulatory deficiency; etiology arises after age 20
Slow, Moderate Robust Pounding	Aerobic exercise (long term)
Slow, Very Tight Hollow Full-Overflowing	Earlier heat from deficiency in vessels
Slow & Tense Ropy	Heat from excess in vessels; 'blood thick' (middle stage arteriosclerosis)
Slow & Tight Ropy	Advanced yin deficiency affects vessels (advanced arteriosclerosis)

        2. EXTERNAL STAGNATION

Slow, Floating, Tense	External cold pathogen

        3. INTERNAL STAGNATION (IMPAIRED QI CIRCULATION)

Slow, Tense (especially left middle position)	Liver qi stagnation (long term); heat pathogen stagnation
Slightly Slow, Tense over entire pulse with slight Robust Pounding	Constitutional 'nervous system tense'

QUALITY	INTERPRETATION
Very Slow, Deep, Tense	Severe internal cold from excess
Tense Hidden (very rare)	Very severe internal cold from excess
Slow and Feeble or Empty	Longstanding internal disease, overwork, overexercise, sex beyond one's energy, and protracted emotional strain cause qi and yang deficiency; etiology begins between age 15-20 with Empty, and after 20 with Feeble qualities
Slow and Slippery	Cold-dampness-phlegm: Spleen qi deficiency; Heart and Kidney qi deficiency
Very Slow, Suppressed Wave	Heart medications: beta blockers
Very Slow, very Deep	Poison over long period of time

QUALITY	SENSATION	INTERPRETATION

III. RATE VARIES

QUALITY	SENSATION	INTERPRETATION
Rate on right and left sides consistently vary (problem began on slower side)	1. Rate on sides differ consistently 2. Feeble at left distal and proximal positions 3. Feeble at left distal position only 4. Feeble on side that is overused	1. Congenital anomaly with blocked vessel 2. Shock during mother's pregnancy 3. Heart qi deficiency, or trauma and heavy lifting 4a. Habitual overuse of that side; 4b. imbalance in digestive and organ 'systems'; 4c. Husband-wife imbalance

VOLUME

I. ROBUST VOLUME

QUALITY	SENSATION	INTERPRETATION
Hollow Full-Overflowing Wave (usually over entire pulse, or a combination of individual positions, especially on left side, or in milder conditions, left middle position)	Forcefully rising from blood depth to above qi depth, with normal sine wave 1. Yielding with pressure (entire pulse) 2. Tense on surface 3. Very Tight on surface 4. Very Tight-Wiry and very Rapid	1. 'Qi wild' 2. Blood heat from excess 3. Heat from blood yin deficiency 4. Imminent stroke
Flooding Excess Wave (entire pulse or individual position)	Rises powerfully and gradually from a strong base at organ depth to above the qi depth, then recedes precipitously to organ depth	Heat from excess in yin organs due to infection (usually acute), or fever (rarely from yang qi constrained internally by cold)

Pounding:
  Robust
  Robust and Suppressed
	Beats against finger w/force
	Only organ depth Pounding
		Heat from excess
		Medication suppressing wave

QUALITY	SENSATION	INTERPRETATION
Suppressed Wave at qi depth (entire pulse)	Wave at top of pulse flat and cut off and/or	Effects of medication
Suppressed Pounding	Pounding at organ depth with no Pounding at blood and qi depths	Effects of medication
Inflated (degrees of tension; individual positions)	Very Tense, round and balloon-like, unyielding to pressure	Trapped qi in organ or area
Yielding Inflated	Yielding Inflated	Improperly talking, breathing and/or singing Unresolved grief
Mildly Tense Inflated	Mildly Tense Inflated	Breech birth
Moderately Tense Inflated	Moderately Tense Inflated	Liver qi attacking upward Breast pathology Trapped heat (invading cold transforms into heat) Emphysema
Tense Inflated	Tense Inflated	Sudden extreme anger and activity One major episode of lifting beyond one's energy Trauma or surgery to upper burner
Very Tense Inflated	Very Tense, round and balloon-like, unyielding to pressure	Trapped blood in organ or area due to trauma to a strong person

II. REDUCED VOLUME

QUALITY	SENSATION	INTERPRETATION
Yielding and Diminished at qi depth (entire pulse or individual position)	Qi depth slightly pliable under gentle pressure	First stage of qi deficiency due to work beyond one's energy, insomnia, and/or mild illness
Reduced Substance at qi depth, Feeble or Absent (entire pulse or individual positions)	Qi depth has Reduced Substance, and is Feeble or Absent	Second stage of qi deficiency (see etiology immediately above)
Spreading at blood depth, Absent at qi depth (entire pulse or individual positions)	Qi depth Absent and blood depth separates to sides of finger with pressure	Third stage of qi deficiency, first stage of blood deficiency (see etiology above)
Yielding Partially Hollow at blood depth	With increased pressure the blood depth separates and then is restored at organ depth	Second stage of blood deficiency
Flooding Deficient Wave (entire pulse)	Rises weakly from organ almost to qi depth and drops precipitously to organ depth	Fourth stage of qi deficiency: 'push pulse' (constantly 'pushing' one's self physically)

Pulse Qualities: Sensation & Interpretation

QUALITY	SENSATION	INTERPRETATION
Reduced Pounding (see below with 'modifiers')	Beats against finger without force, energy, or vigor	Fifth stage of qi deficiency: body is depleted of qi and blood, but still trying to compensate and maintain normal function
Diffuse	Feels like wide, amorphous cheese cloth next to both sides of principal impulse into which it merges without clear boundaries	Sixth stage of qi deficiency
Reduced Substance (see below under modifiers)	Lacks sense of material content and with diminished buoyancy, elasticity, and resilience; feels like threadbare sweater	Seventh stage of qi deficiency
Flat Wave (usually at individual positions)	Wave is suppressed and has very reduced sine curve, usually at organ depth	Stagnant qi cannot reach into organ or area due to emotional and/or physical trauma in a person who was deficient at the time, which has closed off the circulation to this organ or area
Deep (entire pulse or individual positions)	See below under 'depth'	Eighth stage of qi deficiency
Feeble-Absent (entire pulse or individual positions)	Barely or not palpable at organ depth	Ninth stage of deficiency of the 'true qi' and qi and blood of yin organ; very vulnerable to serious illness
Muffled (entire pulse or individual positions)	Qualities palpable but muted and obscure at all depths, as if a towel were placed over artery	All substances chaotic and deficient; active coherent function at cellular/molecular level impaired; tumors; surgery; auto-immune system deficiency; depression (especially at left distal position)
Dead (individual positions)	No sensation, total lack of life or movement in the artery	Usually malignancy and terminal illness

DEPTH
I. SUPERFICIAL

Cotton	Above the qi depth, a spongy, amorphous, formless resistance to pressure	Recent emotional trauma, or physical trauma
Floating --------- Entire pulse or right distal position and/or Special Lung position --------- Entire pulse, left side, or left middle position	Accessed superficially to qi depth, without wave --------- 1. Floating, Tense, Slow 2. Floating, Yielding, Rapid --------- Floating Tight with Normal or slightly Rapid rate	--------- 1. Wind-cold 2. Wind-heat --------- Liver Wind

QUALITY	SENSATION	INTERPRETATION
Empty Entire pulse: Yielding Empty Tense Empty Individual positions	Yielding at qi depth, Separating or Absent at blood and organ depths Tense at qi depth, separating or Absent at blood and organ depths	'Qi wild': separation of yin and yang throughout body Attempt to mobilize qi to cope with extreme sudden emotional stress Separation of yin and yang in organ associated with that position
Yielding Empty Thread-like (entire pulse) Literature (rare): Tight Empty Thread-like	1. Yielding, superficial, and very thin, like a thread floating on water, and Separating or Absent at blood and organ depths 2. Same as above, except Tight rather than Yielding	1. 'Qi wild' due to extreme yin or yang deficiency following severe or terminal illness; difficult parturition 2. Literature (rare): due to damp Spleen
Leather (entire pulse)	Drum-like thick hardness at qi depth, Separating or Absent at blood and organ depths	'Qi wild' due to extreme deficiency of essence, yin, and blood; excessive blood loss
Minute (entire pulse)	Access only at blood depth, as if divided into fragments rather than continuous as one rolls finger from distal to proximal position	Yang, qi, and blood deficiency due to extreme deficiency of yin and yang following serious illness with major loss of fluids and qi; 'ceiling dripping' in AIDS patients
Scattered (entire pulse)	Access only at qi depth; as if divided into fragments rather than continuous, as one rolls finger from distal to proximal position	'Qi wild' due primarily to exhaustion of yang; 'ceiling dripping' in AIDS patients

Hollow
 	
1. Entire pulse
 	
2. Entire pulse
 	
3. Individual position
4. Individual position
 	
5. Entire pulse, left side, or left medial and/or proximal-distal positions
 	
6. Same as no. 5
	Blood depth Diminished, Separating, or Absent:
	
	1. Yielding Hollow Full-Overflowing and:
	    Slow
	    Rapid
	
	2. Yielding Hollow Full-Overflowing, Interrupted-Intermittent
	
	3. Yielding Partially Hollow
	4. Leather-like Hollow
	    Rapid
	    Slow
	
	5. Very Tense Hollow Full-Overflowing
	
	6. Very Tight Hollow Full-Overflowing
		1. 'Qi wild'
		    Gradual development
		    Sudden development
		
		2. Most severe 'qi wild'
		
		3. Mild blood deficiency
		4. Acute severe hemorrhage
		    Imminent
		    Recent past
		
		5. Liver fire-wind; high blood pressure with elevated systolic; heat in blood; potential stroke
		
		6. Liver yin deficiency and wind; advanced high blood pressure; heat from deficiency in blood; imminent stroke

QUALITY	SENSATION	INTERPRETATION

II. SUBMERGED

Deep (entire pulse or individual positions)	Accessed only at organ depth	Internal, serious, or chronic disease. Moderate to severe depletion of all substances, especially qi and yang
Literature (rare): Hidden (entire pulse or individual positions)	Accessed with extreme pressure just above bone	Serious illness
1. Excess	1. Tense Hidden	1. Yang qi trapped internally due to painful obstruction from cold, food, phlegm, blood, and heat transforming into wind
2. Deficiency	2. Yielding Hidden	2. Yang qi too deficient to rise due to severe yang qi deficiency; deterioration of yin organs; neoplasm
Literature: Firm (entire pulse or individual positions [rare])	Deep, Wiry, Long between Deep and Hidden	Stagnation due to cold from excess, neoplasm, and/or exhaustion with 'running piglet' disease

SIZE
I. WIDTH
A. WIDE
1. BLOOD

Blood deficiency	Yielding Partially Hollow; impulse separates between qi and organ depths	Less serious blood deficiency than Thin; slow bleeding (gastro-intestinal ulcer); chronic colitis; mild to moderate menorrhagia
Sudden severe hemorrhage	Completely Hollow and Leather-like	Rapid: imminent Slow: recent
Blood Unclear	Blood depth fills out imperceptibly as one releases pressure from the organ depth	Toxicity in blood from environment, deficient digestion, and inadequate Liver function
Blood Heat	Blood depth fills out significantly as one releases pressure from the organ depth, and decreases on further release of pressure to qi depth	Due to excessive spicy foods, sugar, alcohol; emotional conflict and Liver qi stagnation
Blood Thick	Blood depth expands to qi depth as one releases pressure from the organ depth	Due to excessive fatty and rich foods, emotional conflict, and Liver Qi stagnation
Hollow Full-Overflowing	Blood depth expands above qi depth with sine wave	Heat from excess in blood

QUALITY	SENSATION	INTERPRETATION

2. QI

Wide: (entire pulse or individual positions)	Excess: Robust Pounding, Flooding Excess Deficiency: 1. Yielding at qi depth and Spreading at blood depth 2. Diffuse	Heat from excess in yang ming True qi deficiency: 1. first & second stages of deficiency 2. Sixth stage of qi deficiency

B. NARROW

Qi deficient	Very Thin pulse in young man	Severe auto-immune disease
Yin-essence deficient	Tight-Wiry	Drying of tissues or pain; early diabetes or hypertension at left middle and proximal positions
Blood deficient		Primarily blood deficiency
Thin (entire pulse or individual positions)	1. Thin Tight 2. Thin Yielding	1. Blood and yin deficiency 2. Blood and qi deficiency
Other:		
Yielding Empty Thread-like	Yielding, Superficial, and very Thin, like a thread floating on water; Separating or Absent at blood and organ depths	'Qi wild' due to extreme yin and/or yang deficiency during or following severe or terminal illness; difficult parturition
Restricted (width)	Limited in scope and space either by width, length, or both; used only to describe Special Lung position	While not yet completely defined, this quality is at least a sign of severe stagnation with deficiency; cancer in chest, Lung or other pulmonary obstructive disease

II. LENGTH

Long (entire pulse)	Resilient, continuous, slightly longer than Normal quality	Healthy without symptoms Heat from excess with symptoms and Robust Pounding
Short (between positions)	Sensation is discontinuous between positions; usually two positions feel separated 1. Yielding 2. Tense	Circulation between yin organs is obstructed 1. Due to qi deficiency 2. Stagnation of blood, qi, phlegm, food
Restricted (length)	Limited in scope and space wither by width, length, or both; most commonly used to describe Special Lung position	While not yet completely defined, this quality is at least a sign of severe stagnation with deficiency; cancer in chest, Lung, or other pulmonary obstructive disease

| QUALITY | SENSATION | INTERPRETATION |

SHAPE
    I. FLUID

QUALITY	SENSATION	INTERPRETATION
Slippery (entire pulse or individual positions)	Slides rapidly under finger(s) in one direction "Like a grease ball that slides under the fingers"	Normal in pregnancy; depending on depth and position: damp, phlegm Organ depth: infection Qi depth: due to excess sugar (more Rapid) or qi deficiency (slower) Blood depth: turbulence in blood due to dampness, heat, increased blood viscosity (sugar, lipids); or blood flow in wrong direction, as with Heart valve

    II. NON-FLUID
        A. EVEN

QUALITY	SENSATION	INTERPRETATION
Taut (entire pulse or individual positions)	Resilience and elasticity of a *very wide* rope that is moderately *stretched*	Early sign of qi stagnation
Tense (entire pulse or individual positions)	Resilience and elasticity of a *moderately wide* rope that is *tightly stretched*	Later stage of qi stagnation with heat from excess
Tight (entire pulse or individual positions) 4. Very Tight and Rapid (suddenly, over entire pulse) 5. Floating Tight	1. Rope is *narrower* with *less flexibility* and resilience, and is harder to the touch 2. Biting in some positions 3. Like 'pencil point' in Pericardium position 4. Suddenly extremely Tight over entire pulse 5. Tight above qi depth with no wave	1. Yin deficiency, heat from deficiency, with usual residual qi stagnation and heat from excess 2. Pain, especially abdominal if found in Intestine positions 3. Mild heat from excess or deficiency in Heart 4. Severe emotional shock; severe pain 5. Internal wind
Wiry (entire pulse or individual positions)	Very hard and cutting to the touch, similar to a thin, rigid metal wire	1. Extreme deficiency of yin and essence (diabetes) 2. Absolute yin stage of 6 stages 3. Internal wind (hypertension) 4. Severe pain (from trauma, cold from excess, blood stagnation) 5. Diabetes

QUALITY	SENSATION	INTERPRETATION
Ropy (entire pulse)	Vessel cord-like, large, round, often like twisted rope, distinct from surrounding tissue as if it could be lifted and moved	
Unyielding (hard)	Same as above	Chronic heat from excess or deficiency causing the vessels to thicken and lose elasticity; arteriosclerosis
Yielding	Same as above	Etiology: 1. More common: long-term exercise beyond one's energy 2. Less common: trauma Pathogenesis: vessel walls malnourished Associated condition: neurological disease?

B. UNEVEN

Quality	Sensation	Interpretation
Choppy (individual position)	Rough, uneven and grating like rolling one's finger across a washboard or 'scraping bamboo'	Blood stagnation due to heat from excess; qi, blood, or essence deficiency
Vibration (entire pulse or individual positions)	Buzzing feeling with rapid oscillation 1. Smooth and superficial, light electrical sensation 2. Rougher (coarse buzzing) over entire pulse, all depths 3. Individual position	1. Transient worry when found in a few positions; worrying personality when found in most positions and depths 2. Profound fear and guilt and emotional shock 3. Parenchymal damage

C. MISCELLANEOUS

Quality	Sensation	Interpretation
Nonhomogeneous (individual positions)	Sensation is not accessed uniformly within the area of a particular position. In some parts of position there is consistently more substance than in other parts. It therefore has an uneven, bumpy feeling.	If Robust, stagnation of all substances; if Reduced, deficiency of all substances Function is seriously impaired
Bean (Spinning) (individual positions)	Occupies one position, though often overlaps others. Quality varies: very hard, like a splinter; very Tight-Wiry; like bolt of lightning; bubbles (Literature [rare]: Slippery, Vibrating, and Rapid)	Imbalance from acute chaotic physiology with separation of yin and yang. Associated with severe pain; very great fright; intestinal obstruction; severe neurological disease; metastatic cancer.
Doughy (Neuro-psychological position)	Flabby, amorphous, putty-like 'glob' whose shape is never the same and whose volume varies from very faint to moderately Robust.	Neurological disease; headache, usually of structural etiology; possibly multiple sclerosis

Pulse Qualities: Sensation & Interpretation

QUALITY	SENSATION	INTERPRETATION
D. QUALIFIERS (qualities and sensations that qualify other qualities)		
Rough (entire pulse or individual positions)	Not smooth or level; having bumps, projections; uneven	A Rougher sensation is a sign of a more serious condition than a Smooth sensation
Smooth (entire pulse or individual positions)	A more delicate sensation, as opposed to Rough. Smooth has an even or level surface	Smoothness is associated with a less serious condition than Roughness
Subtle (Vague) (individual positions)	Capable of noticing fine distinctions	In my experience a Subtle quality is generally associated with less disharmony than one that is *not* Subtle
Robust and Reduced Force (entire pulse or individual positions)	Force is defined as strength, energy, vigor, and power, especially the intensity of the power or impetus Robust Pounding: pounds with great force Reduced Pounding: pounds with little force	Most commonly used to modify the depiction of the Pounding quality Signifies attempt by organism to rid itself of excess, usually heat from excess Signifies that depleted organism is still trying to maintain normal function
Robust Substance	Strong material content; experienced as alive and healthy	Normal pulse
Reduced Substance	Lacks a sense of material content, with diminished animation and vitality; feels like threadbare sweater	Seventh stage of qi deficiency; relatively less qi deficient than Feeble quality. E.g., a Thin pulse with Reduced Substance is mildly blood and mildly qi deficient. A Thin Feeble pulse is blood and very qi deficient.
Biting	Very Tight quality with sensation of finger being nipped	Pain, usually at Intestine positions signifying abdominal discomfort
Ephemeral (Transient)	Comes and goes, especially at Neuro-psychological and Valve positions	Signifies less disharmony than with a quality that is more enduring
Separating	On pressure the pulse separates, moving simultaneously in two directions, distal and proximal	Found in early stages of the Spreading, Empty, and Hollow qualities; often confused with the Slippery quality, which moves in only one direction
E. ANOMALOUS QUALITIES		
San yin mai ('three hidden pulse')	Left side Hidden or Absent	Congenital with no clinical significance
Fan quan mai (Transposed)	Pulse primarily found on dorsal aspect of right wrist, or both wrists	Congenital anomalous artery with no clinical significance
Ganglion	Pulse obscured by mucilaginous connective tissue	Synovial or tendon sheath cyst
Trauma	Pulse obscured by scar tissue	Post-traumatic scar due, e.g., to intra-arterial intubati

QUALITY	SENSATION	INTERPRETATION
F. ANOMALOUS VESSELS		
Split vessel	Two vessels in one position; usually left and right middle positions, less often proximal	No established clinical significance; recently found in situations or conditions in which death or annihilation is experienced as imminent, with fear of the unknown, e.g., malignancy, abandonment in infancy
Multiple radial arteries	Radial artery at wrist divides into two or more vessels	No established clinical significance

APPENDIX: 2

Glossary

This glossary contains special terms that were used by Dr. John H.F. Shen, and which are likely to be unfamiliar to other students of traditional Chinese medicine.

'Blood heat'

This is a condition, called heat in the blood in traditional Chinese medicine, in which the thickness of the blood depth is more readily palpable. As one raises one's finger from the organ depth the pulse expands even more in the blood depth than is the case with 'blood unclear.' This is a sign of heat from excess in the blood. Often the blood depth is also Slippery. (According to Dr. Shen, 'blood heat' without Slipperiness is due to overworking the nervous system, while 'blood heat' with Slipperiness is associated with the metabolism of lipids and digestion.) Dr. Shen likens this pattern to a glass containing hot water, in contrast to one containing dirty water, his metaphor for the 'blood unclear' condition.

Two patterns can give rise to this pulse. The first is heat from excess associated with such foods as spices, wine, shellfish, coffee, chocolate and other heat-inducing items. The organs that are usually affected are the Liver, Stomach, Heart, and the Lungs. The second pattern is one of heat from deficiency, which is usually associated with an extremely tense nervous system; from the Chinese perspective, such a system has been working beyond its capacity. Kidney yin depletion usually ensues.

'Blood thick'

With this pattern and its associated quality (Blood Thick), the pulse at the blood depth has become extremely Wide, Slippery (sometimes Rough Vibration) when it is accessed, as described under 'blood heat' and 'blood unclear' conditions. However, with the 'blood thick' condition the pulse continues to widen even to the qi depth. Later, it often develops into a Tense Hollow Full-Overflowing quality, a sign of the later stages of the 'blood thick' process in which the heat from the blood has overflowed into the qi depth, thereby becoming a very prominent feature of the pulse. According to Dr. Shen, an early sign of this condition can be persistent acne after adolescence. The late signs are usually of a cardiovascular nature, such as hypertension.

'Blood thick' has several etiologies and courses. One develops from heat in the blood and is a damp-heat condition involving heat from the Liver and dampness from the Spleen. The causes for this disorder are primarily excessive intake of fat and sugar, leading to elevated levels of serum glucose, cholesterol, and triglycerides. The pulse shows more Slipperiness, especially where the dampness predominates, and less of the very Tense Hollow quality which is characteristic of advancing hypertension associated with the other causes described below. This process gradually interferes with Heart function due to increasing resistance in both the peripheral as well as coronary circulation, which in turn leads to even higher blood pressure, especially the diastolic.

Another contributing factor is a tense nervous system, which causes Liver qi congestion, interfering with the proper digestion and absorption of fats in the alimentary system (Liver attacking Spleen and Stomach), as well as with efficient metabolism of these substances by the Liver. There is a concomitant increase in Liver fire, and later Liver and Kidney yin deficiency along with the development of 'blood thick.' Both processes lead eventually to a Ropy pulse, a sign of arteriosclerosis and atherosclerosis.

'Blood unclear'

This is Dr. Shen's term for a condition in which the blood depth just barely increases (rather than decreases) in size as one raises the finger from the organ depth toward the qi depth. Often the pulse is also slightly Slippery. There is no equivalent term in traditional Chinese medicine.

The most common cause of this quality is exposure to environmental toxins. I first encountered it with artists using highly toxic solvents, often in poorly ventilated rooms, and with the use of acetylene torches, both in art and industry (welders).

Skin symptoms (eczema, psoriasis) are one obvious way in which the body attempts to discharge that toxicity. Another common symptom is fatigue. Dr. Shen likens this condition to a glass of water in which dirt is suspended: the quality of the blood is not good.

A related origin is a stagnant or deficient Liver that does not properly detoxify. In addition to storing the blood itself, the Liver also stores the blood toxins that are not metabolized by the Liver. These toxins contaminate the blood and ultimately the entire organism which it nourishes.

Another cause of this pattern is a qi-deficient Spleen which does not build the blood well due to poor absorption and digestion of food, especially protein. The protein is only partially digested into small chain polypetides the size of viruses, instead of being completely digested down to amino acids. The small chain polypetides are absorbed and the body reacts to them as if they were viruses by inappropriately mobilizing the immune system. Eventually, autoimmune diseases develop.[1]

'Circulatory system'

While all systems are concerned with qi, the 'circulatory system' especially involves the movement of blood, or heavier energy, throughout the channels. There is no known classical source for this connection between Dr. Shen's 'circulatory system' and the lesser yang, except perhaps for its place between the 'nervous system' involving the tai yang and the rapid movement of the most superficial and lightest qi energies, and the 'digestive system' and its logical connection with yang brightness, the deepest of the yang energies.

If the 'circulatory system' is in fact operating at an energetic level between tai yang and yang brightness, this intermediate energy would coincide with the lesser yang level (half interior, half exterior). It is my understanding that Dr. Shen also identifies this level with the muscles.

Because of its involvement with blood, it is especially connected with the function of the Heart. It is particularly affected by the shock of trauma, which tends to diminish the flow. Both overexercise over an extended period of time, and the sudden cessation of heavy, prolonged exercise, may cause a separation of yin and yang in the vessels, resulting in blood out of control, and in turn chaos in the qi ('qi wild'), since the blood nourishes the qi. Milder manifestations are fluctuating symptoms of being easily fatigued, cold hands and feet, migrating joint problems, and being easily angered. More serious manifestations are severe anxiety and depersonalization.

There is no clear equivalent to the 'circulatory system' in traditional Chinese medicine. The *bi* syndrome due to wind describes the migrating aspect of the disorder associated with this system, and Liver qi stagnation is similar to an aspect of its ephemeral nature, but neither of these accounts for the Heart/circulatory aspect of the syndrome.

'Digestive system'

The 'digestive system' (yang brightness) includes the Lungs, the Stomach-Spleen, and the Bladder-Kidneys. According to Dr. Shen, the Lungs digest mucus, the Stomach-Spleen digest food, and the Kidneys digest water. The 'digestive system' can be accessed over the entire right side of the pulse when all of the qualities on that side are approximately the same.

Both Small and Large Intestine are involved. The Small Intestine is reflected at the proximal position on the right side, and the Large Intestine at the proximal position on the left side. Both positions represent the Kidneys, which in conventional traditional Chinese medicine control the lower burner, where each of these organs reside.

Symptoms associated with 'digestive system' disorders include fluctuating appetite and irregular bowel movements (changing from constipation to diarrhea). There is no equivalent term or condition in traditional Chinese medicine.

'Heart closed'

In terms of traditional Chinese medicine, the closest equivalent term to the 'Heart closed' pattern would be Heart qi stagnation. This is a pattern in which a moderately Flat quality is a sign that qi and blood are slightly stagnant in the Pericardium, and cannot freely reach into the Heart. The reason is that circulation of qi, and to a lesser extent blood, to the Heart has been blocked from entering the Heart, usually due to a shock. This ultimately leads to Heart qi deficiency and diminished peripheral blood circulation. While with 'Heart nervous' the shock affects the nervous innervation of the Heart, with 'Heart closed' the substance of the Heart (parenchyma) is slightly affected, though much less so than in the case of either 'Heart small' or 'Heart full.'

The shock is most often an emotional one experienced during childhood while the body's qi is still immature, and usually involves the loss of someone very close, such as a parent. However, it can occur later in life due to a major emotional shock, such as sudden bad news or the sudden breakup of a romance in which the person withdraws their 'heart' feelings. Other causes include Heart qi agitation ('Heart nervous') over a long period of time, or even a physical shock to the chest. The Flat wave associated with a Heart Closed pulse quality usually occurs in a person whose qi is already deficient or undeveloped.

This type of person seems to be in some kind of constant emotional difficulty. By nature the person tends to be vengeful and spiteful. The spirit of the eyes can seem somewhat withdrawn, or angry. The person may experience some chest pain in connection with the closing of qi circulation.

'Heart disease'

By 'Heart disease' Dr. Shen meant, as best I can understand it, Heart yang deficiency. This is the end of the process in the gradual depletion of Heart qi and blood described under the headings of other Heart disorders in this glossary, especially 'Heart weak,' 'Heart full,' 'Heart large,' and 'Heart small.'

Commonly, the entire pulse is very Rapid, arrhythmic (either Interrupted or Intermittent), and sometimes Hollow, with the most serious forms of 'Heart disease.' The left distal position is Deep, shows Changes in Intensity and Qualities, there is constant Deep Rough Vibration and/or an Unstable quality (very serious), and probably Slipperiness. Both proximal positions are almost always Feeble-Absent.

Among the causes are constitutional predisposition, congenital defects, work beyond one's energy as a child, rheumatic fever, extreme abuse of drugs, alcohol and nicotine, prolonged chronic disease, and severe emotional shocks to the Heart and circulation early in life. Repressed anger can always be a contributing factor. All of the etiologies lead to a gradual and ultimately extreme weakening of Heart qi and yang, until the Heart can no longer control the circulation.

The symptoms are the same as those associated with 'Heart large' and 'Heart full,' with the addition of greater chest pain, greater fatigue and shortness of breath on exertion, excessive spontaneous cold or beady perspiration during the day with minimal exertion, coldness in body and especially limbs, dependent pitting edema, and greater need to sleep in a sitting position.

Other symptoms are poor concentration and forgetfulness, palpitation even on mild exertion, numbness of the upper limbs, and a suffocated sensation in the chest. If the etiology is constitutional or congenital, the person will be anxious and vulnerable their entire life.

'Heart full' (trapped qi in the Heart)

This is a condition in which the qi is unable to exit the Heart, which I call trapped qi in the Heart. There is no known equivalent in traditional Chinese medicine, but in quasi-biomedical terms, it would be a very slight energetic enlargement of the heart undetected by x-ray, and might also be accompanied by incipient hypertension.

This condition manifests on the pulse as a Tense Inflated quality at the left distal position. When the condition is less serious, the left distal position can be a little Yielding Inflated, and the rate Normal or a little Rapid. According to Dr. Shen, but outside of my own experience, when the condition is more serious the left distal position is Deep, Thin, and Tight, and the entire pulse rate is Rapid.

A minor cause is sudden and very profound repressed anger at a time when a person is extremely active. A more serious etiology is a prolonged birth with the head inside (breech delivery), because it begins at such an early age. Other causes are trauma to the chest, prolonged grief, or following an episode of sudden extreme lifting beyond one's energy, whose seriousness depends on the events. Uncorrected, 'Heart full' can develop into either an enlarged heart ('Heart large,' see below) or hypertension, or both.

Such individuals will feel tired their entire lives, have little energy, and may be rather depressed. They are frequently very quick to anger. These symptoms are similar to, but more severe than, those associated with Heart blood deficiency ('Heart weak'). The entire body may be uncomfortable. There is more difficulty breathing out than in, and some discomfort when lying down on the left side. In a more advanced stage there may be coughing up of blood, because frequently the Lungs become secondarily stagnant due to cardiopulmonary insufficiency from diminished heart function.

'Heart large'

This is the equivalent of severe Heart qi deficiency in traditional Chinese medicine, or an enlarged heart in conventional medicine, as evidenced by x-ray. Some of the qualities associated with this condition are Change in Intensity or Qualities, and Rough Vibration at the left distal position. There can be a positive response at the Heart Large position in the area between the left distal and left middle positions, which is very Inflated and/or Rough as one moves the finger from distal to proximal, compared to moving from proximal to distal.

Another pulse sign associated with the 'Heart large' condition is a Deep, Thin, and Feeble quality with a rate in excess of 100 beats per minute. Dr. Shen associates this sign with prolonged overwork in a person with constitutionally deficient Heart qi. An Interrupted or Intermittent quality may also be present, and the Mitral Valve position will be Slippery. A Tense Hollow Full-Overflowing quality at the left distal position, with a rate exceeding 100 beats per minute, is another combination associated with the 'Heart large' condition. Dr. Shen associates this with suppressed emotion over a long period of time. An Interrupted or Intermittent quality, and a Slippery quality at the Mitral Valve position, can also be found with both of these latter qualities

The underlying causes are constitutional Heart qi deficiency, any of the other Heart conditions, especially Trapped qi in the Heart ('Heart full') and Heart blood stagnation ('Heart small') with coronary occlusion over a long period of time, and rheumatic heart disease. All of these factors may be exacerbated by chronic, repressed, and profound anger which occurs especially while active.

Also, more common before the advent of child labor laws, but still prevalent in the underdeveloped world, is child labor with excessive physical work at an early age, together with malnutrition. With this etiology there is usually an Interrupted or Intermittent rhythm, and the pulse is Yielding Hollow.

Symptoms include extreme shortness of breath, especially on exertion, difficulty breathing if lying flat on the back or on the left side, and chronic chest discomfort, as well as extensive fatigue. Hypertension is often present.

Heart Vibration

The Vibration quality over the entire pulse or at individual positions is defined by whether it is transient or consistent, superficial or deep, and rough or smooth. Transient, superficial, and smooth characteristics at the left distal position or even over the entire pulse indicate a relatively innocuous process involving passing worries or a tendency to worry, which I define as mild Heart qi agitation (very mild Heart yin deficiency). This sometimes begins with a very mild emotional shock, and often there is a background of very mild Heart qi deficiency.

Consistent Smooth Vibration over the entire pulse is a sign that one is highly susceptible to worry, and will find something to worry about even when there is no reason to.

Consistent Vibration which is rougher and deeper over the entire pulse is a sign of shock, guilt, or fear, and at individual positions indicates parenchymal damage.

'Heart nervous'

This is a condition, and associated pulse quality (Heart Nervous), in which the Heart yin is deficient and the qi is consequently agitated, erratic, and mildly deficient. I refer to this condition as Heart qi agitation. There is often a predisposition toward constitutional Heart qi deficiency.

There are two types of 'Heart nervous.' Less serious is the one due to prolonged worry, either a 'Heart vibration' or 'Heart tight' condition in which the pulse rate tends to be somewhat rapid, 80-84 beats per minute. With this type of condition, the individual will report feeling nervous.

With the second, more serious type, which is due to emotional shock, physical trauma (often at birth and sometimes in utero), there is Occasional Change in Rate at Rest, with no missed beats. When the change in rate is significant, there will be a propensity to panic. If the cause is trauma, there may be a horizontal line under the lower eyelid, a small purple blister on the tongue, and a bluish-green color at the chin and around the mouth. A large change in rate tends to accompany a propensity to panic.

A 'Heart weak' condition (see below) may also lead to the more serious 'Heart nervous' pattern in which case the pulse will generally be Deep and Thin, and the rate on exertion will increase by more than 8-12 beats per minute. On the other hand, a 'Heart nervous' disorder may lead to 'Heart weak.' Smooth Vibration at the Neuropsychological positions accompanies and is another sign of the 'Heart nervous' condition.

The 'Heart nervous' person will complain of easy fatigue, especially in the morning when awakening. Sleep is restless, marked by frequent wakening, so that one is in and out of an agitated state of sleep throughout the night. Palpitations may occur occasionally. The person will report frequent and disturbing mood swings, changes of mind about others and the chosen course of one's life, and as if they are on a "roller coaster" and mildly out of control. There will also be increased irritability, of a relatively mild nature.

'Heart small'

In terms of traditional Chinese medicine, the closest equivalent term to 'Heart small' would be Heart blood stagnation, and in conventional medicine, the closest equivalent condition would be coronary artery spasm and angina. There are mild and temporary, and serious and enduring, varieties.

With the mild and temporary forms, the pattern is usually the result of a sudden shock during which the heart contracts, thereby constricting the arteries of the heart. The constriction of these vessels due to shock deprives the Heart of qi and blood, leading to transient blood stagnation in the coronary arteries and capillaries, and an insufficient oxygen supply to the coronary muscles. The cardiac muscles are tense, the coronary arteries are in spasm, and breathing is difficult. In Dr. Shen's terms, the Heart is "suffocating." The left distal position can be extremely Flat.

With the more serious form the pulse becomes very Deep, Thin, and Feeble. The rate is Normal, slightly Rapid, or slightly Slow. Less often, a Choppy quality has been observed here in the presence of this condition. 'Heart Small' is permanent unless treated, and is equated by Dr. Shen with what he calls "true heart disease," by which he means coronary artery disease.

The etiology of the more serious 'Heart small' disorder is a profound shock at birth when there is prolonged labor and the head has already reached the outside of the birth canal, but is being held back by something like the cord around the neck of the infant. Prolonged fear and unexpressed anger may also lead to this condition, though these emotions may also be the consequence, since one finds in people with the 'Heart small' condition a lifelong, unexpressed, and unexplained fear, as well as some anger and tension. Night terrors and being easily startled are common complaints. There is shortness of breath, in which it is easy to expel air and difficult to take it in. There may be chest pain, usually of a needle-like or stabbing quality in one spot, in the left shoulder and/or down the left arm. Other symptoms are palpitations and cold extremities.

'Heart tight'

This is both a condition ('Heart tight') and the pulse quality associated with that condition (Heart Tight). It is equivalent to mild to moderate Heart qi agitation, which is initially a condition of heat from excess of the Heart (Heart fire flaring up), and subsequently Heart yin deficiency. With heat from excess the left distal position will at first feel Tight in the Pericardium position, as if a strong, sharp point is sticking the middle of the finger with each beat. If the heat becomes overwhelming, the entire position can feel Tense with Robust Pounding. This heat usually has its origins in the Liver, Gallbladder, and Stomach.

With heat from deficiency, Tightness is felt over the entire left distal position. If the condition has existed for a short period of time owing to an emotional shock, the pulse is usually relatively Rapid, between 84-90 beats per minute. Over a much longer period of time, the pulse rate will be Slower, as this condition weakens Heart qi and affects overall circulation. There may also be some coincidental transient, superficial Vibration at the left distal position from time to time, reflecting episodes of worry.

The Heart Tight quality can also be associated with heat from yin deficiency due to overwork of the Heart as it tries to balance the heat from excess in the Liver, Gallbladder, and Stomach associated with worry, shock, Grave's disease, and the manic phases of bipolar disease, and from stimulating drugs and herbs such as cocaine or Herba Ephedra *(ma huang)*.

The 'Heart tight' condition associated with excess is marked by symptoms of irritability, tension, and difficulty getting to sleep. With the yin-deficient variety, one is more restless and complains of constant worry, a "racing mind," and sleep marked by constant awakening throughout the night. With both there is mild to moderate anxiety.

Occasionally, there will be some discomfort in the left side of the chest over a relatively large area. This discomfort is an early form of mild angina, which is due to heat from excess or stagnant qi migrating to the Pericardium from the Liver, Gallbladder, or Stomach, and causing a mild spasm of the coronary arteries. There may also be some shortness of breath during episodes of anxiety.

'Heart weak'

This condition, and associated pulse quality (Heart Weak), is one in which the Heart blood is deficient, with some consequent Heart qi deficiency, both of which cause a deficit in Heart function. The pulse shows a large Change in Rate on Exertion, more than 20 beats per minute if the Heart is very blood deficient, and a lesser change (12-20 beats) if the Heart is only slightly blood deficient. The rate may be a little Rapid, Normal, or Slow, depending upon the chronicity of the condition: the longer the condition has lasted, the Slower the pulse. The left distal position is often Thin when the blood deficiency is more severe, accompanied by Reduced Substance if the Heart qi is also deficient.

While constitutional Heart qi deficiency is sometimes a predisposing factor, Heart blood deficiency is most often due to prolonged and severe Heart qi agitation ('Heart nervous,' see above). If the 'Heart nervous' condition continues, the pulse will generally be more Tight and the vessels under the eyes will be normal. However, Heart blood deficiency can be due to one or any combination of the following: Kidney essence deficiency, Spleen qi deficiency, and gradual blood loss over time. When blood deficiency is the cause, the entire pulse is Thin and a little Feeble and the vessels inside the lower eyelid are pale.

The patient may experience palpitations throughout the day, especially with activity, because there is not enough blood in the Heart. There is also a general feeling of weakness, depression, poor concentration, and forgetfulness. The sleep pattern is one of steadily sleeping for a few hours and then waking, unable to return to sleep. One will be tired in the morning. A prolonged 'Heart weak' pattern can lead to serious 'Heart disease,' with manifestations such as congestive heart failure.

'Nervous system'

The 'nervous system' is associated by Dr. Shen with the lightest and quickest energy, which would be closest to the surface of the body and therefore identified with greater yang, and especially the Bladder channel whose outer course is accessed for the treatment of psychological disorders. 'Nervous system' messages are by far the most rapidly conducted compared to the speed of the endocrine or circulatory systems.

The equivalent of the 'nervous system' in traditional Chinese medicine would be one of the singular organs, the sea of marrow, which is engendered and maintained by Kidney essence; this refers to the substance of the brain, the spinal cord, and the central nervous system.

'Nervous system tense'

When Tension is found uniformly over the entire pulse, I refer to it as the 'vigilance' pulse because it appears constitutionally in ethnic groups whose survival through the centuries has required extraordinary vigilance. A similar pulse quality can be found today in almost anyone living in a large city, or living constantly with the need to be vigilant. Therefore, a differential diagnosis is required between a constitutional 'nervous system tense,' and one that is due to ongoing chronic stress. Making this distinction is important since individuals whose tension is related to their current life situation can alter their lifestyle as part of treatment, which is not true for those for whom the etiology is constitutional.

The principal symptom is an ongoing tension that may or may not be related to a particular life stress. The tension can be in the family over several generations. Accompanying symptoms depend on the vulnerability of other organ systems that are affected by the heat from excess, and especially stasis, which can be a consequence of this condition when it persists over a long period of time.

'Nervous system weak'

Another condition in which this quality is found uniformly over the entire pulse is termed 'nervous system weak' by Dr. Shen. Again, this is a constitutional condition in which the pulse goes through a series of stages, ending eventually in a generally Feeble-Absent pulse quality with a Tight quality at the surface of the pulse, especially on the left side, and sometimes with concomitant Smooth Vibration. This type of pulse is often found in a person who has a lifelong history of neurasthenia, one whose symptoms are always changing and who is highly vulnerable, unstable, and easily disturbed or stressed, and subject to constantly fluctuating allergies. The pulse does not represent illness as much as physical and mental instability and vulnerability to illness.

The closest (but imperfect) equivalents in traditional Chinese medicine would be Kidney qi/yang/essence deficiency and Heart qi/yang deficiency.

'Organ system'

The 'organ system' (greater, lesser, and absolute yin) includes the yin solid organs, especially the Heart, Liver, and Kidneys, which are accessed on the left side of the pulse when all of the qualities on the left side are approximately the same.

The condition associated with this system is primarily yang deficiency, but includes yin-deficient symptoms as well. Symptoms include spontaneous sweating, being easily fatigued, frequent pale urination, aversion to cold and preference for warmth, diarrhea with undigested food or infrequent bowel movements, and an extreme vulnerability to chronic illness and infections from which it is difficult to recover. There is no equivalent term or condition in traditional Chinese medicine.

'Push pulse' (Hesitant and Flooding Deficient Wave)

The Hesitant Wave is one of two pulse qualities which Dr. Shen referred to as a 'push pulse,' which he associated with individuals who pushed themselves too hard. The Hesitant quality reflects a person who pushes herself mentally. It occurs over the entire pulse and is found in cases of Heart yin deficiency with agitated qi. Descriptively, the pulse wave has lost its normal sine wave form whereby the flow to and from the wave peak becomes sharp and abrupt, instead of gradually rising and falling. The term Hesitant is used because some practitioners experience this quality as faltering or balking, yet not missing a beat.

By contrast, the Flooding Deficient quality is the form of the 'push pulse' associated with an individual who pushes herself more physically.

In traditional medical terms, the Hesitant quality is closest to mild to moderate Heart yin deficiency. I have found that this quality occurs in one who tends to think incessantly about one subject. In its most extreme form, this would be a monomaniacal obsessive preoccupation with a particular aspect of life, usually work, in which the person's mind never ceases to rest, even when asleep. This is to be distinguished from a tendency to worry about things in general, both real and imaginary, which is expressed over the entire pulse as a superficial Smooth Vibration at all depths.

In the early stages, except for the symptom of worry or difficulty in getting to sleep, there are no other related signs or symptoms. Later, the person will seek help because of a strong sense of malaise and a feeling that one cannot keep up the pace one has set for oneself. Individuals with this pulse quality often collapse suddenly, physically and/or emotionally.

'Qi wild'

This is a condition of extreme functional deficit in which, for one reason or another, the yin and yang have lost operative contact and are unable to support each other.

The yin, which is the material energy of the universe, can be thought of as a gravitational force that holds the more effervescent yang energies in check, and when drained can no longer serve that function. Under these circumstances, the lighter yang energies wander aimlessly to all parts of the organism, unable to function effectively without the organizing force of the yin. The result is physiological disarray, which disrupts the orderly circulation of yang to the channels and organs, impairing their ability to maintain function.

Thus, 'qi wild' is a condition characterized by chaos and represents a very serious physiological disorganization and disruption. A person suffering from this condition is highly vulnerable to serious and fast-spreading, even life-threatening disease within a very short time, including cancer, autoimmine, and degenerative central nervous system disease. Mental illness is another form of this chaos.

The pulse qualities associated with the 'qi wild' condition are Empty Interrupted-Intermittent; Yielding Hollow Interrupted-Intermittent; Empty; Yielding Hollow Full-Overflowing (Rapid or Slow); Leather; Empty and Thread-like; Scattered; Minute; and Change in Qualities. To be pathognomonic of a 'qi wild' condition, the quality must appear over the entire pulse.

'Systems'

Dr. Shen gradually developed the systems model when patients complained of symptoms for which he could find none of the familiar signs on the pulse, tongue, and eye examinations that were associated with disease in the traditional Chinese medical system. Neither were there any biomedical diagnostic findings. The symptoms were somewhat vague and shifting and inconsistent. What Dr. Shen discovered was that, rather than specific organ dysfunction, functional systems in their entirety were disturbed. He reduced these to four major systems—circulatory, digestive, nervous, and organ—drawing upon the layering of energy from superficial to deep, as described by Zhang Zhong-Jing in *Discussion of Cold Damage (Shang han lun)*.

---

1. William Philpott and Dwight Kalita, *Brain Allergies: The Psychosomatic Connection* (New Canaan, CT: Keats, 1980) 71–72.

APPENDIX: 3

Bibliography

Allport, Gordon. *Becoming.* New Haven, CT: Yale University Press, 1955.

Amber, R.B. *The Pulse in Occident and Orient: Its Philosophy and Practice in India, China, Iran, and the West.* New York: Santa Barbara Press, 1966.

Beijing College of Traditional Chinese Medicine. *Essentials of Chinese Acupuncture.* Beijing: Foreign Languages Press, 1980.

Cheung, C.S., Belluomini, J. An overview of pulse types used in traditional chinese medical differential diagnosis. *Journal of the American College of Traditional Chinese Medicine* 1982;1:1

Dale, Ralph Alan. The demystification of chinese pulse diagnosis. *American Journal of Acupuncture* 1993;21(1):63

de Morant, George Soulié. *Chinese Acupuncture,* trans. Lawrence Grinnell et al. Brookline, MA: Paradigm Publications, 1994.

Deng Tietao. *Practical Diagnosis in Traditional Chinese Medicine,* trans. Marnae Ergil. Edinburgh: Churchill Livingstone, 1999.

Donden, Yeshi. *Healing from the Source: The Science and Lore of Tibetan Medicine,* trans. B. Alan Wallace. Ithaca, NY: Snow Lion Publications, 2000.

Eckman, Peter. Korean acupuncture. *Traditional Acupuncture Society Journal* 1990;7:1

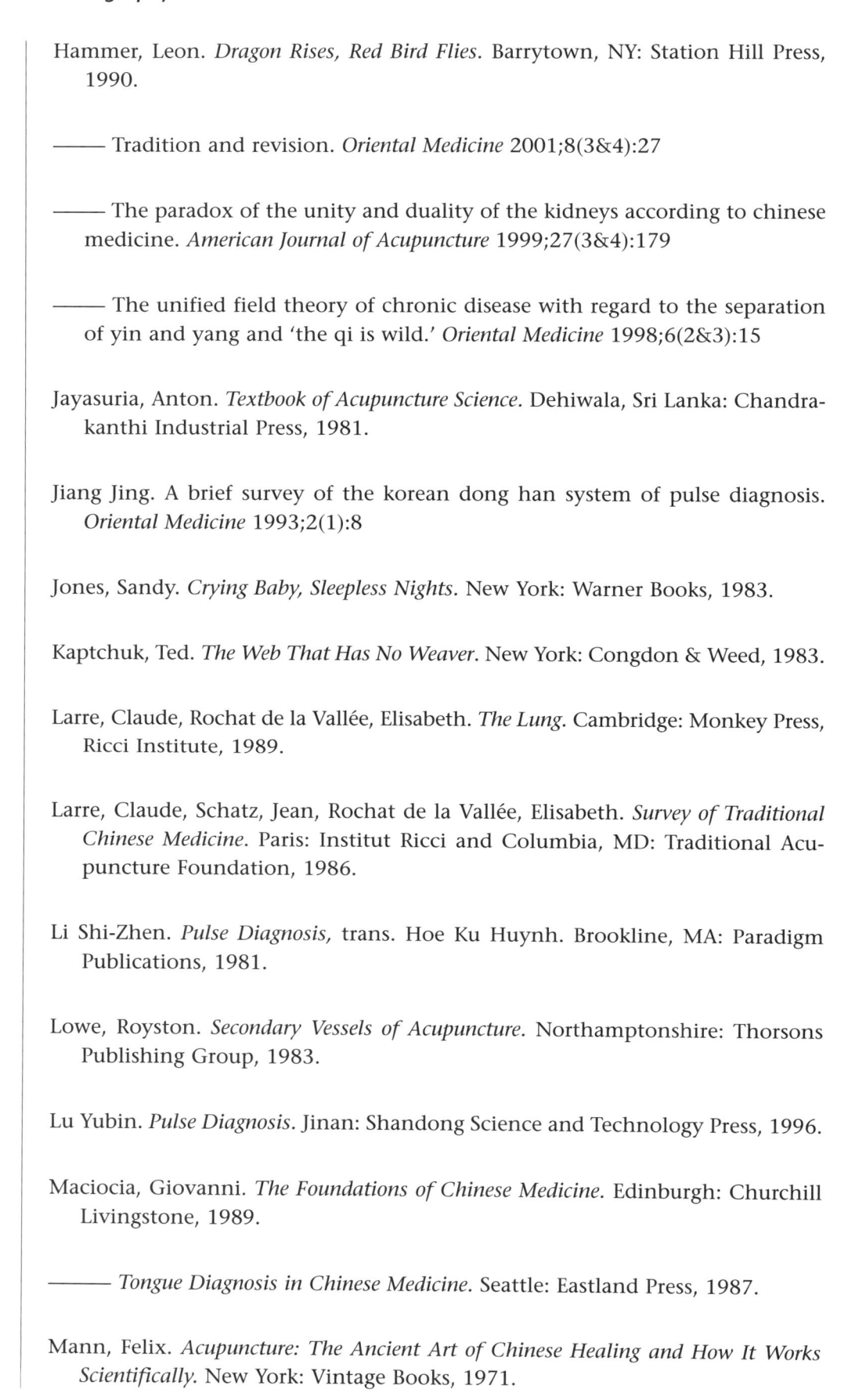

Hammer, Leon. *Dragon Rises, Red Bird Flies.* Barrytown, NY: Station Hill Press, 1990.

—— Tradition and revision. *Oriental Medicine* 2001;8(3&4):27

—— The paradox of the unity and duality of the kidneys according to chinese medicine. *American Journal of Acupuncture* 1999;27(3&4):179

—— The unified field theory of chronic disease with regard to the separation of yin and yang and 'the qi is wild.' *Oriental Medicine* 1998;6(2&3):15

Jayasuria, Anton. *Textbook of Acupuncture Science.* Dehiwala, Sri Lanka: Chandrakanthi Industrial Press, 1981.

Jiang Jing. A brief survey of the korean dong han system of pulse diagnosis. *Oriental Medicine* 1993;2(1):8

Jones, Sandy. *Crying Baby, Sleepless Nights.* New York: Warner Books, 1983.

Kaptchuk, Ted. *The Web That Has No Weaver.* New York: Congdon & Weed, 1983.

Larre, Claude, Rochat de la Vallée, Elisabeth. *The Lung.* Cambridge: Monkey Press, Ricci Institute, 1989.

Larre, Claude, Schatz, Jean, Rochat de la Vallée, Elisabeth. *Survey of Traditional Chinese Medicine.* Paris: Institut Ricci and Columbia, MD: Traditional Acupuncture Foundation, 1986.

Li Shi-Zhen. *Pulse Diagnosis,* trans. Hoe Ku Huynh. Brookline, MA: Paradigm Publications, 1981.

Lowe, Royston. *Secondary Vessels of Acupuncture.* Northamptonshire: Thorsons Publishing Group, 1983.

Lu Yubin. *Pulse Diagnosis.* Jinan: Shandong Science and Technology Press, 1996.

Maciocia, Giovanni. *The Foundations of Chinese Medicine.* Edinburgh: Churchill Livingstone, 1989.

—— *Tongue Diagnosis in Chinese Medicine.* Seattle: Eastland Press, 1987.

Mann, Felix. *Acupuncture: The Ancient Art of Chinese Healing and How It Works Scientifically.* New York: Vintage Books, 1971.

Matsumoto, Kiiko, Birch, Stephen. *Five Elements and Ten Stems.* Brookline, MA: Paradigm Publications, 1983.

Nahman of Bratslav. *The Stories of Rabbi Nachman of Breslov,* trans. Aryeh Kaplan. Brooklyn: Breslov Research Institute, 1983.

Needham, Joseph, Lu Gwei-Djen. *Celestial Lancets.* Cambridge: Cambridge University Press, 1980.

Philpott, William, Kalita, Dwight. *Brain Allergies: The Psychosomatic Connection.* New Canaan, CT: Keats, 1980.

Porkert, Manfred. *The Essentials of Chinese Diagnostics.* Zurich: Chinese Medicine Publications, 1983.

Ramholz, James. An introduction to advanced pulse diagnosis. *Oriental Medicine,* 2000;8(1&2):17

Veith, Ilza (trans.) *The Yellow Emperor's Classic of Internal Medicine.* Berkeley: University of California Press, 1966.

Shanghai College of Traditional Medicine. *Acupuncture: A Comprehensive Text,* trans. & ed. John O'Connor and Dan Bensky. Chicago: Eastland Press, 1981.

Shen, John. *Chinese Medicine.* New York: Educational Solutions, 1980.

Townsend, Graham, DeDonna, Ysha. *Pulses and Impulses.* Northamptonshire: Thorsons Publishing Group, 1990.

Unschuld, Paul. *Forgotten Traditions of Chinese Medicine.* Brookline, MA: Paradigm Publications, 1990.

——— (trans.) *Nan-Ching.* Berkeley: University of California Press, 1986.

Wang Shu-He. *The Pulse Classic,* trans. Yang Shou-Zhong. Boulder, CO: Blue Poppy Press, 1997.

Worsley, J.R. *Acupuncturists' Therapeutic Pocket Book: The Little Black Book.* Columbia, MD: Center for Traditional Acupuncture, 1975.

Wu Shui-Wan. *The Chinese Pulse Diagnosis.* San Francisco: Writers Guild of America, 1973.

Pulse Index

A

Abbreviated (Short), 302
Absence of the blood and qi depths: Deep, 484
Alternating from Tight to Yielding, 340
Amplitude, Change in, 397
    over the entire pulse, 138

B

Bean (Spinning), 374, 399, 475
Bean (Spinning) Tight very Slippery and Rapid, 375
Bean (Spinning) Wiry, 375
Biting, 447
Blood Heat, 430, 480, 747
Blood Thick, 430, 481, 747
Blood Unclear, 292, 430, 479, 748
Bounding, 153

C

Change in Amplitude. *See* Amplitude, Change in
Change in Intensity. *See* Intensity, Change in
Change in Qualities. *See* Qualities, Change in
Change in Rate at Rest. *See* Rate at Rest, Change in
Choppy, 362, 398, 401, 433, 448, 478, 487
Choppy Deep, 273
Choppy Tight or Wiry, 364
Cotton, 236, 394, 404, 470, 511

D

Dead, 227
Deep, 216, 268, 422, 436, 437, 443, 445, 490
    and Rapid, 272
    and Slow, 271
    and Tight or Wiry (very), 274

Deep Choppy, 273
Deep Diffuse, 270
Deep Feeble, 274, 276, 277, 279, 281
    with Increase in Rate on Exertion, 278
    and Slow, 280
Deep Feeble-Absent, 270, 275, 524
Deep Flat, 271, 273, 275, 276
    and slightly Rapid or Slow, 278
Deep Reduced Substance, 270, 490
Deep Separating, 490
Deep Slippery, 271, 274, 275, 276, 278, 279
Deep Slippery Feeble and Slow, 280, 281
Deep Slippery Tense, 280
Deep Slippery Tight and Rapid, 281
Deep Slippery Wiry and Rapid, 280
Deep Tense to Tight with Normal rate, 279
Deep Thin, 272, 276
    and slightly Rapid, 278
Deep Thin Feeble
    with Normal rate, slightly Rapid or Slow, 398
    with rate >100 beats/minute, 398
Deep Thin Feeble-Absent and very Slow, 397
Deep Thin Tight, 274
    and Rapid, 279
    and Rapid, very, 278
    with rate >100 beats/minute, 398
    to Wiry Hollow, 279
Deep Tight, 270, 275, 277, 280
Deep Tight-Wiry and very Rapid, 275
Deep Wide, 273
Deep Wiry, 271, 276, 432
Deep Yielding partially Hollow, 484
Diffuse, 209, 431
    and Reduced Substance, 293

Diminished
    at blood depth, 205
    or Absent at qi depth, 204
Diminished Feeble or Absent at qi depth, 476
Doughy, 375, 401

—— E

Empty, 132, 245, 397, 428, 431, 436, 437, 443, 491, 527
    Change in Intensity and Qualities, 423
    moderately Tense, 249
    at proximal and middle positions, 250
Empty Interrupted, 469
Empty Interrupted-Intermittent, 250, 493
Empty or Yielding Hollow Interrupted or Intermittent, 135
Empty Thread-like, 132, 492
Empty Tight and Rapid, 249
Empty Yielding and Slow, 249
Exuberant blood. *See* Blood Thick

—— F

Feeble, 395
Feeble-Absent, 216, 395, 422, 425, 426, 436, 437, 443, 445, 446, 490
    in both positions, 405
Feeble-Absent Deep and Rapid/Slow, 221
Feeble-Absent Deep Choppy, 221
Feeble-Absent Deep Slippery, 221
Firm, 281
Flat, 209, 396, 421, 436, 487, 514
Flat Tense, 213
Flat Tight and Rapid, 213
Floating, 239, 420, 427, 471, 510
Floating Slippery, 472
Floating Tense
    with Normal or slightly Rapid rate, 244, 510
    and Slow, 244, 425, 510
    and Slow, slightly, 243, 472
Floating Tight, 244, 432, 472
Floating Yielding
    with Normal rate, 243
    and Rapid, 245, 425, 510
    and Rapid, slightly, 243, 471
    and Slow, 510
Flooding Deficient, 205, 477
Flooding Excess, 190, 291, 334, 347, 349, 443, 445, 472, 487, 511
    and Robust Pounding, 432

—— H

Heart Nervous, 751
Heart Tight, 410, 753
Heart Vibration, 751
Heart Weak, 753
Hesitant Wave, 126, 410
Hidden, 282
Hidden Deficient, 284, 491
Hidden Excess, 284, 486
Hidden Normal, 284
Hollow, 259, 529
Hollow Full-Overflowing, 179, 402, 511
Hollow Full-Overflowing Leather-like Hollow and Rapid or Slow, 187
Hollow Full-Overflowing Reduced Pounding, 188
Hollow Full-Overflowing Robust Pounding Bounding and Rapid, 188
Hollow Full-Overflowing Slippery
    over the entire pulse at all depths, 187
    and very Rapid, 188
Hollow Full-Overflowing Tense Hollow and Slippery at the blood depth, 188
Hollow Full-Overflowing Tight or Wiry, 188
    and Slippery, 188

—— I

Inflated, 193, 399, 433, 436, 448, 475, 512
    and Tense, very, 196
Inflated Tense, 195, 196
Inflated Tense-Floating and slightly Rapid or Slow, 196
Inflated Yielding, 196
Inflated Yielding and mildly Tense, 194
Inflated Yielding-Floating and slightly Rapid or Slow, 196
Intensity, Change in, 136, 397, 433, 448, 469
    affecting only one wrist, 138
    undulating from one position to another, 138
    undulating from one wrist to another, 138
Intermittent, 119
    Constantly, 119
    Inconsistently, 120
Interrupted, 121
    Constantly, 121
    Occasionally, 124
    Sudden Transient, 124

—— L

Leather, 132, 255, 492
Leather-like Hollow, 142, 264, 265, 266, 267, 268, 292, 398, 432, 484
    and Rapid or Slow, 262
Left distal
    with a Change in Rate at Rest, 408
    Increase in Rate on Exertion >8-12 beats/min, 408
Left distal and proximal
    Feeble-Absent, and left middle Tense, 407
    Feeble-Absent, remainder Normal, 406
    Thin Feeble, entire pulse Interrupted or Intermittent, 409
Left distal Feeble-Absent
    and left middle very Tense Inflated or Hollow Full-Overflowing, 404
    and left proximal Tight, 406
    and remainder Slippery at blood depth, 407
    and Slow, 408
Left distal Tight
    with Hesitant Wave, 409
    and left proximal Feeble-Absent, 406
    and Rapid or Slow, 408
Long, 301

—— M

Minute, 132, 493
Muffled, 226, 397, 401, 423, 429, 433, 448
    and Dead, 432

N

Nonhomogeneous, 140, 374
Normal Pulse, 89

Q

Qualities
    Change in, 133, 397, 469
Qualities and Intensity
    Change in, 431, 444

R

Rapid, 152, 445
Rate at Rest
    Change in, 115
    Constant Change in, 117
    Occasional Change in, 115
Rate on Exertion
    Constant Large Increase in, 125
    Decrease in, 125
    Occasional Large Increases in, 125
Reduced Pounding, 208
Reduced Substance, 209, 422, 431, 436, 443, 445
Restricted, 429
    length, 302
    width, 301
Right distal Feeble-Absent left middle Tense to Tight, 425
Robust Pounding, 190, 334, 347, 423, 443, 445, 448
    and Bounding with Rapid rate, 474
    and Flooding Excess, 190
    and Hollow Full-Overflowing, 190
    at organ depth, 475
    and Rapid, 349
Robust Pounding Tight
    and slightly Inflated, 403
    and slightly Inflated with Rapid rate, 398
Ropy, 360, 483
Ropy Yielding Hollow, 361
Rough Vibration, 367, 400, 428, 447, 483
    Consistent, 369
    Constant at left distal position at all depths or deep, 397
    deeply or at all depths, 373

S

Scattered, 132, 256, 492
Short (Abbreviated), 302
Short Yielding, 490
Slightly Tight Hollow Full-Overflowing, 268
Slightly Yielding Hollow Full-Overflowing
    and Normal to slightly Rapid, 261
Slippery, 313, 322, 396, 399, 402, 404, 423, 425, 428, 430, 443, 445, 447, 475, 482, 521
    at Esophagus position, 324
    with high fever, 321
    at Mitral Valve position, 321
    moderately to severely, 323
    with Normal rate, 396
    and Rapid, 318, 321, 347, 396
    and Rapid, very, 397
        with high fever, 321
    and Slow, 318, 319, 320, 324
    transiently, 316
    and very Tight Hollow Full-Overflowing, 320
    and Rapid, 321
Slippery Deep (very) and very Rapid, 321
Slippery Deep Feeble, 325
    and Slow, 325
Slippery Deep Tight to Wiry and Rapid, 325
Slippery Feeble, 322
    with Normal rate, 321
    and Slippery Empty, 322
    and Slow, 315, 320, 322, 324
Slippery Inflated, 324
Slippery Tense, 323, 325
    at all depths, 320
    mildly, with Normal to slightly Rapid rate, 323
    and Normal rate, 319
    and Normal to slightly Rapid rate, 320
    at qi depth with Normal or slightly Rapid rate, 320
    and Rapid, 318
    and Rapid, slightly, 322
    and Rapid, slightly to very, 321
    and Rapid, very, 320
    and Slow, 318, 324
Slippery Tense Flooding Excess (and possibly Rapid), 325
Slippery Tight
    and Rapid, 322
    and Rapid, slightly, 318, 324
    and Slow, 322, 323
Slippery Tight Flooding Excess and Rapid, 322, 325
Slippery Tight (Hollow) at Stomach-Pylorus Extension position, 324
Slippery Tight Hollow Full-Overflowing and Rapid, 315
Slippery Tight-Wiry and Choppy or Muffled, 323
Slippery Transient above the qi depth, 318
Slippery Wiry Deep and Rapid, 280
Slippery Yielding (mildly) and Slow, 323
Slow, 162
Smooth Vibration, 367, 371, 372, 400
Spinning (Bean). *See* Bean (Spinning)
Spreading, 205, 431, 484
Superficial, Smooth and Transitory Vibration, 395
Suppressed, 201

T

Taut, 329, 430, 442, 473
    and slightly Rapid or Slow, 330
Taut Choppy, 330
Taut Floating, 329
Taut Inflated, 330
Taut Slippery, 330
Taut-Tense, 486
Taut Wide, 330
Tense, 332, 394, 403, 420, 425, 430, 442, 445, 447, 473, 516
    and Rapid, 333
    and Slow, 333
    very, or Tight Hollow Full-Overflowing, 485
    and very Tense Hollow Full-Overflowing, 263
Tense Choppy, 334
Tense Deep, 333
Tense Floating, 333
Tense Hollow, 263, 265, 267
Tense Hollow Full-Overflowing, 181, 290, 334, 404, 430, 433, 472, 482
    very, 397
Tense Hollow Slippery and Rapid, 262

Tense Inflated, 196, 334, 402, 431, 513, 514
    mildly, 196, 513
    moderately, 197, 513
    very, 195, 197, 398, 479
Tense Inflated Floating, 197
Tense Long, 474
Tense Robust Pounding, 474
Tense Robust Pounding Suppressed, 474
Tense Ropy, 293, 360, 483
Tense Slippery, 334, 433
    with Normal or slightly Rapid rate, 316
Tense-Tight, 436
Tense-Tight Hollow Full-Overflowing, 266
    very, 142
Tense-Tight Inflated at right distal and Special Lung positions, 429
Tense to Tight (deep) with Normal rate, 279
Tense Wide, 334
Thin, 295, 298, 300, 395, 423, 430, 484, 523
    with Increase in Rate on Exertion, 300
Thin Arrhythmic, 298
Thin Deep, 297
    and very Feeble, 297
Thin Deep Feeble, 298
    and Rapid, 301
    and Slow (sometimes Slippery), 299
Thin Deep Tight and Rapid, 298
Thin Deep Tight-Wiry and Slow, 299
Thin Feeble, 299
Thin Feeble Interrupted and Slow, 404
Thin Minute, 297
Thin quality in young man, 294
Thin Slippery, 299
Thin Tight, 299, 489
    and Rapid, 299
Thin Tight-Wiry, 297
Thin Yielding, 296, 488
Tight, 337, 347, 348, 349, 399, 420, 425, 426, 430, 437, 446, 447, 489
    alternating to Yielding, 340
    in both positions, 405
    at Esophagus position, 348
    over entire left distal position, 345
    over entire position and slightly Rapid, 395
    at Pericardium position, 344
    at Pericardium position and moderately Rapid, 395
    at qi depth only, 347
    and Rapid, 338
    with Rate at Rest change, 345
    at Stomach-Pylorus Extension position, 348
    and Thin at qi depth, 477
    and very Tight Hollow Full-Overflowing, 263, 265, 266, 268
    and very Tight-Wiry Hollow-Full-Overflowing, 267
Tight Choppy, 340
Tight Deep, 338, 349
Tight Deep Thin and very Rapid, 345
Tight Deep Thin Feeble and slightly Rapid, 345
Tight Empty at qi depth, 347
Tight Floating, 338, 346
Tight Flooding Excess, 340
Tight Hollow Full-Overflowing, 348
    slightly, 268

Tight Inflated, 340
Tight or Wiry, 428
Tight Robust Pounding and Rapid, 348
Tight Slippery, 433
Tight Slippery Robust Pounding and Rapid, 347
Tight Thin, 338, 346, 348
Tight to Wiry Hollow-Full Overflowing, 184
Tight Wide Slippery, 340
Tight-Wiry, 295, 442, 443, 445, 518
    deep and very Rapid, 275
Tight-Wiry Hollow Slippery, 268
Transiently Slippery, 316

——— U

Unstable, 140, 398

——— V

Vibration, 366, 402, 422, 531. *See also* Rough Vibration; Smooth Vibration
    and Choppy, 431
    at Neuro-psychological positions, 410
    Transitory, 395

——— W

Wide Yielding Hollow Full-Overflowing, with Normal or slightly Rapid rate, 293
Wiry, 349, 397, 421, 430, 433, 489
    and Rapid, 351
Wiry Choppy, 352
Wiry Deep, 351
    and Slow, 352
Wiry Empty and slightly Rapid, 352
Wiry Inflated, 352
Wiry Robust Pounding and Rapid, 352
Wiry Slippery
    at blood depth with Normal or slightly Rapid rate, 351
    and very Rapid, 351
Wiry Thin, 351

——— Y

Yielding, 476
    alternating from Tight, 340
    at qi depth, 203
Yielding Empty Thread-like, 253, 301
Yielding Hollow-Full Overflowing, 181, 261, 262, 264, 265, 267, 268, 469, 472, 493
    and Interrupted-Intermittent, 261
    and Rapid, 187
    with rate >100 beats/minute, 398
    slightly, and Normal to slightly Rapid, 261
    and Slow, 187, 261, 265, 267
Yielding Hollow Intermittent, 135
Yielding Hollow Interrupted, 135, 469
Yielding Hollow Interrupted-Intermittent, 493
Yielding Hollow Ropy, 262
Yielding Inflated, 196, 421, 428, 512, 514
Yielding partially Hollow, 205, 260, 262, 264, 267, 431, 484
    and Slow, 142
Yielding Reduced Pounding, 476
Yielding Ropy, 294, 484
Yielding Ropy Hollow, 133
Yielding Slippery and Slow, 316
Yielding Tense Inflated and slightly Rapid, 395

General Index

Using this index:
d = definition
f = figure
t = table

─── A

Abbreviated (Short), 302
Above the qi depth. *See also* Qi depth
    Cotton, 470
    Excess, 470-472
    Floating, 471
    Floating Slippery, 472
    Floating Tense and slightly Slow, 472
    Floating Tight, 472
    Floating Yielding and slightly Rapid, 471
    Flooding Excess, 472
    Hard, 472
    illustrated, 69f
    qualities (common), 69
    Tense Hollow Full-Overflowing, 472
    Yielding Hollow Full-Overflowing, 471
    Yielding sensations, 470-472
Absence of the blood and qi depths: Deep Yielding partially Hollow, 484
Absent. *See also* Feeble; Feeble-Absent
    defined, 202d
    Feeble vs., 218
    illustrated, 217f
Absent at qi depth. *See also* Qi depth
    about, 204-205
    illustrated, 205f
    Qi deficiency, 476
Abstinence (sexual)
    Taut, 332, 442
    Tense, 336, 337, 518
Accelerated pulse. *See* Rapid
Acute illness (disharmony). *See also* Chronic illness
    the Hard pulse, 35
    in interpretation, 35, 45-47, 640
    Rapid, 160
    Robust and Pounding, 633
    the Yielding pulse, 35
Addiction
    alcohol
        Deep Wiry, 271
        Heart yang deficiency, 416
        as psychological disharmony, 583-584
        Tense, 333
        Tight Thin, 347
    drug abuse
        Empty, 247, 252, 431, 529
        Empty at left middle position, 605
        Feeble-Absent, 614
        Heart yang deficiency, 416
        Muffled, 401
        Muffled at Neuro-psychological position, 610
        as psychological disharmony, 583-584
        'qi wild' condition, 131
        qualities associated with, 45
        Robust Pounding, 474-475
        Robust Pounding Tight and slightly Inflated with

Rapid rate, 398
Taut, 330
Tense, 333
Tight, 341
Tight (including Wiry), 519
Very Tense Inflated, 398
Wiry, 353, 357, 421
nicotine
Heart yang deficiency, 416
Tense, 336
Tense Inflated, 421
Tight, 346, 420, 426, 428
Wiry, 357, 421, 428
Aerobic exercise, Slow pulse, 163, 168-169
Age effects
Feeble-Absent, 220
in interpretation, 40-41, 65, 626
Normal pulse, 95
paradoxical qualities, 631-632
rate, 152
AIDS. *See also* Auto-immune disorders
Scattered, 256, 492, 615
Yielding Empty Thread-like, 253
Alcohol abuse
Deep Wiry, 271
Heart yang deficiency, 416
as psychological disharmony, 583-584
Tense, 333
Tight Thin, 347
Allergies
Feeble-Absent, 426
Floating, 242
Tense-Tight Inflated at right distal, 429
Tense-Tight Inflated at Special Lung, 429
Transiently Slippery, 316
Wiry, 357
Alternating from Tight to Yielding, 340
Amber, R.B., 61-62, 98
Amenorrhea, Choppy, 365
Amplitude, Change in
about, 38
arrhythmia vs., 139
Change in Qualities vs., 139
illustrated, 139f
over entire pulse, 138
position interpretation, 139
Aneurysm
Inflated at Large Vessel position, 614
Slippery, 402
Tense Inflated, 402
Anger, described, 577-578
Anger (qualities)
Feeble-Absent (left distal) and left middle very Tense Inflated, 404

Heart Full, 414
Hollow Full-Overflowing, 404
Inflated, 451, 475
Inflated at Diaphragm position, 578
Inflated Yielding, 194
Slow, 604
Taut, 331
Tense, 332, 337
Tense Hollow, 263, 265, 267
Tense Inflated, 334, 431
Tense Inflated, moderately, 513
Anguish. *See* Emotions/emotional life
Anomalous qualities, 378, 382f, 391
Anomalous vessels, 378-380
Anorexia
Deep Feeble-Absent, 275
Empty, 251, 529
Feeble-Absent Deep, 526
Thin Feeble Interrupted and Slow, 404
Yielding Hollow Full-Overflowing, 266
Anxiety
described, 557-558
Arrhythmic qualities, 562
Empty, 246-247
Exertion, Increase in Rate, 561
Feeble-Absent at left distal position, 561
Heart blood deficiency, 560-562
Heart-Gallbladder deficiency, 562
Heart qi agitation, 558-559
Heart qi deficiency, 560-562
Heart yin deficiency, 560
Heat from excess in Heart, 559
Hollow Full-Overflowing Robust Pounding Bounding and Rapid, 188
Intensity, Constant Change in, over entire pulse, 561
Liver qi stagnation, 407
Mitral Valve position, 402
Pericardium Tight or left distal Tense with Robust Pounding, 559-600
Pounding, 559
Qualities and Intensity, Change in at left distal position, 562
Rapid, 559
Rate at Rest, Change in, occasional, 559
Slippery at Mitral Valve position, 612
Slow, 561
Smooth Vibration, 400, 558, 611
Thin, left distal position, 561
Thin over entire pulse, 561
Tight at left distal position, 559
Vibration and Slippery at Mitral Valve positions, 562
Wiry, 353
Yielding Hollow Full-Overflowing, 561
Yielding Hollow Full-Overflowing and Rapid, 616
Appendicitis
Flooding Excess, 292, 512, 613
Slippery Tense and Slow, 319
Tight, 342

Tight (including Wiry), 520
Wiry, 354
Arrhythmia. *See also* Rhythm
    Amplitude, Change in vs., 139
    anxiety, 562
    classification, 114
    future (distant) disharmony, 604
    future (semi-distant) disharmony, 607
    Heart qi deficiency, 562
    Intensity, Change in vs., 139
    Interrupted or Intermittent, 607
    pseudo, 66, 125-127
    'qi wild' condition, 135
    Rate in Rest, Constant Change in, 604
    true, 65-66
Arteries, multiple radial, 378-379
Arteriosclerosis
    Robust Pounding, Tight, and slightly Inflated, 403
    Rough Vibration at blood depth, 607
    Slippery at blood depth, 607
    Slow pulse, 164
    Tense Ropy, 293, 616
Arthritis
    Blood Unclear, 480, 606
    Slow, 604
Asthma. *See also* Cardiac asthma; Lung disease
    Feeble-Absent, 426
    Floating, 242
    Qi deficiency, 424
    Slippery, 521
    Slippery Tense and Rapid, 318
    Taut, 331
    Tense, 420
    Tense Inflated, 421
    Tense-Tight Inflated at right distal, 429
    Tense-Tight Inflated at Special Lung, 429
    Thin, 523
    Tight, 345, 420
    Tight Deep Thin Feeble and slightly Rapid, 345
    Tight (including Wiry), 519
    Wiry, 353, 357, 421
    yin deficiency, 424
Atherosclerosis
    Choppy, 365
    Robust Pounding, Tight, and slightly Inflated, 403
    Rough Vibration at blood depth, 607
    Slippery at blood depth, 607
    Tense Ropy, 293
    Tight and very Tight Hollow Full-Overflowing, 264
Auto-immune disorders
    Blood Unclear, 292
    Scattered, 256, 492, 615
    Slippery Feeble and Slow, 315
    Thin quality in young man, 294
    Transiently Slippery, 316
    Yielding Empty Thread-like, 253
    Yielding Hollow Full-Overflowing Reduced Pounding, 186

B

Balance
    about, 50
    in Normal pulse, 91, 92f
    between pulses, 503
Barrett's syndrome
    Floating Tight, 618
    qi stagnation, 438
    Rough Vibration, 373
Bean (Spinning)
    about, 374-375
    distal position (left), 399
    future (immediate) disharmony, 617
    qi depth, 475
Bean (Spinning) Tight, very Slippery and Rapid, 372
Bean (Spinning) Wiry, 372
Below the organ depth, 70
Bending forward
    Feeble-Absent, 222
    Flat, 214
    Tense, 335, 517
    Tight, 342
Biting, 376, 447
Bladder position, 82-83, 444
Blood and qi deficiency, Thin, 296-297, 523
Blood and yin deficiency, Thin, 523
Blood deficiency
    absence of the blood and qi depths: Deep, 484
    at blood depth, 484
    Heart and Lung, 523
    Heart, with Heart and Lung phlegm, 524
    Liver, 524
    qualities (common), 628
    Spreading, 484
    Thin, 295-296, 484, 523, 524
    Thin Tight, 489
    Thin Tight-Wiry, 297
    Thin Yielding, 296-297, 488-489
    Yielding Partially Hollow, 484
Blood depth
    about, 477-478
    absence of, 484
    blood deficiency at, 484
    blood excess at, 478-484
    blood instability at, 484-485
    blood stagnation at, 478-479
    Diminished, 205, 207f
    Feeble-Absent, 218
    Flooding Deficient, 205, 207f, 208
    illustrated, 29f, 69f
    in interpretation, 635
    pulse methodology, 70
    qualities (common), 70
    Slippery, 323
    Spreading, 205, 206f
    Yielding partially Hollow, 205, 206f

Blood dycrasias
  Slippery Feeble and Slow, 315
Blood excess at blood depth, 478-484
Blood Heat
  about, 480
  Choppy, 363
  defined, 731d
  future (semi-distant) disharmony, 606
  illustrated, 481f
  Rapid, 157
  Tense Slippery, 334
  Tight Wide Slippery, 340
  Transiently Slippery, 316, 317
  Wiry, 350
  Wiry and Slippery at blood depth with Normal or slightly Rapid rate, 351
Blood instability
  Leather-like Hollow, 484
  Very Tense or Tight Hollow Full-Overflowing, 485
Blood lipids and glucose elevation, Slippery, 315
Blood out of control (reckless blood), 141-142. *See also* Blood instability
Blood stagnation. *See also* Heart blood stagnation
  Blood Heat, 480
  Blood Thick, 481-482
  Blood Unclear, 479-480
  Choppy, 363, 448, 478
  Flat, 606
  at organ depth, 487
  qualities (common), 628
  Ropy, 483
  Rough Vibration, 483
  Slippery, 482-483
  Tense Hollow Full-Overflowing, 482
  Tense Ropy, 483
  Thin, 297
  Tight (including Wiry), 521
  in tissues and body cavities, 478-479
  Very Tense Inflated, 479
  in vessels, 479-484
  Wiry, 355
  Yielding Ropy, 484
Blood Thick
  described, 290, 481-482
  Choppy, 363
  defined, 731d
  future (semi-distant) disharmony, 606
  Hollow Full-Overflowing Tense and Slippery, 188
  illustrated, 482f
  Rapid, 157-158
  Slow pulse, 164
  Tense Slippery, 334
  Tense Wide, 334
  Tight Wide Slippery, 340
  Transiently Slippery, 316
  Wiry, 350
  Wiry and Slippery at blood depth with Normal or slightly Rapid rate, 351
Blood Unclear
  about, 292, 479-480
  defined, 732f
  future (semi-distant) disharmony, 606
  illustrated, 480f
  Tense Slippery, 334
  Transiently Slippery, 316
Bounding, 153
Broken. *See* Scattered
Buddha's pulse, 332, 336, 337, 442
Bulimia
  Deep Feeble-Absent, 275
  Empty, 251, 529
  Feeble-Absent Deep, 526
  Qi stagnation, 438
  Yielding Hollow Full-Overflowing, 266
Buoyancy in Normal pulse, 90, 92f
Burner (middle). *See* Middle position

── C

Cancer
  Choppy, 364, 365, 448
  Deep Feeble, 279
  Empty, 246
  Empty at left middle position, 605
  Feeble-Absent, 614
  Floating Tight, 618
  Muffled, 429
  Muffled and Dead, 432
  Restricted, 429
  Restricted (width), 301
  Rough Vibration, 373, 447
  Slippery at organ depth, 614
  Slippery Empty, 322
  Slippery Feeble, 322
  Wiry, 421
Candidiasis
  Deep Slippery, 276
  Slippery, 323
  Slippery Feeble and Slow, 324
Cardiac asthma
  Tight, 341
  Tight (including Wiry), 519
Cardiopulmonary failure, Slippery Feeble, 322
Cardiovascular system importance, 50-51, 601-602
Ceiling dripping. *See* Scattered
Central nervous system disorders, 584
Cerebral palsy, 401
Cerebrovascular accident. *See* Stroke
Change
  in Amplitude
    about, 38

arrhythmia vs., 139
illustrated, 139f
over entire pulse, 138
principal/complementary individual positions, 139
and in Qualities vs., 139
in Amplitude and Qualities
left distal position, 397
in Intensity
about, 37-38
future (semi-distant) disharmony, 609
Gallbladder position, 433
illustrated, 136f
inconstant over entire pulse, 573
Intestine positions, 448
occasional over entire pulse, 609
'qi wild' condition, 469
shifting back and forth between sides, 585
in interpretation, 633-634
in Qualities
future (immediate) disharmony, 616
illustrated, 134f
'qi wild' condition, 133-135, 469
yin and yang separation and, 37
in Qualities and Intensity
anxiety, 562
bilaterally, 533
left distal position, 397, 562
middle position (left), 431
proximal position, left, 444
uniform on either side, 508
uniform qualities, 532
in Rate at Rest
anxiety, 559
constant, 117-118, 408
future (immediate) disharmony, 610
occasional, 115-117, 408, 559, 610
worry, 564
in rhythm, 114-125
Childbirth. *See* Pregnancy/childbirth
Children/childhood
emotional shock
Deep Flat, 273
Heart Closed, 412
fetal alcohol syndrome
Deep Wiry, 271
malnutrition
Heart qi deficiency, 415
overwork
Heart qi deficiency, 415
qi deficiency, 466
'qi wild' condition, 129
Yielding Hollow Full-Overflowing Reduced Pounding, 187
pulse qualities of, 601
trauma
Deep Flat, 271
Chinese medicine
Chinese physiology, 33-35

the practitioner, 14-15
traditions, 3-6
Western medicine and, 35-36
Cholecystitis
Flooding Excess, 512
Muffled at Gallbladder position, 612
Slippery at Gallbladder position, 612
Tense Slippery at Gallbladder position, 608
Choppy
about, 4, 362-364
blood stagnation, 478, 487
combinations, 364-366
in complementary positions, 393
distal position (left), 398, 401, 617
future (immediate) disharmony, 611, 617
future (semi-distant) disharmony, 609
Gallbladder position, 433, 617
illustrated, 361f
Intestine positions, 448
middle position (left), 617
Neuro-psychological position, 401, 609
Pelvis/Lower Body positions, 617
Vibration vs., 366
Choppy Tight or Wiry, 364
Chronic fatigue syndrome
Feeble-Absent, 220
Feeble-Absent over entire pulse, 614
Slow, 604
Spreading over entire pulse, 604-605
Yielding Hollow Full-Overflowing, 265
Yielding Hollow Full-Overflowing Reduced Pounding, 186
Yielding or Diminished at qi depth, 603
Chronic illness (disharmony)
Feeble-Absent, 220
the Hard pulse, 35
in interpretation, 35, 45, 47, 633, 640
Rapid, 160
stagnation and, 49
Tight, 341
the Yielding pulse, 35
Circulation. *See also* Qi circulation
about, 465-466
of blood
Constant Change in Intensity, 609
Heart and, 468
impaired in the vessels, 479
qi and, 466-469
Heart and, 418-419
Heart blood, Thin, 523-524
stagnant, 407
'Circulatory system', 504, 639, 732d
Cirrhosis of the liver
Tight to Wiry Hollow Full-Overflowing, 184
Wiry, 351
Classification/nomenclature. *See also* Terminology
about, 6-7

Feeble-Absent, 218
Normal pulse, 96-98
qualities, 10, 64, 100-107t
Reduced, 202-203
by sensation/condition, 7
terminology comparison, 8-9t
Weak, 218
Climate and circulation, 467-468. *See also* Seasonal variations
Cold
    Deep Tight, 271
    external, 339
    external that leads to pain, 271
    of overexposure, 521
    stagnation, 443, 445
    Tense, 335, 517
    Tense Inflated, moderately, 513
    Tight, 339
    Tight (including Wiry), 521
    turns to heat, 513
    unresolved, internalized, 335, 517
    Wiry, 350
Cold from deficiency
    Deep and Slow, 272
    qualities (common), 629
    Slow, 163, 167
Cold from excess
    Deep and Slow, 272
    external, 163, 166
    internal, 164, 166, 358
    qualities (common), 629
    Slow, 163, 164, 166
    Stomach, 517
    Tense, 335, 517
    Wiry, 358
Cold (the common)
    Floating Tense and Slow, 611
    Heart condition, 423
Colitis
    Empty, 252, 529
    Feeble-Absent, 223
    Feeble-Absent Deep, 527
    Flooding Excess, 443, 512
    Robust Pounding, 443
    Slippery, 443
    Slippery Deep Tight to Wiry and Rapid, 325
    Slippery Flooding Excess Tense, 325
    Slippery Tight Flooding Excess and Rapid, 325
    Taut, 332
    Tense, 336, 337
    Tight Flooding Excess, 340
    Tight, Flooding Excess, Robust Pounding, Slippery and Rapid, 349
    Tight Hollow Full-Overflowing, 348
    Tight Robust Pounding and Rapid, 348

Tight-Wiry, 443
Wiry, 355, 359
Complementary positions. *See also* specific positions, e.g. Diaphragm
    overview, 23, 26
    Amplitude, Change in, 139
    bilateral similarities, 84
    defined, 6d
    illustrated, 24-25f
    Intensity, Change in, 139
    in interpreting the pulse, 63
    Lung (regular), 79-80
    qualities (common), 393
Consciousness and the three depths, 470
Consistency, 601
Constitution
    Empty, 529
    Feeble-Absent, 224, 443
    Feeble-Absent Deep, 527
    Kidney, 527
    Rapid, 158-159
Cotton
    about, 236-239
    above the qi depth, 470
    distal position (left), 394
    distal position (left) and left middle positions, 404
    distal position (uniform bilaterally), 511
    Floating vs., 242
    future (distant) disharmony, 602
    illustrated, 236f
    middle position (uniform bilaterally), 511
    proximal position (uniform bilaterally), 511
    resignation (emotion of), 580
    uniform quality, 511, 556
Crohn's disease
    Deep Slippery, 277
    Rough Vibration, 373

—— D

Damp-cold
    Reduced (right side) uniformly, 508
    Slippery and Slow, 488
Damp-heat
    Deep Slippery, 276
    Liver-Gallbladder, 319, 522
    Lung, 521
    Robust (right side) uniformly, 507
    Slippery, 487, 521, 522
    Slippery Tense and Slow, 319
    Slow pulse, 165
Damp-phlegm, 628
Dampness (fluid stagnation). *See* Stagnation, of fluids
Dead

about, 227
future (immediate) disharmony, 617
middle position (left), 432
Death indicators
   Choppy, 365
   Dead, 618
   Empty, 247
   Rough Vibration, 373
   Scattered, 257
Deep. *See also* Hidden
   about, 216, 268-269
   combinations, 270-273
   distal position (right), 422
   future (immediate) disharmony, 613
   Hidden compared, 282, 491
   illustrated, 269f
   middle position (right), 436, 437
   positions, 273-281
   proximal position (left), 443
   proximal position (left and right), 443
   proximal position (right), 445
   and Rapid, 272
   and Slow, 271
   and very Tight or Wiry, 274
   withdrawal and, 582
   yin and yang in contact, 490
Deep and/or Feeble-Absent, 631
Deep Choppy, 273
Deep Diffuse, 270
Deep Feeble
   bilaterally at same position, 274, 276
   Exertion, Increase in Rate, 278
   left side, 277
   middle position (left), 279
   middle position (right/left), 279
   proximal position (right), 277, 281
   and Slow, 280
Deep Feeble-Absent, 270, 275
Deep Flat
   about, 271
   bilaterally at same position, 273
   middle position, 275
   proximal position, 276
   and slightly Rapid or Slow, 278
Deep Reduced Substance, 270, 490
Deep Separating, 490
Deep Slippery
   about, 271
   bilaterally at same position, 274
   distal position (right), 278
   middle position, 275
   middle position (left), 279
   middle position (right), 279
   proximal position, 276
Deep Slippery Feeble, 280
   and Slow, 281
Deep Slippery Tense, 280
Deep Slippery Tight and Rapid, 281

Deep Tense to Tight with Normal rate, 279
Deep Thin
   about, 272
   middle position, 276
   proximal position, 276
Deep Thin Feeble-Absent and very Slow, 397
Deep Thin Feeble with Normal rate, slightly Rapid or Slow, left distal position, 398
Deep Thin Tight
   bilaterally at same position, 274
   and Rapid, 279
   Rapid (very), 278
   rate >100 beats/minute, left distal position, 398
   to Wiry Hollow, 279
Deep Tight
   about, 270
   middle position, 275
   proximal position (left), 280
Deep Tight-Wiry and very Rapid, 275
Deep Wide, 273
Deep Wiry
   about, 271
   middle position, 276
   middle position (left) and proximal (left), 432
   proximal position, 276
Denial, 582-583, 601
Depression
   described, 550-551
   agitated, 553
   anaclytic (primary), 553
   anaclytic (secondary), 556
   cyclothymic, 553
   dysphoric, 554-557
   endogeneous, 43, 551-552
   foundational, 43
   hysterical, 553-554
   Kidney energy and, 43, 550-552
   narcissistic, 556
   reactive, 553-554
Depression (qualities)
   Cotton, 556-557
   Empty, 251
   Feeble-Absent, 443, 614
   Flat, 211, 554
   Inflated bilaterally at distal positions, 555
   Intensity, Change in over entire pulse, occasional, 609
   Muffled, 610
   Muffled at left distal, Empty at left middle position, 556
   Muffled at left distal or over entire pulse, 555
   Muffled at left distal position, 613
   Slippery and Slow, 320-321
Depth. *See also* The three depths; The eight depths
   defined, 6d
   in diagnosis, 62-63
   the eight depths, 68-70, 69f, 459, 459f
   flowchart, 286f
   in interpretation, 635

in Normal pulse, 91, 92f
Submerged
    about, 268
    Deep, 268-281, 269f
    Deep and Rapid, 272
    Deep and Slow, 271
    Deep and very Tight or Wiry, 274
    Deep Choppy, 273
    Deep Diffuse, 270
    Deep Feeble, 274, 276, 277, 278, 279
    Deep Feeble-Absent, 270, 275
    Deep Feeble and Slow, 280
    Deep Flat, 271, 273, 275, 276
    Deep Flat and slightly Rapid or Slow, 278
    Deep Reduced Substance, 270
    Deep Slippery, 271, 274, 275, 276, 278, 279
    Deep Slippery Feeble, 280
    Deep Slippery Tense, 280
    Deep Tense to Tight with Normal rate, 279
    Deep Thin, 272, 276
    Deep Thin Tight, 274
    Deep Thin Tight and Rapid, 279
    Deep Thin Tight and very Rapid, 278
    Deep Thin Tight to Wiry Hollow, 279
    Deep Tight, 270, 275, 280
    Deep Tight-Wiry and very Rapid, 275
    Deep Wide, 273
    Deep Wiry, 271, 276
    Firm, 281, 282f
    Hidden, 282-285, 283f
Superficial
    about, 235-236
    Cotton, 236-239, 236f
    Empty, 245-252, 248-249f
    Floating, 239-245, 240f
    Hollow, 259-268
    Leather, 255, 255f
    Minute, 258, 258f
    Scattered, 256, 257f
    Yielding Empty Thread-like, 253-254, 254f
Despair (emotional), 553. *See also* Emotions/emotional life
Diabetes
    Deep Wiry, 271, 276, 432
    Hollow Full-Overflowing, 291, 512
    Hollow Full-Overflowing Tight or Wiry, 188
    Robust (left side) uniformly, 505
    Slippery at qi depth over entire pulse, 607
    Tense and very Tense Hollow Full-Overflowing, 263
    Tense Hollow Full-Overflowing, 433
    Tense Tight (very), or Wiry Full-Overflowing Hollow and Rapid, 615
    Thin-Tight, 605
    Tight, 342, 343, 604
    Tight and very Tight Hollow Full-Overflowing, 264, 265
    Tight and very Tight-Wiry Hollow Full-Overflowing, 267
    Tight Hollow Full-Overflowing, 348
    Tight Hollow Full-Overflowing (very), 530, 531
    Tight (including Wiry), 520
    Tight Thin, 347
    Tight to Wiry Hollow Full-Overflowing, 184
    Wiry, 350, 354, 355, 357, 359, 430, 608
    Wiry Deep, 351
Diaphragm position
    about, 450
    in interpretation, 638
    left, 74-75
    right, 80
    taking the pulse, 74-75, 80
    uniform quality, 532
Diffuse
    about, 209, 293-294
    illustrated, 209f
    middle position (left), 431
'Digestive system'
    circulatory system and, 504
    defined, 733d
    imbalance, rate variation, 170
    in interpretation, 639
    'nervous system' and, 504, 586-587
    'organ system' and, 171, 504-505
    physiology, 506-507
    rate variation, 170
    Robust (uniformly), 507
Diminished
    at blood depth, 205, 207f
    at qi depth, 204, 204f
Diminished Feeble or Absent at qi depth, 476
Disharmony
    acute illness as, 45-47, 633, 640
    chronic illness as, 633
        Feeble-Absent, 220
        interpretation in, 45, 47, 640
        Rapid pulse and, 160
        stagnation and, 49
        Tight, 341
    consistency and seriousness related, 48
    etiology of, 461-463
    and imbalance, left-right, 584-585
    Kidney-Heart, 587-588
    Liver wind, 244
    psychological, 545-547
    qualities (common), 48-50
Distal Liver Engorgement position, 74f
Distal position
    in interpretation, 638
    psychological disharmony, 591
    pulse methodology, 64
Distal position (uniform bilaterally)
    about, 510
    Cotton, 511
    Empty, 527-528
    Feeble-Absent Deep, 525
    Flat, 515
    Floating, 510
    Floating Tense

with Normal or slightly Rapid rate, 510
and Slow, 510
Floating Yielding
and Rapid, 510
and Slow, 510
Flooding Excess, 512
Hollow, 529-530
Hollow Full-Overflowing, 511
Inflated, 512-513
Slippery, 521-522
Tense, 516-517
Thin, 523-524
Tight (including Wiry), 518-519
Vibration, 531
Doughy
about, 375-376
distal position (left), 401
future (semi-distant) disharmony, 606
Neuro-psychological position, 401, 606
Drug abuse
Empty, 247, 252, 431, 529
Empty at left middle position, 605
Feeble-Absent, 614
Heart yang deficiency, 416
Muffled, 401
Muffled at Neuro-psychological position, 610
psychological disharmony, 583-584
'qi wild' condition, 131
qualities (common), 45
Robust Pounding, 474-475
Robust Pounding Tight and slightly Inflated with Rapid rate, 398
Taut, 330
Tense, 333
Tight, 341
Tight (including Wiry), 519
Very Tense Inflated, 398
Wiry, 353, 357, 421
Drum-like quality. *See* Leather
Duodenum position, 82, 439
Dysmenorrhea
Occasional Change in Intensity over entire pulse, 609

――― E

Eating disorders (anorexia)
Deep Feeble-Absent, 275, 526
Empty, 251, 529
Thin Feeble Interrupted and Slow, 404
Yielding Hollow Full-Overflowing, 266
Eating disorders (bulimia)
Deep Feeble-Absent, 275, 526
Empty, 251, 529
Qi stagnation, 438
Yielding Hollow Full-Overflowing, 266

Eating disorders (qualities)
Deep, 437
Deep Feeble-Absent
anorexia, 275, 526
bulimia, 275, 526
Empty, 437, 529
anorexia, 251, 529
bulimia, 251, 529
Feeble-Absent, 437
Thin Feeble Interrupted and Slow from anorexia, 404
Thin Yielding, 488
Yielding Hollow Full-Overflowing, 266
anorexia, 266
bulimia, 266
Eating habits
nervous system and digestive system, 586-587
obscuring interpretation, 45
Eating habits (dieting), 529
Eating habits (irregular)
Cotton, 239
Feeble-Absent, 425
nervous system and digestive system, 586-587
Reduced (right side) uniformly, 508
Tense-Tight, 436
Tight, 425
Eating habits (overindulgence)
Tense Ropy, 360
Eating habits (qualities)
Cotton
irregular habits, 239
rumination, 511
Deep, eating after work, 437
Deep Flat from rumination, 275
Empty
from dieting, 529
rumination, 251, 528
work too soon after eating, 437
Feeble-Absent
irregular habits, 425
work too soon after eating, 222, 437
Feeble-Absent Deep from rumination, 526
Hesitant from rumination, 126-127
Reduced (right side) uniformly
irregular habits, 508
Robust (right side) uniformly, eating too quickly, 507
Tense Ropy from overindulgence, 360
Tense-Tight
irregular habits, 436
work too soon after eating, 436
Tight
eating too quickly, 344
irregular habits, 425
Tight only at qi depth, eating too quickly, 347
Wiry, eating too quickly, 354, 356, 358
Yielding Inflated from rumination, 514
Eating habits (rumination)
Cotton, 511

Deep Flat, 275
Empty, 251, 528
Feeble-Absent Deep, 526
Hesitant Wave, 126-127
Qi stagnation, 438
Yielding Inflated, 514
Eating habits (too quickly)
    Deep, 437
    Empty, 437
    Feeble-Absent, 222, 437
    nervous system and digestive system, 586-587
    Robust (right side) uniformly, 507
    Tense-Tight, 436
    Tight, 344
    Tight only at qi depth, 347
    Wiry, 354, 356, 358
The eight depths, 68-70, 69f, 459, 459f
The eight pulses, 414-415
Emotions/emotional life. *See also* Psychological disorders; Stress; Trauma, emotional
    anger
        described, 577-578
        Feeble-Absent (left distal) and left middle very Tense Inflated, 404
        Heart Full, 414
        Hollow Full-Overflowing, 404
        Inflated, 451, 475
        Inflated at Diaphragm position, 578
        Inflated Yielding, 194
        Slow, 604
        Taut, 331
        Tense, 332, 337
        Tense Hollow, 263, 265, 267
        Tense Inflated, 334, 431
        Tense Inflated, moderately, 513
    anguish, 549
    anxiety
        arrhythmic qualities, 562
        described, 557-558
        Empty, 246-247
        Exertion, Increase in Rate, 561
        Feeble-Absent at left distal position, 561
        Heart blood deficiency, 560-562
        Heart-Gallbladder deficiency, 562
        Heart qi agitation, 558-559
        Heart qi deficiency, 560-562
        Heart yin deficiency, 560
        heat from excess in Heart, 559
        Hollow Full-Overflowing Robust Pounding Bounding and Rapid, 188
        Intensity, Change in (constant) over entire pulse, 561
        Liver qi stagnation, 407
        Mitral Valve position, 402
        panic vs., 558
        Pericardium Tight or left distal Tense with Robust Pounding, 559-600
        Pounding, 559
        Qualities and Intensity, Change in at left distal position, 562
        Rapid, 559
        Rate at Rest, Change in, occasional, 559
        Slippery at Mitral Valve position, 612
        Slow, 561
        Smooth Vibration, 400, 558, 611
        Thin, distal position (left), 561
        Thin over entire pulse, 561
        Tight at left distal position, 559
        Vibration and Slippery at Mitral Valve positions, 562
        Wiry, 353
        Yielding Hollow Full-Overflowing, 561
        Yielding Hollow Full-Overflowing and Rapid, 616
denial, 582-583, 601
depression
    agitated, 553
    anaclytic (secondary), 556
    Cotton, 556-557
    cyclothymic, 553
    described, 550-551
    dysphoric, 554-557
    Empty, 251
    endogeneous, 43, 551-552
    Feeble-Absent, 443, 614
    Flat, 211, 554
    foundational, 43
    hysterical, 553-554
    Inflated bilaterally at distal positions, 555
    Intensity, Change in over entire pulse, occasional, 609
    Kidney energy and, 43, 550-552
    Muffled, 610
    Muffled (left distal), 613
    Muffled (left distal), Empty at left middle position, 556
    Muffled (left distal or over entire pulse), 555
    narcissistic, 556
    primary anaclytic, 553
    reactive, 553-554
    Slippery and Slow, 320-321
despair, 553
explosiveness, 579
fear
    Bean (Spinning), 375, 399, 475
    consistent Rough Vibration over entire pulse at all depths, 565
    Deep Thin Feeble with Normal or slightly Rapid rate, 278
    guilt and, 565-566
    guilt and terror, 565-566
    Heart blood stagnation and, 565
    Kidney qi deficiency, 440
    Rate at Rest, Change in (occasional), 610
    Rough Vibration at Neuro-psychological position, 613
    Rough Vibration over entire pulse, 613
    types of, 564
    Vibration, 369-370
grief
    Cotton, 239

described, 549-550
Empty, 251, 428, 528
Empty Moderately Tense, 250
Heart Full, 414
Yielding Inflated, 421, 512
guilt
   about, 564
   terror and fear, 565-566
   Tight and Rapid, 339
   Vibration, 369-370
horror, 567
indecision, 580
intra-individual failure, 556
irritability
   Occasional Change in Intensity over entire pulse, 609
   Tight, 343
   Tight and Rapid, 339
loneliness, 556
love rejected, 554-555
melancholia, 550
nervous tension
   Tense, 336
   Tense and Rapid, 333
   Tight, 338, 342
   Tight (including Wiry), 519
   Wiry, 350
panic
   anxiety vs., 558
   Slippery at Mitral Valve position, 612
phobia, 558
pulse qualities of, 592-594t
rage, 451, 579
reflection, 580-582
relationships
   husband-wife imbalance, 139, 501-502, 584-585
   Inflated at Diaphragm position, 578-579
   Intestine position, 451
repressed
   Flat, 421, 603
   Heart qi deficiency, 415
   Qi stagnation, 473
   Taut, 430, 473
   Tense, 430
   Tense Long, 474
   Thin, 430
   Tight, 430
   Wiry, 357, 430
resentment
   Taut, 331
   Tense, 332
resignation
   Cotton, 237-238, 580
   Intensity, Change in, between sides, 585
roller-coaster feeling
   described, 567-568
   Occasional Change in Rate at Rest, 610
sadness
   Cotton, 237-238, 239, 404
   Feeble-Absent, 443
spite, Heart closed, 568
stress
   qi stagnation, 438
   Taut, 473
   Tense, 335, 517
   Tight, 338
   Tight and Rapid, 339
   Tight (including Wiry), 519
   Wiry, 353, 354, 358
suppressed
   Cotton, 470-471
   Yielding Hollow Full-Overflowing with rate >100 beats/minute, 398
tension
   Intensity, Change in over entire pulse, inconstant, 573
   Liver qi stagnation and, 573-574
   Taut or Tense at left middle position, 573
   Tense to Tight over entire pulse, 574
   Tight Thin, 346
   Wiry, 355
terror
   Bean (Spinning), 567
   guilt and fear, 565-566
   'qi wild' qualities, 567
   Rough Vibration at Neuro-psychological position, 567, 613
   without guilt, 567
vengefulness
   Flat, 605
   Heart closed, 568
withdrawal, 582
worry
   about, 563
   Cotton, 238
   Heart Tight, 410
   Heart Vibration, 409
   Occasional Change in Rate at Rest, 564
   Smooth Vibration, 371-373, 564, 611
   Tight, 338
   Tightness at Pericardium position and Tense at left distal, 564
   Vibration, 366, 368, 563
Emphysema
   Inflated, 199, 607
   right distal and Special Lung, 424
   Tense Inflated, 421
   Tense Inflated, moderately, 513
   Tense-Tight Inflated at Special Lung, 429
Empty
   about, 245-247
   Change in Intensity and Qualities, 423
   combinations, 249-250
   distal position (left), 397
   distal position (uniform bilaterally), 527-528
   early stage, illustrated, 248f
   Floating vs., 240

future (immediate) disharmony, 615
future (semi-distant) disharmony, 605
Hollow vs., 260
illustrated, 248-249f
at individual positions, 615
later stage, illustrated, 249f
middle position, 250
middle position (left), 431, 605
middle position (right), 436, 437
middle position (uniform bilaterally), 528-529
middle stage, illustrated, 248f
over entire pulse, 615
paradoxical qualities, 631
positions, 250-252
proximal position, 250
proximal position (left), 443
proximal position (uniform bilaterally), 529
'qi wild' condition, 132, 135, 216, 246, 492
Special Lung, 428
uniform qualities, 527-529
yin and yang separation, 491
Empty Intermittent-Intermittent, 493
Empty Interrupted, 469
Empty Interrupted-Intermittent, 250
Empty moderately Tense, 249
Empty Thread-like
    future (immediate) disharmony, 615
    'qi wild' condition, 132
    yin and yang separation, 492
Empty Tight and Rapid, 249
Empty Yielding and Slow, 249
Endometriosis/fibroids, 364, 617
Environmental deprivation
    Empty, 247, 250, 251, 492, 528
    'qi wild' condition, 129
    Yielding Hollow Full-Overflowing, 261
Environmental effects, 40
Ephemeral (Transient), 377
Epilepsy, 614
Equilibrium restoration, 49-50
Esophagus position, 80, 80f, 438
Essence, 94. *See also* Kidney qi
Essence deficiency
    Doughy, 629
    Leather, 629
    Tight (including Wiry), 520
    Wiry, 355, 629
Excess above the qi depth, 470-472
Exercise
    circulation (qi) and, 467
    'qi wild' condition and
        excessive in childhood, 129-131
Exercise (aerobic)
    Slow pulse, 163, 168-169
Exercise (excessive)
    age effects in interpretation, 40-41
    Heart qi deficiency, 415
    Hollow Full-Overflowing Reduced Pounding, 188
    Reduced Pounding, 208
    Ropy Yielding Hollow, 361
    Thin Deep Feeble and Slow, 299
    Yielding Hollow Ropy, 262
    Yielding Ropy, 294, 484
Exercise (excessive in childhood)
    Empty, 247
    'qi wild' condition, 129-130
    Yielding Hollow Full-Overflowing, 261
Exercise (lifting)
    Deep and very Tight or Wiry, 274
    Diaphragm position, 532
    Flat, 212, 214, 215, 422, 515, 516
    Heart Full, 414
    Hollow, 530
    Inflated, 194, 451
    obscuring interpretation, 45
    'qi wild' condition, 131
    rate variation, 170
    Robust Pounding, Tight, and slightly Inflated, 403
    Tense, 335, 517
    Tense Inflated, 513, 514
    Tight, 342
    Vibration, 422
    Wiry, 353
    Yielding Hollow Full-Overflowing, 264
Exercise (qualities)
    Deep and very Tight or Wiry from lifting, 274
    Empty, excessive in childhood, 247
    Flat from lifting, 212, 214, 215, 422, 515, 516
    Heart Full from lifting, 414
    Heart qi deficiency, 415
    Hollow from lifting, 530
    Hollow Full-Overflowing Reduced Pounding from excessive, 188
    Inflated
        lifting, 194, 451
    Rapid pulse from sudden cessation, 161-162
    Reduced Pounding from excessive, 208
    Robust Pounding, Tight, and slightly Inflated from lifting (excessive), 403
    Ropy Yielding Hollow from excessive, 361
    Slow pulse from aerobic, 163, 168-169
    Tense
        lifting, 335, 517
    Tense Inflated
        lifting, 513, 514
    Thin Deep Feeble and Slow from excessive, 299
    Tight
        lifting, 342
    Vibration from lifting, 422
    Wiry
        lifting, 353
    Yielding Hollow Full-Overflowing
        excessive in childhood, 261
        lifting, 264
        sudden cessation of intense, 261
    Yielding Hollow Full-Overflowing and Rapid

sudden cessation of intense, 133, 616
Yielding Hollow Full-Overflowing Reduced Pounding sudden cessation of intense, 187
Yielding Hollow Ropy from excessive, 262
Yielding Ropy from excessive, 294, 484
Exercise (sudden cessation of intense)
   circulation (qi) and, 467
   'qi wild' condition, 130-131
   Rapid, 161-162
   Yielding Hollow Full-Overflowing, 261
   Yielding Hollow Full-Overflowing and Rapid, 133, 616
   Yielding Hollow Full-Overflowing Reduced Pounding, 187
Exertion rate. *See* Rate on Exertion
Exertion, Increase in Rate
   anxiety, 561
   constant, 125
   Deep Feeble, 278
   Feeble, 395
   future (immediate) disharmony, 616
   future (semi-distant) disharmony, 609
   Heart blood deficiency, 408-409, 408-409, 561
   Heart Weak, 408-409, 408-409, 561
   occasional, 125
   paradoxical qualities, 632
   Thin, 300
Explosiveness, 579
Exuberant blood. *See* Blood Thick

F

Failure, 556. *See also* Depression
Fast, 634
Fear
   about, 564-565
   Bean (Spinning), 375, 399, 475
   Deep Thin Feeble with Normal or slightly Rapid rate, 278
   guilt and, 565-566
   guilt and terror, 565-566
   Heart blood stagnation and, 565
   Kidney qi deficiency, 440
   Rough Vibration at Neuro-psychological position, 613
   Rough Vibration consistent over entire pulse at all depths, 565
   Rough Vibration over entire pulse, 613
   types of, 564-565
   Vibration, 369-370
Feeble. *See also* Absent
   described, 202
   Absent vs., 218
   early stage, 216f
   Exertion, Increase in Rate, left distal position, 395
   illustrated, 217f
Feeble-Absent
   about, 216-218, 220, 491
   classification/nomenclature, 218
   combinations, 221
   depth in, 218-219
   distal position (left)
      anxiety, 561
      Normal in remainder, 406
      qualities (common), 395
      remainder Slippery at blood depth, 407
      Tense (left middle), 407
      Tight (left proximal), 406, 588
   distal position (right), 422
   distal and middle positions (left), and Hollow Full-Overflowing, 404
   distal and middle positions (right), 425
   distal and middle positions (left), and left middle very Tense Inflated, 404
   distal and proximal position (right), 426
   distal and proximal positions (left)
      combinations, 405-406
      Normal at left middle with a Slow or Rapid rate, 588
      Tense Inflated at left middle position, 588
   distal (right) and proximal position (left), 426
   future (immediate) disharmony, 613-614
   interpretation, 219-220
   middle position (right), 436, 437
   over entire pulse, 613-614
   positions, 219, 221-225
   proximal position (left), 443
   proximal position (left and right), 443
   proximal position (right), 445
   proximal position (right) and right middle and distal, 446
   sensation, 219
   uniform qualities, 524-527
   yin and yang in contact, 490
Feeble-Absent Deep
   distal position (uniform bilaterally), 525
   middle position (uniform bilaterally), 525-526
   proximal position (uniform bilaterally), 526-527
   and Slow or Rapid, 221
Feeble-Absent Deep Choppy, 221
Feeble-Absent Deep Slippery, 221
Feng shui, 47-48
Fibromyalgia, 604
Fine. *See* Thin
Firm, 281-282, 282f
Five-element (phase) system, 20-21, 22
Flat
   combinations, 212-213
   distal position (left), 396, 605-606
   distal position (right), 421, 603, 606
   distal position (uniform bilaterally), 514-515
   future (distant) disharmony, 603
   future (semi-distant) disharmony, 605-606
   illustrated, 211f
   Inflated vs., 212
   middle position (right), 436
   middle position (uniform bilaterally), 515
   positions, 213-215
   proximal position (uniform bilaterally), 516, 603

qi stagnation, 487
Flat Tense, 213
Flat Tight and Rapid, 213
Floating
    about, 239-243
    above the qi depth, 471
    combinations, 244
    Cotton vs., 242
    differentiating types of, 240-242
    disharmony (external), 242-244
    distal position (right), 420
    distal position (uniform bilaterally), 510-511
    Empty vs., 240
    Flooding Excess vs., 242
    Hollow Full-Overflowing vs., 242
    illustrated, 240f
    Inflated vs., 242
    Liver wind, 244
    middle position (uniform bilaterally), 511
    positions, 244-245
    proximal position (uniform bilaterally), 511
    Special Lung position, 427
    Weak-Floating vs., 241
Floating Slippery, 472
Floating Tense
    with Normal or slightly Rapid rate, 244-245
        distal position, bilaterally, 510
    and Slow, 244
        distal position, bilaterally, 510
        distal position (right) and right middle position, 425
        future (immediate) disharmony, 611
    and Slow, slightly, 243, 472
Floating Tight
    above the qi depth, 472
    future (immediate) disharmony, 611
    Liver wind, 244
    middle position (left), 432
Floating Yielding
    with Normal rate, 243
    and Rapid, 245
        distal position, bilaterally, 510
        distal position (right) and right middle position, 425
        future (immediate) disharmony, 611
        slightly, 243, 471
    and Slow, distal position (bilaterally), 510
Flooding Deficient
    at blood depth, 205, 208
    illustrated, 68f, 207f
    in interpretation, 637
    qi depth, 477
Flooding Deficient Diffuse and Reduced Substance, 605
Flooding Excess
    about, 190-193, 291-292
    above the qi depth, 472
    in complementary positions, 393
    distal position (uniform bilaterally), 512
    Floating vs., 242
    future (immediate) disharmony, 613
    heat from excess, 488
    Hollow Full-Overflowing vs., 190-191
    illustrated, 191f
    in interpretation, 637
    middle position (uniform bilaterally), 512
    positions, 192-193
    proximal position (left), 443
    proximal position (right), 445
    proximal position (uniform bilaterally), 512
    and Robust Pounding, middle position (left), 432
    uniform quality, 512
    wave form, 68f
Fluid qualities
    Liver-Gallbladder damp-heat, 319
    Slippery, 313-315, 314f, 317, 322
        at Esophagus position, 324
        at Mitral Valve position, 321
        moderately to severely, 323
        only at organ depth, 325
        and Rapid, 318
        and Slow, 318, 319, 320, 324
        and very Rapid with high fever, 321
        and very Tight Hollow Full-Overflowing, 320, 321
    Slippery Deep Feeble, 325-325
        and Slow, 325
    Slippery Deep Tight to Wiry and Rapid, 325
    Slippery Deep (very) and very Rapid, 321
    Slippery Empty, 322
    Slippery Feeble, 322
        with Normal rate, 321
        and Slow, 315, 320, 322, 324
    Slippery Flooding Excess Tense and possibly Rapid, 325
    Slippery Inflated, 324
    Slippery Tense, 323, 325
        at all depths, 320
        mildly, with Normal to slightly Rapid rate, 323
        and Normal rate, 319
        and Normal to slightly Rapid rate, 320
        at qi depth with Normal or slightly Rapid Rate, 320
        and Rapid, 318
        and Rapid (slightly), 322
        and Rapid (slightly to very), 321
        and Rapid (very), 320
        and Slow, 318-319, 324
    Slippery Tight
        and Rapid, 322
        and Rapid (slightly), 318, 324
        and Slow, 323
    Slippery Tight Flooding Excess and Rapid, 322, 325
    Slippery Tight (Hollow) at Stomach-Pylorus Extension, 324
    Slippery Tight Hollow Full-Overflowing and Rapid, 315
    Slippery Tight-Wiry and Choppy or Muffled, 323
    Slippery Tight-Wiry and Slow, 322
    Slippery Transient above the qi depth, 318
    Slippery Yielding (mildly) and Slow, 323
    Tense Slippery with Normal or slightly Rapid Rate, 316
    Transiently Slippery, 316

Yielding Slippery and Slow, 316
Fluid stagnation, Slippery, 475
Food stagnation
    Choppy, 365
    at organ depth, 487
    psychosis and, 570
    qualities (common), 629
    Slippery, 522
    Slippery at Esophagus position, 324
    Slippery Inflated, 324
    Taut, 330
    Tense, 335, 517
    Wiry, 358
Force, Robust or Reduced, 377
Foundation in interpretation, 42-43
Frail. *See* Feeble; Feeble-Absent
Frustration. *See* Stress
Full-Overflowing, 68f
Function, defined, 6d
Future (distant) disharmony
    Arrhythmia, 604
    Cotton, 602
    Flat, 603
    Rapid, 604
    Rate at Rest, Constantly Changing, 604
    Slow, 604
    Taut, 603-604
    Tight, 604
    Yielding Inflated, 603
    Yielding or Diminished at qi depth, 603
Future (immediate) disharmony
    Bean (Spinning), 617
    Choppy, 611
        Gallbladder position, 617
        left distal position, 617
        middle position (left), 617
        Pelvis/Lower Body positions, 617
    Dead, 617
    Deep, 613
    Empty, 615
    Empty Thread-like, 615
    Exertion, Increase in Rate, 616
    Feeble-Absent, 613-614
    Floating Tense and Slow, 611
    Floating Tight, 611
    Floating Yielding and Rapid, 611
    Flooding Excess, 613
    Hesitant, 610
    Hollow Yielding Full-Overflowing and Slow, 615
    Inflated, 611, 614
    Intermittent or Interrupted Yielding Hollow, 618
    Interrupted or Intermittent, 617
    Leather, 615
    Leather-like Hollow, 615
    Minute, 615
    Muffled, 610, 612, 613
    Qualities, Change in, 616
    Rate at Rest, Change, 610
    Rate at Rest, occasional Change in, 610
    Rough Vibration, 613
    Scattered, 615
    Slippery, 612, 614
    Slippery Tight at Gallbladder position, 612
    Smooth Vibration, 611
        Neuro-psychological position, 611
    Tense Hollow Full-Overflowing, Large Vessel positions, 616
    Tense Ropy, 616
    Tense Tight (very), or Wiry Full-Overflowing Hollow and Rapid, 615-616
    Unstable, 617
    Wiry, 612
    Yielding Hollow Full-Overflowing and Rapid, 616
Future (semi-distant) disharmony
    Arrhythmia: Interrupted or Intermittent, 607
    Blood Heat, 606
    Blood Thick, 606
    Blood Unclear, 606
    Choppy at Neuro-psychological position, 609
    Doughy, 606
    Empty, left middle position, 605
    Exertion, Increase in Rate, 609
    Flat, 605-606
    Flooding Deficient Diffuse and Reduced Substance, 605
    Inflated, 607
    Intensity, Change, 609
    Intensity, Constant Change, 609
    Intensity, Change over entire pulse, occasional, 609
    Muffled at Neuro-psychological position, 610
    Rhythm, 609
    Rough Vibration at blood depth, 607
    Slippery, 607
    Smooth Vibration at Mitral Valve position, 607
    Spreading, 604-605
    Tense, 608
    Tense Hollow Full-Overflowing, 607
    Tense Slippery at Gallbladder position, 608
    Thin-Tight, 605
    Thin Yielding, 605
    Wiry, 608
    Yielding Ropy, 608-609

G

Gallbladder-Heart deficiency, 434
Gallbladder infection/inflammation
    Choppy, 365
    Inflated, 433
    Slippery, 430
    Tight, 342
    Wiry, 358
Gallbladder position
    about, 76
    Choppy, 433

future (immediate) disharmony, 612
illustrated, 76f
Inflated, 433
Muffled, 433, 612
taking the pulse, 76
Tight Slippery, 433
Wiry, 433
Gallstones
    Choppy, 433
    Intensity, Change in, 433
    Muffled, 433
    Rough Vibration, 373
    Slippery Tight-Wiry, 323
    Tight Empty at qi depth, 347
    Wiry, 433
Ganglion, 378
Gastritis/ulcers. *See* Ulcers/gastritis
Gate of vitality *(ming men)*, 449
Gender effects
    in interpretation, 41, 65, 626
    Normal pulse, 95
    paradoxical qualities, 632
Grave's disease
    described, 557
    Flooding Excess, 292
    Heart tight, 410
    Robust Pounding Tight and slightly Inflated with Rapid rate, 398
    Tight, 341
    Wiry, 356
Grief
    described, 549-550
    Cotton, 239
    Empty, 251, 428, 528
    Empty moderately Tense, 250
    Heart Full, 414
    Yielding Inflated, 421, 512
Guilt
    about, 564
    fear and, 565-566
    Tight and Rapid, 339
    Vibration, 369-370
Gynecological disorders
    amenorrhea
        Choppy, 365
    dysmenorrhea
        Occasional Change in Intensity over entire pulse, 609
    endometriosis/fibroids
        Choppy at Pelvis/Lower Body positions, 364, 617
    hemorrhage
        Thin Yielding, 488
    menorrhagia
        Empty, 252
        Feeble-Absent, 220, 223
        Feeble-Absent Deep, 527
        'qi wild' condition, 130
        Thin Yielding, 488
        Tight Thin, 340

Yielding Hollow Full-Overflowing, 261, 267
menstrual irregularities
    Choppy, 611
    Constant Change in Intensity, 609
    Feeble-Absent, 614
    Thin-Tight, 605
pelvic inflammatory disease
    Deep Slippery Feeble and Slow, 281
    Flooding Excess, 292, 443
    left proximal position, 444
    Robust Pounding, 443
    Slippery, 443
    Slippery Deep Tight to Wiry and Rapid, 325
    Slippery Flooding Excess Tense, 325
    Slippery Tight Flooding Excess and Rapid, 325
    Tense, 336, 337
    Tight, 446
    Tight Flooding Excess, 340
    Tight Robust Pounding and Rapid, 348
    Tight-Wiry, 443
    Wiry, 355, 359
PMS
    Intensity, Change in, Constant, 609
'qi wild' condition, 130
uterine bleeding, chronic
    Yielding Hollow Full-Overflowing, 530
    Yielding Hollow Full-Overflowing and Slow, 530

——— H

Habits, rate variation, 170
Hard
    in acute and chronic illness, 35
    in interpretation, 67
    pliable qualities related, 35
Hard Thin qualities, 297-298
Hashimoto's disease, Wiry, 356
Headache
    Blood Unclear, 606
    Choppy, 365, 401, 611
    Choppy at Neuro-psychological position, 609
    Doughy, 376
    Tight, 341
    Tight (including Wiry), 518
    Wiry, 353
Heart
    circulation, 137, 418-419
    'nervous system' and, 417
    Rapid, 156
Heart and Kidney qi deficiency, 407
Heart and Liver disharmony, 183
Heart attack, Hesitant, 610
Heart blood deficiency. *See also* Heart Weak
    about, 412, 560
    depression, 555
    Exertion, Increase in Rate, 408-409, 561

with Heart and Lung phlegm, 524
    sleep patterns affected, 589
    Thin, 524, 555
    Thin over entire pulse, 561
Heart blood stagnation. *See also* Blood stagnation; Heart Small
    about, 413
    Deep Thin Feeble with Normal or slightly Rapid rate, 278
    depression and, 556
    fear and, 565
    Interrupted, constantly, 122
    Rapid, 156
    Thin Feeble and Normal or slightly Rapid, 300
    Wiry, 356
Heart Closed, 278, 412, 733d
Heart disease/conditions. *See also* Trapped qi in the Heart
    arrhythmia, 604, 607
    defined, 734d
    Heart blood deficiency, 412
    Heart blood stagnation, 413
    Heart qi agitation, 409-412
    Heart qi deficiency, 414-415
    Heart qi stagnation, 412-413
    Heart qi-yang deficiency, 417
    Heart yang deficiency, 416
    Heart yin deficiency, 417-418
    myocarditis, 399
    'nervous system' and, 417-418
    rhythm, 609
    Robust Pounding, Tight, and slightly Inflated, 403
    Slippery, 399
    Unstable, 398
    Yielding Hollow Intermittent, 121
Heart Enlarged position
    distal position (left), 403
    illustrated, 74f
    taking the pulse, 74
Heart fire, 589
Heart Full
    about, 414
    anger qualities in, 577-578
    Deep Thin Tight, 278
    defined, 734d
    Thin Deep Tight and very Rapid, 300, 345
Heart-Gallbladder qi deficiency, 404, 562
Heart heat from excess, 589
Heart Large, 278, 414-415, 735d
Heart Nervous, 120, 411-412, 735d
Heart qi agitation
    about, 409
    anxiety and, 558-559
    Heart Nervous, 411-412
    Heart Tight, 410
    heat from excess, 116
    heat from yin deficiency, 116
    Hesitant Wave, 410-411
    Inconsistently Intermittent, 120
    Rapid, 156

    severe, 411-412
    sleep patterns affected, 589
    Smooth Vibration, 564
    Tight (left distal) and Rapid, 408
    Vibration at Neuro-psychological positions, 411
    worry and, 564
Heart qi and yang deficiency, 163, 169
Heart qi deficiency
    anxiety and, 560-562
    Arrhythmic qualities, 562
    depression and, 555
    Feeble-Absent (left distal), 407, 561
    Heart Large, 414-415
    Intensity, Change in, constant over entire pulse, 561
    Intermittent, constantly, 119
    Qualities and Intensity at left distal position, Change in, 562
    Rate at Rest, Constant Change, 117-119
    rate variation, 170
    Rough Vibration vs., 566
    Slippery, 315
    Slow, 561
    Thin, 523
    Transiently Slippery, 317
    Vibration and Slippery at Mitral Valve positions, 562
    Yielding Hollow Full-Overflowing, 561
Heart qi stagnation. *See also* Qi stagnation
    Flat, 605-606
    Heart Closed, 412-413
    Rapid, 156
Heart qi-yang deficiency
    about, 417
    Constantly Intermittent, 120
    Interrupted, constantly, 121
    Yielding Hollow Intermittent, 121
Heart Small. *See also* Heart blood stagnation
    about, 413
    childbirth and, 417
    Deep Flat, 278
    Deep Thin Feeble with Normal or slightly Rapid rate, 278
    defined, 736d
    depression, 556
    fear and, 565
    Interrupted, constantly, 122-123
    Thin Feeble and Normal or slightly Rapid, 300
    Tight Deep Thin Feeble and slightly Rapid, 345
Heart Tight
    about, 410
    defined, 737d
    Heart qi agitation, 410
Heart Vibration, 409, 735d
Heart Weak. *See also* Heart blood deficiency
    about, 412, 560
    defined, 737d
    Exertion, Increase in Rate, 408-409, 561
    Inconsistently Intermittent, 120
    sleep patterns affected, 589
    Thin, 524, 525

Heart yang deficiency, 416
Heart yin deficiency
    'nervous system' and, 417-418
    sleep patterns affected, 589
    Tight at left distal position, 560
Heartbeat. *See* Rhythm
Heat and Toxicity in the Blood, progression of, 478f
Heat from deficiency
    Deep and Rapid, 272
    qualities (common), 629
    Rapid, 159-160
    Tight, 342
    Tight Deep Thin Feeble, 345
    Tight (including Wiry), 520
    Tight to Wiry Hollow Full-Overflowing, 184
Heat from excess
    in the blood, 183-184
    Deep and Rapid, 272
    followed by heat from yin deficiency, 184-185
    in Heart, 559
    Heart qi and, 116
    internal, 164
    at organ depth, 488
    qualities, 629
    Rapid, 156
    Slow, 164, 167
    Tense Hollow Full-Overflowing, 182-183, 183-184
    Wiry, 355
Heat from yin deficiency
    etiology of, 337-338
    Heart qi and, 116
    Tight, 342
    Tight to Wiry Hollow Full-Overflowing, 184
Heat in the blood. *See* Blood heat
Heat in the qi level, 156-157
Heat, invasion of external, 442
Heat pernicious influence (internal), 165
Heatstroke/exhaustion
    circulation and, 468
    Hollow Full-Overflowing Robust Pounding Bounding, 188
    Rapid, 153
    Slow pulse, 165
    Tense, 518
Hemorrhage
    Leather-like Hollow, 141, 160, 262, 264, 266, 267, 268, 292, 432, 484-485, 529, 530, 615
    Rapid, 160
    Thin Yielding, 488
    Very Tense-Tight Hollow Full-Overflowing, 142
    Yielding Partially Hollow and Slow, 142
Hepatitis
    Deep Slippery, 276
    depression, post, 556
    Empty, 247, 252, 431
    Empty at left middle position, 605
    Feeble-Absent, 614
    Flooding Excess, 292, 512

    Flooding Excess and Robust Pounding, 432
    Slippery, 430
    Slippery at organ depth, 614, 618
    Slippery Tense and Normal to slightly Rapid rate, 320
    Slippery Tense and Slow, 319
    Slippery Tense and very Rapid rate, 320
    Slippery Tight and Slow, 323
    Slippery Tight Flooding Excess and Rapid, 322
    Tense, 333
    Tense Slippery, 334
    Tight, 342
    Tight Flooding Excess, 340
    Tight, Flooding Excess, Robust Pounding, Slippery and Rapid, 347
    Wiry, 350, 357
    Wiry Robust Pounding and Rapid, 352
Hernia
    Choppy, 365
    Inflated, 451
Hesitant Wave. *See also* Push pulse
    about, 126-127
    defined, 739d
    Flooding Deficient and, 208
    future (immediate) disharmony, 610
    Heart qi agitation, 410-411
    illustrated, 68f, 126f
    in interpretation, 637
    obsessive thinking, 581
    as push pulse, 410
Hidden, 282-285, 283f, 491. *See also* Deep
Hidden Deficient, 283f, 284, 491
Hidden Excess, 283f, 284, 486
Hidden Left Pulse, 378
Hidden Normal, 285
Hollow
    about, 259-260
    combinations, 264-268
    distal position (uniform bilaterally), 529-530
    Empty vs., 260
    individual positions, 262-264
    middle position (uniform bilaterally), 530
    proximal position (uniform bilaterally), 530-531
    qualities (common), 260-262
    Slippery vs., 260
    uniform qualities, 529-531
    Yielding Inflated vs., 260
Hollow Full-Overflowing
    about, 179-180
    combinations, 187-188
    conditions associated with, 182-186
    distal position (left), 402
    distal position (uniform bilaterally), 511
    Floating vs., 242
    Flooding Excess vs., 190-191
    illustrated, 180f
    in interpretation, 181, 637
    Large Vessel position, 402
    middle position (uniform bilaterally), 511

positions, 189-190
proximal position, 512
Robust qualities
types, 181
uniform quality, 511-512
Hollow Full-Overflowing Leather-Like, and Rapid/Slow, 187
Hollow Full-Overflowing Reduced Pounding, 188
Hollow Full-Overflowing Robust Pounding Bounding and Rapid, 188
Hollow Full-Overflowing Slippery, 187
Hollow Full-Overflowing Slippery and very Rapid, 188
Hollow Full-Overflowing Tense and Slippery at the blood depth, 188
Hollow Full-Overflowing Tight or Wiry, 188
Hollow Full-Overflowing Tight or Wiry and Slippery, 188
Hollow Yielding Full-Overflowing, 615
Hollow Yielding Full-Overflowing and Slow, 615
Horror, 567
Hot flashes, 338
Hunger. *See* Environmental deprivation
Hurried rate with missed beats, 118-119
Husband-wife imbalance, 139, 501-502, 584-585
Hyperacidity
    Deep Slippery, 279
    Slippery Tight and slightly Rapid, 324
    Yielding Hollow Full-Overflowing, 265
Hyperactivity, 339
Hypertension
    Blood Heat, 606
    Blood Thick, 481-482, 606
    Deep Wiry, 271, 276, 432
    fixed (true), 182, 186
    Hollow Full-Overflowing, 291, 402, 404, 511, 512
    Hollow Full-Overflowing Tight or Wiry, 188
    labile (not true), 185-186
    Left distal Feeble-Absent and left middle very Tense Inflated, 404
    Robust (left side) uniformly, 505
    Robust (right side) uniformly, 507
    Slippery Tight Hollow Full-Overflowing and Rapid, 315
    Tense and very Tense Hollow Full-Overflowing, 263
    Tense Hollow Full-Overflowing, 182, 334, 404, 433, 607
    Tense Hollow Full-Overflowing at Large Vessel positions, 616
    Tense Ropy, 293
    Thin-Tight, 605
    Tight, 341, 342, 344, 604
    Tight and very Tight Hollow Full-Overflowing, 264, 265
    Tight and very Tight-Wiry Hollow Full-Overflowing, 267
    Tight Hollow Full-Overflowing, 348
    Tight (including Wiry), 518, 520
    Tight Thin, 346
    Tight to Wiry Hollow Full-Overflowing, 185-186
    Very Tense Tight, or Wiry Full-Overflowing Hollow and Rapid, 615
    Very Tight Hollow Full-Overflowing, 530, 531
    Wiry, 350, 353, 354, 355, 356, 430, 608
    Wiry Deep, 351
    Wiry Robust Pounding and rapid, 352
Hypothermia
    circulation affects Heart, 418, 468
    circulation and, 468
    Deep and Slow, 272
    Hidden Excess, 486
    Intensity, Change in, 137

―― I

Iatrogens. *See* Medications
Inconsistently Intermittent, 119-120
Incontinence
    Deep Feeble, 281
    Slippery Deep Feeble, 325
    Tight Deep, 349
Increase in Rate on Exertion. *See* Exertion, Increase in Rate
Indecision, 580. *See also* Emotions/emotional life
Individual positions. *See* Pulse positions
Infection (abdomen)
    Wiry, 354
Infection (acute)
    Tense, 337
    Tight, 346
    Wiry, 355
Infection (acute, fulminating)
    Flooding Excess, 488
    Tense Slippery, Flooding Excess, Robust Pounding, 334
Infection (bacterial)
    Slippery Flooding Excess Tense, 325
    Slippery Tense, 320
    Tight, 346
Infection (bladder)
    Deep Slippery Feeble and Slow, 281
    Slippery Tight Flooding Excess and Rapid, 325
    Tight, Flooding Excess, Robust Pounding, Slippery and Rapid, 349
Infection (blood)
    Flooding Excess, 613
    Hollow Full-Overflowing Tight or Wiry and Slippery, 188
    Slippery, 315
    Tense Slippery, 334
    Wiry Slippery and very Rapid, 351
Infection (chronic)
    Deep Slippery Feeble, 280
    Flooding Excess, 292
    Slippery and Slow, 488
    Slippery only at organ depth, 325
    Slippery Tense and Normal to slightly Rapid rate, 320
    Slippery Tense and slightly Rapid, 322
    Slippery Tense and Slow, 319
    Tight, 343
    Wiry Slippery and very Rapid, 351
Infection (early stage)

Tense, 518
Infection (Gallbladder)
 Flooding Excess, 292
 Slippery, 430
 Tight Empty at qi depth, 347
 Wiry, 358
Infection (intestinal tract)
 Tense, 442
Infection (Kidney)
 Deep Slippery Feeble, 280
 Slippery Deep Tight to Wiry and Rapid, 325
 Slippery only at organ depth, 325
Infection (Liver)
 Deep Thin Tight and Rapid, 279
 Deep Tight Slippery, 279
 Slippery, 430
Infection (localized)
 Tight, 339
 Tight (including Wiry), 520
 Tight Slippery and Rapid, 342
 Wiry, 350
 Wiry Robust Pounding and Rapid, 352
Infection (lower burner)
 Slippery, 522
Infection (organs)
 Deep Slippery, 275
Infection (pelvic area)
 Tense, 442
Infection (Pericardium)
 Slippery and Rapid with high fever, 321
Infection (qualities)
 Deep Slippery Feeble
  chronic, 280
  Kidney, 280
 Deep Slippery Feeble and Slow, Bladder, 281
 Deep Slippery, organs, 275
 Deep Thin Tight and Rapid, Liver, 279
 Deep Tight Slippery, Liver, 279
 Floating Yielding and Rapid, respiratory, 611
 Flooding Excess
  acute fulminating, 488
  blood, 613
  chronic, 292
  Gallbladder, 292
 Hollow Full-Overflowing Tight or Wiry and Slippery, blood, 188
 Slippery
  blood, 315
  Gallbladder, 430
  Liver, 430
  lower burner, 522
  systemic, 315
 Slippery and Rapid with high fever, pericardium, 321
 Slippery and Slow, chronic, 488
 Slippery Deep Tight to Wiry and Rapid, Kidney, 325
 Slippery Flooding Excess Tense, bacterial, 325
 Slippery only at organ depth

 chronic, 325
 Kidney, 325
 Slippery Tense and Normal to slightly Rapid rate, chronic, 320
 Slippery Tense and slightly Rapid, chronic, 322
 Slippery Tense and Slow, chronic, 319
 Slippery Tense, bacterial, 320
 Slippery Tight and slightly Rapid, Stomach, 324
 Slippery Tight Flooding Excess and Rapid, Bladder, 325
 Tense
  acute, 337
  early stage, 518
  intestinal tract, 442
  pelvic area, 442
 Tense Slippery, blood, 334
 Tense Slippery, Flooding Excess, Robust Pounding, acute fulminating, 334
 Tight
  acute, 346
  bacterial, 346
  chronic, 343
  localized, 339
 Tight Empty at qi depth, Gallbladder, 347
 Tight, Flooding Excess, Robust Pounding, Slippery and Rapid, bladder, 349
 Tight (including Wiry), localized, 520
 Tight Slippery and Rapid, localized, 342
 Wiry
  abdomen, 354
  acute, 355
  Gallbladder, 358
  localized, 350
  urinary, 359
 Wiry and Rapid, viral, 351
 Wiry Robust Pounding and rapid, localized, 352
 Wiry Slippery and very Rapid
  blood, 351
  chronic, 351
Infection (respiratory)
 Floating Yielding and Rapid, 611
Infection (Stomach)
 Slippery Tight and slightly Rapid, 324
Infection (systemic)
 Slippery, 315
Infection (urinary)
 Wiry, 359
Infection (viral)
 Wiry and Rapid, 351
Inflammation (Bladder)
 Tense, 445
 Tight, 348
 Tight Deep, 349
Inflammation (Intestines)
 Tight, Flooding Excess, Robust Pounding, Slippery and Rapid, 349

Inflammation (Liver)
    Deep Thin Tight and Rapid, 279
    Deep Tight Slippery, 279
    Slippery, 430
Inflammation (localized)
    Tight, 339, 343
Inflammation (pelvic)
    Tense, 445
    Tight, Flooding Excess, Robust Pounding, Slippery and Rapid, 349
Inflammation (qualities), 364
    Choppy, 364
    Deep Thin Tight and Rapid, 279
    Deep Tight Slippery, 279
    Slippery, 430
    Tense, 445
    Tight, 339, 343, 348
    Tight Deep, 349
    Tight, Flooding Excess, Robust Pounding, Slippery and Rapid, 349
    Wiry and Rapid, 351
Inflammation (viral)
    Wiry and Rapid, 351
Inflated
    in complementary positions, 393
    at Diaphragm position, 578-579, 611, 614
    distal position bilaterally, 555
    distal position (left), 399
    Flat vs., 212
    Floating vs., 242
    future (immediate) disharmony, 611, 614
    future (semi-distant) disharmony, 607
    Gallbladder position, 433
    illustrated, 193f
    Intestine positions, 448
    Large Vessel position, 614
    middle position (right), 436
    Pericardium position, 399
    positions, 196-201, 198-202
    qi depth, 475
    types, 194-196
    uniform bilaterally, 512-513
    and very Tense, 196
Inflated Tense, 194-195, 196. *See also* Tense Inflated
Inflated Tense-Floating and slightly Slow, 196
Inflated Yielding, 194-195, 196
Inflated Yielding-Floating and slightly Rapid, 196
Influenza, 424
Inner Classic (Nei jing) on Normal pulse, 91, 93
Instability. *See also* Husband-wife imbalance; Stability; Unstable
    Amplitude, Change in, 138-139, 139f
    blood out of control (reckless blood), 141-142
    Intensity, Change in, 136-138
    in interpretation, 67
    Nonhomogeneous quality, 140
    over entire pulse, 136-138
    Robust and Reduced, 139

    Unstable quality, 140-141
    yin and yang separation, 140
Intensity, Change in
    about, 37-38, 136
    alternating between sides, 68
    arrhythmia vs., 139
    constant over time, 136-137
    future (semi-distant) disharmony, 609
    illustrated, 136f
    inconstant over time, 137-138
    in interpretation, 637
    one wrist affected, 138
    over entire pulse, 561, 573
    over entire pulse, occasionally, 609
    position interpretation, 139
    'qi wild' condition, 469
    Qualities, Change in vs., 139
    shifting back and forth between sides, 585
    undulating from one position to another, 138
    undulating from one wrist to another, 138
Intermittent
    constantly, 119-120
    described, 119
    Inconsistently, 119-121
    rate measurable with missed beats, 118-119
Intermittent or Interrupted Yielding Hollow, 617
Interpretation. *See also* Pulse diagnosis
    acute illness, 45-47, 633
    age effects, 40-41, 631-632
    body condition in, 41-43
    chronic illness, 45-47, 633
    data integration, 626-627
    degree of presence, 627
    the disease process, 625-626
    environmental effects in, 40
    findings summary, 641
    focus, 46
    focus stages, 633-641
    formulation, 641
    foundation and, 42-43
    gender effects, 41, 632
    healing strategies, 642
    life record in the pulse, 34-35, 43-44, 626
    location, 627
    management strategies, 642-643
    methodology
        advanced, 629-633
        beginner, 628-629
        outline, 643-645f
        systematic approach, 633-641
    obscuring factors, 45
    paradoxical qualities, 631-633
    pathologies and qualities overlapping, 46
    position's role in, 44-45
    prediction and, 34-35
    qualities and, 40-45
    rate, 632
    sensation and position in, 44-45

seriousness, 627
size (weight and height), 632
temperature, 632
vulnerability in, 41
Interrupted
　constantly, 121-124
　described, 121
　occasionally, 124
　Sudden Transient, 124
Interrupted-Intermittent, 631
Interrupted or Intermittent, 617, 634
Intestine disorders, 444, 446, 447-448
Intestine position
　Biting, 447
　Choppy, 448
　Inflated, 448
　Intensity, Change in, 448
　Muffled, 448
　Robust Pounding, 448
　Rough Vibration, 447
　Slippery, 447
　Tense, 447
　Tight, 447
Intestine position (Large)
　proximal positions (left and right), 444
　qualities (common), 77
　taking the pulse, 77, 77f
Intestine position (Small)
　proximal positions (left and right), 446
　qualities (common), 83
　taking the pulse, 83, 83f
Irritability
　Intensity, Change in, occasional, over entire pulse, 609
　Tight, 343
　Tight and Rapid, 339

——— K

Kaptchuk, Ted, 97
Kidney deficiency, 223, 527
Kidney essence, 42-43, 550-552
Kidney-Heart disharmony
　about, 405-406, 587-588
　Feeble-Absent in both positions, 405
　Feeble-Absent (left distal) and left proximal Tight, 406
　sleep and, 590
　Tight in both positions, 405
　Tight (left distal) and left proximal Feeble-Absent, 406
Kidney qi, 42-43, 439-441. *See also* Essence
Kidney stones
　Deep Slippery, 276
　Deep Slippery Feeble and Slow, 281
　Deep Slippery Tense, 280
　Deep Slippery Wiry and Rapid, 280
　Deep Wiry, 276
　Slippery, 522

Slippery Deep Tight to Wiry and Rapid, 325
Slippery Tense and Slow, 319
Tight, 343
Tight (including Wiry), 521
Tight-Wiry, 442
Wiry, 355, 359
Kidney yang deficiency, 272
Kidney yin and yang in foundation, 42-43
Kidney yin deficiency, 520
Knotted, measurable rate, 118-119

——— L

Large Intestine position, 77, 77f
Large Vessel position
　Hollow Full-Overflowing, 402
　illustrated, 73f
　Inflated, 614
　Robust Pounding, Tight, and slightly Inflated, 402
　taking the pulse, 73
　Tense Inflated, 402
Leather
　about, 255
　future (immediate) disharmony, 615
　illustrated, 255f
　'qi wild' condition, 132
　yin and yang separation, 492
Leather-like Hollow
　about, 292-293
　bilaterally at same position, 264
　blood instability, 484
　blood out of control, 142
　in complementary positions, 393
　distal position (left), 398
　future (immediate) disharmony, 615
　illustrated, 263f
　middle position (left), 432
　middle position (right), 268
　proximal position (left), 267
　proximal position (right), 266
　and Rapid or Slow, 262
　Stomach-Pylorus Extension position, 268
Left distal position. *See also* Distal position
　about, 393-394
　Choppy, 398, 401
　complementary positions, 399-403
　Cotton, 394, 403
　Deep Thin Feeble, 398
　Deep Thin Feeble-Absent and very Slow, 397
　Deep Thin Feeble with Normal rate, 398
　Doughy, 401
　Empty, 397
　Exertion, Increase in Rate, 408-409
　Feeble-Absent, 395, 404, 406
　Feeble-Absent and Rapid, 408
　Feeble-Absent and Slow, 408

Flat, 396
Heart Enlarged position, 403
Heart-Gallbladder qi deficiency, 404
Hollow Full-Overflowing, 402
Inflated, 399
Large Vessel complementary position, 402-403
Leather-like Hollow, 398
Mitral Valve complementary position, 401-401
Muffled, 397, 401
qualities
    combinations, 403-409
    common, 73, 394-399
    rare, 398
    uncommon, 397
rate and rhythm, 408-409
Rest, Change in Rate, 408
Robust Pounding Tight, 398
Robust Pounding, Tight, and slightly Inflated, 402
Slippery, 396, 399, 402
taking the pulse, 73, 73f
Tense, 394, 403
Tense Hollow Full-Overflowing, 404
Tense Hollow Full-Overflowing, very, 397
Tense Inflated, 402
Tense Inflated, very, 398
Thin, 395, 561
Tight, 399, 406
Tight and Rapid, 408
Tight and Slow, 408
Tight in Pericardium position and moderately Rapid, 395
Tight over entire position and slightly Rapid, 395
Tight with Hesitant Wave, 409
Unstable, 398
Vibration, 402
Wiry, 397
Yielding Hollow Full-Overflowing, 398
Yielding Tense Inflated and slightly Rapid, 395-396
Left distal and left middle positions
    Cotton, 404
    Slippery, 404
    Tense, 403
    Tense Hollow Full-Overflowing, 404
Left distal and left proximal positions
    Feeble-Absent, 405
    Thin Feeble, entire pulse Interrupted or Intermittent, 409
    Tight, 405
Left distal and right middle positions
    Slippery, 404
    Thin Feeble Interrupted and Slow, 404
Left middle and left proximal positions
    Deep Wiry, 432
    Tense Hollow Full-Overflowing, 432
Left middle position. *See also* Middle position
    about, 430
    Blood Heat, 430
    Blood Thick, 430
    Blood Unclear, 430
    combinations, 432-433
    Diffuse, 431
    Empty, 431
    Floating Tight, 432
    Gallbladder, 433-434
    illustrated, 75f
    Leather-like Hollow, 432
    Liver Engorgement, 434
    overwork, 430
    qualities
        common, 75, 430-431
        less common, 431-432
    Reduced Substance, 431
    Slippery, 430
    Spreading, 431
    taking the pulse, 75, 75f
    Taut, 430
    Tense, 430
    Tense Hollow Full-Overflowing, 430
    Tense Inflated, 431
    Tense Inflated, very, 404
    Tense Slippery, 433
    Tense to Tight, 424-426
    Thin, 430
    Tight, 430
    Wiry, 430
    Yielding Partially Hollow, 431
Left Neuro-psychological position, 72, 72f
Left Pelvis/Lower Body position, 78, 78f
Left proximal position. *See also* Proximal position
    about, 441
    combinations, 444
    Deep, 443
    Empty, 443
    Feeble-Absent, 406, 443
    Flooding Excess, 443
    illustrated, 77f
    qualities (common), 76-77
    Reduced Substance, 443
    Robust Pounding, 443
    Slippery, 443
    taking the pulse, 76-77, 77f
    Taut, 442
    Tense, 442
    Tight, 406
    Tight-Wiry, 442, 443
Left side: 'organ system'
    deficient, 506
    in interpretation, 636
    Reduced (uniformly)
        organ system deficient, 506
        qi stagnation with a Cotton quality, 506
    Robust (uniformly)
        Diabetes, 505
        Hypertension, 505
        Liver wind, 506
        Pain, 505
        Stroke, 505
        Toxicity, 505

Left Special Lung position, 71-72, 71f
Length
    Diminished, 302-303
    Extended, 301-302
    flowchart, 305f
    Long, 301-302, 301f
    Restricted, 303
    Short (Abbreviated), 302-303, 303f
Lesser yin heat pattern, 161
Level, defined, 6d, 63
Li Shi-Zhen, 21, 97
Lifting (after eating)
    Tense Inflated, 514
    Tight, 342
Lifting (excessive)
    Diaphragm position, 532
    Flat, 212, 214, 215, 422, 515, 516
    Heart Full, 414
    Hollow, 530
    Inflated, 451
    rate variation, 170
    Robust Pounding, Tight, and slightly Inflated, 403
    Tense, 335
    Tight, 342
    Vibration, 422
Lifting (sudden, extraordinary)
    Deep and very Tight or Wiry, 274
    Inflated, 194
    obscuring interpretation, 45
    'qi wild' condition, 131
    Tense, 517
    Tense Inflated, 513
    Wiry, 353
    Yielding Hollow Full-Overflowing, 264
Liver and qi circulation, 468
Liver attacks Spleen
    Empty, 251, 528
Liver attacks Stomach-Spleen
    Feeble-Absent Deep, 526
Liver attacks upward
    Tense Inflated, moderately, 513
Liver blood and qi deficiency, 300
Liver blood and yin deficiency, 300
Liver blood deficiency, 524
Liver disharmony, 183
Liver Engorgement position
    distal, 74-75, 74f, 434
    lateral, 75-76
    medial, 75-76
    radial, 76f, 434
    taking the pulse, 74-76
    ulnar, 434
Liver-Gallbladder damp-heat, 319
Liver qi 'attacks', 434
Liver qi deficiency, 165
Liver qi stagnation
    left distal and proximal Feeble-Absent, and left middle
        Tense, 407
    Slow pulse, 163, 166
    Taut or Tense at left middle position, 573
Liver Ulnar position, 75f
Liver wind
    Floating Tight, 244, 611
    Robust (left side) uniformly, 505
    Thin-Tight, 605
    Tight Floating, 339
    Very Tense Tight, or Wiry Full-Overflowing Hollow and
        Rapid, 615
    Wiry, 350
Loneliness, 556. *See also* Depression
Long, 301-302, 301f
Love rejected, 554-555
Lower burner. *See* Proximal position
Lung disease. *See also* Asthma
    chronic
        Restricted, 429
    emphysema
        Inflated, 198-202, 607
        Tense Inflated, 421
        Tense Inflated, moderately, 513
        Tense-Tight Inflated at Special Lung, 429
    obstructive
        Restricted (width), 301
        Tight, 346
    pneumonia
        Flooding Excess, 512
        right distal and Special Lung, 424
    tuberculosis
        Tight Deep Thin Feeble, 345
Lung disease (qualities)
    Flooding Excess, 512
    Inflated, 198-202, 607
    Restricted, 429
    Tense Inflated, 421
    Tense Inflated, moderately, 513
    Tense-Tight Inflated at Special Lung, 429
    Tight, 346

—— M

Malnutrition, 488
Masturbation
    Thin Deep Feeble and Rapid, 300
    Thin Deep Feeble and Slow, 299
    Thin Deep Tight-Wiry and Slow, 299
Medications/pharmaceuticals
    corticosteroids, 488
    Cotton, 238
    damp-cold, 488
    Normal pulse and, 96
    obscuring interpretation, 45
    qualities and, 45, 57, 66-67
    Robust Pounding, 474-475
    serotonin uptake inhibitors, 238

Slow, 164, 169
stimulants, 57
Tight, 346
Wiry, 353
Melancholia, 550. *See also* Depression
Menopause
    Muffled at left distal or over entire pulse, 556
    Tight, 338
    Tight Thin, 340
Menorrhagia
    Empty, 252
    Feeble-Absent, 220, 223
    Feeble-Absent Deep, 527
    'qi wild' condition, 130
    Thin Yielding, 488
    Tight Thin, 340
    Yielding Hollow Full-Overflowing, 261, 267
Menstrual irregularities
    Choppy, 611
    Constant Change in Intensity, 609
    Feeble-Absent, 614
    Intensity, Change in, constant, 609
    Thin-Tight, 605
Mental illness
    bipolar disease, 571-573
    disassociated states, 569-571, 616
    Empty, 246
    Flooding Excess, 292
    Heart tight, 410
    obsessive thinking, 580-582
    paranoia, 568-569
    psychosis, 569-571
    'qi wild' condition, 572-573
    Robust Pounding Tight and slightly Inflated with Rapid rate, 398
    schizophrenia, 569-571
    Slippery, 399
    Slippery and Slow, 320-321
    Slippery Tense and slightly to very Rapid, 321
    Slippery Tight and slightly Rapid, 318
    Tight, 341
    Vibration, 370
    Wiry, 353
    Yielding Hollow Full-Overflowing and Rapid, 616
Middle burner. *See* Middle position
Middle position. *See also* Left middle position; Right middle position
    in interpretation, 639
    overflow onto other positions, 392
    psychological disharmony, 591
    qualities (common), 27, 63-64
Middle position (uniform bilaterally)
    about, 509-510
    Cotton, 511
    Empty, 528-529
    Feeble-Absent Deep, 525-526
    Flat, 515-516
    Floating, 511
    Flooding Excess, 512
    Hollow, 530
    Hollow Full-Overflowing, 511
    Inflated, 514
    Slippery, 522
    Tense, 517
    Thin, 524
    Tight (including Wiry), 519-520
    Tight Inflated (very), 514
    Vibration, 531
Mildly Slippery Tense, with Normal to slightly Rapid rate, 323
Mildly Slippery Yielding and Slow, 323
Minute
    about, 258
    future (immediate) disharmony, 615
    illustrated, 258f
    'qi wild' condition, 133
    yin and yang separation, 493
Miscarriage
    Choppy, 364
    Hollow Full-Overflowing Slippery and very Rapid, 188
Mitral Valve position
    illustrated, 74f
    Slippery, 402
    taking the pulse, 73-74
    Vibration, 402
Mitral Valve prolapse
    Mitral Valve position, 402
    Slippery at Mitral Valve position, 321, 612
    Smooth Vibration at Mitral Valve position, 607
Monk's pulse, 332, 336, 337
Mononucleosis
    depression, post, 556
    Empty, 247, 252, 431
    Empty at left middle position, 605
    Feeble-Absent, 614
    Flooding Excess and Robust Pounding, 432
    Slippery, 430
    Slippery Tense and very Rapid rate, 320
    Slippery Tight and Rapid, 322
    Slippery Tight and Slow, 322, 323
Muffled
    about, 226-227
    in complementary positions, 393
    distal position (left), 397, 401, 610, 613
    distal position (right), 423
    future (immediate) disharmony, 610, 612, 613
    future (semi-distant) disharmony, 610
    at Gallbladder position, 433, 612
    illustrated, 226f
    Intestine positions, 448
    at left distal position, Empty at left middle position, 556
    at left distal position or over entire pulse, 555
    middle position (left), 432
    at Neuro-psychological position, 401, 610
    at Special Lung position, 429
Multiple sclerosis, Doughy, 375-376, 401, 606

Musculoskeletal disorders, 28-29, 84, 451, 532

N

Narrow group
    qi deficiency, 294
    Restricted (width), 301
    Thin, 298, 300
    Thin Arrhythmic, 298
    Thin Deep, 297
    Thin Deep and very Feeble, 297
    Thin Deep Feeble, 298
    Thin Deep Feeble and Rapid, 300
    Thin Deep Feeble and Slow, 299-300
    Thin Deep Tight and Rapid, 298
    Thin Deep Tight-Wiry and Slow, 299
    Thin Feeble, 299
    Thin Minute, 297
    Thin Slippery, 299
    Thin Tight, 299
    Thin Tight and Rapid, 299
    Thin Tight-Wiry, 297-298
    Thin with Increase in Rate on Exertion, 300
    Thin Yielding, 296-297
    Tight-Wiry, 295
    Yielding Empty Thread-like, 301
Nausea/vomiting, 438
'Nervous system'
    'circulatory system' and, 504
    defined, 738d
    'digestive system' and, 504, 586-587
    disorders, Doughy, 606
    Heart conditions and, 417-418, 546-547
    in interpretation, 639
    'organ system' and, 224, 503-504, 576, 586
'Nervous system' overworked
    Thin Deep Tight-Wiry and Slow, 299
    Thin Tight and Rapid, 298
'Nervous system' tense
    about, 574-576
    alternating from Tight to Yielding, 340
    Deep Tight, 277
    defined, 738d
    etiology, 574-576
    Heart qi-yang deficiency, 417
    Heart yin deficiency, 417
    Normal pulse and, 96
    Rapid, 158
    Taut, 329, 331, 603
    Taut and slightly Rapid, 330
    Taut and Slow, 330
    Tense, 332, 474
    Tense and Slow, 333
    Tense Ropy, 293
    Tense to Tight over entire pulse, 574
    Tight, 489
    Tight and Slow (left distal), 408
    Tight Thin, 340
    Transiently Slippery, 317
'Nervous system' weak
    defined, 738d
    etiology, 576-577
    Feeble-Absent, 220
Nervous tension
    Tense, 336
    Tense and Rapid, 333
    Tight, 338, 342
    Tight (including Wiry), 519
    Wiry, 350, 356
Neurasthenia. *See* Nervous system weak
Neuro-psychological position
    Choppy, 401, 609
    Doughy, 401
    left, 72, 72f
    Muffled, 401, 610
    right, 78, 78f
    Rough Vibration, 400, 567, 613
    Smooth Vibration, 400, 611
    Vibration, 411, 531, 564
Nicotine addiction
    Heart yang deficiency, 416
    Tense, 336
    Tense Inflated, 421
    Tight, 346, 420, 426, 428
    Wiry, 357, 421, 428
Night sweats
    Thin-Tight, 605
    Tight, 338
Nine principal categories of qualities, 98, 100-107f
Nomenclature. *See* Classification/nomenclature;
  Terminology
Nonfluid qualities, 326-329
Nonfluid qualities (even)
    positions, 352-359
    Taut, 329-332
    Tense, 332-337
    Tight, 337-349
    Wiry, 349-352
Nonfluid qualities (uneven)
    Choppy, 361f, 362-366
    Ropy, 360, 360f
    Ropy Yielding Hollow, 361
    Tense Ropy, 360
    Vibration, 366-373, 366f
Nonhomogeneous, 140, 374
Normal pulse
    aberrations, 96
    age and, 95
    attributes, 90-91, 92f
    characteristics, 464
    classification/nomenclature, 96-98
    essence and, 94
    gender variation, 95
    Hollow Full-Overflowing Reduced Pounding, 188

Inner Classic (Nei jing), 91, 93
   medications/pharmaceuticals and, 96
   'nervous system' tense and, 96
   pregnancy and, 95
   rate and, 90, 92f, 151
   seasonal variation, 94
   spirit and, 93-94
   Stomach qi and, 93
   Taut, 329
   wave form, 38, 38f, 68f, 91f

— O

Obsessive thinking. *See* Rumination
Obstructive lung disease
   Restricted (width), 301
   Tight, 346
Occasionally Interrupted, 124. *See also* Interrupted
Onionstalk. *See* Hollow
Organ depth
   about, 485-486
   below, 70
   blood deficiency, 488-489
   deficiency at, 488-493
   Feeble-Absent, 219
   heat from excess at, 488
   illustrated, 29f, 69f
   in interpretation, 635
   pulse methodology, 70
   qi and yang deficiency, 490-491
   qi stagnation, 486-487
   qualities (common), 70
   Slippery, 323
   yang qi at, 460-461
   yin and essence depletion, 489-490
   yin qi at, 460-461
'Organ system'
   'circulatory system' and, 504
   deficient, 506, 585
   defined, 738d
   'digestive system' and, 171, 504-505
   imbalance, rate variation, 170
   in interpretation, 639
   'nervous system' and, 224, 503-504, 576, 586
   pulse position correlations, 20t
   rate variation, 170
   Reduced (uniformly), 506
   Robust (uniformly), 505-506
   terminology, 6
   vulnerability in interpretation, 41
Overexposure, 336
Overwork. *See also* Work habits
   age effects in interpretation, 40-41
   in childhood
      Heart yang deficiency, 416
      qi deficiency, 466

'qi wild' condition, 129
Deep Feeble, 274
Deep Thin Feeble with rate >100 beats/minute, 398
Diminished Feeble or Absent at qi depth, 476
Empty, 247, 250, 252
Feeble-Absent, 224, 443
Flat, 212
Flooding Deficient Diffuse and Reduced Substance, 605
Heart qi deficiency, 415
Lungs
   Empty, 250, 527
   Feeble-Absent, 222, 422
   Feeble-Absent Deep, 525
   Flat, 214, 515
   Tense, 335, 517
   Tight, 346
   Yielding Inflated, 421, 512
Mildly Slippery Yielding and Slow, 323
qi deficiency, 204, 206, 466
Reduced Pounding, 208
Rough Vibration, 373
Scattered, 257
Spreading, 484
Tense, 333
Thin Tight, 297
Tight to Yielding, alternating, 340
Tight-Wiry, 442
Yielding Hollow Full-Overflowing Reduced Pounding, 187

— P

Pain
   angina, 356, 399
   chest, 353
   chronic, 352
   hernial, 343, 355, 521
   intense/severe, 350, 351, 352, 354, 355, 356, 375, 489, 519
   kidney stones, 442
   localized, 351, 505, 612
   low back, 359
   menstrual, 358
   physical, 583
   qi stagnation, 339
   trauma as cause, 344
   tumor as cause, 341, 342
Pain (qualities)
   Bean (Spinning), 375
   Robust (left side) uniformly, 505
   Tight, 339, 341, 342, 343, 344, 399, 489
   Tight (including Wiry), 519, 520, 521
   Tight-Wiry, 442
   Wiry, 350, 353, 354, 355, 356, 358, 359, 489, 583, 612
   Wiry and Rapid, 351
   Wiry Choppy, 352

Wiry Deep and Slow, 352
Wiry Inflated, 352
Pancreas position, 439
Pancreatic failure, 252
Pancreatitis
    Flooding Excess, 292, 512
    Tight, 342
    Tight (including Wiry), 520
    Wiry, 354
Panic, 558, 612
Parasites
    Deep Slippery, 276
    Deep Slippery Feeble, 280
    Empty, 252, 431, 529
    Feeble-Absent, 223
    Feeble-Absent Deep, 526
    Slippery, 323, 430
    Slippery at organ depth, 614, 618
    Slippery Tense and Normal to slightly Rapid rate, 320
    Slippery Tense and very Rapid rate, 320
    Tense Slippery, 334
    Tight, 342
Parenchymal damage, 629
Parkinson's disease, 294
Patient,
    denial and, 601
    instructions, 59
    position of, 59
Pelvic inflammatory disease
    Deep Slippery Feeble and Slow, 281
    Flooding Excess, 292, 443
    Robust Pounding, 443
    Slippery, 443
    Slippery Deep Tight to Wiry and Rapid, 325
    Slippery Flooding Excess Tense, 325
    Slippery Tight Flooding Excess and Rapid, 325
    Tense, 336, 337
    Tight, 446
    Tight Flooding Excess, 340
    Tight Robust Pounding and Rapid, 348
    Tight-Wiry, 443
    Wiry, 355, 359
Pelvis/Lower Body position
    about, 448
    in interpretation, 638
    left, 78, 78f
    right, 83, 84f
Pericarditis, 398
Pericardium position
    Inflated, 399
    Slippery, 399
    taking the pulse, 72-73
    Tight, 399
    Tight or left distal Tense with Robust Pounding, 559-600
Peritoneal position, 82, 439
Peritonitis
    Flooding Excess, 292, 512, 613
    Slippery Tense and Slow, 319

    Tight (including Wiry), 520
    Wiry, 354
Phlegm
    confuses the Heart, 522, 571
    disturbs the Heart, 570-571
    excess, 425
    Heart and Lung, 524
    and the Heart orifice, 122
    stagnation, 487
    with wind-cold or wind-heat, 243
Phlegm-cold, 571
Phlegm-dampness, 165
Phlegm-fire disturbing the Heart, 521-522, 570-571
Phobia, 558. *See also* Fear
Pleura position, 80, 80f, 429
Pleurisy, 429
Pliable qualities related to hard, 35
Pliable Thin qualities, 296-297
PMS, 609
Pneumonia/pneumonitis, 346, 512
Poisoning. *See also* Toxicity
    Deep and Slow, 272
    Slow pulse, 164, 169
Porkert, Manfred, 98
Positions. *See also* Complementary positions; Individual positions; specific positions, e.g. Diaphragm
    in Normal pulse, 91, 92f
    principal impulse location, 391
    relationships among, 392
Post-traumatic stress syndrome
    Empty, 568
    Empty Moderately Tense, 249
    Empty over entire pulse, 615
    Rough Vibration, 568
Pounding, 190d, 208, 559
Poverty. *See* Environmental deprivation
Pregnancy/childbirth
    breech birth
        Heart Full, 414
        Heart Large, 416-417
        Inflated, 194, 475
        Tense Inflated, mildly, 513
        Yielding Inflated, 603
    Choppy with miscarriage, 364
    cord around neck at delivery
        Flat, 212, 213, 214, 421, 515, 555, 603
        Heart Small, 413, 417
        Yielding Inflated, 428
    ectopic, 373
    Feeble-Absent, 220
    Flat with cord around neck at delivery, 212, 213, 214, 421, 515, 555, 603
    Heart Full with breech birth, 414
    Heart Large with breech birth, 416-417
    Heart Small with cord around neck at delivery, 413, 417
    Hollow Full-Overflowing Slippery and very Rapid with miscarriage, 188
    Hollow Full-Overflowing Slippery over entire pulse, 187

Inflated with breech birth, 194, 475
miscarriage
    Choppy, 364
    Hollow Full-Overflowing Slippery and very Rapid, 188
multiple, 484
Normal pulse and, 95
qi deficiency, 204
Rough Vibration with ectopic, 373
Slippery, 314
Spreading with multiple, 484
Tense Inflated, mildly with breech birth, 513
Yielding Inflated
    breech birth, 603
    cord around neck at delivery, 428
Prevention and prognosis
    cardiovascular system importance in, 601-602
    denial (patient) and, 601
    the disease process, 625-626
    future (distant) disharmony
        Arrhythmia, 604
        Change in Rate at Rest, constant, 604
        Cotton, 602
        Flat, 603
        Rapid, 604
        Slow, 604
        Taut, 603-604
        Tight, 604
        Yielding Inflated, 603
        Yielding or Diminished qi depth, 603
    future (immediate) disharmony
        Bean (Spinning), 617
        Change in Qualities, 616
        Choppy, 611
        Choppy at Gallbladder position, 617
        Choppy at left distal position, 617
        Choppy at left middle position, 617
        Choppy at Pelvis/Lower Body positions, 617
        Dead, 617
        Deep, 613
        Empty at individual positions, 615
        Empty over entire pulse, 615
        Empty Thread-like, 615
        Exertion, Increase in Rate < 8 beats/minute, 616
        Feeble-Absent at individual positions, 614
        Feeble-Absent over entire pulse, 613-614
        Floating Tense and Slow, 611
        Floating Tight, 611
        Floating Yielding and Rapid, 611
        Flooding Excess, 613
        Hesitant, 610
        Hollow Yielding Full-Overflowing and Slow, 615
        Inflated at distal aspect of left Diaphragm position, 614
        Inflated at distal aspect of right Diaphragm position, 611
        Inflated at Large Vessel position, 614
        Intermittent or Interrupted Yielding Hollow, 617
        Interrupted or Intermittent, 617
        Leather, 615
        Leather-like Hollow, 615
        Minute, 615
        Muffled, 610
        Muffled at Gallbladder position, 612
        Muffled at left distal position, 613
        Occasional Change in Rate at Rest, 610
        Rough Vibration at individual positions, 613
        Rough Vibration at Neuro-psychological position, 613
        Rough Vibration over entire pulse, 613
        Scattered, 615
        Slippery at left distal position, 614
        Slippery at Mitral Valve position, 612
        Slippery at organ depth, 614
        Slippery Tight at Gallbladder position, 612
        Smooth Vibration, 611
        Tense Hollow Full-Overflowing at Large Vessel positions, 616
        Tense Ropy, 616
        Unstable, 617
        Very Tense Tight, or Wiry Full-Overflowing Hollow and Rapid, 615-616
        Wiry, 612
        Yielding Hollow Full-Overflowing and Rapid, 616
    future (semi-distant) disharmony
        Arrhythmia: Interrupted or Intermittent, 607
        Blood Heat, 606
        Blood Thick, 606
        Blood Unclear, 606
        Choppy at Neuro-psychological position, 609
        Constant Change in Intensity, 609
        Doughy, 606
        Empty at left middle position, 605
        Excessive Increase in Rate on mild Exertion, 609
        Flat, 605-606
        Flooding Deficient Diffuse and Reduced Substance, 605
        Inflated, 607
        Muffled at Neuro-psychological position, 610
        Occasional Change in Intensity over entire pulse, 609
        Rhythm, 609
        Rough Vibration at blood depth, 607
        Slippery at blood depth, 607
        Slippery at qi depth over entire pulse, 607
        Smooth Vibration at Mitral Valve position, 607
        Spreading over entire pulse, 604-605
        Tense, 608
        Tense Hollow Full-Overflowing, 607
        Tense Slippery at Gallbladder position, 608
        Thin-Tight, 605
        Thin Yielding, 605
        Wiry, 608
        Yielding Ropy, 608-609
    long-range view, 599
    positive signs, 619-620
    seriousness, 600-601
    symptom arrival estimation, 600
    time components, 600-602

time lag, 599-600
Principal positions
    overview, 23
    Amplitude, Change in, 139
    defined, 6d
    distal (left), 72-73, 73f
    distal (right), 79-80, 79f
    hand placement in diagnosis, 71f
    illustrated, 24-25f
    Intensity, Change in, 139
    interpreting the pulse, 63
    middle (left), 75, 75f
    middle (right), 81, 81f
    proximal (left), 76-77, 77f
    proximal (right), 82-83, 83f
Principal impulse location, 391
Prognosis. *See* Prevention and prognosis
Progression of heat and toxicity in the blood, 478f
Prostatitis
    Choppy, 364
    Flooding Excess, 292, 443, 512
    Robust Pounding, 443
    Slippery, 443
    Slippery Deep Tight to Wiry and Rapid, 325
    Slippery Flooding Excess Tense, 325
    Slippery Tight Flooding Excess and Rapid, 325
    Taut, 332
    Tense, 336, 337
    Tight, 446
    Tight Flooding Excess, 340
    Tight, Flooding Excess, Robust Pounding, Slippery and Rapid, 349
    Tight Robust Pounding and Rapid, 348
    Tight-Wiry, 443
    Wiry, 355, 359
Proximal position. *See also* Left proximal position; Right proximal position
    about, 43, 439-440
    deepness of, 392-393
    in interpretation, 639
    origin of disorders and, 43
    psychological disharmony, 590-591
    qualities (common), 442-444
Proximal position (uniform bilaterally)
    about, 509
    Cotton, 511
    Empty, 529
    Feeble-Absent Deep, 526-527
    Flat, 516
    Floating, 511
    Flooding Excess, 512
    Hollow, 530-531
    Hollow Full-Overflowing, 512
    Inflated, 514
    Slippery, 522-523
    Tense, 517-518
    Thin, 524
    Tight (including Wiry), 520-521

Vibration, 531
Proximal pulses and the foundation, 43
Psychological disorders. *See also* Emotions/emotional life
    bipolar disease, 557
    borderline, 610
    in interpretation, 639
    the pulse and, 545-547
    qualities (common), 548, 592-594t
Pulse diagnosis. *See also* Interpretation; Pulse methodology; Pulse positions
    absence of qualities, 27-28
    in children, 601
    Chinese (contemporary), 3-6, 27-29
    Chinese physiology in, 33-35
    complementary diagnostic methods, 13
    data integration in, 627
    interpretations, 19-22
    the life record in the pulse, 34-35, 626
    limitations, 12-13
    in modern practice, 10-15
    of musculoskeletal disorders, 28-29, 451, 532
    potential, 11
    the practitioner, 14
    as predictor, 460
    quantity vs. quality, 39
    the senses role, 14-15
    the sounds/tones of, 15
    terminology, 6, 6-9, 731-740
    theory, 15
    Western physiology and, 35-36
Pulse methodology (taking the pulse). *See also* Pulse diagnosis
    Amber technique, 61-62
    Chinese technique (contemporary), 60-61
    depth, 62-63
    finger placement, 62
    finger pressure, 62-63
    focus stages, 60, 65, 65-70, 71-83
    hand placement, 71f
    level, 63-64
    of middle position (burner), 63-64
    patient instructions, 57, 59
    patient positioning, 59
    practitioner positioning, 59
    principal impulse location, 59-60, 391
    process, 10, 12, 26-28, 60, 60-61, 64-65, 85
    pulse record, 58f
    qualities classification, 64
    rate checking, 84, 151
    rolling the fingers, 26-28, 60, 62
    Shen technique, 61-62
    the three depths, 62-63
    time required for, 10, 57
    of upper burner (distal position), 64
Pulse positions
    by Hammer, 24f
    historical comparisons, 19-22
    illustrated, 24f

interpretation, 28
organ correlations, 19-22, 20t, 28
by Shen, 25f
Pulse record, 58f
Pulse signs
large segment, 36-39
rate, 36-37, 65-66
rhythm, 36, 65-66
small segment, 39
stability, 37-38
wave form, 38, 38f
Push pulse, 127, 739d. *See also* Hesitant Wave

Q

Qi. *See also* Trapped qi in the Heart
blood circulation and, 466-469
external qualities, 628
internal qualities, 628
Stomach, 93
trapped (Inflated), 475
trauma and, 154-155
Qi agitation, Heart. *See* Heart qi agitation
Qi and blood deficiency, 296-297, 523
Qi and blood stagnation, 353
Qi and yang deficiency. *See also* Heart qi and yang deficiency
Deep, 490
Deep Reduced Substance, 490
Deep Separating, 490
Empty, 491-492
Empty Intermittent-Intermittent, Yielding Hollow Interrupted-Intermittent, 493
Empty Thread-like, 492
Feeble-Absent, 490
Hidden Deficient, 491
Leather, 492
Minute, 493
Scattered, 492
Short Yielding, 490
Slow pulse, 167, 169
Tight to Wiry Hollow Full-Overflowing, 185
Yielding Hollow Full-Overflowing, 493
Yin and yang in contact, 490-491
Yin and yang separation, 491, 491-493
Qi circulation, 468. *See also* Circulation
Qi deficiency. *See also* Heart qi deficiency
about, 476
Absent at qi depth, 476
age effects, 40
anxiety, 560-562
asthma, 424
Deep, 216
Diffuse, 209
Diffuse and Reduced Substance, 293-294
Diminished Feeble or Absent at qi depth, 476
Feeble-Absent, 218-219, 222

Feeble-Absent Deep, 525-526
Flooding Deficient, 477
Heart and Kidney, 407
Heart-Gallbladder, 404
Kidney, 524, 552
from overwork, 204, 206
pregnancy and, 204
pulse types, 463
qualities (common), 628
Reduced Pounding, 208
Slippery, 522
Spleen, 514, 522, 524
Spleen and Stomach, 222, 525-526
Thin, 295-296, 524
Tight to Wiry Hollow Full-Overflowing, 185
Width, 294
Yielding, 476
Yielding Inflated, 514
Yielding Reduced Pounding, 476
Qi depth. *See also* Above the qi depth; Absent at qi depth
about, 472-473
absence of, 484
Absent, 205f
agitation at, 475
Bean (Spinning), 475
Diminished Feeble or Absent, 476
Diminished or Absent, 204
Feeble-Absent, 218
Flooding Deficient, 477
fluid stagnation, 475
illustrated, 29f, 69f
Inflated, 475
in interpretation, 635
Mildly Slippery Tense, 323
Mildly Slippery Yielding and Slow, 323
pulse methodology, 70
qi deficiency, 476-477
qi stagnation, 473-475
qualities (common), 70
Robust Pounding and Bounding with Rapid rate, 474
Robust Pounding at organ depth, 475
Slippery, 475
Taut, 473
Tense, 473
Tense Long, 474
Tense Robust Pounding, 474
Tense Robust Pounding Suppressed, 474
Tight and Thin at qi depth, 477
Trapped qi, 475
Yielding at, 476
Yielding Reduced Pounding, 476
Yin deficiency, 477
Qi stagnation. *See also* Heart qi stagnation
Barrett's syndrome, 438
Bean (Spinning), 475
Cotton, 237-238, 470, 506, 511
eating disorders, 438
emotional shock, 438

emotional stress, 438
Esophagus position, 438
Floating, 471
Floating Slippery, 472
Floating Tense and Slow, 472
Floating Tight, 472
Floating Yielding and slightly Rapid, 471
Flooding Excess, 472
hard sensations above the qi depth, 472
Intestinal, 521
from invading cold, 345
lifting, 438
Liver, 407, 573
Liver and Stomach, 514
nausea/vomiting, 438
psychosis and, 569-570
pulse types, 462-463
qualities (common), 628
Robust Pounding and Bounding with Rapid rate, 474
Robust Pounding at organ depth, 475
from rumination, 438
Taut, 473
Taut or Tense at left middle position, 573
Tense, 473
Tense Hollow Full-Overflowing, 472
Tense Inflated, 514
Tense Long, 474
Tense Robust Pounding, 474
Tense Robust Pounding Suppressed, 474
Thin, 524
the three depths, 486-487
Tight Deep Thin Feeble, 345
Tight (including Wiry), 521
Yielding Hollow Full-Overflowing, 472
Yielding (pliable) sensations, 470-472
'Qi wild'
  about, 128
  Arrhythmic rate, qualities of, 135
  defined, 739d
  depression and, 556-557
  described, 466-467
  Empty, 132, 135, 216, 246, 247
  Empty Intermittent-Intermittent, 250, 493
  Empty Thread-like, 132, 615
  Empty Tight and Rapid, 249
  etiology, 129-131
  Hollow Yielding Full-Overflowing and Slow, 615
  Leather, 132, 615
  Minute, 133, 615
  paradoxical qualities, 631
  psychosis and, 572-573
  Qualities, Change in, 616
  qualities (common), 128-130, 567, 615
  Scattered, 132, 256, 615
  three depth qualities, 468-469
  Wide Yielding Hollow Full-Overflowing, 293
  Yielding Empty Thread-like, 301
  Yielding Hollow Full-Overflowing, 133, 187
  Yielding Hollow Interrupted-Intermittent, 493
  Yielding Ropy Hollow, 133
  Yin and yang separation, 491-492
Qi-yang deficiency, 417, 629
Qualifying terms (shape)
  Biting, 376
  Ephemeral (Transient), 377
  flowchart, 382f
  Reduced Force, 377
  Robust, 377
  Rough, 376
  Separating, 378
  Smooth, 376
  Subtle (Vague), 377
Qualities. *See also* individual qualities, e.g. Floating
  absence of, 27-28
  at all positions simultaneously and three depths, 463-464
  balance, 50
  in children, 601
  classification, 10, 64, 100-107t
  by condition, 102-107t
  congruence of, 61
  consistency related, 48
  disharmony in, 48-50
  equilibrium restoration, 48-50
  feng shui and, 47-48
  interpretation of, 40-45, 46, 65-67, 637
  obscuring factors, 45, 391
  overlapping pathologies, 46
  paradox in, 33-34, 61, 619, 631-633
  as pathology predictors, 34-35
  quantity vs. quality, 39
  relationships, 627
  by sensation, 44, 64, 100-102t
Quick pulse. *See* Rapid

——— R

Racing pulse. *See* Rapid
Radial pulse, 460
Rage, 451, 579. *See also* Anger
Rapid
  about, 152-153
  etiology categorization, 153-162
  flowchart, 172-173f
  future (distant) disharmony, 604
  proximal position (right), 445
  seasonal variations, 155
Rate. *See also* Rhythm
  about, 151, 464-465
  age ranges and, 152
  Bounding quality, 153
  distal position (left), 408-409
  in interpretation, 36-37, 65-66, 632, 634
  measurable
    with missed beats, 117-121

no missed beats, 114-117
    unmeasurable, 121-124
Normal pulse and, 90, 92f, 151
Rapid, 152-153, 153-162, 172-173f
Slow, 162-170, 174f
the three depths, 465
unmeasurable, 121-124
variations between wrists, 170-171
Rate at Rest
    Change in
        about, 115
        constant, 117-119, 408
        future (immediate) disharmony, 610
        occasional, 115-117, 408, 564, 610
    in interpretation, 633-634
Rate on Exertion
    decreases, 125
    in interpretation, 634
    paradoxical qualities, 632
    pulse methodology, 84
    stays the same, 632
Reckless blood. *See* Blood out of control
Reduced
    about, 202-203
    Absent at qi depth, 204-205, 205f
    at blood depth, 205-208
    classification/nomenclature, 202-203, 377
    Dead, 227
    Deep, 216
    Diffuse, 209, 209f
    Diminished at blood depth, 205, 207f
    Diminished at qi depth, 204, 204f
    Feeble-Absent, 216-225
    Feeble-Absent Deep and Slow/Rapid, 221
    Feeble-Absent Deep Choppy, 221
    Feeble-Absent Deep Slippery, 221
    Flat, 210-216, 211f
    Flooding Deficient Wave, 205, 207f, 208
    left side: 'organ system' uniformly, 506
    Muffled, 226-227, 226f
    Spreading, 205, 206f
    Substance, 210f
    Yielding at qi depth, 203-204, 203f
    Yielding Partially Hollow, 205, 206f
Reduced Pounding, 208, 631
Reduced Substance
    about, 209-210, 293-294
    distal position (right), 422
    illustrated, 210f
    middle position (left), 431
    middle position (right), 436
    proximal position (left), 443
    proximal position (left and right), 443
    proximal position (right), 445
Reduced (uniformly) left side
    'organ system' deficient, 506
    qi stagnation with a Cotton quality, 506
Reduced (uniformly) right side

damp-cold, 508
    eating habits (after labor), 508
    eating habits (irregular), 508
Reflux, esophageal, 373, 618
Relationships
    divorce/separation
        Inflated at Diaphragm position, 578-579
        Intestine position, 451
    husband-wife imbalance, 139, 501-502, 584-585
Replacement. *See* Intermittent
Repressed emotions
    Flat, 421, 603
    Heart qi deficiency, 415
    qi stagnation, 473
    Taut, 430, 473
    Tense, 430
    Tense Long, 474
    Thin, 430
    Tight, 430
    Wiry, 357, 430
Resentment
    Taut, 331
    Tense, 332
Resignation (emotional), Cotton, 237-238, 580, 585
Restricted
    length, 303
    at Special Lung position, 429
    width, 301
Rheumatic fever, 416
Rhythm. *See also* Arrhythmia; Rate
    about, 113, 464-465
    changes in
        rate measurable with missed beats, 118-121
        rate measurable without missed beats, 114-118
        rate not measurable, 121-124
    flowchart, 143-145f
    future (semi-distant) disharmony, 609
    in interpretation, 36, 65-66, 633-634
    in Normal pulse, 90, 92f
    the three depths, 465
Right distal position. *See also* Distal position
    about, 419-420
    Deep, 422
    Empty, Change in Intensity and Qualities, 423
    Feeble-Absent, 422, 424-426
    Flat, 421
    Floating, 420
    Muffled, 423
    qualities (common), 79-80
    Reduced Substance, 422
    Robust Pounding, 423
    Slippery, 423
    taking the pulse, 79-80, 79f
    Tense, 420
    Tense Inflated, 421
    Thin, 423
    Tight, 420
    Vibration, 422

Wiry, 421
Yielding Inflated, 421
Right distal and left proximal positions
    Feeble-Absent, 426
    Tight, 426
Right distal and right middle positions
    Feeble-Absent, 425
    Floating Tense and Slow, 425
    Floating Yielding Rapid, 425
    Slippery, 425
    Tense, 425
    Tight, 425
Right distal and right proximal positions
    Feeble-Absent, 426
Right middle position. *See also* Middle position
    about, 434
    combinations, 437
    complementary positions
        Duodenum, 439
        Esophagus position, 438
        Pancreas position, 439
        Spleen position, 438-439
        Stomach-Pylorus Extension position, 439
    Deep, 436
    Empty, 436
    Feeble-Absent, 436
    Flat, 436
    illustrated, 81f
    Inflated, 436
    over entire left side, 437-438
    qualities (common), 81
    Reduced Substance, 436
    taking the pulse, 81, 81f
    Tense-Tight, 436
    yang organ and, 434
Right middle and right proximal positions
    Feeble-Absent, 437
    Tight, 437
Right Neuro-psychological position, 78, 78f
Right Pelvis/Lower Body position, 83, 84f
Right proximal position. *See also* Proximal position
    about, 441
    Bladder position, 444
    combinations, 444, 446
    Deep, 445
    Feeble-Absent, 445
    Flooding Excess, 445
    qualities (common), 82-83
    Rapid, 445
    Reduced Substance, 445
    Robust Pounding, 445
    Slippery, 445
    taking the pulse, 82-83, 83f
    Tense, 445
    Tight-Wiry, 445
Right proximal and right middle and distal positions
    Feeble-Absent, 446
    Tight, 446

Right side: 'digestive system'
    in interpretation, 636
    physiology, 506-507
    Reduced (uniformly)
        damp-cold, 508
        eating habits (irregular), 508
    Robust or Reduced (uniformly)
        eating habits (after work), 508
    Robust (uniformly)
        damp-heat, 507
        eating habits (too quickly), 507
        hypertension/stroke, 507
Right Special Lung position, 26f, 78, 78f
Robust
    Flooding Excess, 190-193, 191f
    Hollow Full-Overflowing, 179-180, 180f
    Hollow Full-Overflowing Leather-Like, and Rapid/Slow, 187
    Hollow Full-Overflowing Reduced Pounding, 188
    Hollow Full-Overflowing Robust Pounding Bounding and Rapid, 188
    Hollow Full-Overflowing Slippery
        over entire pulse, 187
        and very Rapid, 188
    Hollow Full-Overflowing Tense, and Slippery at the blood depth, 188
    Hollow Full-Overflowing Tight or Wiry, 188
        and Slippery, 188
    Inflated, 193-201, 193f
        and very Tense, 196
    Inflated Tense, 195, 196
    Inflated Tense Floating and slightly Slow, 196
    Inflated Yielding, 194-195, 196
    Inflated Yielding Floating and slightly Rapid, 196
    left side: 'organ system' uniformly, 505-506
    as qualifying term, 377
    Suppressed, 201-202, 201f
    Tense Hollow Full-Overflowing, 181
    Tense Inflated
        mildly, 196
        moderately, 197
        very, 195, 197-198
    Tense Inflated Floating, 197
    Tight to Wiry Hollow Full-Overflowing, 184-186
    Yielding Hollow Full-Overflowing, 181
        and Rapid, 187
        and Slow, 187
    Yielding Hollow Full-Overflowing Reduced Pounding, 186-187
    Yielding Inflated, 196
Robust Pounding
    about, 190
    and Bounding with Rapid rate, 474
    and Flooding Excess, 190
    and Hollow Full-Overflowing, 190
    Intestine positions, 448
    at organ depth, 475
    paradoxical qualities, 631

positions, 190
proximal position, left, 443
proximal position, right, 445
Robust Pounding, Tight, and slightly Inflated, 402
Robust Pounding, Tight, and slightly Inflated with Rapid rate, left distal position, 398
Robust (uniformly) left side
    diabetes, 505
    hypertension, 505
    Liver wind, 506
    pain, 505
    stroke, 505
    toxicity, 505
Robust (uniformly) right side
    damp-heat, 507
    eating habits (after physical labor), 508
    eating habits (too quickly), 507
    hypertension, 507
    stroke, 507
Roller-coaster feeling, 567-568, 610
Rolling the fingers (on the pulse), 26-28, 60, 62
Root. *See* Essence
Ropy
    about, 360
    illustrated, 360f
    paradoxical qualities, 631
Ropy Yielding Hollow, 361
Rough (qualifying term), 376
Rough Vibration. *See also* Vibration
    about, 367
    at blood depth, 607
    blood stagnation, 483
    Choppy vs., 363
    consistent, 369-370
    consistent over entire pulse at all depths, 565
    deep or at all depths, 372
    distal position (left), 397, 400
    future (immediate) disharmony, 613
    future (semi-distant) disharmony, 607
    Heart qi deficiency vs., 566
    illustrated, 366f
    at individual positions, 613
    Intestine positions, 447
    Neuro-psychological position, 400, 567, 613
    over entire pulse, 613
    Special Lung position, 428
    Tight and Rapid, 339
Rumination (thinking)
    Cotton, 511
    Deep Flat, 275
    Empty, 251, 528
    Feeble-Absent Deep, 526
    Hesitant Wave, 126-127
    qi stagnation, 438
    Yielding Inflated, 514
Running pulse. *See* Rapid

S

Sad pulse. *See* Cotton
Sadness
    Cotton, 237-238, 239, 404
    Feeble-Absent, 443
Scattered
    about, 256
    future (immediate) disharmony, 615
    illustrated, 257f
    'qi wild' condition, 132
    yin and yang separation, 492
Seasonal variations
    circulation and, 467, 468
    Normal pulse, 94
    Rapid, 155
The senses (five) role in diagnosis, 14-15
Separating, 378
Seriousness
    Feeble-Absent, 220
    in interpretation, 627, 629-630
    in literature, 600-601
    Vibration, 368
Sexual
    abstinence
        Taut, 332, 442
        Tense, 336, 337, 518
    abuse
        Tight with Change in Rate at Rest, 345
        Vibration, 370
    excess
        Empty, 529
        Feeble-Absent, 223, 224, 443
        Feeble-Absent Deep, 526
    excess (masturbation)
        Thin Deep Feeble and Rapid, 300
        Thin Deep Feeble and Slow, 299
        Thin Deep Tight-Wiry and Slow, 299
Shape
    anomalous qualities, 378, 391
    anomalous vessels, 378-380
    flowchart, 381f
    fluid qualities
        Slippery, 313-315, 314f, 317, 322
        Slippery and Rapid, 318
        Slippery and Slow, 318, 319, 320, 324
        Slippery and very Rapid with high fever, 321
        Slippery and very Tight Hollow Full-Overflowing, 320, 321
        Slippery at Esophagus position, 324
        Slippery at Mitral Valve position, 321
        Slippery Deep Feeble, 325-325
        Slippery Deep Feeble and Slow, 325
        Slippery Deep Tight to Wiry and Rapid, 325
        Slippery Deep (very) and very Rapid, 321
        Slippery Empty, 322
        Slippery Feeble, 322

Slippery Feeble and Slow, 315, 320, 322, 324
Slippery Feeble with Normal rate, 321
Slippery Flooding Excess Tense and possibly Rapid, 325
Slippery Inflated, 324
Slippery (moderate to severe), 323
Slippery only at organ depth, 325
Slippery Tense, 323, 325
Slippery Tense and Normal rate, 319
Slippery Tense and Normal to slightly Rapid rate, 320
Slippery Tense and Rapid, 318
Slippery Tense and slightly Rapid, 322
Slippery Tense and slightly to very Rapid, 321
Slippery Tense and Slow, 318-319, 324
Slippery Tense and very Rapid, 320
Slippery Tense at all depths, 320
Slippery Tense at qi depth with Normal or slightly Rapid rate, 320
Slippery Tense (mildly) with Normal or slightly Rapid rate, 323
Slippery Tight and Rapid, 322
Slippery Tight and slightly Rapid, 318, 324
Slippery Tight and Slow, 323
Slippery Tight Flooding Excess and Rapid, 322, 325
Slippery Tight (Hollow) at Stomach-Pylorus Extension position, 324
Slippery Tight Hollow Full-Overflowing and Rapid, 315
Slippery Tight-Wiry and Choppy or Muffled, 323
Slippery Tight-Wiry and Slow, 322
Slippery Transient above the qi depth, 318
Slippery Yielding (mildly) and Slow, 323
Tense Slippery with Normal or slightly Rapid rate, 316
Transiently Slippery, 316
Yielding Slippery and Slow, 316
miscellaneous qualities
    Bean (Spinning), 374-375
    Doughy, 375-376
    Nonhomogeneous, 374
nonfluid qualities
    about, 326-329
    classification, 326-327
nonfluid qualities (even)
    positions, 352-359
    Taut, 329-332
    Tense, 332-337
    Tight, 337-349
    Wiry, 349-352
nonfluid qualities (uneven)
    Choppy, 361f, 362-366
    Ropy, 360, 360f
    Ropy Yielding Hollow, 361
    Tense Ropy, 360
    Vibration, 366-373, 366f
in Normal pulse, 90, 92f
qualifying terms
    Biting, 376
    Ephemeral (Transient), 377
    flowchart, 382f
    Reduced Force, 377
    Robust, 377
    Rough, 376
    Separating, 378
    Smooth, 376
    Subtle (Vague), 377
Shelter needs unmet. *See* Environmental deprivation
Shen, John H. F.
    age and body condition, effect on pulse, 40-41, 95, 152
    arrhythmia, 113-114
    blood stagnation qualities, 479-481
    Cotton, 236-237
    Feeble-Absent, 216-217
    Heart conditions and qualities, 409-418
    Hollow Full-Overflowing, 179-180
    'nervous system,' 546
    pulse positions, 21-23
    qi stagnation qualities, 462, 466
    'qi wild' and instability, 127-128
    rate, 152
    Slow, 162
    special terms defined, 747-756
    'systems' model and qualities, 502-506
    taking the pulse, 61-62
    Tight, 313, 337
    Vibration qualities, 366
Shock. *See also* Trauma
    to circulation
        Slippery, 315
    circulation and, 467
    emotional
        Bean (Spinning), 399
        Deep and Rapid, 272
        Feeble-Absent Deep, 525
        Flat, 215, 487
        Heart Closed, 412-413
        Heart Nervous, 411
        Heart yang deficiency, 416
        left distal Tight and Rapid, 408
        qi stagnation, 438
        Smooth Vibration, 371
        Tense and Rapid, 333
        Tight, 338
        Wiry, 353
    emotional in childhood
        Deep Flat, 273
        Feeble-Absent, 222
    physical
        Flat, 487
        Tense, 336
    in pregnancy, 170
    rate variation from, 170
    rhythm affected by, 113
    Slow pulse, 163, 164
    Vibration, 366, 369-370
Short, 303f
Short (Abbreviated), 302-303

Short Yielding, 490
Singing/talking (excessive). *See* Overwork, of Lungs
Sinking. *See* Deep
Sitting bent forward
    Deep Feeble-Absent, 275
    Deep Flat, 275
    Empty, 251, 528
    Feeble-Absent Deep, 526
    Flat, 515-516
    Tight, 342
    Tight (including Wiry), 520
Sitting (prolonged)
    Cotton, 511
    Flat, 214
    Yielding Hollow Full-Overflowing, 265
Skin diseases
    Blood Thick, 606
    Blood Unclear, 606
Sleep, 589-590
Slightly Yielding Hollow Full-Overflowing and Normal to slightly Rapid, 261
Slippery
    about, 313-315
    at blood depth, 323, 607
    blood stagnation, 482-483
    combinations, 315-326
    distal and middle positions (left), 404
    distal and middle positions (right), 425
    distal position (left), 396, 397, 399, 402, 614
    distal position (left) and right middle position, 404
    distal position (right), 322, 423
    distal position (uniform bilaterally), 521-522
    at Esophagus position, 324
    future (immediate) disharmony, 612, 614
    future (semi-distant) disharmony, 607
    Hollow vs., 260
    illustrated, 314f
    Intestine positions, 447
    middle position (left), 430
    middle position (uniform bilaterally), 522
    at Mitral Valve position, 321, 402, 562, 612
    moderate to severe, 323
    with Normal rate, 396
    at organ depth, 614
    at organ depth only, 325
    Pericardium position, 399
    proximal position (left), 443
    proximal position (right), 445
    proximal position (uniform bilaterally), 522-523
    at qi depth, 475
    at qi depth over entire pulse, 607
    and Rapid, 318, 396
    and Rapid (very), 397
    and Slow, 318, 319, 320, 324
    at Special Lung position, 428
    at Special Lung position, bilaterally, 522
    uniform qualities, 508, 521-523
    and very Rapid with high fever, 321
    and very Tight Hollow Full-Overflowing, 320, 321
Slippery Deep Feeble, 325-325
    and Slow, 325
Slippery Deep Tight to Wiry and Rapid, 325
Slippery Empty, 322
Slippery Feeble
    with Normal rate, 321
    and Slow, 315, 320, 322, 324
Slippery Flooding Excess Tense and possibly Rapid, 325
Slippery Inflated, 324
Slippery Tense
    at all depths, 320
    Gallbladder position, 323
    mild, with Normal to slightly Rapid rate, 323
    with Normal rate, 319
    with Normal to slightly Rapid rate, 320
    proximal position (right), 325
    at qi depth with Normal or slightly Rapid rate, 320
    and Rapid, 318
    and Rapid (slightly), 322
    and Rapid (slightly to very), 321
    and Rapid (very), 320
    and Slow, 318-319, 324
Slippery Tight
    future (immediate) disharmony, 612
    at Gallbladder position, 612
    and Rapid, 322
    and Rapid (slightly), 318, 324
    and Slow, 323
Slippery Tight Flooding Excess and Rapid, 322, 325
Slippery Tight (Hollow) at Stomach-Pylorus Extension, 324
Slippery Tight Hollow Full-Overflowing and Rapid, 315
Slippery Tight-Wiry
    and Choppy or Muffled, 323
    and Slow, 322
Slippery Transient above the qi depth, 318
Slippery Yielding and Slow, mildly, 323
Slow
    about, 162
    etiology categorization, 163-165
    flowchart, 174f
    future (distant) disharmony, 604
    Hollow Full-Overflowing Reduced Pounding, 188
    in interpretation, 634
    by rate, 165-169
Small. *See* Thin
Small Intestine position, 83, 83f
Smoking. *See* Nicotine addiction
Smooth (qualifying term), 376
Smooth Vibration. *See also* Vibration
    about, 366
    combinations, 371-373
    distal position (left), 399, 400, 611
    future (immediate) disharmony, 611
    future (semi-distant) disharmony, 607
    illustrated, 366f
    at Mitral Valve position, 607
    Neuro-psychological position, 400, 611

progression from left distal to other positions, 372-373
  superficial, 372, 563
  superficial and deep, 372
Social factors affecting qualities, 47-48
Soft. *See* Empty Thread-like
Soggy. *See* Empty Thread-like
Special Lung position
  about, 23, 26, 426-427
  conditions associated with, 423-424
  Empty, 428
  Floating, 427
  left, 71-72, 71f
  Muffled, 429
  Restricted, 429
  right, 26f, 78, 78f
  Slippery, 428, 522
  Tight, 428
  Tight, bilaterally, 519
  Wiry, 428
  Yielding Inflated, 428
Spinning. *See* Bean (Spinning)
Spirit measurement. *See* Amplitude
Spite, 568
Spleen dampness, 319
Spleen disharmony, 183
Spleen position, 81-82, 81f, 438
Spleen-Stomach position, 581
Spreading
  blood deficiency, 484
  future (semi-distant) disharmony, 604-605
  illustrated, 206f
  middle position (left), 431
  at qi depth, 205
Stability. *See also* Instability
  about, 127, 464-465
  flowchart, 145f
  in interpretation, 37-38, 67
  in Normal pulse, 90, 92f
  'qi wild' condition, 128-135, 468-469
  the three depths, 464-465, 468-469
Stagnant. *See* Flat
Stagnation. *See also* Blood stagnation; Food stagnation; Qi stagnation
  between burners, 531-532
  essence, qualities of, 629
  fluids, 475, 487-488
  phlegm, 487
  qualities (common), 48-49
  yang, qualities of, 628
  yin, qualities of, 628
Standing on hard surfaces/prolonged
  Deep Flat, 276
  Flat, 214, 516
Stomach disorders, 434-436
Stomach-Liver yin deficiency, 342
Stomach prolapse, 439
Stomach-Pylorus Extension position, 82, 82f, 439
Stomach qi, 93

Stress. *See also* Emotions/emotional life
  chemical
    Taut, 330, 473
    Tense, 333
  daily/life
    'nervous system' tense, 574
    Rapid pulse, 158-159
    Tense and Rapid, 333
    Thin Tight, 489
  emotional
    qi stagnation, 438
    Taut, 473
    Tense, 335, 517
    Tight, 338
    Tight and Rapid, 339
    Tight (including Wiry), 519
    Wiry, 353, 354, 358
  post-traumatic stress syndrome
    Empty, 568
    Empty moderately Tense, 249
    Empty over entire pulse, 615
    Rough Vibration, 568
  Thin Tight, 297
  Tight, 341
Stroke
  Blood Heat, 606
  Blood Thick, 606
  Choppy, 365
  Floating Tight, 244, 432, 611
  Hollow Full-Overflowing Leather-Like, 187
  Robust (left side) uniformly, 505
  Robust (right side) uniformly, 507
  Slippery and very Tight Hollow Full-Overflowing, 320
  Slippery Feeble and Slow, 315
  Slippery Tight and slightly Rapid, 318
  Slippery Tight Hollow Full-Overflowing and Rapid, 315
  Tense Hollow Full-Overflowing, 291, 607
  Tight, 344
  Tight and very Tight Hollow Full-Overflowing, 264, 266
  Very Tense Tight, or Wiry Full-Overflowing Hollow and Rapid, 616
  Wiry, 350, 356
Submerged
  about, 268
  Deep, 268-281, 269f
  Deep and Rapid, 272
  Deep and Slow, 271
  Deep and very Tight or Wiry, 274
  Deep Choppy, 273
  Deep Diffuse, 270
  Deep Feeble, 274, 276, 277, 278, 279
  Deep Feeble-Absent, 270, 275
  Deep Feeble and Slow, 280
  Deep Flat, 271, 273, 275, 276
  Deep Flat and slightly Rapid or Slow, 278
  Deep Reduced Substance, 270
  Deep Slippery, 271, 274, 275, 276, 278, 279
  Deep Slippery Feeble, 280

Deep Slippery Tense, 280
Deep Tense to Tight with Normal rate, 279
Deep Thin, 272, 276
Deep Thin Tight, 274
Deep Thin Tight and Rapid, 279
Deep Thin Tight and very Rapid, 278
Deep Thin Tight to Wiry Hollow, 279
Deep Tight, 270, 275, 280
Deep Tight-Wiry and very Rapid, 275
Deep Wide, 273
Deep Wiry, 271, 276
Firm, 281, 282f
Hidden, 282-285, 283f
Subtle (Vague), 377
Sudden Transient Interrupted, 124
Superficial
    about, 235-236
    Cotton, 236-239, 236f
    defined, 236d
    Empty, 245-252, 248-249f
    Floating, 239-245, 240f
    Hollow, 259-268
    Leather, 255, 255f
    Minute, 258, 258f
    Scattered, 256, 257f
    Yielding Empty Thread-like, 253-254, 254f
Superficial Smooth and Transitory Vibration, 395
Suppressed
    about, 201-202
    illustrated, 201f
    in interpretation, 638
Suppressed emotions
    Cotton, 470-471
    Yielding Hollow Full-Overflowing, 398
Suppressed Pounding, 638
Systems, defined, 740d

— T

Talking (excessive). *See* Overwork, of Lungs
Taut
    about, 329-330
    future (distant) disharmony, 603-604
    illustrated, 328f
    middle position (left), 430
    proximal position (left), 442
    proximal position (left and right), 442
    qi depth, 473
    and Rapid (slightly), 330
    and Slow, 330
Taut Choppy, 330
Taut Floating, 330
Taut Inflated, 330
Taut or Tense at left middle position, 573
Taut Slippery, 330
Taut-Tense, 486
Taut Wide, 330
Tense
    about, 332-333
    combinations, 333-334
    distal position (left), 394
    distal position (right), 420
    distal and middle positions (left), 403
    distal and middle positions (right), 425
    distal position (uniform bilaterally), 516-517
    future (semi-distant) disharmony, 608
    illustrated, 328f
    Intestine positions, 447
    middle position (left), 430
    middle position (uniform bilaterally), 517
    over entire pulse, 474
    positions, 335-336
    proximal position (left), 442
    proximal position (left and right), 442
    proximal position (right), 445
    proximal position (uniform bilaterally), 517-518
    qi depth, 473
    and Rapid, 333
    and Slow, 333
    uniform quality, 516-518
    and very Tense Hollow Full-Overflowing, 263
Tense Choppy, 334
Tense Deep, 333
Tense Floating, 333
Tense Hollow, 263, 265, 266
Tense Hollow Full-Overflowing
    about, 181, 290-291
    above the qi depth, 472
    blood stagnation, 482
    conditions associated with, 182-184
    future (semi-distant) disharmony, 607
    illustrated, 483f
    middle position (left), 430
    middle and distal positions (left), 404
    middle and proximal positions (left), 432
Tense Hollow Full-Overflowing at Large Vessel positions, 616
Tense Hollow Slippery and Rapid, 262
Tense Inflated. *See also* Inflated Tense
    about, 334
    distal position (left), 402
    distal position (right), 421
    distal position (uniform bilaterally), 513
    Large Vessel position, 402
    middle position (left), 431
    middle position (uniform bilaterally), 514
    mild, 196-197, 513
    moderate, 197, 513
    very, 195, 197-198
Tense Inflated Floating, 197
Tense Long, 474
Tense Robust Pounding, 474
Tense Robust Pounding Suppressed, 474
Tense Ropy
    blood stagnation, 483

Wide Moderate, 293
Tense Slippery, 334, 433
    at Gallbladder position, 608
    with Normal or slightly Rapid rate, 316
Tense Slippery, Flooding Excess, Robust Pounding, 334
Tense-Tight, 436
Tense-Tight Hollow Full-Overflowing, 266, 631
Tense-Tight Inflated, at right distal and Special Lung positions, 429
Tense to Tight over entire pulse, 574
Tense Wide, 334
Tension
    Change in Intensity, inconstant, over entire pulse, 573-574
    etiology, 574-576
    Taut or Tense at left middle position, 573
    Tense to Tight over entire pulse, 574
    Tight Thin, 346
Terminology, 6, 8-9t, 731-740. See also Classification/nomenclature
Terror
    Bean (Spinning), 567
    guilt and fear and, 565-566
    'qi wild' qualities, 567
    Rough Vibration at Neuro-psychological position, 567, 613
    without guilt, 567
Thin
    about, 295-296
    bilaterally at same position, 298
    blood deficiency, 295-298, 484
    in complementary positions, 393
    distal position (left), 395, 561
    distal position (right), 423
    distal position (uniform bilaterally), 523-524
    Exertion, Increase in Rate, 300
    gender effects, 41
    illustrated, 295f
    individual positions, 300
    in a man, 41, 294, 632
    middle position (left), 430
    middle position (uniform bilaterally), 524
    over entire pulse, 561
    pliable, 296-297
    positions, 298-301
    proximal position (uniform bilaterally), 524
    qi deficiency, 295-296
    uniform qualities, 523-524
Thin Arrhythmic, 298
Thin Deep, 297
    and very Feeble, 297
Thin Deep Feeble
    bilaterally at same position, 298
    and Rapid, 300
    and Slow, 299
Thin Deep Tight-Wiry and Slow, 299
Thin Feeble, 299, 409
Thin Feeble Interrupted and Slow, 404

Thin Minute, 297
Thin Slippery, 299
Thin Tight, 605
    bilaterally at same position, 299
    and Rapid, 298, 299
    yin and essence depletion, 489
Thin Tight-Wiry, 297-298
Thin Yielding
    about, 296-297
    blood deficiency, 488
    future (semi-distant) disharmony, 605
Thready. See Thin
The three depths
    about, 29
    above the qi depth
        hard sensations, 472
        qi stagnation, 470-472
        Yielding sensations, 470-472
    blood depth
        about, 477-478
        blood excess, 478-484
        blood instability, 484-485
    classification/organization, 457-458
    consciousness and, 470
    the eight depths and, 459
    illustrated, 29f, 458f
    interpretation, 459
    location, 469-470
    model, 458
    organ depth
        about, 485-486
        deficiency at (blood), 488-493
        heat from excess at, 488
        stagnation at, 486-488
    pulse methodology, 62-63
    qi depth
        agitation at qi depth, 475
        fluid stagnation, 475
        qi deficiency, 476-477
        qi stagnation, 473-475
        trapped qi, 475
        yin deficiency, 477
    qualities, 469
    qualities found simultaneously at all positions, 463-464
    two depths and, 458
Three yin (san yin mai), 378, 391
Thyroid deficiency, 300
Tight
    about, 337-339
    combinations, 339-340
    in complementary positions, 393
    distal and middle positions (right), 425
    distal and proximal positions (left), 405
        and slightly Rapid, 588
    distal position (left), 399, 559
        Feeble-Absent at left proximal position, 588
        with Hesitant Wave, 409
        and left proximal Feeble-Absent, 406

distal position (right), 420
distal position (right) and proximal position (left), 426
at Esophageal position, 348
future (distant) disharmony, 604
historical note, 4-5
illustrated, 328f
Intestine positions, 447
middle position (left), 430
only at qi depth, 347
over entire left distal position, 345
over entire position and slightly Rapid, 395
at Pericardium position, 344, 399
positions, 340-349
proximal (right) and right middle and distal positions, 446
Rapid, 339
Rate at Rest, Change, 345
right middle position, 437
Special Lung position, 428
at Stomach-Pylorus Extension position, 348
very, 631
and very Tight Hollow Full-Overflowing, 264, 265, 266, 268
and very Tight-Wiry Hollow Full-Overflowing, 267
yin and essence depletion, 489
Tight and Thin at qi depth, 477
Tight Choppy, 340
Tight Deep, 339, 349
Tight Deep Thin and very Rapid, 345
Tight Deep Thin Feeble and slightly Rapid, 345-346
Tight Empty at qi depth, 347
Tight Floating, 339, 346
Tight Flooding Excess, 340
Tight, Flooding Excess, Robust Pounding, Slippery and Rapid, 347, 349
Tight Hollow Full-Overflowing, 348
    slightly, 268
Tight in Pericardium position and moderately Rapid, 395
Tight (including Wiry)
    distal position (uniform bilaterally), 518-519
    middle position (uniform bilaterally), 519-520
    proximal position (uniform bilaterally), 520-521
    uniform qualities, 518-521
Tight Inflated, 340
    very, 514
Tight Robust Pounding and Rapid, 348
Tight Slippery at Gallbladder position, 433
Tight Slippery Robust Pounding and Rapid, 347
Tight Thin, 339, 346-347, 348
Tight to Wiry Hollow Full-Overflowing, 184-186
Tight to Yielding, alternating, 340
Tight Wide Slippery, 340
Tight-Wiry
    about, 295
    proximal position (left), 442, 443
    proximal positions (left and right), 442
    proximal position (right), 445
    yin-essence deficiency, 445

Tight-Wiry Hollow Slippery, 268
Tightness at Pericardium position and Tense at left distal, 564
Tobacco. *See* Nicotine addiction
Touch in diagnosis, 14-15
Toxicity. *See also* poisoning
Toxicity (blood)
    Blood Unclear, 606
    Robust (left side) uniformly, 505
Toxicity (chemical)
    Tight Thin, 347
    Wiry, 351, 357-358
Toxicity (chronic)
    Deep and Slow, 272
    Deep Wiry, 271
Toxicity (environmental)
    Blood Unclear, 292, 479-480
    Feeble-Absent, 614
Toxicity (qualities)
    Blood Unclear, 292, 479-480, 606
    Deep and Slow, 272
    Deep Wiry, 271
    Feeble-Absent, 614
    Robust (left side) uniformly, 505
    Tense, 333
    Tight Thin, 347
    Transiently Slippery, 316
    Wiry, 351, 357-358
Transient (ephemeral), 377
Transposed pulse *(fan quan mai),* 378, 391
Trapped heat
    Flat, 514
    Tense Inflated, 514
Trapped qi. *See also* Qi stagnation
    Inflated, 194-195, 475
    Yielding Inflated, 512, 514
Trapped qi and heat, 513
Trapped qi in the Heart. *See also* Qi
    about, 414
    anger qualities in, 577-578
    defined, 734d
    Rapid, 156
    Thin Deep Tight and very Rapid, 300
Trauma. *See also* Emotions/emotional life; Shock
    circulation and, 467
    rate variation, 170
Trauma (abdomen)
    Empty, 528
    Flat, 515-516
    Tense, 335, 517
    Tight, 342
Trauma (birth)
    Rough Vibration, 400
Trauma (chest)
    Deep Flat, 273
    Feeble-Absent, 222
    Tense, 335, 517
    Tight, 341

Trauma (childhood)
    Deep Flat, 271
Trauma (emotional)
    Cotton, 238, 470-471, 511
    Diaphragm position, 532
    Empty, 251, 528
    Flat, 211, 213, 515
    Flat Tight and Rapid, 213
    Heart circulation, 418
    Intensity, Change in, 137
    obscuring interpretation, 45
    Rapid, 154-155
    Taut, 331
    Tight, 343
    Tight (including Wiry), 521
Trauma (general)
    Tight, 339
    Wiry, 353, 354
Trauma (head)
    Choppy, 365, 401
    Choppy at Neuro-psychological position, 609
Trauma (old)
    Choppy, 365
Trauma (pelvic)
    Smooth Vibration, 371
    Tense, 336, 518
Trauma (physical)
    Cotton, 238
    Empty, 250, 251, 527
    Feeble-Absent Deep, 525
    Flat, 214, 422, 515
    Flat Tight and Rapid, 213
    Heart circulation, 418
    Heart Full, 414
    Intensity, Change in, 137
    Leather-like Hollow, 264
    Rapid, 154-155
    Taut, 330, 331
    Tense, 336
    Tense Inflated, 514
Trauma (qualities)
    Choppy
        head, 365, 401, 609
        old, 365
    Cotton
        emotional, 238, 470-471, 511
        physical, 238
    Deep Flat
        chest, 273
        childhood, 271
    Diaphragm position, emotional, 532
    Empty
        abdomen, 528
        emotional, 251, 528
        physical, 250, 251, 527
        surgical, 528
    Feeble-Absent, chest, 222
    Feeble-Absent Deep, physical, 525
    Flat
        abdomen, 515-516
        emotional, 211, 213, 515
        physical, 214, 422, 515
        surgical, 515-516
    Flat Tight and Rapid
        emotional, 213
        physical, 213
    Heart Full, physical, 414
    Leather-like Hollow, physical, 264
    Rough Vibration, birth, 400
    Smooth Vibration, pelvic, 371
    Taut
        emotional, 331
        physical, 330, 331
    Tense
        abdomen, 335, 517
        chest, 335, 517
        pelvis, 336, 518
        physical, 336
        surgical, 335, 517, 518
    Tense Inflated
        physical, 514
        upper burner, 513
    Tight
        abdomen, 342
        chest, 341
        general, 339
        unresolved, 343
    Tight (including Wiry)
        with pain, 518
        unresolved, 521
    Vibration, rape, 370
    Wiry, general, 353, 354
Trauma (rape)
    Vibration, 370
Trauma (surgical)
    Empty, 528
    Flat, 515-516
    Tense, 335, 517, 518
Trauma (upper burner)
    Tense Inflated, 513
Trauma (with pain)
    Tight (including Wiry), 518
Triple Burner, 449
Tuberculosis
    Deep and very Tight or Wiry, 275
    Feeble-Absent, 224-225
    Feeble-Absent Deep, 525
    Tight, 345
    Tight Deep Thin Feeble and slightly Rapid, 345
    Tight (including Wiry), 519
    Wiry, 354, 357, 421
Tumor
    breast, 513, 515
    Choppy at Neuro-psychological position, 609
    Flat, 422, 487, 515
    mediastinal, 513, 515

Muffled, 612
Tense Inflated, moderately, 513
Tight, 341
Tight (including Wiry), 520
Wiry, 354
Turbid blood. *See* Blood unclear
The two-depth model, 458
Tympanic quality. *See* Leather

—— U

Ulcers/gastritis
Bean (Spinning), 375
Choppy, 364
Cotton, 239
Deep Thin Tight to Wiry Hollow, 279
Deep Wiry, 276
Floating Tight, 618
Slippery, 522
Slippery Tight (Hollow) at Stomach-Pylorus Extension position, 324
Taut Slippery, 331
Tense Hollow Slippery and Rapid, 262
Tense-Tight, 436
Tight, 342
Tight at Stomach-Pylorus Extension position, 348
Tight, Flooding Excess, Robust Pounding, Slippery and Rapid, 349
Tight (including Wiry), 520
Tight-Wiry Hollow Slippery, 268
Wiry, 354, 358
Uniform qualities
bilaterally at same position
about, 509-510
Change in Qualities and Intensity, 532
comparison table, 533-538t
Inflated, 512
Diaphragm position, 532
distal position bilaterally
overview, 510
Change in Qualities and Intensity, 533
Cotton, 511
Empty, 527-528
Feeble-Absent, 525
Floating, 510-511
Floating Tense and Slow, 510
Floating Tense with Normal or slightly Rapid rate, 510
Floating Yielding and Rapid, 510
Floating Yielding and Slow, 510
Flooding Excess, 512
Hollow, 529-530
Slippery, 521-522
Tense, 516-517
Tense Inflated, 513
Tense Inflated, mild, 513
Tense Inflated, moderate, 513
Thin, 523-524
Tight (including Wiry), 518-519
Vibration, 531
Yielding Inflated, 512-513, 514
entire pulse interpreted, 66-67
husband-wife imbalance, 139, 501-502, 584-585
in interpretation, 66-68, 635
left side: 'organ system'
Change in Intensity and Qualities, 508
diabetes, 505
hypertension, 505
in interpretation, 67
Liver wind, 506
'organ system' deficient, 506
pain, 505
qi stagnation with a Cotton quality, 506
Reduced (uniformly), 506
Robust (uniformly), 505-506
Slippery, 508
stroke, 505
toxicity, 505
very Tense or Tight Hollow Full-Overflowing, 508
middle position bilaterally
overview, 509-510
Change in Qualities and Intensity, 533
Empty, 528-529
Feeble-Absent, 525-526
Floating, 511
Flooding Excess, 512
Hollow, 530
Hollow Full-Overflowing, 511-512
Slippery, 522
Tense, 517
Tense Inflated, 514
Thin, 524
Tight (including Wiry), 519-520
Vibration, 531
musculoskeletal disorders, 532
Neuro-psychological position bilaterally, 531
between positions
Diaphragm, 532
musculoskeletal disorders, 532
proximal position bilaterally
overview, 509-510
Change in Qualities and Intensity, 533
Empty, 529
Feeble-Absent, 526-527
Flat, 514-516
Floating
Flooding Excess, 512
Hollow, 530-531
Hollow Full-Overflowing, 512
Slippery, 522
Tense, 517-518
Thin, 524
Tight (including Wiry), 520-521
Vibration, 531-532
right or left side

about, 501-505
    Change in Intensity and Qualities, 508
    emotional disharmony, 584-585
right side: 'digestive system'
    Change in Intensity and Qualities, 508
    damp-cold, 508
    damp-heat, 507
    eating habits (irregular), 508
    eating habits (too quickly), 507
    hypertension, 507
    in interpretation, 68
    Reduced (uniformly), 508
    Robust (uniformly), 507-508
    Slippery, 508
    stroke, 507
    Very Tense or Tight Hollow Full-Overflowing, 508
Unstable. *See also* Instability
    distal position (left), 398
    future (immediate) disharmony, 617
    quality described, 140-141
Upper burner. *See* Distal position
Urogenital disorders
    Choppy, 365-366
    Deep Feeble, 281
    Deep Slippery Feeble and Slow, 281
    Flooding Excess, 512
    incontinence, 281, 325, 349
    Slippery Deep Feeble, 325
    Tense, 445
    Tense Hollow Full-Overflowing, 433
    Thin Yielding, 605
    Tight Deep, 349
    Wiry, 359
Uterine bleeding, chronic, 530

V

Vague (subtle), 377
Vengefulness, 568, 605
Very Slippery Deep and very Rapid, 321
Very Tense Hollow Full-Overflowing, 397
Very Tense Inflated, 398, 479
Very Tense or Tight Hollow Full-Overflowing, 485, 508
Very Tense-Tight Hollow Full-Overflowing, 142
Very Tense Tight, or Wiry Full-Overflowing Hollow and Rapid, 615-616
Vessels
    anomalous, 378-379
    split, 379
Vibration. *See also* Rough Vibration; Smooth Vibration
    about, 366, 367-369
    and Choppy at left middle position, 431
    Choppy vs., 366
    distal position (left), 402
    distal position (right), 422
    distal positions (uniform bilaterally), 531

Heart, 409
Heart qi agitation, 411
middle position (uniform bilaterally), 531
Mitral Valve position, 402
Neuro-psychological position, 411, 531, 564
positions, 371-373
proximal position (uniform bilaterally), 531
and Slippery at Mitral Valve positions, 562
uniform qualities, 531-532
Vibration qualities, Smooth and Rough, 366f
Vigilance pulse, 158-159, 329, 332, 574
Violin, 328f
Volume
    about, 179
    Absent at qi depth, 204-205, 205f
    at blood depth, 205-208
    Dead, 227
    Deep, 216
    Diffuse, 209, 209f
    Diminished at blood depth, 205, 207f
    Diminished at qi depth, 204, 204f
    Feeble-Absent, 216-225
    Feeble-Absent Deep and Slow/Rapid, 221
    Feeble-Absent Deep Choppy, 221
    Feeble-Absent Deep Slippery, 221
    Flat, 210-216, 211f
    Flat Tense, 213-214
    Flat Tight and Rapid, 213
    Flooding Deficient Wave, 205, 207f, 208
    Flooding Excess, 190-193, 191f
    flowchart, 228f
    Hollow Full-Overflowing, 179-180, 180f
    Hollow Full-Overflowing Leather-Like and Rapid or Slow, 187
    Hollow Full-Overflowing Reduced Pounding, 188
    Hollow Full-Overflowing Robust Pounding Bounding and Rapid, 188
    Hollow Full-Overflowing Slippery
        over entire pulse, 187
        and very Rapid, 188
    Hollow Full-Overflowing Tense, and Slippery at the blood depth, 188
    Hollow Full-Overflowing Tight or Wiry, 188
        and Slippery, 188
    Inflated, 193-201, 193f
        and very Tense, 196
    Inflated Tense, 195, 196
    Inflated Tense-Floating and slightly Slow, 196
    Inflated Yielding, 194-195, 196
    Inflated Yielding-Floating and slightly Rapid, 196
    Muffled, 226-227, 226f
    in Normal pulse, 90, 92f
    Reduced
        about, 202-203
        Absent at qi depth, 204-205, 205f
        blood depth, 205-208
        classification/nomenclature, 202-203
        Dead, 227

Deep, 216
Diffuse, 209, 209f
Diminished at blood depth, 205, 207f
Diminished at qi depth, 204, 204f
Feeble-Absent, 216-225
Flat, 210-216, 211f
Flooding Deficient Wave, 205, 207f, 208
Muffled, 226-227, 226f
Reduced Pounding, 208
Reduced Substance, 209-210, 210f
Spreading, 205, 206f
Yielding at qi depth, 203-204, 203f
Yielding partially Hollow, 205, 206f
Reduced Substance, 209-210, 210f
Robust
    Flooding Excess, 190-193, 191f
    Hollow Full-Overflowing, 179-180, 180f
    Hollow Full-Overflowing Leather-Like, 187
    Hollow Full-Overflowing Reduced Pounding, 188
    Hollow Full-Overflowing Robust Pounding Bounding, 188
    Hollow Full-Overflowing Slippery, 187, 188
    Hollow Full-Overflowing Tense, 188
    Hollow Full-Overflowing Tight or Wiry, 188
    Inflated, 193-201, 193f
    Robust Pounding, 190
    Suppressed, 201-202, 201f
    Tense Hollow Full-Overflowing, 181
    Tight to Wiry Hollow Full-Overflowing, 184-186
    Yielding Hollow Full-Overflowing, 181, 187
    Yielding Hollow Full-Overflowing Reduced Pounding, 186-187
Robust Pounding, 190
    and Flooding Excess, 190
    and Hollow Full-Overflowing, 190
Spreading, 205, 206f
Suppressed, 201-202, 201f
Tense Hollow Full-Overflowing, 181, 182
Tense Inflated, 196, 196-197
Tense Inflated Floating, 197
Tight to Wiry Hollow Full-Overflowing, 184-186
Yielding at qi depth, 203-204, 203f
Yielding Hollow Full-Overflowing, 181
    and Rapid, 187
    and Slow, 187
Yielding Hollow Full-Overflowing Reduced Pounding, 186-187
Yielding Inflated, 196
Yielding Partially Hollow, 205, 206f
Vomiting, 438
Vulnerability to disease
    Feeble-Absent, 219-220
    in interpretation, 41
    Scattered, 257
    Slow, 604

W

Walking barefoot
    Tense, 336, 442, 445
Walking on hard surfaces
    Deep Flat, 276
    Flat, 214, 516
Wave form
    abnormal, 126-127
    described, 67
    Hesitant, 126-127, 126f
    illustrated, 38f, 68f
    in interpretation, 67, 637
    in Normal pulse, 90, 92f
    as pulse sign, 38
Weak. *See* Feeble; Feeble-Absent
Weak-Floating, 241
Weather and circulation, 467, 468. *See also* Seasonal variations
Western medicine, 12, 35-36
Wide (pulse) in a woman, 41, 632
Wide Deficient qualities
    Diffuse, 293-294
    Reduced Substance, 293-294
    Wide Yielding Hollow Full-Overflowing with Normal or slightly Rapid rate, 293
    Yielding Ropy, 294
Wide Excess qualities
    about, 289-290
    Flooding Excess, 291-292
    Tense Hollow Full-Overflowing, 290-291
Wide Moderate qualities
    Blood Unclear, 292
    Leather-like Hollow, 292-293
    Tense Ropy, 293
Wide Yielding Hollow Full-Overflowing with Normal or slightly Rapid rate, 293
Width
    about, 289
    flowchart, 304f
    hard Thin qualities, 297-298
    in interpretation, 67
    Narrow group
        Restricted (width), 301
        Thin, 295-296, 298, 300
        Thin Arrhythmic, 298
        Thin Deep, 297
        Thin Deep and very Feeble, 297
        Thin Deep Feeble, 298
        Thin Deep Feeble and Rapid, 300
        Thin Deep Feeble and Slow, 299-300
        Thin Deep Tight-Wiry and Slow, 299
        Thin Feeble, 299
        Thin Minute, 297
        Thin quality in young man, 294-298
        Thin Slippery, 299
        Thin Tight, 299

Thin Tight and Rapid, 298, 299
Thin Tight-Wiry, 297-298
Thin with Increase in Rate on Exertion, 300
Thin Yielding, 296-297
Tight-Wiry, 295
Yielding Empty Thread-like, 301
pliable Thin qualities, 296-297
positions, 298-301
qi deficiency, 294
Restricted (width), 301
Thin, 300
Thin Deep Feeble and Rapid or Slow, 299-300
Thin Deep Tight-Wiry and Slow, 299
Thin Feeble, 299
Thin quality in young man, 294
Thin Slippery, 299
Thin Tight, 299
  and Rapid, 299
Wide Deficient
    Diffuse and Reduced Substance, 293-294
    Wide Yielding Hollow Full-Overflowing, 293
    Yielding Ropy, 294
Wide Excess
    Flooding Excess, 291-292
    Tense Hollow Full-Overflowing, 290-291
Wide Moderate
    Blood Unclear, 292
    Leather-like Hollow, 292-293
    Tense Ropy, 293
Yielding Empty Thread-like, 301
yin-essence deficiency, 295
Wind-cold, 243
Wind-heat, 243
Wind qualities, 243, 629
Wiry
    about, 4-5, 349-352
    in complementary positions, 393
    distal position (left), 397
    distal position (right), 421
    future (immediate) disharmony, 612
    future (semi-distant) disharmony, 608
    Gallbladder position, 433
    illustrated, 328f
    middle position (left), 430
    positions, 352-359
    and Rapid, 351
    and Slippery at blood depth with Normal or slightly
     Rapid rate, 351
    Special Lung position, 428
    yin and essence depletion, 489
Wiry Choppy, 352
Wiry Deep, 351
  and Slow, 352
Wiry Empty and slightly Rapid, 352
Wiry Inflated, 352
Wiry Robust Pounding and Rapid, 352
Wiry Slippery and very Rapid, 351
Wiry Thin, 351

Withdrawal (emotional), 582
Work habits. *See also* Overwork
    labor after eating
        Cotton, 511
        Empty, 251, 528
        Feeble-Absent Deep, 526
        middle position (right), 436
        nervous system and digestive system, 587
        Reduced (right side) uniformly, 508
        Robust (right side) uniformly, 508
        Tense, 336, 517
        Yielding Hollow Full-Overflowing, 530
    lifting after eating
        Tight (including Wiry), 520
Worry
    about, 563
    Cotton, 238
    Heart Tight, 410
    Heart Vibration, 409
    Rate at Rest, occasional Change, 564
    Smooth Vibration, 371-373, 564, 611
    Tight, 338
    Tight at Pericardium position and Tense at left distal position, 564
    Vibration, 366, 368, 563
Wu Shui-Wan, 98

—— Y

Yang deficiency
    Heart, 416, 523
    qualities, 628
    Thin, 523
    Tight to Wiry Hollow Full-Overflowing, 185
    Yielding qualities related, 35
    yin deficiency simultaneous, 35
Yang-essence deficiency, 552
    Absent, 94
    Doughy, 94
    Empty, 94
Yang excess, 628
Yang organ, defined, 6d
Yang qi at organ depth, 460-461
Yielding, 35
Yielding at qi depth, 203-204, 203f, 476
Yielding Empty Thread-like, 253-254, 254f
Yielding Hollow, 393
Yielding Hollow Full-Overflowing
    about, 181
    above the qi depth, 471
    anxiety, 561
    bilaterally at same position, 264, 265
    entire pulse, 261
    individual positions, 262
    and Interrupted-Intermittent, 261
    Large Intestine position, 267

proximal position (right), 268
'qi wild' condition, 469
and Rapid, 133, 187, 616
with rate >100 beats/minute, left distal position, 398
slightly, and Normal to slightly Rapid, 261
and Slow, 187, 261, 265, 267
yin and yang separation, 493
Yielding Hollow Full-Overflowing Reduced Pounding, 186-187
Yielding Hollow Intermittent, 121, 135
Yielding Hollow Interrupted, 135, 469
Yielding Hollow Interrupted-Intermittent, 493
Yielding Hollow Ropy, 262
Yielding Inflated
    distal position (bilaterally), 196
    distal position (right), 421
    distal position (uniform bilaterally), 512-513
    future (distant) disharmony, 603
    Hollow vs., 260
    middle position (uniform bilaterally), 514
    Special Lung position, 428
Yielding or Diminished qi depth, 603
Yielding partially Hollow
    bilaterally at same position, 265
    blood deficiency, 484
    entire pulse, 260
    illustrated, 206f
    middle position (left), 262, 267, 431
    at qi depth, 205
    and Slow, 142
Yielding Reduced Pounding, 476
Yielding Ropy
    about, 294
    blood instability, 484
    future (semi-distant) disharmony, 608-609
Yielding Ropy Hollow, 133
Yielding Slippery and Slow, 316
Yielding Tense Inflated and slightly Rapid, 395-396
Yin and blood deficiency
    Thin, 523
    Tight, 338
Yin and essence deficiency (Kidney), 524
Yin and essence depletion
    Tight, 489
    Wiry, 489
Yin and qi deficiency, 353
Yin and yang deficiency
    about, 42
    Restricted (width), 301
    Yielding Empty Thread-like, 301
Yin and yang distribution, 501
Yin and yang in contact
    Deep, 490
    Deep Reduced Substance, 490
    Deep Separating, 490
    Feeble-Absent, 490
    Hidden Deficient, 491
    Short Yielding, 490
Yin and yang separation
    Empty, 247, 431, 443, 491, 491-492, 615
    Empty Intermittent-Intermittent, Yielding Hollow Interrupted-Intermittent, 493
    Empty Thread-like, 492, 615
    Floating, 240
    in the Heart, 548
    Hollow Yielding Full-Overflowing and Slow, 615
    Leather, 492, 615
    Minute, 493, 615
    Qualities and Intensity, Change in, 431
    Qualities, Change in, 616
    Scattered, 492, 615
    stability/instability, 37, 140
    Yielding Hollow Full-Overflowing, 493
Yin deficiency
    about, 477
    asthma, 424
    Deep Tight, 270
    hard qualities related, 35
    of Heart and Lungs, Tight (including Wiry), 519
    of Lung, Thin, 523
    qualities, 628
    Slow, 164, 167
    Stomach-Liver, 342
    Thin, 523
    Thin Tight-Wiry, 297
    Tight, 342
    Tight and Thin at qi depth, 477
    Tight at left distal position, 560
    Tight (including Wiry), 519
    to yang deficiency, 442-443
    yang deficiency simultaneous, 35
Yin-essence deficiency
    Kidney, 552
    Tight-Wiry, 295, 442, 445
    Wiry, 94, 350
Yin excess, 628
Yin organ, defined, 6d
Yin organ systems deficient, 407
Yin qi at organ depth, 460-461